206.00

Hinman's Atlas of Pediatric Urologic Surgery

Hinman's Atlas of Pediatric Urologic Surgery

2nd Edition

Frank Hinman, Jr., MD, FACS, FAAP, FRCS (Eng) (Hon)
Clinical Professor of Urology
University of California School of Medicine
San Francisco, California

Laurence S. Baskin, MD, FACS, FAAP
Chief of Pediatric Urology
Professor of Urology and Pediatrics
University of California School of Medicine
San Francisco, California

Illustrated by the late Paul H. Stempen, MA, AMI
Illustrations supplemented by Jeanne Koelling, MS, AMI

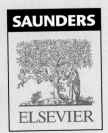

SAUNDERS

ELSEVIER

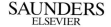

SAUNDERS
ELSEVIER

1600 John F. Kennedy Blvd.
Ste 1800
Philadelphia, PA 19103-2899

HINMAN'S ATLAS OF PEDIATRIC UROLOGIC SURGERY   ISBN: 978-0-7216-0645-3
SECOND EDITION

Notice

Knowledge and best practice in this field are constantly changing. As new research and experience broaden our knowledge, changes in practice, treatment, and drug therapy may become necessary or appropriate. Readers are advised to check the most current information provided (i) on procedures featured or (ii) by the manufacturer of each product to be administered, to verify the recommended dose or formula, the method and duration of administration, and contraindications. It is the responsibility of the practitioner, relying on his or her own experience and knowledge of the patient, to make diagnoses, to determine dosages and the best treatment for each individual patient, and to take all appropriate safety precautions. To the fullest extent of the law, neither the Publisher nor the Authors assume any liability for any injury and/or damage to persons or property arising out or related to any use of the material contained in this book.

Library of Congress Cataloging-in-Publication Data

Hinman's atlas of pediatric urologic surgery / Frank Hinman Jr., Laurence S. Baskin ; illustrated by Paul H. Stempen ; illustrations supplemented by Jeanne Koelling.—2nd ed.
    p. ; cm.
  "Portions of this book, including both text and illustrations, have appeared previously in the Atlas of urologic surgery, 2nd Edition, by Frank Hinman, Jr., published by W.B. Saunders Company, 1998."
  Includes bibliographical references and index.
  ISBN 978-0-7216-0645-3
  1. Genitourinary organs—Surgery—Atlases. 2. Children—Surgery—Atlases. 3. Pediatric urology—Atlases. I. Baskin, Laurence S. II. Hinman, Frank, Atlas of urologic surgery. III. Title. IV. Title: Hinman's atlas of pediatric urologic surgery. V. Title: Pediatric urologic surgery.
  [DNLM: 1. Urologic Diseases—surgery—Atlases. 2. Child. 3. Female Urogenital Diseases—surgery—Atlases. 4. Infant. 5. Male Urogenital Diseases—surgery—Atlases. WS 17 H663a 2009]
  RJ466.H57 2009
  617.4'6—dc22
                          2008011018

Acquisitions Editor: Scott Scheidt
Developmental Editor: Arlene F. Chappelle
Project Manager: Bryan Hayward
Design Direction: Gene Harris

Printed in Canada

Last digit is the print number: 9   8   7   6   5   4   3   2   1

Dedication

*This atlas is dedicated to the pioneers who developed the
procedures of the now established subspecialty of pediatric urology,
to the clinicians and teachers who practice and teach them,
and to the children who have gained so much from their efforts.*

Special thanks to my family, Miriam, Joshua, Avi, and Rachel.

LAURENCE S. BASKIN

Commentators

Mark C. Adams, MD
   Department of Urologic Surgery
   Vanderbilt University
   Nashville, TN
28: Pediatric Heminephrectomy

Julian S. Ansell, MD, FACS
   Professor Emeritus, Urology
   University of Washington
   Seattle, WA
75: Modern Staged Reconstruction for Vesical Exstrophy

Darius J. Bagli, MDCM, FRCSC, FAAP, FACS
   Associate Professor of Surgery
   Faculty of Medicine
   University of Toronto
   Division of Urology
   The Hospital for Sick Children
   Toronto, Ontario, Canada
38: Distal Tunnel Reimplantation
58: Psoas Hitch Procedure

John M. Barry, MD, FACS
   Division of Urology
   Oregon Health & Science University
   Portland, OR
31: Renal Transplant Recipient
44: External Tunnel Method

Julia Spencer Barthold, MD
   Division of Urology
   A.I. duPont Hospital for Children
   Wilmington, DE
64: Gibson Incision
107: Testis Biopsy

Laurence S. Baskin, MD, FACS, FAAP
   Chief of Pediatric Urology
   Professor of Urology and Pediatrics
   University of California School of Medicine
   San Francisco, CA
23: Ureterostomy in Situ
133: Penile Curvature

Stuart B. Bauer, MD, FACS, FAAP
   Department of Urology
   Children's Hospital Boston
   Boston, MA
67: Pubovaginal Sling
72: Insertion of Artificial Sphincter

Mark F. Bellinger, MD
   Professor of Urology
   University of Pittsburgh School of
      Medicine
   Pediatric Urology Associates
   Pittsburgh, PA
14: Supracostal Incision
101: Ureterocystoplasty

A. Barry Belman, MD, MS, FAAP
   Chair Emeritus, Urology
   Children's National Medical Center
   Washington, DC
126: Abdominal and Inguinal Approaches to Varicocele
   Ligation
143: Transverse Preputial Onlay Island Flap
153: Closure of Urethrocutaneous Fistula

James M. Betts, MD, FACS, FAAP
   Attending Pediatric Urologist and
      Surgeon
   Director of Trauma Services
   Children's Hospital Oakland
   Clinical Professor of Urology and Surgery
   University of California, San Francisco
   San Francisco, CA
   Pediatric Surgical Associates
   Oakland, CA
16: Repair of Pleural Tear
17: Splenorrhaphy and Splenectomy
18: Repair of Flank Incisional Hernia
120: Repair of Testicular Injury
169: Repair of Penile Injuries

Adrian Bianchi, MD, FRCS
   Department of Paediatric Urology
   Royal Manchester Children's Hospital
   Manchester, United Kingdom
114: Microvascular Orchiopexy

David A. Bloom, MD
   Professor
   Department of Urology
   Division Chief, Pediatric Urology
   University of Michigan Health System
   A. Alfred Taubman Health Center
   Ann Arbor, MI
54: Calycoureterostomy
155: Meatotomy

Guy A. Bogaert, MD
Chief, Pediatric Unit
Department of Surgery
University Hospital
Leuven, Belgium
41: Extravesical Trough Technique
115: Laparoscopic Orchiopexy Techniques

Joseph G. Borer, MD
Assistant Professor of Surgery (Urology)
Harvard Medical School
Children's Hospital Boston
Boston, MA
37: Transvesical Advancement Technique
79: Cloacal Exstrophy

Aivar Bracka, MBChB, FRCS
Russells Hall Hospital
Dudley, United Kingdom
150: Two-Stage Revision Buccal Mucosa Hypospadias Repair

Claire M. Brett, MD
Pediatric Anesthesiologist
University of California, San Francisco
San Francisco, CA
119: Reduction of Testicular Torsion

John W. Brock, III, MD
Professor and Director
Division of Pediatric Urology
Surgeon-in-Chief
Monroe Carell Jr. Children's Hospital at Vanderbilt
Vanderbilt University Medical Center
Nashville, TN
39: Transtrigonal Technique
49: Ureteroneocystostomy for Duplicated Ureters

Mark P. Cain, MD
Professor of Pediatric Urology
Indiana University School of Medicine
Indianapolis, IN
62: Lower Midline Extraperitoneal Incision
73: Closure of Vesical Neck
85: Pediatric Vesicostomy

Anthony Caldamone, MD, FACS, FAAP
Director of Pediatric Urology
Hasbro Children's Hospital
Professor of Surgery (Urology) and Pediatrics
The Warren Alpert Medical School of Brown
University
Department of Urology
Rhode Island Hospital
Providence, RI
82: Excision of Urachus
109: Scrotal Orchiopexy
152: Foreskin Preservation

Douglas A. Canning, MD
Professor of Surgery (Urology)
University of Pennsylvania School of
Medicine
Chief, Division of Urology
The Children's Hospital of Philadelphia
Philadelphia, PA
74: Vesical Exstrophy Primary Complete Closure
129: Vascularized Pedicle Flaps
146: Transverse Tubularized Preputial Island Flap
157: Repair of Circumcision Injuries

Patrick Cartwright, MD
Primary Children's Medical Center
Salt Lake City, UT
15: Dorsal Lumbotomy
63: Lower Abdominal Transverse Incision
102: Autoaugmentation

Anthony J. Casale, MD
Chair, Department of Urology
University of Louisville School of
Medicine
Louisville, KY
92: Ileovesicostomy
93: Continent Vesicostomy

Pasquale Casale, MD
Assistant Professor of Surgery (Urology)
University of Pennsylvania School of
Medicine
Philadelphia, PA
21: Pyeloureteroplasty

Marc Cendron, MD, FAAP
Associate Professor of Surgery (Urology)
Children's Hospital Boston
Harvard School of Medicine
Boston, MA
40: Sheath Approximation Technique
141: Perimeatal-Based Flap Repair

Earl Y. Cheng, MD, FAAP
Associate Professor of Urology
Children's Memorial Hospital
The Feinberg School of Medicine at Northwestern
University
28: Pediatric Heminephrectomy
97: Ileocystoplasty

Bernard M. Churchill, MD, FRCS(C), FAAP
Professor of Urology
Chief, Division of Pediatric Urology
University of California, Los Angeles
Los Angeles, CA
88: Transverse Colon Conduit

Arnold H. Colodny, MD, FACS, FAAP[†]
Clinical Professor of Surgery
Harvard Medical School
Pediatric Surgeon
Children's Hospital Boston
Boston, MA
163: Vaginoplasty

Douglas Coplen, MD
Director of Pediatric Urology
St. Louis Children's Hospital
Washington University School of Medicine
St. Louis, MO
57: Endoscopic Ureterocele Decompression

Roberto De Castro, MD
Chief, Pediatric Urology
Director, Department Pediatric Surgery
Ospedale Maggiore
Bologna, Italy
170: Construction of the Penis: Phalloplasty in Infants

Ross M. Decter, MD
Thomas J. and Jesse I. Rohner, Jr., MD, Professor
of Surgery
Chief, Division of Urology
Director, Pediatric Urology
The Milton S. Hershey Medical Center
Hershey, PA
*134: Dorsal Tunica Albuginea Plication (TAP Procedure)
and Elliptical Excision Technique*
144: Tubularized Plate Urethroplasty

Charles Devine, Jr., MD, FACS[†]
Professor Emeritus
Eastern Virginia Medical School
Norfolk, VA
148: Free Tube Graft

Paddy Dewan, PhD, MD, FRACS
Head of Paediatric Surgery
Sunshine Hospital
Parkville, Victoria, Australia
102: Autoaugmentation
174: Posterior Urethral Valves

David A. Diamond, MD
Department of Urology
Children's Hospital Boston
Boston, MA
161: Epispadias Repair
171: Female Urethrovaginal Fistula

Michael DiSandro, MD
Associate Professor
Department of Urology
University of California, San Francisco
UCSF Medical Center
San Francisco, CA
122: Inguinal Hernia Repair
159: Penile Torsion
164: Vaginoplasty Using Urogenital Sinus

Steven G. Docimo, MD
Professor and Director, Pediatric Urology
Vice-Chair, Department of Urology
The University of Pittsburgh Medical Center
Vice President, Medical Affairs
The Children's Hospital of Pittsburgh
Pittsburgh, PA
*43: Laparoscopic Extravesical Ureteroneocystostomy (Lich-Gregoir
Adaptation)*
115: Laparoscopic Orchiopexy Techniques

John W. Duckett, Jr., MD, FACS, FAAP[†]
Professor of Urology in Surgery
University of Pennsylvania School of Medicine
Director, Pediatric Urology
Children's Hospital of Philadelphia
Philadelphia, PA
85: Pediatric Vesicostomy
104: Ileal Cecal Colonic Reservoir
138: Meatoplasty and Glanuloplasty (MAGPI Repair)
146: Transverse Tubularized Preputial Island Flap

Jack Elder, MD, FAAP, FACS
Chair, Department of Urology
Henry Ford Health System
Associate Director, Vattikuti Urology Institute
Division of Urology
Children's Hospital of Michigan
Detroit, MI
26: Simple Nephrectomy
86: Fetal Interventon Vesicoamniotic Shunt
154: Excision of Male Urethral Diverticulum
171: Female Urethrovaginal Fistula
175: Excision of Utricular (Mullerian Duct) Cyst

Amicur Farkas, MD
Professor and Chair Emeritus
Department of Urology
Share Zedek Medical Center Jerusalem
The Ben Gurion University of the Negev
Be'er Sheva, Israel
164: Vaginoplasty Using Urogenital Sinus

Fernando A. Ferrer, MD
Associate Professor
Urologic Surgery and Oncology
Surgeon-in-Chief and Director
Department of Pediatric Urology
Connecticut Children's Medical Center
Hartford, CT
35: Excision of Neuroblastoma
118: Radical Orchiectomy

Casimir F. Firlit, MD, PhD
Cardinal Glennon Children's Medical Center
Saint Louis University
St. Louis, MO
55: Ileal Ureteral Replacement

Israel Franco, MD, FAAP
Associate Professor of Urology
New York Medical College
Valhalla, NY
151: Penoscrotal Transposition Repair
158: Concealed (Buried) and Webbed Penis

Qiang Fu, MD, PhD
Vice Professor
Department of Urology
Shanghai 6th Hospital
Shanghai Jiaotong University
Shanghai, China
130: Bladder Epithelial Grafts

John P. Gearhart, MD, FAAP, FACS
Professor and Chief
Pediatric Urology Service
The Johns Hopkins Hospital
Baltimore, MD
75: Modern Staged Reconstruction for Vesical Exstrophy
166: Vaginal Reconstruction: Skin Inlay
168: Thigh Flap Vagina and Tissue Expansion

Kenneth I. Glassberg, MD
Professor of Urology
Director, Division of Pediatric Urology
Morgan Stanley Children's Hospital of
New York–Presbyterian
Columbia University Medical Center
New York, NY
127: Laparoscopic Varicocelectomy
147: Onlay Urethroplasty with Parameatal Foreskin Flap

James Glenn, MD, FRCS Eng(Hon)*
Professor of Surgery
University of Kentucky College of Medicine
Lexington, KY
38: Distal Tunnel Reimplantation

Edmond T. Gonzales, Jr., MD
Director of Pediatric Urology
Texas Children's Hospital
Houston, TX
138: Meatoplasty and Glanuloplasty (MAGPI Repair)
145: Incision of the Urethral Plate (Snodgrass Modification)

Ricardo González, MD, FAAP
Professor of Urology
Thomas Jefferson University
Philadelphia, PA
A.I. duPont Hospital for Children
Wilmington, DE
15: Dorsal Lumbotomy
34: Surgical Approaches to the Adrenals
72: Insertion of Artificial Sphincter
99: Colocystoplasty and Sigmoidcystoplasty
161: Epispadias Repair
163: Vaginoplasty

David C. S. Gough, FRCS, FRACS, DCH†
Department of Paediatric Urology
Royal Manchester Children's Hospital
Manchester, United Kingdom
120: Repair of Testicular Injury

Richard Grady, MD
Associate Professor of Urology
The University of Washington School of Medicine
Acting Chief, Pediatric Urology
Children's Hospital and Regional Medical Center
Department of Surgery/Division of Urology
Seattle, WA
76: Plastic Correction of Exstrophy Suprapubic Defect
77: Umbilicoplasty
79: Cloacal Exstrophy

Saul P. Greenfield, MD
Director, Division of Pediatric Urology
Department of Pediatric Surgical Services
Women & Children's Hospital of Buffalo
Clinical Professor of Urology
State University of New York at Buffalo School of Medicine
Buffalo, NY
149: Two-Stage Primary Skin Repair
153: Closure of Urethrocutaneous Fistula

Willy Gregoir, MD†
Professor Emeritus
Department of Urology
University of Brussels
Brussels, Belgium
41: Extravesical Trough Technique

*Retired

†Deceased

Moneer K. Hanna, MD, FRCS, FACS

Clinical Professor of Urology
Weill Medical College of
   Cornell University
Attending Pediatric Urologist
New York Hospital—Cornell
Attending Pediatric Urologist
Schneider Children Hospital
New York, NY
10: Anterior Transverse (Chevron) Incision
76: Plastic Correction of Exstrophy Suprapubic Defect
129: Vascularized Pedicle Flaps
170: Construction of the Penis: Phalloplasty
*   after Puberty*

David A. Hatch, MD

Professor of Urology & Pediatrics
Loyola University, Chicago
Department of Urology
Loyola University Medical Center
Maywood, IL
31: Renal Transplant Recipient
60: Renal Autotransplantation

W. Hardy Hendren, III, MD

Department of Surgery
Children's Hospital Boston
Boston, MA
47: Ureteroneocystostomy with Tailoring
172: Female Urethral Construction

Terry W. Hensle, MD, FAACP, FACS

The Given Foundation Professor of Urology
Vice Chair
Department of Urology
Children's Hospital of New York
New York, NY
82: Excision of Urachus
167: Sigmoid Vaginal Reconstruction

Adam Hittelman, MD, PhD

Pediatric Urology Fellow
University of California, San Francisco
San Francisco, CA
63: Lower Abdominal Transverse Incision
156: Circumcision

Norman B. Hodgson, MD, FAAP†

Clinical Professor of Urology
Medical College of Wisconsin
Milwaukee, WI
128: Introduction to Hypospadias Repair

Nicholas Holmes, MD

Director, Pediatric Urology Division
Children's Specialist of San Diego
Rady Children's Hospital
San Diego, CA
86: Fetal Intervention Vesicoamniotic Shunt
123: Correction of Hydrocele

†Deceased

Charles E. Horton, MD

Eastern Virginia Medical School
Norfolk, VA
141: Perimeatal-Based Flap Repair

Stuart Howards, MD

Department of Urology
University of Virginia Health System
Charlottesville, VA
125: Subinguinal Varicocelectomy

Douglas Husmann, MD

Professor of Urology
Chair Mayo Clinic
Rochester, MN
51: Ureteropyelostomy
55: Ileal Ureteral Replacement

John M. Hutson, AO, MD, DSc, FRACS, FAAP

Chair of Paediatric Surgery
University of Melbourne
Department of Urology
Royal Children's Hospital
Melbourne, Victoria, Australia
108: Inguinal Orchiopexy (Open Technique)
111: High Ligation Orchiopexy

Anette Jacobsen, MBBCh, MMed, FAMS

Senior Consultant and Acting Head
Chair, Division of Surgery
Department of Paediatric Surgery
KK Women's and Children's Hospital
Singapore
156: Circumcision

David B. Joseph, MD, FACS, FAAP

Professor of Surgery
University of Alabama at Birmingham
Chief of Pediatric Urology
Children's Health System
Children's Hospital
Birmingham, AL
25: Repair of Renal Injuries

George W. Kaplan, MD

Clinical Professor of Surgery and Pediatrics
University of California, San Diego School of Medicine
Chief of Surgery
Rady Children's Hospital, San Diego
San Diego, CA
50: Ureteroureterostomy for Duplicated Ureters
119: Reduction of Testicular Torsion
148: Free Tube Graft

Evan J. Kass, MD, FACS, FAAP

Chief, Pediatric Urology
William Beaumont Hospital
Royal Oak, MI
54: Calycoureterostomy
126: Abdominal and Inguinal Approaches to Varicocele Ligation
144: Tubularized Plate Urethroplasty

Michael A. Keating, MD
  Clinical Professor of Urology
  University of South Florida
  Chief of Pediatric Urology
  Nemours Children's Clinic
  Orlando, FL
87: Cutaneous Ureterostomy, Transureteroureterostomy, and
  Pyelostomy
137: Skin Coverage
140: Pyramid Procedure for Repair of the Megameatus: Intact
  Prepuce Hypospadias Variant

Antoine E. Khoury, MD, FRCSC, FAAP
  Chief of Urology
  The Hospital for Sick Children
  Professor
  Department of Surgery
  The University of Toronto
  Toronto, Ontario, Canada
14: Supracostal Incision

Lowell R. King, MD
  Albuquerque, NM
75: Modern Staged Reconstruction for Vesical Exstrophy
89: Ureteroileostomy (Ileal Conduit)

Andrew J. Kirsch, MD, FAAP, FACS
  Clinical Professor of Urology
  Children's Healthcare of Atlanta
  Emory University School of Medicine
  President
  Georgia Urology, PA
  Atlanta, GA
46: Endoscopic Reflux Correction

Stephen A. Koff, MD
  Professor and Chief
  Pediatric Urology
  The Ohio State University
  Nationwide Children's Hospital
  Columbus, OH
112: Low Ligation Orchiopexy
142: Balanitic Groove Hypospadias Repair
147: Onlay Urethroplasty with Parameatal Foreskin Flap

Barry A. Kogan, MD
  Falk Chair in Urology
  Professor, Surgery and Pediatrics
  Albany Medical College
  Albany, NY
17: Splenorrhaphy and Splenectomy
27: Partial Nephrectomy
52: Transureteroureterostomy
139: Glans Approximation Procedure

Stanley J. Kogan, MD, FAAP, FACS
  Clinical Professor
  New York Medical College
  Valhalla, NY
56: Ureterocele Repair
110: Orchiopexy for Abdominal Testes
165: Clitoroplasty

Martin A. Koyle, MD, FAAP, FACS
  Professor of Surgery and Pediatrics
  University of Colorado Denver School
    of Medicine
  Department of Pediatric Urology
  The Children's Hospital
  Denver, CO
30: Excision of Wilms' Tumor
94: Malone Antegrade
  Continence Enema

Anand Krishnan, MD
  Attending Physician
  Pediatric Urology
  Kaiser Permanente Medical Center
  Oakland, CA
24: Open Renal Biopsy
45: Revision Transplant Ureter

Bradley P. Kropp, MD, FAAP, FACS
  Professor and Chief, Pediatric Urology
  Children's Hospital of Oklahoma
  University of Oklahoma Health
    Science Center
  Oklahoma City, OK
58: Psoas Hitch Procedure
91: Appendicovesicostomy

Kenneth A. Kropp, MD
  Professor and Chair
  Department of Urology
  Medical College of Ohio
  Toledo, OH
70: Intravesical Urethral Lengthening

Eric A. Kurzrock, MD, FAAP
  Associate Professor of Urology
    and Pediatrics
  Chief, Pediatric Urology
  Director, Urology Outpatient Services
  University of California, Davis Children's Hospital
    and School of Medicine
  Sacramento, CA
59: Bladder Flap Repair
71: Bladder Neck Wraps
95: Colon Flap Continence Channel
98: T-Pouch Hemi-Kock Procedure

Guy W. Leadbetter, MD, FACS, FAAP†
  Professor Emeritus of Surgery and Chief
    of Urology
  University of Vermont Medical School
  Medical Center Hospital of Vermont
  Burlington, VT
68: Trigonal Tubularization

Henri Lottmann, MD
  Consultant in Pediatric Urology
  Hôpital Necker-Enfants Malades
  Paris, France
66: Posterior Midline Approach to the
  Bladder Neck

†Deceased

Richards P. Lyon, MD
Clinical Professor
Department of Urology
University of California, San Francisco
San Francisco, CA
53: Transureteroureterostomy with Cutaneous Stoma
119: Reduction of Testicular Torsion

Antonio Macedo, Jr., MD, FNUPEP
Chief, Pediatric Urology
Associate Professor of Urology
Federal University of São Paulo
São Paulo, Brazil
105: Ileal Reservoir with Ileal Catheterizable Channel
170: Construction of the Penis: Phalloplasty in Infants

Max Maizels, MD
Professor of Urology
Northwestern University School of Medicine
Attending Urologist
Children's Memorial Hospital
Chicago, IL
21: Pyeloureteroplasty

Padraig S. J. Malone, MCh, FRCSI, FRCS
Consultant Paediatric Urologist
Southampton University Hospitals
Southampton, United Kingdom
94: Malone Antegrade Continence Enema

Jack McAninch, MD, FACS
Professor of Urology
Chief of Urology
San Francisco General Hospital
San Francisco, CA
25: Repair of Renal Injuries

Gerald C. Mingin, MD
Director of Pediatric Urology
Department of Surgery
Vermont Children's Hospital
Burlington, VT
64: Gibson Incision

Michael E. Mitchell, MD
Children's Hospital of Wisconsin
Milwaukee, WI
74: Vesical Exstrophy Primary Complete Closure
99: Colocystoplasty and Sigmoidcystoplasty
100: Gastrocystoplasty
104: Ileal Cecal Colonic Reservoir
160: Epispadias Repair: Penile Disassembly

Paul Mitrofanoff, MD*
Department of Pediatric Urology
Rouen University Hospital
Rouen, France
91: Appendicovesicostomy

Paulo R. Monti, MD
Head of Urology Department
School of Medicine
Universidade Federal do Triângulo Mineiro
Uberaba, Brazil
92: Ileovesicostomy

Pierre D. E. Mouriquand, MD, FRCS(Eng), FAPU
Department of Pediatric Urology
Claude-Bernard University
Lyon, France
29: Radical Nephrectomy
52: Transureteroureterostomy

Hiep T. Nguyen, MD, FAAP
Assistant Professor in Surgery (Urology)
Harvard Medical School
Director of Robotic Surgery and
    Research
Department of Urology
Children's Hospital
Urological Diseases Research Center
Boston, MA
73: Closure of Vesical Neck

John M. Park, MD
Associate Professor
Chief, Division of Pediatric Urology
Department of Urology
University of Michigan Medical School
Ann Arbor, MI
122: Inguinal Hernia Repair

Thomas S. Parrott, MD, FAAP, FACS†
Clinical Associate Professor of
    Surgery (Urology)
Emory University School of Medicine
Atlanta, GA
29: Radical Nephrectomy

Alberto Peña, MD
Director, Colorectal Center
Department of General and
    Thoracic Surgery
Cincinnati Children's Hospital
    Medical Center
Cincinnati, OH
81: Closure of Rectourethral Fistula

Sava Perovic, MD, PhD
Professor of Urology and Surgery
Belgrade University School of
    Medicine
Belgrade, Serbia
47: Ureteroneocystostomy with Tailoring
101: Ureterocystoplasty
151: Penoscrotal Transposition Repair

Craig A. Peters, MD
Professor of Urology
University of Virginia Health System
Charlottesville, VA
19: Laparoscopic Renal Surgery
*43: Laparoscopic Extravesical Ureteroneocystostomy
(Lich-Gregoir Adaptation)*
175: Excision of Utricular (Mullerian Duct) Cyst

J. L. Pippi Salle, MD, PhD, FRCSC, FAAP
Professor
Division of Urology
Hospital for Sick Children
University of Toronto
Toronto, Ontario, Canada
70: Intravesical Urethral Lengthening

Victor A. Politano, MD*
Formerly Professor
Department of Urology
Leonard M. Miller School of Medicine
University of Miami
Miami, FL
37: Transvesical Advancement Technique

John Pope, MD
Department of Urologic Surgery
Vanderbilt University
Nashville, TN
22: Nephrostomy
51: Ureteropyelostomy

Dix P. Poppas, MD, FACS, FAAP
Professor and Chief
Institute for Pediatric Urology
New York–Presbyterian Hospital
Weill Medical College of Cornell University
New York, NY
102: Autoaugmentation
125: Subinguinal Varicocelectomy
165: Clitoroplasty

John F. Redman, MD, FACS, FAAP
Professor of Urology and Pediatrics
University of Arkansas College of Medicine
Arkansas Children's Hospital
Department of Pediatric Urology
Little Rock, AR
136: Glansplasty
142: Balanitic Groove Hypospadias Repair

Alan B. Retik, MD
Department of Pediatric Urology
Children's Hospital Boston
Boston, MA
104: Ileal Cecal Colonic Reservoir
119: Reduction of Testicular Torsion
149: Two-Stage Primary Skin Repair

Richard C. Rink, MD
Riley Hospital for Children
Indiana University Medical Center
Indianapolis, IN
93: Continent Vesicostomy
100: Gastrocystoplasty
164: Vaginoplasty Using Urogenital Sinus

Mike Ritchey, MD
Professor of Urology
Mayo Clinic College of Medicine
Phoenix, AZ
10: Anterior Transverse (Chevron) Incision
30: Excision of Wilms' Tumor

Jonathan H. Ross, MD
Head of Pediatric Urology
Glickman Urological Institute
The Children's Hospital at Cleveland Clinic
Associate Professor of Surgery
Cleveland Clinic Lerner College of
Medicine
Case Western Reserve University
Cleveland, OH
118: Radical Orchiectomy

H. Gil Rushton, MD, FAAP
Professor of Urology and Pediatrics
The George Washington University
School of Medicine
Chief, Division of Pediatric Urology
Children's National Medical Center
Washington, DC
21: Pyeloureteroplasty
116: Simple Orchiectomy
117: Laparoscopic Orchiectomy

Ellen Shapiro, MD
Professor of Urology
Director, Pediatric Urology
New York University School
of Medicine
New York, NY
26: Simple Nephrectomy
84: Suprapubic Cystostomy

Stephen R. Shapiro, MD, FAAP, FACS
Pediatric Urologist
Sacramento, CA
24: Open Renal Biopsy
89: Ureteroileostomy (Ileal Conduit)

Yoshiyuki Shiroyanagi, MD, PhD
Clinical Instructor
Department of Urology
Kanagawa Children's Medical Center
Yokohama, Japan
62: Lower Midline Extraperitoneal Incision

---

*Retired

Linda M. Shortliffe, MD
Stanford University School of Medicine
Stanford Hospital and Clinics
Santa Clara Valley Medical Center
Stanford, CA
10: Anterior Transverse (Chevron) Incision
50: Ureteroureterostomy for Duplicated Ureters
80: Prune-Belly Syndrome: Reduction Cystoplasty, Abdominal Repair, and Umbilicoplasty

Steven J. Skoog, MD, FAAP, FACS
Professor of Surgery and Pediatrics
Oregon Health & Science University
Director, Pediatric Urology
Doernbecher Children's Hospital
Portland, OR
22: Nephrostomy

E. Durham Smith, MD, MS, FRACS, FACS†
Emeritus Consultant Surgeon
Royal Children's Hospital
Melbourne, Australia
128: Introduction to Hypospadias Repair

Grahame H. H. Smith, MB, BS, FRACS
Head of Department of Urology
The Children's Hospital at Westmead
Westmead, Australia
174: Posterior Urethral Valves

Warren Snodgrass, MD
Children's Medical Center
University of Texas Medical Center
Dallas, TX
145: Incision of the Urethral Plate (Snodgrass Modification)

Brent W. Snow, MD, MBA, FACS, FAAP
Professor of Surgery and Pediatrics
University of Utah
Pediatric Urology
Primary Children's Medical Center
Salt Lake City, UT
154: Excision of Male Urethral Diverticulum

Howard M. Snyder, III, MD
Professor of Urology
University of Pennsylvania School of Medicine
Pediatric Urology
The Children's Hospital of Philadelphia
Philadelphia, PA
12: Subcostal Incision
40: Sheath Approximation Technique
56: Ureterocele Repair
113: Redo Orchiopexy

Harry M. Spence, MD, FACS†
Clinical Professor of Urology
Southwestern Medical School
University of Texas Health Science Center
Dallas, TX
11: Midline Transperitoneal Incision

Raimund Stein, MD
Department of Urology
Johannes Gutenberg University of Mainz
Mainz, Germany
106: Ureterosigmoidostomy

George Steinhardt, MD, FAAP, FACS
Director, Pediatric Urology
DeVos Children's Hospital
Grand Rapids, MI
157: Repair of Circumcision Injuries

F. Douglas Stephens, MB, MS, FRACS, FAAP (Hon)*
Emeritus Professor
Urology and Surgery
Northwestern University
Honorary Senior Research Fellow
Royal Children's Hospital
Research Foundation
Melbourne, Australia
111: High Ligation Orchiopexy

Ronald Sutherland, MD
Department of Pediatric Urology
Kapi'olani Medical Center for Women and Children
Honolulu, HI
117: Laparoscopic Orchiectomy
135: Dermal Graft

Hubert S. Swana, MD
Clinical Assistant Professor
University of South Florida
Pediatric Urology
Nemours Children's Clinic Orlando
Celebration, FL
116: Simple Orchiectomy
121: Insertion of Testicular Prosthesis

Emil A. Tanagho, MD
Professor Emeritus
Department of Urology
University of California, San Francisco Medical Center
San Francisco, CA
69: Vesical Neck Tubularization

†Deceased

*Retired
†Deceased

Saburo Tanikaze, MD
Surgeon-in-Chief
Aichi Children's Health and Medical Center
Obu, Japan
65: Mobilization of the Omentum
108: Inguinal Orchiopexy (Open Technique)
147: Onlay Urethroplasty with Parameatal Foreskin Flap

Richard Turner-Warwick, CBC, BSc, MCh, DM (Oxon), DSc (Hon), FRCP, FRCS, FRCOG, FACS, FRACS (Hon)*
Emeritus Surgeon
Middlesex Hospital
London, United Kingdom
65: Mobilization of the Omentum

Katsuhiko Ueoka, MD
Pediatric Urology
National Research Center for Child Health
and Development
Tokyo, Japan
13: Transcostal Incision
27: Partial Nephrectomy
77: Umbilicoplasty

Julian Wan, MD
Clinical Associate Professor
Department of Urology
University of Michigan
Ann Arbor, MI
67: Pubovaginal Sling
173: Urethral Prolapse

Ming-Hsien Wang, MD
Pediatric Urology Fellow
Department of Urology
University of California, San Francisco
Medical Center
San Francisco, CA
46: Endoscopic Reflux Correction
110: Orchiopexy for Abdominal Testes

Robert Whitaker, MD, MChir, FRCS*
University of Cambridge
Cambridge, United Kingdom
21: Pyeloureteroplasty

Duncan Wilcox, MBBS, MD
Associate Professor
Department of Urology
UT Southwestern Medical Center
Children's Medical Center Dallas
Dallas, TX
66: Posterior Midline Approach to the Bladder Neck
77: Umbilicoplasty
78: Cloacal Repair

Jason Wilson, MD
Assistant Professor of Surgery (Urology)
University of New Mexico School of Medicine
Albuquerque, NM
19: Laparoscopic Renal Surgery
123: Correction of Hydrocele

John R. Woodard, MD, FACS, FAAP*
Clinical Professor of Surgery (Urology)
Emory University School of Medicine
Atlanta, GA
108: Inguinal Orchiopexy (Open Technique)

Hsi-Yang Wu, MD
Assistant Professor of Urology
University of Pittsburgh School of Medicine
Children's Hospital of Pittsburgh
Pittsburgh, PA
107: Testis Biopsy
113: Redo Orchiopexy

Yuichiro Yamazaki, MD, PhD
Chief, Department of Urology
Kanagawa Children's Medical Center
Yokohama, Japan
62: Lower Midline Extraperitoneal Incision

Mark R. Zaontz, MD, FACS, FAAP*
Urology for Children
Voorhees, NJ
42: Detrusorrhaphy (Modifications of the Lich-Gregoir Technique)
139: Glans Approximation Procedure
158: Concealed (Buried) and Webbed Penis

Stephen A. Zderic, MD
Professor of Surgery (Urology)
University of Pennsylvania School of Medicine
Attending Urologist
The Children's Hospital of Philadelphia
Philadelphia, PA
32: Living Donor Nephrectomy
48: Ureteral Tailoring (Folding) Technique

*Retired

*Retired

Foreword to the Second Edition

Former Surgeon General C. Everett Koop is sounding another theme in his multifaceted career: that the country must produce a "new kind of doctor for the 21st century." By strengthening each new physician's awareness of the tenets of Hippocratic medicine, we can elevate the ethics of the physician of the future. He wants to provide opportunities in the curriculum to reintroduce students to the humanistic values that have been forgotten in modern health care delivery. "We have got to find a way of having better listeners and better communicators in the medical profession."

That "new kind of physician" has been serving as a role model for our generation of urologists, and several before, in the person of Frank Hinman, Jr. To say that Frank has balanced the art and science of medicine is an understatement. He has taken the practice of urology to the ultimate rewards of personal satisfaction, a "true Renaissance man." In the private practice of urology in the San Francisco area for his lifetime, he has an army of devoted patients who recognize the confidence of his great scientific knowledge and the art of caring and providing that human element to their relationship.

Frank Hinman is the son of a pioneer in urology; his father clearly had a significant influence as a role model for becoming the "complete urologist." After an impeccable school experience at Stanford and Johns Hopkins, he moved into a medical internship at Hopkins and a surgical residency at Cincinnati; this was interrupted by active duty in the Navy on the carrier Intrepid in the Pacific. After his discharge in 1946, he returned to the University of California, San Francisco for urology training under his father.

Besides every important urologic organization in the world, he has served as a Trustee for the American Board of Urology, with the Residency Review Committee for Urology, and on the Advisory Council at the National Institutes of Health. He received the Pediatric Urology Medal from the American Academy of Pediatrics Urology Section and the St. Paul's Medal from the British Association of Urologic Surgeons. He has also served as a Regent of the American College of Surgeons. He has been recognized by his peers with the Hugh Hampton Young Award, as well as the Ramon Guiteras Award from the American Urological Association and the Barringer Medal from the American Association of Genitourinary Surgeons.

Besides *Hinman's Atlas of Pediatric Urologic Surgery*, he has produced *Atlas of Urologic Surgery*, an atlas of urological anatomy, a tome on benign prostatic hypertrophy, and one on hydrodynamics of micturition.

His expertise in urology has been so varied that nearly every subspecialty ranks Frank Hinman as one of its "founders." His contributions to the advancement of our urologic knowledge are legend. Among the topics are BPH, reconstruction, urodynamics, voiding dysfunction, hydronephrosis, infection, and nearly every issue in pediatric urology.

This atlas is compiled in a unique manner that only Frank Hinman could direct. Those who have contributed to the individual procedures have added their comments, especially the "pitfalls." The clarity of Paul Stempen's illustrations provides a sequenced approach to accomplishing our surgical goals. This should prove to be a most useful addition to the future dispersion worldwide of pediatric urology, a subspecialty of urology that is now firmly established thanks to the advice, leadership, wisdom, and caring of a great man: Frank Hinman, Jr.

John Duckett, 1992

Foreword to the First Edition

In every area of surgical practice, there is a balance to be struck between the generalist and the specialist; between those with a broad experience of many aspects of disease and those who, by narrowing their field, gain a deeper understanding; between those who, when faced with newly emerging problems, adapt the techniques developed in previously encountered circumstances and those who would study them de novo. Modern surgery has inexorably progressed toward specialization despite the very justifiable warnings issued at every stage by an older generation of the dangers of fragmentation and surgical tunnel vision. As a specialty, pediatric urology has been little more than 40 years in the making; its emergence now seems inevitable even though there have been many attempts to keep it within a wider fold. It has grown less by the giving off of a segment of general urology than by the discovery of new opportunities for the correction of disorders previously unrecognized or deemed untreatable. A generalist perusing this book cannot fail to be impressed by the rapidly expanding scope, and the excitement, of this specialty.

It is a truism that the techniques of operative surgery cannot be learned from books alone, that practical experience in the operating theatre is indispensable. But for those who have already acquired the basic skills and already have knowledge of urinary tract disease, there is an enormous amount that can be learned from the precise descriptions and lucid illustrations in this volume. Even those engaged primarily in the practice of pediatric urology will find there is much their colleagues can teach them; the general urologists will find much more.

This is a very specialized treatise, but we must still preserve the balance; the amount of operative surgery required for children will always be small compared to that needed for adults. Urologists devoting their whole time to pediatrics will always be relatively few, meaning they cannot be everywhere available when a child's condition demands intervention; knowledge of the techniques employed in the specialty must be widely accessible. There is no one better to meet this challenge and strike the proper balance between the general and the special than the author of this book. Frank Hinman has been in the business of pediatric urology since its earliest days, but he has never lost touch with the mainstream of his department. As an able clinician he has taught successive generations of urologists and has represented the interests of the specialists amongst the generality of surgeons. He is a statesman in our profession. As an old friend and admirer, I congratulate him and Paul Stempen, his incomparable artist, on yet another achievement. I warmly recommend this book to all who would embark on the fascinating task of setting to rights the developing urogenital tract.

David Innes Williams

Preface to the First Edition

Fewer than 500 urologists worldwide limit their practice to children. However, most other urologists perform some pediatric operations, and an appreciable number cite pediatric urology as a field of special interest. A source of surgical instructions is not currently at hand either for the simpler pediatric procedures performed by the generalist or for the more complicated ones by the subspecialist. Because of the preponderance of the 1989 *Atlas of Urologic Surgery,* which served as a guide for adult operations, it seemed logical to develop a work focusing on the pediatric aspects of urologic surgery.

Many of the procedures and precautions described in this volume were learned while the author was Chief of Urology at the Children's Hospital of San Francisco and San Francisco General Hospital, and many have come from publications, presentations, and discussions with colleagues in the Urology Section of the American Academy of Pediatrics (AAP) and the Society for Pediatric Urology (SPU). The chapters were selected to include all of the common procedures plus many of the new techniques coming into use in children's centers. Each is presented in a step-by-step manner, with an illustration drawn as viewed at the table by a surgically oriented illustrator, Paul H. Stempen. The result is that each operative step has both an illustration and straightforward directions on what to do as well as what not to do.

A preliminary section explains the structural and functional differences between adults and children, with the special problems associated with fluid balance, anesthesia, and intraoperative care. Another describes the special techniques involved in operating on neonates and infants and the problems of postoperative care. The remainder of the volume is divided into sections for each organ, each containing detailed illustrations accompanied by a description of the operation, extending from procedures for the kidney to those for the penis. Most of the new pediatric operations are included, and, in addition, much of the relevant material from our 1989 *Atlas* has been appropriately adapted.

The authority of the book is guaranteed by the inclusion of commentaries for each operation written by prominent pediatric urologists selected from the membership of the SPU and the Urology Section of the AAP. These commentators have reviewed and corrected the text and illustrations, verified the accuracy of the description, and written a critique from the perspective of their own experience.

Although the descriptions of operations in this volume are as accurate as possible, the surgeon cannot put the book on a Mayo stand at the operating table and just follow directions. Pediatric surgery is demanding. It requires special training and special skills, both because of the complexity of the operations and because of the size and delicacy of the tissues in children. For genital operations in particular, training must be gained under the guidance of an accomplished pediatric urologist.

The book should be especially useful for the experienced subspecialist confronted with an operation done infrequently, for the young urologist in training, and for the other urologists who are interested in expanding their pediatric repertoire with new procedures and with new insights into older ones.

Frank Hinman, Jr.
February 15, 1994

Acknowledgments

The value of this atlas to the practicing urologist, whether just starting in training or later in the midst of a career, when confronted with a new surgical problem, owes much to the late Paul Stempen. He illustrated every step of each operation so clearly with his attractive line drawings that, when you combine them with the straightforward instructions in the text, the operation must run smoothly. We also thank Jeanne Koelling for continuing in the brilliant tradition of Paul Stempen in adding new illustrations as our specialty evolves with new operations.

For the final accuracy of both the figures and the descriptions, we thank the outstanding cadre of commentators, drawn from the top rank of the subspecialty. Their supervision makes this atlas "authoritative."

We appreciate the generous assistance given us by all the members of the Department of Urology at the University of California, San Francisco, first under Emil A. Tanagho and, more recently, under Peter A. Carroll. Thanks go to our former Chief of Pediatric Urology, Barry A. Kogan, now chief in Albany, New York, as well as our inquisitive urology residents and fellows. A special thanks to Claire Brett, Professor of Anesthesia at UCSF for extensive help revising the perioperative and anesthetic sections. Finally, special thanks to Arlene Loui and Jeanne Dea for their tireless assistance.

Laurence S. Baskin

Frank Hinman, Jr.

Contents

Section 1

PREPARATION FOR
PEDIATRIC OPERATIONS

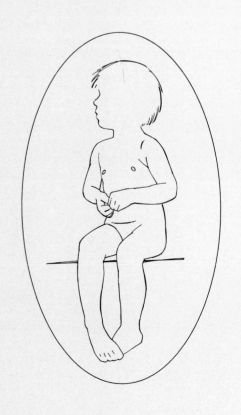

Chapter 1

Preoperative Evaluation

Ideally, the pediatric urologist participates actively in all aspects of the preoperative evaluation of the infant or child. A general or subspecialty pediatrician and/or anesthesiologist may provide supplementary data and offer critical analysis and input for managing the perioperative care of an infant or child who has a complicated medical history, requires a prolonged or complex surgical procedure, or has encountered an unexpected intraoperative event in the past. Nonetheless, the history and physical examination performed by the responsible urologist contributes to defining a comprehensive, focused surgical plan and establishing rapport with the family. If warranted, the urologist must generate a plan for additional cardiorespiratory, hematologic, renal, or hepatic evaluation as the timeline for surgery is initially introduced to the family. On the other hand, in the absence of any abnormal medical or family history and with no unexpected physical findings, the surgical preoperative evaluation is complete and a definitive plan for surgical intervention can be discussed. Specifically, no preoperative laboratory, electrocardiogram, or radiologic studies are indicated in the well child scheduled for simple, elective surgery (e.g., circumcision, hypospadias repair).

The child with abnormal renal function may require intense preoperative evaluation and/or treatment coordinated across several subspecialists. In most cases, these patients are under meticulous ongoing care by both a pediatric urologist and nephrologist so that fluid and electrolyte balance is maintained as an outpatient. However, in some cases, children with chronic renal dysfunction may benefit from inpatient monitoring to ensure adequate preparation for surgery. As an inpatient, fluid balance (total fluid intake versus urine/other output) can be meticulously documented and correlated with serum electrolytes. These data may provide critical guidelines for intraoperative fluid management. Of particular significance, hyperkalemia or uncompensated metabolic acidosis can be corrected and electrolyte balance documented for at least 24 to 48 hours preoperatively. If dialysis is indicated, surgery can be timed appropriately. In the setting of chronic renal failure, identifying and defining the appropriate treatment of various sources of coagulopathy and anemia are vital. Hemoglobin concentration, platelet count, bleeding time, prothrombin time, and partial thromboplastin time should be measured and corrected as needed. Of importance, laboratory results must be interpreted from the standpoint of normal developmental changes in coagulation and other hematologic values. For example, the neonate has a specific set of "normal" laboratory values and these change dramatically over the first year of life, mostly during the first 1 to 2 months. A pediatric hematologist should be consulted in complex clinical scenarios. Defining an adequate level of hemoglobin, total protein, and clotting function preoperatively must be based on age, current nutritional status (e.g., total serum protein and albumen), hemodynamic status (e.g., heart rate, blood pressure, acid-base status), coexisting cardiorespiratory dysfunction, underlying hematologic abnormalities, and complexity of the surgical procedure, such as anticipated length and type of surgery (e.g., intra-abdominal with intense fluid requirements) and predicted blood loss.

Children with a history of urinary tract infection should have sterile urine confirmed prior to elective surgery. The system for collecting urine for culture must be carefully controlled to avoid contamination and a false-positive culture. Until a child is old enough to provide a midstream urine sample, the most common method for collecting urine involves applying a "bag" to the perineum. However, unless meticulous technique is followed, these urine samples are commonly contaminated with organisms from skin and genitalia. To minimize contamination, the genitalia should be washed and dried, tincture of benzoin compound applied to the area, and then the urine collection bag positioned over the genitalia. Cutting out an opening in the adhesive area of the bag that is just large enough to surround the genitalia for both boys and girls may increase the likelihood of obtaining an accurate urine sample for culture. In addition, the bag should be removed as soon as possible after the sample enters the bag. That is, the goal is to collect only one voiding to minimize contamination. The sample should be immediately emptied into a sterile container. If an indwelling catheter is in place, clamp the tubing close to the urethra, wipe the wall with an alcohol sponge, and aspirate a sample with a syringe and a fine needle. Avoid disconnecting the tube from the urinary collection bag to avoid introducing infection into the sterile system.

EVALUATION BY THE PEDIATRIC ANESTHESIOLOGIST

In the setting of outpatient procedures, the pediatric anesthesiologist often evaluates the patient on the day of surgery. At times, a phone conversation is held 1 to 2 days preoperatively. If the patient is healthy and the family has received appropriate nothing-by-mouth (NPO) instructions, discussing plans for and risks from anesthesia (general, regional) and plans for monitoring, premedication, and parental presence during induction can all be adequately addressed the day of surgery. In the setting of complex medical problems or a history of complications during prior surgery/anesthesia, or in planning for a high-risk surgery, the pediatric urologist should advise the anesthesia team about the projected procedure and transmit any information about the child's status to allow a more intense preoperative discussion with the family. Of significance, in the setting of a history of prior intraoperative problems, a family history of malignant hyperthermia, or a complex medical history, records can be obtained from other medical centers, other physicians involved in the patient's care can be consulted, and a detailed, coordinated approach defined to present to the family.

The system for relaying information about NPO guidelines varies among medical centers. In general, the age-dependent guidelines established by the American Society of Anesthesia should be followed. Infants may have a higher risk for hypotension on induction of anesthesia after a prolonged fast, so that surgery is ideally scheduled earlier in the day for the youngest patients. Although the guidelines clearly prohibit solids and milk for 6 hours prior to the induction of anesthesia (age > 6 months), clear liquids may be given up to 2 hours before induction of anesthesia. Thus, the appropriate preoperative instructions should not only emphasize when to stop feeding, but should also clearly remind families that clear liquids can be given up to 2 hours before arrival at the hospital/surgery center. Some medical centers will ask that clear liquids be discontinued 3 hours before arrival to allow modifying the surgical schedule (e.g., patients canceling on the day of surgery).

NUTRITION

Enteral Nutrition

Nutritional status should be evaluated and, in the case of elective procedures, be a major factor in timing of surgery. Underlying nutritional status plays a vital role in perioperative metabolism and wound healing. A simple tactic is to document that weight gain has been normal (Table 1-1).

NORMAL WEIGHT GAIN

TABLE 1-1

Age	Growth Rate (g/kg)
8–28 days	10
1–2 mo	6.5
3–4 mo	3.5
1 yr	1

If nutritional status seems inadequate, a serum total protein and albumin may provide evidence for either inadequate intake or excessive losses. Preoperatively, supplemental oral feeding may be indicated. Postoperatively (except after intra-abdominal procedures), oral nutrition should be introduced as soon as possible with the same formulas tolerated before surgery. For example, most infant formula contains 50% fat and 10% to 20% protein, and delivers 0.67 calories/mL. Often, these formulas are adjusted to provide a higher concentration of calories and an appropriate concentration of protein in the setting of renal failure or malnutrition. Such infants also are supplemented with vitamins and minerals.

Parenteral Nutrition

Chronically ill children may require parenteral nutrition to provide adequate caloric intake to avoid poor wound healing, immunologic deficiencies (total lymphocyte count should be above 1500 mm^3), and excessive catabolism postoperatively. Premature infants often require specific ratios of protein, fat, and glucose and are particularly susceptible to acid-base imbalance perioperatively. One goal for premature infants is to mimic breast milk with respect to the relationship of protein, glucose, and fat to total calories delivered.

Infusions of total parenteral nutrition consist of glucose, amino acids, emulsified fat, minerals, vitamins, and trace elements that are adjusted in response to metabolic profiles, weight gain, and acid-base balance. Protein and caloric requirements are listed in Table 1-2.

PROTEIN AND CALORIE REQUIREMENTS

TABLE 1-2

Age	PROTEIN (g/kg/day)		CALORIES PER KILOGRAM PER DAY	
	Enteral	Parenteral	Enteral	Parenteral
Premature	4–6	2.5–3.5	150	85–130
Neonate	1.8–2	2.5	100–110	100–110
1 Year	1.5	1.5–2	80–135	80–135
Adolescent	0.85–1	1–1.5	50–60	50–60

PREPARATION OF THE CHILD AND FAMILY

Although preparation of the child and the family starts at the initial visit, the specific events on the day of surgery require a focused set of anticipatory guidance. Often the pediatric anesthesiologists and/or a separate team designated to prepare children for surgery, provide handouts for families to provide general information about surgery.

"Play therapy" is frequently integrated into the preoperative process for older children and their families. These services provide parents and children details about what to expect before (e.g., premedication, waiting areas), during (how families are informed about progress during surgery), and after surgery (e.g., recovery areas, admission versus discharge, pain and treatment). A child-friendly "prepare" clinic visit prior to surgery is now offered routinely to families. Handouts for specific surgical procedures describing the operation and postoperative course have been developed by surgical subspecialties. Despite this wide variety of standard material available, parents require a private conversation with the surgeon to ask their own questions and to receive information in a manner that is easy to understand and that acknowledges their specific concerns. Parents often need guidance about what to share with their child and benefit from reassurance that they should transmit information in their own style to reassure their child. The preoperative anxiety varies with age and as a function of prior experiences. For example, the central anxiety for older infants and young children is often the initial separation from their parents, but for the adolescent, the primary stress is related to fear of harm to body image, pain, death, and awakening during surgery. Clearly, providing families with several venues to discuss the emotional aspects of surgery is critical to an overall successful and effective outcome.

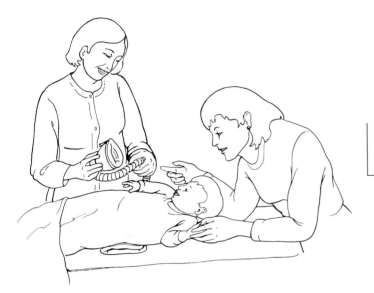

FIGURE 1-1. Preoperative pediatric urology patient in child-friendly "prepare" clinic. Child development staff show child an anesthesia mask.

Chapter 2

Preparation for Surgery

PREMEDICATION

Providing a preoperative environment to facilitate calm separation of a child from his or her parents plays a critical role in fostering a supportive relationship with a family on the day of surgery. Anticipatory guidance for the day of surgery should begin during the surgeon's initial interaction with the family, outlining a clear road map from the preoperative evaluation to discharge home. This allows several opportunities for rediscussion of risks and alternatives, scheduling expert consultations, realigning of specific goals, and revising of timelines. Of note, some parents present with a vast array of experience, knowledge, and/or opinions; others arrive with few preconceived ideas. Each requires a formal orientation to the practices of the current surgeon and medical center and an invitation to take an active role in planning for the child's care. Integrating parents into the plans for surgery and anesthesia fosters confidence and mutual respect, allowing a family to adapt to a specific medical center.

Parents frequently have acquired abundant knowledge about premedication and about "induction rooms" where families remain with their child during induction of general anesthesia, and, therefore, often present to the surgeon and anesthesiologist with definite opinions and expectations that may or may not be consistent with all practices at all medical centers. A close working relationship among the presurgical evaluation clinic (e.g., the PREPARE clinic at the University of California, San Francisco), the surgeons, and the anesthesiologists should minimize disseminating conflicting information to parents as they maneuver the numerous points for preoperative assessments.

In general, the focus of the presurgical evaluation clinic should be to present all possible options for the day of surgery and to set the stage for the family to make final decisions with the anesthesiologist who will be caring for the child on the day of surgery. Clearly, if a specific plan is made during a preanesthesia visit, changing this on the day of surgery can be unsettling to a family.

Premedication is one of several effective mechanisms to allow a calm separation of a child from his or her family (Table 2-1). However, premedication is not appropriate for all pediatric patients. Age, underlying medical problems, preoperative setting, and length of the procedure are several of the factors that must be analyzed to safely design an appropriate plan. Infants less than 9 to 12 months of age rarely require premedication, since separating from parents does not elicit crying or discomfort. Transporting the child directly into the operating room eliminates the small but definite risk of sedating at one site and then moving to another for surgery.

For children between the ages of 1 to 5 years, premedication plays a major role in allowing a calm separation of a child from his or her caregivers, especially if the child has had prior surgical experiences. Oxygen, airway support devices and related medications, suction devices, pulse oximeter/other monitors, and resuscitation equipment and related medications must be immediately available. Another common alternative (or supplement) to premedication involves parental presence in a designated induction area. In this case, the parents remain with their child during a "mask induction." This may be an inappropriate option for some families.

Children older than 5 years vary enormously in their requirements for premedication. In fact, an anesthesiologist who commonly interacts with pediatric patients and who can establish rapport by clearly communicating with family and child may then effect a calm transition from preoperative site to the operating room without either premedication or parental presence. On the other hand, some 5- to 8-year-old children are fearful by nature or secondary to prior operative experiences or developmental delay, and these patients benefit from either sedation and/or parental presence.

In all cases, sedation may be contraindicated because of coexisting medical problems (e.g., craniofacial deformity with an abnormal upper airway). In the setting of short outpatient procedures, the parents should be advised that a premedication may delay discharge to home because of a longer recovery room stay.

Most children prefer inhaled rather than intravenous (IV) induction of anesthesia. Even with healthy, nonobese older children and adolescents, pediatric anesthesiologists negotiate this request readily. Of note, some children who require repeated surgical interventions request an IV induction. Inserting a small-gauge catheter into a site where local anesthetic cream (e.g., eutectic mixture of local anesthetics [EMLA]) has been applied at least 30 minutes earlier minimizes trauma. Of importance, apply the local anesthetic cream to several sites to allow options when attempting to place an IV catheter painlessly.

Providing a calm, seamless separation of a child from his or her parents is time consuming. To avoid frustrating

PEDIATRIC PREMEDICATION IN CURRENT USE AT UNIVERSITY OF CALIFORNIA, SAN FRANCISCO

TABLE 2-1

Agent*	Oral	Intranasal	Rectal	IM
Midazolam maleate	Yes	Yes	Rarely	Yes
Ketamine	Yes	—	Rarely	Yes (best use)
Benzodiazepine (Valium)	Rarely	—	—	—
Sufentanil	—	Rarely	—	Rarely
Methohexital	—	—	Rarely	—

*The dose of the drug will vary with the route of administration.

delays in the flow of a busy operating room, systems must be established to evaluate children at least 1 hour before the anticipated time for induction of anesthesia, so that premedication (any route other than IV) can be delivered and local anesthetic cream applied at least approximately 30 minutes before the effects are required. In some cases, a family can be instructed to apply the local anesthetic before arriving in the preoperative area. On the other hand, providing oral sedation to children before arrival to the medical facility introduces an undesirable level of risk.

NOTHING BY MOUTH

Guidelines for discontinuing nonclear fluids and solids and clear liquids have been established by the American Society of Anesthesiologists. A schedule of preanesthetic NPO (nothing by mouth) directions for families consistent with these should be given to families by the surgeon when surgery is initially scheduled and then reinforced during a preanesthetic visit or phone call a day or two before the surgery (Table 2-2).

FASTING (NPO) GUIDELINES AT UNIVERSITY OF CALIFORNIA, SAN FRANCISCO

TABLE 2-2

8 hr before surgery	Discontinue nonclear liquids and solids (this includes food and also hard candy or gum)
6 hr before surgery	Discontinue formula
4 hr before surgery	Discontinue breast milk
2 hr before surgery	Discontinue clear liquids (water, clear apple juice)

BOWEL PREPARATION

Urologic reconstruction using intestine requires bowel preparation before surgery. A general approach includes the following:

• Admit the child to the hospital to ensure compliance with a liquid diet, to measure serial electrolytes, and to document fluid balance while delivering a continuous balanced bowel preparation solution (e.g., GoLYTELY) via a nasogastric tube. Children will not reliably drink an adequate volume of this solution.
• Reconstruction is typically done in patients older than 5 years of age with the majority being young adolescents or teenagers.
  Children should fast for 2 to 4 hours prior to initiating GoLYTELY. For children, the infusion rate using a nasogastric tube is 25 to 40 mL/kg/hour until effluent is clear (usually 4 to 10 hours). Please note, children with neurogenic issues to their bowel require longer infusions to obtain clear effluent than children who are neurogenically normal. For adults or older teenagers the rate is 20 to 30 mL/minute (1.2 to 1.8 L/hour) until 4 L is reached or effluent is clear. Older teenagers and adults may also drink the GoLYTELY; 240 mL every 10 minutes until 4 L or rectal effluent is clear.
• Serum electrolytes and body weight should not be affected as GoLYTELY is isoosmotic and not exchanged across the barrier of the bowel wall.

VASCULAR ACCESS

Unless the child has had an IV catheter placed during the process of a bowel preparation, the most common practice is to induce general anesthesia before vascular access is achieved. Occasionally, an older child may request an IV induction. In some cases, central venous access may be indicated in the setting of coexisting medical problems or a complex surgery (e.g., anticipated large blood loss). In most cases, a percutaneous subclavian or internal or external jugular approach is preferable over a femoral vein catheterization.

PERIOPERATIVE INFECTION

The following precepts have been incorporated into routine surgical practice:

1. As much as possible, perform procedures in an outpatient setting to reduce the risk for hospital-acquired infections.
2. Treat infections (e.g., urinary tract, cutaneous) aggressively before surgical intervention.
3. Ensure complete bowel preparation in relevant surgery.
4. Provide antibacterial prophylaxis in the setting of major surgery.

Antibacterial Prophylaxis

Surgical infections are classified according to the nature of the wound of origin: Category 1 refers to infections arising from clean, uncontaminated wounds; category 2 refers to those from clean but contaminated wounds; and category 3 refers to infections at the site of frankly contaminated wounds. Prophylaxis in the setting of major surgery but in the absence of infected urine or tissue is only indicated if the intra- and/or postoperative periods are associated with a high risk for contamination. Of note, trimethoprim/sulfamethoxazole is contraindicated during early infancy (first 3 months of age). Instead, amoxicillin or penicillin G (with or without an aminoglycocide) is an appropriate agent for perioperative prophylaxis. Specific recommendations for each category of wounds include:

Category 1: Prophylactic antibiotics are not indicated except during insertion of prosthetic devices.
Category 2: Prophylactic antibiotics are indicated intraoperatively to extend coverage for 3 or 4 hours postoperatively.
Category 3: Antibiotics assume a therapeutic rather than a prophylactic role and are selected based on the bacteria commonly encountered in a specific surgical intervention. For example, for abdominal contamination, clindamycin plus gentamicin or a third-generation cephalosporin serves as an effective combination.

Although delivery of prophylactic antibiotic regimens is commonly discussed, the evidence for specific benefits of perioperative antibiotics has yet to be established, except in a few carefully defined clinical scenarios. The following are examples of well-established indications for delivery of prophylactic antibiotics:

- Placement of a balloon catheter or for cystoscopy (cephalosporin [cephalexin] 25 mg/kg IV)
- Existence of a ventriculoperitoneal shunt or valvular heart disease (for nonurinary tract–related operations, vancomycin IV immediately before surgery and for 2 days postoperatively; gentamicin should be added if the urinary tract is involved)
- Intra-abdominal surgery (follow a bowel preparation protocol; deliver ampicillin, gentamicin, and metronidazole intraoperatively and continue for 48 hours postoperatively)

The following is an example of a specific perioperative prophylactic regimen:

- Deliver gentamicin intravenously 1 hour before operation and repeat at 8-hour intervals for 2 more doses. In the presence of an indwelling urinary catheter, ampicillin also should be delivered intravenously (i.e., to provide prophylactic coverage of *Enterococcus*).
- Trimethoprim with sulfamethoxazole is often given for several days following removal of a urinary catheter.

ADJUNCTS TO SURGICAL PLANNING

The widespread availability of radiologic imaging and minimally invasive diagnostic studies allows the surgeon to meticulously define anatomy and pathology preoperatively. This provides the opportunity to plan the operative procedure in detail well ahead of the day of surgery. This allows for consulting with other experts, recruiting of a surgical colleague to assist intraoperatively as needed, eliciting input from the pediatric anesthesiologist, and/or arranging for appropriate postoperative monitoring/supportive care. Such comprehensive evaluation and analyses should facilitate preoperative planning with the family and patient as well as streamline intraoperative care and improve efficiency.

OUTPATIENT SURGERY

The pediatric population requiring urologic surgery is commonly made up of ideal candidates for the "come-and-go" setting. The patients are healthy and many of the procedures are simple and of short duration. Often the outpatient surgery center provides a more circumscribed environment (e.g., smaller, less complicated) with fewer personnel and less opportunity to get lost. The pace is often less hectic and the acuity of the patients is lower than in the larger, busy in-hospital setting. Similarly, the recovery area is often open to families. This combination of factors may decrease the psychological impact of surgery by minimizing the time a child is separated from his or her family. Also, with minimal exposure to the in-hospital setting, the risk for infection may decrease.

On the other hand, the overall success of outpatient surgery is linked to the ability of parents or guardians to understand the surgical procedure, meticulously follow the perioperative instructions, and accept the responsibility to ask questions. Identifying patients and their families as well as selecting procedures (e.g., inguinal and scrotal surgery, many endoscopic procedures, hypospadias repair) that are appropriate for come-and-go status are critical responsibilities of the surgeon and other members of the operative team.

LATEX ALLERGY

Spina bifida syndromes are associated with a high incidence of acquiring an allergy to latex. To avoid this sensitization, infants with myelomeningocele are protected from unnecessary exposure to latex immediately after birth. That is, exposure to latex from gloves, tourniquets, and other equipment is avoided. If an older child has been sensitized to latex, in addition to meticulous protection from latex, he or she should receive an H_1 blocker such as diphenhydramine and an H_2 blocker such as ranitidine preoperatively. If the patient is inadvertently exposed to latex, an anaphylactic reaction may develop, as manifested by cutaneous lesions (e.g., hives), bronchoconstriction, and/or cardiovascular collapse. Aggressive resuscitation with fluids, vasopressors (e.g., epinephrine), oxygen, and vigorous bronchodilatation and ventilation may be required. Hydrocortisone and serial doses of diphenhydramine and an H_2 blocker may be necessary. If response to the supportive therapy is not prompt, surgery should be discontinued.

HYPOTHERMIA

Newborns, especially premature infants, cannot maintain core body temperature as effectively as older infants and children, in part because of an inability to shiver. Thus, controlling the environmental temperature is essential to avoid the consequences of hypothermia (e.g., hypoglycemia, apnea, arrhythmias, acidosis, hypotension). Newborns are capable of metabolizing brown fat to maintain core temperature, but this source of energy is rapidly depleted. Maintaining a warm temperature in the operating room, covering the infant's head, providing a warming device on the operating room bed, using overhead warmers until surgery begins, and warming IV fluids and inspired anesthetic gases are among the interventions commonly used during surgery on newborns and small infants.

POSITIONING DURING PEDIATRIC SURGERY

This atlas includes detailed diagrams recommending appropriate positioning for each surgical procedure. However, protecting from excessive pressure or hyperextension also must be evaluated for each patient after final positioning for the surgery. The surgeon, anesthesiologist, and nurse should meticulously ensure that foam rubber padding protects bony prominences to avoid damage to adjacent nerve trunks (e.g., the ulnar nerve or brachial plexus). After final positioning for the surgery, the patient should be examined to eliminate excessive stretch on muscles, ligaments, and joints.

PREOPERATIVE CHECKLIST

A preoperative checklist consistent with requirements of the medical center, Joint Commission on Accreditation of Healthcare Organizations, and other regulatory agencies should be generated to facilitate and document completion of required practices before each surgery (Table 2-3).

TABLE 2-3

PREOPERATIVE CHECKLIST

Informed consent and permit

Confirm the patient identification, diagnosis, and site/side of the pathology

Preanesthetic medication

Allergies recorded

Medications

Blood availability

Antibiotics

Mark site "Time-out"

Skin preparation

Section 2

OPERATING ON NEONATES, INFANTS, AND CHILDREN

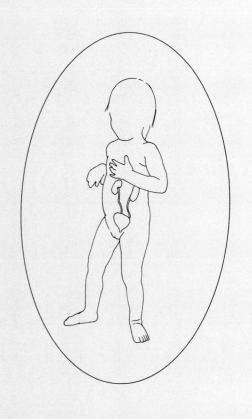

Chapter 3

Intraoperative Monitoring

Currently, national and medical regulations require the presence of the attending urologist in the operating room before general anesthesia is induced. This allows for the time-out needed to confirm the patient's name, planned surgical procedure, and allergies and to ensure that any specific equipment or tools are available. More informally, this early appearance in the operating room provides another opportunity to update the anesthesiologist and other members of the surgical team about the surgical plan. For older children, the presence of the surgeon is reassuring. The surgeon serves as a resource if any problems arise during induction of anesthesia. First-hand encounters with events during induction are critical to provide analysis and recommendations to a family either intra- or postoperatively.

The American Society of Anesthesia (ASA) standards for routine intraoperative monitoring include electrocardiogram, blood pressure, oxygen saturation, and end-tidal carbon dioxide. In most cases blood pressure is measured via an automated device, such as a Dinamap monitor. In the setting of long, complex surgical procedures and/or coexisting medical problems, direct arterial cannulation provides beat-to-beat monitoring of blood pressure and allows easy access for blood sampling. A precordial stethoscope allows the anesthesiologist to monitor heart and/or breath sounds continuously.

Body temperature should be measured via a rectal (or esophageal) probe to ensure appropriate environmental temperature to avoid hypo- or hyperthermia. The loss of body heat can be significant in newborns and young infants who have a large surface area to body mass ratio. In addition, especially in the premature infant, diminished, inefficient mechanisms for maintaining core temperature over a wide range of environmental temperatures predisposes to developing clinically important hypothermia. The setting of anesthesia and surgery exaggerates the susceptibility to heat loss secondary to vasodilation and other cardiovascular changes, pharmacologic effects of medication, exposure of the large surface area of the peritoneal cavity, and a high rate of intravenous (IV) fluid delivery. Commonly, the anesthesiologist attempts to counteract these phenomena by ensuring that inspired gases are heated and humidified, placing a warming device on the operating room bed, warming IV crystalloid and colloid, covering the infant's head, and controlling the room temperature in response to the patient's core temperature. An overhead radiant warmer should be used before draping and after the drapes are removed (i.e., during induction and prepping skin, during positioning, and again after the surgery is completed, while preparing to transport the patient to the recovery room or intensive care unit). During surgery, the sterile adhesive drapes provide some protection from excessive heat loss. The surgeon contributes to protecting the patient from hypothermia by using warm irrigation, minimizing the time of surgical exposure of body cavities, and cooperating with requests for higher environmental temperature.

POSITIONING OF THE CHILD

Appropriate positioning of small infants for some procedures may require modifying the standard recommendations depicted in the atlas (see specific illustrations for each surgery). In general, the same common precautions employed for adults apply to patients with a small body mass. That is, avoid hyperextension of muscles and joints (e.g., predisposes to nerve injury), minimize prolonged compression to dependent areas, protect the endotracheal tube and other airway devices from surgeons, ensure access to IV and/or arterial ports, and so on.

SKIN PREPARATION

Techniques to prepare the skin and to isolate the operative field via draping contribute to the goal of maintaining core temperature, especially in young infants. Warming prep solutions, avoiding agents that evaporate on the skin (povidone-iodine applied as a scrub with stick sponges is preferable to soap and water), and performing the scrub rapidly are simple systems for avoiding hypothermia secondary to presurgical scrub.

In addition to the surgical scrub, the quantity and quality of drapes must also be considered to minimize the impact of temperature loss during the presurgical period. Adhesive drapes function as a barrier to bacteria and heat. Covering the areas adjacent to the site of the incision with sterile dry towels and stabilizing with small clips may contribute to protecting the patient from heat loss, but only if the towels remain dry. Fold the covering drape on itself to form a lateral pocket to hold instruments.

An overhead heater should be focused over the child during the interval between placement on the table and application of the drapes. During lengthy operations, the IV fluids should be warmed to body temperature.

FLUID REPLACEMENT AND ELECTROLYTES

Meticulously evaluating an infant's cardiorespiratory and metabolic status preoperatively is critical, especially in the newborn. For example, if the birth has been traumatic or the infant asphyxiated, cardiovascular instability may persist for hours or, rarely, days. Electrolytes may be abnormal secondary to renal, hepatic, or cardiac dysfunction. Thus, reviewing the trends in blood pressure, heart rate, respiratory rate, and acid-base status and then correlating these data with the amount of IV fluid, blood products, electrolytes (sodium, potassium, calcium), vasopressors, and medications is essential to understand the physiologic status, correct as many abnormalities as possible, and develop an intraoperative plan for surgery and anesthesia. On physical exam, a dehydrated newborn/young infant may have depressed fontanels, delayed capillary refill, and abnormal skin turgor. Older infants and children also manifest decreased intravascular volume on physical exam. Dry mucous membranes, abnormal skin turgor, and mental status are some of the common indicators of dehydration.

Evaluating abnormalities of fluid and electrolyte status and repleting intravascular volume preoperatively contributes to an uneventful induction of anesthesia and stable intraoperative course. Fluid management intraoperatively is challenging in the setting of ongoing losses and extravascular extravasation so that establishing a normal baseline status is essential.

At any time, fluid delivery is calculated based on four considerations: deficit (e.g., secondary to preoperative nothing-by-mouth [NPO] status), maintenance needs, ongoing losses, and special requirements (e.g., calcium, glucose in a diabetic). The increased fluid losses during surgery vary with the procedure, the metabolic state (e.g., fever, sepsis), and other factors (e.g., third spacing secondary to tissue injury). In general, open-abdominal procedures often require infusing normal saline or lactated Ringer's solution at a rate of 4 to 10 mL/kg/hour, in addition to maintenance fluid (4 mL/kg/hour, for 1 to 10 kg + 2 mL/kg/hour; 10 to 20 kg + 1 mL/kg for >20 kg). For simplicity, lactated Ringer's solution or normal saline (rather than the usual 0.25% normal saline) is used to deliver maintenance fluid to avoid a second IV solution. Depending on the length of the NPO period and the status of the patient, the "deficit" may or may not be included in the fluid regimen during surgery. That is, a 2- to 4-hour period of NPO has little effect on a normal infant or child, and does not necessarily need to be replaced. In the setting of some intracranial surgery, fluid restriction may supersede the routine practice of replacing the "deficit" secondary to NPO precautions.

In most cases, colloid is not routinely delivered intraoperatively. In the setting of large surgical blood loss, underlying physiologic instability or disease, or unexplained intraoperative bleeding or cardiovascular instability, packed red blood cells or other blood products (e.g., platelets, fresh-frozen plasma) may be required. In general, until the blood loss exceeds 15% to 20% of the blood volume and with a hematocrit of 25%, transfusion is not initiated. On the other hand, a newborn or young infant may not tolerate a loss of 10% (or less) of the blood volume or a hematocrit less than 35% to 40%. Patients with cyanotic congenital heart disease may require maintaining the hematocrit above 45% (or higher). Children who have hepatic or hematologic disease may require specific blood component therapy. Thus, establishing precise rules or protocols for blood administration is impossible. Of importance, each operating room must establish a system to measure/monitor blood loss, to allow obtaining prompt and serial laboratory values, and to ensure easy communication with the blood bank. The task of intraoperative evaluation of blood loss is challenging for small infants and during surgery, especially when losses inside body cavities can be easily underestimated and the absolute value of blood volume is small (i.e., 100 mL/kg = 100 mL for a premature infant who weighs 1 kg).

In general, if blood loss exceeds 20% of the blood volume and/or the hematocrit is less than 25% and continued surgical blood loss is anticipated, a packed blood cell infusion should be considered. If cardiovascular instability or rapid losses are encountered, transfusion is initiated earlier. Devising systems to collect blood from the wound in a small trap in the drapes, storing discarded surgical sponges in a pan, and including small-volume collection devices in the suctions allows more accurate tracking of blood loss. The surgeon and anesthesiologist should negotiate the topic of blood loss, as the surgeon frequently has a more accurate view of the surgical field, should be able to predict trends in ongoing/future losses, and should estimate the time frame for completing the procedure.

GLUCOSE DELIVERY

Intraoperative glucose delivery must be adjusted to avoid hypoglycemia but avoid the central nervous system side effects and osmotic diuresis that may accompany glucose loading. In general, three groups of patients require meticulous monitoring and delivery of glucose intraoperatively. First, newborns (especially prematures) may have limited ability to avoid hypoglycemia without continuous substrate delivery. After a traumatic delivery and in the setting of continued stress (e.g., hypothermia, sepsis, congenital anomalies) newborns are predisposed to developing hypoglycemia. On the other hand, renal tubular immaturity and physiologic stress (e.g., sepsis) precipitate glucosuria at serum levels as low as 70 to 80 mg/dL. Second, any patient receiving IV alimentation may not tolerate an abrupt discontinuation of the glucose solution. Third, diabetic patients are predisposed to both hyper- and hypoglycemia depending on the interplay of insulin and substrate delivery. The intraoperative management of these three groups of patients must include a mechanism to measure glucose as needed.

Of note, the so-called "maintenance glucose" requirement of a normal newborn is approximately 4 mg/kg/minute

(240 mg/kg/hour) while that of older infants and children decreases to about 2 mg/kg/minute. Since 5% dextrose contains 50 mg/mL and the maintenance fluid rate for 1 to 10 kg of body weight is 4 mL/kg/hour (200 mg/kg/hour), delivering higher rates or concentrations of dextrose may precipitate hyperglycemia. Similarly, if a patient is accustomed to a higher rate of IV glucose from hyperalimentation (e.g., D10 to D25), sudden withdrawal of this source of glucose can precipitate hypoglycemia.

Thus, glucose is not routinely infused intraoperatively in older infants and children who are neither diabetic nor receiving IV alimentation. For newborns and patients receiving IV alimentation, intraoperatively obtaining a blood sample to measure serum glucose should be anticipated. In general, IV alimentation is either slowly weaned over hours to days preoperatively or maintained at a stable, chronic rate and adjusted only in response to a specific intraoperative serum glucose level. Of course, rare syndromes such as insulinomas or other pancreatic or endocrinologic disorders will require specific management devised in consultation with subspecialists such as pediatric endocrinologists.

REGIONAL AND LOCAL ANESTHESIA

Lidocaine hydrochloride (Xylocaine) is effective within 5 minutes and for between 1.5 and 2.5 hours after administration. For ilioinguinal and penile and caudal blocks, 0.5 to 1 mL/kg of 0.25% bupivacaine (Marcaine) is the most commonly used agent (see Chapter 6). Suggested maximum doses (with or without epinephrine) are as follows: procaine (Novocain), 14 to 18 mg/kg; lidocaine, 7 to 9 mg/kg; and bupivacaine, 2 to 3 mg/kg. Short-beveled needles are less apt to encounter and injure nerves and, therefore, are often recommended for regional anesthesia. In the setting of complex intra-abdominal surgery (e.g., ureteral reimplantation), an epidural should be considered to produce postoperative pain relief.

Adding epinephrine (1:200,000, 5 µg/mL) induces vasoconstriction and as a result may decrease local blood flow, the rate of absorption and serum concentration of the agent, and therefore, the side effects of the anesthetic. On the other hand, absorption of epinephrine rarely can elicit hemodynamic side effects (e.g., arrhythmias, hypertension). Of particular importance, bupivacaine can induce severe cardiovascular collapse in the setting of an IV injection. Central nervous system toxicity secondary to local anesthetics includes minor, transient symptoms (e.g., slurred speech, disorientation) but can also progress to seizures. Treatment of all complications primarily includes cardiorespiratory support, including oxygen and ventilatory support, IV fluids, and vasopressors. Seizures may also require IV barbiturates (e.g., thiopental, methohexital, pentobarbital) or benzodiazepines IV (e.g., diazepam, midazolam, lorazepam). Such treatment of seizures may also induce respiratory depression.

In the setting of surgery involving young infants, regional and local anesthesia usually serves as an adjunct to general anesthesia. That is, in addition to decreasing the depth of general anesthesia required, field blocks and caudals provide postoperative analgesia for both inpatients and outpatients.

One-eighth to one-quarter bupivacaine induces a sensory block without a dense motor blockade. Nonetheless, infants and children should be meticulously evaluated for motor function before discharge to the ward or home. If a urinary catheter is not in place postoperatively, urinary retention could be a complication of caudal (epidural) anesthesia and should be evaluated before discharge.

GENERAL ANESTHESIA

Most anesthesiologists recommend general anesthesia to provide appropriate conditions for urologic surgery on infants and children. These general anesthetics include inhaled (e.g., nitrous oxide, sevoflurane, isoflurane, halothane, desflurane) and IV (e.g., midazolam, propofol, fentanyl, morphine, other narcotics) agents. In many cases, the agents are introduced in various combinations of inhaled and IV substances, depending on the prior anesthetic history of the patient, requests of the patient or family, and choice of the anesthesiologist. The length of the procedure, plans for postoperative recovery, and coexisting medical problems also factor into the design of the general anesthetic.

For a majority of urologic procedures, an appropriately sized laryngeal mask airway (e.g., 1, 1.5, 2, 2.5, 3) provides excellent airway support during general anesthesia. For more complex, lengthy, and/or intra-abdominal surgery, endotracheal intubation with or without muscle reaxation may be safer. In addition, coexistent medical problems or critical acute physiologic developments may demand endotracheal intubation.

The laryngeal mask airway (LMA) is a combination mask and airway with a conventional silicone tracheal tube that has been cut off diagonally to remove the cuff and an inflatable cuff in the shape of a pediatric face mask attached to the distal end. In all cases, the LMA must be positioned properly to allow both effective spontaneous and mechanical ventilatory support. Rarely, the LMA does not seat properly at the larynx, so that effective ventilation is impossible. In all such cases, depending on the surgical procedure, either a face mask or an endotracheal tube must be used instead.

Because of the physiologic effects of inhaled anesthetics, lung mechanics, and gas distribution, and due to the respiratory depressant effects of both inhaled and IV agents, a fractional concentration of inspired oxygen (FIO_2) greater than 0.21 is required during general anesthesia. Of additional significance, although the functional residual capacity (FRC) of infants is similar to the older child and adult, their oxygen consumption is higher. An FIO_2 of greater than 0.21 provides a "reserve" of oxygen in the setting of apnea, airway obstruction, or increased oxygen consumption. For example, if FRC is 30 mL/kg, an FIO_2 of 1 will provide 5 times the amount of oxygen uptake as an FIO_2 of 0.21, if the oxygen consumption is the same. In the setting of total airway obstruction, the length of time before hypoxemia ensues will be 5 times as long if the FRC contains an FIO_2 of 1 (30 mL/kg of oxygen) versus an FIO_2 of 0.21 (21% of 30 mL/kg).

In those premature infants having a history of periodic breathing, apnea can be a special problem postoperatively;

they must be monitored closely even the day following surgery. In addition, these infants are more liable to aspiration, infection, and hypothermia.

MONITORING

Morbidity and mortality attributed to anesthesia continue to be greater in the youngest age group. On the other hand, an inhaled induction of anesthesia seems to be less apparent in the young infant. Overall, the significantly increased risks directly attributable to anesthesia in newborns and young infants can be distributed to several physiologic factors:

1. Apnea and bradycardia constitute a type of "common pathway" of response in the newborn. That is, metabolic abnormalities (e.g., hypoglycemia, hypocalcemia), sepsis, hypoxia, anemia, hypo- or hyperthermia, and so on, may all elicit apnea and/or bradycardia.
2. Ventilatory excursion is primarily dependent on the diaphragm rather than the intercostals, so that ventilation may be compromised secondary to intra-abdominal events more commonly than in older infants and children.
3. The central nervous system's control of ventilation is unpredictable. For example, hypoxia may elicit a short burst of hyperventilation but is quickly followed by apnea.
4. Oxygen consumption is high so that the functional reserve capacity is exhausted more quickly in the setting of airway obstruction.
5. The gastroesophageal junction is incompetent even in normal infants so that gastroesophageal reflux is common. In the presence of abdominal distention, the young infant is at high risk for regurgitation and aspiration of gastric contents.

Routine monitoring to meet the ASA standards includes EKG, blood pressure, oxygen saturation, end-tidal carbon dioxide, and temperature. Invasive monitoring should be justified and initiated in response to the patient's underlying medical status and the complexity of the surgical procedure.

Malignant Hyperthermia

Malignant hyperthermia (MH) is a rare disorder (1:20,000 to 1:40,000) now classified as a pharmacogenetic abnormality of calcium regulation in skeletal muscle. That is, in most cases, unequivocal familial MH has been linked to mutations in the gene encoding the calcium release channel (the ryanodine receptor) in skeletal muscle, predisposing to abnormal calcium homeostasis during excitation-contraction coupling, characterized by increased intracellular free-ionized calcium and the need for intracellular ATP (adenosine triphosphate) to drive calcium pumps. An episode of MH is recognized clinically by the signs of an increased metabolic rate after exposure to a "triggering agent" (e.g., succinylcholine, halothane). The clinical markers of MH are variable, initially nonspecific, and include masseter spasm, total body rigidity, increased partial pressure of carbon dioxide (PCO_2) with a high minute ventilation, dysrhythmias

(inappropriate sinus tachycardia, ventricular tachycardia/fibrillation), inappropriate and/or rapid rise in body temperature, sweating, and mottling of skin. At the same time, laboratory findings include respiratory and metabolic acidosis, hyperkalemia, elevated creatine kinase, and myoglobinuria/myoglobinemia. In fulminant cases, the metabolic acidosis and hyperthermia develop rapidly. With current standards of monitoring, the clinical diagnosis of MH is entertained before the fulminant clinical state develops.

Administering dantrolene (repeated doses of 2.5 mg/kg) and discontinuing all triggering agents are the critical components of treatment. Simultaneously, ventilating aggressively with an FIO_2 of 1, and treating arrhythmias, metabolic acidosis (e.g., fluids, sodium bicarbonate), hyperkalemia (e.g., insulin/glucose), and myoglobinuria (e.g., mannitol, furosemide) are critical (Table 3-1). Cooling (i.e., remove drapes, eliminate heated inspired gases, initiate cooling via a mattress, deliver iced saline into an orogastric tube, irrigate open body cavities with cool, sterile solutions, deliver cool IV fluids, place ice packs into the groin/axilla and cool cloths to the body surface, direct a fan close to the patient to facilitate heat loss via evaporation) should be initiated promptly to reduce muscle metabolism and the associated hyperthermia. Extracorporeal bypass with a heat exchanger is an extreme but well-described system for controlling body temperature. Dantrolene should be administered repeatedly until the physical and laboratory evidence of the hypermetabolic state is reversed. Dantrolene (1 mg/kg) should be delivered approximately every 6 hours until the creatine kinase has consistently decreased.

To monitor and treat during an episode of MH, an arterial and multiple peripheral/central IV catheters should be inserted. A urinary catheter is essential. After effective treatment in the operating room, monitoring and treatment must be continued in an intensive care unit. Recurrence of MH is not uncommon, especially in the first few hours after the initial episode. Monitoring of cardiovascular, acid-base, and electrolyte status, as well as aggressive supportive care are critical. Treating rhabdomyolysis must be aggressive. Disseminated intravascular coagulopathy and nonspecific systemic, multisystem organ failure (especially respiratory failure) are highly associated with fatal MH.

TABLE 3-1 TREATING MALIGNANT HYPERTHERMIA

Discontinue triggering agents	Administer bicarbonate
Hyperventilate, FIO_2	Administer diuretics
Administer dantrolene	Treat arrhythmias
Initiate cooling procedures	Insert arterial, intravenous, urinary catheters

Chapter 4

Operative Management

PEDIATRIC SURGICAL TECHNIQUE

The techniques and maneuvers in pediatric surgery are much the same as those in adults but are carried out more precisely because of the size of the patient and the friability of the tissues. The operation must be planned in advance so that it can be completed with the fewest steps, even if the findings are different from those expected. Keep in mind possible complications, noted in the text, so that they may be avoided.

The skin of children is malleable so that incisions may be made along Langer's lines. Choose a transverse incision over a vertical one if the exposure will be the same, because there is less chance for dehiscence. For major operations, make marks across the incision with a skin pen to assure realignment of the skin. If you and your assistant press along the margins of the incision, fewer small vessels will need fulguration, and the skin will become everted to expose the bleeders remaining in the subcutaneous tissue. Divide muscles with the cutting current, and fulgurate the vessels with the coagulating current through a needlepoint stylus. Dissect vessels by opening the scissors parallel to them to avoid tearing and to allow fulguration or ligation before division.

Develop your operative technique for work on children by making your movements delicate and precise. As you work, think ahead to what you will need for the next step; then you will not have to wait for an instrument or suture because the scrub nurse will have it ready.

The tissue of young children is tenuous, requiring care as each instrument is applied. Dependence on antibacterial agents to avoid infection is not the same as handling tissues gently to allow healthy cells to resist it. The tools of the careful surgeon are stay sutures, skin hooks, and delicate forceps. Needle or bipolar electrodes are used for point fulguration. Fine ligatures and sutures are important. Also, keep the tissues covered with moist gauze to protect them.

PEDIATRIC SURGICAL INSTRUMENTS

A set of instruments designed for operations on neonates and infants must be organized, with size and weight being the most important features. The needlepoint electrosurgical unit divides fascia and muscle with minimal injury and allows immediate control of small vessels by coagulation.

With the help of the operating room nurse or technician, make out a card for each operation you commonly perform, listing the position of the patient, the instruments needed, and the sutures to have ready. In this atlas, lists of special instruments are given for many operations; these may be copied on your cards. Keep these cards up to date, and check them with the scrub nurse at the instrument table when you arrive to be sure everything is at hand.

A pediatric genitourinary (GU) cart is a necessity because of the special needs of children. Set up a five- or six-drawer roll-around shop-cart, outfit it with the required special sutures, stents, and special instruments, and have it in the operating room during the operation.

VISIBILITY

Visual acuity is directly related to the intensity of the light in the wound. At least two light sources are required, with one shining over the surgeon's right shoulder. Focused beams should reach the bottom of the wound without interference from heads. For deep wounds in children, a head lamp will help.

Magnification also increases the ability to see what you are doing and is particularly important for pediatric operations. Every pediatric urologic surgeon needs to have a personal pair of binocular loupes permanently attached to plain or prescription glasses. Be sure the glasses fit well behind the ears so that they do not end up in the wound. For the occasional assistant, less expensive, industrial-type loupes on plastic headbands can be kept in the operating room to be slipped on when needed.

INCISION

A single stroke through the skin and subcutaneous tissue using a good-sized scalpel blade does the least damage. Multiple small cuts cause more injury to the vulnerable subcutaneous tissue and promote infection. Do not use the cutting current in the subcutaneous tissue because it damages a wider path than does the knife. Select a very sharp knife for the same reason. Let the scalpel float down through the fat until it meets the fascia. You do not need to discard the skin knife unless it is dull; it has been shown that it does not pick up bacteria from the skin.

For incising muscle and fascia, select the undamped cutting current delivered through the smallest available electrode, a needle electrode. A foot pedal leaves the hand free to grasp the handle of the stylus in any position. Realize that the surgical electrode is similar to a ray gun; it does not cut or coagulate through contact but rather through the arc that emanates from its tip. Avoid burrowing under a muscle before dividing it; this only opens more tissue planes. Rather, cut through the muscle progressively with the cutting current, using long strokes while taking care not to go deeply in any one area. As the muscle retracts, its vessels are seen and the next layer is exposed. It is therefore not necessary to clamp, cut, and ligate muscles, a process that causes more necrosis than does electrosurgery.

DISSECTION

All forceps cause some injury to tissue. If a forceps grasping your skin can cause you pain, it also will damage tissue. Hemostats held inverted between the thumb and third finger keep the bulk of the hand away from the wound.

HEMOSTASIS

Control vessels less than 2 mm in diameter by pinpoint coagulation with damped current rather than suture ligature, because it produces less local destruction. Special bipolar coagulating forceps operated by the first assistant speeds up the operation and produces minimal damage to delicate tissues. An insulated knife or scissors connected to monopolar current also may reduce time. In any case, do not wave the electrode back and forth but be precise and coagulate only the bleeding vessel. For small bleeders in retractile muscle, insert the electrode first and then apply the current. For larger vessels, do not fulgurate but clamp first and then divide and ligate. These methods damage less tissue than when the vessel is cut and then clamped. Electrocoagulation, similar to electroincision, increases the chance of infection threefold; therefore, avoid its use in the skin and subcutaneous tissue. Finally, use only bipolar coagulation on the penis; monopolar current is more penetrating and so increases the risk of urethral injury and fistula, even at low power.

ASSISTANTS AND ASSISTANCE

Always perform major surgery with a competent assistant. This assistant should review the operative steps and be familiar with the procedure to not only be of more help but also learn more. Teaching as you operate makes you more aware of anatomic details and is invaluable for the assistant. The main function of an assistant is to provide exposure. This is accomplished not just by retraction, which is really the job of a self-retaining ring retractor or of the second assistant if you have one. A good first assistant, by anticipating the next move and exposing or grasping the appropriate tissue layer at the right time and place, can essentially perform the operation, with the surgeon merely following the lead.

PROTECTION OF THE SURGICAL TEAM FROM INFECTION

It is the responsibility of the surgeon to operate on all patients, regardless of their HIV status. The result is that caution must be constantly exercised by all the team members as they are exposed to blood or secretions. This means that surgeons, anesthetists, and scrub personnel should wear protective glasses during invasive procedures in the operating room and routinely wear protective boots or impervious shoe coverings. Exposed skin surfaces should be washed with detergent immediately after contamination with blood or body fluid. Hands should be washed immediately after gloves are removed at the end of a procedure.

Extreme caution should be exercised with needles and sharp instruments. Meticulous technique is required both in the immediate operative field and the entire operating room to minimize accidental HIV exposure.

Have the scrub nurse place sharp instruments on a tray from which you can pick them up. Although needles are the greater hazard, a scalpel in the hand of the surgeon or the assistant can puncture through two layers of glove. Take extreme care to avoid needle sticks. Needles should not be recapped, bent, or broken. After use, needles and disposable sharp instruments should be immediately placed in puncture-resistant containers for disposal.

Personnel scrubbing in the middle of a case should put on their own gowns and gloves to prevent contamination of the inside of the garments with blood or bodily fluids. If a gown becomes contaminated with blood, it should be changed as soon as possible.

SELECTION OF SUTURES

The wounds of infants and children heal faster than those of adults, but only after a lag phase of 5 days when they are dependent on the holding power of sutures. Major fibrous repair occurs for 2 weeks, followed by a slow increase in strength.

We each have our own preferences for sutures, but two important variables must be considered in their selection: persistence of strength and tissue reactivity. The initial strength is proportional to size, but the rate of loss of strength is a function of the suture material itself. Sutures are absorbed at variable rates, but the strength of the sutures is lost much more rapidly than it is absorbed. Reactivity of the tissue to the foreign body depends on the amount and type of reaction it invokes. The larger the size, the greater the reaction. Natural sutures incite a greater immunologic reaction than synthetic sutures. Also, greater suture size with larger knots creates increased reactivity. (The knots contribute most to the mass for reaction.)

Absorbable and nonabsorbable sutures have different effects. Plain catgut and chromic catgut sutures stimulate a large macrophage response with resultant proteolysis leading to significant tissue reactivity and to a variable absorption time. Synthetic absorbable sutures, in contrast, are removed by acid hydrolysis and thus have moderate tissue reactivity and more predictable absorption times.

Those made from monofilament polyglycolic acid (Dexon, Vicryl) retain only 20% of their strength at 14 days, whereas those made from polydioxanone (PDS) retain 50% of their strength at 4 weeks. Dexon and Vicryl in the gastrointestinal tract are absorbed in 3 to 4 weeks. In infected urine, monofilaments (Maxon) and PDS sutures retain the most strength. Nonabsorbable sutures such as Maxon stimulate the least reaction in the tissues and have the least attraction for bacteria. In contrast, braided sutures are easier to handle and tie more securely, but are unsuitable in the presence of bacteria or urine. Silk and cotton rapidly lose their strength after the second month but probably are useful in the outer layer of an intestinal anastomosis and in the mesentery. Nylon is a polyamide, Dacron is a polyester, and polyethylene and polypropylene are polyolefins; of these, nylon loses its strength first.

In general, Dexon and Vicryl sutures are preferable to plain or chromic catgut for urologic surgery, except in cases of infected urine and for the skin. Because of expense, as few different sizes and kinds of sutures as possible should be opened in any given case. Although suture selection is an individual matter, certain practical guidelines can be followed. The composition and trade names of the most used sutures are listed in Table 4-1, and their application is described in Table 4-2.

Fascia

Regardless of what suture is used, the immediate strength of the wound is only between 40% and 70% of the intact structure. With nonabsorbable sutures, this reduced strength persists at least for the 3 months or so that it takes for the wound to heal completely. For an absorbable suture, the strength initially is the same as that of a nonabsorbable one if an equivalent size is used, but in 1 or 2 weeks, its strength will have declined appreciably. The exceptions are PDS and Maxon, which are still strong at 2 weeks. By this time, however, the wound itself will have gained enough strength to balance the diminished strength derived from the sutures. Thus, it is during the second week that the wound is most vulnerable to separation. For this reason, sutures of nonabsorbable material often are used for closure of wounds subjected to stress, such as those in the abdomen and flank.

In clean wounds, PDS is absorbed by 26 weeks but maintains adequate strength for 6 weeks. However, it is stiff, and firm knots are hard to tie. Be sure to invert these sutures to avoid bumps on the outside. Vicryl and Dexon sutures maintain their strength and are eventually resorbed; they are preferable to PDS because they are easier to handle, and the knots will hold if they consist of a surgeon's knot with a square knot superimposed or four square knots.

For contaminated wounds, macrophage activity is stimulated by the process of absorbing the sutures, with resultant low tissue oxygen tension. This activity also reduces endothelial migration and capillary formation, thus providing a suitable environment for anaerobic bacterial growth. Polyglycolic acid sutures foster the least inflammatory response of absorbable sutures, and the degradation products themselves may be antibacterial. Conversely, nonabsorbable sutures, especially monofilaments, produce

SUTURE TYPES

TABLE 4 - 1

Material	Coated	Name of Suture
Absorbable		
Synthetic braided		
Polyglactin	Yes	Vicryl*
	No	Dexon "S"†
Polyglycolic acid	Yes	Dexon plus†
Synthetic monofilament		
Polyglyconate	—	Maxon†
Polydioxanone	—	PDS*
Gut		
Plain gut	—	Plain gut*,†
Chromic gut	—	Chromic gut*,†
Nonabsorbable		
Synthetic braided		
Polyester	No	Merseline,* Dacron†
Nylon	Yes	Surgilon†
Synthetical monofilament		
Nylon	—	Ethilon,* Dermalon†
Polypropylene	—	Prolene,* Surgilene†

*Manufactured by Ethicon, Somerville, NJ.
†Manufactured by U.S. Surgical, Norwalk, CT.
Adapted from Edlich R, Rodeheaver Gy, Thacker JG: Considerations in the choice of sutures for wound closure of the genitourinary tract. *J Urol* 137:373, 1987.

the least reaction, but once infected they may stay infected because they remain in the wound. Polypropylene is the best choice in contaminated wounds; it is much better than silk or cotton. For a debilitated patient in whom poor healing is expected, use either a nonabsorbable suture or the absorbable suture that retains its strength the longest (i.e., PDS). Retention sutures of heavy, nonabsorbable material (polypropylene or wire) may be needed in a debilitated patient, especially if the wound is contaminated. Bolsters cut from a red rubber catheter reduce damage to the skin.

Subcutaneous Tissue

This layer is the site of most wound infections because of the weak defense mechanisms in this fatty areolar tissue. Do not use sutures here unless truly necessary to obliterate a dead space, and then use the finest minimally reactive absorbable suture of polyglycolic acid. Avoid plain or chromic catgut.

SUGGESTED TYPE AND SIZE OF SUTURE FOR VARIOUS TISSUES

TABLE 4-2

Tissue	ADULT		PEDIATRIC	
	Type	Size	Type	Size
Skin				
Cosmetic closure	Absorbable	4-0	Absorbable	5-0
Noncosmetic closure	Staples	4-0	Nonabsorbable	5-0
	Nonabsorbable	3-0		4-0
Fascia	PDS	Zero	PDS	3-0
	Maxon, silk	1-0	Maxon, silk	2-0
Muscle	Absorbable	1-0	Absorbable	3-0
		2-0		3-0
Bladder	Absorbable	3-0	Absorbable	4-0
		2-0		3-0
Ureteropelvic junction	Absorbable	5-0	Absorbable	5-0
		4-0		6-0
Urethra	Absorbable (Maxon, PDS, Monocryl)	4-0	Absorbable	5-0
		5-0		6-0
Bowel	Staples		Staples	
	Absorbable (inner layer)	3-0	Absorbable (inner layer)	5-0
		4-0		4-0
	Nonabsorbable (outer layer)	3-0	Nonabsorbable (outer layer)	4-0
Vascular	Nonabsorbable	4-0	Nonabsorbable	4-0
		5-0		5-0

Skin

Tape is best to approximate skin edges if they are not subjected to too much tension. Skin clips, if not too tight, are the next best choice, because they do not penetrate the wound, but they cost more and are a nuisance because they require subsequent removal, to the distress of the child. Monofilament nonabsorbable material leaves a better wound but must be removed. Polyglycolic acid sutures placed subcuticularly can remain until resorbed, while producing little reaction. By means of a skin hook, the subcutaneous layer can be pulled forward to aid in placing each stitch. This material is not suitable when placed as interrupted sutures in the skin because it depends on hydrolysis for absorption and so will persist on the dry surface.

Urinary Tract

Urothelium covers the suture line within 3 days. Ureteral and vesical wounds gain strength more rapidly than those in the body wall; normal strength is reached in 21 days. The type of suture material is not as critical here, but absorbable sutures cause less reaction than nonabsorbable ones in the long term. Although more subject to encrustation, absorbable sutures usually are gone before stones can form. PDS sutures last too long to be of use in the urinary tract. Polyglycolic acid sutures are less reactive than chromic catgut sutures, and they have a more predictable rate of absorption. Although polyglycolic acid sutures are not completely absorbed before 28 days, they are usually the better choice, with one exception: In the presence of infection with *Proteus*, resorption is much too rapid, and catgut should be used.

Intestine

Use interrupted nonabsorbable sutures, reaching well into the submucosa. If a hemostatic layer is desired, place a running absorbable suture in the mucosa. Chromic catgut is suitable for sutures penetrating the lumen; otherwise, use synthetic absorbable sutures. Controlled-release needles speed the process of suturing.

Vascular Sutures

Monofilament, synthetic nonabsorbable sutures are strongest and least reactive.

POSITION AT SURGERY

Decide on which side of the table to stand for each operation. In this atlas, position is shown for right-handed surgeons, and the exposure and procedure also are illustrated from that point of view.

Start with the table at a height that allows your elbows to be flexed at right angles when your hands are resting on the surface of the patient. The operative field is small, so avoid putting your head down; your naked eyes (or with corrective glasses) have a reading distance of greater than 30 cm. A loupe will provide needed magnification. Infants have short legs, so the surgeon and assistants can work best while standing, even when operating on the perineum.

INTRAOPERATIVE BLEEDING

Although screening has been carried out preoperatively, abnormal bleeding may occur intraoperatively. Vitamin K deficiency occurs if the neonate has received only breast milk without prophylactic vitamin K supplement at birth. This deficiency should be picked up by a disproportionately prolonged prothrombin time and is readily treated by giving 1 to 2 mg of intravenous (IV) vitamin K oxide. The cause of bleeding may be disseminated intravascular coagulation secondary to hypoxemia, trauma, and infection.

Thrombocytopenia can be improved with IV gamma globulin. Packed red blood cells are a direct answer to intraoperative bleeding, given along with fresh-frozen plasma, although whole blood is better if the bleeding is rapid.

BLOOD LOSS AND TRANSFUSIONS

Because 7% of body weight is blood, a child weighing 10 kg has a circulating blood volume of approximately 700 mL. A loss at operation of up to 15% of this volume will not affect blood pressure, pulse pressure, respiration rate, or capillary blanch test results. Unless other fluid losses are occurring, count on transcapillary refill and other compensatory mechanisms to restore blood volume.

A volume loss between 15% and 30%, however, representing 100 to 200 mL of blood in a child (class II hemorrhage according to trauma surgeons), causes tachycardia, tachypnea, and, most significantly, a decrease in pulse pressure. Realize that the systolic pressure may be fairly well sustained, but the rise in diastolic pressure is ominous. The capillary blanch test results become positive, and the urinary output falls moderately to between 20 and 30 mL/hour. Patients with this condition require transfusion.

A volume loss of over 30% produces a measurable drop in systolic blood pressure (class III hemorrhage).

Blood loss in the postoperative period can be recognized by clinical signs. Hematocrit determinations are unreliable and inappropriate to estimate acute blood loss. A child who is cool and tachycardic is in shock and needs immediate transfusion. Septic shock produces a wide pulse pressure, an important differentiating point.

Use lactated Ringer's solution for initial replacement, giving a bolus of 20 mL/kg in a child. Observe the response. If the signs are not reversed or are only transiently improved, and if urinary output remains low, give packed red blood cells if already matched, and establish a central venous pressure (CVP) line, best done by percutaneous subclavian vein puncture. Crystalloid is replaced in a ratio of three volumes for each volume of blood lost. In an emergency, use type-specific or type O blood. Matched whole blood, of course, is best, if it can be obtained.

After 700 mL of blood replacement in a 10-kg child, coagulopathy becomes a problem, mainly because of hemodilution. Should abnormal bleeding appear after replacement, obtain a clotting screen and give a platelet pack. If clotting factors are found to be significantly deficient, give at least 400 mL of fresh-frozen plasma.

Be concerned about possible fluid overload, even when the CVP has not reached normal levels. Instead of depending on the CVP, watch for return of adequate perfusion by the urinary output, skin color, and return of pulse rate and blood pressure toward normal. However, if overload does occur, avoid diuretics because they render measurement of urine output useless as a guide and may precipitate hypovolemia.

FIXATION OF ORGANS AND TISSUES BEFORE CLOSURE

All structures should be restored to a position as near normal as possible. Pull the omentum down and spread it out to separate the intestines from the wound. In the flank, tack Gerota's fascia and the perirenal fat together with fine plain catgut sutures to isolate pelvic and ureteral repairs from the body wall. If the kidney has been freed, it must be repositioned with one or two nephropexy stitches taken into the psoas muscle. After reconstruction with intestinal segments, be sure to close the proximal edge of the mesentery against the retroperitoneal surface to prevent an internal hernia in the "trap."

OPERATIVE CONTAMINATION AND INFECTION

Washing the fat and tissue debris from the wound with sterile water by repeatedly filling and aspirating the wound bed is good practice. It will effectively reduce the inoculum and allow primary closure in contaminated wounds because an inoculum must contain at least 10^6 bacteria to cause infection, no matter what the species. If contamination of the wound is especially feared, use a solution of bacitracin, 500,000 units, and neomycin, 0.5 g, in 1000 mL of saline as extraperitoneal irrigation. Erythematous infected wounds or those grossly contaminated should be left open, covered with gauze, and then closed secondarily 3 or more days after the operation. For invasive infections, supplement antibiotic therapy with nasal oxygen.

DRAINS

The harmful effects of drainage tubes are usually outweighed by their benefits after urologic operations, especially those that enter the urinary tract. Drains render the tissue more susceptible to bacterial invasion and provide the route for bacterial entry from the skin and external environment, but they do facilitate the exit of potentially contaminated serum and blood, as well as collections of pus. Most important, they allow egress of urine that may leak from the tract. The most common purpose of a drain is prophylaxis, to prevent the accumulation of potentially infected blood, serum, or urine. Any surgical wound is susceptible to infection, and hematomas increase that risk. The indications for drainage are still controversial; neither drains nor antibiotics are substitutes for an atraumatic surgical technique. Make a decision about drainage at the end of the operation based on the pros and cons. For example, after a retroperitoneal operation, a drain allows trapped air and blood to escape; it may be removed the next day. When the urinary tract has been opened, a drain placed extraperitoneally through the fascial layers is especially important to provide an escape route for urinary leakage; remove it 2 or 3 days after you are sure the drainage has stopped.

Two types of drains are in current use: passive drains, such as the Penrose, and the more expensive, active-suction drains, such as the closed (Jackson-Pratt or Hemovac) or open (sump) drains. Passive drainage depends on intra-abdominal or wound pressure; active drainage, on suction. Passive drainage is adequate for most urologic wounds because it permits escape of air and any accumulated blood. If the urinary passages have been opened, it prevents formation of urinomas because urine as a dilute fluid will follow any route of escape through the body wall if such is provided. Stated another way, urine does not require suction for drainage. However, active, closed suction drainage is valuable in more superficial operations, such as inguinal node dissection and, with miniaturization, in certain cases of hypospadias, to obliterate the space beneath the skin flaps. It also may be useful after major pelvic operations to detect postoperative bleeding and reduce the incidence of lymphoceles. It is not effective for urine leaks, because the holes are easily plugged. If urinary leakage is a good possibility, two Penrose drains exiting through the wound, rather than through a stab wound, will ensure the best drainage.

Be careful to keep the end of the drain away from contact with the site of repair or from an anastomosis, but suture the Penrose drain to an adjacent structure so that it will not be displaced during closure. In all cases, but especially in children, suture the drain to the skin. Pierce it with a safety pin so that it cannot be lost, except in young children for whom

the safety pin itself could be a hazard. A drain causes less harm to the wound if brought out through a separate stab wound; however, if significant urinary leakage or gross contamination is anticipated, it is much more efficient to have it come through the wound itself. In children, stab wounds become unsightly with growth.

CATHETERS AND TUBES

Catheters are placed transurethrally before an operation to empty the bladder and get it out of the way, to fill the bladder preparatory to its incision, to instill antibacterial or antineoplastic agents, or to allow identification of the urethra and vesical neck. For these purposes, an 8- or 10-F catheter is usually satisfactory in children. One made of silicone is preferable, even if it is to remain only a few days. For a given external size, a balloon catheter has a smaller drainage channel than a straight tube or catheter. Intraoperatively, the catheter may be replaced with one of a smaller size, also made of silicone, so that it will be better tolerated by the urethral wall as it is left indwelling. If clots are anticipated, a larger catheter is necessary. In complicated cases, the catheter should be stitched to the glans and taped to the penis and abdomen or leg, because its inadvertent removal could be disastrous.

Waterproof tape applied over tincture of benzoin is required to hold catheters or tubing. Once applied, it must be checked regularly.

A good alternative to a balloon catheter for bladder operations, especially in children, is to place a suture in the end of a Robinson catheter with a curved Keith needle, then insert both ends of the suture in the eye of the needle and run them out through the bladder and body walls. Tie them together over a bolster. Remember at the end of the operation to connect the drainage tube to the catheter while the patient is still on the table to prevent contamination at the connector.

Suprapubic drainage has several advantages over the transurethral route. It allows cystography for a trial of voiding before removal. This type of drainage is preferred in a patient who is expected to have difficulty emptying the bladder postoperatively, as after sling procedures and bladder augmentation. It is less likely than a balloon catheter to fall out, because it is routinely stitched to the skin, and may be less likely to introduce infection than one through the urethra. The disadvantages are the need to create a wound in the bladder and body wall and the tendency to irritate the trigone if the tip is not held in the dome of the bladder.

STENTS

Stents are useful for several purposes: to relieve obstruction, to align the ureter and its connections, to facilitate closure of fistulas, and to provide a scaffold for repair. They may be placed retrogradely, antegradely by a percutaneous route, or intraoperatively on a temporary or permanent basis. However, they should not be used without a definite indication, and they do not obviate meticulous surgical technique.

Available stents range from straight silicone rubber tubing to double pigtail stents with fixed curves on either end that are self-retaining. Certain polymers are stiffer than silicone and so can be placed either retrogradely or antegradely. By preliminary insertion of guide wires, passage is facilitated. Drainage holes may be located at the proximal end or at both ends.

WOUND CLOSURE

Before closing the incision, search for bleeding, and at the same time, look for sponges. Irrigate the wound copiously with water to flush out free tissue and clots. Place drains so that they drain the space without making contact with the site of repair.

DRESSINGS

An occlusive dressing is less desirable than one porous enough to allow skin products and wound secretions to move away from the wound.

Apply tincture of benzoin to the skin before placing tape. Realize that in newborns the skin barrier is fragile and easily disrupted. Montgomery straps are useful if appreciable drainage is expected and abdominal pads are to be applied. Leave the dressing in place for at least 2 days. By that time, the incision will be sealed and no longer susceptible to contamination.

POSTOPERATIVE ANTIBACTERIAL PROPHYLAXIS

For the first 3 months of life, avoid trimethoprim/sulfamethoxazole. Use penicillin G, if it can be obtained, or amoxicillin. After 3 months, when the liver has matured, switch to trimethoprim/sulfamethoxazole.

Chapter 5

Postoperative Care and Pain Management

After the surgical procedure is complete, attention is focused on ensuring that the patient's cardiorespiratory status is stable and suitable to allow transport to the postanesthesia care unit (PACU). Overhead warming should be reintroduced if more than a few minutes are required to achieve extubation, to ensure cardiovascular stability, and to transfer the patient to the transport bed. For most pediatric urologic surgery, the anesthesiologist should have established an anesthetic plan that allows extubation of the trachea—or removal of the laryngeal mask airway (LMA)—before (or shortly after) transport to the PACU. That is, as the surgery is completed, the patient should be hemodynamically stable, sustaining spontaneous ventilation, and maintaining an adequate oxygen saturation. Allowing for any underlying medical dysfunction, the age of the patient, and residual effects of anesthetic agents, the level of consciousness of the patient should be consistent with maintaining an independent airway. Alternatively, transport and admission to a critical care unit (CCU) should have been discussed with both the attending surgeon and the appropriate critical care physician pre- or intraoperatively.

The patient's medical history, intraoperative course, intra-arterial/intravenous (IV) access, and requirements for postoperative monitoring should be communicated to the appropriate staff in the PACU/CCU to allow smooth transition of care. In most cases, supplemental oxygen and a system for delivery of positive pressure ventilation (e.g., Jackson Rees circuit) should be available for the transport. In most cases, oxygen saturation and cardiovascular monitoring are essential during a transport to a distant CCU but not required for transfer to a nearby PACU. A surgeon should remain in the operating room with the anesthesiologist and other operating room staff until outcome of emergence is clear. In many cases, a surgeon may be needed to transport the patient to the PACU or CCU (local policies prevail). Postoperative orders for the PACU/CCU should be immediately available to the staff of these units on admission. Oversight of cardiorespiratory status and treatment of pain in the PACU is usually the primary responsibility of the anesthesiologist, but close communication with the primary team and appropriate consultation with other caregivers are critical. Communicating with the family about the specific details of the operative procedure resides with the surgeon, but other specific aspects of care (e.g., ventilatory support, pain control) may be relegated to the anesthesiologist or others.

POSTOPERATIVE RESPIRATORY SUPPORT

The newborn and young infant present unique challenges for postoperative supportive care. In many cases, the underlying disorders that are associated with surgical intervention in the newborn (e.g., extrophy) require long, intra-abdominal procedures, including intraoperative neuromuscular blockade and at least moderate doses of narcotics intra- and/or postoperatively to adequately treat pain. The newborn's immature neurologic, respiratory, cardiac, renal, and hepatic systems predispose to apnea, airway obstruction, and prolonged effects from neuromuscular blockers, narcotics, and sedatives. Often, newborns and young infants are transported to a CCU postoperatively to provide 24 to 48 hours (or longer) mechanical ventilatory support. If the trachea of a newborn/young infant is extubated in the operating room, meticulous monitoring of cardiorespiratory function is essential, especially during the first 24 hours postoperatively. For example, cold temperature, hypoglycemia, hypocalcemia, hypoxia, hypercarbia, or a "normal" dose of narcotic (morphine, 0.05 to 0.1 mg/kg) may induce apnea or periodic breathing in this age group. Underlying acid-base/renal dysfunction may exacerbate the persistent effects of the operative intervention and general anesthesia. Thus, even if the newborn/young infant tolerates extubation of the trachea in the operating room, admission to a setting that ensures intense cardiorespiratory monitoring may be indicated (e.g., intensive care nursery, pediatric ICU, step-down or intermediate care unit).

Even after complex, invasive, lengthy surgery, older infants and children rarely require postoperative ventilatory support or admission to a CCU for cardiorespiratory monitoring without preexisting disorders or unexpected intra- or postoperative events. Supplemental oxygen and continuous oxygen saturation monitoring may be required for as long as 24 to 48 hours, but this is usually readily accomplished in a step-down unit or in a monitored setting on an inpatient ward. In some cases, requiring postoperative supplemental oxygen can be correlated with overhydration or transient renal insufficiency.

POSTOPERATIVE FLUIDS

After major intra-abdominal procedures, IV fluid delivery is calculated by monitoring of intake versus output, evaluating

24

cardiorespiratory function (blood pressure, heart rate, central venous pressure), and measuring electrolytes and blood gases serially, commonly for at least 24 to 48 hours (or longer). In addition to normal maintenance fluid (5% dextrose in 0.25% to 0.5% normal saline, 4 mL/kg/hour), third-space losses (or gastrointestinal drainage) are often replaced with lactated Ringer's solution or normal saline. In some cases, electrolyte output in urine or gastrointestinal drainage may be measured to more carefully guide fluid delivery. Hypotension and/or tachycardia must be evaluated and treated aggressively, and may require vigorous crystalloid, colloid, or vasopressor support. In such cases, the underlying etiology (beyond routine postoperative hypovolemia) must be considered and evaluated systematically (e.g., physical examination, laboratory studies, radiologic imaging).

Although evaluating fluid requirements may be intense in the immediate postoperative period, the staffing and monitoring in the PACU provides an ideal environment for this process. The subsequent 24 to 48 hours may be challenging for the surgical and ward teams, as serially modifying fluid and medications in response to physical examination, cardiorespiratory status, body weight, and laboratory results (e.g., electrolytes, blood urea nitrogen [BUN], creatinine) is critical.

If enteral feeds cannot be reintroduced within 24 to 48 hours, IV nutrition should be initiated within 2 to 3 days postoperatively, especially if a prolonged nothing-by-mouth (NPO) period is likely. Placing a central venous catheter during surgery should be discussed in the setting of major procedures, especially in newborns/young infants and in malnourished patients of any age.

Determining if a young infant requires transfusion of red blood cells and/or other blood products requires simultaneously interpreting the physical examination and laboratory values in the context of the patient's age, current

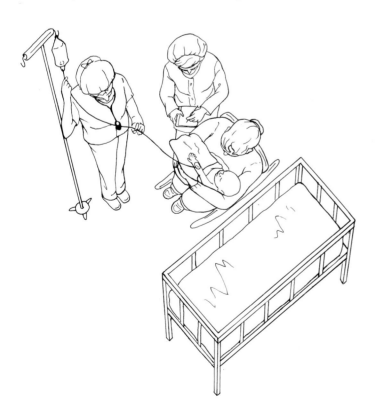

hemodynamic status, anticipated postoperative course, and underlying cardiorespiratory, metabolic, renal, and hepatic function. For example, a hemoglobin of 8 to 9 g/dL may be acceptable in a 6-month-old after a ureteral reimplantation who had a preoperative hemoglobin of 11 g/dL, who is hemodynamically stable in the PACU, and who has no medical problems and is developing and growing normally after a full-term delivery. A hemoglobin of 8 g/dL may prompt a red blood cell transfusion in a 6-month-old after the same surgical procedure if the patient was a 28-week-gestation premature who currently weighs 6 kg, is oxygen dependent secondary to chronic lung disease, and has mild congestive heart failure secondary to a ventricular septal defect.

POSTOPERATIVE ORDERS

Child and Mother in the Recovery Room

After most noninvasive urologic surgeries/procedures with unremarkable intraoperative courses, patients without underlying medical problems are discharged home directly from the PACU. The only postoperative orders are for routine cardiorespiratory monitoring and maintenance IV fluid. Heart and respiratory rates, and oxygen saturation, are measured continuously and blood pressure noted every 15 to 30 minutes for the first 1 to 2 hours after arrival in the recovery area or until the child is fully awake. Supplemental oxygen is weaned in response to the oxygen saturation. When the patient is awake and without nausea/vomiting, clear liquids are introduced. If the child is nauseated, pharmacologic treatment may be given, according to local protocols (e.g., dolasetron mesylate [Anzemet]). In some cases, urine output may be a critical factor to determine discharge home. In other cases, pain control may be the critical factor.

After more invasive procedures, especially in the presence of coexisting medical problems, the PACU serves three functions: monitoring for immediate complications (e.g., bleeding, bowel perforation), monitoring during cardiorespiratory recovery from general anesthesia, and aggressively treating pain in a monitored setting. In such cases, postoperative orders should include the routine monitoring of heart and respiratory rates, blood pressure, and oxygen saturation. However, IV fluids must include maintenance as well as replacement of ongoing losses. Types of fluids must be defined in terms of the intraoperative course, immediate postoperative status (e.g., blood pressure, heart rate, urine output), and certain specific goals (e.g., maintaining a certain urine output, treating hematuria). The results of postoperative laboratory studies often prompt a change in fluid therapy. Orders related to stents, drainage devices, and other uncommon devices should be documented in writing but also discussed in detail with the staff. Supplemental oxygen may be weaned but often is continued after transfer from the PACU.

The anesthesiologist usually manages postoperative treatment of pain in the PACU. IV agents are titrated in small but frequent doses while monitoring cardiorespiratory status and while delivering supplemental oxygen. After discharge from the PACU, the primary surgical team is usually responsible for orders to treat pain and should be based on the patient's requirements in the PACU and chronically, as well as on underlying medical status (e.g., respiratory, renal, and hepatic function). Orders related to infusion of specific agents in epidural catheters are often under the direction of an inpatient pain service (process varies among medical centers).

POSTOPERATIVE INFECTIONS

Fevers during the first or second postoperative day are often attributed to atelectasis and other nonspecific respiratory dysfunction. However, careful physical examination of the patient is essential to ensure that other etiologies are absent (e.g., infected IV sites, intra-abdominal process). After 48 to 72 hours, infections of the urinary tract, surgical wounds, and intra-abdominal sites must be evaluated more intensely. At this later stage, in addition to the history and physical examination, laboratory and imaging studies may play a vital role in assessment of postoperative fever. Pharmacologic treatment may be initiated before results of cultures are available, depending on the patient's current status, the history of the recent course, and the site of the infection (e.g., wound versus urinary tract). Therapy is based on local prevalence of microbial agents and their response profiles, and then adjusted when/if a definitive infectious agent is identified.

Infection in the newborn may be difficult to evaluate. Fever may be absent or minor and physical findings may be nonspecific (tachycardia, tachypnea, irritability, apnea). Often, evaluating a newborn with a low-grade fever or non-specific symptoms may include cultures of blood, urine, and cerebrospinal fluid (CSF) followed by prompt treatment with antibiotics. Initial therapy varies among medical centers, depending on various local profiles of specific infectious agents.

TREATMENT OF PAIN

Regional anesthesia plays a central role in treating pain associated with urologic procedures, primarily because of the site of surgery and the ease of performing the block. These techniques often supplement general anesthesia, but at times are employed as the only anesthetic. The advantages are obvious: minimal side effects, profound pain relief, decreased requirements for narcotics, clear mental status, decreased bladder spasm, early ambulation, excellent patient and parent satisfaction.

The pain associated with the common urologic procedures (circumcision, hypospadias repair, herniorrhophy, orchiopexy, hydrocelectomy) is particularly amenable to a caudal block (see Chapter 6). In most cases, the anesthesiologist induces general anesthesia with an inhaled or, less commonly, an IV agent, an IV catheter is placed, an LMA (or endotracheal tube) is inserted, and then the caudal performed. In general, 0.125% to 0.25% bupivacaine (0.75 to 1 mL/kg) is inserted into the caudal space. The 0.125% solution is reserved for older children (who are walking) to minimize motor blockade. Various needles, catheters,

and positioning techniques have been recommended. This block has an excellent safety profile in experienced hands. Uncommonly, an inadvertent subarachnoid injection may lead to apnea, but hemodynamic effects are uncommon. The sensory blockade (i.e., pain relief) commonly persists from 2 to 6 hours and may last as long as 12 hours. Of significance, with this early profound pain relief, patients often require only acetaminophen to alleviate pain. However, in other cases, IV or oral narcotics are required after the block has receded. After a procedure longer than 4 hours, the caudal block can be repeated either with the same or a lower dose.

Alternatively, an ilioinguinal/iliohypogastric block (0.25% to 0.5% bupivacaine, up to 2 mg/kg) is also effective to prevent/treat pain associated with an inguinal incision (see Chapter 6). A penile block is effective during and after a circumcision or other penile surgery (see Chapter 6). Local infiltration of the wound should be considered if a block has not been conducted or seems ineffective.

In the setting of major intra-abdominal surgery, epidural catheters are frequently placed (usually in children older than 1 year) both to provide intraoperative anesthesia and postoperative analgesia. Similar to the caudal block, epidural anesthesia is conducted during general anesthesia and serves as a supplement to general anesthesia. This technique is particularly useful during urologic procedures, as the urinary retention as a side effect is irrelevant because bladder catheters are invariably in place after surgery. A variety of agents are effective; bupivacaine or rupivacaine plus fentanyl are most commonly infused during and after surgery. The local anesthetic may be eliminated in the postoperative period, depending on the preferences of the pain service. This technique requires precise protocols and continuous availability of appropriate expertise if employed outside the operating room and PACU.

If a regional technique is not performed or is inadequate, rectal acetaminophen (30 mg/kg), IV ketorolac (Toradol), IV nonsteroidal agents, and narcotics (IV, oral, intramuscular) commonly combine to provide postoperative pain relief both in the PACU and while hospitalized. Patient-controlled analgesia (PCA) should be integrated into the care of older children, coordinated in many cases by a pain service but, in some cases, by the primary surgical team. Transition to oral agents provides analgesia for patients without IV access both as inpatients and after discharge (see previous sections).

POSTOPERATIVE PROGRAM

Especially in the case of extensive, complicated procedures, a postoperative checklist/protocol introduces a system to facilitate postoperative care. For example, some centers may follow the practice of obtaining an abdominal X-ray to evaluate for retained needles, instruments, and sponges. Obtaining specific laboratory profiles or imaging studies may be integrated into routine postoperative care after certain surgical procedures (Table 5-1).

The attending surgeon should dictate the operative report to ensure specific vital or unusual aspects of the procedure for the medical record. In particular, each surgeon may have preferences for certain details that are critical

CHECKLIST FOR POSTOPERATIVE ORDERS

T A B L E   5 - 1

Vital signs every 15 min until awake in the postanesthesia recovery unit; then every 4 hr for 8–12 hr postoperatively

Mobilize, ambulate

Monitor intake and output

Incorporate experts for treatment of pain, as needed

Deliver antibiotics according to local protocols

Monitor nutrition

Review laboratory values/studies to define daily monitoring needs

Respiratory care: suctioning, supplemental oxygen, monitoring

Care of catheters and drains

Monitor intravenous access sites

Order special monitoring (wound, circulation, neurologic)

Request notification for hypotension, oliguria, etc.

for future surgery or in interpreting follow-up evaluations. Of note, the attending surgeon should educate residents and fellows about the style and content of such reports. In some cases, a senior trainee may conduct this vital responsibility but the attending surgeon must meticulously review and concur with the report.

As with any surgical intervention, clearly communicating with family seems to foster recovery and postoperative care. Parents/caregivers should be integrated into postoperative care as soon as possible, often starting in the PACU. If the family seems to encounter problems in understanding information about the surgery or postoperative care, a single source of information should be established, most commonly the attending surgeon.

Designing detailed protocols and education for the nursing staff elevates the postoperative care to a smooth, interactive system that involves the family and patient, nurses, and physicians. Such protocols should include approaches to various routes of urinary drainage, whether from the urethra or from a transcutaneous tube; labels and diagrams are critical in complicated cases. These protocols should also include an approach to securing the catheters, requirements for volume of output, and methods for troubleshooting if drainage decreases/stops. Anticipatory guidance about pain, feeling of bladder fullness/urgency, and level of activity are essential. A protocol for evaluating urinary stream, urine output, and care of tubes and surgical sites after catheters and dressings are removed should be discussed in detail before discharge home.

MANAGEMENT OF COMPLICATIONS

Many postoperative complications associated with each surgical procedure can be anticipated and, in some cases, predicted based on the intraoperative course. Analyzing the common complications pre- and intraoperatively may contribute to decreasing their incidence. Complications should be discussed with the family early in the course, especially if the family has not been informed about the incidence of a particular complication as part of the consent process.

In this atlas, key postoperative problems are described after each surgical protocol. Bleeding, ischemia, and infection should be identified readily if protocols for meticulous postoperative monitoring are followed.

Chapter 6

Perioperative Techniques

Surgeons performing urologic operations on children not only need the skills and techniques common to all urologists, such as the approximation of tissues and the anastomosis of bowel, they need skill in handling fragile tissue in small subjects. They also must perform procedures not strictly in the field of urology: they may be required to repair a laceration of the spleen or a vessel, or to create a colostomy for fecal diversion. Although a pediatric surgeon, if available, can help, the urologist operating on children should have an adequate repertoire of suitable procedures in general pediatric surgery and have the ability to apply them without outside help.

VASCULAR ACCESS

Percutaneous Cannulation

The use of plastic cannulas with an inner metal needle stilet facilitate placement in the antecubital vein of the forearm in children and the dorsal surface of the hand in infants. First, place the arm on a padded board held with roller gauze to hyperextend it, and tape the board to the mattress. Apply a Penrose drain tourniquet. Wipe the site and the surgeon's palpating finger with antiseptic solution, then dry the area. Use an 18- to 22-gauge needle to make an initial puncture a centimeter distal to the vein, and then insert the cannula very slowly with the bevel down, at the same time palpating it and the vein with a finger of the other hand. Slowly advance it toward the vein while aspirating with the syringe. When blood appears in the chamber, aspirate a small amount into the syringe, then reinject it to dilate the vein ahead of the

needle, while advancing the cannula. Withdraw the stilet and advance the cannula until the hub meets the skin. If blood does not flow, slowly withdraw the cannula until flow starts, then rotate and advance it. Fix the cannula permanently with waterproof tape applied over tincture of benzoin, and fasten the arm firmly to the arm board so that flexion is not possible. In neonates, the cannula may be placed in a dorsal vein of the hand by grasping the fist to stretch the vein.

Central Venous Catheterization, Internal Jugular Cut-Down Technique

With the development of percutaneous techniques for venous catheterization, an open procedure rarely is used. Standard of care is placement of catheters percutaneously via the subclavian or jugular route.

Placement of a central venous catheter is also possible either by cutting down on the basilic vein in the antecubital fossa or by use of the standard procedure, which is by way of the jugular vein in the neck, particularly the deep jugular vein.

SUTURE TECHNIQUES

The objectives of suturing are to approximate the tissues with the least impairment of their blood supply. Use the technique most suitable for the tissue, with sutures of the smallest size and of the fewest types. Tie the suture while holding it near its free end, so that it may be used twice, saving both suture material and time.

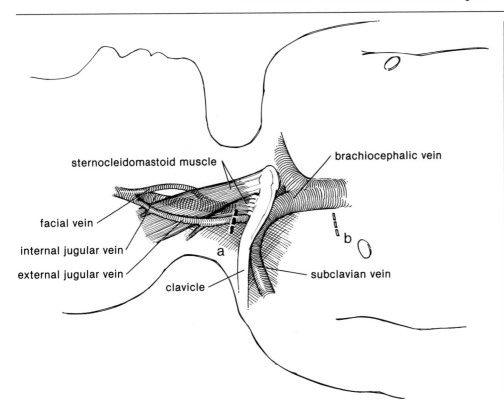

FIGURE 6-1. With the child under general anesthesia in a 20-degree Trendelenburg position to eliminate the possibility of introducing air, elevate the infant's shoulders, and extend the neck to the left. Prep the neck, chest, and upper arm. Make a 1.5-cm transverse incision above the clavicle over the right external jugular vein (a). If this incision is not adequate, usually because of previous utilization, extend the skin incision medially to expose the internal jugular vein between the heads of the sternocleidomastoid muscle. (The anterior facial vein, an excellent alternative, is reached through an incision 1.5 cm below the angle of the jaw over the medial border of the sternocleidomastoid muscle.) Make a second transverse incision on the chest below (b).

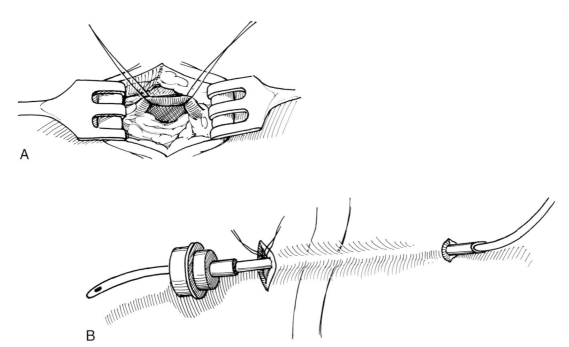

FIGURE 6-2. A, Free the vein, and loop it with fine sutures. If the internal jugular vein is used, it is advisable to put a purse-string 5-0 or 6-0 polydioxanone suture at the proposed venotomy site. Alternatively, use the anterior facial vein by making an incision 1.5 cm below the angle of the jaw over the medial border of the sternocleidomastoid muscle. **B,** Select a catheter suitable for the age and weight of the child. The smaller Broviac catheters (beginning at 2.7 F) can be used in newborns and infants; the larger Hickman catheters (up to 9.6 F) can be used in older children. Insert a large hollow (ventricular) needle with a bore equal to the diameter of the venous catheter to extend from the upper to the lower incision, and draw the tip of the catheter up through the tunnel. Position the monofilament knitted polypropylene cuff from 2 to 5 cm deep to the site of entry. Trim the catheter to the appropriate length to lie at the junction of the superior vena cava and right atrium. Estimate the length by following the external landmarks.

   Elevate the vein, and cut it on a tangent with fine scissors. Flush the catheter with heparinized saline (1 unit/mL), and insert its tip into the vein (a small vein introducer may facilitate this maneuver).

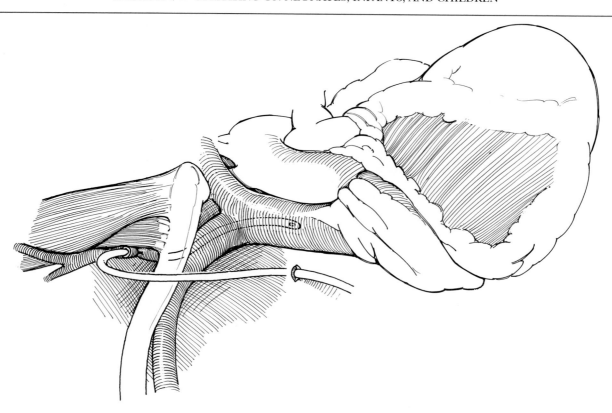

FIGURE 6-3. Advance the catheter into the superior vena cava toward the right atrium. The position of the catheter can be checked fluoroscopically. Be sure the catheter irrigates freely and that blood can be readily withdrawn. Ligate the vein above with the upper suture and tie the catheter in place with the lower one. Infuse the catheter with heparinized saline solution (100 units/mL), and cover the end with the Luer Lock cap.

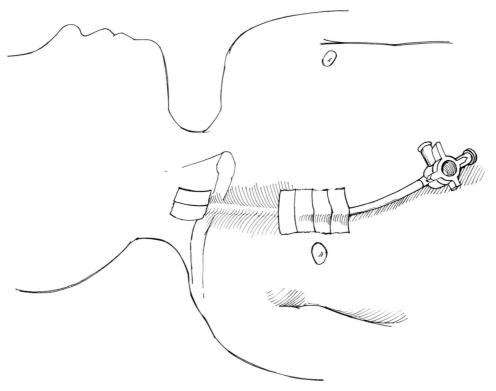

FIGURE 6-4. Suture the catheter to the skin and cover it with sterile strips.

Skin

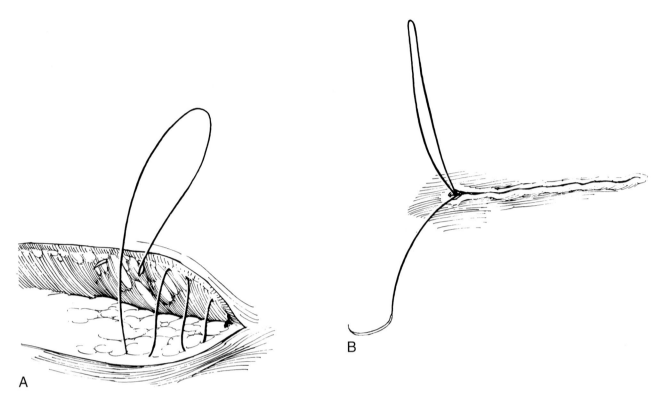

A

B

FIGURE 6-5. Subcuticular closure: Use a 5-0 synthetic absorbable suture or a pullout suture of monofilament nonabsorbable suture material. **A,** Start the stitch with a buried knot at one end. Pull the subcutaneous tissue forward with a fine skin hook, and drive the needle point well into the dermis in a plane parallel to the surface, entering exactly opposite the exit site of the last bite. **B,** Bury the last knot with a deep stitch. Alternatively, use absorbable interrupted sutures placed subcuticularly, inverted to bury each knot.

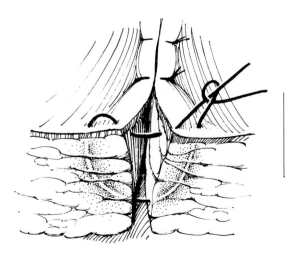

FIGURE 6-6. Vertical mattress suture: A double stitch that forms a loop about the tissue on both sides produces eversion of the skin. Use monofilament nonabsorbable sutures and catch only the very edge of the skin in the second bite. Alternatively, use a subcuticular closure, skin staples in older children, or tapes.

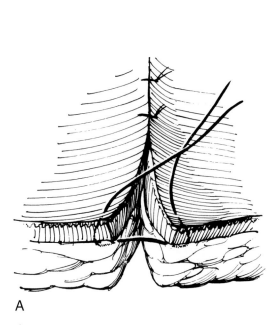

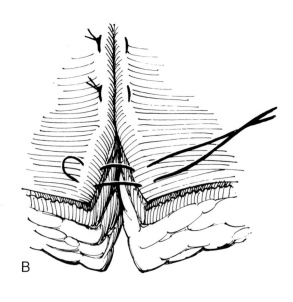

FIGURE 6-7. **A,** Everting interrupted suture: For plastic procedures, penetrate the skin close to the edge of the incision, then encircle a larger amount of tissue beneath. **B,** Halsted mattress suture. Invert the edges.

Fascia

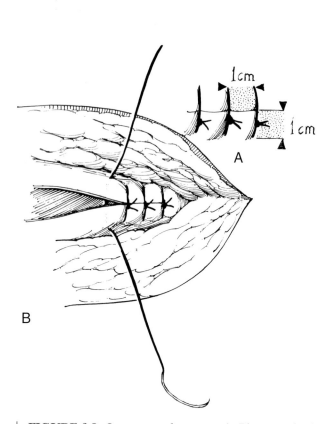

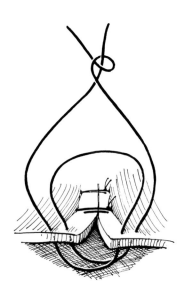

FIGURE 6-9. Far-and-near sutures: Use synthetic absorbable sutures at 1-cm intervals.

FIGURE 6-8. Interrupted sutures: **A,** Place synthetic absorbable sutures 1 cm deep and 1 cm apart. **B,** Tie them only tight enough to bring the fascial edges in contact. Throw at least four square knots. An alternative to absorbable sutures is nonabsorbable monofilament sutures made from polypropylene. In thin adolescents and in children, be sure that the knot is well buried to avoid wound discomfort.

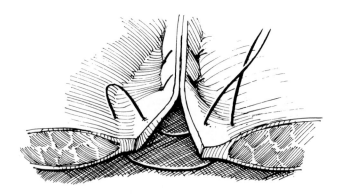

FIGURE 6-10. Near-and-far sutures: For mass closure of the abdomen, use nonabsorbable sutures.

Bowel

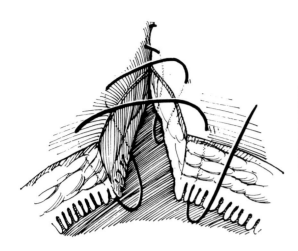

FIGURE 6-11. Connell suture: A continuous suture that inverts the inner wall of the intestine. The stitch enters and exits the bowel on each side successively. It may include only the mucosa and submucosa. Use 3-0 synthetic absorbable sutures. This stitch is an especially useful technique for closing the angles of a bowel anastomosis.

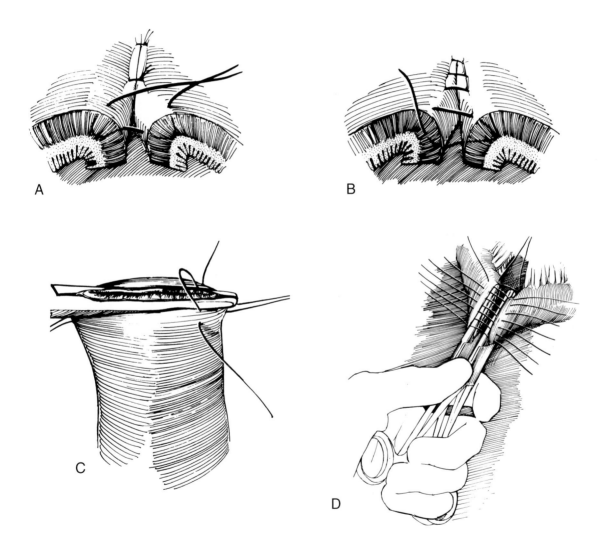

FIGURE 6-12. Lembert suture: An inverting suture that produces serosal apposition by including most of the muscular layer. It may be interrupted (**A**) or placed continuously (**B**). It is useful for closing the end of the bowel or to anastomose two ends. Use 4-0 braided nonabsorbable sutures. Each bite should reach into but not through the tough submucosal layer.

To close the end of the bowel, use interrupted Lembert sutures over a clamp. First, place a traction suture at each end and lay all the sutures. Remove the clamp carefully and tie each suture successively as your assistant inverts the mucosa (**C**). For a one-layer bowel anastomosis, place interrupted Lembert sutures; then have your assistant gently withdraw the clamps as you successively tie each suture. Your assistant should insert the tip of a clamp under the loop to invert the edges as you tie each suture (**D**).

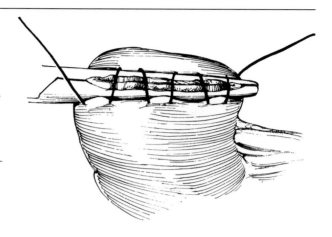

FIGURE 6-13. Parker-Kerr suture: An inverting suture that is used to close the end of the intestine. It may be laid continuously or may be interrupted. Use a 4-0 nonabsorbable suture, with bites taken parallel to the edge, rather than across it as is done in the Lembert stitch.

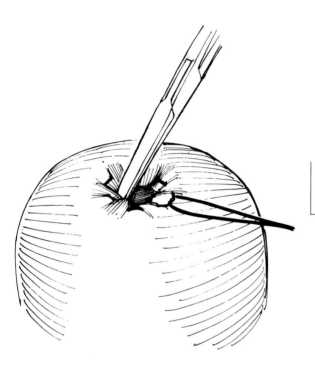

FIGURE 6-14. Purse-string suture: A continuous suture that is placed around a defect for inversion (appendix) or closure (hernia sac).

FIGURE 6-15. Lock-stitch suture: A continuous suture used for closure of mucosal edges in which every third or fourth stitch is passed under the previous one. Select it when puckering must be avoided.

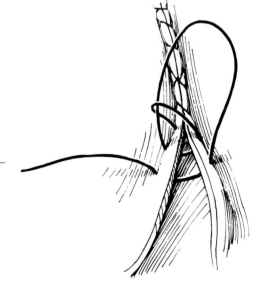

BOWEL STAPLING TECHNIQUES

See Section 6 for application of these techniques to noncontinent and continent diversion.

Stapled anastomoses are less likely to leak than sutured ones, but they are more likely to bleed because they do not devascularize the margins as thoroughly. It is important to check the staple line for bleeding from both the mucosal and the serosal sides, although it is not always possible to check the mucosal surface. Placement of a figure-eight stitch of 4-0 synthetic absorbable suture will usually control the bleeding.

Several automatic staplers should be available: models TA 55, TA 30, EEA, and GIA.

End-to-End Anastomosis

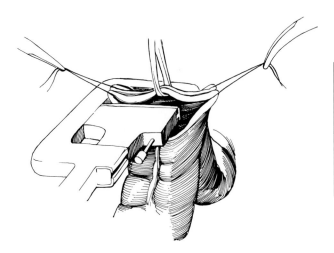

FIGURE 6-16. Clear the mesentery from the ends of the bowel for a distance of 1 cm. Place a stay suture through the full thickness at the mesenteric and antimesenteric edges. Grasp and elevate both median walls with an Allis clamp. Place the jaws of the TA 55 stapler to include the bowel beneath the Allis clamp and the stay sutures. Approximate the blades by turning the thumbscrew until the black lines on them are aligned. Push the pin firmly in place. Release the safety catch and fire the staples.

FIGURE 6-17. Shave off the excess bowel wall with a knife. Cut as close as possible to the anvil and cartridge to prevent retention of necrotic tissue.

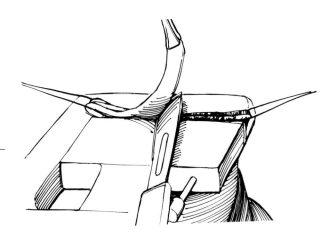

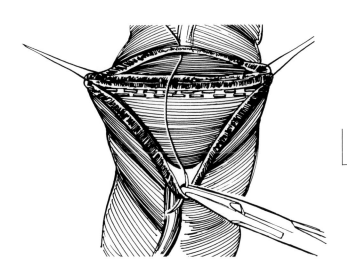

FIGURE 6-18. Insert an everting stay suture through the midpoint of both free edges to triangulate the defects.

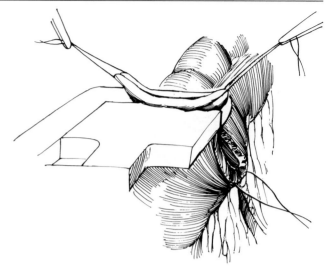

FIGURE 6-19. Place half of the remaining edge into the TA 30 stapler. Be certain to overlap the original row of staples at the angle. Push the pin in place and fire the staples. Trim the excess bowel wall, but preserve the central suture. Reinforce the mucosal edges with figure-eight sutures at any bleeding sites.

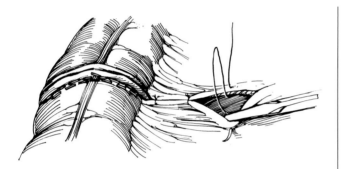

FIGURE 6-20. Staple the remaining half similarly, being sure that the rows overlap both in the center and at the angle. Shave the excess bowel. Check the anastomosis visually to be certain no gaps remain. Cut the stay sutures and close the mesenteric defect. Alternatively, triangulate the bowel with three everting stay sutures, staple the mesenteric border first, and then close the other two sides of the triangle. Take care not to catch the back wall, and be sure to incorporate the end of the previous line of staples. Check the staple line for bleeding, placing a figure-eight stitch, if necessary.

End-to-Side Anastomosis of Ileum to Ascending Colon

FIGURE 6-21. Make a window in the antimesenteric border of the ascending colon 3 cm from the open end. Through it, insert the EEA stapler into the ileum and clamp the stapler. After firing and removing the stapler, check the anvil to be sure the tissue button is complete. Achieve hemostasis and close leaks in the suture line with horizontal, inverting mattress sutures of 4-0 silk from the serosal side.

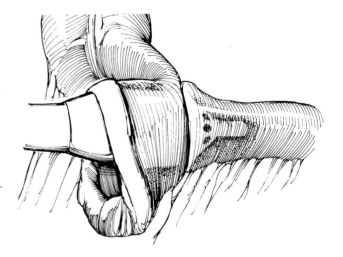

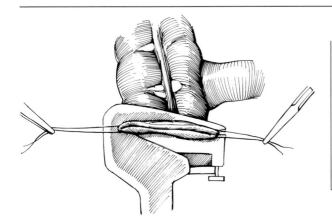

FIGURE 6-22. To close the end of the colon, place two stay sutures in the mesenteric and antimesenteric borders. Apply the TA 55 stapler proximal to them. Turn the thumbscrew clockwise to approximate the blades so that the black lines are aligned. Release the safety catch and clamp the handles. Trim the excess and close the mesentery. Reinforce the mucosal edges with figure-eight sutures at any bleeding sites. Check for viability because the blood supply may be attenuated here. The same closure technique can be used for the ileum.

Side-to-Side Anastomosis of Ileum

FIGURE 6-23. A, Clear the mesentery from the distal ends of the bowel for a distance equal to the length of the limbs of the GIA stapler. Place stay sutures in the mesenteric and antimesenteric edges of both bowel ends to maintain alignment. Insert the limbs of the GIA stapler so that they lie in line with the mesentery. Lock the stapler together, and push the driver that inserts the staples and activates the knife. **B,** Remove the driver, unlock the limbs, and remove the stapler. Check for viability of the distal mucosa and for hemostasis. Reinforce the serosal edges with horizontal, inverting mattress sutures of 4-0 silk as required.

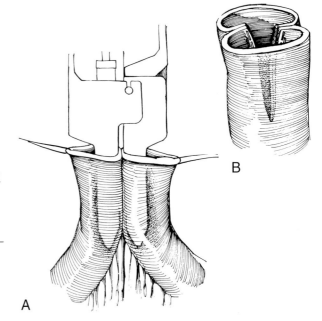

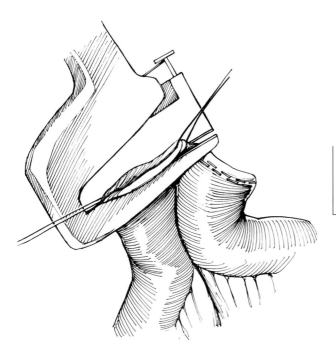

FIGURE 6-24. Apply the TA 55 stapler to each side of the common opening, as described previously in the section "End-to-End Anastomosis." Check for viability because the blood supply may be attenuated here. Close the mesentery.

Formation of an Ileal Conduit (see Chapter 89)

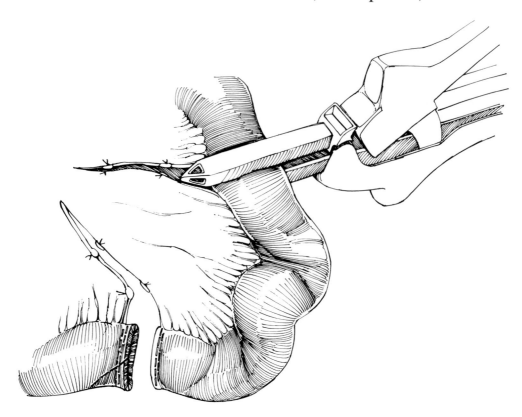

FIGURE 6-25. Select a segment of ileum and divide the mesentery. Place the GIA stapler at the appropriate site and push the lever home, placing two rows of staples and dividing the bowel between. Repeat the procedure at the other end.

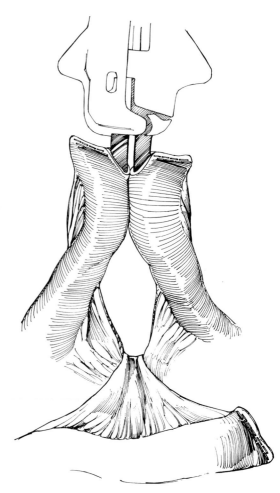

FIGURE 6-26. For ileal reanastomosis, trim the antimesenteric corner from both staple lines. Rotate the bowel 180 degrees, and insert a blade of the GIA stapler all the way into each lumen. Connect the handles of the blades together and push the lever to make two rows of sutures with an opening between. Check the serosal side of the staple lines for hemostasis, and reinforce it with horizontal, inverting mattress sutures of 4-0 silk as needed.

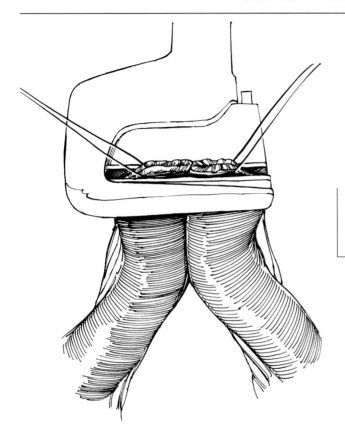

FIGURE 6-27. Place a stay suture at the end of each row of staples. Then apply the TA 30 stapler over the remaining opening to overlap the original rows of staples; drive in the staples. Close the mesentery.

FIGURE 6-28. Complete the procedure by anastomosing the ureters to the loop, drawing the distal end of the bowel through the abdominal wall, trimming the end proximal to the staples, and suturing the edge to the skin.

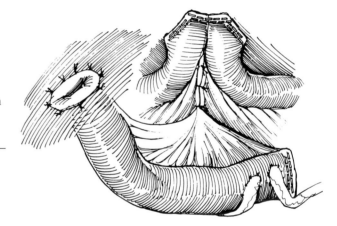

MICROVASCULAR SURGICAL TECHNIQUES

Instruments

Wear a 2.5× surgical loupe equipped with a headlight to expose and trim the vessels, and then use the operating microscope for the delicate anastomosis. Provide a non-locking spring-handle needle holder with a curved tip long enough to fit in the hand like a pen, a #5 jeweler's forceps for vascular work (be sure the tips are aligned), both sharp-tipped and blunt-tipped slightly curved scissors, nontraumatic vascular clamps (both straight and curved, which may be mounted on a bar), a bipolar coagulator set at low power, microsurgical sponges, a suction tip (3 F), a 30-gauge blunt-angled needle for delivery of heparin-saline irrigating solution, and plastic background material. Select a 10-0 monofilament nylon suture on a triangular cutting needle.

Arterial Anastomosis

For arteries with diameters less than 2 mm, use the operating microscope. For larger vessels, a 3.5-power loupe is adequate. Have your assistant sitting opposite.

Dissect the severed ends of the artery adequately in both directions. Coagulate any fine branches with the bipolar current, and divide them 1 mm away from the vessel. Place a piece of blue background material behind the vessel. Looking through the microscope or loupe, carefully trim the perivascular connective tissue. Reverse vasospasm with a few drops of 1% lidocaine solution, and then keep the vessel moist with drips of warm saline solution. Apply the fixed arm of the vascular clamp to the less mobile end of the vessel; then move the second arm to grasp the more mobile end, leaving the arms of the clamp approximately 1 cm apart.

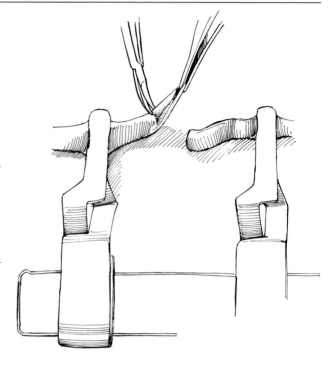

FIGURE 6-29. Cut the end of the vessel cleanly across with scissors. Pick up the adventitia at the cut and tease it out over the end in several places to form a stocking. Trim this tissue flush with the end of the vessel (circumcision technique). It will withdraw; even a small tag projecting into the lumen can initiate a thrombus. Alternatively, carefully lift the adventitia from the vessel wall, and trim it circumferentially with the microscissors. Be careful when cleaning the adventitia of small delicate vessels not to be too thorough and injure the vessel itself. Irrigate the lumen with heparinized saline to clear it of blood.

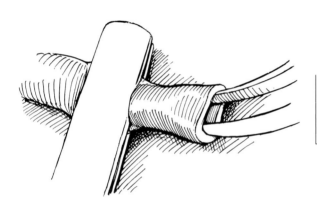

FIGURE 6-30. Dilate the lumen with #5 jeweler's forceps. Repeat these steps on the opposite stump, and bring the two ends together to lie approximately one vessel diameter apart by adjusting the movable arm.

FIGURE 6-31. Place the first guide suture (G1) of monofilament nylon through the vessel edge on the right at 10 o'clock. Grasp the needle again, pass it through the vessel to the left, and pull it until only 3 or 4 mm remain free. Tie it with a double-throw (surgeon's) knot and then with two square single-throw knots. Cut the short end near the knot, and then cut the long end to a length of 1.5 cm to use for traction. For small vessels, use 25× magnification for placing the sutures and 16× for tying them.

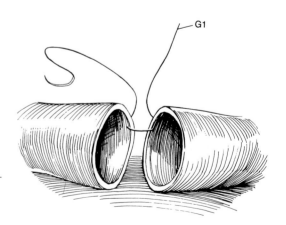

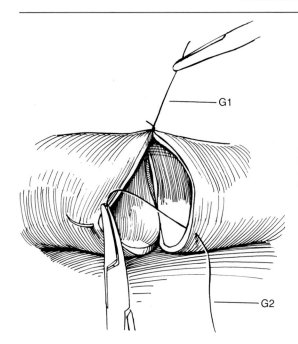

FIGURE 6-32. Have your assistant put slight traction on the first suture, G1. Place the second guide suture (G2) at a point one third of the way around; tie and cut it in the same way as described in Figure 6-31.

FIGURE 6-33. Place one or two approximating sutures (A1) between the guide sutures (G1, G2). Use a single-throw technique, and then cut both ends of the suture.

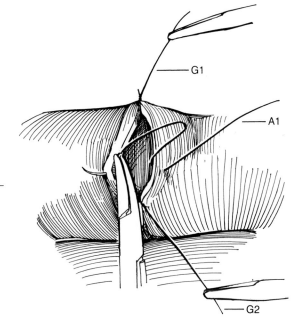

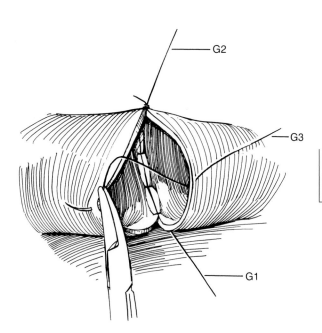

FIGURE 6-34. Invert the vessel and its holder, and inspect the interior for defects in the anterior suture line. Place the third guide suture (G3) equidistant from the other two (G1, G2).

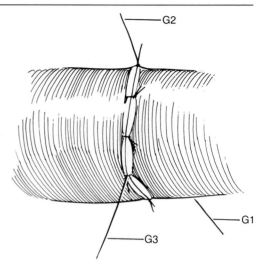

FIGURE 6-35. Insert one or two approximating sutures between G1 and G2 and between G2 and G3, while your assistant manipulates the guide sutures appropriately.

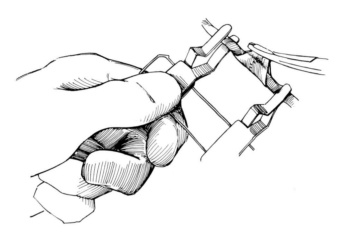

FIGURE 6-36. Remove the distal clamp first, and make sure that reverse blood flow immediately fills the entire segment. If it fails to fill, the anastomosis must be revised. If it fills slowly, apply papaverine solution to remove any factor of spasm. Release the proximal clamp and observe for pulsation beyond the repair. In case of doubt, Doppler ultrasound may be helpful in assessing flow. Irrigate away any blood that leaks out which might initiate formation of a thrombus or cause spasm. If there is a leak, it is wise to replace the clamps and place a suture at that site to get a tight seal.

Patency test: Pulsation alone does not mean that the anastomosis is open. In very small vessels in which the flow cannot be visualized, test for patency 20 minutes after completing the anastomosis by gently pressing the blood from a segment of vessel just below the anastomosis and seeing that it refills rapidly when the more proximal clamp is released. Be careful not to injure the intima by too much force. Do not hesitate to do the anastomosis over again if you are at all concerned about a technical detail, because even a small error can result in failure.

Venous Anastomosis

Use maximum illumination. Dissect a small vein using round-tipped microscissors to avoid damage to the media or inadvertent puncture. Avoid grasping the edge of the vein with forceps. Place the vessel clamp arm on the body side first to avoid overstretching the vein. Clear the periadventitial tissue carefully using two pairs of #5 jeweler's forceps simultaneously and working longitudinally. To see the lumen, float the walls open with saline irrigation. This must be done with each stitch to avoid catching the opposite wall. The technique of suturing small veins is the same as that for small arteries, but requires constant visualization of the thin vessel wall and the tip of the needle to avoid incorporation of the opposite wall. Wrapping the anastomosis as shown may be done but is probably not necessary. Release the proximal clamp and then the distal clamp, and perform a patency test.

URETERAL STENTS

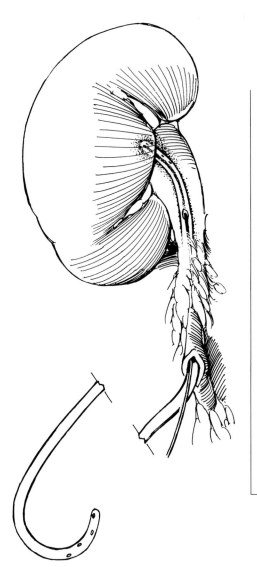

FIGURE 6-37. Double pigtail stent: Select a stent of the proper length and with the largest caliber that will fit easily inside the ureter without stretching it. Provide for low-dose antibiotic coverage. For intraoperative insertion, the required length can be determined by passing a calibrated ureteral catheter to the renal pelvis and then into the bladder and adding the measured lengths together. Aspiration and irrigation may be used to prove that the tips of the catheter are in the renal pelvis and in the vesical lumen.

To place the stent, cut an extra hole in its midportion or gently enlarge an existing drainage hole with a mosquito clamp. Insert a guidewire or stilet to straighten the curve. Feed the stent into the renal pelvis and remove the wire. Repeat the process for passage to the bladder.

Alternatively, place the stent on two guidewires. Pass one wire into the bladder, and feed the stent over it; do the same for the renal end. For easy, early removal in boys, make a small opening in the dome of the bladder, grasp the tip of the balloon catheter that had been inserted previously transurethrally, and tie the stent to it so that the stent will come out the urethra with the urethral catheter. Close this cystotomy in two layers. In girls, tie a long suture to the catheter end in the bladder, draw it out of the meatus with a clamp, and fasten it to the labia. Close the ureterotomy and drain the area, or proceed with ureteral anastomosis if the ureter has been divided.

If the stent is to remain long term, check its position occasionally by roentgenography, and follow with regular urine cultures and with serum creatinine determinations to detect obstruction. In a child at risk for stone formation, change the stent at least every 6 weeks. When removing a stent, do not try to pull it out with a sharp clamp; this might shear off the end.

FIGURE 6-38. Stents for ureteroureterostomy (see Chapter 50). In performing the anastomosis, place a stent unless you are sure that the ureters are of good caliber and vascularity, with no suspicion of constriction or tension at the anastomosis. Before completing the anastomosis, select the largest-caliber silicone-rubber tubing, infant feeding tube, or pigtail catheter that will fit loosely in the normal ureter. Measure the distance to the donor pelvis and to the bladder with a 5 F ureteral catheter. If you use a feeding or silicone rubber tube, cut holes in it at 1-cm intervals and mark it with a removable suture at the length required to reach the renal pelvis. Cut the other end at the length needed to reach the bladder, but add 3 cm so that it will lie well within the bladder to allow transvesical retrieval. First pass it up the donor ureter to the pelvis, then down into the bladder. Fix it in place with a 5-0 chromic catgut suture through the edge of the ureteral wall and the tubing, tied loosely. Complete the anastomosis. If the recipient ureter is large, pass a second stent up and down it, as described previously for the pigtail and straight catheters.

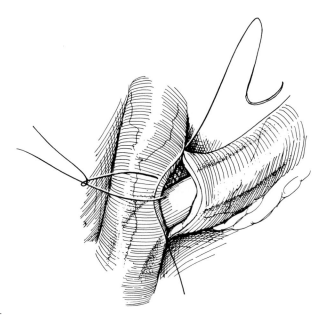

Problems Associated with Stents

Dysuria, urinary frequency, and nocturia are common, especially early after placement of stents. Give antispasmodic drugs and wait for subsidence of the symptoms. Flank pain or pain in the lower abdomen is a frequent complaint. Reflux sometimes results in flank pain during micturition but is buffered by leakage of urine through the side holes. Urinary tract infections will intervene less frequently if prophylactic antibiotics are given, especially in girls, but at the risk of selecting for resistant organisms. Culture the urine at semimonthly intervals. If results are positive and antibacterial therapy does not eradicate the infection, change the stent, culture the urine, and provide appropriate antibiotics.

Severe complications may evolve silently. Calculous obstruction is a common and serious sequela, usually occurring some 2 months after insertion. In a child known to form stones, good practice is to schedule regular stent replacement. For others, checking every month by roentgenography and serum creatinine level determinations may be adequate. However, a program of regular replacement every 6 to 8 weeks may be safest, but the interval must be adjusted to the conditions of the individual child, who in turn (with the parents) must be kept informed of the need for follow-up. Stent migration toward the bladder occurs if the initial placement was faulty. Migration into an upper calyx is due to too short a stent, or if the curvature on the proximal end of a J stent is less than 180 degrees. Proximal migration is relatively rare but is difficult to correct, requiring procedures under anesthesia. Removal may be done using a ureteroscope, a stone basket, a Fogarty catheter, a ureteral dilating balloon, or flexible forceps. A short retrieval suture inserted at the distal end is useful, and more frequent stent changes help. Breakage of a stent occurs because it had been acutely angulated during traction or was damaged by grasping (biopsy) forceps. If a stent is not easily withdrawn, do not pull on it but try again in 24 hours. Sometimes weak rubber band traction will gradually withdraw a recalcitrant stent. Fragmentation of the stent can occur if left in place over several months. These types of accidents require cystoscopic, ureteroscopic, or even percutaneous retrieval.

A blocked balloon in a catheter may be deflated by injecting mineral oil, by running a wire into the inflation port, by hyperinflation, or by percutaneous puncture. Retrieve the fragments.

Intraoperative Injury to the Ureter

Ureteral injury during a difficult abdominal operation may be less likely to occur if the ureters are stented for identification. A plugged balloon catheter in the bladder during the procedure will allow detection of hematuria secondary to injury if ureteral catheters are not in place. Cross-clamping the ureter in situ for an appreciable length of time results in ischemia, warranting insertion of a double-J stent for at least 10 days. If the ureter had already been isolated, resection of the ischemia segment with reanasto-mosis is advisable, along with insertion of a Penrose drain. Inadvertent ligation of a ureter, even if recognized immediately, usually requires ureteral stenting. If that segment is obviously and persistently ischemic, it is better to excise it, with reanastomosis. Should the ureter be inadvertently cauterized, look for damage to the adventitial vessels, because ischemic tissue must be excised. A severed ureter requires spatulation and anastomosis over a stent, but avulsion or extensive damage makes a psoas hitch (V-23) or bladder flap (V-24) necessary.

Suspect ureteral injury postoperatively in the presence of flank pain and tenderness in the costovertebral angle, with a low-grade fever, and especially with ileus. Ultrasonography and urography may reveal the site and extent. Retrograde passage of a double-J stent should be tried first, with or without a guidewire. Percutaneous nephrostomy is an alternative, with drainage maintained awaiting the dissolution of obstructing absorbable sutures. If the child is in good condition, consider immediate surgical correction.

PLASTIC SURGICAL TECHNIQUES

Important Grafting Concepts

The skin in grafts and flaps is viscoelastic. Traction for 10 or 15 minutes will enlarge a flap, because of stress relaxation and creep. However, a compromise must be made between tension and resultant loss in vascularity.

Blood is supplied to the skin either through a longitudinal artery lying deep to the muscle that supplies perforators to the subdermal and dermal plexus in the overlying skin, or through longitudinal vessels lying superficial to the muscle that connects directly to the plexus in the skin, beneath the dermis, or in the periadnexal dermis. These channels are extremely delicate and cannot withstand compression in forceps. Skin hooks and stay sutures are essential tools.

Grafts for the first 24 hours pick up nutrients from the bed, then establish vascular connections during the next 2 days. Thus, the graft must remain immobilized and closely applied to the bed, which in turn must be well vascularized. Seromas or hematomas block these steps, as does infection and preexisting scar tissue.

Full-thickness grafts are made up of all the skin layers and must be cleared of underlying fatty tissue before application. They contract only 15% to 25%, and provide durable skin covering. However, because fewer vessels are available for vascularization, they have a greater incidence of failure. Split-thickness skin grafts, composed of only part of the dermis along with the epidermis, will take better but do provide a more fragile covering. They contract 50% or more in loose areas. Dermal grafts, free of epidermis, are more elastic and can become vascularized on both sides. If skin is not available for urethral construction, consider grafts of bladder mucosa.

Flaps, in contrast to grafts, bring in their own blood supply. They may be random (or peninsular) flaps, without special orientation of the blood supply; these require a 1:1 ratio between base and flap. An axial flap has a defined, self-contained blood supply. An island flap is a form of axial flap that has dangling blood vessels and may also be used as a free flap with microvascular anastomosis. A pedicle flap is actually a misnomer because pedicle and flap mean the same thing. A musculocutaneous flap is composed of muscle and skin; in a fasciocutaneous flap the fascia and skin are elevated together.

Flaps may be used simply for cover or can be used for structure and revascularization (muscle), sensation (fasciocutaneous flaps), and function (muscle).

Choose a flap with size and ability to arc into place, with adequate vasculature, accessibility, proper composition, and an acceptable donor site.

Split-thickness grafts cut with an electrical dermatome may be thin (0.08 to 0.10 inches), medium (approximately 0.18 inches), or thick (over 0.18 inches). For a medium-thickness graft, put two thirds of the bevel of a #15 knife between the blade and the cutting block. Meshing the graft in a cutter will provide greater coverage and allow the escape of serum and blood; however, the graft will contract more. These grafts must be placed with good hemostasis, be free of contamination, and be immobilized. Mesh grafts are placed with the slits parallel to the skin line. They can be expected to contract 30% to 60% except on the back of the hand, on the scrotum, and on the penis.

Stretch the graft in place to overcome the pull of the elastic fibers in the skin. Secondary contraction occurs with maturation of the scar tissue, lying between the skin graft and its bed, beginning after the 10th day and continuing for 6 months. Thin grafts, flexible vascular beds, and complete take of grafts all reduce the chances for contraction. Skin grafts require good contact with the recipient bed. Tension, serum or blood beneath, and movement prevent adherence by preventing revascularization by capillary ingrowth.

Avoid causing suture marks in the skin as a result of tension. Tie the suture just tight enough for the edges to make contact and no tighter. Subcutaneous sutures can reduce it, as does placing the incision parallel to the skin lines. The length of time the sutures remain is also a factor; 6 or 7 days are usually adequate, but allow 10 to 14 days on the back. Small bites of tissue close to the edge are followed by less apparent skin marks; infection is accompanied by more prominent ones. Of course, a patient prone to keloid formation is at greatest risk.

Slight eversion of the skin edges results in a flat scar; inverted edges leave a depressed scar. Thus, in some areas, a vertical mattress suture is necessary to stabilize the skin edges. If skin clips are used, they should grasp the skin with equal bites and should be angled so that they slightly evert the skin. Microporous skin tape, used in conjunction with buried sutures, may be placed initially as primary skin closure or applied at the time of suture or clip removal. (It helps adherence to wipe the skin with alcohol or acetone before application.) Skin tapes have the advantages of quick application, prevention of suture marks, and provision of better tensile strength. But they do not evert the skin edges, and may come off while support is still needed.

Sensation returns to a graft beginning in 3 weeks if dense scarring does not occur. Fortunately, skin grafts and flaps grow as the patient grows, stimulated by tension from the surrounding skin.

For local anesthesia in adolescents, use 1% lidocaine with 1:200,000 epinephrine; for a child, use 0.5% lidocaine with 1:400,000 epinephrine. Inject it slowly while explaining the procedure to the child. Stop for a minute if the injection is causing pain. Regional block often may be better than local infiltration.

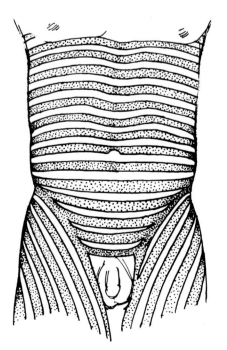

FIGURE 6-39. Use Langer's lines of minimal tension along skin folds by making incisions parallel to them to reduce contracture and formation of keloids.

CORRECTION OF SCARS AND CONTRACTURES

Z-Plasty (Horner)

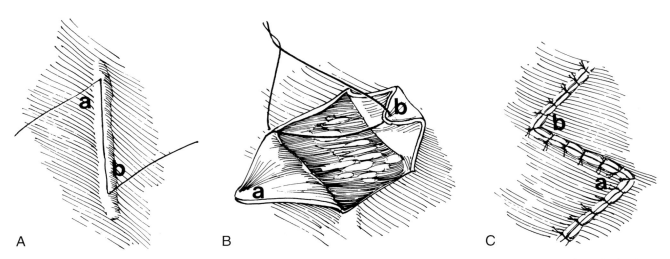

A   B   C

FIGURE 6-40. **A,** Incise along the length of the scar. Make a cut at a 30-, 45-, or 60-degree angle at each end of this incision. The gain in length will be 25%, 50%, and 75%, respectively. The length of the two angle incisions should be the same as that of the vertical incision, and they should lie along the lines of minimal tension (Langer's lines). **B,** Mobilize the two triangular flaps. **C,** Move one flap (a) down and the other (b) up, and suture them in place. Expect an almost twofold increase in length.

V-Y Advancement

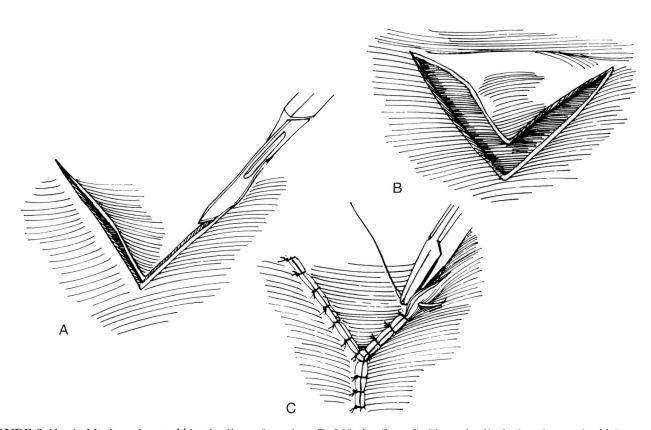

A   B   C

FIGURE 6-41. **A,** Mark and cut a V in the line of tension. **B,** Lift the flap. **C,** Close the limb that forms the Y first.

Rhomboid Flap (Limberg)

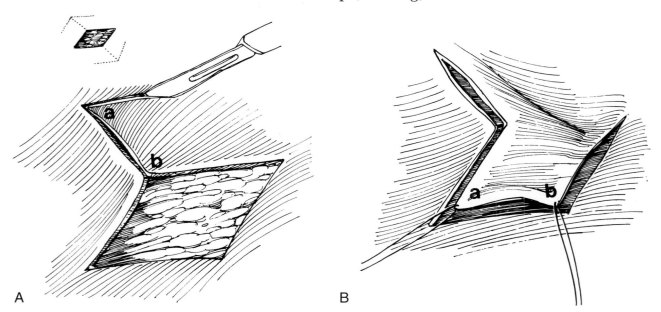

FIGURE 6-42. A, Pinch the skin between the thumb and forefinger to determine in which direction the excess skin lies. Draw a line at a 60- to 120-degree angle across this excess skin. Excise the lesion in the rhomboid. Draw a line perpendicular to the long axis of the defect equal to the length of one side of the rhomboid. Draw a second line at a 120-degree angle, making it parallel to a side of the rhomboid. (The other three optional incisions are shown by dotted lines.) **B,** Raise the flap, rotate it, and suture it in position.

Flap Rotation

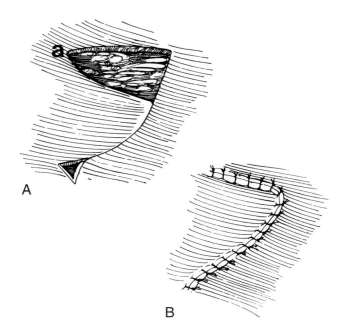

FIGURE 6-43. A, Trim a piece of suture paper the size of the defect. Rotate it on the pivot point of the flap (a) to check the arc of rotation of the flap. Mark and incise the skin. Excise a small triangle at the base of the flap on the outside of the arc. **B,** Raise and rotate the flap. Note: Cutting paper models of skin defects will often help the surgeon visualize the needed cuts and rotations.

Flap Advancement by Perpendicular Basal Incisions

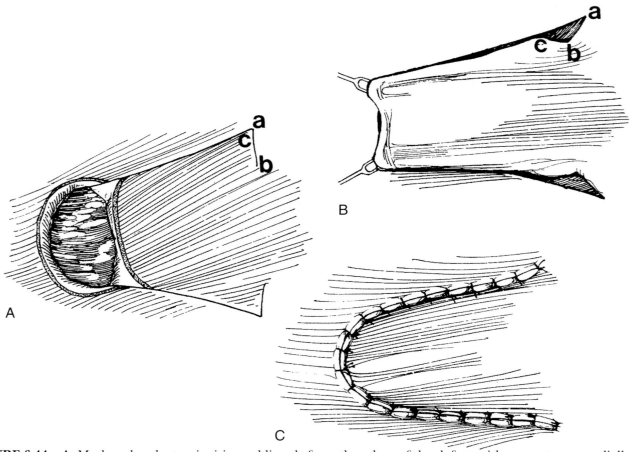

FIGURE 6-44. **A,** Mark and make two incisions obliquely from the edges of the defect, with an acute cut medially at the end at c. **B,** Advance the flap to form triangular defects cba. **C,** Close the gaps while suturing the flap in place.

Correction of Dog Ear

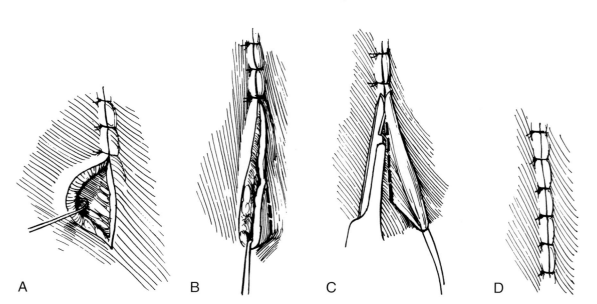

FIGURE 6-45. **A,** Retract the longer edge from a point that equalizes the length of the two sides of the incision. **B,** Divide the skin on the other side of the line of the incision. **C,** Excise the flap of excess skin. **D,** Close the wound.

Problems after Grafting

Loss of a skin graft results from poor adherence, most often caused by a hematoma, but improper immobilization of the graft is next in importance, making perfect hemostasis and proper fixation the keys to success in skin grafting. Hematomas can compromise the dermal-subdermal circulation and lead to necrosis not only by pressure-blocking neovascularization but by a direct toxic effect. They indicate a technical error that should be corrected at once. Aspiration of the hematoma early (within 24 hours) may salvage the flap. Fixation is dependent on the quality of the dressing. Infection can arise in a poorly vascularized wound after bacterial contamination. Deficiency in the size of a flap is the result of improper selection of the site or design of the flap. Rarely, failure is the result of putting the graft on upside down.

Ischemia results in necrosis of the flap and can come from direct damage to the blood supply or from overstretching the skin through failure to use a back cut or a long enough pedicle. Release a few of the sutures at once. However, it may be necessary to redesign the closure or even replace the flap to its original position and use it at a later time. Deficient arterial inflow is the principal cause, although poor venous drainage with stasis can be an important factor. Appropriate techniques applied during the procedure will preserve the blood supply but not completely eliminate the risk of ischemia. Tension is especially harmful when the blood supply is marginal.

CORRECTION OF LARGE DEFECTS

Gracilis Musculocutaneous Flap

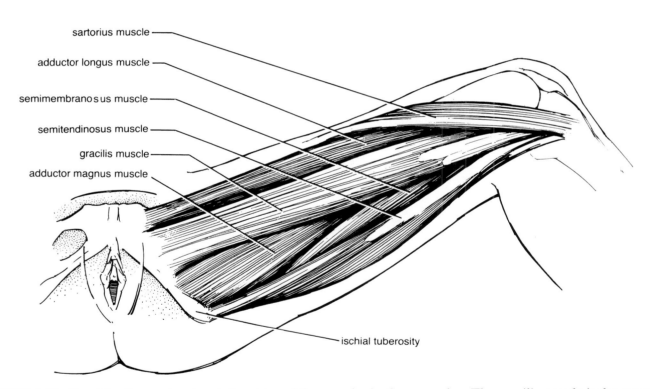

FIGURE 6-46. Consider the anatomic relationships of the muscles in the upper leg. The gracilis muscle is the most medial of the superficial muscles when the leg is abducted, lying medial to the adductor longus muscle. It originates on the inferior ramus of the pubis and the ischial ramus and inserts on the medial shaft of the tibia below the medial condyle.

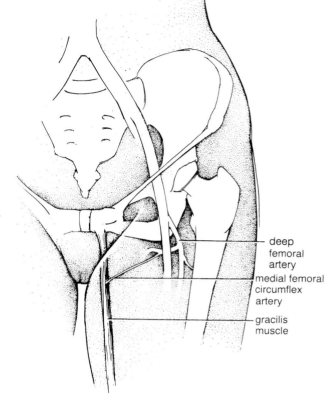

FIGURE 6-47. The medial femoral circumflex artery, arising from the deep femoral artery, provides the blood supply to the gracilis muscle.

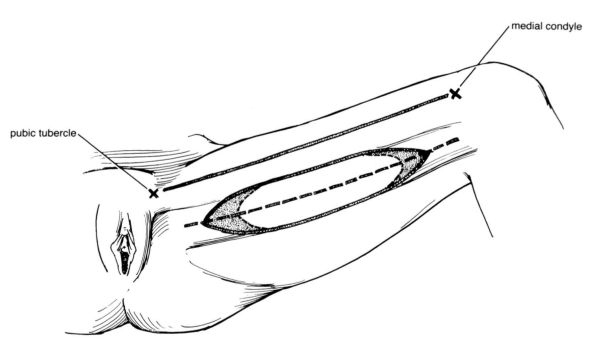

FIGURE 6-48. Position: Place the child in the dorsal lithotomy position and establish the normal anatomic relationships before abducting the leg. Incision: The adductor longus tendon, inserting on the tubercle, is on tension as the leg is abducted; this is the key to locating the gracilis muscle, which lies medial to it. Mark the pubic tubercle and the medial condyle at the knee, because the flap will be raised from the skin and muscle below a line between these two structures. Palpate the soft area below the pubic tubercle where the gracilis muscle originates. Now mark an ellipse 6- or 7-cm wide, beginning 10 cm below the tubercle and ending approximately 18 cm distally. It can be as wide as the 12 cm needed for a neovagina. Mark the length of this ellipse longer than required for the flap to allow provision for a tapering closure of the defect; the ends of the graft will be trimmed later. Prepare the left (or right) leg from the lower abdomen to below the knee. Also prepare the vulva and vaginal area. Drape the area appropriately.

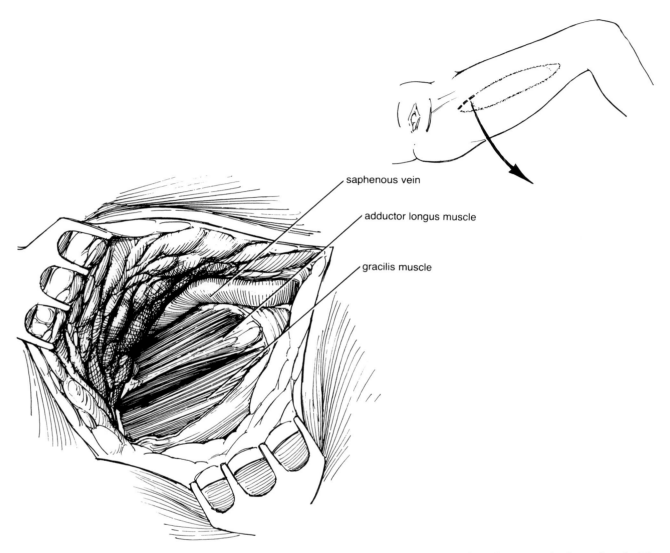

saphenous vein

adductor longus muscle

gracilis muscle

FIGURE 6-49. First opening: Incise the skin along the lateral superior portion of the ellipse marked previously. The saphenous vein will be encountered; stay behind it. Cut first onto the adductor longus muscle, which, similar to the adductor magnus muscle beneath, is a broad muscle. Then enter the cleft between the adductor longus and the medially lying gracilis muscles. It is now possible to run a finger around the gracilis muscle, because the vessels lie more distally. Be certain that you have correctly identified the gracilis muscle, because you can easily be mistaken. Divide the saphenous vein, keeping it anterior.

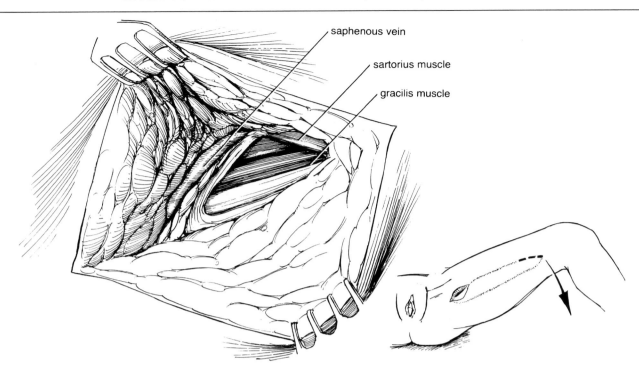

saphenous vein

sartorius muscle

gracilis muscle

FIGURE 6-50. Second opening: Make this incision along the lateral inferior portion of the ellipse. The sartorius muscle and the saphenous vein will be found lying anterior to the gracilis muscle. Dissect to the deep fascia, and punch through it to pass a finger under the gracilis muscle inferiorly. Note that the sartorius muscle crosses obliquely from below, running in a lateral direction, and that it is composed exclusively of muscle fibers, in contrast with the distal end of the gracilis muscle, which is half muscle and half tendon. You will not confuse the gracilis muscle with the semimembranosus and semitendinosus muscles that lie behind, because they are made up entirely of tendon.

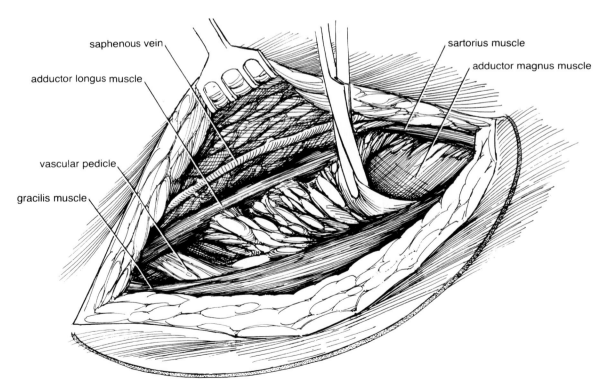

saphenous vein

adductor longus muscle

vascular pedicle

gracilis muscle

sartorius muscle

adductor magnus muscle

FIGURE 6-51. Dissect against the adductor longus muscle. The branches from the saphenous vein to the gracilis muscle can be divided. Continue cutting on the medial side of the adductor longus muscle, exposing the belly of the gracilis muscle until the vascular pedicle of the gracilis muscle is approached.

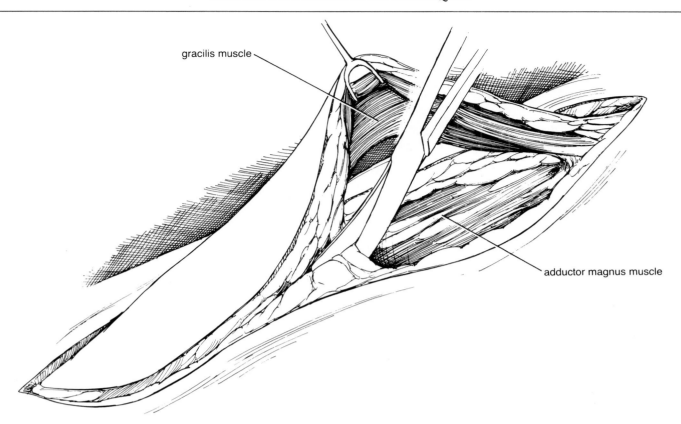

gracilis muscle

adductor magnus muscle

FIGURE 6-52. Complete the elliptic incision of the skin down the medial border, and cut the deep fascia medial to the gracilis muscle.

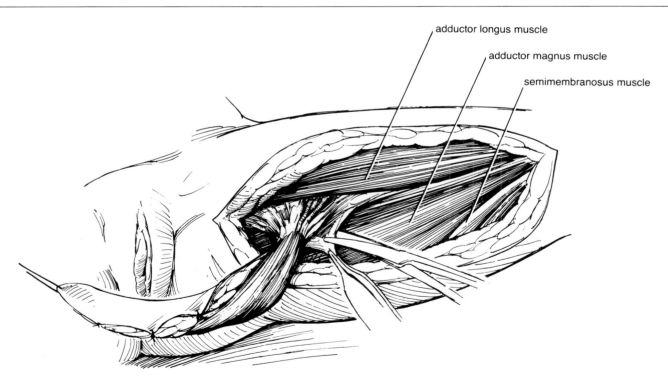

adductor longus muscle

adductor magnus muscle

semimembranosus muscle

FIGURE 6-53. Elevate the flap from below after cutting the gracilis muscle on the tendon. Insert a silk suture for traction, but take care not to pull on the flap, which can induce spasm of the entering artery. Tack the skin edges to the muscle. The vascular pedicle will be encountered approximately 9 cm below the pubic tubercle, with the motor (obturator) nerve to the gracilis muscle lying above it. A minor pedicle, arising from the superficial femoral artery, must be divided. (This artery is the blood supply to the distal skin, which will be discarded.) Use Stevens scissors for this dissection; a loupe is not necessary. Skeletonize the small vessels lying behind the pedicle, and watch out for branches of the obturator nerve. Do not do too much dissecting. Continue freeing the proximal end of the muscle, but leave its origin intact. The flap is now ready for rotation into position to cover perineal defects or for vesicovaginal reconstruction.

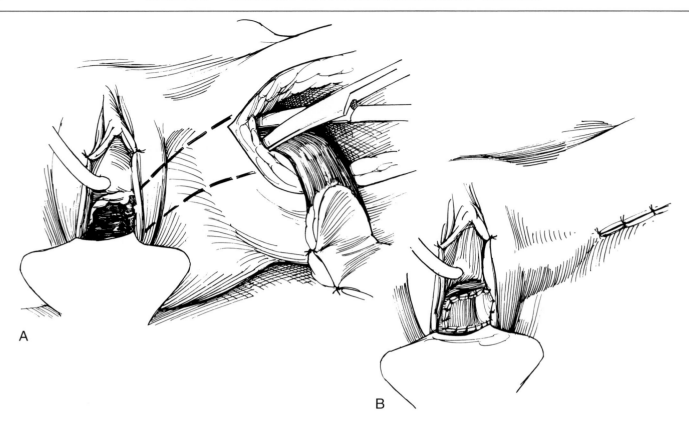

FIGURE 6-54. A, Tunnel (or divide) the bridge of skin and subcutaneous tissue in the groin; rotate the flap clockwise, counterclockwise for the right. **B,** Suture the muscle in position with 3-0 chromic catgut sutures. Approximate the skin edges with the same suture.

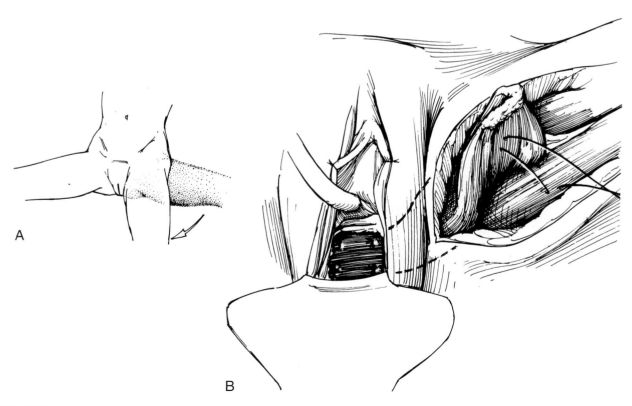

FIGURE 6-55. A and **B,** For a muscular flap, raise the gracilis muscle as a flap without overlying skin, as previously described, but without overlying skin. Adduct the leg, pass the flap through a tunnel, and suture it in place. Fix the base of the flap to the adductor magnus muscle.

Inferior Rectus Abdominis Flap

This operation is a good selection if the largest possible flap is needed both to fill a defect and to provide a vascularized base of skin. The donor site is readily closed. Either rectus muscle may be used depending on the quality of the common femoral arteries. The center of rotation of the flap allows placement into the perineum for reconstruction of the vagina and for repair of defects of the base of the bladder.

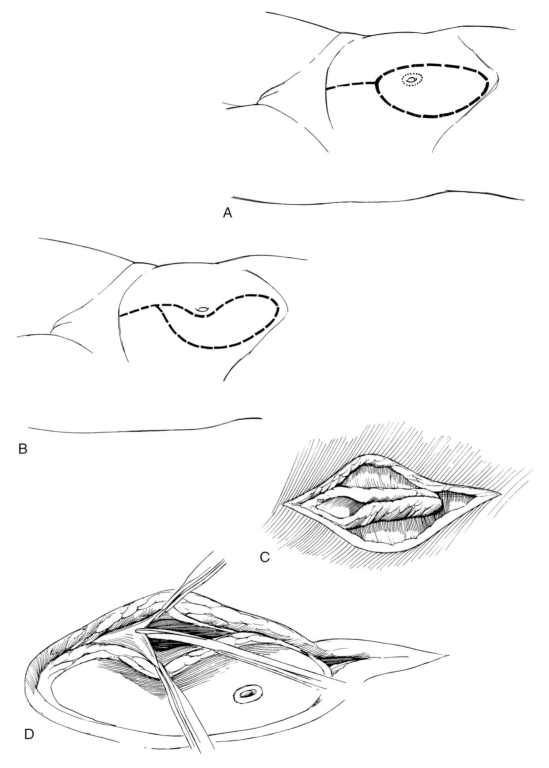

FIGURE 6-56. Prepare the recipient site first. If there is any question about the integrity of the common femoral artery on one side, use the contralateral rectus muscle. **A,** Outline an asymmetric flap extending well below the umbilicus to include the perforating vessels entering there. The width depends in part on the size needed for coverage of the defect and also on the laxity of the abdominal wall for closure. Incise the skin and subcutaneous tissue down to the rectus sheath. Circumscribe the umbilicus so that it may remain behind, adherent to a part of the rectus sheath. **B,** Alternatively, incise beside the umbilicus for a better cosmetic appearance. **C,** Elevate the skin edges. **D,** Divide the fascia beneath the skin edges, beginning along the lateral border. Leave 1 to 1.5 cm of the anterior sheath laterally for closure.

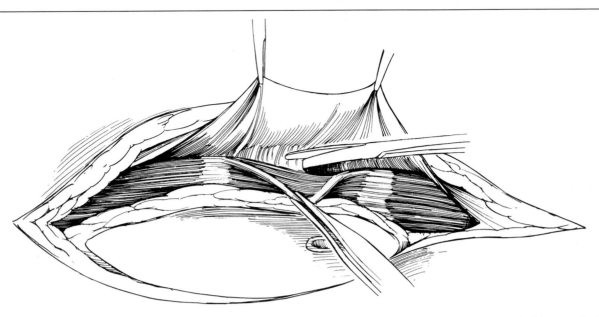

FIGURE 6-57. Dissect the rectus muscle from its sheath, again starting laterally, freeing its upper half posteriorly to the midline.

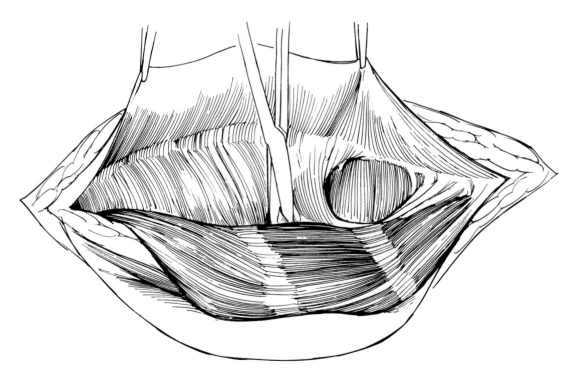

FIGURE 6-58. First take the anterior sheath and then the posterior sheath off of the muscle. The dissection inferiorly, below the arcuate line, will be directly on the peritoneum. Preserve the major perforating vessels that join fascia to skin. Place silk-tacking sutures to hold the skin edges to the muscle. During this dissection, be cautious not to injure the muscle or small vessels, although the separation of muscle from sheath is usually not difficult, except at the tendinous inscriptions.

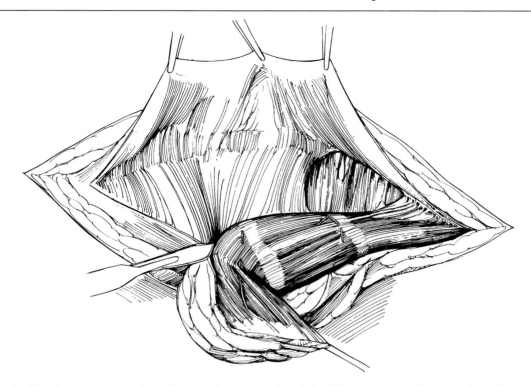

FIGURE 6-59. Divide the rectus muscle at its attachment to the xiphoid, and secure the superior epigastric artery. Insert a traction suture of 2-0 silk in the end of the muscle. Continue freeing the muscle posteriorly, while dividing and clipping the segmental motor branches.

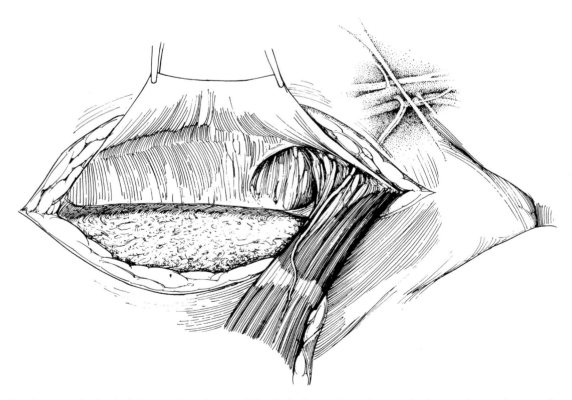

FIGURE 6-60. Approach the inferior end with care. The inferior epigastric vessels that make up its vascular pedicle arise somewhat laterally to enter into the lower fifth of the muscle. Dissect the vessels and encircle them with a vessel loop. Divide the inferior end of the rectus muscle to allow freer rotation of the flap and to reduce concern that it will be compressed when placed in a tunnel. Or leave that end attached to provide a margin of safety against harmful traction during placement. If it is divided, insert a stay suture in that end to aid in positioning.

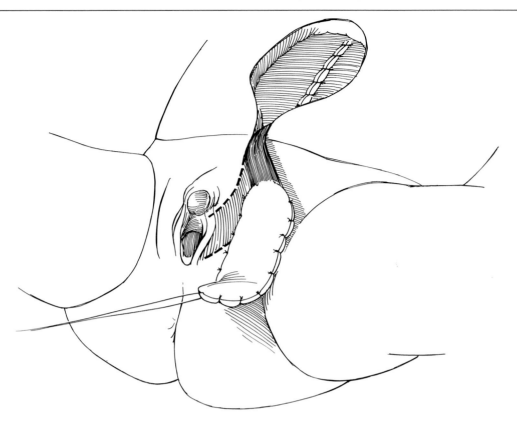

FIGURE 6-61. Tunnel the flap into position in the perineum or the groin, making sure that the pedicle is not kinked or constricted and fasten it in place with two layers of sutures after inserting a suction drain beneath it. Close the rectus sheath with a running doubled #0 nylon suture. Because the posterior wall is weak in the distal third where the sheath is absent, a sheet of synthetic material (GORE-TEX) may be cut to size and sutured in place with heavy synthetic sutures, each tied with eight or nine knots. Insert a suction drain within the rectus sheath, which may drain lymph. Close the skin of the abdomen with running sutures of 2-0 Vicryl subcutaneously and with 4-0 synthetic absorbable suture on PC3 needles intracuticularly. Postoperatively, give methylprednisolone (SoluMedrol) twice to reduce the inflammatory reaction. Provide simethicone to reduce intestinal gas. The child will find it hard to walk but should not be allowed to sit for more than a few minutes (e.g., either stand, or lie down, perhaps on an air-cushioned bed).

Other musculocutaneous flaps may be useful in urologic repair: (1) the rectus femoris muscle can fill large defects, but terminal knee extension may be limited; (2) the inferior half of the gluteus maximus muscle not only can provide filling for closure of a vesicovaginal fistula but also can support the vaginal wall; and (3) a gluteal thigh flap also will perform much the same function.

NERVE BLOCK TECHNIQUES

Nerve blocks in children are typically performed for post-procedure pain control under general anesthesia. Avoid an overdose of the agent as well as inadvertent intravascular injection. When aspirating, allow sufficient time for the blood to become visible in the syringe. Do it gently so that the vessel wall will not occlude the lumen. Should toxic symptoms appear, it may not be necessary to treat them, as long as respiration and circulation are adequate. Have at hand a nasopharyngeal tube for an obstructed airway, a bag and mask for assisted breathing, a blood pressure cuff to monitor arterial pressure and pulse, and preparations for possible cardiopulmonary resuscitation.

Intercostal Nerve Block

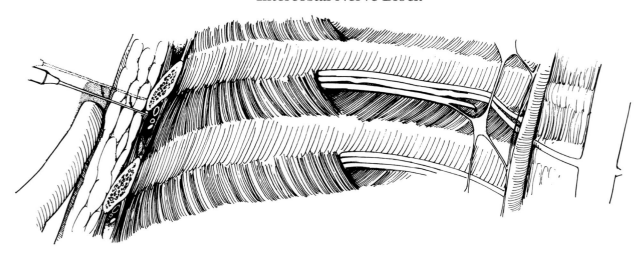

FIGURE 6-62. Anatomic relations: The intercostal nerves run segmentally under the respective ribs external to the endothoracic fascia. After passing the angle of the rib, the nerve continues below the artery and vein in the costal groove between the internal and external intercostal muscles.

Procedure: Place the child in a lateral position with the ipsilateral arm extended over the head. Palpate the lower margin of the rib just beyond the angle. Insert a fine needle vertically until it touches the lower half of the rib. With the free hand, pull the skin caudally until the needle point slips off the rib. Push it 3 mm deeper until a click is felt. Then angle the needle upward and advance it under the lower edge of the rib. Aspirate for air or blood. Inject 5 mL of anesthetic agent, preferably bupivacaine 0.5% with epinephrine. Pneumothorax, even tension pneumothorax, can result if the rib is difficult to palpate and the needle is inserted too deeply.

Penile Nerve Block

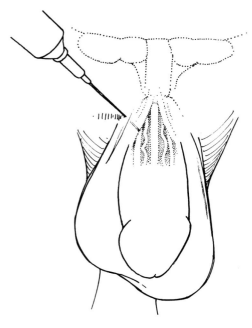

FIGURE 6-63. The right and left dorsal nerves of the penis arise from the pudendal nerves, pass under the symphysis, and penetrate the suspensory ligament of the penis to continue under the deep (Buck's) fascia.

Procedure: Palpate the symphysis pubis. Insert a short 22-gauge needle to one side of the midline at the 10-o'clock position to reach the caudal border of the symphysis. Withdraw it slightly and move it so that it just clears the bone. Pop it through Buck's fascia. Aspirate and inject up to 10 mL of 1% lidocaine solution. Repeat the procedure at the 2-o'clock position.

Iliohypogastric, Ilioinguinal, and Genitofemoral Nerve Blocks for Orchiopexy and Hernia Repair

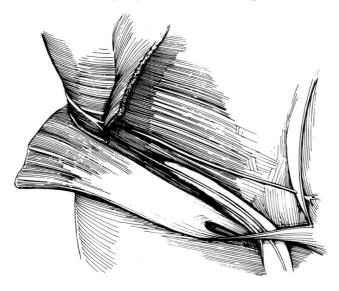

FIGURE 6-64. Anatomic relationships: The iliohypogastric nerve, from T12 and L1, exits through the transversalis muscle just medial to the anterior superior iliac spine and runs between the transversalis muscle and the internal oblique muscle 2 to 3 cm medial to the spine. The ilioinguinal nerve, from L1, arises slightly below and runs parallel to the nerve and continues between the internal and external oblique muscles. The genitofemoral nerve, from L1 and L2, runs over the surface of the psoas major muscle to divide just above the inguinal ligament into the genital and femoral branches. The genital branch enters the inguinal canal behind the cord.

Pudendal Nerve Block

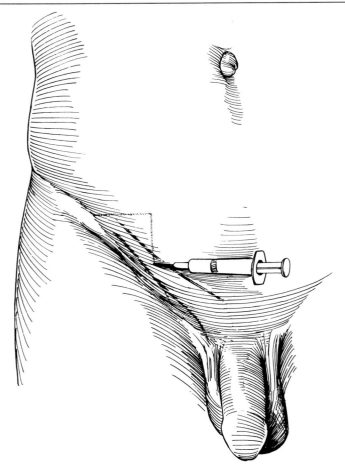

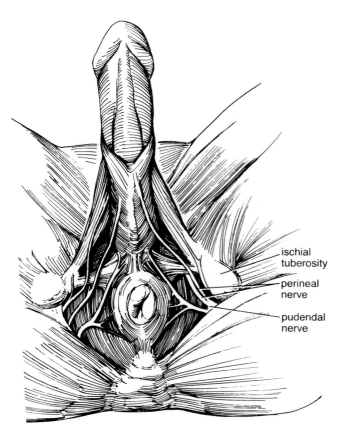

FIGURE 6-65. Procedure: Palpate the anterior superior iliac spine, and mark a point 2.5 to 3 cm medial and 2 to 3 cm caudal to it. Insert a 22-gauge needle to touch the inner surface of the iliac bone and inject 5 to 7 mL of a solution of bupivacaine 0.5% with epinephrine as the needle is withdrawn. Repeat the procedure more medially, injecting 5 to 7 mL of solution just beneath the fascia of the three muscle layers. For block of the genitofemoral nerve, palpate the pubic tubercle, and inject 5 to 7 mL of the anesthetic solution in the muscle layers laterally, cranially, and medially. Supplement the nerve block with subcutaneous injections fanned out to the inguinal fold laterally and the midline medially.

FIGURE 6-66. Anatomic relationships: The pudendal nerve arises from S2, S3, and S4, runs laterally and dorsally to the ischial spine and sacrospinous ligament, and divides into the perineal nerve and the inferior rectal nerve. Plan to block the nerve as it passes the ischial spine.

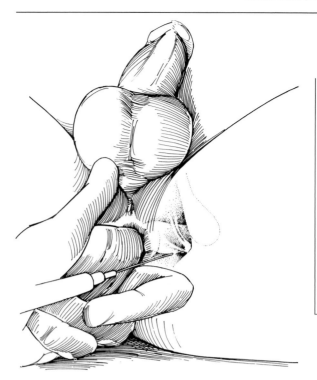

FIGURE 6-67. Procedure: With the boy in the lithotomy position, insert the index finger in the rectum and palpate the ischial spine. Make a skin wheal 2 to 3 cm posteromedially to the ischial tuberosity. Insert a 12- to 15-cm, 20-gauge needle on a 10-mL syringe in a posterior and lateral direction and pop it through the sacrospinous ligament. Use the index finger as a guide to determine that the needle comes in contact with the bony prominence of the ischial tuberosity. Aspirate and inject 5 to 10 mL of local anesthetic laterally and under the tuberosity to anesthetize the inferior pudendal nerve. Move the needle to the medial side of the tuberosity and inject another 10 mL after aspiration. Then advance the needle 2 to 3 cm into the ischiorectal fossa and inject 10 mL. Finally, guide the needle dorsolaterally to the ischial spine and pop the needle through the sacrospinous ligament there. Aspirate for blood and inject 5 or 10 mL of the agent. Repeat the procedure on the other side.

Trans-sacral Nerve Block

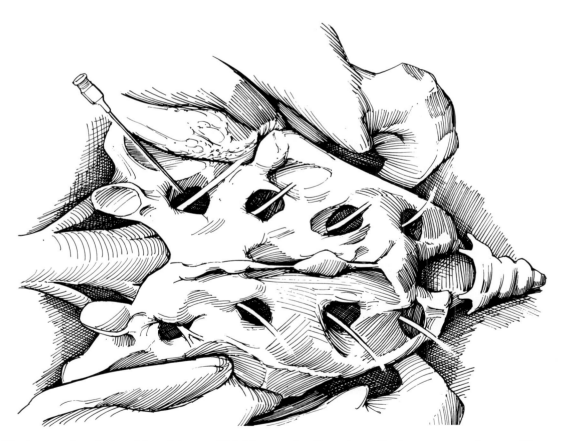

FIGURE 6-68. Anatomic relationships: A layer of highly vascular fatty tissue lies between two layers of bone. This continuation of the lumbar epidural space contains the posterior primary divisions of the sacral nerve, which exit through the posterior foramina to supply the buttocks, and the anterior primary divisions, which exit through the ventral foramina to innervate the perineum and part of the leg.

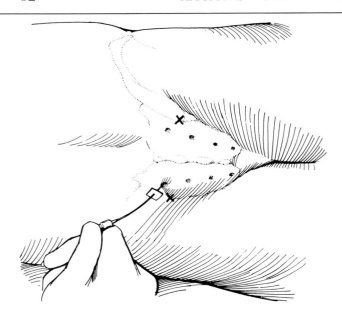

FIGURE 6-69. Procedure: Place the anesthetized child prone with a pillow under the hips. Palpate and mark both posterior superior iliac spines. Mark a point 1.5 cm medial and 1.5 cm cephalad to the posterior superior iliac spine to locate the first sacral foramen. Draw a line from this point to the lateral surface of the sacral cornua. Mark successive points 2 cm apart below the first foramen for locating the other three foramina.

Inject the agent subcutaneously to raise wheals. Insert a 12-cm, 22-gauge spinal needle containing a stilet perpendicular to the surface to contact the rim of the selected foramen. Move the rubber marker on the needle to a point 1.5 cm from the skin surface. Withdraw the needle slightly and angle it 45 degrees caudally and 45 degrees medially to insert it into the foramen up to the marker, for a depth of 1.5 cm. Inject 1.5 to 2 mL of anesthetic agent. For total caudal anesthesia, inject 15 to 25 mL (see Figs. 6-70 and 6-71). Hazards include producing a subarachnoid block and injecting the agent intravascularly into the large venous plexus.

Caudal Epidural Block

A single-shot caudal epidural block is used to provide perioperative analgesia for genital and groin surgery.

FIGURE 6-70. After general anesthesia the patient is placed in a lateral decubitus position with the knees drawn up to the chest or in a prone position with a roll under the hips for caudal epidural block placement. After initially identifying the coccyx continue to palpate in the midline in a cephalad fashion to identify the sacral cornua on either side of the midline approximately 1 cm apart. The sacral hiatus is felt as a depression between two bony prominences of the sacral cornua.

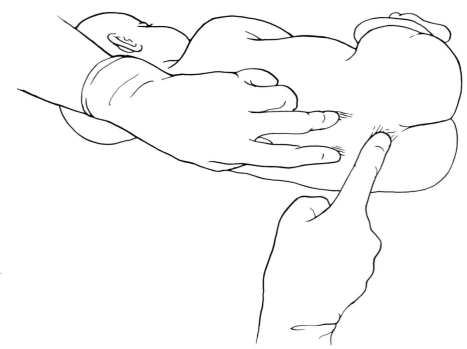

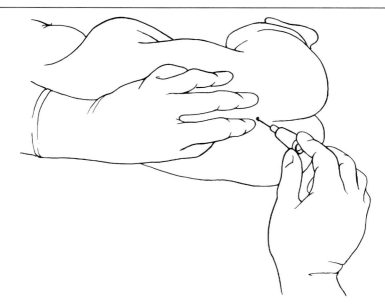

FIGURE 6-71. Under sterile conditions, the needle is inserted and advanced into the sacral hiatus at approximately a 70-degree angle to the skin until a distinctive "pop" is felt as the sacrococcygeal ligament is punctured. Following this puncture, the angle of the needle should be reduced to approximately 20 to 30 degrees while the needle is advanced 2 to 4 mm into the caudal canal. Any advancement past this point risks an inadvertent dural puncture. The classic "pop," felt as the sacrococcygeal membrane is pierced, confirms proper caudal needle placement. The absence of subcutaneous bulging and the lack of resistance upon injection of local anesthetic are additional signs of proper needle placement. Aspiration of the needle should be clear of blood and cerebrospinal fluid (CSF).

Formulas exist for the volume of local anesthetic required to achieve a given dermatomal spread. In practice, a dose of 1 mL/kg of 0.25% bupivacaine with epinephrine will give 4 hours of postoperative analgesia with a low incidence of motor block. The only additives that have been shown to prolong analgesia without increasing side effects are clonidine, 1 to 2 μg/kg (approximately 8 hours postoperative analgesia) and ketamine (preservative free), 0.5 mg/kg (up to 12 hours postoperative analgesia).

REPAIR OF VASCULAR INJURIES

Control the bleeding with digital pressure. Immediately increase the exposure; obtain blood; provide a second intravenous (IV) line and suction set; and obtain appropriate instruments, sutures, and assistance.

Venous Injuries

LACERATION OF THE VENA CAVA

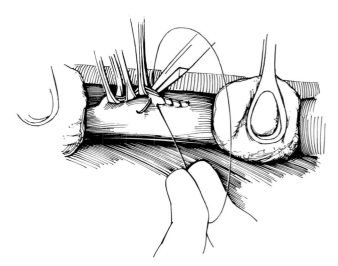

FIGURE 6-73. Grasp the edges of the laceration with several fine Allis clamps. This will allow dissection for better exposure. Run a 6-0 vascular suture down the laceration as the clamps are removed successively. If this fails to stop the bleeding, keep pressure on the bleeding site while freeing the circumference of the vena cava from both sides. Close the end of the laceration with a 2-0 silk suture, then oversew it with the same suture.

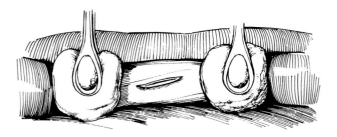

FIGURE 6-72. Have your assistant compress the vena cava digitally at the site of injury. Free the vena cava from the aorta and have the flow blocked above and below with sponge sticks.

INJURY TO THE PELVIC VENOUS PLEXUS

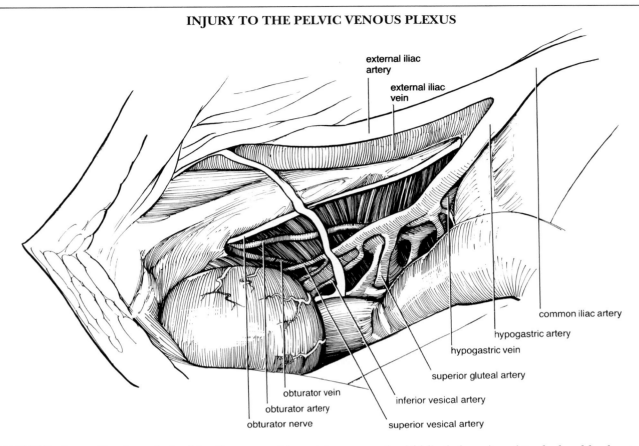

external iliac
artery

external iliac
vein

common iliac artery

hypogastric artery

hypogastric vein

superior gluteal artery

inferior vesical artery

obturator vein

obturator artery

superior vesical artery

obturator nerve

FIGURE 6-74. Immediately pack the bleeding area with moist sponges. Avoid blind clamping. Attach shoulder braces, and tilt the child into the steep Trendelenburg position to empty the pelvic veins. Orient yourself to the anatomic distribution of the pelvic veins before attempting repair. Slowly remove the pack. Clamp and tie the bleeding vein, or compress it distal to the tear with a sponge stick, and suture it with a 5-0 arterial monofilament suture (Prolene). Blind clamping and suture ligation can result in an arteriovenous fistula. If exposure is still not adequate, expose the ipsilateral internal iliac artery and clamp it with a vascular clamp at its origin from the common iliac artery. You may have to clamp both internal iliac arteries for control. Now remove the pack and control the vessel. If control still is not obtained and help is not available from the vascular team, permanently ligate the internal iliac arteries and place a pack to be removed 48 hours postoperatively.

INJURY TO THE COMMON AND EXTERNAL ILIAC VEINS

Note: Collaterals are numerous and can dilate in a few days after acute occlusion of a major vein.

Maintain direct pressure over the site. Visualization of these veins is better because of their more superficial location, compared with the hypogastric and pelvic veins, so that Trendelenburg tilt and proximal occlusion of the common iliac artery usually are not needed. Obtain proximal and distal control with sponge sticks and vascular clamps.

FIGURE 6-75. Repair the vein after a longitudinal or transverse laceration or after complete division if tension and constriction can be avoided. Carefully suture the edges of the defect with a 5-0 or 6-0 monofilament suture, placed as a continuous over-and-over stitch. Take small bites (1 to 2 mm deep and 1 mm apart). Inspect the vein for constriction.

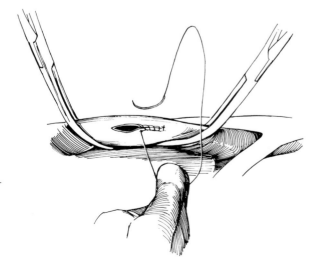

VENOUS PATCH GRAFT

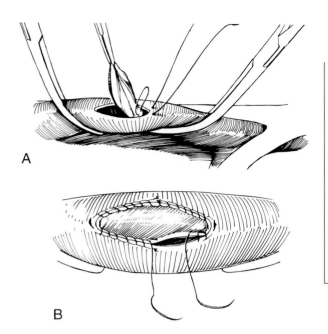

FIGURE 6-76. When the caliber of the vein would be significantly reduced by closure with a suture, interpose a venous patch graft. **A,** Expose the saphenous vein in the opposite leg. Resect a suitable length, open it longitudinally, and excise the valves. Trim one end of it to fit the defect. Manipulate the patch by the edges that will be trimmed to avoid intimal trauma and later platelet deposition and thrombosis. Suture the trimmed end to one end of the defect with a double-armed 5-0 or 6-0 monofilament mattress suture. **B,** Fasten the midportions of the patch to the corresponding part of the laceration with monofilament sutures. Trim the distal end and coapt it with a second double-armed mattress suture. Complete the anastomosis by running the two mattress sutures. Start suturing at each end on each side of the patch, tying the sutures to each other in the middle. Release the vascular clamps one at a time.

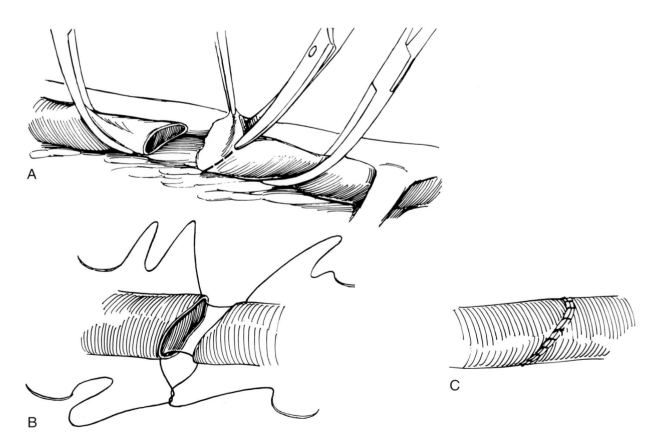

FIGURE 6-77. A, For repair after transection of a vein, trim the ragged edges obliquely, but do not spatulate them. Mobilize the vein proximally and distally so that it will come together without tension. If tension is inevitable, resort to ligation unless the pelvic collaterals have been so disrupted that gangrene is inevitable. In this case, place a vein graft. **B,** Insert a double-armed 5-0 monofilament suture. **C,** Run one end down each side.

INJURY TO THE LUMBAR VEINS

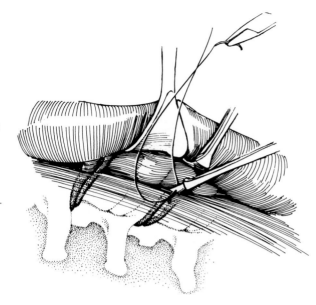

FIGURE 6-78. For a severed vein, as you slowly remove the pack, gently grasp each end of the lumbar vein with an Allis clamp. Suture ligate them with a 6-0 monofilament suture. If the cut end has retracted into the intervertebral space, pack the site for a longer period until the bleeding stops. Then expose it and sew over the end of the vein.

Arterial Injuries

AORTIC LACERATION

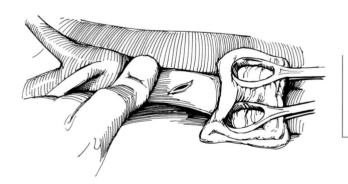

FIGURE 6-79. Control proximal flow by quickly preparing two sponge sticks to hold a tightly folded (4 × 8 inches) sponge between them. Have your assistant apply firm pressure with this loop of gauze without entering the field. Control back-bleeding yourself with digital pressure.

LACERATION OF THE BRANCHES OF THE INTERNAL ILIAC ARTERY

FIGURE 6-80. Temporarily occlude the abdominal aorta just above its bifurcation with one hand to reduce the bleeding. Clamp and ligate the cut artery. This can be done without risk of ischemia. Alternatively, maintain pressure on the bleeding point with a stick sponge while you free up the artery proximally and distally for several centimeters. Apply an arterial clamp proximally only tightly enough to stop blood flow. Divide and ligate the vessel. When diffuse pelvic bleeding is present, consider ligation of the internal iliac artery.

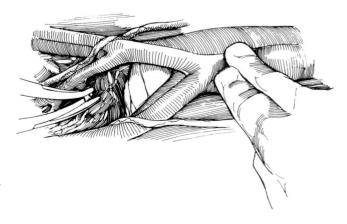

EXTERNAL ILIAC ARTERY LACERATION

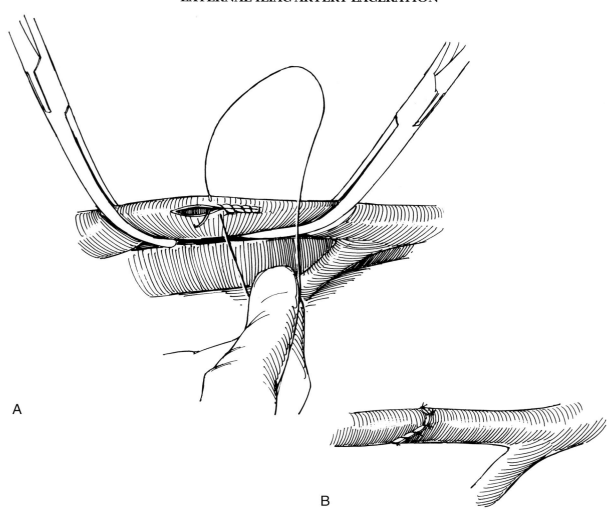

FIGURE 6-81. A, Maintain compression over the defect with a sponge stick or fingers. Free the vessel proximally and distally. Apply vascular clamps, closed minimally. Place a running, over-and-over 4-0 or 5-0 monofilament suture. **B,** If the laceration is tangential or irregular, divide, trim, and reanastomose the artery. In adolescents, up to 1 cm can be lost without serious tension. Check the anastomosis for a strong pulse and absence of a thrill. If questionable, redo the anastomosis. You can insert an arterial graft, although this is seldom necessary in children.

LOSS OF CONTROL OF A RENAL ARTERY

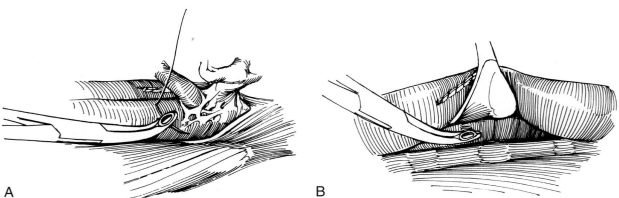

FIGURE 6-82. Left renal artery: **A,** With loss of control of the left renal artery during flank nephrectomy, compress the pedicle area. Expose the aorta just below the diaphragm and compress it. Identify, clamp, and suture ligate the stump of the artery. Right renal artery: **B,** Before clamping the right renal artery, dissect the vena cava away from the aorta above and below so that the aorta may be clamped in an emergency. If aortic clamping has not been done, control the stump with sponge stick or digital pressure. Clamp and suture ligate the stump.

CLOSURE OF BOWEL LACERATION

Small Bowel Closure

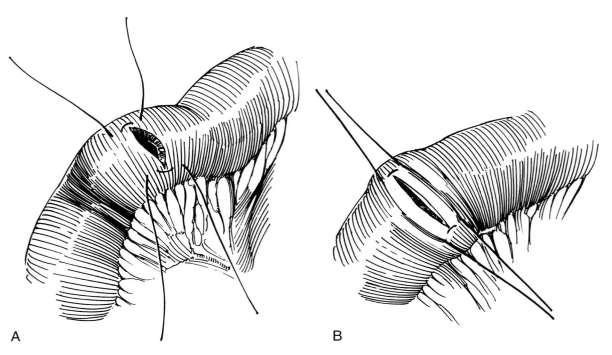

A   B

FIGURE 6-83. A, For a transverse cut, place Lembert sutures of 4-0 silk at the mesenteric and antimesenteric ends of the laceration. **B,** Place traction on the sutures to draw the cut edges together for Lembert suturing.

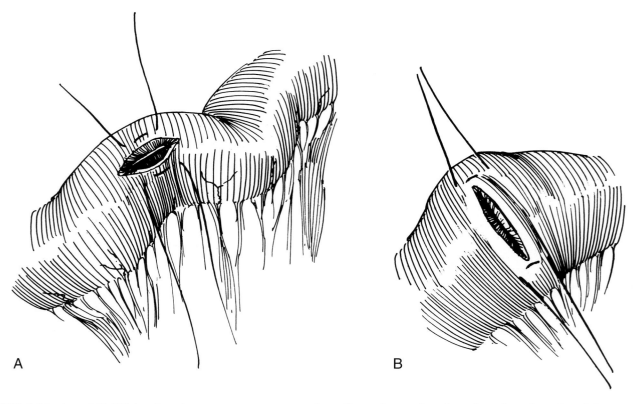

A   B

FIGURE 6-84. A and **B,** With a Lembert suture, convert a short linear laceration (one less than 3 cm long) into a transverse one to avoid narrowing the lumen. Tag the sutures and have your assistant put gentle traction on them.

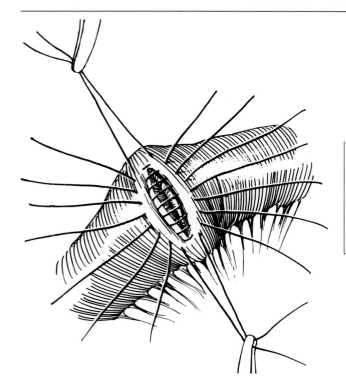

FIGURE 6-85. Place additional Lembert sutures, first at the midpoint, then midway between those already placed, dividing each remaining gap in half. Take bites of 3 to 4 mm through serosal-muscularis-serosal layers on each side. The sutures should penetrate the tough submucosa (evidenced by overlying blanching) but not enter the intestinal lumen. Next, place sutures 4 mm apart to close the remainder of the defect.

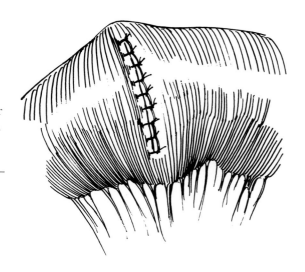

FIGURE 6-86. Have your assistant depress the edges with a clamp under the sutures as you tie them. For lacerations longer than 3 cm, close them longitudinally. Very long lacerations require resection and end-to-end anastomosis.

Closure of Large Bowel Laceration

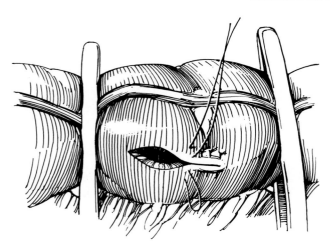

FIGURE 6-87. Occlude the bowel above and below the lesion with intestinal clamps (not with tapes, which could harm the vessels) passed through the mesentery. Trim the edges of the defect. Place a row of vertical mattress 4-0 synthetic absorbable sutures.

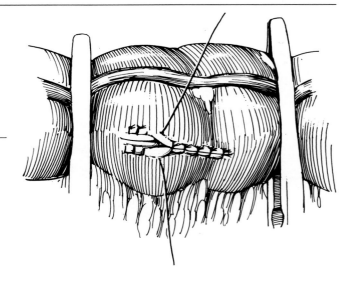

FIGURE 6-88. Place a second row, using Lembert sutures to invert the bowel over the first row.

Chapter 7

Laparoscopic Techniques in Children

SPECIAL CONSIDERATIONS IN CHILDREN

The following is a list of special considerations when using laparoscopic techniques in children:

1. The abdominal cavity in children is shallow; use care with inserting needles and trocars to avoid the great vessels.
2. The fascia is thinner, so apply less pressure during insertion of instruments.
3. The bladder lies high (in infants outside the pelvis) and must be drained before the needle is inserted for pneumoperitoneum.
4. The capacity of the peritoneal cavity is much smaller in infants and children, requiring a smaller volume of gas.

PLACEMENT OF THE VERESS NEEDLE

Place the child in a 30-degree head-down position to move the abdominal contents cephalad. Stand on the left side of the child (right-handed surgeon) and make a small subumbilical incision. Elevate the lower lip of the umbilicus with a towel clip. Hold the needle in the right hand. Have only a small length exposed to avoid penetrating too deeply. Aim the needle toward the pelvis at an angle of 30 degrees. With a 10-mL syringe containing 5 mL of saline, test for position by first aspirating for blood or bowel contents. Instill 5 mL of saline, which should enter without resistance. Aspirate again; no fluid should return. Remove the syringe and observe the fluid remaining in the hub of the needle disappear. Finally, advance the needle 1 to 2 cm, without resistance. Connect the insufflation line, reset the CO_2 volume indicator to 0, and insufflate at a rate of 1 L/minute to establish an intraperitoneal pressure of 15 mmHg. Percuss over the liver; loss of dullness indicates insufflation. If there is no flow or the 15-mmHg limit is reached, rotate the needle or slightly retract it to check for contact. If that does not correct the problem, withdraw the needle and repeat the insertion (multiple passes are permissible). Be aware that infants are especially sensitive to higher pressures, which produce respiratory problems, reduce venous return, and cause excessive absorption of gas. You may find that a volume of only 300 or 400 mL is needed.

INSERTION OF TROCARS

Avoid injury to "deep" structures, which are not so deep in children. It may help to elevate the abdominal wall with towel clips at each port site. Because of thinness of the fascia about the umbilicus in infants, which fosters leakage of gas, place this port slightly more caudally. If available, use pediatric laparoscopy instruments; they come in smaller sizes, with shorter sheaths for easier manipulation.

Insert the camera and look for injury from placement of the needle or trocar. Insert the other trocars under vision. In infants, the transmitted light from the trocar lets you avoid significant vessels in the body wall. Fix each trocar to the abdominal wall.

ANESTHESIA

Administer anesthesia endotracheally, using a cuffed tube to combat increased intra-abdominal pressure. The child must remain motionless during laparoscopic procedures.

To detect hypercarbia, monitor by pulse oximetry and end-tidal CO_2 (a sudden drop indicates obstruction of the pulmonary vasculature; change to the deep Trendelenburg position, release the pneumoperitoneum, and aspirate through a central line). Avoid halothane because of the possibility of cardiac dysrhythmia, and also nitrous oxide because of its effect of dilating the bowel. Be sure the anesthesia is adequate so that the child does not move during the procedure. Because the respiration of a child is sensitive to inflation pressure, use mechanical ventilation and keep intra-abdominal pressure low, about 15 mmHg.

LAPAROSCOPIC TRAINING

Because of differences in the techniques in laparoscopic surgery for exposure, hemostasis, and suturing, special training is needed. There is a steep learning curve, but once the basic manipulations have been mastered, increasing skill will come from practice.

PEDIATRIC CASES NOT SUITABLE FOR LAPAROSCOPY

Laparoscopy is a poor approach for operations on children who have had extensive abdominal or, especially, retroperitoneal surgery or previous generalized peritonitis. Other possible contraindications are abdominal wall infection, large abdominal hernia, abdominal distention, and coagulopathies. Children with severe cardiopulmonary disease are not good candidates because pneumoperitoneum can obstruct venous return to the heart.

Section 3

KIDNEY

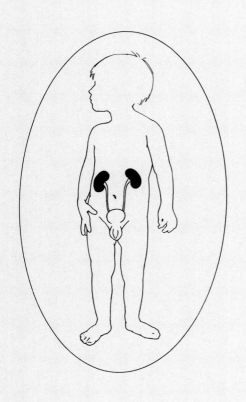

Chapter 8

Selection of the Incision

The kidneys lie centrally in the upper abdomen, and thus may be approached anteriorly, laterally (flank), or posteriorly.

ANTERIOR APPROACH

An anterior transperitoneal route will provide maximum exposure for major procedures on the kidney, ureter, and adrenal gland in infants and young children, in part because of their protuberant bellies and wide rib cages. For localized lesions, access can be gained from an anterior *subcostal* incision. For better exposure, use an anterior *transverse* incision (the chevron incision), which is ideal for excision of bilateral Wilms' tumors and for excising a neuroblastoma or pheochromocytoma. Generous access is also gained with a midline incision, an approach that is usually reserved for trauma or renal transplantation in small children that also requires nephrectomy. Because the costal margin in children is high, a midline incision provides a more direct approach to the kidneys than in an adult. In addition, an anterior or midline incision (1) provides an opportunity to evaluate other intra-abdominal organs, (2) gives superior access to the renal vessels, and (3) allows better control of the great vessels should they be injured. The disadvantages are the risk of generating intestinal adhesions and the limited access that can be obtained in obese older children.

An anterolateral extraperitoneal approach through an anterior subcostal incision provides greater exposure in infants than it does in adults because of their wide costal flare and the more accommodating abdominal musculature. In debilitated children, a firm closure is assured because stress is distributed among all three fascial layers of the anterior abdominal wall. This approach induces fewer problems with ventilation than the standard flank incision, reduces postoperative pain, and allows earlier mobilization. The pediatric extended anterior incision benefits from its extension onto the anterior abdominal wall. It is a valuable incision for the removal of Wilms' tumor.

LATERAL/FLANK APPROACH

A flank or an extraperitoneal lateral approach that runs first below the ribs subcostally, then through the rib bed transcostally, or between the lower ribs as a supracostal incision, reaches the kidney where it lies closest to the surface. The higher trans- and supracostal routes are especially useful in obese adolescents. If wider exposure becomes necessary for more extensive surgery on the kidney, such a lateral incision can be extended into a thoracoabdominal incision. The price for the superior access provided by these lateral incisions is (1) the division of large muscles, (2) the greater risk of injuring nerves, (3) the need to make a relatively long incision, and (4) the greater difficulty in controlling the renal vascular pedicle, which lies on the opposite side of the kidney. In spite of these limitations, lateral incisions may be safer in neonates even for bilateral pyeloplasties, which require two flank incisions, by avoiding the intestinal adhesions with possible intestinal obstruction that are associated with a transperitoneal approach.

POSTERIOR APPROACH

The lumbar approach may be ideal for more limited, reconstructive operations in children. A dorsal lumbotomy entirely avoids division of muscles and nerves and heals quickly with minimal pain. Although it gives limited exposure, this incision provides the most direct approach to the ureteropelvic junction for localized lesions. Because it avoids crossing muscles and nerves, it assures a quicker recovery. In adolescents, it is suitable at least for renal biopsy. The skin incision is placed obliquely to follow Langer's lines, easily accomplished in a child.

LAPAROSCOPIC APPROACH

Laparoscopic approach to the kidney is now appropriate for both ablative surgery and reconstructive surgery. The two main approaches are transperitoneal and retroperitoneal (see Chapter 19).

INCISIONS SUGGESTED FOR SPECIFIC OPERATIONS

TABLE 8 - 1

Operation	Incision
Wilms' tumor	Anterior subcostal
Bilateral Wilms' tumor	Anterior transverse (chevron)
Pyeloplasty	Dorsal lumbotomy Flank incision (from tip of 12th rib running anterior parallel to intercostal nerves, an alternative to dorsal lumbotomy)
Upper pole nephrectomy/ reconstruction	Flank incision

Chapter 9

Anterior Subcostal Incision

EXTRAPERITONEAL APPROACH

The extraperitoneal approach provides early access to the renal pedicle. For bilateral Wilms' tumors, use a chevron incision (see Chapter 10).

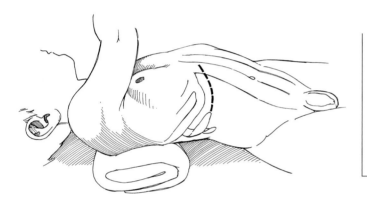

FIGURE 9-1. Position: Place the child supine in the semi-oblique position, with the buttocks flat and the shoulders turned up 30 to 40 degrees. For infants, place a folded towel under the sacroiliac joint, but for adolescents, use a sandbag and also flex the table.

Incision: Start the incision in the midline, at a point one third of the distance from the xiphoid to the umbilicus. End the incision at the tip of the 11th rib, near the anterior axillary line. Curve it to avoid the costal margin.

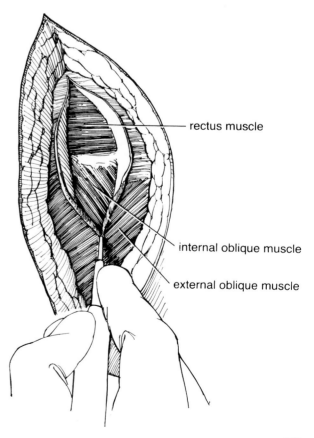

rectus muscle

internal oblique muscle

external oblique muscle

FIGURE 9-2. Divide the left side of the anterior rectus sheath and the external oblique muscles for a short distance in the line of the incision. If the rectus muscle itself must be divided, divide and ligate the underlying superior epigastric artery.

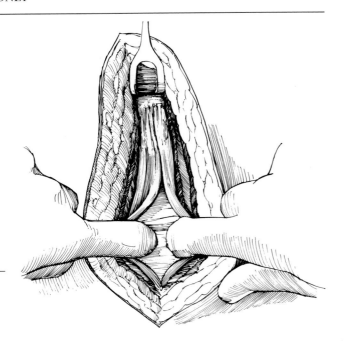

FIGURE 9-3. Divide or bluntly split the internal oblique muscle and digitally separate the fibers of the transversus abdominis muscle. Start as far posteriorly as possible, where the peritoneum is less adherent. Incise the transversalis fascia, and also its condensation at the lateral margin of the rectus muscle, while bluntly stripping the peritoneum down from that area of the transversalis fascia, which covers the inferior portion of the anterior abdominal wall. Free the peritoneum superiorly as well.

For more exposure, divide some of the contralateral rectus sheath. For further exposure, extend the incision posteriorly as a flank incision (see Chapter 12), or cut across both rectus muscles to open the peritoneum as a chevron incision (see Chapter 10).

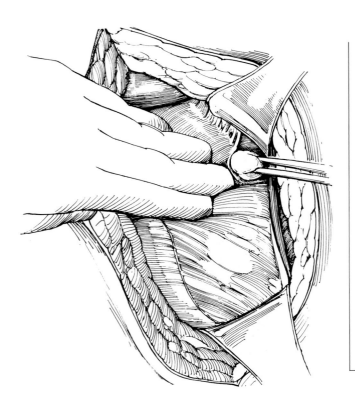

FIGURE 9-4. Use one hand in the extraperitoneal space to sweep far posteriorly to reach the lateral edge of the psoas muscle, and then bluntly strip the peritoneum from the overlying muscle layer. The peritoneum will be quite adherent here; use a peanut dissector or a sponge stick to avoid tearing it. Some sharp dissection with the scissors may also be required. Make a transverse incision through the transversalis fascia where it passes behind the posterior rectus sheath and a sagittal incision through it where it descends into the pelvis.

Free the peritoneum from the transversalis fascia for at least a few centimeters above and below the wound so that it may be mobilized anteriorly to expose the posterior lamella of Gerota's fascia.

Limitations in exposure are not primarily of muscular origin but are from the envelopment of the peritoneum by the transversalis fascia. Thus, the broadest exposure can be gained by incising the fascia in two directions: a transverse incision through its condensation as the posterior rectus sheath and a sagittal incision through it as it descends into the pelvis beneath the lower musculature, after separating the peritoneum from it medially.

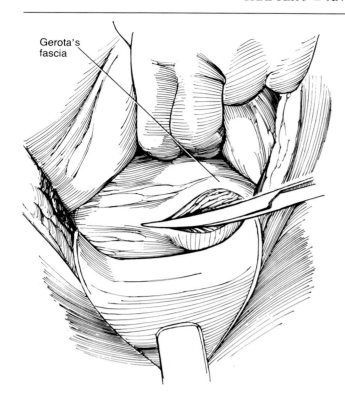

Gerota's
fascia

FIGURE 9-5. Enter Gerota's fascia over the lateral aspect of the kidney; reflect the fascia anteriorly. Avoid the pancreas and the superior mesenteric artery.

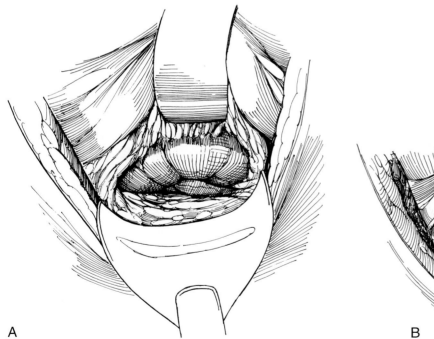

A

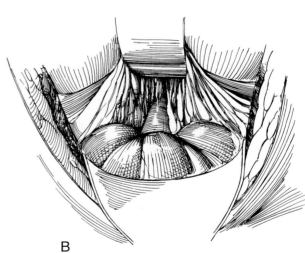

B

FIGURE 9-6. A and **B,** Carry the peritoneum anteriorly with Gerota's fascia. Dissect the perirenal fat so that the posterior portion of it remains under the kidney, to provide isolation from the posterior body wall after repair. Expose the posterior and anterior surfaces of the kidney. Proceed with the renal procedure. Close the wound in layers, usually around a Penrose drain.

Intraoperative problems may arise with this incision if the upper renal pole is large or is adherent, but initial control of the pedicle reduces the risks. For bleeding from an accessory vessel, extend the incision across the midline. Pressure of the retractor on the 10th and 11th intercostal nerves may produce temporary postoperative hypesthesia.

TRANSPERITONEAL APPROACH

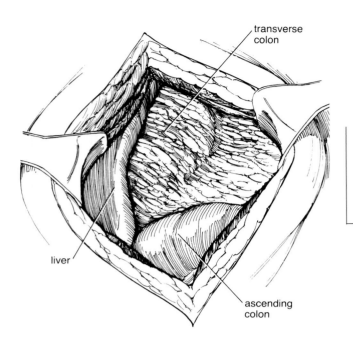

FIGURE 9-7. For exposure of the liver, the ascending colon, and that portion of the greater omentum covering the transverse colon, make a subcostal incision (see Fig. 9-1); then bluntly separate the fibers of the internal oblique and transversus muscles to expose the outer surface of the peritoneum. Divide the peritoneum in the line of the incision.

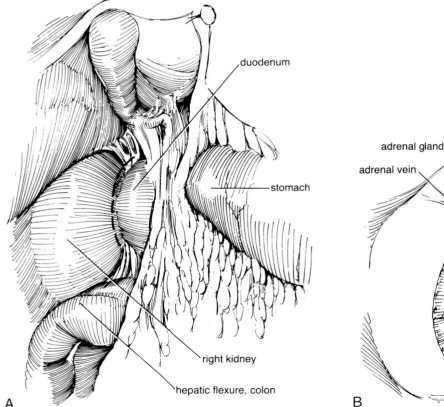

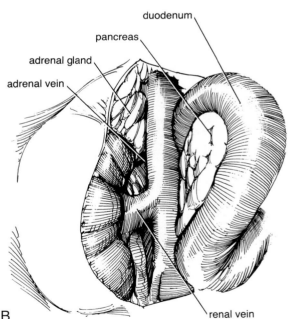

FIGURE 9-8. A, Right kidney. The Kocher maneuver allows a direct approach to the renal hilum on the right side. Make the incision in the posterior peritoneum lateral to the second portion of the duodenum (dashed line) to expose the anterior surface of the vena cava, posterior to the portal vein and anterior to the renal vein. **B,** Identify the right gonadal vein emptying anterolaterally into the vena cava, as well as any accessory polar veins, and also the large adrenal vein that enters posterolaterally cephalad of the renal vein.

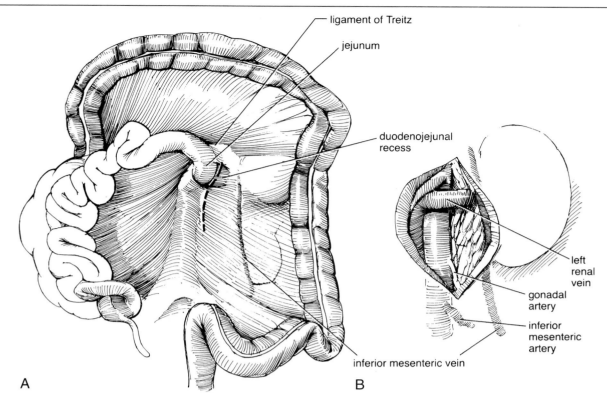

FIGURE 9-9. A, Left kidney. For approach to the left renal hilum, make a vertical incision in the posterior peritoneum just caudad to the ligament of Treitz and beside the fourth portion of the duodenum. Expose the anterior surface of the aorta. **B,** Identify the left renal vein as it crosses the aorta, and the left gonadal artery that lies anteriorly, as well as the inferior mesenteric vein and the superior mesenteric artery.

ANTERIOR APPROACH TO THE LEFT ADRENAL GLAND

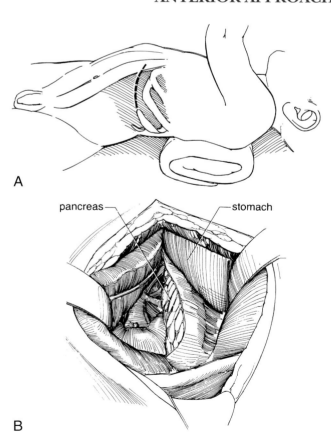

FIGURE 9-10. Position: Semioblique. Incision: Anterior subcostal (see Figs. 9-2 to 9-6).

A, As an alternative, the adrenal may be approached anteriorly through the lesser sac. **B,** Divide the gastrocolic portion of the omentum to enter the lesser sac anterior to the pancreas and behind the stomach. Retract the transverse colon inferiorly. Incise the retroperitoneum just below the pancreas, and divide the splenocolic and renocolic ligaments to allow exposure of the left renal hilum.

Before closure, insert a drain to allow release of trapped air and bring it out extraperitoneally through a stab wound. It is not essential that the peritoneum be reattached behind the colon.

Place a running synthetic absorbable suture to join the edges of the peritoneum and posterior rectus sheath. Approximate the transversalis and internal oblique muscles with interrupted sutures. Close the external oblique fascia and anterior rectus sheath similarly. Complete the closure of the subcutaneous layer and the skin.

Chapter 10

Anterior Transverse (Chevron) Incision

The chevron incision is an extension of an anterior subcostal incision across the midline (see Chapter 9). It can provide generous simultaneous access to both sides of the retroperitoneum as required for bilateral Wilms' tumors. It is valuable for removing large renal or adrenal masses on the left side, because of the greater exposure for division of the splenocolic ligament, thus avoiding injury to the spleen. Avulsion of the right adrenal vein from the vena cava is avoided by the improved access to the upper retroperitoneum. The exposure allows the caudate lobe of the liver to be lifted from the cava to allow safe division of the small hepatic veins. This incision is most valuable when access to both sides of the retroperitoneum is required: for left renal neoplasms invading the cava, for bilateral renal or adrenal tumors, or for large residual abdominal masses after chemotherapy for metastatic testis tumor.

Convert the chevron incision to a thoracoabdominal approach by extending either limb upward below the corresponding 11th rib and dividing the diaphragm to expose intrathoracic extension of the neoplasm. Alternatively, by splitting the sternum at the apex, a wide V incision is formed that allows pursuit of renal neoplasm with caval involvement extending to the suprahepatic level.

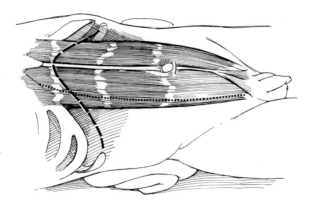

FIGURE 10-1. Position: Place the child supine and hyperextended over a folded towel. Incision: Incise the skin toward the midline below the costal margin from the tip of the 11th rib to a point just below the xiphoid process. Continue down the opposite side to the tip of the other 11th rib. If you are uncertain about operability or the need for such an extensive incision, make only half of it first.

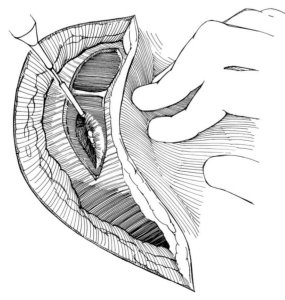

FIGURE 10-2. Incise the subcutaneous tissue, and divide both sides of the anterior rectus sheath. It helps to first insinuate a finger under the rectus muscle and then divide it with the cutting current. Ligate the superior epigastric artery as it is encountered.

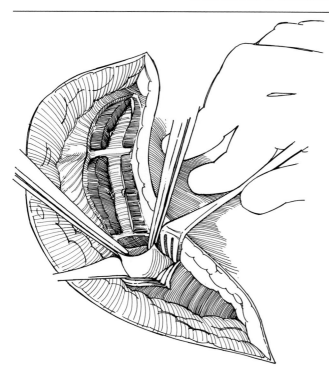

FIGURE 10-3. Divide the external and internal oblique investing fascia and muscles, and split the fibers of the transversus abdominis muscle. Incise the transversalis fascia and enter the peritoneal cavity just lateral to the edge of the posterior rectus sheath.

FIGURE 10-4. Complete the incision with cutting current or scissors against one or two fingers inside the abdomen. Divide the round ligament of the liver between clamps and ligate each end.

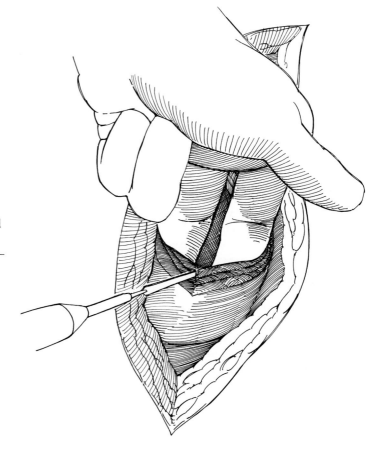

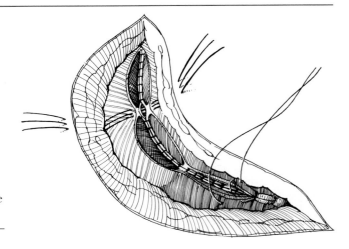

FIGURE 10-5. Closure: Have the towel removed from under the back and the table straightened. Reapproximate the round ligament of the liver. Place three heavy sutures through the skin and linea alba at the apex of the incision to secure the linea alba in the midline, but tie them when the rest of the closure is completed. Close the peritoneum, transversalis fascia, posterior rectus sheath, and linea alba in one layer with a running suture. Approximate the internal and external oblique muscles and the anterior rectus sheath with interrupted stitches of the same material. Alternatively, the fascial and muscular layers may be closed quickly with a Prolene running suture through all layers. Close the subcutaneous tissue and skin and tie the three midline retention sutures over bolsters.

Commentary by
MONEER HANNA

What is essential to open renal surgery is adequately wide exposure; a simple operation can be rendered more difficult and complicated if there is inadequate surgical access. The chevron incision provides excellent exposure for both large and bilateral Wilms' tumors. It is the perfect approach to a left Wilms' tumor: the duodenum is kocherized, and reflected medially, thus exposing the aorta. The left renal artery can then be identified and ligated as it branches off the aorta. It can also be used for bilateral partial nephrectomies.

Commentary by
MIKE RITCHEY

A generous, transverse transperitoneal incision is the most common incision used for removal of renal tumors in young children. This provides excellent exposure for unilateral or bilateral tumors. The chevron incision is more useful for larger teenagers or young adults.

A thoracoabdominal incision is rarely necessary for management of a Wilms' tumor. Tumors that are so massive such that adequate exposure cannot be obtained through the standard transverse transperitoneal incision usually would benefit from preoperative chemotherapy to shrink the tumor. A typical abdominal incision will usually suffice after chemotherapy. For very large non-Wilms' tumors that cannot be treated with preoperative chemotherapy, a thoracoabdominal incision may afford excellent exposure as described by Dr. Hinman.

Those patients with known inferior vena cava extension above the level of the suprahepatic veins will typically be treated with preoperative chemotherapy. If the tumor thrombus fails to shrink after preoperative therapy, there are several operative approaches that can be used. If cardiopulmonary bypass is being considered for surgical extraction of the tumor, a midline abdominal incision with median sternotomy will provide good exposure and access for cardiopulmonary bypass.

It is important to mention that when opening the peritoneal cavity in children with renal tumors, the bowel is often compressed between the tumor and abdominal wall. Care must be taken on entering the peritoneal cavity to avoid an inadvertent enterotomy. With unilateral tumors, it is best to open the peritoneum opposite the tumor where the bowel is less likely to be compressed.

An acceptable closure of the abdominal incision is to close the individual fascial layers with a running polydioxanone (PDS) suture. I neither use interrupted sutures nor do I routinely use retention sutures. Dehiscence of the wound is a rarely reported complication in children who have undergone surgery for Wilms' tumor.

LINDA M. DAIRIKI SHORTLIFFE

Commentary by

With minimally invasive laparoscopic techniques currently available, this incision is used less commonly and thus one may be less familiar with details of this incision. Current body imaging techniques allow better surgical planning so that the anterior transverse incision needs only to be used for renal, adrenal, or perirenal surgery requiring more extensive exposure and mobilization of tissues and organs in the area of the renal and great vessels rather than for exploratory surgery. I have found that one of the advantages of the anterior transverse incision is its easy extension into the chevron incision, which is useful when mobilization of the great vessels may be necessary, or, commonly, when bilateral renal exploration may be needed.

For bilateral pyeloplasties or other surgery not requiring vascular isolation, I usually prefer a retroperitoneal approach. In my experience, careful incision with adequate fascial margin between the costal margin and 11th rib, as well as incision and good exposure of fascial layers so that they may be seen readily as one is suturing closed the incision, is important in preventing incisional hernias or wound problems. I have closed all three fascial layers separately with large polydioxanone or polyglycolic acid sutures, unless chemotherapy, radiation therapy, or the need for reoperation has been anticipated.

Chapter 11

Midline Transperitoneal Incision

The midline transperitoneal incision allows exposure of the entire urinary tract. The classic use is for urinary reconstruction when both the upper and lower urinary tracts need to be accessed simultaneously. A midline approach allows direct access to the bowel for bladder augmentation and for the creation of continent catheterizable channels. A midline approach can be from the pubic bone to the xiphoid process allowing maximum exposure in the case of pelvic or retroperitoneal tumor. When associated injury is expected in the trauma setting, the midline approach facilitates evaluation of other abdominal contents. In smaller children the midline transperitoneal approach is also used for renal transplantation.

The midline approach is also useful for patient with horseshoe and/or rotation renal anomalies where the kidney does not lie in the normal position in the retroperitoneum.

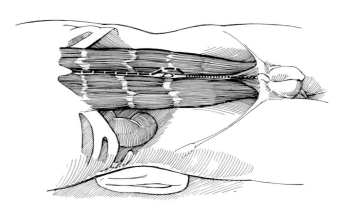

FIGURE 11-1. Position: Place the child supine over a rolled towel, positioned to elevate the side of the lesion. Incision: Make an incision in the midline from the xiphoid to a point just below the umbilicus, after first pulling the umbilicus to one side with an Allis clamp to allow making a straight skin incision that is at right angles to the surface. For greater exposure, continue the incision to the symphysis.

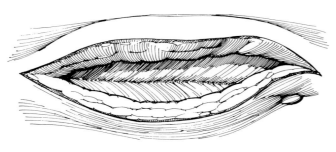

FIGURE 11-2. Divide the subcutaneous tissue and identify the midline by the fine decussations of the fused aponeuroses of the anterior abdominal wall muscles that form the linea alba. The rectus sheath here is covered with a delicate investment that may be opened to be certain of the position of the midline.

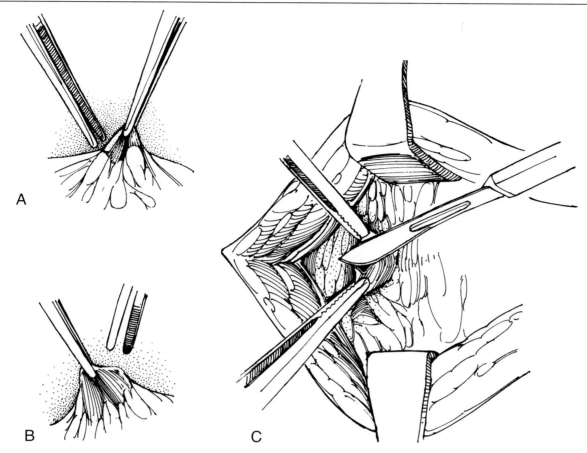

FIGURE 11-3. A and **B,** Incise the rectus sheath through the linea alba into the very loose preperitoneal fat covering the peritoneum. Elevate the areolar tissue and fat with two forceps successively applied by you and your assistant to tent the peritoneum, taking care with each grasp not to include any bowel, and then incise the preperitoneal tissue between them. **C,** After three or four such maneuvers with the forceps, only the peritoneum will be tented up. Penetrate the peritoneum with the knife. Air will enter, allowing the bowel to fall away.

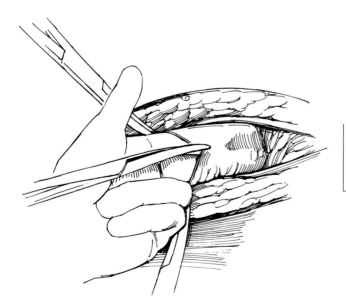

FIGURE 11-4. Grasp the edges of the peritoneum in curved clamps, and open it in both directions with curved scissors while protecting the abdominal contents with the finger of the left hand. Divide and ligate the ligamentum teres.

HARRY M. SPENCE

Having long been a devotee of transperitoneal nephrectomy for Wilms' tumor in children and hypernephroma in adults, I feel qualified to express some thoughts on the indications and technique for transperitoneal renal surgery. I am prompted to make these remarks in view of the current, somewhat overly enthusiastic trend that all operations on the kidney be done using this approach. Please regard my remarks as personal opinions and not ex cathedra.

First and foremost, there is no better approach for a Wilms' tumor or hypernephroma, big or little. The advantages are that the renal pedicle can be ligated and cut early, obviating to some extent manipulative metastases and cutting down on bleeding from the fragile distended veins, usually found with kidney tumors. Operability (i.e., movability) can be determined early, as well as the presence or absence of metastasis. The entire mass with its fatty capsule intact can be removed in toto. Thus, this appeals to me as a good cancer operation.

I formerly used the Hugh Cabot T- or L-incision, combining a vertical midline and a transverse component from the midline incision to the flank. This gives unexcelled exposure, but the lateral portion is time consuming, both to make and close. After watching the aortic graft experts, I have come to prefer the midline incision from xiphoid to pubis. To be truly adequate it must extend from ensiform to pubis. Closure with interrupted cotton or wire gives a sound wound. Neither the simple transverse nor the subcostal incision has given me the type of exposure I like. Furthermore, they are both more tedious to close.

Apart from tumors, I restrict the transperitoneal approach to the horseshoe kidney and the ectopic kidney. In both of these conditions, it facilitates handling the blood supply, which so often is anomalous. In the case of horseshoe kidney, it permits one to section the isthmus, do any necessary revision of the ureteropelvic junction, and anchor each lower pole outward at one operation.

Beyond these three specific indications for the transperitoneal approach, I believe the conventional flank route gives superior exposure for nephrectomy, pyelolithotomy, nephrolithotomy, nephrostomy, upper and lower pole resection, and pyeloplasty, as well as decortication of large cysts. Of course, one must have adequate exposure so that the necessary manipulation can be done under vision and not by feeling blindly. These requirements in turn demand proper position on the table, good light, and a relaxed patient.

Chapter 12

Subcostal Incision

A subcostal incision provides limited access to the upper pole of the kidney and the renal pedicle. This incision is best used for severe ureteropelvic junction obstruction where the obstructed pelvis extends inferiorly toward the bladder. The incision is also useful for lower pole ureteropelvic junction obstruction in a duplex system. A variation of the incision off the tip of the 12th rib is appropriate for exposure in the majority of pyeloplasties.

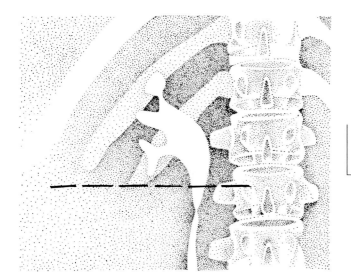

FIGURE 12-1. To evaluate access draw a horizontal line on an imaginary urogram from the lateral border of the rib cage. Only structures below that line will be adequately exposed.

FIGURE 12-2. Position: Place the child in the flank position, with a rolled towel under the 12th rib. In an adolescent, use the kidney lift in conjunction with table flexion, but watch for hypotension from poor venous return, mediastinal shift, and displacement of the liver. Incision: Start the incision at the lateral border of the sacrospinalis muscle, 1 cm below the lower edge of the 12th rib. Follow the lower border of the rib anteriorly. Curve the incision caudally as it crosses the anterior abdominal wall to avoid the subcostal nerve. End it near the lateral border of the rectus abdominis muscle. If the 12th rib is rudimentary, place the incision well below the 11th rib.

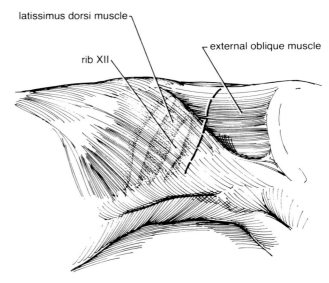

latissimus dorsi muscle

rib XII

external oblique muscle

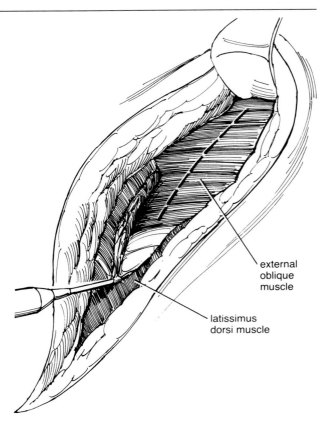

FIGURE 12-3. Incise the latissimus dorsi and serratus posterior inferior muscles, cutting back from their anterior free borders. Use the cutting current to minimize the blood loss and the trauma to the tissue that would occur with the application of multiple clamps and ligatures.

external oblique muscle

latissimus dorsi muscle

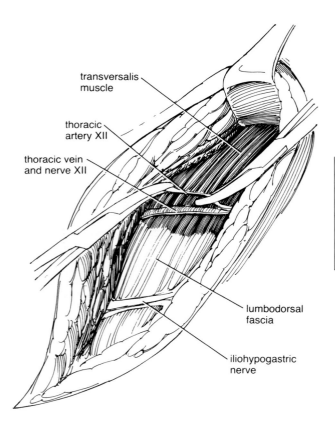

transversalis muscle

thoracic artery XII

thoracic vein and nerve XII

lumbodorsal fascia

iliohypogastric nerve

FIGURE 12-4. Incise the external and internal oblique muscles, starting at their posterior free border. Then incise the serratus posterior inferior muscle. Watch for the 12th intercostal neurovascular bundle that lies between the internal oblique and transversus abdominis muscles. Free the bundle and push it upward. Divide and ligate the small and fragile intercostal veins accompanying the bundle.

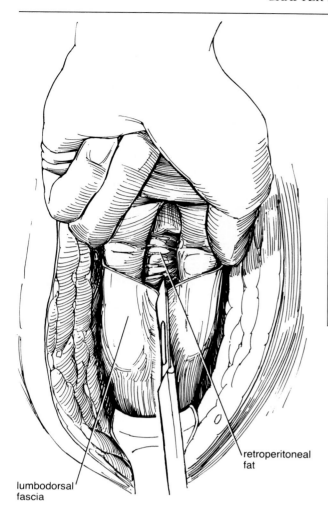

FIGURE 12-5. Identify the firm white lumbodorsal fascia and incise it in mid-incision enough to allow insertion of two fingers. Push the peritoneum forward to avoid cutting into it while completing the incision through the muscle. The fingers will also aid hemostasis. Sharply cut the fascia up to its junction with the anterior musculature. Incise and digitally split the transversus abdominis muscle. This exposes the peritoneum, which can be bluntly freed and pushed anteriorly.

lumbodorsal
fascia

retroperitoneal
fat

FIGURE 12-6. Incise the posterior layer of the lumbodorsal fascia, along with a few fibers of the serratus posterior inferior, working back from the anterior border of the sacrospinalis muscle. Divide the sacrospinalis muscle with cutting current to expose the costotransverse ligament.

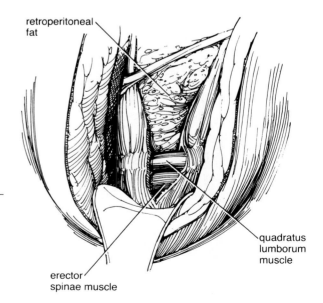

retroperitoneal
fat

quadratus
lumborum
muscle

erector
spinae muscle

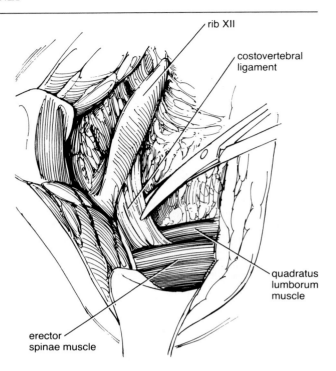

FIGURE 12-7. While elevating the 12th rib, cut the costovertebral ligament with partially opened Mayo scissors. Keep the curved side down to avoid cutting the intercostal artery or entering the pleura, which lies beyond the tip of the transverse process. Free the subcostal nerve further to be able to move it superiorly. Insert a self-retaining retractor and proceed with entry into Gerota's fascia.

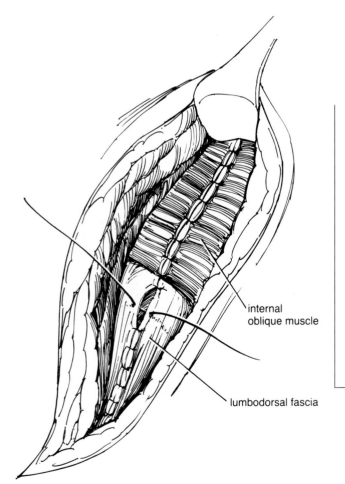

FIGURE 12-8. Closure: Lower the kidney rest and flatten the tabletop. Insert a Penrose drain to exit through a stab wound below the incision and also an infant feeding tube to supply bupivacaine analgesia postoperatively. Start anteriorly to close the transversus abdominis and internal oblique muscles in one layer with interrupted 2-0 synthetic absorbable sutures. Alternatively, close the flimsy transversus muscle first. Work posteriorly and close the lumbodorsal fascia by approximating the aponeurotic portion of the transversus abdominis muscle and the posterior layer of the lumbodorsal fascia. Approximate the external oblique muscle beginning anteriorly, and suture the serratus posterior inferior and latissimus dorsi muscles, beginning posteriorly, with interrupted 2-0 synthetic absorbable sutures. Close the subcutaneous tissues with plain catgut and approximate the skin.

To allow observation of the kidney bed for any oozing during closure, before lowering the kidney lift, insert figure-eight sutures through all layers of the body wall. Clamp the ends. Now lower the lift and tie the sutures in sequence.

HOWARD SNYDER

Commentary by

Staying lateral to the rectus muscle lowers the morbidity of muscle injury seen with a broader incision. When freeing up the 12th nerve, remember that it is embedded in the filmy fascia over the transversalis muscle and is frequently displaced upward with mobilization and division of the internal oblique musculature, risking division of the nerve. Being aware of this enables the nerve to be better protected. Usually the nerve can be freed up superiorly and inferiorly and displaced laterally so that the surgery can be accomplished anterior to the nerve without injury. In small children it is usually not necessary to do a 12th rib excision because the ribs are more flexible and can be more easily retracted than in adults. In freeing up the peritoneum to displace it medially to expose Gerota's fascia, it is quite easy to enter the peritoneum in small babies. The secret to avoiding peritoneal entry is to use your finger to push against the musculature of the interior abdominal wall, which will protect the peritoneum while giving broad mobilization.

Chapter 13

Transcostal Incision

Where functioning renal tissue is to be retained, such as during partial nephrectomy and/or heminephrectomy, a lateral retroperitoneal incision may be appropriate. The choice between a subcostal 12th rib incision or supracostal 11th rib incision depends on the position of the kidney, the location of the lesion, previous surgical incisions in the flank, and the experience of the surgeon. The transcostal incision approaching the upper retroperitoneum through the bed of the 12th rib may also be used for simple nephrectomy and for simple adrenalectomy in older children and adolescents,

although a supracostal incision (see Chapter 14) may be easier to make and give equal or better exposure.

INSTRUMENTS

Special rib instruments used by thoracic surgeons are necessary: Snyder and Alexander periosteal elevators, Matson and Doyen rib strippers, guillotine rib cutters, rongeurs, and self-retaining laminectomy (Sheldon) or chest (Finochietto) retractors.

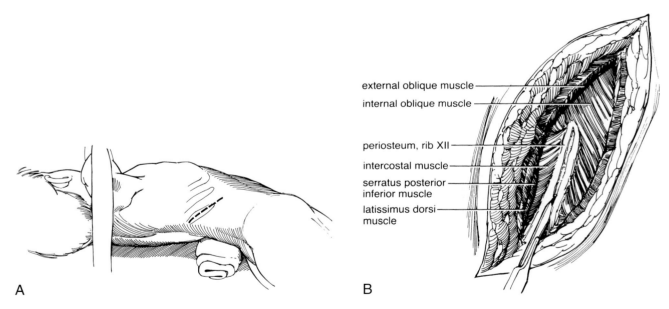

external oblique muscle

internal oblique muscle

periosteum, rib XII

intercostal muscle

serratus posterior inferior muscle

latissimus dorsi muscle

A

B

FIGURE 13-1. Position: Place the child in the flank position, over the break in the table, and elevate the kidney rest. Palpate the 12th and 11th ribs, and then scratch the skin vertically in several places along the course of the 12th rib to guide the incision and to help align the skin at the time of closure. **A,** Incise the skin starting at the margin of the erector spinae muscles, running obliquely following the 12th rib and ending at the lateral border of the rectus abdominis muscle. If the rib cannot be felt through a thick body wall, estimate its site and cut through enough of the subcutaneous tissue so that it can be palpated. **B,** Once the rib can be felt, divide the external oblique muscle and the latissimus dorsi muscle directly over its center line with the electrosurgical blade to expose the periosteal surface. Incise the periosteum sharply with a knife blade.

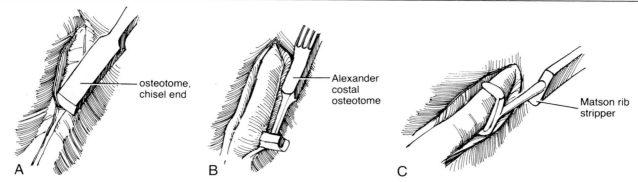

FIGURE 13-2. A, Scrape the periosteum from the rib with the chisel end of the Alexander periosteal elevator, beginning at the junction with the neck. Use small strokes to free the periosteum from the convex surface of the rib, and then free the upper and lower edges. A dry sponge may also be used to strip back the muscle and periosteum. Finally, run the elevator along both edges at an angle to free the periosteum under the rib. **B,** The curved blades on the other end of the Alexander elevator are useful here to free the periosteum from the edges of the rib. **C,** Apply the Matson rib stripper. Because of the oblique angle of attachments of the intercostal muscles, push the stripper anteriorly on the upper edge of the rib and posteriorly on the lower.

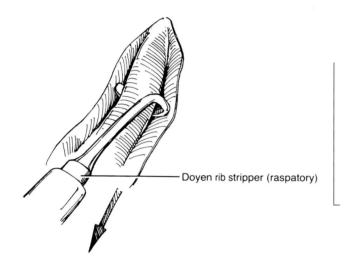

FIGURE 13-3. Insinuate the Doyen rib stripper under the rib inside the periosteum. Lift up on the shaft and pull back along the undersurface to the angle of the rib. Depress the handle and push forward to the tip of the rib, thus using each of the cutting edges effectively. Alternatively, but not as cleanly or easily done, the rib may be excised extraperiosteally. To do this, omit incising and freeing the periosteum, but proceed immediately to insertion of the Doyen rib stripper superficial to the transversalis fascia, forcibly separating the rib from the muscles and fascia inserting on it.

FIGURE 13-4. Grasp the rib with a Kocher clamp to steady it. Insert the rib cutter with the blade on the medial side and slide it well posteriorly to divide the rib as far back as possible. After division, use the rongeurs to trim away more of the rib if needed and to round the edges. Press bone wax into the cut end if it is bleeding (rare from the 12th rib). After lifting up the posterior end, cut the anterior fibrous attachments of the rib with Mayo scissors and remove it.

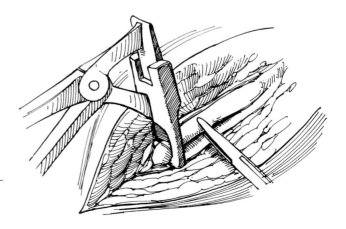

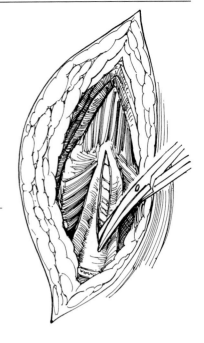

FIGURE 13-5. Incise the posterior layer of periosteum at the anterior end under the site of the rib tip to enter the retroperitoneal space. Insert a finger to depress the pleura and peritoneum; then extend the incision both ways with scissors. Spare the branches of the 12th intercostal neurovascular bundle by palpating them and letting them move caudally. Watch out for a vessel joining the 12th and 11th bundles anteriorly.

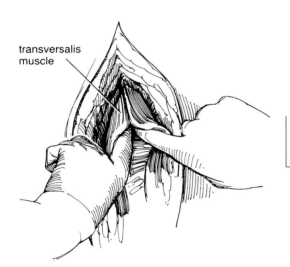

transversalis
muscle

FIGURE 13-6. Divide the internal oblique muscle electrosurgically. Incise the thin fascia over the transversalis muscle and then digitally split the muscle up to the anterior end of the wound.

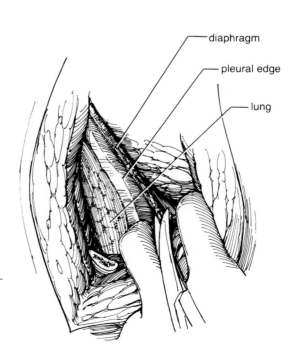

diaphragm

pleural edge

lung

FIGURE 13-7. Identify the pleura posteriorly; have the anesthetist inflate the lung for easy visualization. (For the repair of pleural tears, see Chapter 16.) Gently dissect the pleura from the endothoracic fascia beneath the 11th rib. At the same time, cut the attachments of the diaphragm against the body wall with Metzenbaum scissors. Separate the diaphragm from the retroperitoneal connective tissue to allow its displacement superiorly. By blunt dissection, free the peritoneum thoroughly from the transversalis fascia on the undersurface of the abdominal wall, not only medially but superiorly and inferiorly as well. This will facilitate placement of retractors to achieve optimal exposure.

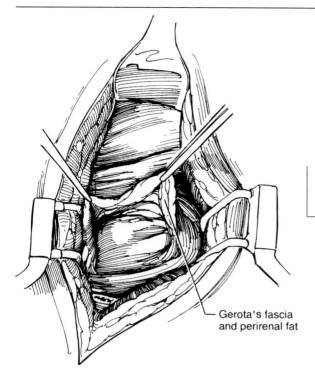

FIGURE 13-8. Insert a self-retaining retractor. Enter Gerota's fascia bluntly to displace part of the perirenal fat posteriorly and expose the kidney.

Gerota's fascia
and perirenal fat

FIGURE 13-9. Closure: Insert a Penrose drain through a separate stab wound. (Only if heavy, infected drainage is expected should the drain exit through the wound itself.) Have the anesthetist lower the kidney rest and flatten the table. Pull the child's shoulder back if it has fallen forward. (Note that rotation of the hip and shoulder in opposite directions opens or closes a flank incision.)

Approximate the anterior layer of the cut periosteum, beginning posteriorly. At the superior margin, catch it superficially to avoid the intercostal bundle. Then close the combined transversus and internal oblique muscles; begin anteriorly using interrupted synthetic absorbable sutures. Close the external oblique muscle along with the posterior inferior serratus muscle and approximate the latissimus muscles with the same suture material. Do not cinch the sutures too tightly. Approximate the subcutaneous tissue obliquely so that the caudal part of the wound does not sag posteriorly. Close the skin guided by the scratches made originally. Suture the drain to the skin; in young children, do not place a safety pin through it.

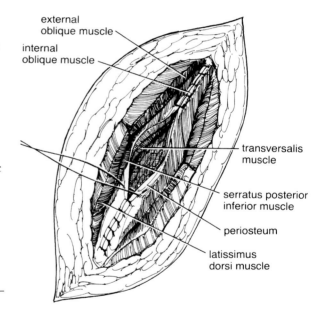

external
oblique muscle
internal
oblique muscle
transversalis
muscle
serratus posterior
inferior muscle
periosteum
latissimus
dorsi muscle

KATSUHIKO UEOKA

Commentary by

Though the transcostal incision is currently only used for a donor nephrectomy in living, related renal transplant in our institution, I believe it would be a good choice for a partial nephrectomy with an extraperitoneal approach in an older patient with bilateral renal tumors. Care must be taken not to injure the pleura during dissecting and cutting the rib. Absence of pneumothrax can be confirmed with chest film after the operation. Also, effort to spare the nerves should be taken when cutting the muscles. The exposure of the transcostal incision is excellent and surgical procedures can be done without limitation and stress. It should be noted, however, that postoperative pain will be quite severe, because the incision is long and muscles are cut. Also bear in mind that misalignment of layers can happen easily during the wound closure.

Chapter 14

Supracostal Incision

This incision placed just above the 12th or the 11th rib is easier to make than a transcostal incision and gives equal or better exposure. This incision allows exposure for nephrectomy and partial nephrectomy as well as reconstructive procedures.

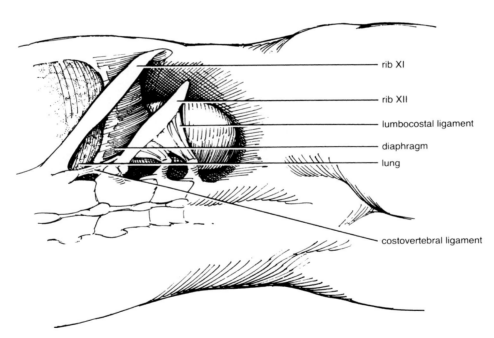

FIGURE 14-1. Anatomic orientation: The opened intercostal space provides wide exposure of the kidney and adrenal gland between the ribs after dividing the intercostal muscles and lumbocostal ligament, followed by detachment of the lateral attachments of the diaphragm. Reserve an incision above the 11th rib for patients with short or absent 12th ribs or for those requiring greater exposure for radical nephrectomy or adrenalectomy.

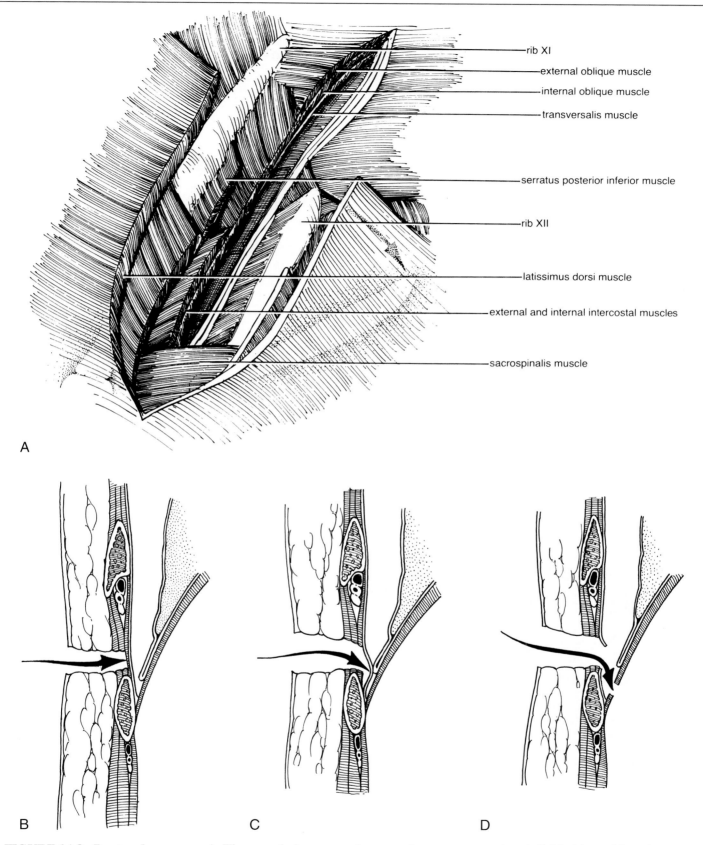

rib XI

external oblique muscle

internal oblique muscle

transversalis muscle

serratus posterior inferior muscle

rib XII

latissimus dorsi muscle

external and internal intercostal muscles

sacrospinalis muscle

A

B   C   D

FIGURE 14-2. Route of exposure: **A,** The muscle layers are shown as they are exposed and divided in making the incision. **B,** The route of the incision is through a skin incision between the 11th and 12th ribs, and then through the latissimus dorsi and serratus posterior inferior muscles and the external intercostal muscles. **C,** The internal intercostals are cut, entering the retrocostal space. By dividing the attachment of the extrapleural fascia to the posterior surface of the rib, the intercostal nerve is left in its own compartment against the rib. **D,** The extrapleural fascia is cut and the diaphragm divided along the posterior body wall.

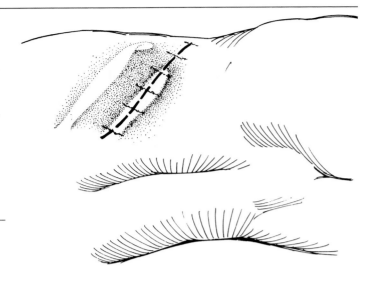

FIGURE 14-3. Position: Use a flank position. If the incision is to be extended to or across the midline, place a folded towel under the chest to displace the child obliquely at an angle of 30 degrees. Incision: Palpate the line of the chosen rib and mark the skin with vertical scratches to facilitate its alignment at the time of closure. Start the skin incision obliquely over the selected rib and extend it anteriorly to its tip. Carry the incision posteriorly to the margin of the sacrospinalis muscle group, exposing the edges of the external oblique and latissimus dorsi muscles.

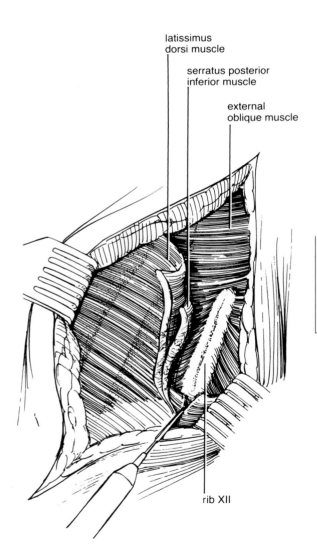

latissimus
dorsi muscle

serratus posterior
inferior muscle

external
oblique muscle

rib XII

FIGURE 14-4. Cut directly down onto the rib through the overlying muscles with the cutting current. This divides the external and internal oblique muscles and the latissimus dorsi muscle, as well as the serratus posterior inferior muscle. Make the cut right *onto* the periosteum. Incise the muscle of the abdominal wall just anterior to the tip of the rib, where its layers coalesce.

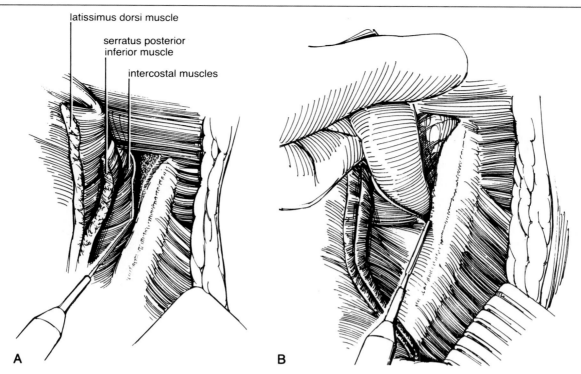

latissimus dorsi muscle

serratus posterior
inferior muscle

intercostal muscles

A   B

FIGURE 14-5. A, Reduce the setting for the cutting current. Divide the external intercostal muscle along the upper margin of the rib. Start at the tip of the rib (which is away from the pleura) by first dividing the muscles for an inch or so. **B,** Insinuate the index finger to displace the extrapleural fascia and the pleura. Progressively divide the inner intercostal muscle against the fingertip, separating it from the rib throughout its length. This leaves the intercostal nerve against the rib.

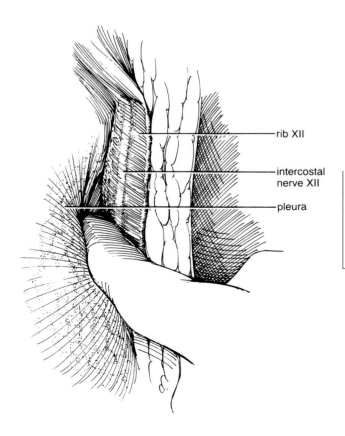

rib XII

intercostal
nerve XII

pleura

FIGURE 14-6. With the fingertip, separate the thin extrapleural fascia from the undersurface of the rib. This fascia splits into two layers to form a tunnel that contains the intercostal nerve (see Fig. 14-2C). Carefully divide its external layer. As the posterior part of the wound is reached, push the pleura down with the index finger, away from the intercostal muscle and the rib.

FIGURE 14-7. Run the pad of the left index finger dorsally along the top edge of the rib until it meets the sharp edge of the costovertebral ligament. Insert slightly opened heavy curved scissors, curve down, over the rib and under the finger. Hug the top of the rib with the scissors to divide the ligament sharply and at the same time avoid the intercostal bundle that lies below the rib above. The lower rib can now pivot on its costovertebral joint (both the 11th and 12th ribs have a single attachment to the vertebra) and be retracted inferiorly to be held with a self-retaining retractor. (To prevent the retractor from becoming levered out of the wound, support the handle with a rolled towel stabilized with towel clips.)

Complete the anterior part of the incision: divide the external and internal oblique muscles and split the transversus abdominis muscle sufficiently to allow the lower rib to be fully retracted downward until it lies alongside the lateral border of the quadratus lumborum muscle. To incise these anterior layers earlier would risk tearing the pleura before it had been freed from the 12th rib.

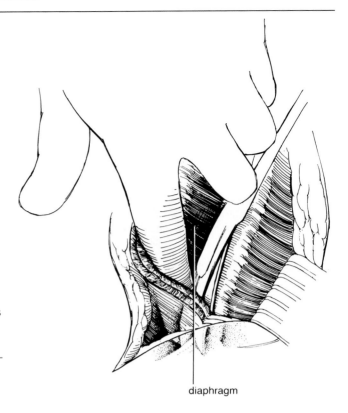

diaphragm

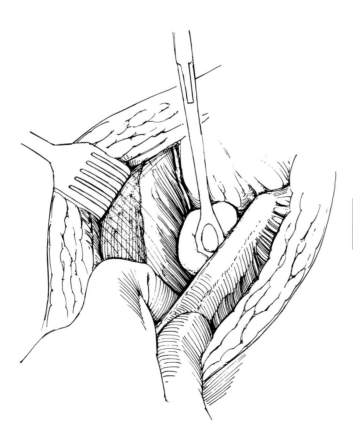

FIGURE 14-8. Push the diaphragm away from the undersurface of the rib and from the lateral arcuate ligament over the quadratus lumborum muscle.

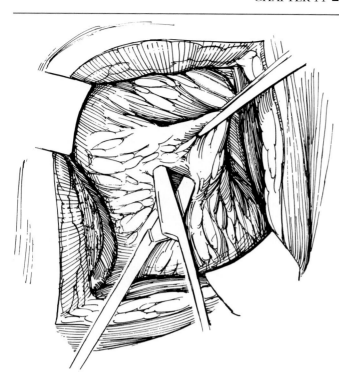

FIGURE 14-9. With the scissors, divide the diaphragm close to its origin. Coagulate those vessels encountered. Stay well away from the pleura, especially as the division is started anteriorly. As the diaphragm is freed, the pleura will now rise out of the way.

For exposure of the renal pedicle, peel the peritoneum from the transversalis fascia with a cherry sponge in one hand while depressing the peritoneum with a lap tape with the other hand. This should be done now even if the incision is to be extended across the midline by dividing one or both rectus muscles, because it is difficult to retract the peritoneum from the body wall once it has been opened.

FIGURE 14-10. Place a retractor, open Gerota's fascia laterally, and expose the kidney through the perirenal fat. Supracostal 11th incision: This incision differs from the supracostal 12th only in that here the pleura extends lower and is more exposed to possible entry during its dissection from the inner aspect of the 12th rib, to which it is somewhat adherent, and during the division of the diaphragm at its origin. Closure: First partially straighten the table, to allow the edges of the wound to come together.

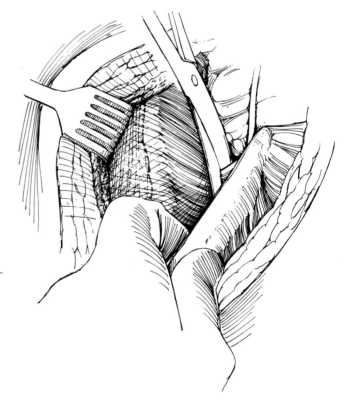

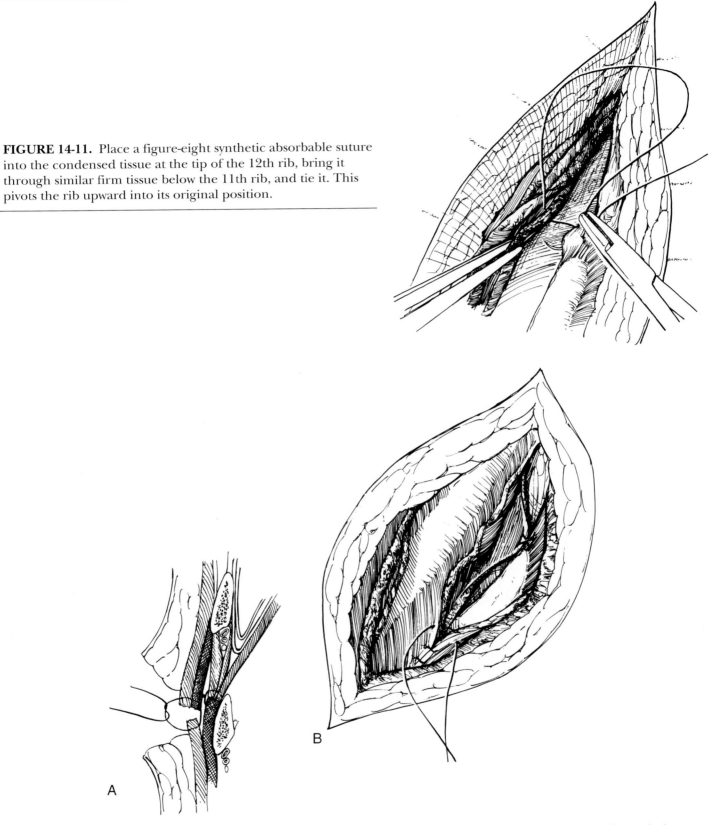

FIGURE 14-11. Place a figure-eight synthetic absorbable suture into the condensed tissue at the tip of the 12th rib, bring it through similar firm tissue below the 11th rib, and tie it. This pivots the rib upward into its original position.

A

B

FIGURE 14-12. A and **B,** Starting posteriorly, pull the detached diaphragm and intercostal muscles out through the intercostal space and stitch them progressively to the edge of the muscles below the incision external to the inferior rib (serratus posterior inferior muscle posteriorly and the latissimus dorsi muscle anteriorly) with interrupted synthetic absorbable sutures. Because this will also close the pleura if it has been inadvertently opened, the anesthetist must expand the lung before the final sutures are tied. Avoid encircling the lower rib with a closure suture—this risks injury to the intercostal vessels in the notch on its inferior surface.

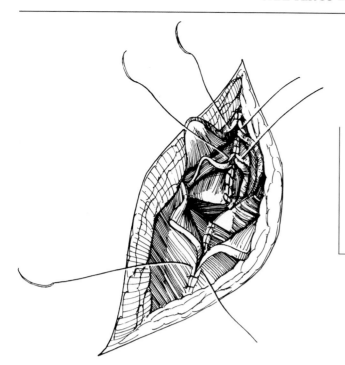

FIGURE 14-13. Stitch the upper margin of the incised latissimus dorsi muscle to the external surface of the serratus muscle, and then to the lower margin of the latissimus dorsi muscle. Place a Penrose drain through a stab wound below the 12th rib to allow the escape of trapped air and exudate, and close the subcutaneous tissue and skin. If the pleura has been entered, place a small catheter in the pleural space and put it under water as a seal during closure.

ANTHONY KHOURY

Commentary by

These three classic incisions (subcostal, transcostal, and supracostal) are effectively described in the preceding chapters. These incisions are associated with potential pitfalls, including injuries to the intercostal neurovascular bundle and entry into the pleura or the peritoneum. The correct approach to these structures is meticulously highlighted in the text and the illustrations to aid the surgeon in avoiding these complications. However, with the evolution of endoscopic and minimally invasive techniques, these incisions have either been abandoned or significantly modified to reduce the morbidity to the child. The miniaturization of endoscopic instruments and the availability of small-caliber energy sources (laser, ultrasound, or lithoclast) have all but eliminated open surgery for stones. In Toronto, the majority of children with ureteral or renal calculi—who are not candidates for, or fail, extracorporeal shock wave lithotripsy—are approached endoscopically. Laser lithotripsy combined with the modern small-caliber, semirigid or flexible ureteroscopes make this an appealing initial option, with percutaneous procedures as a reasonable backup. Open surgery is reserved for the rare child with massive staghorn stones not amenable to sandwich therapy, especially if associated with intrarenal anatomic malformations. The supracostal incision is valuable in these situations to allow complete mobilization of the kidney with excellent control of the pedicle and cooling of the kidney if an anatrophic nephrolithotomy is planned. Occasionally, one encounters an infant with a ureteropelvic junction obstruction and a renal pelvic stone. These stones can be removed during the pyeloplasty whether completed in an open fashion or by laparoscopy.

The selection of incisions for pyeloplasty has also changed significantly in recent years. Many surgeons now prefer a laparoscopic approach, especially in the older child. In infants, open surgery remains the standard, at least temporarily, but I suspect this will evolve with the ongoing progress in instrument development and suturing techniques. The push to minimally invasive surgery has challenged the surgeons who persist with open surgery to use smaller, less morbid incisions such as the muscle-splitting subcostal or dorsal lumbotomy. This has resulted in shorter hospital stays and has reduced the need for postoperative analgesic use.

Although the incisions described in these chapters have been traditionally used for simple and partial nephrectomy, laparoscopic surgery (trans- or retroperitoneal) is rapidly becoming the preferred approach for simple and partial nephrectomy. There are also emerging reports on the use of laparoscopy for surgery for Wilms' tumors in centers where preoperative chemotherapy is routinely used, leading to a smaller, firmer tumor. However, the preferred approach to renal tumors remains the anterior chevron incision (see Chapter 10). This incision provides superior exposure to both kidneys over the midline incision and is very well tolerated by children.

MARK BELLINGER

The supracostal approach to the kidney in pediatric patients is primarily useful for surgical exposure of lesions of the upper pole and posterior aspect of the kidney.

In contrast, the most common approach to lesions of the ureteropelvic junction is through an anterior muscle-splitting incision beginning at the tip of a rib, usually the 12th or 11th rib. In this approach, the incision is made in a radial direction directly off the tip of the rib and in line with it, which usually permits preservation of the intercostal neurovascular bundle. This incision is generally carried out with the patient in the supine position, using a small inflatable lift or rolled towel under the back to elevate the upper abdomen and lower rib cage. In larger patients, the kidney rest of the operating table may be slightly elevated.

When a supracostal approach is to be used, the patient is placed in the lateral flank position, with the kidney rest elevated in older children, or using a rolled towel or inflatable kidney rest in infants. The patient should be rotated slightly off of the true lateral position toward the back, exposing a bit more of the upper abdomen than would be possible in the true lateral position. The skin incision is made directly over the distal 1 to 2 cm of the rib, and carried in a radial fashion off of the tip of the rib as in the anterior muscle-splitting approach. In most cases, a small incision will suffice as the short supracostal extension will allow improved exposure of the upper pole of the kidney over what is possible with an anterior extraperitoneal approach.

The deeper incision through the muscle layers is now made with no attempt made to split the muscle layers in the direction of their fibers. The incision, using cutting current electrocautery with a needle electrode, is taken directly onto the surface of the rib. The anterior incision is then taken down through the external and internal oblique muscles to the transversus abdominis muscle. This muscle and the transversalis fascia are opened by passing a small curved clamp through these layers off the tip of the rib into the retroperitoneal space, being careful to avoid the peritoneum. Once the retroperitoneal space is entered, this opening is enlarged using finger dissection or a pair of peanut dissectors until a finger can be inserted in the retroperitoneal space to sweep the peritoneum in an anterior direction away from the overlying muscle. The transversalis layer can now be split safely toward, but avoiding, the peritoneum. The posterior aspect of the incision can now be opened, disconnecting the muscles from the superior aspect of the rib using the cutting current. Once the incision is opened, Gerota's fascia is identified and opened. The surgeon should be particularly careful in younger children to avoid the peritoneum. Once Gerota's fascia is opened and the kidney exposed, a self-retaining retractor is placed. If enlargement of the incision becomes necessary, either an anterior or a supracostal extension of the incision, or both, may be used.

Chapter 15

Dorsal Lumbotomy

UNILATERAL POSTERIOR LUMBOTOMY

Unilateral posterior lumbotomy provides less access to the kidney than flank approaches, but it has many uses in pediatric urologic surgery including pyeloplasty, open renal biopsy, removal of small kidneys, simultaneous bilateral renal operations, large pelvic stones, and stones fixed in the upper or midureter (rarely indicated if endoscopic equipment is available). It is not suitable for malignancies or malpositioned kidneys. If the incision is made somewhat transversely, the disadvantage of a scar resulting from crossing Langer's lines may be obviated without sacrifice of exposure.

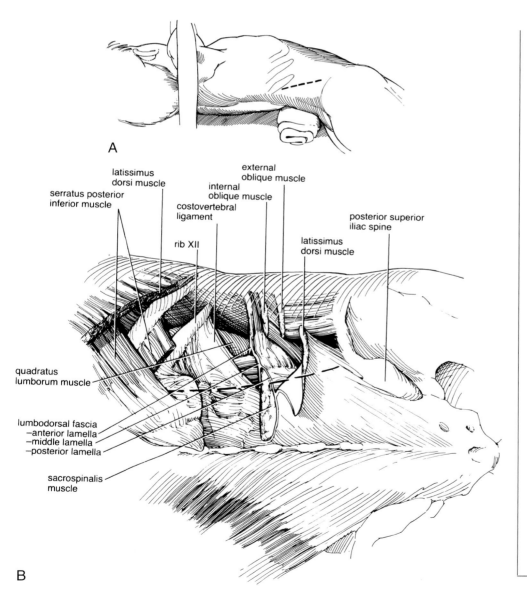

A

latissimus dorsi muscle

serratus posterior inferior muscle

internal oblique muscle

external oblique muscle

costovertebral ligament

rib XII

posterior superior iliac spine

latissimus dorsi muscle

quadratus lumborum muscle

lumbodorsal fascia
—anterior lamella
—middle lamella
—posterior lamella

sacrospinalis muscle

B

FIGURE 15-1. Instruments: For larger children, provide a laminectomy retractor (Sheldon or Lilienthal) and Gil-Vernet retractors, as well as long curved retractors. **A,** Position: After tracheal intubation and insertion of a urethral catheter, place the child in a modified lateral position, rotated forward 30 to 45 degrees. Flexing the table puts tension on the muscles of the back. A prone position is an alternative, placing longitudinal rolls that do not compress the chest and abdomen. (For renal biopsy, the lateral position without flexion with the knees bent keeps the kidney from falling away from the surgeon and is less limiting on respiration.) Incision: Make an oblique skin incision more or less along Langer's lines, one that extends from the angle of the 12th rib, where the lateral border of the sacrospinalis muscle crosses the lower margin of the rib, to the iliac crest at a point one third of the distance from the anterosuperior iliac spine to the spinal process. **B,** View the landmarks in relation to the line of incision (dashed line), especially the iliac crest, the 12th rib, and the vertebral spinous processes.

Continued

FIGURE 15-1, cont'd. C, Make the approach anterior to the sacrospinalis and quadratus lumborum muscles through the lumbodorsal fascia (dotted line). Incision: Follow obliquely more or less along the skin lines (Langer's lines) that extend from the angle of the 12th rib, where the lateral border of the sacrospinalis muscle crosses the lower margin of the rib (in the child this is 2 to 3 cm from the spinal processes). Continue down to the iliac crest to a point one third of the distance from the anterior superior iliac spine to the spinal processes.

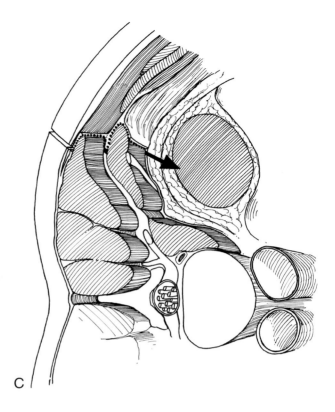

C

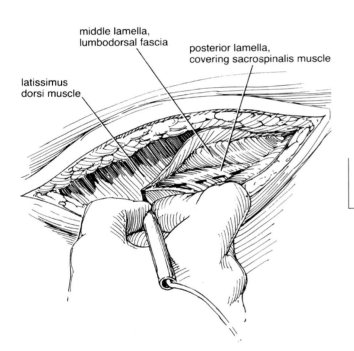

middle lamella, lumbodorsal fascia

posterior lamella, covering sacrospinalis muscle

latissimus dorsi muscle

FIGURE 15-2. Free the subcutaneous tissue and make a vertical incision in the posterior projections of the latissimus dorsi and posterior inferior serratus muscles.

FIGURE 15-3. Divide the posterior lamella of the lumbodorsal fascia in the line of the incision, to expose the sacrospinalis muscle.

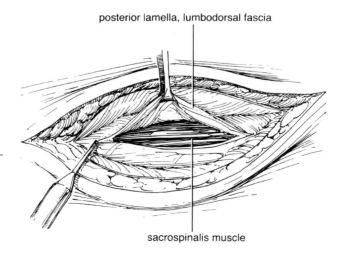

posterior lamella, lumbodorsal fascia

sacrospinalis muscle

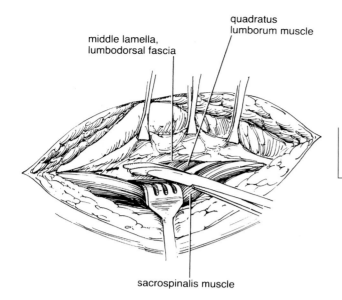

middle lamella,
lumbodorsal fascia

quadratus
lumborum muscle

sacrospinalis muscle

FIGURE 15-4. Elevate the lateral edge of the cut lumbodorsal fascia with Allis forceps and draw the lateral edge of the sacrospinalis muscle medially.

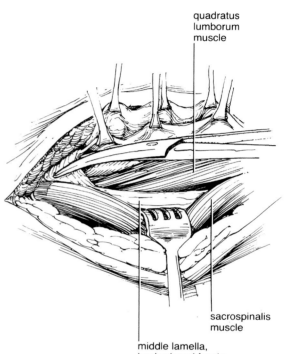

quadratus
lumborum
muscle

sacrospinalis
muscle

middle lamella,
lumbodorsal fascia

FIGURE 15-5. Bluntly dissect the lateral margin of the sacrospinalis muscle to expose the subcostal vessels and the costovertebral ligament. Under vision, divide this ligament with scissors. Incise the exposed fused middle and anterior lamella of the lumbar fascia about 1 cm under the edge of the quadratus lumborum muscle, down to the iliac crest. Watch out for the iliohypogastric nerve under the fascia during exposure and closure.

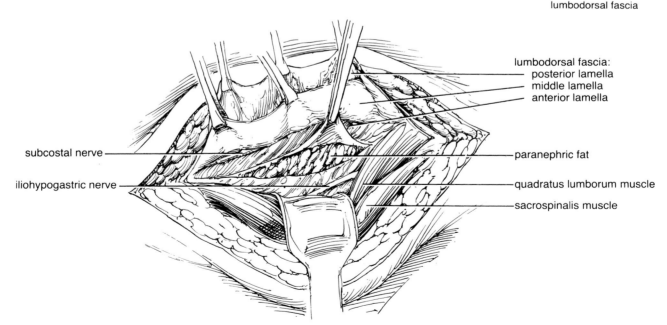

lumbodorsal fascia:
posterior lamella
middle lamella
anterior lamella

subcostal nerve

iliohypogastric nerve

paranephric fat

quadratus lumborum muscle

sacrospinalis muscle

FIGURE 15-6. Retract the quadratus lumborum muscle dorsally and expose the anterior lamella of the lumbodorsal fascia. Incise this lamella between the subcostal and iliohypogastric nerves that course obliquely across it. Extend the incision in the lumbodorsal fascia cephalad to divide the costovertebral ligament and allow upward rotation of the 12th rib.

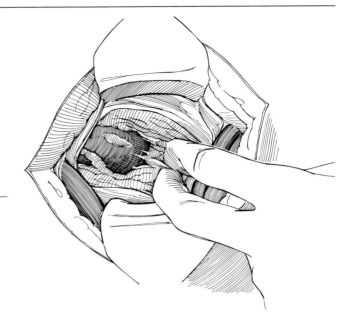

FIGURE 15-7. Pick up Gerota's fascia between two forceps at the cranial end of the wound and incise it. Extend the opening caudad with two fingers. For exposure, have your assistant hold deep Deaver retractors, or insert a laminectomy retractor.

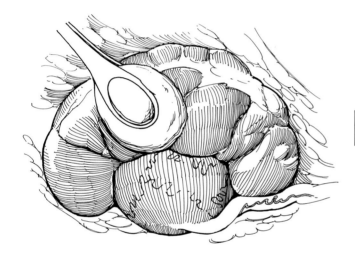

FIGURE 15-8. Pick up the ureter just below the kidney on a tape and begin renal dissection at the hilum.

FIGURE 15-9. For pyelolithotomy, insert a Gil-Vernet retractor to control the position of the kidney, open the hilum, and assist in removal of the stone. After removal of the stone, close the pyelotomy with fine absorbable sutures.

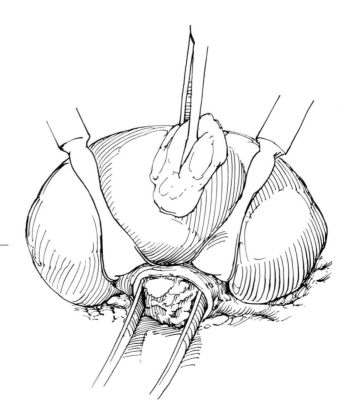

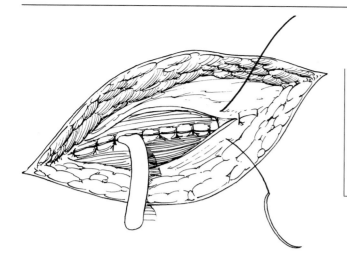

FIGURE 15-10. Insert a Penrose drain. Close the incision with 2-0 or 3-0 synthetic absorbable sutures in the two good layers of the lumbodorsal fascia. (The middle layer is tenuous and closure risks catching the iliohypogastric nerve.) Tie the sutures in the second layer after the kidney rest has been lowered. If the latissimus dorsi and posterior inferior serratus muscles were divided, reunite them with sutures. Approximate the subcutaneous tissue and skin.

Extended Dorsal Lumbotomy

When exposure is limited by the 12th rib above and the iliac crest below, mobilize the 12th rib: Divide the costovertebral ligament and resect a 2-cm segment from the rib posterior to the angle (see Chapter 13), keeping close to the rib to avoid the pleura. The subcostal (12th) nerve and the iliohypogastric nerve now cross the incision. Free them, preserving at least the iliohypogastric nerve. Insert a self-retaining retractor and open Gerota's fascia vertically.

BILATERAL POSTERIOR LUMBOTOMY

For simultaneous nephrectomy in children undergoing renal transplantation, or for bilateral ureteropelvic junction repair, a bilateral posterior lumbotomy is recommended.

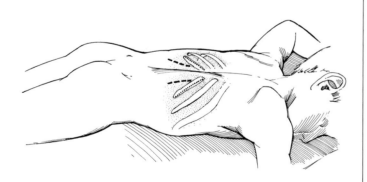

FIGURE 15-11. Position: Place the child prone with bolster support under shoulders and pelvis to avoid compression of the chest and abdomen and to allow diaphragmatic breathing. Flex the table slightly. One surgeon and one assistant on each side of the table allow for simultaneous exposure. Make oblique skin incisions (dashed lines). Start each of them at the angle of the 12th rib where the lateral border of the sacrospinalis muscle crosses the lower margin of the rib (approximately 5 to 6 cm from the spinal processes). Continue down to the iliac crest to a point one third of the distance from the anterosuperior iliac spine to the spinal process. Proceed as described for unilateral dorsal lumbotomy, but arrange the self-retaining retractor to compress the muscles medially.

RICARDO GONZÁLEZ

Commentary by

Before adopting laparoscopic surgery as the preferred approach to pyeloplasty in all age groups, I used the posterior lumbotomy approach almost exclusively for pyeloplasty. I did things somewhat differently from the description in this chapter. Because of the limited exposure it is imperative to be certain of the location of the obstruction and that the kidney is normally rotated. For this reason, I always position the patient prone (even for unilateral cases) and start by inserting a needle in the renal pelvis and performing an antegrade pyelogram. I prefer a transverse incision in the skin and then proceed as in the figures. I do not routinely divide the costovertebral ligament. Once the lower pole of the kidney is identified, it helps to retract it in a cephalad and lateral direction. This maneuver opens the angle between the kidney and the ureter and aids in its identification. Identification of the ureter below the ureteropelvic junction is the first (and often difficult) step in a pyeloplasty using this approach. In rare cases, in which the incision needs to be extended, I prefer to do so toward the flank rather than with a rib resection. I find the dorsal lumbotomy incision also useful for open renal biopsies but not very useful for stone surgery.

PATRICK C. CARTWRIGHT

The dorsal lumbotomy is an excellent incision to gain access to the posterior kidney in children. This has been the standard approach to pyeloplasty in our practice for children 8 years or younger, while older or more thickly muscled children would be considered for a flank or laparoscopic approach. Recovery is quick due to the muscle split with a dorsal approach and it is also good cosmetically.

We generally place the child prone with two longitudinal chest rolls and the table flexed substantially to accentuate the space for dissection. The skin incision follows Langer's lines, usually 1 cm below the 12th rib. To determine the exact position of the incision, it is very helpful to place fingers at the posterior midline and push skin and muscle anteriorly and laterally. This will create a subtle, but distinct, angled longitudinal skin depression where the lateral edge of the sacro-spinalis muscle meets the fused lumbodorsal fascia. I mark this line on the patient. The incision is then split around this line with one third being medial and two thirds lateral to it. Once the skin is incised and fat dissected away from fascia, this maneuver is repeated at the fascial level to determine just where to make the fascial incision, that being just along the edge of the sacrospinalis muscle and through the fused lumbodorsal fascia. I find that the costovertebral ligament can be left intact in many children.

To expose the kidney, I prefer handheld Deaver retractors over fixed retraction as the exposure is ever-changing. Gil-Vernet or vein retractors may be useful to place in the renal sinus and roll the pelvis more posteriorly. Traction sutures into the pelvis and early needle decompression of the particularly large pelvis will facilitate exposure in harder cases. In a difficult circumstance, where more exposure is needed for bleeding, the skin incision may be quickly extended laterally and the fascia may be opened in the same direction by creating a T off the original fascial incision. This will yield much more exposure and mobility of the entire kidney.

Fascial closure can be done in a single layer for most children. As with opening, nerves running along the anterior surface of the psoas muscle must be noted and avoided. The middle lamella of lumbodorsal fascia is often wispy, and I do not attempt to include it in the closure.

Chapter 16

Repair of Pleural Tear

For inadvertent tears of the pleura, have the anesthetist inflate the lung before wound closure to allow identification of a defect. If perforated, have the lung deflated to draw the margin of the lung away from the site. Through the tear, insert a small red Robinson catheter into the pleural space. Start a running 3-0 or 4-0 plain catgut suture by tying it just beyond the anterior end of the pleural defect. Continue it around the catheter and tie it beyond the other end of the defect, leaving the catheter in place for later reinflation. Alternatively, for greater support, include the diaphragm on one side and the intercostal muscles on the other, avoiding the intercostal vessels and nerve.

For small defects, have the anesthetist inflate the lung while you aspirate pleural air through the catheter with a large syringe; then tie the suture in the pleura as the catheter is withdrawn.

For larger defects, leave the catheter in the pleura (taking care not to position a Penrose drain near it) until the wound is entirely closed. Place the end of the catheter under water while the anesthetist fully inflates the lung. Remove the catheter when bubbling stops and complete the closure of the wound. In the recovery room, expose a portable chest film to check for pulmonary inflation.

If there is any possibility that the lung itself has been perforated, do not remove the catheter but place it under water in a sterile vacuum system (Pleur-evac).

Hemopneumothorax results from injury to both the underlying lung and an intercostal vessel in the chest wall. Insert a large right-angle tube, with extra holes that will lie within the chest. Fasten the tube to the chest wall with a nonabsorbable suture that closes the skin firmly around the tube and also holds it so that it cannot be withdrawn inadvertently. Place a strip of Vaseline gauze around the tube for a seal and connect it to continuous drainage using a closed drainage system. Make a portable upright chest radiograph to be sure the lung is expanded and all fluid has been evacuated from the pleura. When no air has been recovered in the suction bottle for 8 hours, remove the tube.

Commentary by
JAMES M. BETTS

Exposure is key to closing a pleural tear. Increase the size of the incision, if necessary. It is important to coordinate work with your anesthesia team for proper lung insufflations and deflations. When using the technique described, closure of the pleura is best facilitated using either vicryl or polydioxanone sutures.

Chapter 17

Splenorrhaphy and Splenectomy

SPLENORRHAPHY FOLLOWING INTRAOPERATIVE INJURY

Intraoperative injury of the spleen usually is the result of capsular avulsion by forcible retraction of the spleen away from the peritoneal surface, where it is held by the splenomental fold that lies between the greater omentum and the medial aspect of the lower pole of the spleen. Splenectomy should be avoided, especially in children; splenorrhaphy or segmental splenectomy usually are achievable alternatives.

Pack the tear with hemostatic gauze, and hold it firmly with a dry lap pad. Avoid using a retractor, which will usually make the tear worse or start a new one. (If the bleeding is brisk and time is needed for repair, open the lesser sac and compress the tail of the pancreas containing the splenic vessels.) Mobilize the spleen by incising the lienorenal ligament to be able to deliver the spleen and tail of the pancreas into the wound. The splenic vessels now may be readily compressed, and the splenic wound itself can be tamponaded and repaired under direct vision.

Cover the defect with hemostatic gauze or omentum. Then place a row of 3-0 synthetic absorbable mattress sutures over it. Bolsters of hemostatic gauze inserted under the loops of suture decrease cutting into the capsule. For gross injury, stretch polyglycolic acid knitted mesh over the spleen and sew the edges of the mesh together either to encase the entire spleen or to cover one pole as a cap (see Chapter 25). Resort to splenectomy only if all conservative measures fail.

SPLENECTOMY

The vasculature of the spleen, somewhat like that of the kidney, allows segmental splenectomy. Selective ligation is possible because the splenic artery, before it reaches the spleen, gives off a superior polar artery supplying the upper segment of the spleen. Near the hilus, the artery divides again into two branches going to the middle and lower polar segments. By preliminary ligation of one of these vessels, a segment of spleen may be removed along a relatively avascular plane.

For partial splenectomy, a Frazier neurosurgical suction tip helps in identification and clipping of intrasplenic vessels.

The argon beam coagulator may be used for parenchymatous dissection, although blunt dissection with pressure hemostasis is usually adequate. The splenic vein pursues a tortuous course above the pancreas, allowing inadvertent ligation at one of the anterior bends. An accessory spleen may be encountered, usually with an independent blood supply, and should be preserved.

Procedure: With the right hand, gently retract the greater omentum and transverse colon inferiorly. With the left hand, reach over the top of the spleen and rotate it anteriorly and medially. First incise the attachments to the peritoneum and then those to the kidney, diaphragm, and colon.

Slide the left hand more laterally to hook the fingertips under the medial edge of the peritoneum that was just divided. (Avoid traction injury to the splenic capsule or vessels.) Incise the posterior parietal peritoneum superiorly and inferiorly to the pancreas and release the final attachments of the splenocolic and splenodiaphragmatic ligaments. Place one or two lap tapes into the bed to ensure hemostasis and to keep the spleen from dropping back into the wound. Identify the gastrosplenic ligament and the short gastric vessels where the spleen abuts the stomach. Be sure to work high on the greater curvature of the stomach in a caudad to cephalad direction to expose and avoid tearing the most cephalad short gastric vessels. Doubly clamp the short gastric vessels sequentially, divide them, and have your assistant tie them beneath the clamps. Be sure not to clamp or ligate any part of the stomach.

Lift the spleen with the left hand. Hold the tail of the pancreas out of the way with the left thumb and index finger during dissection of the vessels under direct vision and during clamping. Dissect the artery from the vein before it divides into its branches. Clamp and ligate the artery first so that contraction of the spleen gives the patient a transfusion. Clamp each vessel with three clamps. If the pedicle is small it may be clamped in toto but with some risk of an arteriovenous fistula.

Cut between the distal clamps. Tie beneath the first clamp with a #1 synthetic absorbable suture and remove the clamp. Repeat for the second clamp. Remove the packs from the bed. If any bleeders are seen, oversew them with 4-0 synthetic absorbable sutures. Drainage is not necessary.

POSTOPERATIVE PROBLEMS

Because of the risk of overwhelming infection, administer pneumococcal polysaccharide vaccine and penicillin.

BARRY KOGAN

Commentary by

Intraoperative splenic injuries in children are even rarer than in adults, perhaps because of the relatively thicker splenic capsule or the pliability of pediatric tissues. When they do occur it is nearly always due to limited exposure of the kidney at the time of transperitoneal nephrectomy. Though not substantiated by data, it appears that this may be even less common in the era of laparoscopic nephrectomy.

Nonetheless, the spleen is of great importance in preventing infection with encapsulated bacteria and, as noted previously, every effort should be made to save the spleen in children unless the injury is severe. The techniques noted, including use of the argon beam coagulator, harmonic scalpel, hemostatic gauze, and, very rarely, partial splenectomy, are all useful. When the spleen must be removed, immunization for *Haemophilus influenzae* and meningococcus should be done as soon as possible.

JAMES M. BETTS

Commentary by

When approaching the control of the splenic vessels, at the level of the tail of the pancreas, the grasping of the tail and vessels, or compression of the vessels at that location, is very effective in gaining control of splenic bleeding. Partial splenectomy can be extremely challenging. The use of Vicryl mesh to "encase" a fragmented but perfused spleen can be successful, coupled with the ligation of any individual bleeding vessels that can be readily identified. Fibrin glue can also be instilled into fractures and into oozing sites to gain control of blood loss. When suturing is attempted, using bolsters of Surgicel soaked in thrombin or gelfoam soaked in thrombin placed over the bleeding lacerations, or fractures, can often facilitate the control of bleeding from those sites.

Chapter 18

Repair of Flank Incisional Hernia

Incisional hernias appearing postoperatively may be the result of a wound infection, malnutrition, postoperative sepsis, use of a vertical incision, use of absorbable sutures, or not placing retention sutures when indicated, and also excessive postoperative coughing. Realize that bulging of the flank after lateral incisions is more often from denervation of the muscles than from herniation of the peritoneum. Thus, repair would be done because of cosmetic indications or local discomfort; the risk of intestinal incarceration is small. Provide prophylactic antibiotics.

AUGMENTED REPAIR OF LARGE DEFECTS USING SYNTHETIC MATERIALS

Clear the fascial surfaces of fat and proceed as described in Figures 18-1 to 18-5. If possible, close the peritoneum separately with 3-0 or 4-0 synthetic absorbable sutures. Cut a piece of polypropylene mesh to shape, making it large enough to overlap the edges by 1 to 2 cm. Suture the mesh to the aponeurosis with interrupted 2-0 or 3-0 non-absorbable sutures. If there is any question about asepsis

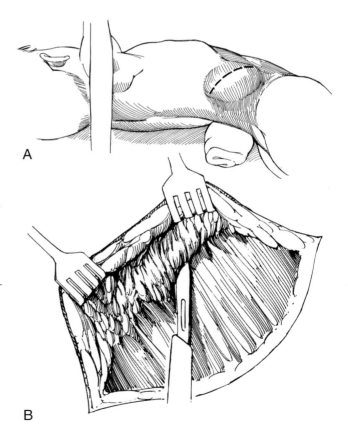

FIGURE 18-1. Position: Lateral or oblique, depending on the site of the hernia. **A**, Incision: Make an elliptical incision to excise the scar. **B**, Extend the incision through the subcutaneous layer circumferentially. Expose normal fascia away from the defect first, as your assistant elevates the wound edges with rake retractors. Mobilize the fascial flaps and define the area of the defect, but do not open the hernia sac prematurely. Hemostasis is important.

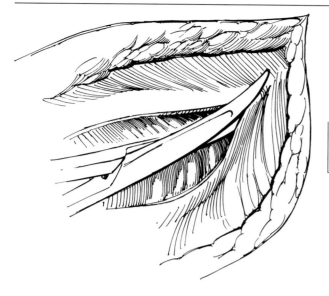

FIGURE 18-2. Deliberately open the sac, composed of attenuated fascia and peritoneum. If the bowel is adherent, free it carefully. Trim the edges of the defect to reach intact fascia.

FIGURE 18-3. Imbricate the fascia in a side-over-side (vest-over-pants) technique with heavy synthetic absorbable sutures placed as interrupted mattress stitches. Do this by entering the upper fascia well back from its edge, then pass through the lower fascia nearer its edge. Exit from the lower flap 1 cm lateral to the stitch; then exit from the upper flap 1 cm lateral to the original site of entry. Clamp the ends of the suture. Repeat placing these stitches 1 cm apart for the length of the defect. Tie them sequentially, as your assistant keeps tension on the rest.

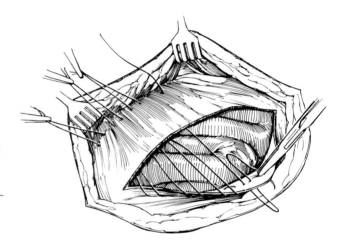

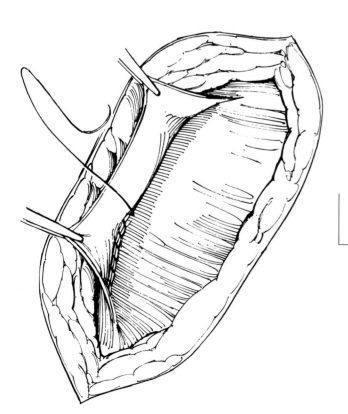

FIGURE 18-4. Run a #1 synthetic absorbable suture under the flap just below the first row of sutures. Take care not to penetrate the fascia and catch the underlying bowel in the stitch.

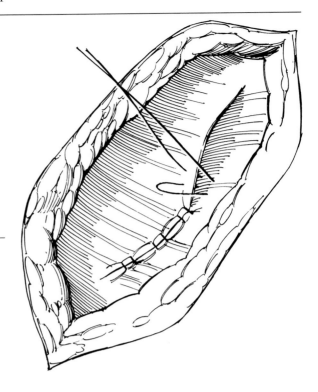

FIGURE 18-5. Place a row of interrupted, figure-eight synthetic absorbable sutures between the upper flap and the adjacent lower (posterior) flap. Insert two suction drains in the subcutaneous space but do not place sutures in that layer. Close the skin with interrupted silk sutures. An abdominal binder may be placed over the dressing.

or hemostasis do not use polypropylene mesh, for should the wound become infected, this mesh would have to be removed. However, tantalum mesh can be substituted if asepsis is in doubt. A stronger repair is obtained by placing the mesh under the fascial layer rather than on top of it. The mesh should extend well beyond the edges of the fascia. Close the subcutaneous tissues and skin over suction drains.

Alternatively, if you were able to close the defect edge to edge with interrupted sutures, strengthen the suture line by running a firmly placed monofilament nylon suture back and forth both vertically and horizontally to "darn" the

defect. (This last technique does encourage closure with tension, which is associated with recurrence. If used at all, place relaxing fascial incisions well lateral to the defect.)

POSTOPERATIVE PROBLEMS

Infection is the greatest concern and must be approached aggressively, both prophylactically and therapeutically. Recurrence of the herniation is not common, but bulging of the area may persist from weakness of the muscle layers.

JAMES M. BETTS

Commentary by

The use of imbricating, or mattress, sutures can be an effective closure method. Simple, interrupted sutures through the fascial and muscle layers, with close, but not strangulating approximation of the tissue planes, are another way to repair the defect. Each individual fascial plane, with its accompanying muscle layer, is closed separately.

A closed Jackson-Pratt type suction drain can be placed in the subcutaneous space if fluid accumulation is expected. The use of synthetic materials should be only as a last resort, when there is tissue loss and a primary repair is not possible. In the pediatric age group, somatic growth is to be expected, and, with a synthetic graft in the place of the defect, with time and growth of the individual, the synthetic material will not "stretch" as such, and a recurrence is probable. "Darning" the wound with a nonabsorbable suture would not be advisable, as the strength would not be enhanced and the amount of foreign material could be a nidus for infection. This "fixed" point of the repair is susceptible to pulling away from the surrounding tissue, with a recurrent hernia resulting.

Chapter 19

Laparoscopic Renal Surgery

LAPAROSCOPIC NEPHRECTOMY

Weight and size permitting, the laparoscopic approach to removal of the nonfunctional renal moiety in children is the preferred method. It offers well-documented advantages in reducing recovery time and the use of postoperative analgesia as well as excellent cosmesis. A transperitoneal or a retroperitoneoscopic approach may be used. Both convey advantages over the open approach in which the retroperitoneal approach is used unless contraindicated.

RETROPERITONEOSCOPIC SIMPLE NEPHRECTOMY

This technique affords adequate and familiar exposure and preserves the principles of open retroperitoneal surgery. In the rare necessity of an open conversion the patient is properly positioned.

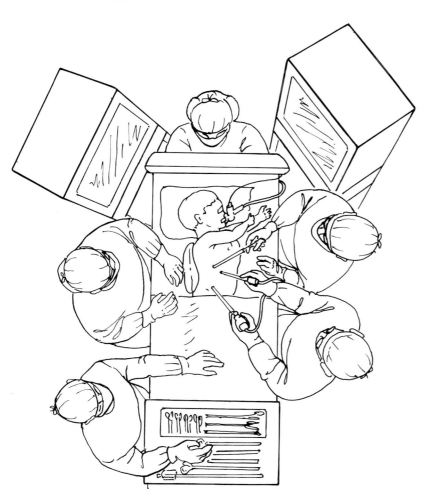

FIGURE 19-1. Laparoscopic environment: The patient is placed in the lateral decubitus position, exposing the involved side as in positioning for an open simple nephrectomy. The operator and first assistant stand on the abdominal side of the patient. Monitors are positioned opposite the surgeons and second assistant (if present) and surgical technician. Extremities and areas of pressure are appropriately padded, and either the kidney rest is used in combination with table flexion or a "bump" can be used for the smaller patient (<15 kg) to achieve maximal distance between the anterior superior iliac crest and inferior aspect of the 12th rib.

FIGURE 19-2. A transverse, 1-cm incision is made at the
costovertebral angle 1 cm inferior to the 12th rib and 1 cm
lateral to the paraspinous muscles. Using a blunt hemostat,
the subcutaneous space is developed until a level of tactile
resistance is encountered at the lumbodorsal fascia.
Alternatively, the surgeon may confirm the correct depth
visually with adequate retraction. The hemostat is then used to
bluntly enter the retroperitoneal space anterior to the psoas
muscle and posterior to Gerota's fascia. Note: no resistance is
encountered except at the lumbodorsal fascia. The entry site is
widened by spreading the hemostat. A blunt forceps is used to
insert the balloon dilation device described in Figure 19-3.

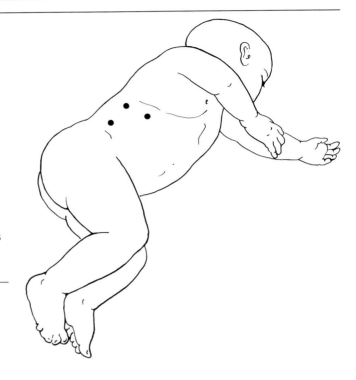

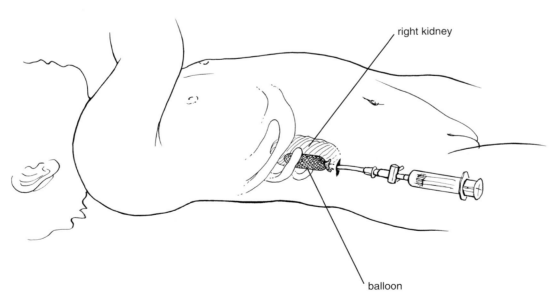

right kidney

balloon

FIGURE 19-3. Balloon dissection device: The finger from a green-colored "indicator" glove is securely fastened to the
distal end of an 8-F feeding tube. Size 0 silk ties may be used to secure the glove finger. Using a 60-mL Luer Lock syringe
and a three-way stopcock, the balloon is tested for its ability to hold air and have the air removed without difficulty. If
there is resistance to either, the process is repeated until the balloon is safely inflated and deflated. Saline may be used,
but air works just as well in the pediatric patient.

 Proper placement is confirmed by the ease with which the air or saline is placed and the appearance of a bulge
anterior and medial. The volume needed is variable. Adequate space creation is achieved when the volume is such that
the balloon device is visible as a mass anterior, medial, and slightly inferior to the tip of the 12th rib.

Accessing the Retroperitoneal Space

Port placement is initiated after a balloon dissection device is used to enlarge the potential retroperitoneal space. A volume between 150 and 300 mL is usually adequate and the balloon should be left inflated approximately 3 minutes to establish the space and achieve hemostasis.

A 5-mm trochar is inserted bluntly and used for CO_2 insufflation to 12 mmHg. The lens can then be inserted confirming dilation of the correct space bordered posteriorly by the paraspinous and psoas muscles and anteriorly by Gerota's fascia and the peritoneum. After confirmation of correct placement, the trochar can be secured with a nylon suture to prevent migration and loss of pneumoretroperitoneum. It is also helpful at this stage to use the distal aspect of the port to increase the space posterior to Gerota's fascia, using it for visually directed blunt dissection, and to gently reflect the peritoneum more medially. Once the space has been enlarged with blunt dissection, the surgeon may proceed with visually directed placement of the second and third ports.

The second port (3, 5, or 10 mm) is placed medial and inferior to the tip of the 12th rib (approximately at the anterior axillary line) and medial to the peritoneal reflection. The light from the lens is used to illuminate the abdominal wall to avoid cutaneous vessels. Local anesthetic with epinephrine is used to control any bleeding that may result from port placement and the needle is used to confirm proper orientation before the trochar is passed. The third port (3 or 5 mm) is placed approximately at the mid-axillary line 1.5 cm superior to the iliac crest, using the same technique of visually directed placement used in securing the second access site. Correct port placement will allow better range of motion and ease of dissection by avoiding port crowding that can be experienced when working in the limited space of the retroperitoneum.

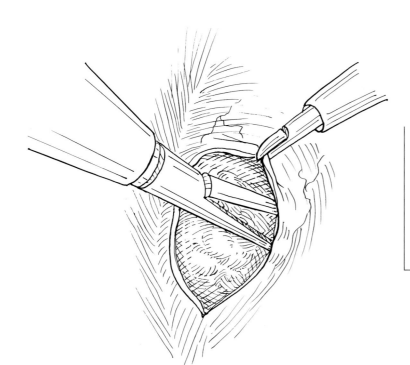

FIGURE 19-4. Standing on the involved side (camera direction opposite), the surgeon first mobilizes the lower pole and attempts identification of hilar vessels posteriorly. This initial portion of the procedure can usually be facilitated before entering Gerota's fascia. If the kidney is extremely dilated, it may be necessary to decompress the pelvis or large cyst before adequate traction and countertraction can be used to facilitate proper identification of the planes of dissection.

FIGURE 19-5. The renal artery is first identified
posteriorly and dissected for application of clips: two
for the patient side and one for the specimen side.
After safe ligation and division of the renal artery,
the technique is repeated for dividing the renal
vein. It is occasionally necessary to divide the ureter
before hilar dissection to gain sufficient traction
and exposure. The remainder of the dissection
can then be completed using the harmonic scalpel
or electrocautery for smaller vessels, taking care
to identify any accessory arteries or veins that may
require formal ligation and division. When the
specimen is fully mobilized and ready for removal,
the second port site is used.

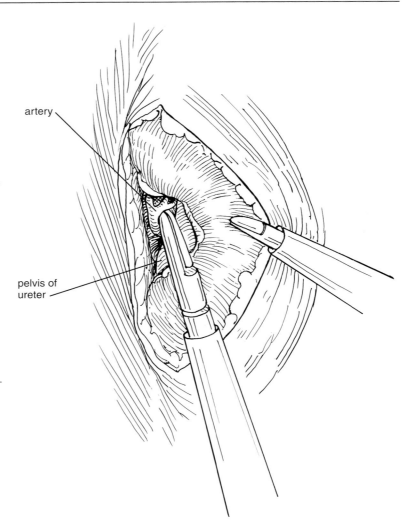

artery

pelvis of
ureter

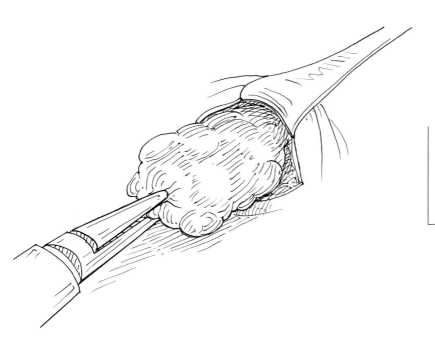

FIGURE 19-6. It may be necessary to lengthen
the fascial incision to allow removal. Alternatively,
a specimen bag can be used to "catch" and
morcellate the specimen. Closure of the fascia at
the second port site is undertaken and the first
and third port site skin incision is closed.

TRANSPERITONEAL TECHNIQUE

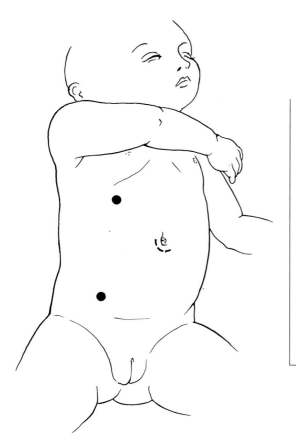

FIGURE 19-7. Place the child with the flank of the involved side elevated at a 30-degree angle to facilitate exposure after reflecting the colon. Insert a 10-mm camera port above the umbilicus and create a pneumoperitoneum. Under vision, insert one 5-mm port about 2 cm below the costal margin in the midclavicular line and a second port above the iliac crest in the anterior axillary line. If liver retraction may be needed, insert a 2-mm port in the epigastrium.

Dissection is initiated by incising sharply in the avascular plane along the white line of Toldt, exposing Gerota's fascia. The ureter is identified and divided as distal as possible. If reflux is present, the ureter is tied with an absorbable suture before dividing. The harmonic scalpel is used to cauterize the vessels and tethering fascia.

Pass the specimen into the 10-mm sheath and remove it with a grasper. Remove a larger specimen through an enlarged umbilical port. Reduce the pneumoperitoneum and look for bleeding. Close the fascia with an absorbable suture and the skin with a running subcuticular absorbable suture. Apply Steri-Strips and a clear occlusive dressing.

LAPAROSCOPIC RESECTION OF NONFUNCTIONING SEGMENT

In patients with complete ureteral duplication and an upper pole, nonfunctioning segment, a partial nephrectomy may be indicated.

A retroperitoneal approach is possible but is usually avoided in favor of the transperitoneal technique in patients requiring resection of the duplicated, dilated ureteral segment. For simple excision of the upper pole with a partial ureterectomy, the extraperitoneal approach can be used. In small children, a transperitoneal approach is preferred over a retroperitoneal one, in spite of a greater incidence of intra-abdominal problems.

Retroperitoneal Technique: Upper Pole

Retroperitoneal access is established as described. For patients in which the involved ureter may not be apparent because of significant size discrepancy, a ureteral catheter may be placed in the normal ureter, causing minimal delay in the procedure and low additional morbidity.

The involved ureter is identified and mobilized as described in the transperitoneal technique. The line of incision is easily defined after the upper pole vessels are identified, clipped, and divided. The harmonic scalpel is used to provide a hemostatic excision of the upper pole. The consistency of the upper and lower poles and the ease with which the harmonic scalpel jaws are approximated provide excellent cues in establishing the proper line of excision as well. The specimen is then removed through the medial and cephalad port site as previously described.

Transperitoneal Technique: Upper Pole

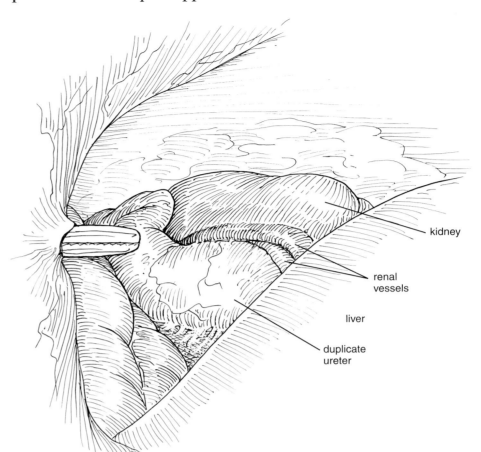

FIGURE 19-8. Dissection is initiated as for simple nephrectomy by incising sharply in the avascular plane along the white line of Toldt, exposing Gerota's fascia. The ureter of the affected segment is identified.

kidney

renal vessels

liver

duplicate ureter

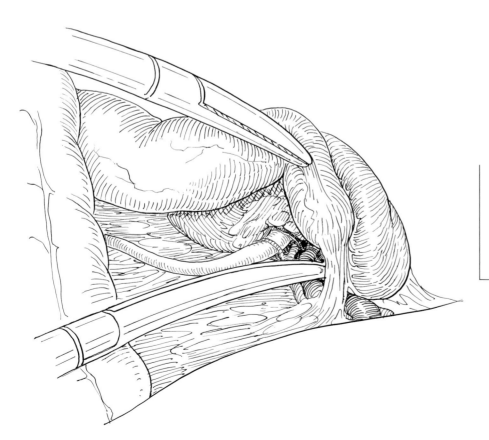

FIGURE 19-9. The upper pole ureter is dissected from the retroperitoneum and divided as distal as possible, avoiding damage to the blood supply of the normal ureter. If reflux is present, the ureter is tied with an absorbable suture before dividing.

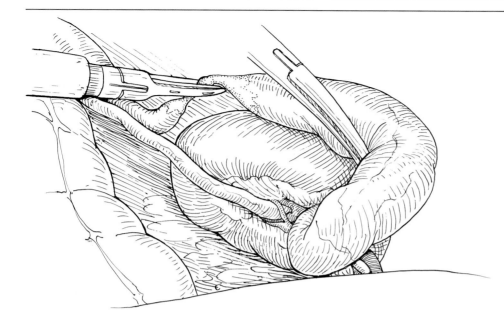

FIGURE 19-10. Dissection along the involved ureter is then continued proximally until it can be safely passed behind the renal hilum.

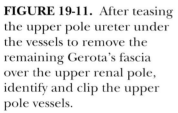

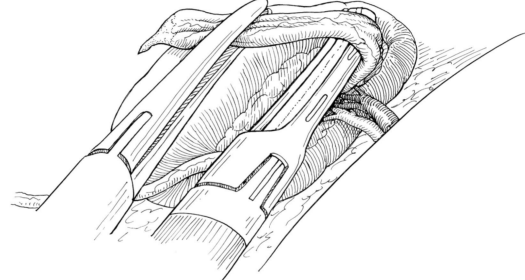

FIGURE 19-11. After teasing the upper pole ureter under the vessels to remove the remaining Gerota's fascia over the upper renal pole, identify and clip the upper pole vessels.

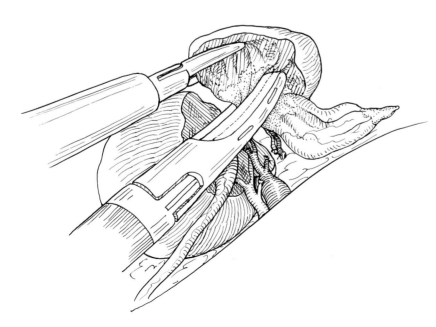

FIGURE 19-12. Transect the parenchyma at the site of blanching, using a cautery or harmonic scalpel. Cauterize bleeding vessels and cover the raw area with Gerota's fascia. Remove the specimen as previously described and close the port sites.

CRAIG A. PETERS

Retroperitoneoscopic nephrectomy in children has several advantages over transperitoneal approaches. There is less risk of injury to adjacent organs such as the bowel, liver, or spleen. There is little risk of formation of intraperitoneal adhesions, and the retroperitoneum can be drained more effectively than the peritoneum. In contrast, a transperitoneal approach offers a wider working space and a more direct view of intra-abdominal organs to avoid, and the umbilical port is well concealed, particularly for specimen removal. The traditional approaches to the kidney are retroperitoneal and this has become our favored access for nonrobotic laparoendoscopic procedures, while robotic procedures are performed transperitoneally.

Retroperitoneal access to the kidney may be by the prone or lateral approach, each having specific advantages and applications. For simple nephrectomy and partial nephrectomy, the prone approach offers direct access to the kidney in an anatomic orientation, with gravity facilitating exposure of the renal hilum. When the dissecting balloon can be inflated within Gerota's fascia, the posterior aspect of the kidney will be exposed prior to any manipulation and the renal vessels are usually rapidly exposed for control. The artery lies posteriorly so it can be controlled without manipulating the vein. The renal pelvis is posterior as well, facilitating mobilization and exposure as needed. If open access to the kidney becomes urgent, it can be performed through a lumbotomy incision, which may give slightly less exposure than the lateral flank incision, but in the one case where this has been needed, exposure was readily accomplished. The lateral approach does provide slightly more working room and gives access to the lower ureter, but requires traction on the kidney to expose the renal hilum. It is probably more efficient in the obese child, and in an adult in whom the posterior musculature can be quite thick. Both approaches should be part of the laparoendoscopist's armamentarium with recognition of their particular applications.

For each approach, several factors deserve comment. Port position is very important in retroperitoneal access to maximize working room. To avoid obstruction between them, working instruments should not be too close to each other and the camera port should be between the line of action of the two working ports. A fourth port may be placed if needed for traction.

Instrument size depends on surgeon preference and availability. We have used all sizes from 2 mm to 10 mm. The 2-mm instruments are too fragile for regular use and several have broken. The 3.5-mm instruments have been the best compromise in terms of durability, rigidity, and small size, although some of the available cannulas are bulky. The smallest clip appliers available are 5 mm, so at least one larger port must be placed. While some surgeons prefer developing the working space under vision with the camera, this takes a fair amount of time in contrast to a well-placed inflation balloon. Care should be taken to avoid too rapid or too much inflation of the balloon, which in infants may tear the peritoneum. Infants can accommodate about 120 mL of saline, while older children can accommodate 180 to 200 mL. The secondary ports should be placed carefully under direct vision to avoid injury to the peritoneum. If the peritoneum is inadvertently entered, it may inflate preferentially and reduce the working area. This can be remedied by either venting the peritoneal space with an angiocatheter or by opening the peritoneotomy widely to eliminate the trapping of insufflating gas. During nephrectomy, peritoneotomy occurs most often at the upper pole, near the liver where the kidney surface lies close to the peritoneum.

It is preferable to control the renal hilar vessels first to permit further renal mobilization. Occasionally it will be necessary to mobilize the ureter to lift the kidney and expose the hilum. Care must be taken to ensure that all vessels are controlled and ligated, as small polar vessels may escape detection and be avulsed during further dissection. The gonadal vessels should be identified and controlled to avoid bleeding.

Retroperitoneal drainage is usually not needed unless there is the possibility of a urine leak, as after partial nephrectomy, or the kidney is infected. A drain may be left through one of the port sites. Specimen removal is usually accomplished with the kidney intact in cases of dysplastic kidneys. On occasion, the specimen must be cut up or the incision enlarged slightly for removal. Close all port sites, even the small ones, with a fascial or muscular stitch, aided by injecting local anesthetic into them.

It is important to secure the transected end of the distal ureter in cases with reflux, as several instances of urine leaks have occurred. A metal clip is inadequate and can fall off; double ligation with suture is probably the ideal.

With the advent of robotic technologies for laparoscopic procedures, we routinely perform partial nephrectomy with robotic assistance, but most nephrectomies are performed with conventional laparoscopic tools using a retroperitoneal approach. The advantage of robotic assistance in partial nephrectomy is finer dexterity with the delicate vascular control of the affected pole, as well as the ability to close any defects in the remaining collecting system, as well as suturing the edges of the remaining pole over a fat bolster as is commonly performed in open surgery. This limits the risk of a residual fluid collection.

JASON WILSON

Commentary by

Laparoscopic retroperitoneal nephrectomy offers advantages similar to the retroperitoneal approach for open surgery. Primarily, the peritoneal cavity and its contents are avoided, minimizing risk of injury that may occur when mobilizing bowel and avoiding potential future complications associated with intraperitoneal adhesions. The retroperitoneoscopic approach is difficult in children weighing less than 10 kg and in cases requiring total ureterectomy. Port crowding can prevent adequate dissection and countertraction in the small patient. The limited space in the retroperitoneum can be troublesome in the extremely hydronephrotic kidney after aspiration of the fluid, as there is limited space to achieve the traction necessary for dissection. There is adequate anterior reflection of the peritoneum in the lateral decubitus position, allowing placement of the initial port after creation of the retroperitoneal space.

Using table flexion and the kidney rest, the space between the inferior costal margin and the iliac crest is maximized. Peritoneal tears are avoided by gradual inflation of the balloon system and careful visualization with subsequent port placements at the mid- and anterior-axillary lines. Peritoneal compromise can decrease the retroperitoneal space and it may be necessary to enlarge the area and perform a transperitoneal technique. If the peritoneal space is entered after control of the hilum and division of the ureter, the procedure can be completed with anterior retraction of the peritoneal reflection. The prone approach has been described as a successful position for retroperitoneoscopic procedures.

Our preferred method of access is in the modified lateral decubitus position with the patient turned approximately 15 degrees toward the prone position. The lateral approach allows maximal area for port placement and is easily and rapidly converted to familiar retroperitoneal nephrectomy in an emergent situation. A described advantage of the prone approach is ease with which the hilum is accessed. With adequate retroperitoneal insufflation and minimal retraction the hilum is easily accessed and controlled with either approach. The renal artery is commonly visualized posteriorly after creation of the retroperitoneal space as a pulsating area of hilar fat. It is worth reiterating that early control of the artery is facilitated by an extraperitoneal approach.

There is a range of ports available as well as working instruments. Surgeons' choices should be based on availability, familiarity, and comfort. The harmonic scalpel and clip appliers require 5-mm ports. It is our preference to use 5-mm ports with radially dilating sheaths to minimize port movement. Port movement, as well as frustrating, can increase operative time and can cause subcutaneous crepitus and repeated loss of pneumoretroperitoneum. Radially dilating sheaths prevent migration and conserve space. Whatever ports chosen should be placed at the maximum distance apart. The anterior port can be placed quite anteriorly if placed after the posterior and inferior. Through the initial ports, blunt dissection can increase the space, allowing anterior placement while avoiding the peritoneal reflection. Adhering to these guidelines can allow a maximal distance between the two working ports.

When creating the retroperitoneal space, attempt placement of the balloon anterior to the psoas muscle and posterior to Gerota's fascia. Frequently, the space dilated is inferior, between the psoas muscle and inferior pole of the kidney, especially in hydronephrotic kidneys or kidneys associated with frequent episodes of pyelonephritis. Visually directed placement of the inferior port is easily accomplished after which time a blunt instrument can be used to gently reflect the peritoneum anteriorly and further develop the space posterior to Gerota's fascia. It is useful to first determine port position by placing local anesthetic with a small needle and confirming the planned point of entry by visualizing the needle entering through the abdominal wall. Illumination of the skin with the lens will help avoid subcutaneous vessels.

Port placement and blunt dissection will maximize the working space and the surgeon may proceed with mobilization of the inferior pole of the kidney. Bluntly dissecting posteriorly from the lower pole in a cephalad direction will allow identification of the renal artery. The ureter can also be identified and divided early if extra traction is needed in identification of the hilum. When removing an upper pole segment it is helpful to place a ureteral catheter in the normal ureter to aid in proper identification of the upper pole ureter. The vessels to the upper pole segment are frequently small and located posteriorly at the ureteropelvic junction of the upper pole segment. It is necessary to mobilize the ureter to determine the upper pole segment and avoid injury to the lower pole collecting system. A large, distended system will often require drainage before the hilum can be located. The renal artery is divided after three clips are placed: two proximal and one distal. The vein can then be accessed and divided in a similar manner. Polar vessels should be identified with careful dissection and the gonadal vein may be controlled early as well to avoid unnecessary blood loss. Superiorly, careful and controlled dissection avoids liver and peritoneal injury.

The specimen can easily be removed through the anterior port after visually confirmed placement of a clamp through the port site with which the port site can be slightly enlarged (by spreading) and the specimen securely grasped. It is rarely necessary to extend the fascial and/or skin incision to remove the specimen. The fascia should be closed at this site and it is not necessary to close muscle or fascia at the other port sites, as they are small (5 mm) incisions. After removal of the specimen, a second look confirms hemostasis and complete specimen removal. Drainage is not necessary unless injury to the remaining kidney is suspected in the case of upper pole nephrectomy. A Penrose drain can be placed through the posterior port site. Skin incisions are closed with absorbable suture in an inverted subcuticular fashion.

Part II

Kidney Reconstruction

Chapter 20

Introduction to Kidney Reconstruction

Indications for repair of an obstructive ureteropelvic junction (UPJ) causing hydronephrosis and the estimation of potential for recovery are recurrent controversies. With fetal ultrasonography, a decision may be made soon after birth. Assess the degree of hydronephrosis and caliectasis, renal size, and the thickness of the parenchyma, as well as the presence of a corticomedullary junction. Evaluate the ureters, and check the bladder for wall thickness and a ureterocele to confirm an accurate diagnosis. Although no test will predict which kidney will deteriorate, rely on a renal scan to give differential renal function. Assess contralateral compensatory hypertrophy as a measure of obstruction.

UPJ obstruction is the most common obstructive lesion, but also consider obstruction at the ureterovesical junction, obstructive ureterocele, posterior urethral valves, urethral atresia, and hydrometrocolpos. Also look for nonobstructive lesions that include physiologic hydronephrosis, vesicoureteral reflux, megacalicosis, and the prune belly syndrome.

Unilateral pelvicalyceal dilation detected prenatally or in a newborn infant does not necessarily develop into hydronephrosis requiring surgical correction. Closely follow these infants for progression, which is suspected if the glomerular filtration rate falls more than 10% or if progressive hydronephrosis is shown by ultrasonography or diuretic renography.

Infants have great ability for recovery of lost function by pyeloplasty, even when intervention is delayed.

Perform ultrasonography to detect dilation (either ureteral dilation, as megaureter, or renal dilation, as UPJ obstruction), and also to evaluate the quality of the renal parenchyma. A dilated ureter suggests either vesicoureteral reflux or ureterovesical junction obstruction.

Grade the hydronephrosis according to the Society of Fetal Urology:

Grade 0—normal kidney with no hydronephrosis
Grade 1—slightly dilated renal pelvis with mild caliectasis
Grade 2—moderately dilated pelvis with mild caliectasis
Grade 3—large renal pelvis, dilated calyces, and normal renal parenchyma
Grade 4—very large renal pelvis, and large dilated calyces with thinning of the renal parenchyma

Finding a pelvis with an anterior–posterior diameter over 2 cm suggests that repair will be needed but do not rush to operation because of diagnostic inaccuracy—there is the small risk that the kidney will be injured by delay, but many such kidneys rapidly improve in function with spontaneous reduction of dilation.

129

Expect improvement during the postnatal period. Many children may subsequently show little or no obstruction. In an older child, a renal scan may be useful in identifying a nonsalvageable kidney.

Note: An intravenous urogram is not a reliable way to estimate renal function. Retrograde or antegrade studies seldom add useful information, although such anatomic studies may help in directing the surgical approach if a lumbotomy incision is being considered.

In infants, even though renal damage may appear severe, choose repair rather than nephrectomy because every nephron may be needed in later life should single-nephron hyperperfusion supervene.

METHODS FOR REPAIR

Two techniques are applicable for primary repair: open pyeloplasty and laparoscopic pyeloplasty. Endopyelotomy, either retrograde or antegrade, should be reserved for revision procedures.

Open Pyeloplasty

The traditional dismembered pyeloplasty has the highest documented long-term rate of success. A dismembered pyeloplasty (see Chapter 21) is most applicable to all children with a blockage at the UPJ but is particularly suitable for patients with crossing vessels or with high insertion of the ureter.

Laparoscopic Pyeloplasty

An alternative to open pyeloplasty is laparoscopic pyeloplasty. The steps and the results are similar, but the incisions and instrumental techniques can be more difficult and time-consuming and the learning curve high. Moreover, the special problems encountered, such as intrinsic ureteral obstruction, high insertion anomaly, crossing vessels, or a redundant renal pelvis, may be more difficult to cope with laparoscopically.

Retrograde or Antegrade Endopyelotomy

Endopyelotomy, that is, incising the UPJ by either a retrograde or an antegrade route, is a minimally invasive approach. The success rate is not as high as primary repair and therefore should be reserved for secondary procedures. As primary therapy it is not suitable for a child with (1) a redundant renal pelvis, (2) a high ureteral insertion, (3) a crossing vessel, or (4) a long stricture.

Chapter 21

Pyeloureteroplasty

OPEN DISMEMBERED PYELOPLASTY

The Anderson-Hynes dismembered pyeloplasty technique is applicable to almost all variations of ureteropelvic junction (UPJ) obstruction. Place a bladder catheter and administer intravenous antibiotics prior to beginning the procedure.

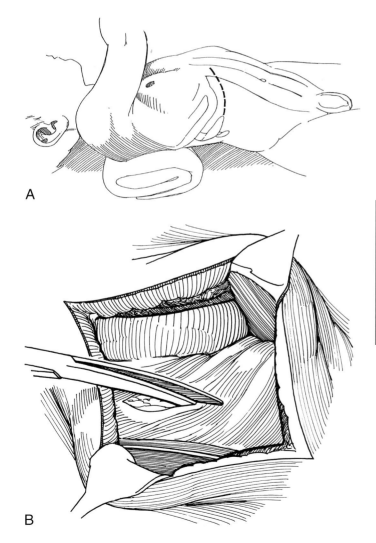

A

B

FIGURE 21-1. A, Approach the pelvis through a dorsal lumbotomy incision in infants; in older children, use an incision off the tip of the 12th rib or an anterior subcostal incision, taking care to stay out of the peritoneal cavity. **B,** Open Gerota's fascia and approach the surface of the pelvis. Free as little as possible of the kidney itself, and leave fat attached for traction and manipulation. Have your assistant hold the lower pole up and anteriorly with a sponge stick to expose the UPJ posteriorly.

FIGURE 21-2. A, Expose the ureter below the UPJ first and place a small Penrose drain or vessel loop around it. For secondary operations, locate the normal part of the ureter distally and dissect up from normal to abnormal. Dissect as short a length of the ureter as possible and preserve its adventitial vessels. **B,** Palpate and look for aberrant lower-pole vessels; division will result in segmental ischemia and hypertension.

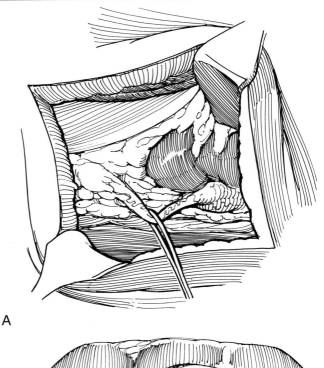

A

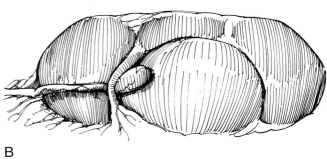

B

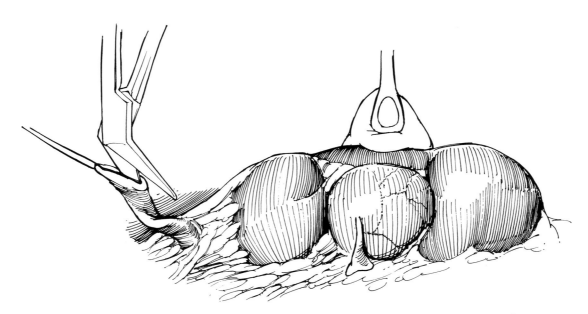

FIGURE 21-3. After exposure of the UPJ, make a decision as to what type of operation to use. It is necessary to ask: Is the ureter long enough to allow dismemberment and excision of the UPJ? A modified Anderson-Hynes pyeloplasty is suitable in the overwhelming majority of repairs. Only in the rare circumstance will the ureter not have sufficient length requiring a flap repair from the pelvis. Place a stay suture in the ureter at its junction with the pelvis; divide the ureter obliquely and spatulate on its less vascularized lateral surface for a distance equal to the length of the proposed V-shaped flap, a step often more accurately done after the pelvic flap is formed.

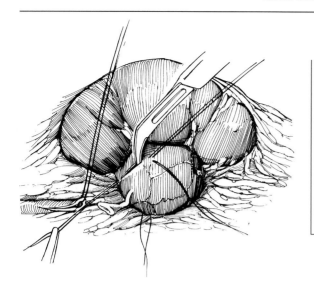

FIGURE 21-4. With the pelvis full, map out the proposed diamond-shaped incision with a skin-marking pen, angling the caudal triangle medially to form a **V**-flap. The kidney can be brought up into the wound with vein or Gil-Vernet retractors or rotated with a sponge stick. Place 6-0 stay sutures at the angles of the diamond. Since considerable pyelectasis is the rule, include a portion of the pelvis, as reduction pyeloplasty is part of the repair. Caution: Do not remove too much pelvis, especially in a bifid system, and keep well away from the calyceal necks, which can be surprisingly close to the edge; otherwise, closure will be difficult and infundibular stenosis could result. Incise for a short distance along one of the planned lines with a #11 hooked blade.

FIGURE 21-5. Use Lahey, Iris, or Potts scissors to complete the resection, cutting from inside one stay suture to inside the next. Remove the specimen.

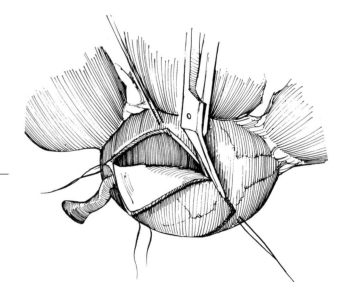

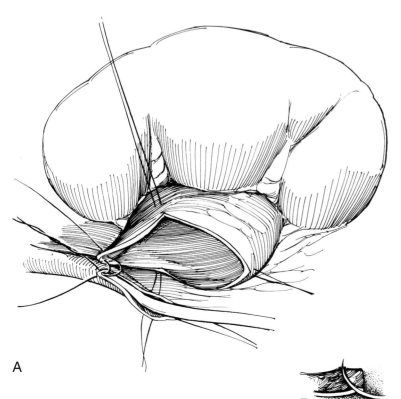

FIGURE 21-6. A, Insert an infant feeding tube of suitable size into the ureter to prevent catching the far wall in a suture. Using loupes, place one 5-0 or 6-0 synthetic absorbable suture adjacent to the apex of the V-shaped flap from outside in, and then out through the apex of the ureteral slit. Place a second suture 2 mm away from the first. Tie both sutures with four knots and cut the short ends. Use the ureteral stay suture for manipulation; do not use forceps. **B,** Catch the mucosa minimally to include more muscularis and adventitia in the stitch.

A

B

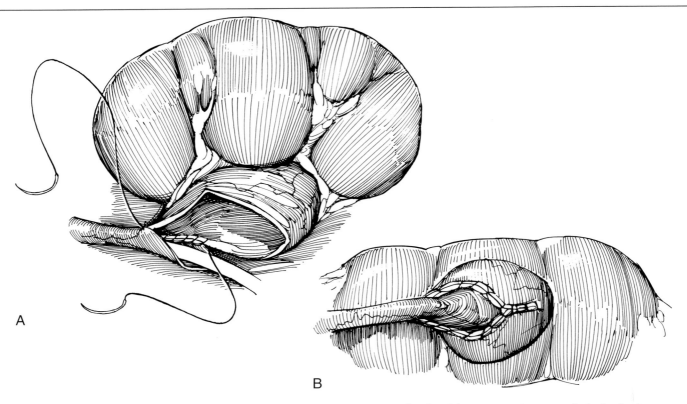

A

B

FIGURE 21-7. A, Continue the first suture to the tip of the ureter on the far side as a continuous stitch, locked at every four or five bites. Do the same for the second suture on the near side. Remove the feeding tube and irrigate the pelvis and calyces free of clots, which is especially important with an anterior approach. **B,** Tie the two sutures together, cut one, and continue with the other to close the pelvic defect.

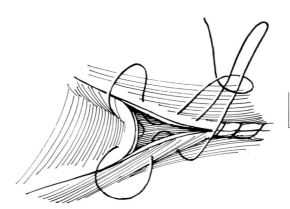

FIGURE 21-8. Alternatively, form a purse string around the central defect by starting a third suture from the upper end.

FIGURE 21-9. Inject saline with a fine needle through the pelvic wall to test for watertightness and for patency of the anastomosis. Add a suture or two if needed to close a leak. Use an omental wrap (see Chapter 65) if the tissues appear hypovascular or if the operation is the second one.

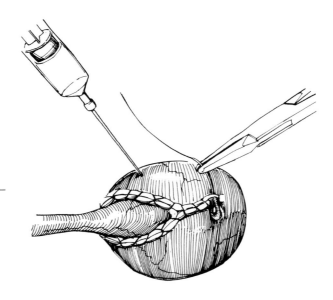

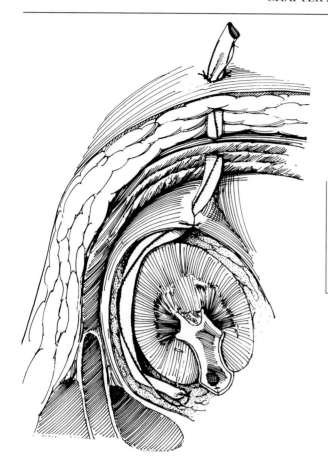

FIGURE 21-10. Insert a Penrose drain near but not touching the anastomosis. Alternatively, use a suction drain; accurate drainage is important. Tack the two edges of Gerota's fascia together around the kidney with fine plain catgut. Close the wound in layers, leading the drain laterally so that the child will not lie on it. An adhesive stomal bag may be applied if leakage warrants, but it should very rarely be necessary.

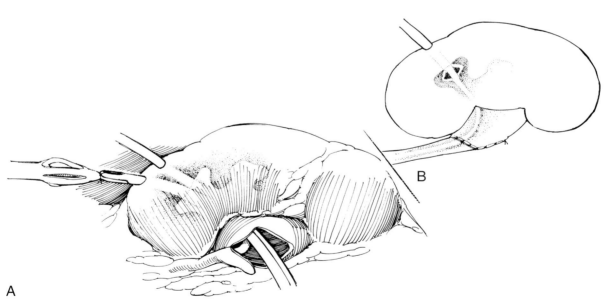

FIGURE 21-11. **A,** If the repair appears tenuous or the kidney is infected, insert a nephrostomy tube (see Chapter 22), or a nephrostomy tube along with a double-J stent or soft silicone tubing, before closing the pelvis. **B,** Combining a nephrostomy and stent is an alternative; if a double-J stent is too long, it may enter the bladder and siphon off the bladder contents, which can be very disturbing. In general, avoid placing a stent, although it may prevent kinking by a large floppy pelvis. A compromise may be to place a nephrostomy tube in an infant, and to use both the tube and a double-J stent in any difficult repair.

Consider giving suppressive antibiotic therapy. Avoid irrigating a nephrostomy tube. Discharge an infant in 48 hours with the drain in place. Shorten the drain 2 days after drainage stops and then remove it. If a stent has been placed, take it out in 10 to 12 days when a nephrostogram shows the anastomosis to be watertight, unless repair was difficult. Remove the nephrostomy tube if it drains readily when filled while held vertically or after a trial of intermittent clamping and checking for residual urine.

PELVIC FLAP PYELOPLASTY

Use the Culp procedure (oblique flap) for a long ureter
defect at the UPJ.

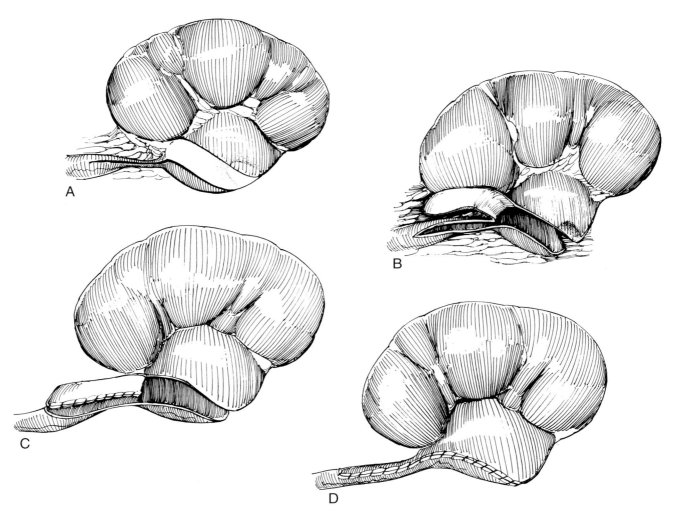

FIGURE 21-12. A, Culp technique: Mark a spiral flap running obliquely around the enlarged pelvis and extending
the incision down the ureter for a distance equal to the length of the flap. **B,** Incise the flap and insert a stay suture to
deflect it down. **C,** Approximate the posterior edge of the flap to the lateral edge of the ureter with a running 4-0 or 5-0
synthetic absorbable suture. **D,** Close the anterior edge of the flap and the pelvis with similar sutures. It helps to suture
over a small infant feeding tube.

POSTOPERATIVE PROBLEMS

Urinary leakage may occur within the first 24 hours because
of an overfull bladder (a reason for an indwelling catheter
for the first 24 to 48 hours). Stents and nephrostomy tubes
are usually not required; an accurately placed drain is sufficient. However, leakage persisting for over a week should
be investigated because the consequent peripelvic and periureteral fibrosis may affect the anastomosis. First, be sure the
drain is not in contact with the anastomosis or with the adjacent ureter. Try shortening the drain, or subsequently remove
it and replace it with a soft catheter with extra holes to prevent pooling of urine. Manage persistent leakage by passing

a stent either from below or from above, or by inserting a
percutaneous nephrostomy.

Alternatively, as soon as obstruction is suspected or
when leakage continues, insert a double pigtail stent from
below. (In an infant, place it antegradely.) Before removing
a stent, test for leakage by gravity-filling the system with contrast medium. Also determine that the repair is intact before
withdrawing the drain.

A urinoma may form if the drain is removed prematurely. Passing a curved clamp down the drainage tract
will usually relieve the collection of urine. If the drain
falls out, to prevent pooling of urine, replace it by passing
a small Robinson catheter, cut off and with extra holes,

through the fascia and transfix it with a safety pin taped to the skin.

Obstruction at the UPJ after the stent removal may be managed by (1) leaving the nephrostomy tube in place and waiting for edema to subside, (2) inserting a tube into the pelvis percutaneously to remain until a film shows the tract to be open, or (3) passing a double pigtail stent from above or below.

This last alternative may be best because stenting prevents scar tissue from obliterating the anastomosis, which would require reoperation. To detect silent obstruction, check the renal status by sonography 4 to 6 weeks postoperatively, by diuretic renography.

Pyelonephritis after pyeloplasty is typically related to the prolonged need for a nephrostomy tube and stent. Appropriate intravenous antibiotics will resolve the acute crisis. It is important to determine that the kidney is adequately drained, that is, the nephrostomy tube is not blocked or displaced.

FOLLOW-UP AFTER PYELOPLASTY

Obtain a sonogram at 1 month. If conditions are stable or are better than on the preoperative sonogram, repeat the sonogram at 1 and 2 years, and then every 2 to 3 years to age 18. If the first sonogram shows increased hydronephrosis, perform a diuretic renogram to be sure there is no obstruction requiring further surgical measures. A renogram half-time of less than 20 minutes 3 months after pyeloplasty predicts surgical success. After 6 months, expect no further improvement in drainage, but the dilation viewed by sonogram may not be reduced before 1 or 2 years. Children exhibit good catch-up growth of the parenchyma after repair, but do not expect parallel improvement in the pyelographic appearance.

RECURRENT URETEROPELVIC JUNCTION OBSTRUCTION

After open pyeloplasty, recurrence of obstruction is a rare complication, but it does require repair. After endopyelotomy, children with persistent obstruction are candidates for reoperation, usually by an open method. Also reoperate on children who, after open or laparoscopic repair, have increased drainage from the Penrose drain, who form a large urinoma, or in whom a postoperative renal scan shows a significant decrease in function from the preoperative state. In such cases, place a percutaneous nephrostomy and perform an antegrade pyelogram to locate the site of obstruction.

Open repair after failure of the primary procedure is more certain of success than repair by a closed method. At reoperation, the typical finding is a dense collection of fibrous tissue that resulted from inaccurate drainage with obstruction, from leaving too much pelvis behind (a 1-cm rim from the entrance to a calyx is optimum), or from a kink at the UPJ.

Technique: Approach the site from a previously unexposed area by extending the incision anteriorly from the flank or by opening the peritoneum. Pick up the ureter below the scar and dissect it carefully (and tediously, as you preserve its vessels) to the UPJ. Resect the stenotic section and perform a dismembered pyeloplasty, taking special care to avoid any tension on the anastomosis. If the ureter is atretic but sufficient pelvis remains, apply a spiral flap. As a last resort, if the pelvis has already been reduced, perform ureterocalicostomy. In any case, insert a stent through the anastomosis and place a nephrostomy tube. Provide an omental wrap. After 2 or 3 weeks, make a gravity nephrostogram to check the repair. Remove the tube if (or when) the pelvis empties at low pressure.

Acucise endopyelotomy is an alternative technique for postpyeloplasty strictures in children where instrumentation is of appropriate size. Under fluoroscopic control, advance the active end of the Acucise device over a guidewire until it straddles the UPJ. Have the cutting wire facing posterolaterally. Apply a 75-watt cutting current for 5 seconds while the balloon is inflated. Check the effect with a retrograde ureteropyelogram, looking for relief of the obstructive waist and for extravasation of the contrast medium. Insert a double pigtail stent to remain for 6 weeks. Alternatively, the procedure can be performed in antegrade fashion.

If redo pyeloplasty is not successful, alternatives are autotransplantation of the kidney to the true pelvis with anastomosis of the renal pelvis to healthy distal ureter. Less ideal is the interposition of an ileal ureter.

ROBERT H. WHITAKER

Commentary by

A pyeloplasty is a most agreeable operation in the urologist's armamentarium, and it is unusual to complete the operation without a feeling of satisfaction. Thus, it is all the more disconcerting when a complication occurs; a surgeon who has not seen such a problem perhaps has not done enough pyeloplasties.

We must not encourage the age-old, dangerous habit of a nephrostomy tube without a stent, as this is asking for trouble in terms of the anastomosis' bridging across internally with neither tube nor urine through it. In the United Kingdom, we do not use Penrose drains (as is done in the United States). We use a round silicone tube drain that can be attached to a bag. We feel they are much easier to manage.

Using the techniques in this section, excessive leakage should not occur and obstruction should be a rarity. Early insertion of a double-J splint in all but a small child as soon as obstruction is suspected may work well. You should be in no hurry to remove it. Remember, also, that residual dilation for months or even years is not unusual after a pyeloplasty for a chronically obstructed hydronephrosis, so always prove with renography or pressure flow studies before assuming that the operation has been less than fully successful.

MAX MAIZELS

Commentary by

It is disappointing that our specialty has yet to objectify the performance of pyeloplasty for newborns with hydronephrosis and renographic obstruction. Currently, the best that can be done is to identify instances of obstruction, and to understand the need to predict which cases might reasonably resolve over time while maintaining inherent function. While the performance of retrograde pyelography prior to pyeloplasty is controversial, I perform it routinely. The images confirm the nature of the obstruction and the likelihood of extended ureteral mobilization that will be needed to effect the ultimate result of a pelvis and ureter contiguous as one linear axis.

To perform pyeloplasty on infants, I modify the traditional flank position with rotation of the child toward the edge of the bed, so that the intestines tend to fall away from the field. The skin incision is kept small and the surgery can be done single-handed using self-retaining retractors. The renal pelvic incision may be made more easily with serrated scissors rather than with a knife blade. The serrations maintain the tissue position without slippage that may be noted in nonserrated scissors. A technique that I have relied on over the years was suggested by my friend Dr. Ricardo Gonzales. He suggested that pyeloplasty may be started with a double-armed 6-0 absorbable polydioxanone suture rather than requiring placement of two apical sutures. I still rely on looped KISS catheter drainage of the kidney postoperatively: closed drainage for 1 week, clamp the catheter for 1 week, and then remove both stent and drain. For cosmesis, rather than exiting the catheters via a stab skin incision, the catheters may exit the flank using a 16-gauge angiocatheter trocar. Cases of nephrogenic diabetes insipidus should be maintained on catheter drainage until the color of the urine improves from "tap water" darkening after overnight dehydration during sleep.

My experiences with reoperative pyeloplasty show that exposure is well attained by an anterior extraperitoneal approach, which will prove to be devoid of reaction from surgery that has been done via a posterior approach. Should a closed approach using endopyelotomy be chosen, exercise caution regarding penetration of an unrecognized accessory renal hilar vessel. Empiric practices dictate the manner of postoperative follow-up. My practice is to employ ultrasonography every 5 years until adulthood. It takes about 2 years for preoperative Society for Fetal Urology hydronephrosis grade 3–4 to downgrade to grade 1–2. Discrepancy in renal polar length normalizes about 5 years postoperatively. It is paradoxical, but empiric practice confirms that cases of gigantic kidneys caused by UPJ obstruction that are treated by preemptive nephrostomy when the patient is a newborn show the most dramatic recovery.

H. GIL RUSHTON

Commentary by

This chapter provides an excellent description of open, operative pyeloplasty in children and the management of potential complications of this procedure. Open pyeloplasty can be one of the more rewarding reconstructive procedures in pediatric urology with excellent success rates when performed correctly.

I have frequently taught residents that the most difficult part of management of patients with hydronephrosis suggestive of UPJ obstruction is determining who actually needs surgery, particularly now that the majority of cases of hydronephrosis are detected incidentally by prenatal sonography. Historically, the majority of patients with UPJ obstruction presented between the ages of 6 to 15 years with symptoms of flank or abdominal pain or urinary infection. In this scenario, the presence of symptoms combined with the finding of hydronephrosis on intravenous pyelography made the decision to operate an easy one.

However, with prenatally detected hydronephrosis in an asymptomatic infant, the decision to operate is much less straightforward. Despite advances in imaging technology with sonography, renal scintigraphy, and MRI urography, all of which provide more quantitative information regarding the function and drainage of the hydronephrotic kidney, a universally accepted diagnosis of obstruction remains elusive. Most would agree that those hydronephrotic kidneys with both reduced, relative renal function and delayed drainage warrant surgical intervention. However, the majority of kidneys with prenatally detected hydronephrosis have good preservation of measurable renal function, even in the face of significant hydronephrosis and delayed drainage parameters. Furthermore, longitudinal follow-up of these kidneys demonstrates that most maintain good function and that, in most cases of mild and moderate hydronephrosis, both drainage and hydronephrosis spontaneously improve. This has led to a more conservative initial approach of expectant management with serial imaging in those kidneys with good function, even in the presence of significant hydronephrosis and delayed drainage. Whereas some would recommend intervention only if there is a decrease in renal function or urinary infection, others would recommend pyeloplasty if worsening hydronephrosis and/or drainage is observed over time with the hope of preventing loss of function. Indeed, experience with this approach of expectant management has shown that deterioration in drainage almost always precedes a significant decrease in renal function, as long as upper tract infection does not occur.

Recognizing that at this time there is no study that can predict with certainty which kidneys will deteriorate or develop symptoms, we currently recommend pyeloplasty for prenatally detected hydronephrosis when there is initial high-grade obstruction (defined as a flat or rising drainage curve that does not improve significantly in the upright or prone position associated with Society for Fetal Urology grade 4 hydronephrosis), initial, reduced split renal function (less than 35%), worsening drainage or deteriorated renal function on serial diuretic renography, and/or subsequent development of symptoms of urinary infection.

Once the decision to operate has been made, most controversy related to operative pyeloplasty revolves around the use of retrograde pyelography and/or the use of stents or nephrostomy tubes. We have reported our long-term experience with success rates of 98% without the use of routine retrograde pyelography or stenting of uncomplicated pyeloplasties. Others who do routinely employ one or both of these procedures have reported similar success rates. Thus, to a large extent, the routine use of retrograde pyelography and/or postoperative stenting is based on surgeon preference, rather than relative superiority of one approach over another. One caveat is that antegrade passage of ureteral catheters or cannulation of the ureter down through the ureterovesical junction should be avoided in small infants, as there is a recognized risk of creating iatrogenic obstruction at the ureterovesical junction.

Another area of controversy surrounds the postoperative imaging protocol used to evaluate the success of pyeloplasty. Even with a successful pyeloplasty, hydronephrosis may take up to 1 to 2 years to improve, making sonography a less-than-ideal imaging modality for early follow-up. In contrast, our experience with postpyeloplasty MAG-3 (mercapto acetyl triglycine) renal scans has demonstrated that over 85% of patients demonstrate early surgical success evidenced by a renogram half-time of less than 20 minutes at 3 months and 98% by 12 months. Furthermore, none of these patients developed delayed failure, obviating the need for long-term imaging follow-up in patients who demonstrate unobstructed drainage 2 to 3 months following pyeloplasty.

A final comment regarding recurrent UPJ obstruction: Several years ago Dr. Robert Jeffs suggested to me that I would likely find missed crossing vessels in a patient of mine who required a redo pyeloplasty. To my surprise and chagrin, he was absolutely correct. Since that patient, I have encountered the same pathology in a few cases referred to me for redo pyeloplasties. Undoubtedly, the crossing vessels were present the first time but were likely missed when the peripelvic tissues were retracted superiorly to expose the region of the UPJ.

PASQUALE CASALE

Commentary by

When a patient is diagnosed with a UPJ obstruction, a decision needs to be made as to whether that patient is a candidate for a minimally invasive approach or requires open surgery. The decision is typically based on the patient's age and the degree of expertise the surgeon has with minimally invasive surgery. I have found during the physical examination in the office, if the child has a distance of approximately 7 cm between the anterior superior iliac spine and umbilicus as well as a 7- to 8-cm distance between the umbilicus and xiphoid process, he or she would be an excellent candidate for a minimally invasive approach such as laparoscopy or robotics.

Both transperitoneal and retroperitoneal approaches have been used for laparoscopic intervention to repair UPJ obstructions. It has been my experience that in the younger child, the transperitoneal approach facilitates laparoscopic intracorporeal suturing, as the limited space of the retroperitoneum does make it difficult to navigate, especially when teaching residents who are new at the laparoscopic approach. I have also found that the intraoperative complications regarding CO_2 absorption and hemodynamic instability have been greater with the retroperitoneal approaches. The transperitoneal approach is best suited for robotic intervention as well. If the retroperitoneum restricts movement, then robotic manipulation is just not feasible. The arms collide, making the procedure extremely taxing.

Prior to laparoscopic insufflation, the bladder should be emptied. The patient is then placed in a modified lateral position, slightly rolled between 30 and 60 degrees depending on the child's body habitus. Port placement will also vary with the body habitus of the child. For the thinner, shorter patient a more linear approach to the port sites with less triangulation has been optimal. Usually this would require that the camera port not be placed in the umbilicus; rather, it has to be placed about 1 or 2 cm above it. The more obese patient should be placed more obliquely as the colon may need to be fully mobilized. Obesity can make the transmesenteric approach difficult and, if you need to mobilize the colon, a more exaggerated lateral approach is best. If the child is not obese, a transmesenteric approach has been quite beneficial due to the decreased bowel manipulation. I like to use a transmesenteric approach when possible to repair the UPJ.

Whether using robotics or pure laparoscopy, our anastomosis is performed with a 6-0 absorbable monofilament suture. If an indwelling ureteral stent is placed we prefer a percutaneous approach. I use a 16-gauge angiocatheter that is placed

Continued

subcostal and lateral, and then a guidewire is manipulated antegrade down to the level of the bladder. The stent is then placed in an antegrade fashion over the guidewire traversing the ureter. This, however, is performed after the posterior anastomosis has been completed. I find it imperative to use a stent early on during the learning curve to prevent postoperative urinary leakage that can be encountered during that period.

There are times when I feel a hitch stitch may be helpful. Typically a hitch stitch is placed in the renal pelvis prior to transecting the ureter to help remove the area of surgery from either a pool of urine after the ureter is transected at the level of the UPJ or from a deep hole that may be encountered with a transmesenteric approach. The hitch stitch also aids in performing the posterior anastomosis. I find that the majority of the time I do not need a hitch stitch, but it is very helpful especially when you are first learning to do these minimally invasive procedures. The hitch stitch comes through the abdominal wall on a large needle that should have a monofilament suture so as to avoid any drag of tissue. Once the needle is brought through the abdominal wall, it is placed through the renal pelvis, well above the area requiring transaction near the UPJ, and then once again brought through the anterior abdominal wall near the area of entry. Both ends of the suture are then pulled to allow enough tension to raise the area of interest from the surrounding tissue and urine within the field.

If needed an accessory port can be placed typically midline subxiphoid between the cephalad working port and the camera port. This accessory port can be used for passing suture as well as a suction device. The accessory port might become extremely important when a pyelolithotomy needs to be performed. I like to place a flexible ureteroscope through the 5-mm port and manipulate the stones out of the collecting system using a Nintol basket. The stones are then extracted from the port. If the stones are larger than the port, they are typically left in place and put in an endoscopic bag at the end of the case. They are then all extracted simultaneously.

Typically, in the laparoscopic and robotic approach, flank drainage is not necessary. If a drain is placed, a separate stab wound traversing the retroperitoneum should be used. As the Foley catheter is placed to empty the bladder at the beginning of the procedure, we usually leave it in until the next morning after surgery. A Foley catheter does not always have to be used for a child who has not been potty trained, but the potty-trained child tends to hold his or her urine after surgery because he or she does not want to get up because of the immediate postoperative discomfort.

The question of which analgesic is the best for the laparoscopic and robotic approach is always asked. The use of intrathecal opioids has been proven to be beneficial in children undergoing laparoscopic and other minimally invasive procedures. The intrathecal opioid would require the catheter to stay overnight. We typically use this approach for our minimally invasive procedures. We find that the vast majority of these patients do not require oral opioids once they are discharged from the hospital. We restrict them from heavy physical activity for 2 weeks. They can resume all normal activity afterward with no restrictions at all.

If a stent is used the child should be placed on prophylactic antibiotics during that time. Reflux and some aspect of voiding dysfunction are inherent with stent placement in children. Stents, if placed, are typically removed 4 weeks postoperatively. Different time frames are used by different doctors and vary from a couple of a days with a dangler string as far out as 8 weeks for complex reconstructions.

The same type of approach, laparoscopically or robotically, can be employed if a duplex system is encountered. An upper-pole to lower-pole ureteroureterostomy can be performed in the same manner as the open approach. If the upper pole needs to be anastomosed to the lower pole, typically an upper-pole to lower-pole ureteropyelostomy is used. The stent is then placed via the lower pole, traversing the anastomosis into the upper pole to keep the area drained. If the reconstruction is more amenable at the level of the bladder then a lower reconstruction can be performed. Always remember to have the stent traverse the anastomosis to help maximize drainage in that area.

The most daunting task we have at the academic institutions is the ability to pass minimally invasive surgery skills on to our residents and fellows. The surgical demand required compared to the time needed to teach these complex reconstructions to each and every resident on a new learning curve just does not match up. I have found it useful to have the residents master simple and basic laparoscopic and robotic techniques using a pelvic trainer and inanimate exercises. And, although expensive, I also have the residents attend minimally invasive porcine workshops. With the advent of simulation training and laparoscopic and robotic simulators, we can augment the learning experience. Until these simulators become more available, we need to exercise extreme patience with our doctors in training to maximize their education and give our patients the best possible outcomes in the process.

Chapter 22

Nephrostomy

Percutaneous nephrostomy is the better temporary alternative to open nephrostomy. In the case of open renal surgery in which a nephrostomy tube is indicated, this technique is safe and effective.

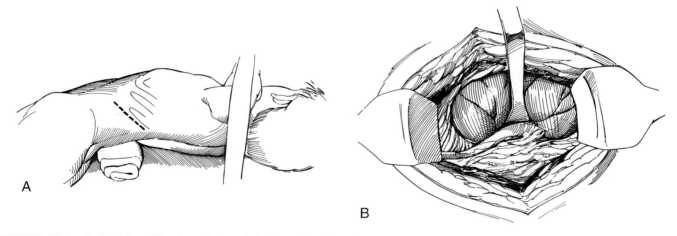

FIGURE 22-1. A, Position: Flank position with the table flexed. **B,** Incision: Make a subcostal (see Chapter 12) or transcostal incision (see Chapter 13). Expose the renal pelvis and hold the edge of the hilum steady with vein or Gil-Vernet retractors. Place two 5-0 synthetic absorbable sutures in the pelvis well away from the uteropelvic junction (UPJ). Make a 1- to 2-cm incision parallel to the border of the hilum with a hooked knife blade. Prepare a small Malecot catheter by transfixing the tip with a #1 silk suture. An alternative: Use a whistle-tip, plastic Foley catheter that may be replaced by merely passing a guidewire through it down the ureter.

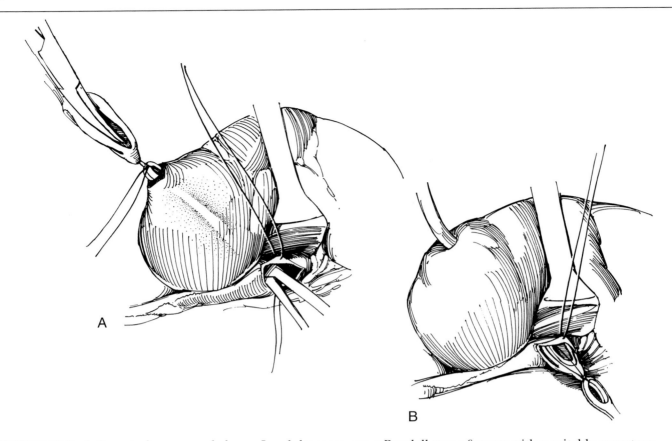

FIGURE 22-2. A, Insert a long curved clamp. In adolescents, use a Randall stone forceps with a suitable curvature. Pass the tip into a lower calyx and press it firmly into the parenchyma while palpating for it through the capsule. Cut the capsule in a radial direction over the clamp to allow it to exit. Open the clamp slightly to dilate the tract. Grasp the suture on the catheter in the clamp. **B,** Have your assistant steady the kidney. Stretch the tip of the catheter by pulling on the clamp with one hand and the catheter with the other, or by inserting a curved clamp from outside between the wings to reduce their diameter. Gradually move both hands in concert to draw the catheter through the tract and into the pelvis. Cut the suture, and then draw the catheter back until it fits in or near the lower calyx.

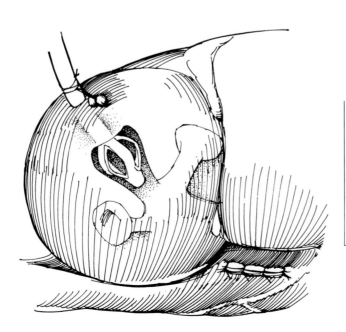

FIGURE 22-3. Suture the catheter to the capsule with a figure-eight, 3-0 synthetic absorbable suture over bolsters of fat. Bring the tube out through a separate stab wound in the flank, placed well anteriorly so that the child will not lie on it. Be sure that the nephrostomy tube runs in a straight course from the renal pelvis through the parenchyma and body wall to allow replacement. Fix it to the skin with a #1 silk suture. Close the pyelotomy incision with a running 6-0 synthetic absorbable suture. Place a Penrose drain and replace the perirenal fat and Gerota's fascia.

ALTERNATIVE TECHNIQUE

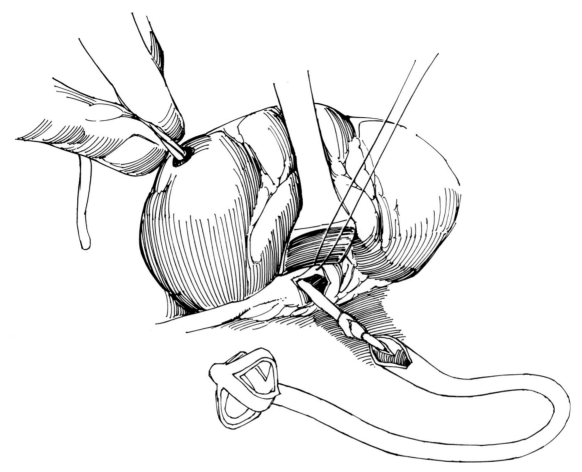

FIGURE 22-4. Prepare a Malecot catheter by cutting the distal end obliquely and making a vertical slit in it to create an eye. Insert the clamp into the pelvis and out through the parenchyma. Grasp the end of a length of moistened umbilical tape and draw it out through the pelvis. Pass a mosquito clamp through the eye of the catheter, bring the tape through, and tie it. Draw the tape with the attached catheter out through the cortex and position the catheter as described. Take care not to "saw" the parenchyma.

STEVEN J. SKOOG

Open placement of a nephrostomy tube has become a lost art, but it is one that needs to be retained. Internal drainage with a double-J stent is far more commonly performed. I have used open nephrostomy drainage in two circumstances: in young infants with UPJ obstructions requiring pelvic reduction in whom a stent will not easily pass and in trauma cases.

The four most important aspects of placement of the nephrostomy tube are (1) keep it away from your UPJ repair, (2) ensure the wings of the Malecot catheter are not impacted into a calyx, (3) fix the tube to the renal capsule, and (4) when bringing the catheter out to the skin, take the patient out of the flexed flank position first; otherwise, the catheter can be displaced.

Commentary by

JOHN C. POPE IV

Commentary by

Percutaneous placement of a nephrostomy tube is now the treatment of choice when acute, prompt drainage of the kidney is needed, primarily in emergent situations such as acute renal obstruction or obstructive urosepsis. Open nephrostomy tube placement is reserved for the rare situation when a percutaneous tube (due to size limitations) will not provide adequate drainage or when nephrostomy tube placement is needed as an adjunct to a reconstructive procedure, such as pyeloplasty or ureterocalycostomy. While rarely used in this day and age, this classic procedure should still be a part of the urologist's armamentarium.

I only have a couple of comments on the excellent description given herein. First, in this day and age of latex-free operating rooms, it is now often hard to find a latex Malecot catheter. From my experience and from what I have heard from others, the silastic alternative to the Malecot catheter leaves a lot to be desired in terms of its propensity to stay in place long term. A Foley catheter also can be used in this situation but be careful to not overfill the balloon within the renal pelvis. Doing so could cause obstruction as well as pressure necrosis of the pelvis and/or renal parenchyma. To hold the catheter in place without causing the above complications, 1 to 2 mL in a 5-mL Foley balloon is usually sufficient. Also, in this situation, I find it easier to first bring the catheter in through a separate stab incision inferior to the surgical incision, and then insert it into the kidney as described previously. This is easier than trying to bring both the drainage port and the balloon port of the Foley catheter through the skin from inside to outside.

If bleeding occurs after the tube is passed through the renal parenchyma, it will usually stop spontaneously. Gentle traction on the catheter will aid in this hemostasis. I rarely find it necessary to sew the catheter to the kidney but if your nephrotomy is too large for the catheter, certainly a purse-string suture may be placed in the capsule around the catheter to hold it in place. It is also important to be sure the catheter is pulled back far enough in to the calyx so as not to obstruct the UPJ. Finally, in some cases, you may desire a stent across an anastomosis (i.e., for pyeloplasty or ureterocalycostomy), in addition to the nephrostomy tube. In this situation, a 3- or 4-F whistle-tip ureteral catheter can be passed down the catheter's drainage port and out the tip. The distal end can then be fed down the ureter while the proximal end can be placed with the nephrostomy tube into a catheter drainage bag. This ureteral stent can then be removed independently of the nephrostomy tube if so desired.

Chapter 23

Ureterostomy in Situ

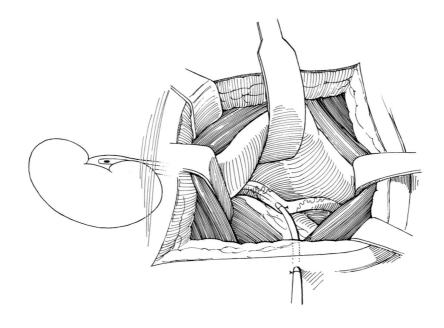

For temporary diversion, expose the upper ureter retroperitoneally. Make a short ureterotomy and insert an infant feeding tube into the renal pelvis. Fix it in place with a suture in the ureteral wall. Make a stab wound in the anterior axillary line, draw the tube out, and stitch it to the skin with a nylon suture. At operation, ureterostomy in situ is a simple, quick procedure and the catheter emerges in a more comfortable position for the child.

LAURENCE BASKIN

Commentary by

Ureterostomy in situ is rarely needed in primary surgery but is a welcome addition in redo ureteral surgery. This is especially true in the unusual situation in which the ureter may be not be accessible via endoscopic techniques, for example, in patients that have had previous transtrigonal ureteral reimplant or bladder neck reconstruction with ureteral reimplant secondary to an ectopic ureterocele.

I find the technique especially useful in the rare situation when a ureter is obstructed after complex reconstruction and the best solution is a transureteroureterostomy into the contralateral unobstructed ureter. Ureterostomy in situ allows temporary placement of a stent without having to open a previously operated bladder or instrument a potentially complex reconstructed urethral or catheterizable stoma.

Chapter 24

Open Renal Biopsy

Sonographic-guided renal biopsy is the preferred technique for children with renal disease. Open renal biopsy is indicated in children and adolescents with solitary or small, contracted kidneys and those with very poor renal function, or who are very obese or have some bleeding tendency. Open

renal biopsy is also indicated if the kidney is accessible during a simultaneous procedure.

Avoid biopsies in children with severe hypertension and uncorrected coagulopathies. Use general anesthesia.

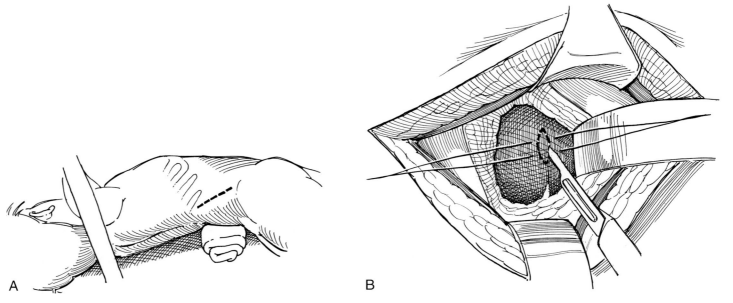

A   B

FIGURE 24-1. A, Incision: Approach the kidney through a dorsal lumbotomy incision (see Chapter 15). An alternative is the subcostal (see Chapter 12) or tip-of-the-12th rib incision (see Chapter 13). **B,** Incise Gerota's fascia over the lower pole of the kidney, and mobilize the perirenal fat caudad to expose the renal capsule. Insert a narrow Deaver retractor between the kidney and the fat to draw the kidney down. (Realize that such a small incision can lead to biopsy of the wrong organ.) Retract the wound with other Deaver retractors. Insert two fine chromic catgut stay sutures in the parenchyma on either side of the intended biopsy site. Make a deep elliptical incision into the cortex on each side of the suture and remove the specimen. Place it on saline-moistened coated gauze (not into formalin). Close the capsule by tying each suture to itself and then the sutures to each other. If bleeding continues, carefully rotate a taper-cut needle swaged with 5-0 chromic catgut through the renal cortex at the depth of the incision on both sides as a horizontal mattress suture. Incorporating oxidized cellulose may help hemostasis. Tie the suture carefully with two-handed square knots to avoid tearing it from the tissue. Place a second suture if necessary. Then obtain a needle biopsy specimen under direct vision to obtain tissue from the deep cortical and juxtamedullary levels. If that site bleeds, close it with a figure-eight suture. Alternatively, use the argon beam for hemostasis after removing a wedge of renal tissue. This has been very effective without the need for capsular sutures. Approximate Gerota's fascia, and then the muscles, fascia, and skin in layers. Divide the biopsy tissue directly on the coated gauze and fix the three portions respectively in formalin, in 2% glutaraldehyde, and by quick freezing. Have the pathologist confirm that the renal tissue contains glomeruli and is adequate for analysis prior to closure.

POSTOPERATIVE PROBLEMS

Bleeding occurs, especially in hypertensive children or those with minor coagulation problems. Gross hematuria will usually stop after 24 hours of bed rest. Pain is minimal with a muscle-splitting incision. A retroperitoneal hematoma may form. Wound infection is uncommon.

STEVE SHAPIRO

Commentary by

Indications for open renal biopsy have diminished with the increased use of needle biopsies by pediatric nephrologists.

I continue to favor a small anterior subcostal incision for open renal biopsy, especially when there is a possibility of bleeding (i.e., patient with history of bleeding disorder) because this allows better control. As nearly all of the clotting factors can be tested preoperatively, the patient can usually be prepared appropriately preoperatively by the pediatric hematologists. Hypertension, an additional factor, can also nearly always be controlled medically prior to surgery.

I have not used a suture in the parenchyma and I have not had to use a needle biopsy via open technique. Instead, I use a #11 blade to obtain a deep wedge of renal tissue that can be gently coaxed out without crushing. Bleeding can be controlled with 2-0 chromic catgut sutures. Polyglycolic acid sutures should not be used because they can cut through the renal capsule and renal tissue. Other options for bleeding control include the argon beam coagulator and/or thrombogenic material (e.g., Surgicel).

Good exposure and proper identification of the kidney prior to biopsy must be assured to avoid biopsy of the spleen on the left and the liver on the right side.

ANAND KRISHNAN

Commentary by

Open renal biopsy has largely been replaced by the percutaneous approach. Patients with relative indications (solitary kidney, obesity, coagulopathy) will now routinely undergo several attempts at percutaneous biopsy before proceeding with an open approach. One remaining indication is for suspected malignancy, such as bilateral Wilms' tumor. In this case, when definitive partial or total nephrectomy is deferred until after chemotherapy, we prefer bilateral flank incisions. Vascular control is avoided if possible to facilitate future hilar dissection at the time of definitive extirpation. Uncontrollable bleeding is uncommon and interposition of perinephric fat and reapproximation of the renal capsule with absorbable sutures is usually sufficient. If necessary, hemostatic agents such as oxidized cellulose (surgical), absorbable gelatin (Gelfoam), or gelatin/thrombin matrix (Floseal) can be used adjunctively, though it may make future procedures more difficult. The argon beam coagulator is also a very useful adjunct. It is important in all cases of open renal biopsy of suspicious lesions to include a sufficient amount of normal, adjacent renal parenchyma for the pathologist to make an accurate diagnosis.

Chapter 25

Repair of Renal Injuries

EXPLORATION, EXPOSURE, AND REPAIR

Renal injury in children is usually the result of blunt trauma. A preexisting lesion may be present in as many as a fifth of such injured children.

Obtain urine for microscopic analysis, either by having the child void or by catheterization. In either case, collect the urine after the first 30 mL has passed. More than five red blood cells per high-power field is suggestive of injury, although vascular avulsion may be missed. Obtain a computed tomography (CT) scan to stage the injury.

Decide whether observation or operation is appropriate. With markedly abnormal studies, such as a disrupted ureteropelvic junction (UPJ) or major renal bleeding that is life threatening, proceed to operation.

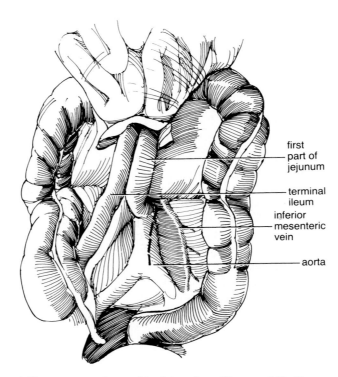

FIGURE 25-1. Incision: Make a midline transperitoneal incision (see Chapter 11). First explore the abdomen for associated injury. Apply laparotomy sponges to the kidney area to help control hemorrhage. Repair injuries to the liver, spleen, and bowel first, unless renal bleeding is more rapid than can be controlled or replaced. Lift the small bowel and place it on the chest in a plastic bag. Identify the aorta if possible. If it is covered by hematoma and cannot be palpated, identify the inferior mesenteric vein and incise the posterior parietal peritoneum medial to it over the site of the aorta, extending the incision superiorly to the ligament of Treitz. Dissect through the medial portion of the hematoma to expose the aorta. Watch out for the inferior mesenteric artery. Avoid disturbing the perirenal hematoma by not dissecting laterally near the kidney.

FIGURE 25-2. Dissect along the aorta superiorly to reach the next landmark, the left renal vein where it crosses the anterior to the aorta. Place a vessel loop around it and retract the vein cephalad to expose first the left and then the right renal artery. Be wary of the posterior lumbar vein that comes off the left renal vein. Place vessel loops around the renal artery of the injured side to be ready for placement of a vascular clamp, but unless bleeding is heavy, do not clamp at this time.

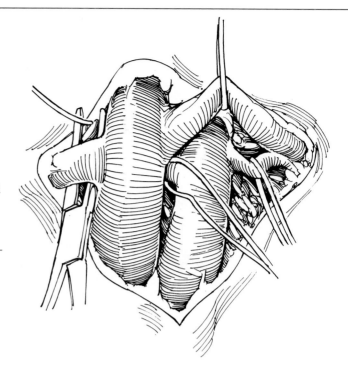

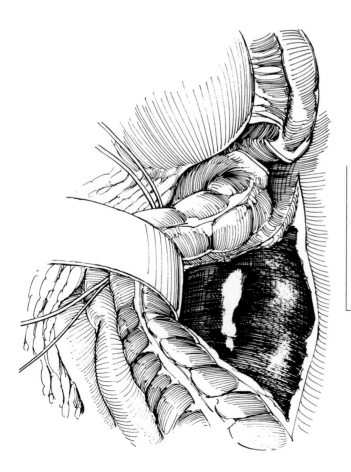

FIGURE 25-3. For left renal injury (as shown), incise the parietal peritoneum lateral to the descending colon and reflect the colon medially to expose the hematoma lying inside Gerota's fascia. Dissect directly into the hematoma through the fascia and the perirenal fat to reach the kidney. Free all aspects of the kidney thoroughly to examine it. If the bleeding warrants, clamp the artery with a vascular clamp before proceeding with definitive repair of the renal defect(s). However, in most cases, compression with the fingers is sufficient.

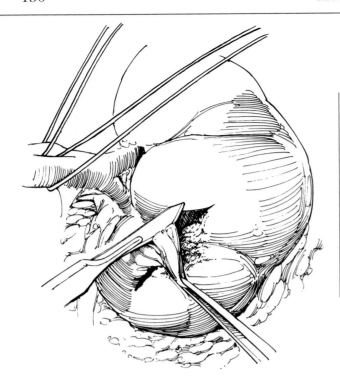

FIGURE 25-4. Remove the intrarenal hematoma from the laceration. Resect any necrotic tissue. If you think reconstruction will take more than 30 minutes, cool the kidney with slush (see Chapter 26). Secure hemostasis by placing fine figure-of-eight 4-0 chromic catgut sutures on the interlobar, arcuate, or interlobular vessels. (Use catgut sutures; they slide through tissue better than do woven, nonabsorbable ones.) Ligate a segmental vessel if it supplies less than 15% of the kidney; if the resulting infarction is greater than that, remove that portion of the kidney. If there is a major injury of the upper or lower pole, elect partial nephrectomy (see Chapter 27). Injured segmental veins can be ligated without concern for renal infarction because of intrarenal collateral circulation.

FIGURE 25-5. Close any open calyces or infundibula watertightly with running 4-0 chromic catgut sutures. Be certain that there is no leakage: pinch the upper ureter closed while injecting a small amount of dilute methylene blue directly into the renal pelvis. Close any residual openings. Apply patches of gelatin sponge or microfibrillar collagen to persistently oozing areas.

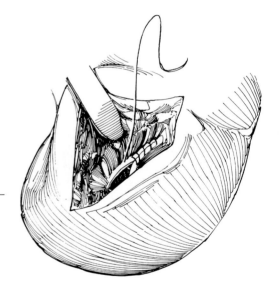

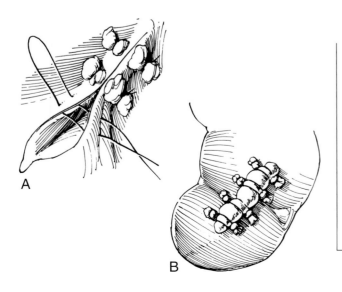

FIGURE 25-6. A, Cover the defect with any available capsule and hold it in place with mattress sutures over fat bolsters. **B,** Alternatively, apply a long bolster of gelatin sponge to the capsule, held with mattress sutures. The capsule often is destroyed; in that case, use a pedicle flap of omentum (see Chapter 65) brought through a window in the mesocolon and tacked in place with interrupted 4-0 chromic catgut sutures. Because the calyces usually have been entered and there is a risk of urinary leakage, insert a closed-system (Jackson-Pratt) drain that exits retroperitoneally from the flank through a stab wound. (Choose closed drainage in preference to Penrose drainage because it decreases the chance for infecting the retroperitoneal hematoma.) Leave the drain in place for 2 days (only) after urinary drainage stops.

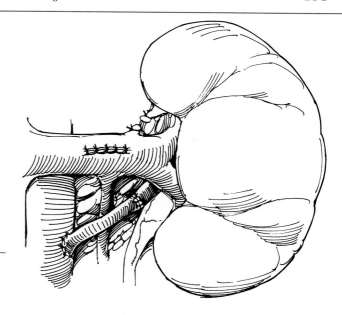

FIGURE 25-7. Renal artery thrombosis: Remove that segment of the artery and replace the defect with vascular graft obtained from the saphenous vein or hypogastric artery. Close lacerations of the main renal vein with fine vascular sutures but ligate a lacerated venous branch and depend on internal collateral circulation. With deceleration injury to the renal artery, the defect is usually at the origin of the artery from the aorta, leaving a length of artery on the kidney suitable for autotransplantation (see Chapter 60). Follow the blood pressure and hematocrit closely and provide intravenous fluids to achieve a high-urine output.

POSTOPERATIVE PROBLEMS

Watch for delayed bleeding, infection with abscess formation, formation of a urinoma, and continued open or closed urinary leakage. Later complications are formation of an arteriovenous fistula, hypertension, renal atrophy, renal calculi, and secondary hydronephrosis. Obtain a renal scan 6 months after injury.

Commentary by JACK W. MCANINCH

In the pediatric age group, renal injuries occur most commonly from blunt trauma. The presence of five red blood cells or more per high-power field in the urine is indicative, and imaging studies should be done (intravenous urogram and/or CT scan) to stage the injury. The major indication for exploration is renal bleeding, but large segments (more than 15%) of nonviable tissue associated with a parenchymal laceration and urinary extravasation constitute relative indications. If the renal vessels on the injured side are isolated before exploration of the kidney, they can then be clamped should heavy bleeding be encountered when Gerota's fascia is entered. Total renal exposure is important, because multiple injuries may be present.

It is important to place vessel loops on the renal vasculature before exploring the hematoma and kidney. Clamping of the renal artery usually is not necessary. Bleeding often can be controlled with finger compression. All clot and nonviable tissue should be removed and hemostasis obtained, as recommended in the text. The use of microfibrin collagen hemostatic sponge is helpful when small amounts of bloody oozing persist on the repaired surface.

Aggressive debridement of nonviable tissue should be done by sharp dissection. Bleeding vessels are individually suture ligated, and the collecting system is closed watertightly. The fracture margins can be approximated by closing the capsule over bolsters. When the capsule has been destroyed, omentum or a free graft of peritoneum can be used to cover the defect. Omentum is my choice because of its viability and support of wound healing.

When the collecting system has been opened, a drain should be placed only until one is certain that urine is not draining and then should be removed (48 hours). This will help avoid infecting the retroperitoneum and the hematoma.

Injuries to the main renal artery seldom can be repaired with adequate return of renal function in approximately 20% of cases; in many of these, multiple associated injuries make renal arterial reconstruction—a time-consuming process—unfeasible. In most cases, renal vein injury can be repaired. Segmental artery injury without parenchymal laceration should be ligated; the infarcted tissue will be reabsorbed, and hypertension seldom occurs.

A watertight closure of the collecting system is important. A simple method to check the closure is to occlude the upper ureter by finger compression and inject 5 mL of dilute methylene blue into the renal pelvis. Any small openings are easily noted and closed; follow with coverage of the defect (e.g., omentum) to provide added security. Closed-system (Jackson-Pratt) drains are preferred to decrease the potential for infecting the retroperitoneal hematoma. These reconstructions should take less than 1 hour in most instances. It is important to move through the process expeditiously; otherwise, the trauma surgeon becomes impatient as the child's temperature drops along with the blood volume.

DAVID JOSEPH

Blunt trauma accounts for more than 90% of pediatric renal injuries, often associated with coexisting intra-abdominal and skeletal injuries. The presence of gross or microscopic hematuria may be misleading when placed in context with the magnitude of the injury. Children have been identified to have renal injuries in the face of a normal urinalysis. Significant gross hematuria may be noted in "minor" trauma, raising suspicion of a congenital abnormality. Pediatric kidneys in general, especially those with a congenital abnormality, are more susceptible to injury due to decreased protective perirenal fat and less protection from the rib cage. This contributes to increased mobility of the kidney while the ureter remains relatively fixed, resulting in a greater association of UPJ disruption.

Most trauma protocols within the United States rely on CT imaging for screening. Ideally renal evaluation requires a triphasic examination that includes precontrast images, a rapid postcontrast injection phase, and delayed images to evaluate parenchymal injury, extravasation, and renal pelvic and ureteral continuity. However, many centers only obtain the rapid postcontrast injection phase as part of their trauma protocol. That provides better imaging of other abdominal organs but only allows for renal parenchymal assessment. Obtaining a delayed study is often deferred because of the radiologist's desire to minimize radiation exposure, or the trauma surgeon's critical need to transport the child to the operating room. Unfortunately, the urologist is often called after the initial imaging has been completed when the child is in the intensive care unit or operating room. Repeat imaging may be required particularly to identify extravasation or a UPJ disruption. A single intravenous urogram image must be obtained in the operating room before exposing the retroperitoneum if renal function has not been confirmed and ureteral anatomy has not been visualized on initial imaging.

I think the greatest operative dilemma regarding pediatric renal trauma is lack of experience for most urologists, due to the infrequent exposure to the initial, emergent evaluation and treatment. Trauma surgeons appropriately have become more conservative with operative intervention of associated internal injuries, limiting the number of children urgently taken to the operating room. With aggressive resuscitation, children remain hemodynamically stable and observation has become the rule even in the face of dramatic grade 3, 4, and 5 injuries. This experience has taught us that major renal injury and extravasation in itself is not the trigger for exploration. The exception is emergent exploration for UPJ transection even with a stable patient. When trauma surgeons take a child to the operating room it usually is a reflection of major associated injuries and hemodynamic instability. When faced with a renal injury rarely do trauma surgeons feel it time-efficient to call the urologist and usually embark on their own, often resulting in a nephrectomy.

When confronted with operative trauma it is usually because the child is unstable. Operative time becomes critical for survival of the kidney and child. Wide exposure of the retroperitoneum is necessary. It is intuitive to gain early access to the renal hilum to assist with control of bleeding but this is usually not an easy task and may not be required or found beneficial in all situations. A compromise is rapid digital compression of the hilum allowing for debridement of the traumatized renal tissue and suture ligature of bleeding vessels. A watertight closure of the collecting system is also appealing but not always possible and could become detrimental if vigorously pursued. The pediatric renal capsule is diminutive to begin with. Most injuries requiring urgent operative intervention are so extensive that covering the injury with a capsule is not feasible. Gelfoam supported by an absorbable mesh wrap placed around the defect and sutured to itself can be beneficial to secure a major renal disruption. The renal bed should be drained preferentially through the flank or back. I place the drain dependently and avoid direct contact with the repair. I typically do not use suction drains because I feel the negative pressure encourages leakage. When faced with a significant vascular injury I would undertake segmental or total nephrectomy, depending on the location of the vascular injury, over any attempt at a vascular repair. Unless you have significant vascular experience, the time required and risk-to-benefit ratio for attempted vascular repair are not favorable.

Chapter 26

Simple Nephrectomy

For retroperitoneal masses, obtain a sonogram. If the mass is renal and cystic do a radioisotope scan. Nonfunction means multicystic kidney or advanced ureteropelvic junction (UPJ) obstruction. If the kidney functions, perform a voiding cystourethrogram. Reflux identifies megaureter and duplication. Absence of reflux can mean UPJ or ureterovesical junction obstruction, duplication, or ureterocele. If the renal mass is solid by sonography, a computed tomography (CT) scan is needed to identify Wilms' tumor, neuroblastoma, or mesoblastic nephroma.

Subject an adrenal mass detected by sonography to CT scan to differentiate solid neuroblastomas from cystic adrenal hemorrhage. The CT scan also will help identify retroperitoneal lymphomas and sarcomas. For Wilms' tumor, if CT scan and sonography show a unilateral tumor, proceed with nephrectomy. If nephrectomy is not possible, perform a biopsy preparatory to chemotherapy and delayed nephrectomy. If tumors are bilateral perform unilateral total and contralateral partial nephrectomy or a bilateral partial nephrectomy; if that is not possible, obtain a biopsy preparatory to chemotherapy. In a solitary or fused kidney, do a partial nephrectomy or a biopsy if partial nephrectomy is not possible. For pyonephrosis, consider percutaneous drainage to clear the infection before removing the kidney.

For renal carcinoma, rare in children, radical excision of the kidney with nodal dissection for malignancy appears not to add to the rate of cure. However, removal of tumor from the vena cava is beneficial.

SELECTION OF INCISION

The selection of incision for a simple nephrectomy should be dictated by the size of the nonfunctional renal unit. A small, nonfunctional kidney secondary to reflux can safely be removed through a dorsal lumbotomy or small modified transcostal incision off the tip of the 12th rib. In contrast, a large, nonfunctional UPJ obstruction may best be removed with an anterior subcostal incision (see "Anterior Subcostal Approach") or transcostal approach. Presently, a laparoscopic approach if available is the least morbid approach for simple nephrectomy.

ANTERIOR SUBCOSTAL APPROACH

Give intravenous crystalloid fluids preoperatively. Have blood available in case of a vascular accident. Provide endotracheal anesthesia and adequate relaxation.

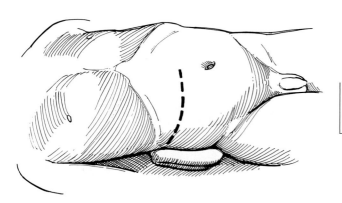

FIGURE 26-1. Position: Place the child on the operating table in a semioblique position, with a folded towel under the flank. Incision: Perform an anterior subcostal incision (see Chapter 12).

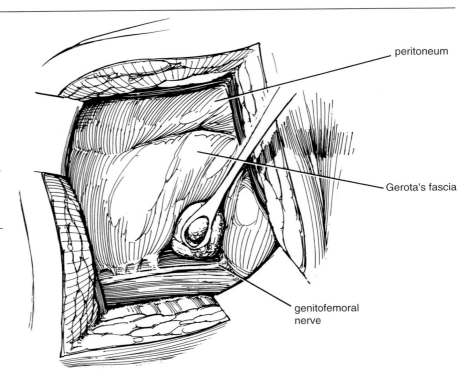

peritoneum

Gerota's fascia

genitofemoral
nerve

FIGURE 26-2. Bluntly push Gerota's fascia medially off of the psoas muscle, carrying the peritoneal reflection with it. Install a self-retaining retractor.

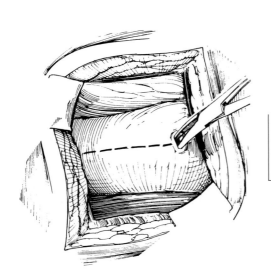

FIGURE 26-3. Insert a Kelly clamp through Gerota's fascia into the pale, lemon-yellow–colored perirenal fat. Open Gerota's fascia longitudinally with scissors through the length of the incision. Fingers may also be used to separate the thin fascia.

FIGURE 26-4. Bluntly and sharply dissect the perirenal fat from the lower pole of the kidney. Do the easy parts first, gradually working toward the more adherent areas. Take care ventrally where the peritoneum may be adherent. Open the peritoneum if adherent bowel is suspected. Gerota's fascia should be held medially in two curved clamps by the assistant. Watch for aberrant blood vessels, especially near the poles. An area resistant to dissection may well contain a vessel. Aspirate the contents of a large hydronephrosis to aid in exposure. Dissect sharply under vision near the pedicle. Fulgurate the emissary veins and do not dissect under the capsule. Identify the ureter on the peritoneal side of the wound. Free it with a right-angle clamp, and encircle it with a Penrose drain to allow it to be freed further. Be aware that the gonadal vein is readily torn.

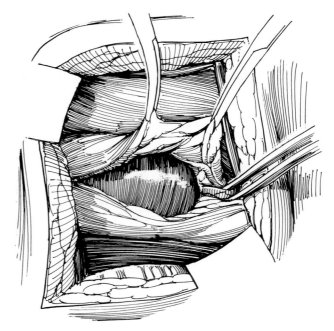

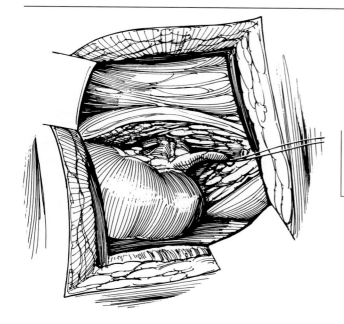

FIGURE 26-5. Doubly clamp and cut the ureter. Ligate both ends with absorbable suture material, leaving the proximal suture long enough for identification and traction. Dissect proximally along the ureter to free the pelvis.

SECURING THE PEDICLE

Complete the dissection of the tissue anterior to the pedicle, trimming it approximately 1 cm away from the hilum. Identify the renal vein anteriorly, dissect it for a short distance, and encircle it with a vessel loop. Below the vein, identify and dissect the artery.

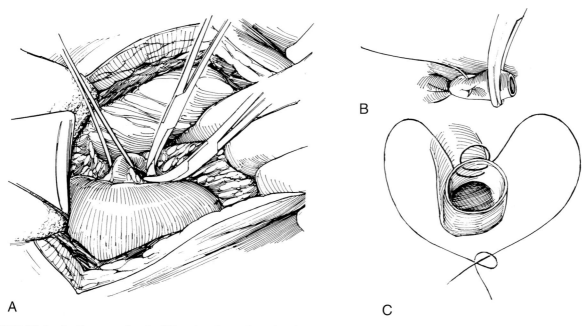

A

B

C

FIGURE 26-6. A, One method of ligation is to doubly clamp the artery and divide it between the clamps; do the same for the vein and remove the specimen. **B** and **C,** Tie the artery with a 1-0 synthetic absorbable suture, reinforced with a second, more distal 1-0 synthetic absorbable suture as a stick tie. Ligate the vein with a 1-0 synthetic absorbable suture.

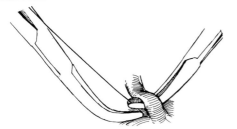

FIGURE 26-7. A preferable method of pedicle ligation, rather than to clamp the vessels, is to pass a right-angle clamp under the artery and draw two ligatures successively around it. Then, doubly ligate the artery. Do the same for the vein. If it is the right renal vein, use two Satinsky clamps on the vena cava and oversew the cuff after removing one clamp.

LOSS OF CONTROL OF THE PEDICLE

Remain calm. Palpate the source of the spurting blood to be able to compress the vessel digitally for 10 minutes. Alternatively, compress the artery and vein with a stick sponge. Take time to obtain a second suction line, more blood, and some 5-0 vascular sutures and vascular clamps. Tell the anesthetist about the situation. First, replace the blood loss. Do not clamp blindly, but get exposure, compress the aorta above the renal artery, and, under vision, clamp the artery with a vascular clamp or try to visualize one end of the hole and put a suture in it. Tie the suture and hold it up as you put a stitch in the part your assistant exposes next. Run the vascular suture up the defect and down again as your assistant slowly rolls the packs away and you apply suction.

Alternatively, hold a finger over the hole and grasp the vessel with the tip of a Kocher clamp. Pulling up on it stops the bleeding so the vessel can be suture ligated. For the vena cava, Allis clamps are adequate.

CLOSURE

Fill the wound with saline solution and look for bubbles, because the pleura might have been breached. If the pleura does require repair proceed as described (see Chapter 16) and expose an upright chest film in the postanesthesia care unit. Beware of tension pneumothorax from either a torn pleural adhesion or an actual laceration of the lung. When the pleura is intact, insert a Penrose drain to be left 24 hours to let the air and serum out of the wound, and allow observation for bleeding. Inject 0.25% or 0.5% bupivacaine into the appropriate intercostal nerve, or insert a small feeding tube adjacent to the wound to allow subsequent bupivacaine administration. Close the wound with 3-0 or 4-0 synthetic absorbable sutures. If this is a secondary operation, first insert the sutures and then tie them successively.

ANTERIOR TRANSPERITONEAL APPROACH

Divide the parietal peritoneum lateral to the descending or the ascending colon. Enter the plane between the peritoneum and Gerota's fascia, and bluntly separate these structures to approach the aorta or vena cava. For nonmalignant conditions, enter Gerota's fascia over the medial border of the kidney and expose the vein and artery. On the left side, secure the renal artery with a heavy silk ligature by retracting the vein caudad. On the right side, secure it between the vena cava and aorta. Now clamp the vein, ligate it, and divide it. Place a second tie, divide the artery, and oversew the end with a 4-0 arterial suture. The kidney is then readily removed within Gerota's fascia. Drain the area through the flank by a stab wound.

SUBCAPSULAR NEPHRECTOMY

Removal of the kidney inside the capsule is rarely performed except in unusual situations such as severe infection or rejection of a transplanted kidney. Be careful because the kidney capsule may lie just below the fascia so that the parenchyma can be entered easily because little pararenal or perirenal fat usually remains in this area. Before concluding that a subcapsular nephrectomy is necessary, try separating the perirenal fat from the capsule with blunt dissection in the usual way. Only if this proves impossible, proceed subcapsularly. Incise the scarred perirenal tissue and the capsule from the lateral border medially to the hilum and grasp the edge with a Mayo clamp. With a finger beneath this layer, bluntly peel the capsule from the parenchyma anteriorly until the hilum is reached.

Draw back on the kidney while retracting the capsule medially. Palpate the renal artery (it is usually small) and incise the turned-back capsule directly in line with it.

Dissect the renal artery first if possible, even though it lies behind the vein. Triply ligate the artery in continuity and divide it. Treat the renal vein similarly. If separation of the vessels is not possible, place two pedicle clamps and divide between them. Rotate the kidney cephalad and place a Penrose drain around the ureter below the scar tissue; then divide and ligate it. Continue the dissection up along the ureter to free the renal pelvis. Remove as much perirenal tissue with the specimen as feasible. Close with adequate drainage, to be continued longer than that usual for an uncomplicated case.

POSTOPERATIVE PROBLEMS

Hemorrhage can arise from the renal artery, aorta, or vena cava. A vessel in spasm may be overlooked during closure. Ileus can be a problem, secondary to retroperitoneal dissection about the celiac axis. Even after a flank approach, the patient should not resume oral intake until peristalsis returns.

JACK ELDER

Simple nephrectomy generally is performed for removal of a nonfunctioning or poorly functioning kidney in a child with hypertension or vesicoureteral reflux, hydronephrosis secondary to a UPJ obstruction or single-system ureterocele, multi-locular cystic nephroma, mesoblastic nephroma, and occasionally a Wilms' tumor, a kidney involved with xanthogranu-lomatous pyelonephritis, or an unusual multicystic, dysplastic kidney. The laparoscopic approach (either transperitoneal or retroperitoneal) is preferred, even in infants, but in selected cases it is performed through a small flank, anterior subcostal, or dorsal lumbotomy. The principles of nephrectomy are similar, however, irrespective of the operative approach.

If the procedure is performed through an incision for removal of a hydronephrotic or multicystic kidney, it can generally be performed through an incision that is only 2 to 2.5 cm, even for a severely hydronephrotic kidney. After Gerota's fascia is opened, most of the urine or fluid in the kidney may be aspirated, allowing the kidney to shrink significantly. This maneuver is helpful also for laparoscopic nephrectomy. The kidney may then be freed up without much difficulty. In a nonfunctioning kidney, the vascular pedicle is attenuated, but nevertheless, control of the pedicle is important. I think it is easiest to place a small right-angle clamp across the pedicle in nonfunctioning kidneys, transect the vessels, remove the kidney, and then tie off the vessels together with two polyglycolic acid sutures; it is unnecessary to separate the artery and vein. On the other hand, if the kidney is functioning, then the vessels should be tied off in continuity, and the artery should be separated from the vein. Although classic teaching is to tie off the artery first, I have not found that tying off the renal vein before the renal artery causes significant renal swelling.

Management of postoperative pain has improved significantly in recent years. Assuming there is minimal oozing during the nephrectomy, intravenous ketorolac, 0.5 mg/kg (maximum 30 mg) is administered at the end of the operation, and 0.25 mg/kg is administered every 6 hours with a maximum of 7 doses. In addition, an intercostal nerve block is quite benefi-cial. A solution composed of 5 mL of 0.25% bupivacaine and 5 mL of 1% xylocaine with 1:100,000 epinephrine (yielding 0.125% bupivacaine with 1:200,000 epinephrine) is injected through a 23-gauge butterfly needle in the T10, T11, and sub-costal spaces into the neurovascular bundle. This block provides pain relief for up to 12 hours postoperatively. Alternatively, a high caudal block may be effective as well. The combination of a short incision and the intercostal block has made it possible to perform outpatient nephrectomy; in our experience, all but one who were scheduled for outpatient nephrectomy were discharged within 1 to 2 hours of the procedure. In the long run, however, the incision tends to grow with the child, whereas the laparoscopic incisions tend to blend in with the skin folds, and I think that the laparoscopic approach is preferable.

ELLEN SHAPIRO

Most simple nephrectomies are currently performed laparoscopically. Nonetheless, when simple nephrectomy is performed open, it is imperative to appropriately pad the axilla and upper and lower extremities. In small infants, the Bovie pad is placed on the contralateral flank before the flank roll is positioned. A subcostal incision is almost always used. I initially mark the anterior and posterior axillary line with the patient supine so that the incision is not visible when viewing the patient from the front. Once the incision is made, Gerota's fascia is opened with the Bovie cautery to minimize bleeding. I start the dissection at the lower pole by identifying the ureter. I leave the ureter patent when there is no demonstrable reflux on a voiding cysto-urethrogram. When the system refluxes, the ureter is oversewn and left as short as possible. If the ureter is ectopic, a preop-erative, cyclic voiding cystourethrogram will determine if there is reflux and whether or not the ureter should be left open or closed. In cases of ureteroceles, I pass an 8-F catheter down the distal ureter and irrigate the ureterocele. The ureterocele is left open for drainage and decompression. The vessels are dissected with a short, blunt-tipped right angle.

I tie all the vasculature structures with small silk sutures. The renal artery and vein usually require a 2-0 or 3-0 silk suture. A double tie is placed on the patient's side for safety. If there is loss of control of the pedicle, pressure should be applied. Do not clamp haphazardly, as the aorta and the inferior vena cava will be small in infants and can be inadvertently ligated. Never hesitate to call for the assistance of a vascular surgeon. Beware of injury to the left renal vein when you are performing a right nephrectomy. Also remember that the right renal vein is short and must be treated with great respect. When I was a resident, my mentor left a small Penrose drain in infants, as unexpected blood loss would not be tolerated. Dextrose water is initially given postoperatively and the diet is advanced as tolerated for age. Most patients are ready for discharge within a 23-hour stay.

Chapter 27

Partial Nephrectomy

Consider partial nephrectomy for children with bilateral tumors or a tumor in a solitary kidney, especially in the presence of compromised renal function. Partial nephrectomy provides functional renal reserve at the cost of a technically more difficult operation, with a greater chance of local recurrence and more manipulation of the tumor.

For bilateral Wilms' tumor, perform a CT scan or an MRI to allow for preoperative planning. Renal arteriography is rarely needed.

Have the child well hydrated before occluding the arterial blood supply. If the operation might become complex, prepare iced slush for renal cooling. With a solitary kidney, which may become severely stressed by intraoperative ischemia, arrange for vascular access preoperatively to be ready for postoperative dialysis.

Extracorporeal surgery for partial nephrectomy is useful with large tumors to avoid spillage and to allow more complete resection, but it is rarely necessary, and it does carry a higher risk. After removing the kidney in toto, flush the main artery with renal preservation solution until clear. Excise the tumor, avoiding injury to the major vessels and ureter. Take special care not to interfere with the vessels supplying the ureter and renal pelvis. Perfusion through the artery or vein helps identify vascular branches. After closing the collecting system and parenchyma, transplant the kidney into the iliac fossa.

Make preparations for cooling even though warm ischemia time seldom exceeds 30 minutes. Start intravenous (IV) mannitol administration.

FIGURE 27-1. **A,** Position: Lateral, over a kidney bolster. Incision: A supracostal incision is best for adolescents (see Chapter 14), but a partial anterior transverse incision (see Chapter 10) is suitable for children, especially if autotransplantation is a possibility. With the flank approach, open Gerota's fascia in the lateral plane, and free up the entire kidney. Leave the perirenal fat around the tumor undisturbed. **B,** Dissect the vascular pedicle sufficiently to allow immediate application of vascular clamps. Place a vascular tape around the renal artery. Identify the hilar vessels leading to the involved portion of the kidney. Palpate for hilar nodes (left para-aortic for left-sided tumors; right paracaval for right-sided tumors) as the operation is for carcinoma, and send suspicious nodes for frozen-section examination.

Inspect the kidney to determine the practicality and the site for heminephrectomy. To find the line of demarcation, place a bulldog clamp temporarily on the identified artery and observe for blanching. Intravenous indigo-carmine dye may give a line for resection. Place a vascular tape around any accessory vessels. Ligate and divide polar vessels that directly supply the segment to be removed. The plane of excision must follow the radial direction of the renal segments.

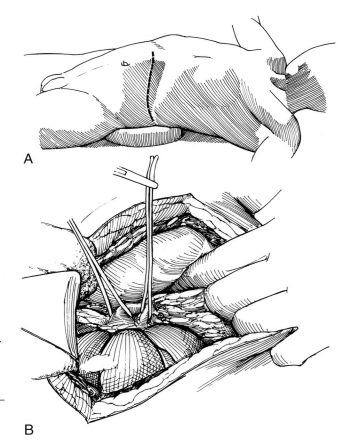

A

B

POLAR PARTIAL NEPHRECTOMY

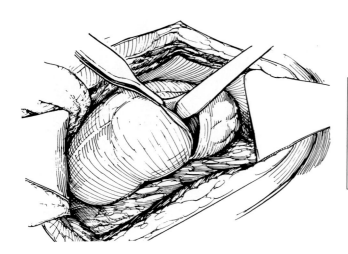

FIGURE 27-2. Apply a padded rubber dam, clamp the artery in a padded clamp, and cool the kidney, unless ischemia time is estimated to be less than 30 minutes. Ask the anesthetist to inject furosemide or give 20% mannitol IV. Incise the capsule 1 to 2 cm distal to the site of the proposed resection unless this is over tumor, in which case, move the incision proximally. Reflect the capsule from the normal parenchyma with the back of the knife.

FIGURE 27-3. Place a rubber-shod bulldog clamp on the artery. In some cases, finger compression of the parenchyma may substitute for vascular clamping. It is not necessary or desirable to clamp the renal vein if the main renal artery is occluded.

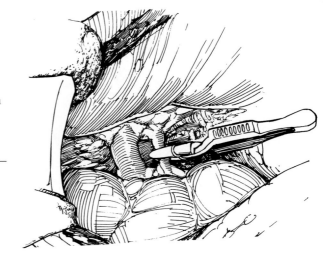

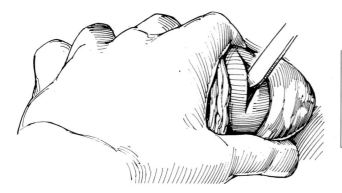

FIGURE 27-4. Bluntly incise the parenchyma, using the knife handle, leaving 1 cm of normal tissue with the side of the tumor. Follow the normal plane (neither guillotine nor wedge) between the renal lobules. Progressive slices may be removed if the disease process extends more proximally, unless dealing with carcinoma, in which case it must be treated by nephrectomy.

FIGURE 27-5. Use the thumbnail as a wedge to help separation.

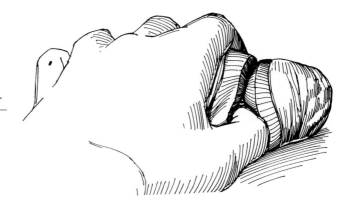

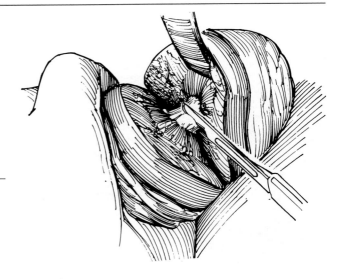

FIGURE 27-6. Sharply divide the arcuate vessels with Lahey scissors and suture-ligate them with figure-eight, 4-0 or 5-0 chromic catgut sutures. Divide each calyceal infundibulum with knife or scissors. Transect them as distally as possible in stone cases.

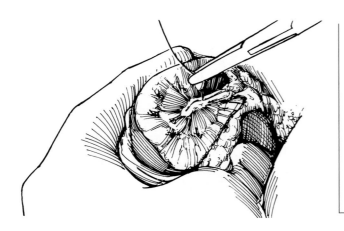

FIGURE 27-7. Suture-ligate all remaining arcuate vessels, paying special attention to the large venous collectors near the hilum. Work rapidly but accurately. Electrocoagulation cannot be used because of the electrolytes in the urine, although argon beam laser coagulation, if available, may be effective. Ligate the interlobar vessels with sutures that include the adjacent infundibulum. Release the bulldog clamp momentarily to help identification and ligation of remaining open vessels. Place a self-retaining ureteral stent if desired. Close the infundibulum with a 4-0 or 5-0 continuous synthetic absorbable suture to make sure the suture line is watertight. If the operation is for a tumor, send specimens of appropriate margins for frozen-section examination.

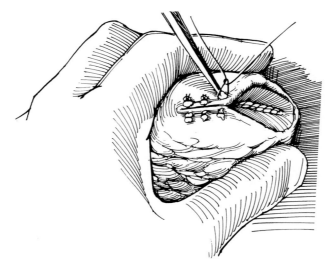

FIGURE 27-8. If possible, close the kidney on itself (it will be limp because the artery is clamped) or close the capsule alone, using 3-0 or 4-0 chromic catgut mattress sutures; enclose fat pads obtained from the properitoneal fat in the loops. A free peritoneal graft can substitute for an inadequate capsule, or pull the omentum through the retroperitoneum and apply it as a wrap. Gelfoam may be applied for hemostasis before closing the capsule over it. Release the bulldog clamp, and compress the kidney at the suture line for several minutes to ensure hemostasis. If urinary output decreases after release of the clamp, give IV furosemide.

Place a closed suction drain to exit through a stab wound. Close Gerota's fascia to cushion the repair inside the perirenal fat. Complete the wound closure. Drain for at least 7 days. If leakage does occur, perform a retrograde ureterogram and place a J stent. Within the first postoperative month, obtain a sonogram and CT study of the kidney as a baseline, and follow with sonograms every 3 months for the first 2 years.

WEDGE RESECTION FOR PERIPHERAL TUMORS

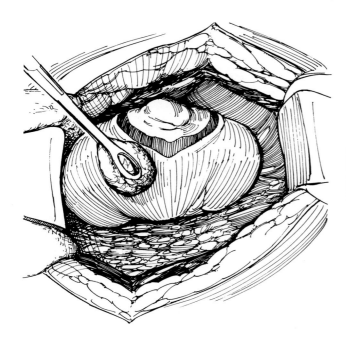

FIGURE 27-9. Incise the capsule 2 cm away from the tumor margin (0.2 cm is minimum). Consider clamping the renal artery if the resection will be extensive.

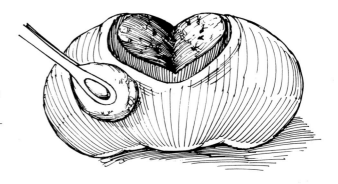

FIGURE 27-10. Remove a wedge by following the plane of the nephrons to include adequate normal parenchyma beyond the tumor. Secure hemostasis by figure-of-eight suture ligation. Before closing the collecting system, place an internal stent.

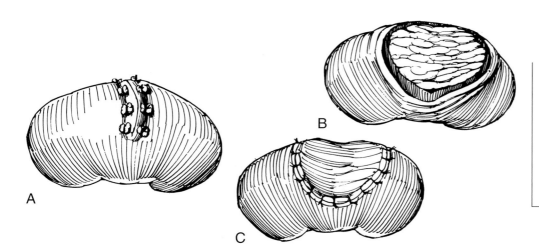

FIGURE 27-11. A, Close the defect with mattress sutures including fat bolsters to the capsule. **B,** If the defect is large, fill it with retroperitoneal or omental fat before closure. **C,** Suture the two poles together, or apply hemostatic gauze or a free peritoneal graft.

A

B

C

ENUCLEATION

Enucleation is done for a very small tumor and is the only possibility for a patient with multiple tumors in a solitary kidney. However, malignant cells may extend into the pseudocapsule and lead to local recurrence. Rather than simply enucleating, remove a layer of normal parenchyma if it can be done without entering a major vessel or calyx. Vascular control is not needed.

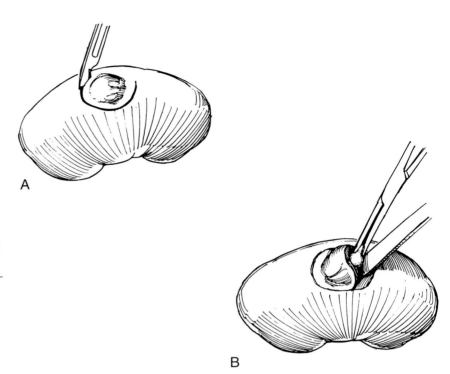

FIGURE 27-12. A and B, Incise the capsule around the tumor. Bluntly enucleate the tumor by following the plane outside of the compressed pseudocapsule, which is composed of relatively avascular renal tissue. Avoid entering a calyx. Fulgurate the false capsule with an argon beam laser and pack it with oxidized cellulose or omentum as necessary to control oozing. Close the capsule as in other techniques.

POSTOPERATIVE PROBLEMS

If urinary leakage persists, look for distal obstruction. Urinomas and fistulas are uncommon but occur with wedge resections that are closed with large mattress sutures. A resection following the plane of the lobules followed by closure of the calyx with a watertight suture is best. Placement of a ureteral catheter rarely is necessary.

Renal artery thrombosis from damage to the intima by traction on the pedicle is a rare complication. Secondary nephrectomy is necessary in fewer than 3% of cases. A brief period of renal insufficiency may follow partial nephrectomy in a solitary kidney, and gradually decreasing renal function may occur later in children with reduced renal parenchyma as a result of hyperperfusion.

BARRY KOGAN

Commentary by

A flank approach is preferred for partial nephrectomy as exposure is better and morbidity less. However, in a patient with bilateral tumors, depending on the clinical situation, a transperitoneal approach may be necessary as it is often appropriate to deal with both kidneys at the same time. The techniques illustrated are excellent and, in addition, laparoscopic instrumentation has allowed for some new modifications. In particular, the harmonic scalpel can be used in an open approach and allows for an almost bloodless dissection of the kidney. Indeed, it is our preferred method of dissection for partial- or heminephrectomy. Control of the hilum is important, but clamping the vessels is rarely needed today, unless the tumor is central or there are multiple vessels.

Commentary by
KATSUHIKO UEOKA

When the size of tumor is large, dissection is performed just outside the tumor capsule. Leaving the capsule intact is more than adequate in such situations. Intraoperative ultrasonography is useful in cases in which the tumor is located inside the kidney and invisible at the operative field. Because even a small amount of blood loss would be relatively substantial in younger children, I would recommend not to hesitate to clamp the renal artery and vein in the difficult dissections.

Chapter 28

Pediatric Heminephrectomy

Heminephrectomy is indicated for excision for a diseased upper pole in a duplicated system. Excision of the refluxing stump is indicated in genital ectopy, in contrast to urinary ectopy in which a secondary procedure is rarely required.

Simple endoscopic incision of the associated ureterocele may allow deferral of heminephrectomy, and also facilitate lower urinary tract reconstruction and reduce the need for partial nephrectomy.

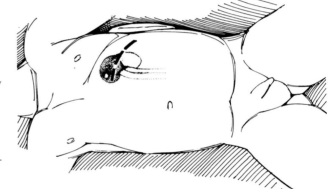

FIGURE 28-1. Position: Place the child supine with the involved side slightly elevated. Incision: Make an anterior subcostal extraperitoneal (see Chapter 9) or transcostal (see Chapter 13) incision. Open Gerota's fascia posteriorly and mobilize the usually scanty fat anteriorly to free the entire kidney. Rotate the kidney anteriorly and expose the upper-pole ureter, pelvis, and the renal pedicle from behind. The line of demarcation will be obvious on inspection and palpation.

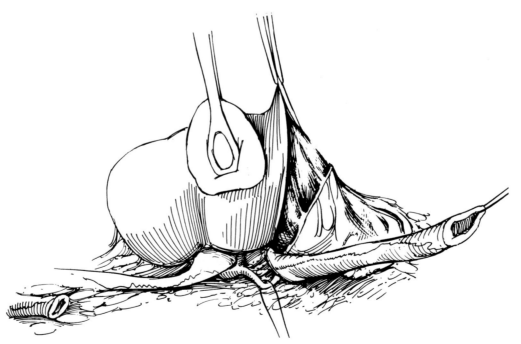

FIGURE 28-2. Identify both ureters and trace the dilated one to the upper pole. Encircle this ureter with a vessel loop or small Penrose drain and free it from its bed as distally as feasible, while avoiding interference with the blood supply to the other ureter. Complete the ureterectomy especially in genital ectopy, which may require a counterincision (see Chapter 63). Divide the ureter but do not ligate the distal stump, especially if the urine is infected. Provide a Penrose drain.

FIGURE 28-2, cont'd. Place a traction suture on the proximal end of the ureter and pass it under (posterior to) the upper-pole vessels. While completing the proximal ureteral dissection into the hilum, lifting the ureter will help identify the vessels before division. Take care not to avulse the small branches to the upper-pole segment. Locate and dissect the blood supply to the upper segment. If a vessel is not clearly separate from those going to the rest of the kidney, pass a 3-0 silk suture around it, occlude it with traction, and note the area of blanching. If you see that all or part of the upper pole becomes ischemic, tie the suture and divide the vessel. It is seldom necessary to occlude the main renal artery; if such occlusion is needed, give intravenous mannitol before applying the clamp.

Note the deep groove between upper and lower moieties and the relative difference in thickness and color of the parenchymas. Feel for the pulsation of the arteries to the lower pole. Incise the renal capsule circumferentially 2 cm distal to the now obvious line of demarcation and peel it back with a knife handle.

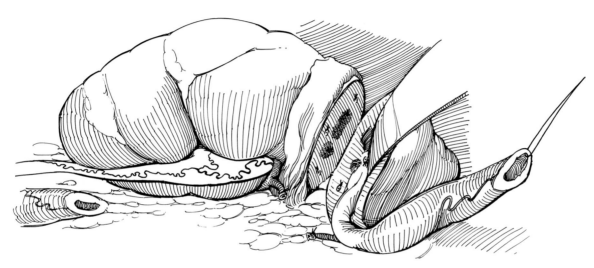

FIGURE 28-3. Transect the renal parenchyma, which will be concave at this site, with knife blade, knife handle, and scissors along the plane of demarcation. Sharp dissection is needed because of the fibrous character of the tissue. Insert the index finger into the upper-pole renal pelvis to help identify the plane between the upper and lower poles. If in doubt, leave some upper-pole tissue behind because any residual upper-pole tissue or portions of calyces may be trimmed later. As the separation proceeds, place a figure-of-eight, 4-0 synthetic absorbable transfixion suture on any major parenchymal vessel, especially on those associated with the calyx or pelvis. Remove the remnants of the calyceal lining, that is, those not already contained in the specimen. Avoid opening into the upper calyx belonging to the lower segment; if opened, close that calyx with a running 4-0 synthetic absorbable suture.

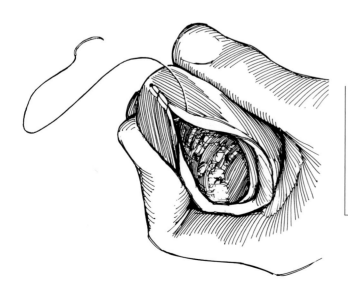

FIGURE 28-4. Close the capsule over the exposed parenchyma with a running 4-0 synthetic absorbable suture. Place a Penrose drain adjacent to the area of transection, reapproximate the perirenal fat and Gerota's fascia, and close the wound in layers. For the rare case requiring lower-pole heminephrectomy, the procedure is similar, except that extreme care must be taken to preserve the vascular supply to the upper pole, which is usually a branch from the main lower-pole vessel.

EARL Y. CHENG

There are numerous options for management of a duplex system when the upper-pole system is associated with either a ureterocele or an ectopic ureter. These include heminephrectomy, ureteroureterostomy, and common sheath reimplantation. When lower-pole reflux does not exist, upper-pole nephrectomy is considered by many to be the most definitive surgical treatment. This can be done both laparoscopically and with traditional open surgery. Although minimally invasive approaches are becoming more applicable to heminephrectomy and other renal surgery due to improved instrumentation, the open approach is still preferred in infants and children with complicated anatomy.

One of the most important aspects of this procedure to ensure surgical success is adequate dissection of the upper-pole ureter behind the main vessels. When this is accomplished appropriately, you can easily pass the upper-pole ureter (following transection) underneath the vessels without difficulty or tethering of adjacent tissue. Be aware of small accessory vessels that can be closely associated with the upper-pole ureter, which can easily be torn and difficult to control when they are not identified prior to passing the ureter behind the vessels. The ureteral stump can then be used as a "handle" to retract the upper-pole segment that can further facilitate exposure for upper-pole excision.

In most cases, identification of the segmental upper-pole vessels is not difficult as long as careful and meticulous dissection of the hilum is undertaken. When there is doubt as to whether an individual vessel is going to the upper pole, you should place a bulldog clamp on the vessel to ensure that it is not supplying the lower pole.

The excision of the upper pole can be done sharply or with electrocautery. When using electrocautery, caution should be exercised to prevent excessive use of the cautery, which can cause unwanted spread of thermal energy with subsequent damage to the lower-pole segment. In cases in which the upper pole is not well demarcated or you anticipate that the excision will encroach on the lower-pole collecting system, placement of an open-ended ureteral stent into the lower-pole system prior to the heminephrectomy can be helpful. The stent can be injected with methylene blue to assist in identification of any injuries to the lower-pole collecting system. Following complete excision of the upper-pole segment, hemostasis is usually not a problem when the upper-pole segment is cystic and nonfunctioning. However, when it is more solid and has some retained function, control of bleeding can be more difficult. In such cases, the argon beam laser is very useful in controlling bleeding. When there is not enough residual capsule to close over the parenchymal defect, a thick bolster of a biodegradable hemostatic material (e.g., Surgicel) can be placed on top of the raw parenchymal surface and sewn into place with chromic mattress sutures.

MARK C. ADAMS

Once heminephrectomy is selected as appropriate treatment for a duplication anomaly, three factors influence the ease of surgery and the result.

First, as with any surgery, good exposure is critical. In infants and children, a subcostal incision is virtually always satisfactory for a safe approach to the upper pole of the kidney. In large teens, a supracostal incision may be better, or such patients may be ideal for laparoscopic approach. The principles of resection should be the same whether the procedure is performed open or laparoscopically. Severe downward traction on the upper-pole ureter is not a suitable means to achieve exposure as it may result in avulsion of upper-pole vessels or trauma to lower-pole blood supply. Light traction on the upper-pole ureter is, however, very helpful. Careful inspection of the two ureters is important to identify the upper-pole one with certainty before either is grasped aggressively with forceps or divided. Once the upper-pole ureter is divided, dissection of that ureter away from the lower-pole one should be done inside the adventitia of the upper-pole ureter to preserve all adventitia and blood supply with the lower-pole ureter, which will remain.

A second important aspect of surgery is accurate determination of the line of demarcation between the upper- and lower-pole segments. It is often obvious when there is dysplasia of the upper-pole segment but may be more obscure when the upper pole is hydronephrotic. When in doubt, it is better to enter the upper-pole collecting system during resection than to injure the lower pole. Any small remaining segments of the upper-pole system can be excised secondarily.

Third, the most significant potential complication of the surgery is vascular injury to the lower-pole segment; thus, the critical part of the resection itself is prospective ligation of the upper-pole blood supply while carefully protecting the lower-pole vasculature. If the upper-pole segment has a separate blood supply or is served by an early bifurcation off the lower-pole vessels, proximal ligation of the dominant vessels may be done with ease. If the bifurcation is more distal, so too must be the ligation. This may mean division of more vessels closer to the upper-pole parenchyma. Small upper-pole renal vessels often run both anteriorly and posteriorly against parenchyma within a groove with the upper-pole ureter. As the ureter is retracted cephalad, those vessels can be noted and suture ligated in situ just proximal to the line of incision into parenchyma for hemostasis. I suspect that most lower-pole infarction after upper-pole heminephrectomy results not from ligation of lower-pole vessels, but from over-zealous stretch or torque on the vessels with subsequent thrombosis. The lower-pole parenchyma should be carefully observed throughout surgery for turgor and color. If ischemia is noted, exposure should be released until color improves and then resumed carefully. I believe from my experience that younger infants are particularly more prone to such transient vasospasm.

Chapter 29

Radical Nephrectomy

CHOICE OF INCISION

For large tumors a useful approach in children is the anterior subcostal incision (see Chapter 9). Although it takes longer to make than a flank incision, it provides better exposure and has the advantage that neither the chest nor abdomen is entered. The anterior subcostal incision can easily be extended into a transperitoneal approach via the chevron or anterior transverse incision (see Chapter 10). This allows maximum exposure facilitating early control of the arterial blood supply and reducing possible blood loss.

RIGHT TRANSVERSE APPROACH

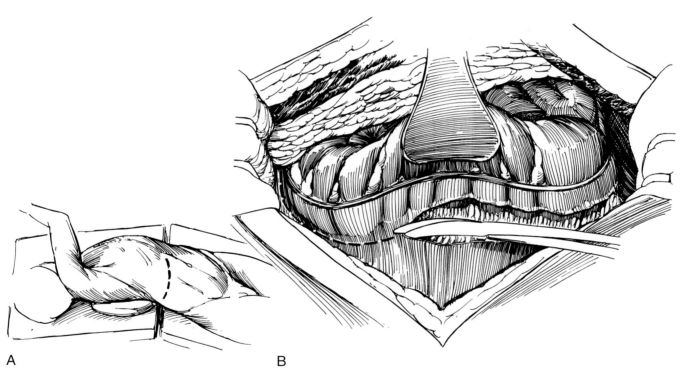

A   B

FIGURE 29-1. A, Position: Right semioblique. Incision: Extended anterior subcostal incision. The surgeon stands on the right. Open the peritoneum fully. Insert a self-retaining retractor while packing the liver and gallbladder superiorly. Palpate the abdominal viscera and the nodes. Shifting the liver medially is made easier by incising the lateral ligaments. Pack the liver superiorly but avoid injury to the underside. **B,** Retract the ascending colon medially. Pick up the parietal peritoneum and incise it over the kidney near the colon. Extend this incision from the aortic bifurcation to above the renal pedicle. With large tumors, the peritoneum covering the kidney is often infiltrated by the tumor and as a consequence, incision there becomes difficult. It may be better to begin the incision at the caudal end of the tumor, where the layers are intact. If the tumor has grown in the direction of the colon, detachment may be difficult. Avoid injury to the mesocolon.

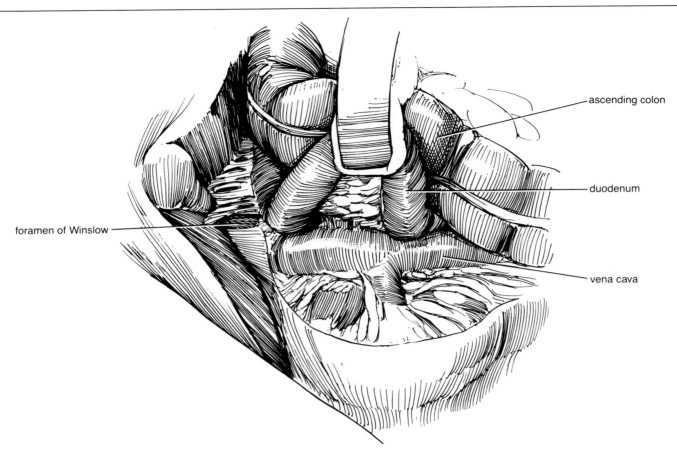

FIGURE 29-2. Mobilize the hepatic flexure of the colon and kocherize the duodenum by blunt dissection (see Chapter 9). The second part of the duodenum may be closely connected to the tumor. Detach it as follows: Carefully divide the connecting fibers by sharp dissection, and only then begin blunt dissection. (There is danger of injury to the vascular supply to the duodenum, with consequent necrosis and perforation.) Do not coagulate in this region; at the most, use only bipolar coagulation. If the duodenum is lacerated, repair it in three layers around a tube brought out through a stab wound. If a duodenal injury produces an expanding intramural hematoma, clamp and ligate the bleeding vessel, then close the serosa. Hold the bowel medially with retractors over moist lap tapes. Place laparotomy tapes over the inferior edge of the wound and hold them with a retractor blade. Beware of injury to the liver with an inadequately padded retractor—repair it with interrupted horizontal mattress sutures. Finally, it is very important to occasionally moisten the bowel and to watch it for compromised circulation.

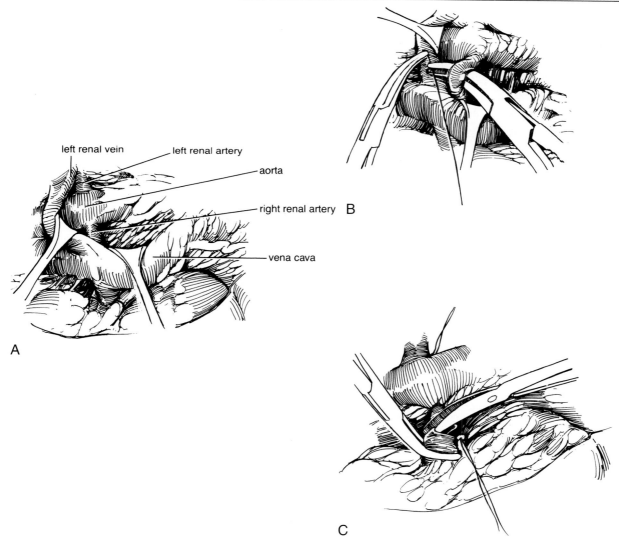

FIGURE 29-3. **A,** Dissect on the left side of the vena cava and free the left renal vein. Keep close to the anterior surface of the aorta to avoid the lumbar veins. Palpate and then expose the right renal artery by elevating the left renal vein and gently drawing the vena cava toward you. For large tumors that overlap the vena cava, it is easier to begin the dissection of the cava in the caudal region, below the lower pole of the kidney, and then slowly work up, while applying clips on the aortic side of the vena cava.

B, Pass a right-angle clamp beneath the right renal artery, grasp a ligature, pull it through, and tie it close to the aorta. Place a second ligature and tie it. Clamp and divide the artery and ligate the distal end. A suture tie may be placed on the proximal stump. A better method may be to put one tie on the artery and proceed to divide the vein to gain exposure before completing ligation of the artery with the second tie.

C, Dissect the right renal vein. If the vein is large, dissection dorsally with a right-angle clamp can be tricky. Beware of injury to the vein by too aggressive drilling on the hidden dorsal side; instead, carefully dissect it by spreading the clamp. Palpate the vein gently for any firmness that could suggest a tumor thrombus. Watch for the entrance of the main adrenal vein into the vena cava. If it is avulsed, grasp the stump with an Allis clamp and close it with a running 5-0 vascular suture. Alternatively, place one Satinsky clamp and then place a larger one beneath it; remove the top one, and oversew the stump. If the adrenal is injured, oversew the edge.

Watch for lumbar veins that enter the renal vein or vena cava at this level. When they are encountered, pass a size 0 silk ligature on a right-angle clamp and tie the renal vein. With any large tumor infiltrating in the region of the hilum, it is advisable to apply a Satinsky clamp to the vena cava proximal to the takeoff of the renal vein and then oversew the cut venous stump secondarily. Dissect the vein distally, and then clamp, divide, and ligate it. Leave the suture on the distal end of the renal vein long enough for identification by the pathologist.

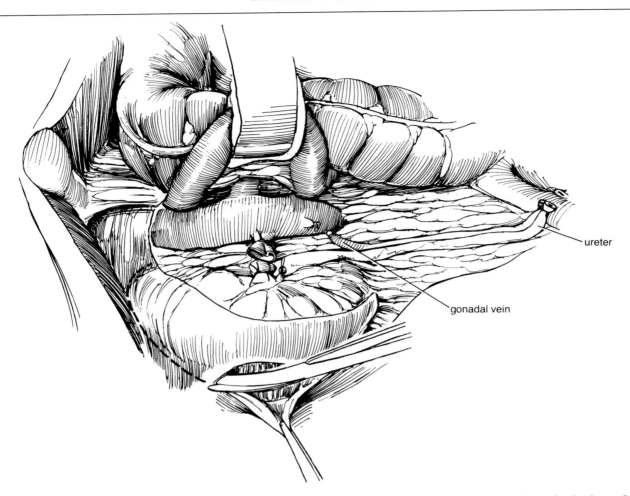

ureter

gonadal vein

FIGURE 29-4. Clear the anterior surface of the vena cava and ligate the gonadal vein. Free the lymphatic tissue from the vena cava, moving it laterally toward the right. Clip all lymphatic vessels. Mobilize the ureter and gonadal vein bluntly to the level of the bifurcation of the aorta. Lift them into the wound; clamp and ligate them with size 0 silk ligatures, leaving the proximal suture long enough for later identification. If total ureterectomy is planned for transitional cell neoplasms, free the distal end as low as is feasible, and then divide and tag it for recovery from below.

FIGURE 29-5. Pick up the lateral edge of the peritoneum below the tumor and incise it vertically up to the liver and then medially to just above the adrenal gland. Lift the lower pole of the kidney with the left hand and mobilize Gerota's fascia enclosing the kidney from the posterior body wall. Clip small vessels as they are encountered, and doubly clamp and ligate large collateral veins with 2-0 silk ligatures. Alternatively, clip these veins with large clips.

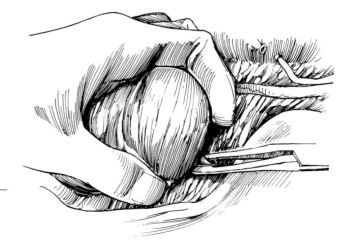

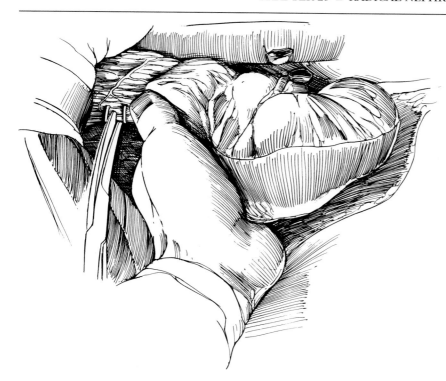

FIGURE 29-6. Pull down on the upper pole of the kidney to expose the adrenal gland while progressively dividing the connective tissue, with the vascular and peritoneal attachments. (For the tumor restricted to the lower pole, adrenalectomy is not necessary, but it is an important step with tumors in the upper part of the kidney.) Dissection is made easier by proceeding laterally along the posterior body wall toward the crus of the diaphragm. The cranial connections to the adrenal gland must be divided carefully between clips, one at a time. Clip the small vessels and especially clip the lymphatics.

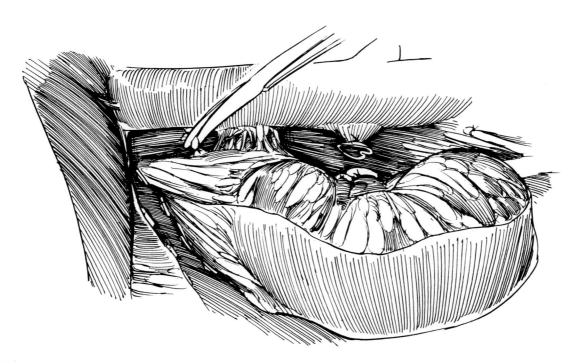

FIGURE 29-7. Displace the kidney caudally and laterally to visualize the vena cava. Expose the right adrenal vein and divide it between 2-0 silk ligatures. Avoid the small veins bridging between the liver and vena cava but clip and divide the lymphatics and the small adrenal arteries.

Unresectable tumors are those with medial extension to the aorta, vena cava, superior mesenteric vessels, and celiac axis. For renal cell carcinoma it is of little use to excise part of these tumors; the patient's only chance is complete removal. For Wilms' tumor ancillary treatment with chemotherapy is efficacious. Remove the tumor mass. It may be sensible to oversew the stumps of the renal artery and vein with 5-0 arterial silk. Close the defects in the mesocolon to prevent internal hernias. Check blood pressure; if below normal, anticipate possible bleeding from small vessels now in spasm.

REGIONAL LYMPHADENECTOMY FOR RIGHT RENAL TUMORS

Generally, it is worthwhile to perform limited, regional removal of hilar, paracaval, and para-aortic lymph nodes with resection of the corresponding interaortocaval nodes, especially for staging. The lymphadenectomy should extend as far above as the suprarenal vein and to the level of the inferior mesenteric artery below.

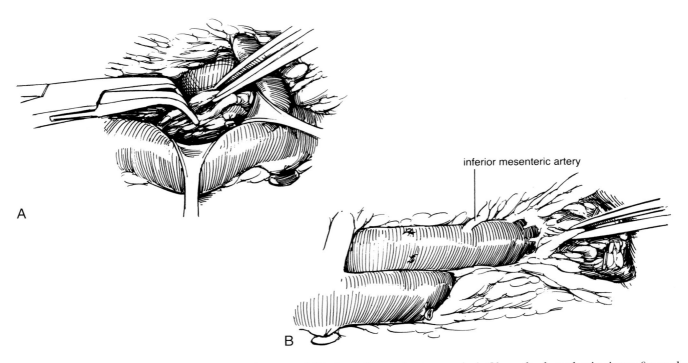

FIGURE 29-8. A, Draw the vena cava toward you and lift the left renal vein caudad. Clear the lymphatic tissue from the aorta and pass it under the stump of the right renal vein. Clip all lymphatic vessels. **B,** Continue dissecting along the aorta to its bifurcation. The lumbar arteries and veins may need division.

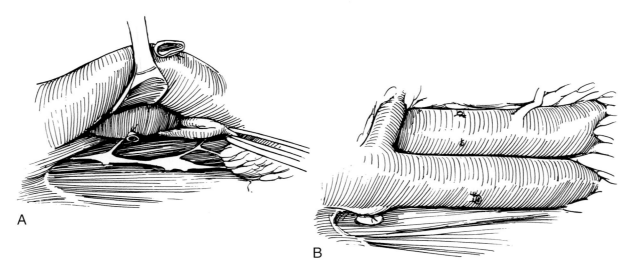

FIGURE 29-9. A, Retract the vena cava to the left, and dissect the tissue from behind it and from the right side of the aorta. **B,** Proceed down to the level of the aortic bifurcation.

LEFT LATERAL APPROACH

This incision may be preferable in obese older children and adolescents.

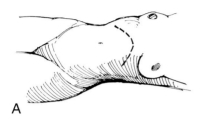

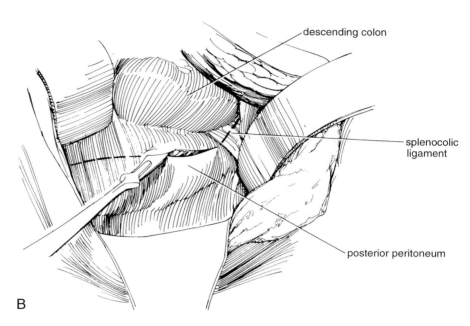

FIGURE 29-10. **A,** Incision: Make an 11th rib supracostal incision, extending anteriorly (see Chapter 14). Alternatively, an anterior transverse chevron incision may be used (see Chapter 10). Open the peritoneum. **B,** Pack the spleen, pancreas, and stomach cephalad and to the right side. (This may not be easy in obese patients.) Place a self-retaining retractor and cover the intestines with a moist pack. Beware of injuring the spleen with a retractor, and be sure to inspect it for injury before closing the abdomen.

Pick up the posterior peritoneum lateral to the descending colon and incise it from the bifurcation of the aorta to a point above the adrenal gland. Divide the lienorenal ligaments to mobilize the pancreas and spleen upward and to the right. The pedicle of the left kidney can be exposed by freeing the greater omentum from the transverse colon and splenic flexure and then retracting it cephalad with the stomach, spleen, and pancreas, while moving the large intestine caudad. Watch for infiltration and invasion of the mesocolon, the colon itself, and the tail of the pancreas. Preoperative studies often do not show involvement of these structures.

If the pancreas is injured, obtain a consultation from a pediatric or general surgeon. Close a simple laceration with mattress synthetic absorbable sutures, and drain the retroperitoneum with a sump drain. If the pancreatic duct also is injured, resect the tail of the pancreas, ligate the duct, close the capsule, and drain freely.

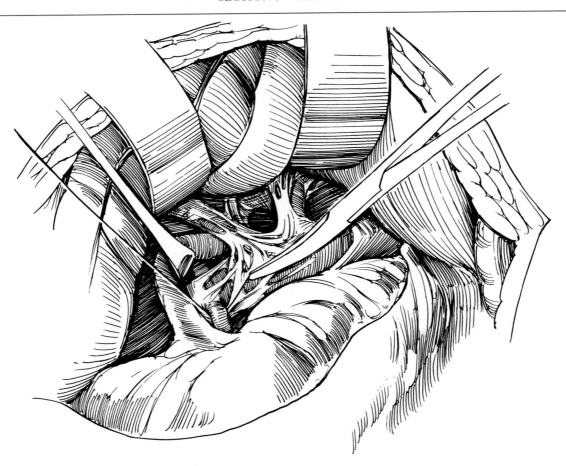

FIGURE 29-11. Dissect medially to expose the aorta. If the tumor is large with medial extension, or if the child is obese, it may be difficult to uncover the aorta. Begin the dissection caudal to the renal hilum and locate the renal vein where it crosses the aorta. For large tumors with involved lymph nodes, the dissection of the renal artery can be difficult because of its dorsolateral junction with the aorta. Remove the connective tissue and lymphatics to expose the left renal artery by downward traction on the left renal vein. In many cases, the mesocolon has attached itself to the anterior surface of the tumor, making this dissection difficult. In addition, look for connections between the tail of the pancreas and the tumor. Also, with a tumor situated cranially, be alert for the neighboring splenic vessels.

   Place a ligature around the renal artery close to its origin and tie it. Generally (and theoretically), it is better to ligate the artery first. However, on approaching the pedicle from the front, it is sometimes easier to ligate and divide the vein first, after which the artery is easily exposed and may be quickly clamped and ligated.

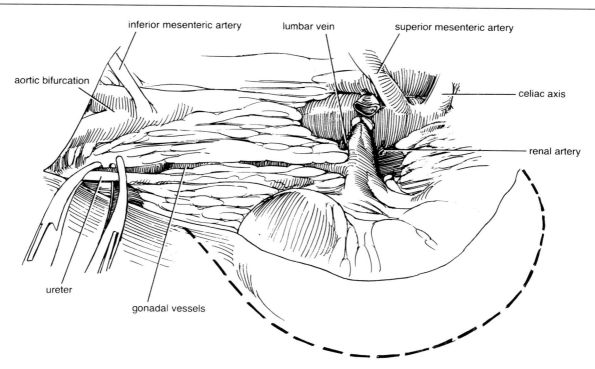

FIGURE 29-12. Dissect the left renal vein as it crosses over the aorta. Palpate it carefully for contained thrombus. Doubly clamp, divide, and ligate it. Dissect it laterally to locate and divide the lumbar vein entering it. You need not expose the adrenal or gonadal veins as they will be included in the en bloc dissection. Complete the dissection of the left renal artery, and clamp it distally. Divide and ligate the left renal artery both proximally and distally.

Free the ureter and the gonadal veins as low as is feasible and divide them between clamps. Ligate the tissue distally and proximally with a 2-0 silk ligature. Leave the sutures long on the side of the specimen. If ureterectomy is planned (for transitional cell carcinoma), dissect the ureter distally as far as possible.

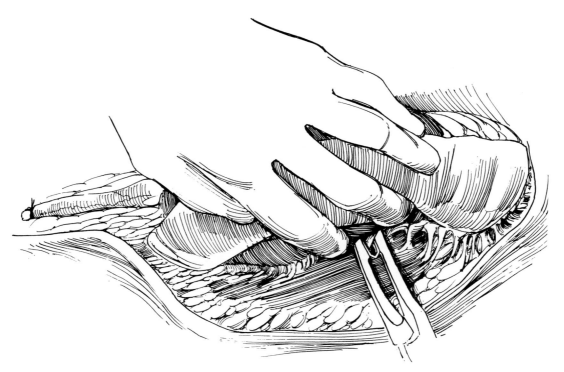

FIGURE 29-13. Divide the peritoneum over the lateral border of the kidney. Free its posterior and lateral surfaces by blunt and sharp dissection keeping outside Gerota's fascia. Work from the caudal end up to the medial border, while dividing any additional vessels so that the lower pole of the kidney can be completely freed. Clip each vessel as it is encountered; use large clips on the large collateral veins.

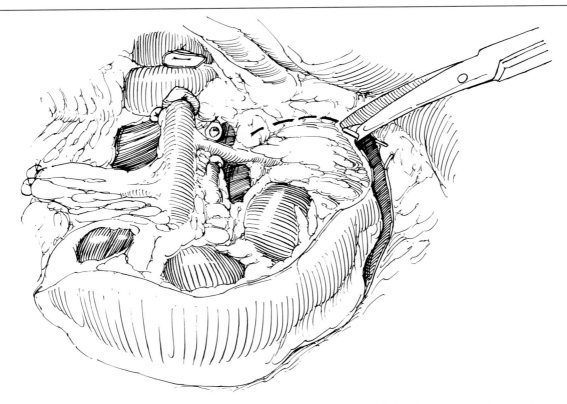

FIGURE 29-14. Complete a step-by-step dissection on the cranial and medial borders by pressing the kidney downward and laterally, working along the crus of the diaphragm and exposing the remaining small vessels and the adrenal artery. Remove the specimen.

REGIONAL LYMPHADENECTOMY FOR LEFT RENAL TUMORS

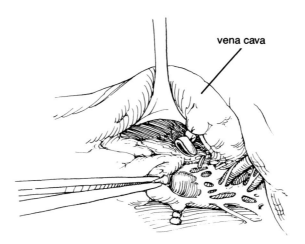

FIGURE 29-15. Retract the vena cava to the right to dissect the lymphatic tissue from the anterior and lateral surfaces of the aorta. Clip or ligate all the lymphatics at the upper margins.

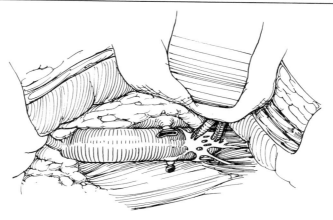

FIGURE 29-16. Dissect down along the aorta, preserving the superior mesenteric artery (SMA) as well as the celiac ganglia and splanchnic nerves, which lie on the aorta at its origin. Continue down between the vena cava and aorta and along the lateral surface of the aorta to the inferior mesenteric artery. Leave the lumbar vessels intact. Remove the specimen after marking it appropriately with silk ties for orientation. Check the spleen for injury (see Chapter 17). Close the wound in layers around a Penrose drain.

Bilateral tumors require preliminary node dissection with frozen-section biopsy examination before proceeding. Perform radical nephrectomy on the most involved side and partial nephrectomy on the other side as previously described. Preserve at least one of the adrenal glands. Alternatively, proceed in two stages, preserving tissue on one side at the first operation and then on the other side later. Note: With asynchronous bilateral tumors, probably one of them represents a metastasis.

POSTOPERATIVE PROBLEMS

For a collapsed lung that fails to expand, arrange for bronchoscopic aspiration. A tension pneumothorax can occur if the lung is inadvertently cut or if an old adhesion separates with a tear. In an emergency, push a needle into the second intercostal space and then insert a pleural drain attached to a water seal (see Chapter 16). Pleural effusions should be aspirated. Bleeding from the wound is usually from a loose vessel in the muscle layers; pressure on the area will often arrest it.

Pancreatic injury may not be recognized intraoperatively. Postoperatively, an elevation of serum amylase levels, an alkaline drainage from the wound, or a retroperitoneal collection of fluid is highly suggestive of such injury. Analyze the fluid for amylase. Obtain a CT scan to identify the pocket and then drain it. Expect spontaneous closure of the fistula, but provide hyperalimentation during the time of drainage. The spleen may be injured if the splenocolic and lienophrenic attachments are not divided to allow the spleen to be swung up out of the way.

Vascular injuries should be minimal if adequate exposure is obtained through a large incision with mobilization of the bowel. On the right side, the adrenal vein is vulnerable to injury where it enters the deep side of the vena cava. If your assistant lifts up the right lobe of the liver and retracts the vena cava while you are dissecting carefully, laceration or avulsion can be avoided. The superior mesenteric artery (SMA) or the celiac vessels are at risk when large tumors create distortion. If one of these major vessels is transected, reanastomosis with a borrowed arterial segment may be necessary.

Pulmonary complications of atelectasis and lobar collapse can be prevented by proper inflation and suctioning. The diaphragm may be injured during retrocrural dissection of nodes lying above the renal hilum, as the crus is being divided and resutured.

THOMAS S. PARROTT

Commentary by

Radical nephrectomy is a very important operation. Anyone dealing with renal malignancies in children should be thoroughly familiar with the concepts outlined in this chapter. Almost all renal tumors in children, especially the most common nephroblastoma, can be satisfactorily approached through a subcostal transperitoneal incision.

Rarely is it preferable to open the chest, because even large upper-pole renal tumors usually can be safely removed with the less-morbid abdominal approach. If more exposure is required when employing the traditional incision, the subcostal incision can be extended to a T shape, carrying the arm of the T into the thorax. However, this should rarely be necessary.

Currently, controversy exists on whether the opposite kidney should be completely mobilized and its anterior and posterior surfaces carefully inspected for tumor. Recent evidence suggests that a normal CT scan is adequate for determining that the opposite kidney is normal, and mobilization should therefore be unnecessary. Whether contralateral mobilization and inspection are undertaken is a surgical choice; however, the need for accurate information is absolutely essential. The surgeon's responsibility is to assess tumor spread accurately to allow for proper staging and precise treatment. This is particularly important in stage 5 (bilateral) disease, because in recent years, the objective of surgery in bilateral Wilms' tumor cases has changed from ablation to preservation of as much renal tissue as possible.

Preliminary ligation of the renal pedicle is desirable but may not be technically possible when large anterior-projecting tumors are encountered. Under such circumstances, the tumor may be mobilized initially and the vessels divided only after the tumor has been satisfactorily encircled, allowing the operator to grasp the pedicle between the thumb and forefinger. At such times, I often find it helpful to stand on the opposite side of the tumor, allowing for adequate retraction of the abdominal wall away from the tumor. On rare occasions, the extent of tumor may be so great as to make the attempt at its total removal hazardous to the immediate survival of the patient. This is especially true with lesions involving the root of the mesentery at the takeoff of the SMA, when the duodenum is significantly involved, or when the head of the pancreas is clearly infiltrated. In such circumstances, it may be prudent to take adequate biopsies, including sampling of regional nodes, and to mark the extent of the tumor with clips prior to closure. Chemotherapy and radiation may reduce the size of the tumor, making second-look procedures technically easier and far less hazardous.

Metastasis to regional lymph nodes occurs in approximately one third of cases, and it is now clearly evident from the National Wilms' Tumor Study that lymph node involvement affects prognosis. Accurate staging requires knowing whether lymph nodes are involved or not; however, there is no good evidence that total lymph node removal influences survival in Wilms' tumor cases. Excision of hilar nodes and selective sampling of paracaval and interaortocaval nodes are essential.

The interested reader should commit to memory the anatomic relationships shown in Figure 29-12. Realizing the proximity of the SMA takeoff to the left renal vein is essential in avoiding damage to the former structure when tumor surrounds the left renal pedicle. Other surgical pitfalls to be avoided when performing nephrectomy on the left side include damage to the pancreas and spleen. Careful retraction and division of the splenorenal ligament should prevent the latter.

PIERRE MOURIQUAND

Commentary by

The transperitoneal approach of the kidney via a transverse supraumbilical incision is the most common way to expose a renal tumor in children. It is therefore quite rare to consider a combined chest approach except when the tumor extends into the vena cava or the right atrium. It is then strongly advised to perform this surgery in combination with a cardiothoracic surgeon in an adequate environment. The situation is more complicated in older patients or in adults where a good exposure requires a more invasive approach.

The main pitfalls I have met in surgery of renal tumors in children were related to the distortion of the anatomic landmarks due to the size of the tumor. It is therefore of paramount importance to start the dissection from the lower medial aspect of the kidney and then carefully follow upward the medial edge of the kidney until the ipsilateral renal vessels are clearly identified. Crossing the midline without noticing it is a significant threat for the opposite sound kidney and its blood vessels.

The place of laparoscopic surgery in pediatric oncology remains to be defined. It is likely that laparoscopic assistance has an important role to take in the initial dissection of the tumor or in its staging.

Urogenital cancers are too rare in children to identify pure pediatric oncologic surgeons in most institutions. This surgery should be dealt with in a pediatric environment by a surgeon who is familiar with the retroperitoneal area and the abdomen. Experience in this field comes from a perfect knowledge of the organ itself and its region.

Bilateral tumors raise the question of conservative surgery, that is, preservation of as much normal parenchyma combined with excision of the tumor nodules with a sufficient margin of tissue around them. This conservative approach is usually performed in situ after controlling the renal pedicle. The possibility of taking out the kidney to remove the tumor areas (bench surgery) has limited indications. Here again, very few surgeons have experience with these rare and difficult cases, which should be operated on in very specific centers.

Chapter 30

Excision of Wilms' Tumor

Stage the tumor carefully before operation with computed tomography (CT) scan of the chest and abdomen. Obtain serum electrolyte, blood urea nitrogen, serum creatinine, and hematocrit levels. A sonogram of the inferior vena cava can exclude vascular extension (4% are positive). CT discloses the extent of renal involvement and assesses the stage of the tumor, and evaluates the liver as well. However, it does not accurately assess the lymph nodes or the venous system. The CT can confirm the presence of a functioning contralateral kidney and usually detects any bilateral involvement with tumor. Should the vena cava not be seen or appear to be involved on ultrasonography, order a magnetic reso-

nance imaging (MRI) examination, which will also pick up the typical variable signal intensities from hemorrhage or necrosis, as well as show the extent of the tumor.

With bilateral synchronous tumors (4% to 6% of cases), first biopsy both tumors (looking especially for those with favorable histology) and then proceed with chemotherapy. Later, excise residual tumor by enucleation, partial nephrectomy, or removal of the entire, still-involved kidney.

Consider obtaining consent for placement of a central line with an infusion port, to be ready for postoperative chemotherapy. With your pediatric and radiation oncology consultants, develop a coordinated treatment plan.

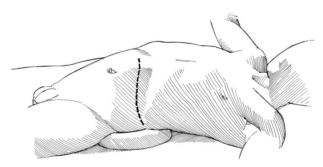

FIGURE 30-1. Position: Tilt the involved side to an angle of 30 to 45 degrees, elevating the flank on a rolled towel. For fluid and blood replacement, establish reliable vascular access in the neck or upper extremities, not in the legs where flow may be blocked by operative interference with the vena cava. Place a nasogastric tube and a urethral catheter.

Incision: Use a modified chevron incision (see Chapter 10), large enough to allow exploration of the contralateral kidney and the assessment and removal of lymph nodes. A flank approach is not suitable; it makes staging impossible. Extend the anterior incision posteriorly into a thoracoabdominal incision through the bed of the 9th or 10th rib for very large upper-pole lesions, especially those associated with ipsilateral pulmonary metastases. The incision may be extended across the midline or be supplemented with a midline sternotomy as an inverted Y to allow control of the suprahepatic inferior vena cava.

Divide the falciform ligament. Use a self-retaining ring retractor. Pack the bowel with moist lap pads. (For large tumors, pack the bowel outside the abdominal cavity but watch it closely for venous congestion.) First assess the extent of the tumor, then cover it with a moist lap pad to prevent injury. Determine if primary excision is possible: Inspect the liver for metastases and look for nodal and vena caval involvement.

Local invasion: If the operation is obviously going to be very difficult because of invasion of surrounding organs, back out and provide chemotherapy, radiation therapy, or both. If the pseudocapsule has been broached, mark the edges with titanium clips to allow the size of the tumor to be followed and to aid in directing radiation. Do not rupture the capsule itself and spill tumor into the peritoneal cavity.

Contralateral exploration: Because 7% of bilateral Wilms' tumors are missed on CT scanning, reflect the colon with the peritoneum covering the contralateral kidney, and open Gerota's fascia. Free the kidney from the fascia, and inspect both anterior and posterior surfaces. Perform a biopsy of any suspicious lesions, because bilateral Wilms' tumors must be managed differently from unilateral ones.

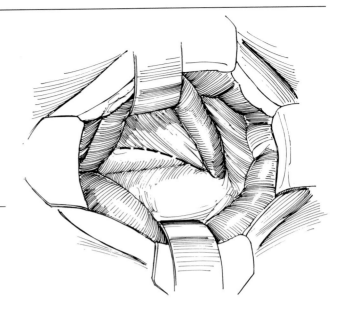

FIGURE 30-2. Displace the small bowel medially. (A bowel bag may be helpful.) Retract the colon laterally. Incise the parietal peritoneum vertically over the aorta along the root of the mesentery. Divide the ligament of Treitz and mobilize the duodenum upward and to the right. An alternative approach is to incise along the white line and mobilize the colon medially.

LEFT-SIDED TUMOR

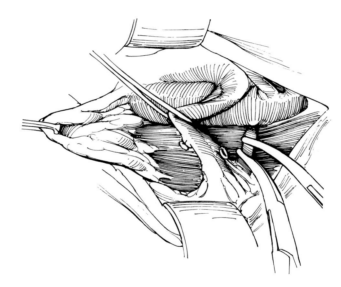

FIGURE 30-3. Dissect the anterior surface of the vena cava to the level of the superior mesenteric artery, which must be identified, and to the origin of the left renal pedicle. Begin by selectively sampling the lymphatics over the vena cava and over the left renal vein for staging purposes. (A formal node dissection does not improve the prognosis.) Dissect the left adrenal vein starting at its crossing of the aorta and then free the left gonadal vein. Tie each vessel in continuity and divide it.

Take care not to injure the left renal vein as it is attenuated over the tumor. With large tumors, the left vein may be confused with the right. Retract the left renal vein downward with a vascular loop and sample the nodal tissue about the renal artery, and then biopsy the hilar, para-aortic, iliac, and celiac nodes. Palpate the renal vein for tumor extension. Thrombi are not usually invasive and are readily extracted. Only 1 thrombus in 10 extends into the vena cava and thus would have been detected on the preoperative imaging. Ligate the renal artery proximally, and then doubly clamp and divide it between the clamps. Ligate each end under the clamp. The tumor will now be softer and less liable to rupture. (If not, suspect a second arterial supply.)

To facilitate arterial ligation, a segment of the inferior vena cava may require mobilization to allow rotation of the tumor and its venous drainage away from the renal artery. To do this requires identification and cautious ligation of the adjacent lumbar veins. Sometimes it is not feasible to reach the renal artery with the renal vein in place, in which case, divide and ligate the vein first, even though this results in severe congestion of the kidney (and blood lost in the specimen).

Now, turn your attention to the friable parasitic veins before they become torn. Dissect enough of each vein to allow ligation, thus avoiding blood loss and a chance of tumor spillage.

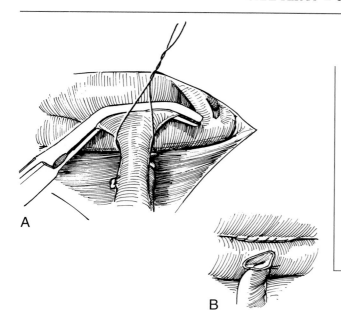

A

B

FIGURE 30-4. A and **B,** Palpate the vena cava for extension of the tumor; if extensive thrombus is present, obtain consultation from a vascular surgeon consultation. Place a small Satinsky clamp across the vena cava just proximal to the insertion of the left renal vein. Ligate the vein distally and divide it proximally. Run a continuous 5-0 or 6-0 vascular suture over the stump and remove the clamp from the vena cava.

Continue dissection para-aortically on the left, as well as between aorta and vena cava, down to the bifurcation. Stay away from the inferior mesenteric artery. Expose and control the lumbar vessels. Dissecting cephalad, ligate the small adrenal arteries, and remove the adjacent nodal tissue. This tissue is sparse in children; do not attempt en bloc dissection.

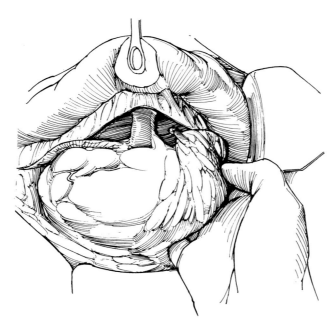

FIGURE 30-5. Hold the descending colon medially and incise the parietal peritoneum laterally along the white line. Bluntly separate the mesocolon from Gerota's fascia. Have your assistant hold the spleen and tail of the pancreas out of the way with padded retractors. Work one hand over the top of the mass and mobilize Gerota's fascia and the kidney. With upper-pole tumors, include the adrenal gland. Be careful to avoid entering the tumor, while removing Gerota's fascia and its attached pararenal fat with the mass. Watch for an engorged accessory vein that may run from the upper pole to the vena cava. Tumor extension into the liver may occur on the right side; it can usually be resected inside a pseudocapsule after the liver has been mobilized. It may be necessary to resect part of the diaphragm if involved. Divide the ureter well below the kidney and remove the specimen.

Complete extirpation may require resection of a segment of spleen, stomach, or colon, the tail of the pancreas, or portions of the diaphragm or psoas muscle. But do not be heroic. Avoid splenectomy because of the risk of pneumococcal sepsis. Tag the nonresected (unresectable) portion(s) of the tumor and any suspicious areas with titanium clips (which do not interfere with the CT beam) to permit following tumor size during chemotherapy and radiation treatment, and to provide guidance in a second-look operation. Irrigate the wound with normal saline and obtain complete hemostasis. Replace the colon to cover the dead space from the tumor, tack the retroperitoneum together anteriorly, and close the wound in layers.

RIGHT-SIDED TUMOR

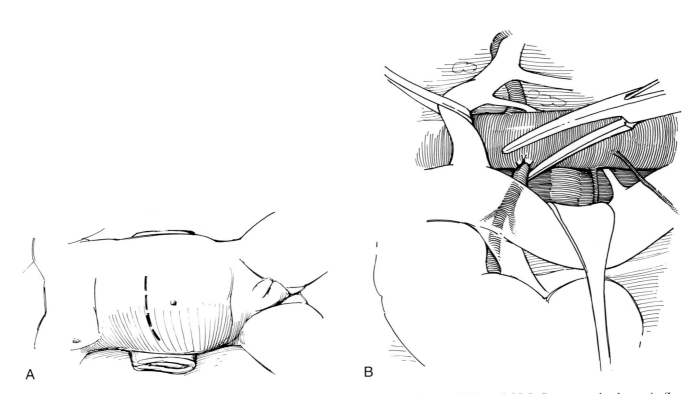

A   B

FIGURE 30-6. A and **B,** Expose the retroperitoneum as described in Figures 30-1 and 30-2. Separate the hepatic flexure of the colon and the right and transverse colon from the duodenum, liver, and gallbladder. Retract the duodenum medially and expose the great vessels. Now selectively sample the nodal tissue over the vena cava and below the renal vein. Draw the cava to the right, and retract the left renal vein cephalad with a vascular tape. Clear the right renal artery, ligate it in continuity, doubly clamp and divide it, and then ligate both ends. Ligate the right renal vein close to the vena cava, and then doubly clamp it, divide it, and ligate both ends. Use a suture ligature on the proximal end because the stump of the vein is short. Continue the nodal sampling caudally, removing some right paracaval tissue while dividing and ligating the gonadal vessels.

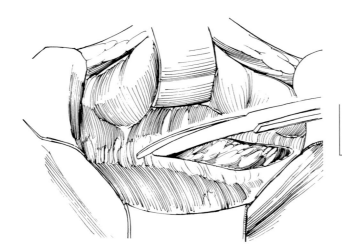

FIGURE 30-7. Incise the parietal peritoneum lateral to the ascending colon, separate the mesentery from Gerota's fascia, and move the duodenum medially over the vena cava.

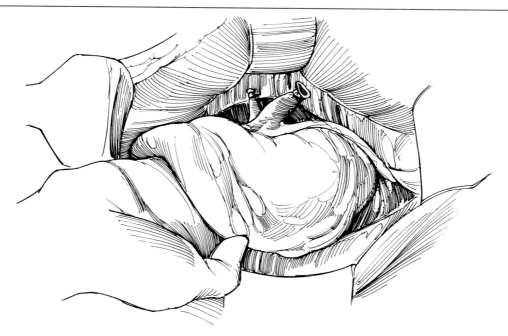

FIGURE 30-8. Dissect and divide the adrenal vein: First draw the renal artery from beneath the vena cava, and then place a hand over the top of the mass and strip Gerota's fascia from the body wall, to include the adrenal gland if the tumor is in the upper pole. Care is needed because the right adrenal vein is short and is situated partially behind the vena cava. The pseudocapsule of a large tumor may be adherent to the undersurface of the liver but it can be dissected free. If the liver is actually involved with tumor, remove a wedge of liver en bloc with the specimen (rarely is hepatic lobectomy required). Divide the ureter as low as is feasible and remove the specimen. Ligate the ureteral stump with an absorbable suture. Close the wound with drainage.

Should hepatic lobectomy be necessary because of extensive involvement, free the coronary and triangular ligaments, and successively dissect the porta hepatis and the right hepatic artery, hepatic duct, and right branch of the portal vein. If the segmental hepatic structures can be identified and resected with the help of an ultrasonic probe and an ultrasonic dissector, less liver need be removed. Proceed with the operation as described for the left side.

POSTOPERATIVE STAGING

Postoperative staging is as follows: stage I, tumor is completely removed with the kidney; stage II, tumor is completely removed but part of it lies outside the kidney; stage III, residual local tumor; stage IV, hematogenous metastases; and stage V, bilateral involvement. Determine favorable or unfavorable histology, and proceed with chemotherapy and radiation therapy (XRT).

BILATERAL TUMORS

For small bilateral tumors at the renal poles, perform partial nephrectomies. For one large and one small tumor, perform total nephrectomy for the more involved kidney and a partial nephrectomy for the other. Preserve at least one of the adrenal glands. Alternatively, proceed in two stages, preserving renal parenchymal tissue on one side at the first operation and then on the other side later.

If both kidneys are extensively involved, take biopsy specimens and obtain representative lymph nodes from each side. Close the incision.

Postoperatively, give chemotherapy. In a case with favorable histology, return for a second look with the intent to conserve as much renal tissue as possible. With unfavorable histology, institute intensive chemotherapy followed by XRT and then take a second look. At that time, if the tumor still cannot be resected, it is reasonable to give further chemotherapy and make a third attempt at removal. Bilateral nephrectomy with renal transplantation is the last resort because immunosuppression fosters return of the neoplasm.

Lung metastases require both chemotherapy and radiation therapy. For persistent lesions found at follow-up, arrange for removal by wedge resection or lobectomy.

POSTOPERATIVE PROBLEMS

Surgical Complications

Vascular injury may occur during the resection. It is important to visualize the contralateral aorta, vena cava, and renal vessels. The celiac axis, the contralateral renal artery, the superior mesenteric artery, and the aorta below the origin of the renal artery must be visualized to prevent inadvertent ligation. Ligation of the inferior mesenteric artery is not harmful in a child, especially if done close to the aorta to preserve the marginal artery. The left renal vein must not be divided during a right-sided operation in a child. If it is cut inadvertently, anastomose it to the vena cava while providing diuresis.

Air embolism or tumor embolism can occur during manipulation of the vena cava. Bowel ischemia and necrosis result from interference with the mesenteric blood supply, which is especially attenuated after XRT. Intestinal obstruction may be a problem. Pancreatic fistulas occur if the resected end of the tail of the pancreas is not carefully oversewn with a running nonabsorbable suture. Splenic injury is secondary to overretraction (see Chapter 17). Chylous ascites can arise if the cisterna chyli is torn, but will usually respond to repeated paracentesis. Atelectasis or pneumothorax may occur if the diaphragm was involved or if wedge resection of the lung was performed.

Complications from chemotherapy or XRT may be anticipated: Bone marrow toxicity, cardiomyopathy/congestive heart failure, gastrointestinal or hepatic toxicity, pneumonitis, renal impairment, and secondary tumors. Be alert for second malignancies from the irradiation or chemotherapy; these may occur in the first 15 years. Followup must be strict, especially for cases with unfavorable histology.

MICHAEL L. RITCHEY

Commentary by

Despite tremendous advances in pediatric oncology, surgical extirpation of Wilms' tumor remains the cornerstone of therapy. It is incumbent on the surgeon, however, to do this safely and completely. In North America most tumors are removed primarily before chemotherapy is administered. It is therefore imperative that surgeons handle the tumors with great care and avoid operative mishaps.

The preoperative assessment of Wilms' tumor has changed over the past few decades. All children now undergo preoperative CT examination of the abdomen and chest. Very small chest lesions will be seen on CT that are not visible on plain chest radiographs. The significance of these small lesions is unclear. There is evidence that most patients treated with limited chemotherapy without chest irradiation will have a favorable outcome. However, at many centers these lesions are biopsied and if found to be metastases, the patient is treated for stage IV disease. The current Children's Oncology Group (COG) protocol will assess the response of these lesions to chemotherapy to determine the need for pulmonary irradiation.

Abdominal imaging has improved very dramatically. CT scan or MRI can provide some information regarding the extent of tumor and (indirectly) its staging. However, there can be overestimation of the extent of tumor, particularly on the right side where it abuts against the liver. The studies are also limited in their ability to detect nodal metastases. The important message is that tumors should not be declared inoperable based on the imaging evaluation alone. Inoperability is generally determined at the time of surgical exploration.

For many years, formal exploration of the contralateral kidney was recommended in children with presumed unilateral Wilms' tumor. Data from the Fourth National Wilms Tumor Study (NWTS-4) revealed that 7% of contralateral lesions were missed on preoperative imaging. However, extended follow-up of this cohort showed that the overall good outcomes of small contralateral lesions missed on modern-day imaging obviates the need for routine contralateral renal exploration. Imaging modalities have continued to improve and even very small lesions should be detected on the preoperative CT or MRI scans. The current COG Wilms' tumor protocols do not require exploration of the contralateral kidney if the preoperative CT or MRI demonstrates a normal kidney.

There are some circumstances in which preoperative chemotherapy should be employed. As outlined previously, patients with bilateral tumors will benefit from chemotherapy. Also, those patients detected to have extension of tumor into the vena cava that rises above the hepatic veins are recommended to have preoperative chemotherapy. This is predominantly due to the increased surgical morbidity of managing these patients. Preoperative chemotherapy can shrink the intravascular component to a level below the hepatic veins, simplifying the surgical task. Shrinkage of the primary tumor will improve visualization of the great vessels. Preoperative chemotherapy is also recommended for those patients determined to be inoperable.

At the time of surgery, if the tumor cannot be removed without resecting other visceral organs, biopsy is performed and the patient is closed. Prior studies from the National Wilms Tumor Study Group (NWTSG) have shown that in most cases the tumor does not invade these other organs but is very adherent. After shrinkage of the tumor, surgical resection is facilitated. There are occasions when removal of a small portion of the diaphragm or the tip of the pancreas may be advisable if it allows the surgeon to remove the tumor intact without spillage. The incidence of operative complications is also reduced when managing these bulky tumors after preoperative therapy. In virtually all instances the tumor is resectable within 6 to 12 weeks of initiating chemotherapy.

The main disadvantage of preoperative chemotherapy is that staging of tumors after chemotherapy is less accurate. This is most noted for evidence of lymph node metastases. Small tumor deposits in lymph nodes can be eradicated by preoperative chemotherapy. The International Society of Pediatric Oncology (SIOP) has extensive experience with preoperative chemotherapy. They have formulated guidelines for the pathologic and surgical staging postchemotherapy and for postoperative chemotherapy treatment regimens. In the NWTSG protocol, all patients who receive preoperative chemotherapy for inoperability of the tumor are considered stage III, which mandates increased therapy.

During the course of the operation, the surgeon must take extreme care to avoid spillage of tumor. These tumors are often very soft and friable and even with care, rupture of the tumor capsule may occur. The importance of avoiding tumor spill has been recently documented. Tumor spill that was deemed to be local or confined to the region of the tumor was not thought to have an adverse impact on tumor recurrence. These patients have always been treated as stage II lesions without the use of XRT. However, a recent review by the NWTSG noted that there is an increased risk for local tumor recurrence in patients with local tumor spill. Although the survival of these patients is quite good, patients that develop abdominal recurrence require an intensive retrieval regimen. The current COG Wilms' tumor protocol now considers children with local tumor spill to have stage III disease.

It is also imperative that the regional lymph nodes be sampled. Formal lymph node dissection is not required. Determination of lymph node involvement is important so that patients receive appropriate therapy. Data from the NWTSG has shown that patients that fail to have lymph node sampling have a much higher rate of intra-abdominal recurrence. Presumably this is due to inadequate staging and the failure to detect nodal involvement.

All children with bilateral Wilms' tumors should undergo preoperative chemotherapy prior to tumor resection. This will offer maximum reduction in the size of the tumors prior to surgery. At the time of complete excision of the tumors, the maximum amount of renal parenchyma can be preserved. The duration of chemotherapy prior to definitive surgery should be brief. Experience from SIOP has shown us that maximum reduction of tumor burden occurs within 4 weeks after initiation of therapy. Repeat imaging is performed after the initial round of chemotherapy. If the tumors are amenable to partial resection, surgery should be performed. If there has been a good response to the tumor, but it does not appear that a partial resection is feasible, an additional 6 weeks of therapy can be employed. Tumors that do not respond to the initial course of chemotherapy should be biopsied. This is needed to assess histology. The tumor may be an unfavorable histology that requires a different chemotherapy. However, not all tumors that fail to shrink have an unfavorable histology. Some Wilms' tumors have very mature stromal elements and skeletal muscle. These tumors often fail to shrink and may even increase in size. However, they have a good prognosis after complete excision. Such tumors may also be amenable to enucleation with salvage of a portion of the kidney despite their massive size.

One concern in patients with bilateral Wilms' tumors is that an increased incidence of anaplasia has been noted. Many of these cases are detected after prolonged courses of preoperative chemotherapy. Anaplastic tumors do not respond to chemotherapy and complete surgical excision is necessary. For most of these patients, a complete nephrectomy will probably provide the best local tumor control to avoid leaving residual disease. Some small lesions may be amenable to partial nephrectomy with a margin of normal tissue. Try to preserve as much renal parenchyma as possible to avoid the late occurrence of renal failure. This is not an uncommon occurrence in patients with bilateral Wilms' tumor. Renal failure occurs in 15% of patients at 15 years from diagnosis. However, if bilateral nephrectomy is needed for patients with nonresponding tumors, their outcome is good.

The postoperative chemotherapy regimens continue to evolve. The Fifth National Wilms Tumor Study (NWTS-5) evaluated the need for postoperative chemotherapy in patients less than 2 years of age with tumors less than 550 g. If a tumor was completely excised and was stage I, and the histologic findings were favorable, these patients did not receive any adjuvant therapy. It was noted that relapse occurred in 13% of the patients. This portion of the NWTS-5 study was suspended due to the rate of tumor relapse. However, these patients were successfully treated with chemotherapy after relapse with nearly 100% survival. This approach is currently being reevaluated in the current COG Wilms' tumor study. The SIOP group has also eliminated therapy for a subset of their patients. After receiving 4 weeks of preoperative therapy, the tumors are removed. If the tumor is completely necrotic with no viable elements, then no further adjuvant chemotherapy is administered.

The underlying principle in treating children with tumors is to try and maximize outcome while limiting the intensity of therapy. Late effects of both chemotherapy and XRT are significant. The significant impact of radiation on growing tissues in the child was recognized early. However, over time, other late consequences such as second malignancies and congestive heart failure due to chemotherapy and XRT become evident. Even longer follow-up will be needed to note if there are any consequences for successive generations in these cancer survivors. Continued support of the pediatric cooperative groups who study these rare solid tumors is essential.

MARTIN KOYLE

Surgery still maintains an important role in the child with Wilms' tumor, especially as it pertains to therapy/staging and ultimately to choosing the appropriate adjuvant therapeutic regimens that will be instituted in each case. Regardless, for lower-stage, favorable histology tumor, chemotherapy is mandated, and in anaplastic and advanced-stage tumors, both chemotherapy and radiotherapy are used. The improvement in survival in children with Wilms' tumor over the past half century clearly is related to advances in chemotherapy. Preoperative chemotherapy should be considered in cases with caval involvement where tumor extends above the hepatic veins; with contemporary protocols, primary chemotherapy also is instituted in cases of radiologically identified bilateral disease, without the need for mandatory exploration and tissue diagnosis beforehand.

Radiologic evaluation of the child with an abdominal mass has continued to evolve. Often an initial ultrasound will differentiate a cystic from a solid renal mass and is an excellent tool to evaluate the patency of the inferior vena cava. A contrast-enhanced CT or MRI is usually obtained to further define the anatomy. Nodal disease, liver involvement, and the possibility of tumor extension into contiguous organs may be suspected by these studies. Whereas CT may be superior in suggesting lymphadenopathy, MRI is preferred if delineation of the vena cava is indicated. Attention should be directed to the function and integrity of the contralateral kidney. Currently, however, surgical exploration is still indicated to assess lymph nodes and confirm inoperability in those cases with suspected local extension. As noted previously, however, patients with suspected bilateral disease now should receive primary chemotherapy rather than undergo routine surgical staging and tissue confirmation.

At surgery, initially, a lifeline (chemotherapy line) should be placed for subsequent chemotherapy and also to ensure large-bore vascular access for fluid/blood products if necessary. Blood is usually typed and screened but only rarely required. However, in patients with suprahepatic venous involvement, be prepared for blood product transfusion. We have been pleased with our anesthesiologists placing an epidural catheter for perioperative analgesia before making the incision. We place a Foley catheter, but now rarely place a nasogastric tube, although many have an orogastric tube placed temporarily during the procedure. I like to elevate the affected side with appropriate padding, 25 to 30 degrees, in the case of unilateral tumors.

In most cases, the standard chevron incision is used. In small tumors, rather than placing a self-retaining retractor, I place a heavy suture (#1 Prolene) through each part of the upper and lower rectus flaps, and fix them to the drapes. I prefer to pack exposed bowel and keep it within the abdominal cavity, rather than exteriorizing it and allowing it to become dusky and edematous. In complex cases, especially if access to the cava is necessary, this may not be possible. I thus make a point of replacing the bowel in the abdomen periodically if I feel that it is becoming engorged and congested.

The contralateral kidney is exposed and palpated and visually inspected. If there is a small tumor that can be enucleated safely with a good margin, I do so; if it is a large, unsuspected lesion, it is just biopsied. Likewise, if there appears to be invasion of contiguous organs or resectability appears unsafe, it is better to biopsy, treat with postoperative chemotherapy, and come back for a second look.

It is paramount to identify essential anatomic structures before proceeding with resection. We have encountered the inadvertent complications of complete vena cava excision and ligation of the superior mesenteric artery performed during nephrectomy elsewhere, neither of which was recognized until the patient reached the recovery room. I find it safest to work from the known to the unknown by identifying the ureter first and working my way up cranially, along the great vessels, identifying the inferior mesenteric artery along the way. Even if there is no gross lymphadenopathy, I make a point of including lymphatic tissue with my en bloc specimen. This may upstage the tumor and hence change the adjuvant therapy, if lymph nodes are involved. On the left, the gonadal and adrenal veins and any accessory lumbar veins are ligated and divided. (I use absorbable sutures, usually 4-0 vicryl for smaller vessels.) The renal artery(ies) are identified and ligated. If the kidney does not become less engorged and the main vein is still full, suspect an accessory renal artery.

Once the arteries are controlled, the renal vein can be ligated and divided. I tend to use 2-0 and 3-0 Vicryl sutures to tie off the renal vessels rather than use suture ligatures. Although it has been argued that primary vascular control should be accomplished prior to renal mobilization, with the hopes that spill can be minimized, this sometimes is just not possible. If the kidney does require primary mobilization, Gerota's fascia should not be opened, and any unnecessary manipulation of the kidney itself should be kept to a minimum. It should be mentioned that there are no data to support that traditional radical nephrectomy is superior to simple nephrectomy in the patient with Wilms' tumor, but as noted, I do take local lymphatic tissue and Gerota's fascia and try to touch the mass as little as possible. The adrenal, if easy to identify and clearly not involved, can be preserved, and obviously, if bilateral tumors are defined, at least one adrenal must be preserved.

With respect to partial nephrectomy, angiography generally is not required. The patient should be well hydrated preoperatively. With larger lesions, it may be advantageous to have a central venous pressure and even arterial line placed. Oftentimes, when preoperative chemotherapy has been employed, a plane will be evident between the tumor and normal parenchyma. I have been impressed that even when imaging suggests little viable normal kidney, that once the tumor is removed, almost like an accordion, the compressed tissue will expand. Thus, if possible, I give the benefit of the doubt to the kidney segment, not the tumor, and proceed with partial nephrectomy. I place a vessel loop around the artery and vein individually, rarely using vascular clamps, even though always prepared to do so. Most of the time, bleeding can be controlled using manual compression of the vessels. If clamps are used, "gentle" bulldogs are used. Iced slush is always available in the event of a difficult tumor, in which formal, prolonged clamping of the renal vessels is indicated and ischemia is thus anticipated. In such instances, we do not heparinize the patient, but do give an osmotic diuretic such as mannitol before placing the clamps, and give a loop diuretic such as furosemide when the clamps have been removed.

Cautery is used to circumscribe the lesion with a rim of contiguous normal tissue. If electrocautery cannot control the bleeding from the base, the argon beam coagulator or harmonic scalpel can be used. A thrombin-Surgicel sandwich packs the base. If the parenchyma can be gently sutured over bolsters to bring the tissue together, I will do so with 3-0 vicryl horizontal mattress sutures. Be prepared to place a stent if the collecting system has been opened—only if I cannot control the collecting system well do I place a drain as well as a stent.

It must be reemphasized that unlike the patient with neuroblastoma, a patient with Wilms' tumor rarely, if ever, needs to undergo heroic extirpative surgery. Thus, unless all medical therapy has been exhausted, if proposed surgery could lead to significant morbidity or jeopardize the patient's life, it is best to defer to further chemotherapy, and return for another or second-look surgery when indicated.

Although laparoscopy has now successfully been used in the management of the child with Wilms' tumor in countries outside of North America, such techniques have not yet been embraced on this continent. Still, the role and extent of surgery for the child with Wilms' tumor continues to evolve. The goal of mutimodality therapy is to minimize the morbidity for each given patient and to maximize his or her outcome.

Chapter 31

Renal Transplant Recipient

RENAL TRANSPLANTATION ON ADOLESCENTS AND TEENAGERS

Optimize the overall health of the patent. Avoid pretransplant nephrectomy unless hypertension cannot be controlled or chronic infection is present. Confirm normal bladder function by history in patients with medical renal disease. In those children with voiding dysfunction or prior urinary diversion, perform formal urodynamic studies. Perform bladder augmentation, if necessary, at least 6 weeks before transplantation and then check to make sure the storage and evacuation systems work. In children with prior urinary diversion, it is important to determine that the bladder has adequate capacity, empties without residual urine, and has a functioning continence mechanism. In children postdiversion with adequate capacity but with incomplete emptying, intermittent catheterization may be necessary. If the native bladder is not suitable, drainage of the new kidney into an augmented bladder or urinary conduit is feasible, but will have a higher incidence of complications, with perforation of the augmented bladder being the most serious.

To prepare the patient just before operation, dialyze to ensure metabolic and electrolyte balance.

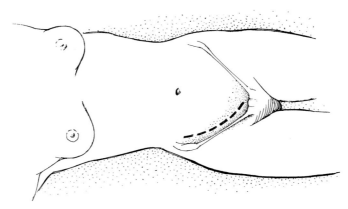

FIGURE 31-1. Position: Supine; break the table slightly to hyperextend the abdomen. The kidney is most commonly placed in the right side of the pelvis. Shave and prepare the abdomen. Insert an 18-F, 5-mL silicone balloon catheter. Instill 100 mL or more of sterile saline that contains 1 ampule of bacitracin-neomycin solution to partially fill the bladder. Immediately before preparing the abdomen, place a 20-F, 5-mL balloon catheter into the bladder, which is drained. Fill the bladder with antibiotic solution to facilitate an extravesical ureteroneocystostomy. This is best done by gravity using the barrel of a Toomey syringe, attached to the balloon catheter. Once the bladder is filled, clamp the catheter and attach it to sterile drainage. Clamp the tubing at an accessible site to allow release at the time of the cystostomy.

Incision: Make a curved, right-lower-quadrant (Gibson) incision (see Chapter 64), beginning below the lower thoracic cage, running 2 cm medial to the anterior superior iliac spine, and staying at least 2 cm above the iliac crest, to reach a point just above the symphysis pubis. Incise the external and internal oblique muscles and the transversus abdominis muscle. If necessary for more exposure, divide part of the rectus sheath and muscle for access to the bladder, and extend the incision up to the tip of the 12th rib.

Instruments: Provide a general laparotomy set with vascular instruments; Gemini-Mixter forceps; a bent-handled, curved DeBakey aortic clamp, an angled DeBakey clamp, three pediatric vascular clamps; a curved DeBakey endarterectomy scissors; an 8-F Robinson catheter; heparinized saline solution, bacitracin-neomycin irrigant; 3-0 silk arterial sutures; 4-0 absorbable sutures; 1-0 silk arterial sutures; 1-0 or 2-0 braided nylon; 5-0, 6-0, and 7-0 cardiovascular sutures; and 4-0 nylon skin sutures.

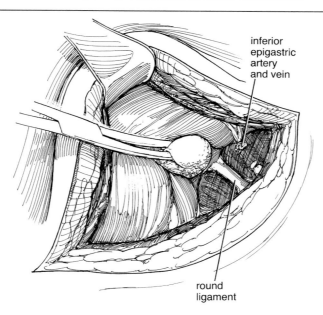

FIGURE 31-2. Free the inferior epigastric vessels; divide and ligate them. Divide the thin inner layer of the transversalis fascia and enter the extraperitoneal space. Sweep the peritoneum medially from the iliac vessels. In the female, transect and ligate the round ligament. In the male, identify the spermatic cord and free it to its entry into the inguinal canal. It can then be surrounded by a Penrose drain and pulled medially, to be retracted with the medial portion of the incision. Division of vessels or vas deferens is not usually required.

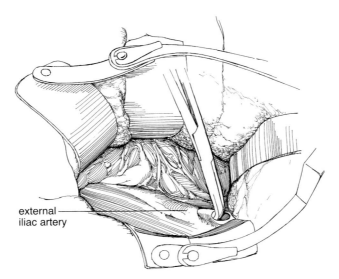

FIGURE 31-3. Insert a self-retaining Buchwalter retractor. A ring retractor with fixation to the operating table via a post permits many different exposures using a variety of fixed and adjustable blades. Be certain that a blade does not compress the femoral nerve. Develop the extraperitoneal space over the iliac fossa to expose the distal common and external iliac artery. Start the dissection over the distal iliac artery, elevating the tissue anteriorly with right-angle forceps. Post-transplant lymphocele formation is often due to leakage from donor kidney lymphatics, but it is well to avoid large, visible lymphatic trunks from the femoral canal by staying 2 to 3 cm proximal to the canal. Ligate overlying lymphatics before they are divided. Ties are better than clips to prevent lymphoceles. Continue up onto the common iliac artery. Skeletonize and elevate the iliac artery with sharp dissection. Iliac preparation should extend several centimeters proximal to the bifurcation of the hypogastric artery. Try to place the renal artery, especially from the right kidney, on the anterior wall of the common iliac artery.

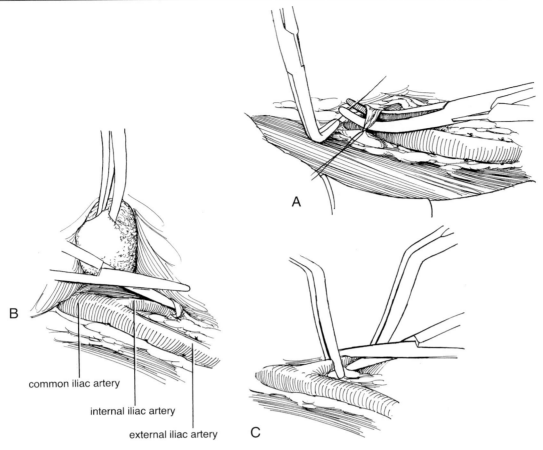

common iliac artery

internal iliac artery

external iliac artery

FIGURE 31-4. A, Palpate the vessel walls at the bifurcation of the common iliac artery and internal iliac artery. Carefully tie the lymphatics over the distal side of the bifurcation, and divide them to allow skeletonization of the internal iliac artery. **B,** Expose the internal iliac artery. **C,** Clamp the internal iliac artery proximally and distally with artery clamps. Divide it, and ligate the distal stump.

End-to-Side Anastomosis to External Iliac Vein

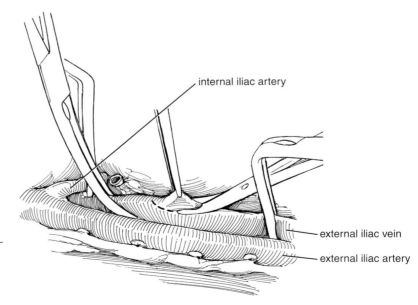

internal iliac artery

external iliac vein

external iliac artery

FIGURE 31-5. Skeletonize the iliac vein, taking care to tie and divide all the overlying lymphatics and connective tissue. Look for tributaries posteriorly; when they are found, doubly ligate and divide them. Avoid double clamping, which may avulse these delicate vessels. Place a bent-handled, curved DeBakey aortic clamp on the vein proximally and an angled DeBakey clamp distally. Cut a smooth ellipse from the vein with the curved DeBakey endarterectomy scissors. Irrigate the lumen with heparinized saline.

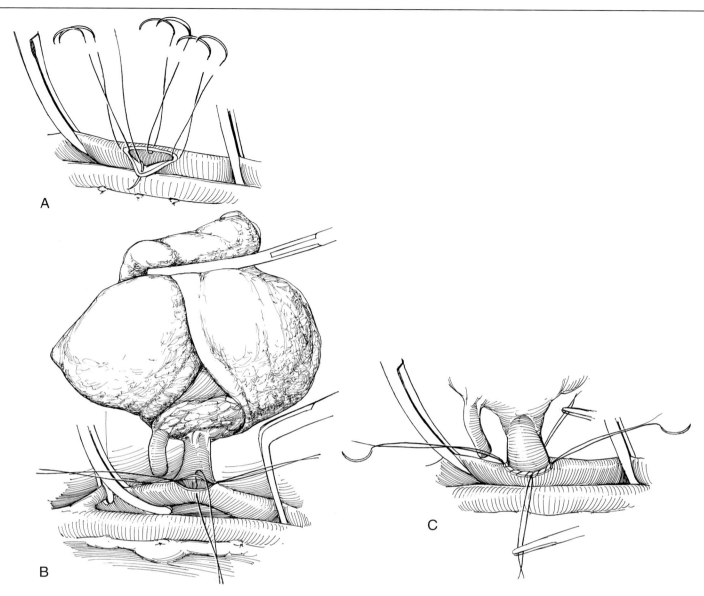

FIGURE 31-6. A, Place four 5-0 or 6-0 double-swaged cardiovascular sutures, two at each end and two at each side of the venotomy (quadrant technique). **B,** Have the cadaver or living donor kidney brought to the room packed in iced slush, and secure it in a sling formed from a laparotomy tape with a hole cut in it for the vessels, held in a clamp. Avoid warming the kidney by touching it with the fingers. Check that all branches from the renal vein are ligated. Pass the four sutures from the iliac vein through the wall of the renal vein in the appropriate quadrants, and tie them. Pull on the medial and lateral sutures with mosquito clamps to draw the front suture line away from the back wall of the iliac vein. **C,** Run the superior suture down the lateral side and the inferior suture up the medial side; tie the sutures to their partner's free end. Cut all four sutures.

End-to-End Anastomosis to Internal Iliac Artery

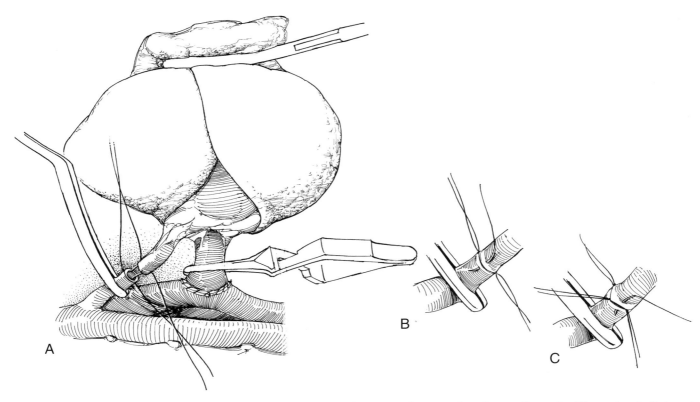

FIGURE 31-7. Place a bulldog clamp on the renal vein, and remove the vascular clamps from the iliac vein. **A,** Bring the renal and internal iliac arteries together in a gentle curve. Place a 5-0 or 6-0 cardiovascular suture in the opposite walls of both vessels and tie them, leaving the ends long. **B,** Continue closure with interrupted sutures by putting the first one at the midpoint between the apical sutures anteriorly, then approximating each of the two quadrants. Cut these sutures. **C,** Rotate the vessels by traction on the apical sutures. Place the posterior sutures in the same manner as the anterior ones. Avoid a continuous suture. Even if it is placed by the quadrant method described for the venous anastomosis, it may act as a purse string and partially occlude the vessel.

Alternative: End-to-Side Anastomosis

FIGURE 31-8. A, Occlude the iliac artery above the level of the renal vein anastomosis with a bent-handled, curved DeBakey aortic clamp. Place an angled DeBakey clamp below, avoiding discernible atheromatous plaques. Make a longitudinal incision on the anterior or anterolateral surface of the artery with a #11 knife blade. Instill 80 mL of heparinized saline (1000 units/ l00 mL) into the distal limb of the artery. **B,** Remove half an ellipse from the arterial wall on each side of the incision with the curved DeBakey endarterectomy scissors to produce a smooth oval arteriotomy. Alternatively, use a 4- or 5-mm aortic punch to make the opening in the iliac artery.

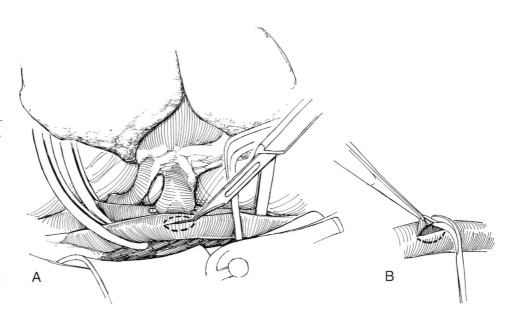

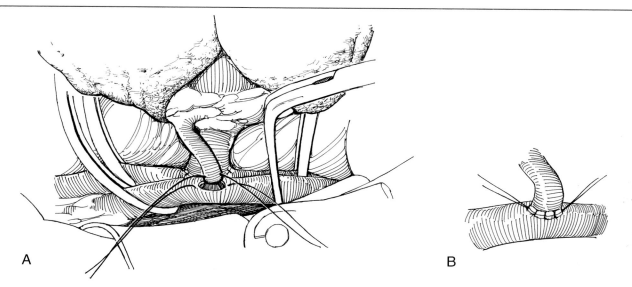

A   B

FIGURE 31-9. A, Insert a superior and an inferior suture of 5-0 or 6-0 cardiovascular silk through the iliac and renal arteries and tie them. **B,** Close the remaining defect with interrupted sutures, first on the posterior surface and then anteriorly. Alternatively, place running, double-armed sutures of 6-0 Prolene, taking care not to create a purse-string effect.

Remove the sling from the kidney. Release the vascular clamps, venous side first. If cold agglutinin titers were moderate to high preoperatively, warm the kidney in situ by applying warm saline solution over its surface before reestablishing circulation. Failure of the kidney to become pink and firm immediately suggests a technical occlusion of the renal vein or artery that requires review of the anastomoses. Check for perfect hemostasis. Be certain that the circulation is good in the ipsilateral leg.

Multiple Renal Arteries

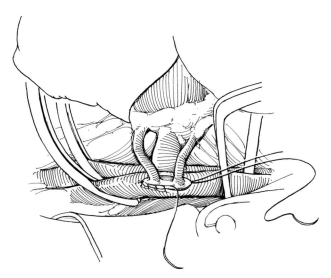

FIGURE 31-10. For cadaver kidneys harvested with a Carrel patch, make an oval arteriotomy the width and length of the patch with a knife and DeBakey endarterectomy scissors. Err on the small side because the patch can be trimmed slightly. Pass the vein back through the arterial cleft, if necessary, before making the venous anastomosis. Fix the patch in place with one 5-0 cardiovascular suture at each apex. Run the suture from the superior end down the lateral side, and tie it to the free end of the inferior suture. Run the inferior suture up the medial side and tie it.

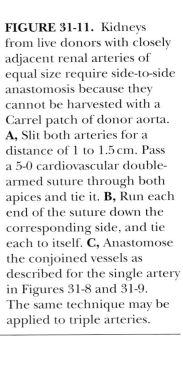

FIGURE 31-11. Kidneys from live donors with closely adjacent renal arteries of equal size require side-to-side anastomosis because they cannot be harvested with a Carrel patch of donor aorta. **A,** Slit both arteries for a distance of 1 to 1.5 cm. Pass a 5-0 cardiovascular double-armed suture through both apices and tie it. **B,** Run each end of the suture down the corresponding side, and tie each to itself. **C,** Anastomose the conjoined vessels as described for the single artery in Figures 31-8 and 31-9. The same technique may be applied to triple arteries.

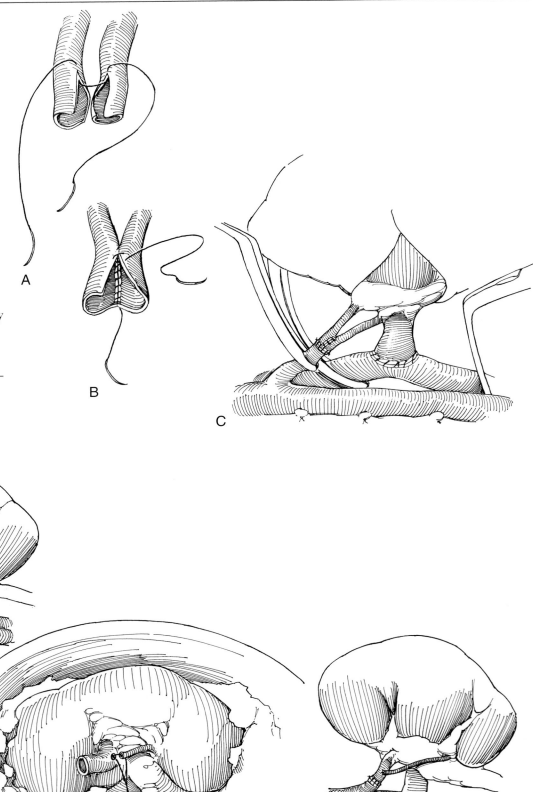

FIGURE 31-12. A, Alternatively, anastomose the superior renal artery end to end to the internal iliac artery and the inferior renal artery end to side to the external iliac artery. **B** and **C,** Another alternative: Before implanting the kidney, perform an ex vivo anastomosis in iced slush of the small polar vessel to the larger main renal artery with interrupted 6-0 or 7-0 cardiovascular sutures, using a loupe. It is important to preserve circulation in the polar vessels because they often supply the pelvis.

SHORT RIGHT RENAL VEIN

Kidneys recovered during excision of the liver may suffer from a short right renal vein when the inferior vena cava is transected through the cephalic portion of the renal vein to provide a wide inferior vena cava cuff for caudal inferior vena caval anastomosis. To fill the defect, use a patch graft from the vena cava distally to patch the superior defect, and use a portion of the cava to extend the lower margin of the renal vein. Alternatively, create a rotation flap from the inferior vena cava, discarding the excess cava. The right renal vein of a cadaver kidney may be unduly short. When harvesting it, split the attached length of vena cava longitudinally into halves, and fold the proximal and distal ends together, thus converting the caval segment to a clamshell configuration. Alternatively, excise a segment of donor external iliac vein and interpose.

Children's Kidneys in Adults

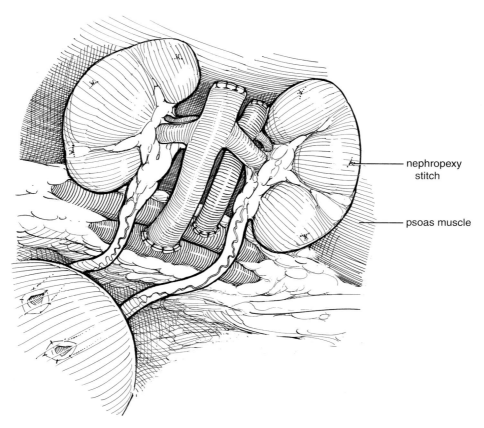

nephropexy stitch

psoas muscle

FIGURE 31-13. Resect the kidneys en bloc, and close the proximal end of the aorta and the vena cava. Anastomose the aorta to the external iliac artery and the vena cava to the external iliac vein.

RENAL TRANSPLANTATION IN SMALL CHILDREN

Because an adult kidney is used for renal transplantation in small children (those weighing 20 kg or less), a vertical midline transperitoneal (see Chapter 11) approach is practical, and the kidney can be positioned posterior to the cecum.

An adult kidney usually requires venous anastomosis to the inferior vena cava and arterial anastomosis to the aorta or common iliac artery. Ureteral implantation may be difficult because of multiple previous procedures. If ureteroneocystostomy is not possible, anastomose the ureter or renal pelvis directly to the bladder, or anastomose the renal pelvis or ureter to the native ureter.

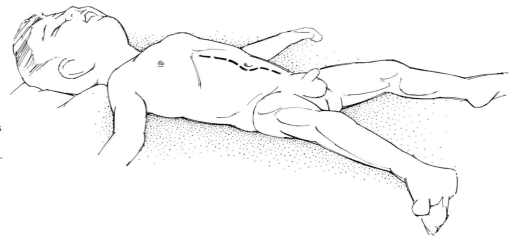

FIGURE 31-14. Position: Supine. Incision: Make a midline incision from the xiphoid to the symphysis pubis.

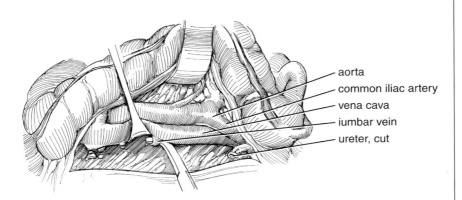

aorta
common iliac artery
vena cava
iumbar vein
ureter, cut

FIGURE 31-15. Reflect the right colon medially by incising the lateral posterior parietal peritoneum and develop the retroperitoneal space down to the lateral aspect of the bladder. Remove the native right kidney and ureter, if necessary. Free the vena cava from the level of the right renal vein to its bifurcation. Sometimes it is necessary to mobilize both proximal iliac veins. Divide the lumbar veins above, below, and in the area of the proposed renal vein anastomosis. Mobilize the aorta distally from just below the renal arteries to the bifurcation of the right common iliac artery and the proximal left common iliac artery. Consider blood transfusion now to compensate for the relatively large volume of blood that will be required to fill the adult kidney.

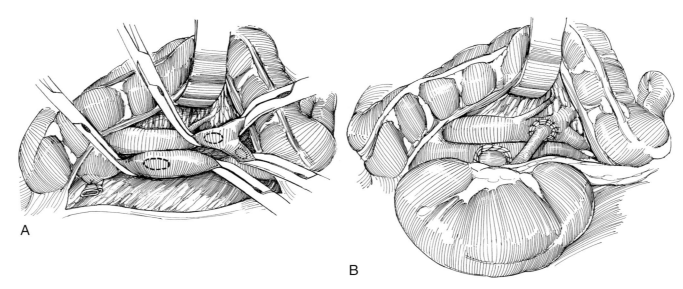

A

B

FIGURE 31-16. **A,** Isolate a segment of aorta or right common iliac artery between vascular clamps. Perform an arteriotomy. Consider enlarging it with a 6-mm aortic punch to prevent coaptation of the recipient artery and renal artery thrombosis in the event of subsequent hypotension. Perform an end-to-side anastomosis of the spatulated renal artery to the distal aorta or right common iliac artery with running or interrupted 5-0 or 6-0 cardiovascular sutures. **B,** Isolate a segment of inferior vena cava between vascular clamps, perform a longitudinal venotomy, and anastomose the shortened renal vein to the inferior vena cava with running or interrupted 5-0 or 6-0 cardiovascular sutures. Remove the superior clamp on the inferior vena cava first, then the aortic and common iliac clamps, and finally the remaining clamp on the inferior vena cava.

URETERAL REIMPLANTATION

Extravesical Ureteroneocystostomy

An extravesical reimplantation technique (see Chapter 43) is associated with fewer leaks and is preferable in most cases to a transvesical approach (see "Transvesical Ureteral Implantation"). When the donor ureter is short or its circulation is compromised, an alternative is to anastomose the recipient ureter to either the donor pelvis or to the shortened donor ureter.

TRANSVESICAL URETERAL IMPLANTATION

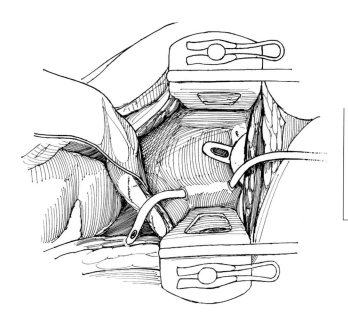

FIGURE 31-17. Open the partially filled bladder on the anterior aspect. Select a site on the floor of the bladder as near and as lateral to the recipient ureteral orifice as possible. Make a short transverse incision through the mucosa. Make a second transverse incision proximally and dissect a submucosal tunnel between them with curved scissors. The length of the tunnel is usually about 2 to 3 cm.

FIGURE 31-18. Pass a right-angle clamp obliquely though the bladder from the outside just above the upper end of the submucosal tunnel. Stretch the hiatus enough to prevent it from obstructing the ureter. Draw an 8-F Robinson catheter through the tunnel and bladder wall with a clamp and fasten it to the tip of the ureter with a suture. Pull the ureter gently into the bladder, leaving a little redundancy outside the bladder. The transplant ureter should lie behind the spermatic cord.

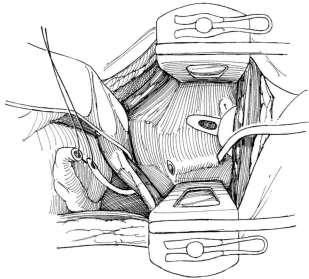

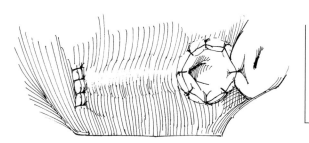

FIGURE 31-19. Trim and spatulate the end of the ureter. Anchor the apex with a 5-0 synthetic absorbable suture to the bladder muscle and mucosa. Place several interrupted mucosal sutures to anastomose the full thickness of the ureter to the bladder mucosa. Test for absence of constriction with an infant feeding tube. Close the proximal mucosal incision. A stent is usually not needed.

FIGURE 31-20. Close the cystotomy in one layer with a running full-thickness suture of 3-0 or 4-0 synthetic absorbable suture by catching just the edge of the mucosa but taking a good bite of the muscularis. Carry the stitches beyond the ends of the incision to avoid leakage. Free up the lateral peritoneal margin posteriorly to be able to approximate it to the lateral peritoneal reflection of the ascending colon with a running 4-0 plain catgut suture. This will maintain the position of the kidney and extraperitonealize the kidney transplant and its ureter. To prevent lymphoceles, some surgeons make an incision in the peritoneum below and medial to the kidney. Flood the wound with bacitracin-neomycin solution, and then aspirate it. Obtain perfect hemostasis because these patients may bleed from azotemic coagulopathy as a spastic vessel opens. Close the abdomen appropriately. Place a balloon catheter through the urethra into the bladder.

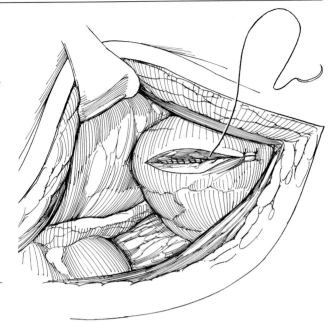

POSTOPERATIVE PROBLEMS

Hyperacute rejection is indicated by swelling and discoloration of the kidney soon after circulation is restored. First check the circulation of the kidney by temporarily obstructing the renal vein and watching for swelling of the kidney. Arterial obstruction could be due to tension on the running suture, a flap from the edge of the artery, or a film of adventitia in the donor artery. Take a biopsy specimen to confirm the diagnosis of rejection. If the results are positive, it may be advisable to remove the kidney; if doubtful, leave the kidney in place and hope for reversal.

Try not to confuse the signs and symptoms of rejection with those of urologic complications. Use ultrasonography and renal scintigraphy to differentiate among acute tubular necrosis, rejection, and urinary obstruction. Percutaneous nephrostomy is diagnostic for total or partial obstruction and moreover is therapeutic.

Renal rupture is an unusual complication, secondary to acute rejection, and requires emergency nephrectomy.

Urinary infection may appear later, with or without pyelonephritis, especially if reflux persists. Urinary leakage may occur at the ureterovesical anastomosis or from the bladder closure. It may be the result of ischemic necrosis of the distal ureter.

Ureteral obstruction, when seen in the first week or so, is usually a consequent of edema, but may be due to hematoma, lymphocele, or ureteral ischemia from improper harvesting. Later, periureteral fibrosis or contraction of the ureter from partial ischemia can cause obstruction. In any case, the diagnosis of obstruction must be made at once; the alternative is sepsis and loss of the graft. Insert a stent transurethrally or percutaneously. Some cases may respond to percutaneous transluminal ureteroplasty. If these measures are inapplicable or if they fail, reoperate. Reimplant the ureter, or resort to pyeloureterostomy, ureteroureterostomy, or crossed ureteropyelostomy.

Lymphoceles, possibly confused with extravasation, appear several weeks after surgery rather than at once. Look for reduced renal function, local swelling, genital edema, ipsilateral thrombophlebitis, and increased blood pressure and weight. Aspiration with the aid of ultrasonography will identify lymph, which has lower levels of creatinine and potassium than does urine. At the same time, a small tube can be placed for drainage if the lymphocele is large, symptomatic, and obstructive. If it recurs, marsupialize it into the retroperitoneum.

Renal artery stenosis results from a defective anastomosis, chronic rejection, or kinking or torsion due to excessive length. In children, the inadequate size of the recipient vessels may be the cause. It can occur both early and late. Look for hypertension, although this may be due to rejection or renal disease. Obtain an angiogram, especially if you find a diastolic bruit or a decrease in renal function. Use selective renin determinations to be sure the kidney is the cause of the hypertension and locate the lesion with anteroposterior and oblique views on digital substraction imaging. Delay treatment if renal function is stable and hypertension can be controlled medically. In any case, try transluminal angioplasty before proceeding with a difficult surgical procedure that carries a real chance for loss of the graft.

Arterial thrombosis usually results from either tearing of the intima while the kidney is being secured or during perfusion, but rejection and poor anastomotic technique may be factors, as well as hypercoagulability, arteriosclerotic disease in the recipient artery, or embolus. Treatment is usually prompt nephrectomy.

Venous thrombosis is secondary to such errors as kinking of the graft when the kidney is put in place. It is hard to distinguish the signs of swelling of the graft, oliguria, and proteinuria from those of rejection. Perform renal venography when suspicion is aroused, and reexplore immediately to do a thrombectomy.

Nephrectomy after transplantation can be difficult because of the rejection reaction and the resultant adherence of the kidney to the recipient artery and vein. The operation should be done by the original transplant surgeon, who can most effectively clear these vessels. Allograft nephrectomy more than a week or two after transplantation to minimize dissection should best be done subcapsularly because of perinephric fibrosis.

It may be advisable to remove the host kidneys before or during transplantation in cases with poorly controlled renin-mediated hypertension, persistent urinary tract infection, prior urinary diversion, or severe reflux. Laparoscopic nephrectomy is the preferred approach. In small children who will require a midline transperitoneal approach for transplantation, the kidneys can be removed at the time of transplant through the same midline incision.

JOHN BARRY

Commentary by

A Y-connector system with each of the limbs hooked up to the bladder catheter, an inflow system of antibiotic solution, and an outflow tube to the drainage bag, respectively, allow for the bladder to be rinsed and filled for identification in a scarred pelvis and to select the best site on the bladder for ureteroneocystostomy.

A straight mid-symphysis pubis incision carried cephalad toward the costal margin in the line of the external oblique fascia is used in our program. The rectus muscle never has to be cut; it is easily retracted after the anterior rectus sheath has been incised. If there is a possibility that a separate lower-pole segmental renal artery will have to revascularized separately from the main renal artery, we leave the inferior epigastric stump long so it can be used for an end-to-end anastomosis to that segmental renal artery.

Avoid the use of clips on lymphatics. They have a tendency to be removed with suction if there is bleeding after removal of the vascular clamps.

Place the kidney in the wound and choose the recipient vessels for revascularization on the basis of a "best fit."

Cutting an ellipse from the recipient's common or external iliac vein or inferior vena cava prior to the venous anastomosis is unnecessary; a simple longitudinal incision is satisfactory.

A surgical glove with a finger cut out of it and filled with slush and the kidney transplant can be a substitute for a laparotomy tape sling with a hole cut in it.

We have found systemic heparinization prior to vascular occlusion to be preferable to infusing a heparin solution into the external iliac artery distal to the vascular clamp.

A continuous suture for an arterial anastomosis in a child is quite acceptable when the renal artery is spatulated and when the anastomosis will be greater than 5 mm in diameter.

After performing a pair-of-pants renal arterioplasty to join two renal arteries together, check the lumens for patency with a vessel dilator or a plastic catheter.

The transplantation of en bloc kidneys from a small child into an adult can be accomplished by longitudinally splitting the donor aorta and inferior vena cava and anastomosing the vascular patches onto the recipient's iliac vessels, or by excising a segment of external iliac artery and sewing the donor aorta into the defect as an interposition graft.

The transplantation of an adult kidney into a small child can be performed through an extraperitoneal approach by extending a Rutherford Morison or a modified Gibson incision from the pubis to the right costal margin.

DAVID HATCH

Commentary by

End-stage renal disease affects 1 in 65,000 children and teenagers. When renal replacement therapy is necessary, kidney transplantation offers several advantages over dialysis. Kidney transplant recipients show more normal growth and development patterns, typically have more energy, and have considerably more freedom compared to those on dialysis. Nevertheless, kidney transplantation carries its own complications, including an increased risk of infection and malignancy as well as the surgical complications of the procedure itself. Current immunosuppression protocols have decreased the risk of infection and complications of steroid use (e.g., acne, hirsutism, aseptic necrosis of the hip, cataracts) while also decreasing the risk of rejection.

Optimal vascular anastomosis techniques depend on the individual situation and the anatomy of the renal vasculature and the recipient vessels. Especially in younger recipients, transplant surgeons should, whenever possible, preserve options for future transplantation in case the allograft fails. Some surgeons prefer to use an end-to-end anastomosis of the renal artery to the internal iliac artery for the first allograft. This preserves the external iliac artery for subsequent use. It is best not to use the internal iliac artery in patients with diabetes and those with an increased risk of vascular disease. Use of the internal iliac artery in such patients increases the risk of later complications (e.g., impotence in males).

In younger patients with smaller arteries, growth can be expected. Therefore, the arterial anastomosis must accommodate this change. For recipients of cadaver kidneys, use of a Carrel (aortic) patch will provide a wide anastomotic line. When two renal arteries are present on a common patch, excision of a segment of the intervening aorta will shorten the patch, decreasing the length of the arteriotomy in the extra iliac artery. When one of two renal arteries is smaller, another option is to use an end-to-end anastomosis between the smaller renal artery and the inferior epigastric artery.

Extravesical ureteroneocystostomy has become the procedure of choice for anastomosing the ureter to the bladder. It can be accomplished in almost all recipients and it is simpler to perform and more rapidly completed than a transvesical ureteroneocystostomy. Ureteric stents are not necessary and have not been shown to decrease complication (e.g., urine leak or stenosis) rates.

Current cross-matching techniques have virtually eliminated hyperacute rejection. Typical immunosuppression protocols currently in use include a calcineurin inhibitor (cyclosporine or tacrolimus) combined with an inhibitor of lymphocyte proliferation (mycophenolate mofetil) and steroids. Using these regimens, rates of acute rejection have dropped and allograft survival has increased. Nevertheless, immunologic rejection remains the most common cause of allograft loss.

Lymphocele is the most common surgical complication following kidney transplantation. When a lymphocele is of sufficient size to cause symptoms (pain or vascular or urinary obstruction), marsupialization by creation of a peritoneal window is indicated. This is usually best accomplished using laparoscopic techniques, placing ports in the peritoneum, confirming the location of the lymphocele by aspiration, and by cutting a large hole in the peritoneum overlying the lymphocele.

Chapter 32

Living Donor Nephrectomy

The left kidney is preferred over the right because of its longer vein, unless multiple renal arteries are located on that side. Perform renal arteriography and/or an MRI or CT angiography to detect abnormal vasculature. Prepare the donor by giving 1000 to 2000 mL of lactated Ringer's solution beginning either the evening before or 2 hours before surgery. Give prophylactic antibiotics with the preoperative medications, and continue for 3 days postoperatively. Do not anesthetize the donor until a good diuresis results from intravenous fluids given in the operating room. Place a 16-F, 5-mL balloon catheter into the bladder.

Three approaches are in use, one extraperitoneal and the other transperitoneal, either open or laparascopic. Open-donor nephrectomy is typically performed via an extraperitoneal approach and laparascopic nephrectomy via a transperitoneal approach with the kidney removed through a lower abdominal transverse incision (see Chapter 63).

SUPRACOSTAL 11TH- OR 12TH-RIB APPROACH

Left Nephrectomy

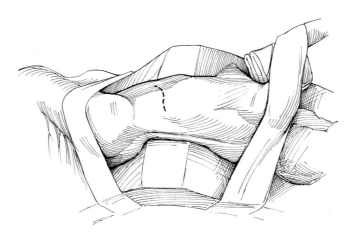

FIGURE 32-1. Instruments: Provide Sheldon, Balfour, Harrington, and two Deaver retractors; a Satinsky clamp; size 0 silk ties; surgical clips; 5-0 silk arterial sutures; and a basin with cold electrolyte solution.

Incision: Follow the plan outlined for the supracostal incision (see Chapter 14), but curve the anterior part of the incision toward the symphysis to allow better access to the lower ureter. Open Gerota's fascia over the lateral curvature of the kidney. Fulgurate small capsular branches, but watch for a polar artery that also supplies the renal pelvis. If the artery is inadvertently severed, reanastomose it, using a loupe.

FIGURE 32-2. Locate the ureter and gonadal vessels as they cross the iliac vessels. Place a 5-0 absorbable stay suture in the ureter at the level of the iliac vessels and divide it. Ligate the stump with a 3-0 silk arterial suture. Insert an infant feeding tube in the severed ureter to monitor urinary output. Dissect the gonadal vessels, ureter, and intervening areolar tissue en bloc up to the lower pole of the kidney. (The periureteral and peripelvic areolar tissues are not shown in order to depict the underlying structures.) Divide the gonadal vein where it crosses the ureter.

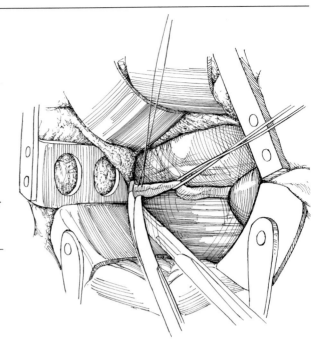

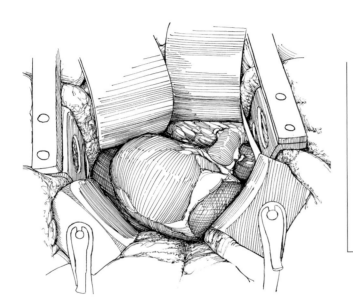

FIGURE 32-3. At the level of the kidney, dissect as much as possible outside Gerota's fascia. Expose the left renal vein by rotating the kidney posteriorly. Dissect the tissue angle where the renal vein and artery join the vena cava and aorta. Give mannitol in divided doses during the dissection. Clear the areolar tissue below the vessels as well as above them, mobilizing the tissue toward the hilum and ligating and dividing the lymphatics. To reduce vascular spasm, avoid approaching the hilum until completion of the dissection. If the kidney becomes soft from vasospasm, stop dissecting until it is again firm. Ligate and divide the adrenal vein. Locate, ligate, and divide the lumbar vein that enters the left renal vein posteriorly.

FIGURE 32-4. Shift the kidney anteriorly, and dissect the tissue laterally from the aorta, moving it toward the pelvis and hilum.

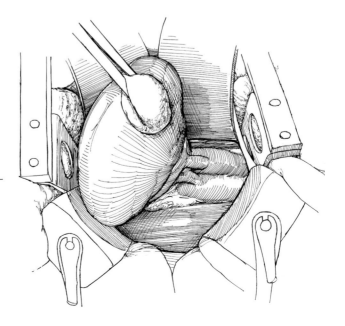

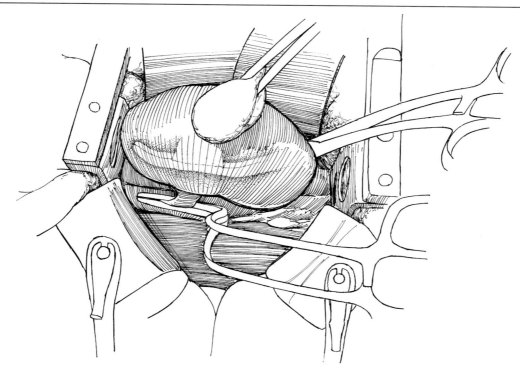

FIGURE 32-5. When the recipient has been prepared to receive the graft, give the donor mannitol and furosemide maximal diuresis, as monitored from the ureteral catheter. Clamp the renal artery with a vascular clamp near the aorta, and divide it distal to the clamp. Clamp the renal vein and divide it. Free the remaining areolar and lymphatic tissue. If the renal vein is torn, reclamp it or suture the tear. Remove the specimen and place it in a bowl of chilled electrolyte solution, ready to be perfused and transferred to the operating room of the recipient.

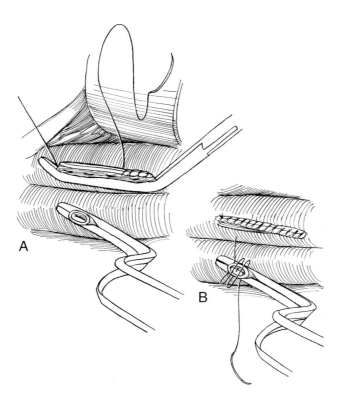

FIGURE 32-6. A, Place a 6-0 silk mattress suture in the renal vein distal to the clamp, and run it as a continuous suture back over the suture line ("baseball stitch"). Remove the clamp from the renal vein. **B,** Close the renal artery with a running stitch, beginning at one side and returning to that side. Remove the arterial clamp.

Right Nephrectomy

For right nephrectomy proceed as described in Figures 32-1 to 32-6, with a similar incision but in the right flank.

MULTIPLE RENAL ARTERIES

An aortic patch, such as a Carrel patch, cannot be taken from a living donor as it can from a cadaver donor. When multiple arteries are present, divide them at their point of exit from the aorta in the ampullary portion. If double arteries are nearly the same size, spatulate them and insert them under magnification side to side to form a single ostium. If the vessels are of unequal size, anastomose the spatulated polar branch end to side to the main renal artery after excising a small patch. This makes it essentially a primary branch of the renal artery. With three or more vessels, apply a combination of these two techniques to form a single ostium. The incidence of late thrombosis in a vessel 1 to 2 mm in diameter is much less by making it a primary branch of the renal artery than by attempting to anastomose it separately into a recipient external iliac artery. Ligate accessory veins with impunity.

After removal of the kidney, inspect the wound to make certain that hemostasis is complete. Reperitonealize the posterior parietal peritoneum with a running 2-0 absorbable suture, using a continuous suture or short sections of continuous suture as needed. Perform a layered closure of the abdominal wall with slowly absorbed suture material, such as polydioxanone suture (PDS) or Prolene. The latter is preferred because it has no interstices, is associated with minimal blood loss from the wound, and has, because of its homogeneity, a low incidence of infection. Close the internal oblique and transversus muscles together with the peritoneum with running 2-0 PDS or Prolene sutures. Close the rectus sheath with interrupted Prolene sutures anteriorly and posteriorly, along with the linea alba. Make no attempt to reconstitute the falciform ligament. Use no drains in the usual case. If oozing appears from cut edges of a structure, make every effort to control the oozing prior to closure. Close the anterior rectus sheath with interrupted 0 or 2-0 PDS or Prolene sutures. Close the subcutaneous fat, including Scarpa's fascia, in a single layer with running 4-0 vicryl or 4-0 absorbable sutures, and close the skin with staples.

POSTOPERATIVE PROBLEMS

Complications after extraperitoneal donor nephrectomy are those of simple nephrectomy (see Chapter 26). The most frequent problem is pneumothorax, treated by observation or aspiration. Rarely is a chest tube required. Wound infections, aspiration pneumonia, and urinary retention may be seen. Complications after transperitoneal nephrectomy are more frequent and include splenic injury, incisional hernias, and bowel obstruction.

STEVE ZDERIC

Commentary by

In busy transplant centers, living related donors often come from far away, as do recipient families. It may be tempting to arrange for meeting the prospective donor at the last minute; this is unwise. In our practice, donors arrive for consultation only after a formal evaluation carried out by an adult nephrologist has given them a medical clearance. Meeting in person in a relaxed and calm atmosphere allows time for the donor surgeon to review the radiographic studies with the patient and explain what lies ahead. It is important to offer them an explanation of the major details and small but real risks they face. Donors must be reminded that there is absolutely no medical benefit to them from this proposed procedure. It is also important to remind donors that on rare occasions the remaining kidney may be put at risk from stone disease, malignancy, or medical renal disease.

We feel that the recipient and donor should be admitted to the hospital the day before surgery for the final cross match. In addition the donor will benefit from a mechanical bowel prep with GoLYTELY; while unpleasant the night prior to surgery, constipation 1 week later with a flank incision is worse. In addition intravenous fluids should be initiated so as to ensure good hydration at the beginning of the procedure. Compression boots with their cycling pump should be ordered for the operating room so as to be ready for application as soon as the patient is asleep. It is also critical to assess the recipient's medical and surgical history for this will influence the order of induction. A recipient who has had multiple reconstructive procedures and requires native nephrectomies should be given a head start so as to minimize the amount of time a donor is kept under anesthesia.

The use of an up-front epidural anesthetic has been very helpful for these patients. By inserting this at the beginning of the case, the anesthesia staff can assess the effectiveness of the placement and charge the epidural catheter. This approach allows for a more effective intraoperative anesthetic and greatly enhances postoperative pain control; we tend to leave the epidural catheter in for 2 to 3 days postoperatively. It has been my observation that the few patients who refused an epidural or whose back problems proved a contraindication experienced a slower postoperative recovery.

Once the patient is asleep a Foley catheter is placed to monitor urine output, and attention is turned to positioning the patient. The importance of proper positioning cannot be underestimated. I will spend a good deal of time getting the positioning just right, and assuring the padding is placed to protect critical areas. For the right or left kidney, I favor using a 10th- to 11th-interspace incision. In my experience, optimal exposure of the hilum is assured by placing the patient in a

45-degree torque position, which is maintained with a beanbag, and flexing the table as much as is allowed. Taping the patient to the bed with 2-inch silk tape is recommended in case of the need for sudden shifts in position. Generously padding the shoulders, free arm, legs, and feet will avoid neural compression syndromes later on.

The 10th- to 11th-interspace incision works well in this setting. I favor angling the incision upward following the curve of the rib cage. I prefer this approach because it gives the surgeon maximal exposure over the hilum and the upper pole. This approach does not compromise our ability to dissect out the ureter distally and achieve a ligation close to the iliac vessels. I have found it is much easier to perform a distal ureteral dissection with less optimal exposure than suffer the consequences of an upper pole that is hard to see with the threat of renal artery branches lurking in the perinephric fat.

The use of a self-retaining Buckwalter retractor allows for outstanding exposure; the accessory ratchets to which the various blades can be attached offer a wide range of retraction and can be in-toed nicely so that the surgeon can really set up a stable operative field. I rarely use the post in this set, preferring to allow the opposing retraction to provide the stability; this speeds up the process of readjusting the exposure as the dissection proceeds.

On entering the retroperitoneal space, I will enter Gerota's fascia distally and identify the ureter, which can then be traced distally followed by a proximal dissection up to the renal hilum. However, I never divide the ureter until the recipient is ready to accept the kidney—urine output is monitored by the Foley output and by direct observation and palpation of the kidney.

On further entering Gerota's fascia, the upper and lower poles of the kidney can be cleared of perinephric fat and a cradle can be fashioned using the loops from the ends of lap pads to snare the upper and lower poles of the kidney. This maneuver allows you to position the kidney to get the best angle in dissecting out the renal hilum. As the hilum is dissected out, it is crucial to monitor the urine output and assess the color and firmness of the kidney. Loss of a healthy coloration or softening of the kidney calls for stopping the dissection and often requires a fluid bolus. This is the time when administration of mannitol may begin. If arterial spasm has resulted in diminished renal perfusion, the use of topical papaverine can rapidly reverse this.

Prior to any irreversible maneuvers, direct communication with the recipient surgeon is reestablished to assure that the recipient is ready, and, at that point, the ureter is ligated distally and divided. On the left side, Satinsky clamps are placed around the artery first and then the vein. I favor the use of an angled Potts scissors to make a clean cut in the presence of these clamps. As soon as the kidney is passed off to the recipient surgeon at the side table, it is flushed with EuroCollins solution. The artery is tied off with a 0 silk tie, followed by a 2-0 silk stick tie. The vein is oversewn with a 5-0 Prolene running suture. On the right side my preference is to place the Satinsky clamp as far back on the artery as possible, and then tie a size 0 silk behind this followed by a 2-0 silk stick tie. Two paired Satinsky clamps are then placed on the right renal vein, taking with this a cuff of vena cava. At this point the right artery is divided, followed by division of the vein. As soon as the kidney is passed off to the side table, the first Satinsky clamp is removed, exposing a cuff of vena cava that is oversewn with a running and locking 5-0 Prolene suture in two layers. Only at that point is the second Satinsky clamp slowly removed.

If you enter the pleural space that occurs in about half of the cases, keep moving and allow the lung to collapse until the kidney is removed. Early on I order a 24-F chest tube and a Pleur-evac with water seal so they will be ready as the closure is about to begin. The pleura is closed around the chest tube, which is threaded into the pleural cavity. Take generous bites of the diaphragm with these sutures so as to get a better seal. Once the pleura is closed, apply a vacuum to the Pleur-evac, and let this run continuously while closing. Run the transversalis layer first, followed by the internal obliques layers. Then thread the chest tube out between the internal and external oblique layers such that it exits at 6 to 9 inches away from where it penetrates the transversalis layer, and close the external oblique layer over the tube. As the skin is being closed with a running 4-0 PDS subcuticular suture, ask the anesthetist to shut off the suction and monitor the Pleur-evac for signs of residual pneumothorax. If the water seal holds, the tube may be pulled. Whether one has entered the pleura or not, a chest film is always checked in the recovery room. Using this protocol, none of our patients have required subsequent reinsertion of a chest tube.

Section 4

ADRENAL GLAND

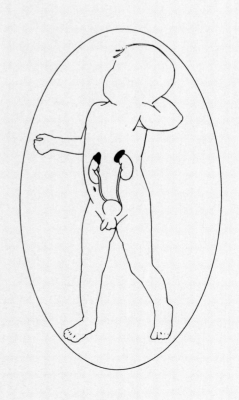

Chapter 33

Preparation and Approaches to Adrenal Surgery

PHEOCHROMOCYTOMA

Measure total and individual plasma catecholamines, epi- nephrine (adrenal source), and norepinephrine (extra-adrenal source). Plasma-free metanephrines or 24-hour urine total metanephrines (metanephrine and normeta-nephrine) may be the best single test. Use an oral clonidine suppression test in doubtful cases.

Localize the tumor in children preoperatively, because 10% are bilateral, 10% are multiple, and 10% are extra-adrenal. Localize the tumor by (1) abdominal CT scan, (2) MRI, using both T1 and T2 images (pheochyomocytomas light up on T2-weighted images; adenomas are hypodense compared with metastatic lesions), (3) radionuclide studies with meta-iodobenzylguanidine (^{131}MIBG) scan, (4) positron emission tomography scan, or, rarely, (5) venous sampling.

Preparation

Avoid stimulating diagnostic procedures. Preoperative and intraoperative adrenergic blockade with prozasin, phenoxy-benzamine, or a catecholamine-synthesis inhibitor such as alpha-methyltyrosine, while preventing hypertensive crises, does make the detection of small extra-adrenal tumors more difficult by blunting the sudden rise in blood pressure during exploration, which may be the only indication of their presence. For dysrhythmia during the operation, use intravenous lidocaine or propranolol. To be safe, have two experienced anesthesiologists at the table, with adequate monitoring equipment.

Place one intravenous catheter to monitor central venous pressure. Insert a second intravenous catheter for fluid administration. Attach the tubing from the bottle containing the drug used for control of excess blood pressure to the connector next to the vein. (Keep this connection close to the vein to avoid dead space and resultant delay in getting the drug into the circulation.) Monitor intra-arterial pressure with a cannula in the radial or brachial artery. Monitor electrocardiogram tracings continuously. Induce anesthesia with thiopental sodium. For an anesthetic agent, avoid halothane and tubocurarine chloride. Methoxyflurane is preferred, along with succinylcholine

and nitrous oxide. Use sodium nitroprusside or phentol-amine to reverse a hypertensive crisis that occurs during intubation or manipulation of the tumor. In any case, stabilize the patient before beginning the operation. A hypotensive episode during surgery requires the vigorous administration of whole blood and plasma volume expanders to fill the vascular spaces consequent to removal of alpha-adrenergic stimuli. Sympathomimetic amines can be used as backup. Vasoconstrictors, however, have the risk of precipitating renal shutdown and cerebral ischemia. For hypotension after removal of the tumor, expand the blood volume with fluids and whole blood.

Localization has become so exact that exploration with bilateral exposure is rarely necessary. However, the endocrine support and supplementation critical to a successful outcome requires a team approach that includes several specialists.

Incision

For pheochromocytoma, an anterior transabdominal incision through a high modified chevron-shaped incision (see Chapter 10) is the approach of choice because of the high incidence of extra-adrenal sites, especially in children in whom these tumors may be bilateral, multiple, or extra-adrenal (20% to 30%). A radical adrenalectomy is required to remove adjacent neural crest tissue.

However, newer imaging techniques for localization of pheochromocytoma make a lateral approach tempting because it results in far fewer complications. A good rule is to avoid a lateral approach in children whom you suspect to have extra-adrenal pheochromocytomas. An anterior approach is also preferred in infants for excision of neuro-blastoma, which often is infiltrating and thus not confined to the adrenal. For the same reason, an approach anteriorly through a modified chevron incision is suitable for tumors greater than 10 cm in diameter in patients of any age. Also, for a child undergoing reoperation for adrenal disease, the exposure will be much better through the peritoneum than through the flank. However, the disadvantages of an anterior incision are several: The exposure takes longer to obtain, and the approach to the adrenal is not as direct.

Further, the adrenals are usually found to lie surprisingly deep and high. Postoperatively, ileus is common and intestinal adhesions may become a problem.

A laparoscopic approach is attractive because it results in far fewer complications. For adrenal excision laparoscopy is often preferable to open routes, excepting primary adrenal cancer or bulky metastatic disease, which requires extensive en bloc resection.

Postoperative Support

Continue monitoring blood pressure because acute hypotension remains a risk, especially if the child is moved. Correct it with fluids. Check the blood glucose level to detect hypoglycemia before it can become fatal. Follow up with metanephrine and vanillylmandelic acid levels every 6 months for 3 years and yearly for another 4 years. Recurrent (residual) tumors, with recurrence of symptoms, are not infrequently found in the opposite adrenal gland but are small and easily excised.

OTHER ADRENAL TUMORS

Preparation for surgery and the surgical approach to an adrenal lesion other than pheochromocytoma and neuroblastoma depend on the lesion type and function. Localization has become so exact that exploration using bilateral exposure is rarely necessary. Endocrine support and supplementation are critical to a successful outcome.

To prevent adrenal insufficiency during and after such a stressful procedure, prepare the child or adolescent scheduled for adrenal excision with steroids by giving cortisone acetate in appropriate doses orally for 2 days preoperatively. Supplement this with an intravenous dose given both immediately before and immediately after the operation. Subsequent therapy depends on the amount of adrenal tissue left after surgery.

Chapter 34

Surgical Approaches to the Adrenals

The posterior approach (see Chapter 15) is ideal for the small, well-localized, benign adrenal tumor, providing adequate access with the lowest morbidity. But do not use it for a large adrenal tumor with its parasitic blood supply or for a malignant tumor, which has potential for intra-abdominal extension. Use the wider exposure of an anterior approach (see Chapter 10).

Preoperatively, complete biochemical diagnostic tests. Correct hypokalemic acidosis and plan for replacement of adrenal steroids. Localize an aldosterone tumor by (R)-N-methyl-3-(2-iodophenoxy)-3-phenylpropanamine (MIPP) scintillation scanning (with or without dexamethasone suppression), CT scanning at 0.5-cm intervals, and adrenal vein aldosterone levels. Adrenal venography is rarely indicated. If the tumor cannot be localized,

which is a rare occurrence, realize that adenomas arise three times more frequently on the left side and use the bilateral posterior approach described here or an anterior approach. Consider that hyperplasia is best treated medically.

ANTERIOR APPROACH

Approach to the Left Adrenal for Pheochromocytoma

Localize the tumor with MRI and also with a metaiodobenzyl guanidine (^{131}MIBG) scan. Remember that in children multiple tumors are not rare.

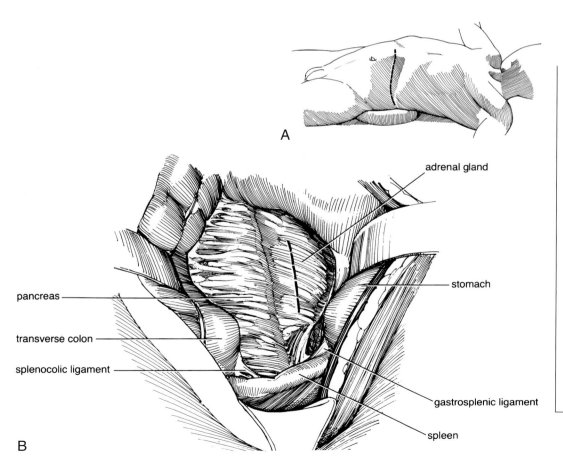

FIGURE 34-1. **A,** Position: Place the child supine. Incision: Make an extended anterior incision (shown) or a chevron (see Chapter 10) incision. **B,** Approach the adrenals through the lesser sac, rather than by reflecting the splenic flexure. Incise the splenocolic ligament to mobilize the colon medially. For more exposure, ligate the inferior mesenteric vein and divide the ligament of Treitz. Dissect the pancreas from the surface of the adrenal gland. Incise the retroperitoneum just below the lower border of the pancreas and open the Gerota's fascia.

adrenal gland

stomach

pancreas

transverse colon

splenocolic ligament

gastrosplenic ligament

spleen

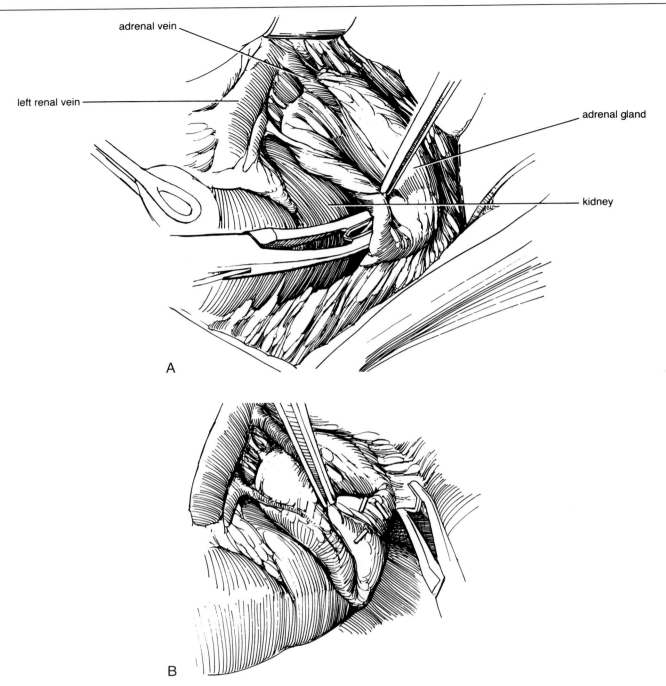

FIGURE 34-2. Place retractors; use an appropriate-sized ring retractor, if available. Realize that pheochromocytomas, especially large ones, are soft and friable, and some are malignant, so that any break in the capsule can cause recurrence. **A,** Carefully free the gland from its bed inferiorly. **B,** Dissect it laterally to the superior margin of the left renal vein and locate the adrenal vein, which may empty into the inferior phrenic vein or even directly into the vena cava.

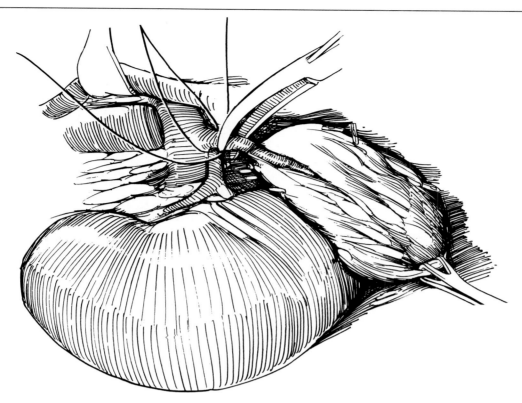

FIGURE 34-3. Dissect out the vein. Notify the anesthesiologist. Pass a 2-0 silk ligature to be ready to ligate the vein proximally. If the child is stable, avoid venous congestion (which increases friability) by delaying venous ligation until the arterial inflow is controlled. Otherwise, clamp and divide the vein and ligate it beneath the clamp. Leave the distal ligature long for traction. Bluntly free the gland posteriorly. Retract the splenic vein with a padded retractor to expose the upper pole. Clip the fascial attachments. Pull the gland laterally and inferiorly to clip and divide the one or more arteries from the aorta and from the inferior phrenic artery. Do not try to tie them until after removal of the adrenal gland and tumor.

For either a left or right pheochromocytoma, if malignancy is suspected as evidenced by fixation or by invasion of local tissues, proceed with regional lymphadenectomy. For tumors that appear smaller than predicted by the vanillylmandelic acid level, look for another tumor in the para-aortic region. Open the posterior peritoneum over the aorta and palpate the renal pedicle on both sides and the groove between the aorta and vena cava to a point below the bifurcation. Close the retroperitoneal incision. Reapproximate the gastrocolic ligament and close the abdominal wound.

Bluntly free the gland posteriorly. Retract the splenic vein with a padded retractor to expose the upper pole. Clip the fascial attachments. Pull the gland laterally and inferiorly to clip and divide the one or more arteries from the aorta and from the inferior phrenic artery. Do not try to tie them until after removal of the adrenal gland and tumor.

APPROACH TO THE RIGHT ADRENAL FOR PHEOCHROMOCYTOMA

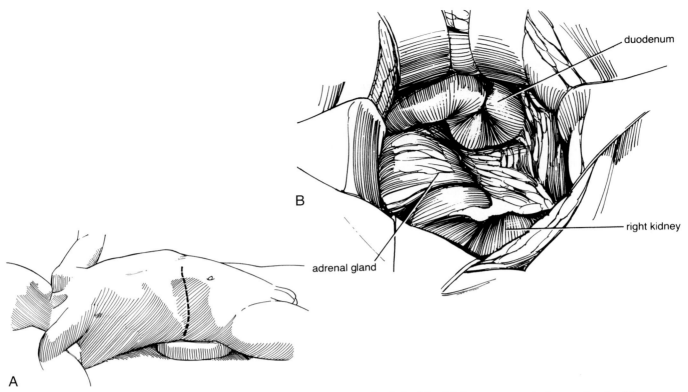

FIGURE 34-4. A, The exposure here need not be as wide as on the left side. Make an extended anterior incision (shown). **B,** Retract the liver and perform a wide Kocher maneuver to mobilize the duodenum. Free the hepatic flexure of the colon (using clips as needed) to expose the right colic artery. Continue the incision in the parietal peritoneum to the level of the cecum.

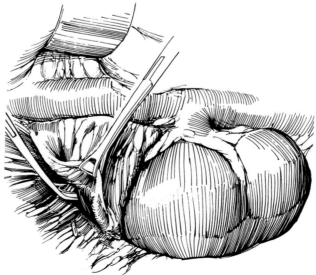

FIGURE 34-5. Pull the kidney down and dissect the right adrenal laterally, as described for the left adrenal.

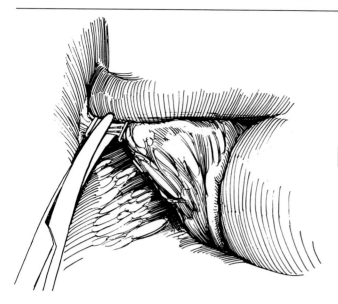

FIGURE 34-6. Clip the branch from the phrenic artery.

FIGURE 34-7. Expose the adrenal vein entering the vena cava by dissecting from above downward. Take great care not to injure the thin-walled vein or tear the vena cava, gently retracting the vena cava with a long vein retractor. Notify the anesthesiologist and place a 2-0 silk suture around the vein and ligate it near the vena cava. If the vein is short and wide, insinuate a Satinsky clamp onto the cava and use that for control instead of using a ligature alone. Place a tie or a hemoclip distally. Clip the small arteries from the aorta individually (do not try to tie them). Remove the specimen. Close the retroperitoneum and the wound.

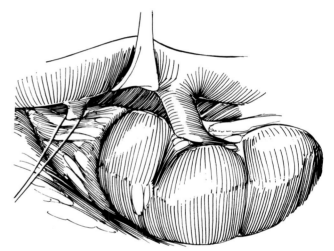

SIMULTANEOUS BILATERAL EXPOSURE

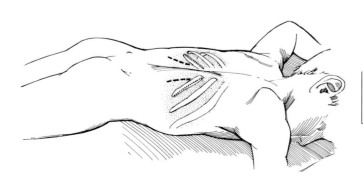

FIGURE 34-8. With the child prone and a pillow under the abdomen (not shown), make a bilateral lumbotomy incision, or resect the 12th rib on both sides.

POSTOPERATIVE PROBLEMS

Adrenal insufficiency and hypotension are related to the preoperative diagnosis and the amount of adrenal tissue remaining. Appropriately monitored therapy will replace the deficits. Other complications are similar to those after nephrectomy. Pneumothorax and injury to the pancreas and spleen are not uncommon, nor are wound infection and retroperitoneal hemorrhage and hematomas. More particular to adrenalectomy are injuries to the portal vein, to the vena cava at the entrance of the adrenal vein, and to the hepatic vein—all of which are managed intraoperatively. Subdiaphragmatic abscess can be an additional complication.

Commentary by
RICARDO GONZÁLEZ

I agree with the use of the anterior approach to the adrenal in children, since the principal indication for adrenalectomy is the removal of tumors. The transperitoneal laparoscopic approach can be used as well. To approach the left adrenal through the lesser sac, it is not necessary to reflect the splenic flexure of the colon. On the contrary, the lesser sac is approached dividing the gastrocolic mesentery, and then accessing the tumor or the gland as depicted. Alternatively, the splenic flexure can be reflected medially. This approach may be better for larger tumors or when doing the operation laparoscopically.

Chapter 35
Excision of Neuroblastoma

Localize the tumor with MRI and perhaps also with a metaiodobenzyl guanidine (^{131}MIBG) scan. Such localization may make the traditional, complete transabdominal exposure unnecessary. In children, however, multiple tumors are more common.

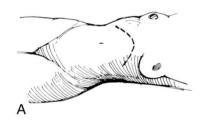

A

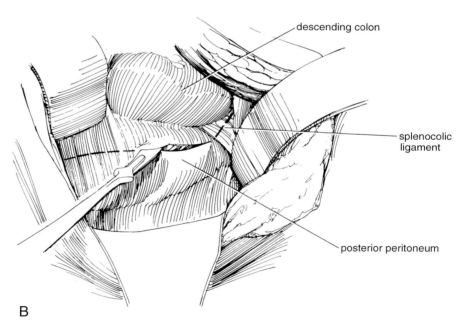

B

FIGURE 35-1. A and **B,** Expose the tumor via a chevron incision (see Chapter 10). After entering the abdomen, gently palpate the adrenal and para-aortic areas while the anesthetist monitors the blood pressure to search for previously undetected tumors. On the left mobilize the colon medially by incising the splenocolic ligament. On the right the ascending colon should be reflected inferiorly. An alternative is to approach the adrenals through the lesser sac rather than reflecting the splenic flexure.

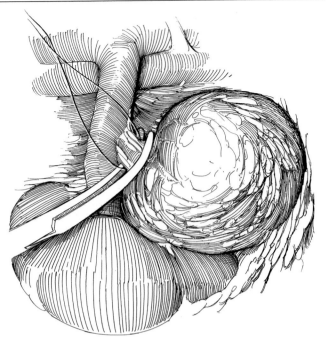

FIGURE 35-2. Place retractors; a large ring retractor is best. Carefully free the tumor from its bed inferiorly. Dissect it laterally to the superior margin of the renal vein. Take care to separately ligate the adrenal vein, which may empty into the inferior phrenic vein or even directly into the vena cava. Parasitic vessels are common. Unresectable tumor should be managed with postoperative chemotherapy and MIBG-tagged therapy.

DR. FERNANDO A. FERRER

Commentary by

Given that many pre- or perinatally diagnosed adrenal neuroblastomas have a benign course, the Children's Oncology Group has an open study with an observation-only arm for this group of patients. Inclusion criteria include age less than 6 months and a tumor volume less than or equal to 16 mL. The patients are watched carefully by sonography and biochemical testing.

    The surgical principles for most patients at initial diagnosis include the establishment of a diagnosis, resection of as much of the primary tumor as is safely possible, and lymph node assessment. If a tumor can safely be resected it should be removed. Procedures that require removal or compromise of other organs should not be undertaken at the initial procedure. Commonly, an open-wedge biopsy is the initial procedure. The surgeon should anticipate and prepare for the possibility that significant bleeding may result from the biopsy. Hemostatic agents should be available, as should blood. The patient must be carefully monitored postbiopsy. After chemotherapy, definitive surgical resection at a second procedure is usually performed. Detailed surgical guidelines are available in the Children's Oncology Group protocols.

    One of the more controversial subjects related to surgery for neuroblastoma is the importance of a complete resection of the tumor at the time of definitive surgery. Some authors have suggested that a complete resection is not necessary. This is based on data suggesting that local recurrence rates are low and that distant failure is the principle determinant of outcome. Others have disputed this, suggesting that complete resection is preferable. Until conclusive data are available, it seems prudent to strive for a complete resection.

Section 5

URETER

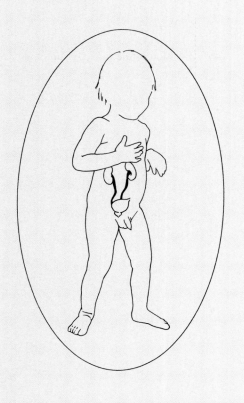

Part I

Ureteroneocystostomy

Chapter 36

Introduction to Ureteroneocystostomy

Indications for antireflux surgery continue to remain the same. They include breakthrough upper-tract infection on suppressive antibiotics, pyelonephritis due to poor patient compliance with prophylactic antibiotics, and persistent high-grade reflux.

Reimplant the ureter directly into the bladder with an antireflux mechanism. In the rare case that this is not possible, alternatives include insertion into a mobilized wing of the bladder or anastomosis to the other ureter. If the ureter is too short, the kidney may be mobilized, or even "transplanted" with its vasculature. In rare circumstances, a segment of bowel may be placed as a ureteral substitute.

Grade I and II reflux most likely will resolve spontaneously and will rarely require intervention. Children with grades III and IV can be followed safely with observation and suppressive medication until resolution or an indication for surgery. Grade V reflux should be corrected after 1 year of age or at the time of diagnosis if older than 1 year. Resolved contralateral reflux that recurs or reflux appearing after unilateral repair need not be managed immediately with ureteroneocystostomy because it will probably resolve with time. In infancy, reimplantation has a high rate of technical success with low postoperative morbidity.

A voiding cystourethrogram is used to establish the presence and degree of reflux. Reflux at low bladder pressure or capacity is a poor prognostic factor. The patient should be followed with ultrasonography, a valuable screening procedure. It is especially useful to assess renal scarring in children who are asymptomatic and have low-grade reflux. A child with higher grades of reflux, a history of infection, and an abnormal ultrasound study can be assessed for renal scarring with a dimethylsuccinic acid (DMSA) scan. A normal DMSA study is an excellent prognostic indicator for reflux resolution and low chance of recurrent infection. In contrast, abnormalities consistent with renal scarring predict poor reflux resolution and higher risk of recurrent urine infection.

If the urine is infected, the patient should be given antibiotics, especially during diagnostic procedures requiring catheterization. Anticipate spontaneous resolution of the reflux in a high proportion of cases; the younger the child, the more likely resolution will occur. Treating associated bladder dysfunction is important. For resistant cases, use behavioral intervention to correct voiding dysfunction. But after 5 years of observation and supervision, do not expect resolution, especially in children with persistent high-grade reflux. Prophylactic antibiotic coverage may be discontinued after time with little chance for scarring. These children also become more resistant to infection as they grow older.

FORMS OF REFLUX

Primary Reflux in a Single System

Grade the reflux. Observe the orifice cystoscopically, although this adds little to the diagnosis or prediction of spontaneous resolution. A paraureteral (Hutch) diverticulum, if present, will have been seen on cystography. Treat reflux of grades I through IV conservatively with antibiotics and expect a high rate of resolution. But intervene if infection persists or parenchymal loss from scarring appears. Reserve reimplantation for grade V. Do not reimplant the contralateral ureter unless reflux has been demonstrated at some time on that side. Contralateral reflux seldom appears de novo after unilateral repair; if it does, it usually resolves spontaneously.

Primary Reflux in a Duplex System

Alternatives to standard common sheath reimplantation include ureteropyelostomy (see Chapter 51) or ureteroureterostomy (see Chapter 50).

Secondary Reflux

Assess the urodynamic status of the bladder for evidence of neurogenic or nonneurogenic bladder dysfunction. Correct the dysfunction with drugs and training before treating the reflux surgically because implantations into such bladders are more prone to fail. Make every attempt to obtain normal detrusor dynamics before operation.

Ureteropelvic junction obstruction, due in part to repeated overload from refluxed urine, can be present in a small percentage of cases. Perform pyeloplasty before ureteroneocystostomy because correcting reflux first does not appear to protect against the eventual need for pyeloplasty. Ureteral duplication may be associated with reflux into the lower-pole segment. Surgically implant both ureters in their common sheath. Injection techniques are less successful in these cases.

Of particular note, it is rarely necessary to remove the refluxing ureteral stump after nephrectomy and partial ureterectomy for a nonfunctioning kidney due to reflux nephropathy.

SELECTION OF TECHNIQUE

The aim of the operation is construction of a submucosal tunnel with a length five times the diameter of the ureter over a firm backing and without tension.

An extravesical approach (see Chapter 41) has fewer complications than a transvesical approach. However, for infants and children with small trigones and/or large ureters, a transvesical approach (see Chapter 37) may be better. Use a transvesical approach for bilateral reimplantation; it interferes less with the perivesical nerves and thus results in less postoperative urinary retention.

REIMPLANTATION TECHNIQUES

Transvesical techniques—the simple advancement (Politano-Leadbetter), the distal tunnel advancement (Glenn-Anderson), or the popular transtrigonal (Cohen) techniques—are methods for advancement that can be done with minimal dissection. Extravesical techniques—such as the Lich-Gregoir adaptation and the external tunnel (Barry) method—are associated with significantly less morbidity and are useful not only for the unilateral, "fresh" case, but also for more complicated ones, such as in children with thick-walled bladders. Voiding problems are more common with extravesical techniques, especially if done bilaterally; however, they usually resolve with time. For megaureter, use ureteral tapering or folding techniques (see Chapters 47 and 48).

In the thick-walled bladder, dissect the ureter extravesically, pull it through the original hiatus, and then advance it submucosally. For duplicated ureters, common sheath reimplantation is practical even if tapering is required, although this does require construction of a larger tunnel.

Relative Advantages and Disadvantages

Blind extravesical passage of the ureter, as in the Politano-Leadbetter technique, carries some risk of obstruction by kinking. The Glenn-Anderson advancement technique avoids this problem and may be a good choice for the laterally placed (ectopic) ureteral orifice, even though persistent reflux is more likely. The Cohen technique is safe and easily performed, but does make future ureteral catheterization difficult, even with a flexible cystoscope. An advantage of an extravesical reimplantation is that it may be done on an outpatient basis.

INTUBATION

Ureteral intubation is a personal decision. A ureteral stent provides free urinary flow, which is especially important in children with impaired renal function or a solitary kidney. However, a tube inflames the ureter, especially at the orifice, which may cause obstruction on removal. In any case, after an intravesical procedure, drain the bladder with a ureteral or suprapubic catheter for 4 or 5 days. Placement of a perivesical Penrose drain is optional.

REIMPLANTATION FOR URETERAL STENOSIS OR INJURY

If the lesion in the ureter is low, perform ureteroneocystostomy with or without a psoas hitch (see Chapter 58). In the lower ureter, ureteroureterostomy is usually technically difficult and is prone to failure. If the ureter has only been crushed, stent it. Realize that a fibrotic or contracted bladder may be unsuitable for either implantation or a flap procedure. Instead, consider performing transureteroureterostomy (see Chapter 52). Interposing the appendix, or transplanting the kidney (see Chapter 60) may bridge the gap in some cases. As a last resort, perform ureteroileostomy (see Chapter 55), or cutaneous ureterostomy (see Chapter 87). Nephrectomy is rarely indicated. For transureteroureterostomy, do not mobilize the ureter more than necessary or leave tension on the anastomosis. In the teenager, it may not be essential to provide a nonrefluxing anastomosis, thus making the operation technically easier.

ANESTHESIA

General anesthesia is preferred. Continuous epidural anesthesia may be used for postoperative pain control.

POSITION

Place the child supine with a rolled towel under the small of the back. Insert a silicone urethral catheter and partially fill the bladder through a Y-tube arrangement.

INCISION

For primary operations, make a small, lower abdominal transverse (Pfannenstiel) incision (see Chapter 11); for secondary operations, a vertical abdominal incision may be required for adequate exposure.

Chapter 37

Transvesical Advancement Technique

A standard procedure with a high rate of success, the transvesical, or Politano-Leadbetter, technique has a lower incidence of transient voiding problems postoperatively than extravesical approaches but results in more de novo contralateral reflux.

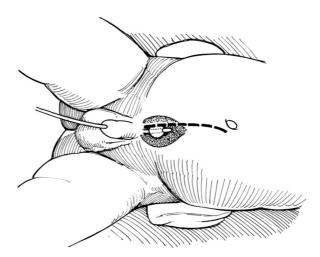

FIGURE 37-1. Position: Place the child supine in the frog-legged position, and insert a small silicone catheter into the bladder. Incision: For primary operations, make a small transverse abdominal incision (see Chapter 63). For secondary operations, a vertical abdominal incision may occasionally be required. Place a ring retractor. Incise the bladder vertically, and then bluntly enlarge the opening with the index fingers. Place a figure-eight suture where the incision approaches the retropubic space to prevent further extension during retraction.

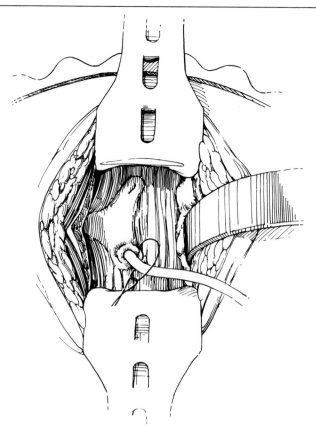

FIGURE 37-2. Insert four stay sutures to support the edges of the bladder, and drape them over the retractor for exposure (not shown), or place lateral retractor blades inside the bladder to retract the bladder edges. Hold a moist pack in the bladder dome with a Deaver retractor. Do not rub the bladder wall; this will induce edema and distortion. Insert a 5-F infant feeding tube into the ureter and suture it at the orifice with a purse-string 4-0 synthetic absorbable suture. Consider donning a headlamp.

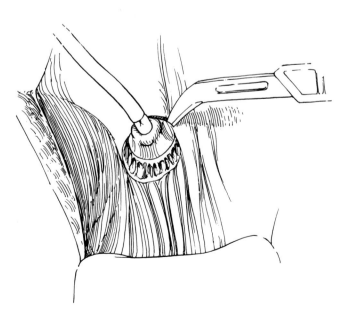

FIGURE 37-3. Gently lift the feeding tube to draw the ureteral orifice into the bladder. Cut through the mucosa around the orifice with a hooked blade or a needle-tipped electrocautery.

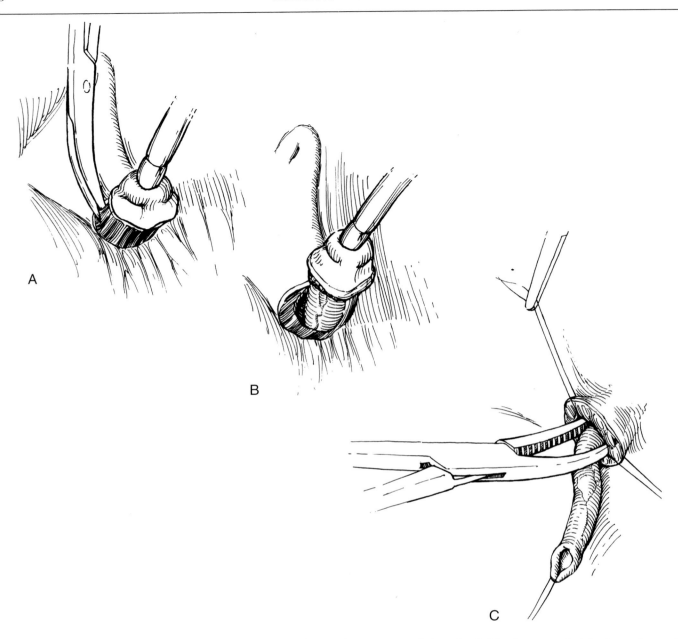

FIGURE 37-4. A, Hold tenotomy scissors at right angles to the ureter and sharply divide the superficial trigonal muscles, which are exposed medially and inferiorly as the ureter is elevated. **B,** With a Küttner dissector (or a cotton swab in infants), develop a plane inferiorly next to the ureteral adventitia, and then bluntly and sharply free the ureter of all attachments to Waldeyer's sheath. Periureteral injection of 1% lidocaine with a 1:100,000 epinephrine solution decreases bleeding and facilitates dissection by defining this plane. A small retractor in the hiatus may help dissection. To ensure tension-free repositioning, mobilize enough ureter by pushing the adherent peritoneum away with a peanut dissector. Be careful to preserve the vascular ureteral adventitia; stripping it results in ureteral ischemia, necrosis, and stricture. Look both intra- and extravesically to avoid kinking, twisting, or J-hooking the ureter. **C,** Insert traction sutures through the bladder wall medially and laterally to open the hiatus. Elevate the hiatus with a narrow retractor. (Do not use forceps.) Bluntly dissect between the ureter and bladder wall to free the peritoneal attachments under vision, using a right-angle clamp or a Küttner dissector. Again, take care not to devascularize (or perforate) the ureter.

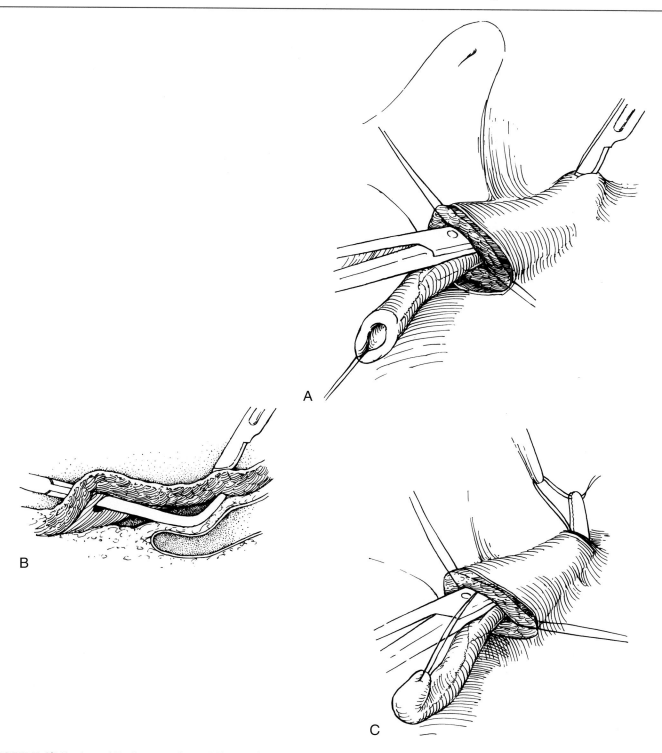

FIGURE 37-5. A and **B,** Insert a long Mixter clamp into the hiatus and dissect directly along the outer surface of the bladder wall cephalad to the meatus. Be careful that the tip of the clamp does not pass through peritoneum or bowel. In boys during this dissection, identify and protect the vas deferens. At a point at least 2.5 cm cephalad and slightly medial to the hiatus, elevate the tip of the clamp against the overlying wall. (For larger ureters, make the distance longer; a 5:1 ratio of tunnel length to ureteral diameter is needed.) Avoid placing the new hiatus any more laterally than the original one and be sure the new opening is large enough to accommodate the ureter. If a longer tunnel is needed for a large ureter, incise the hiatus cephalolaterally and close the bladder wall below the ureter after anastomosis. **C,** Catch the ureteral traction suture (and also the stent if it has not yet been removed) in a right-angle clamp and draw it through the tunnel and out the new hiatus. Now draw the ureter into the bladder through the new retrovesical tunnel. Again, check to be certain that it is neither kinked nor under tension. Close the bladder wall behind the original hiatus with interrupted 3-0 or 4-0 synthetic absorbable sutures.

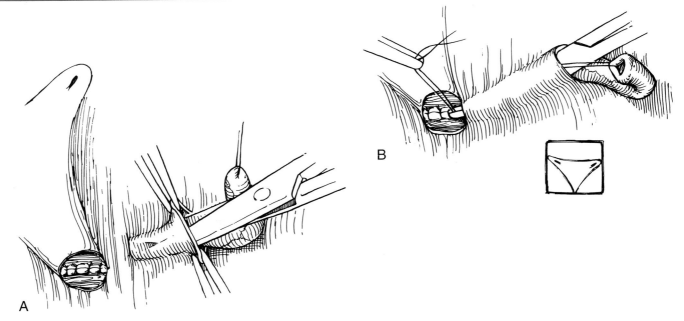

FIGURE 37-6. A, Dissect a suburothelial tunnel from the new hiatus to the old one by cutting and spreading with small, curved tenotomy scissors. The plane may be better defined and bleeding decreased by injecting 1% lidocaine with 1:100,000 epinephrine solution through a fine needle around the ureteral orifice and along the site of the proposed tunnel. In some cases, it may be easier to dissect from distal to proximal. If the roof is torn, complete the implantation, and then tack it back with a fine suture. It is even acceptable to incise the intervening mucosa and dissect it back as two flaps and subsequently approximate them over the ureter. In that case, check the size of the entrance to the tunnel by inserting the tip of a Mixter clamp. **B,** Pass the clamp, holding the stay suture down through the tunnel, grasp the suture, and draw the ureter through with it. Again, check the caliber of the tunnel and hiatus. As depicted in the insert, the tunnel should lie within a square outlined from the trigone.

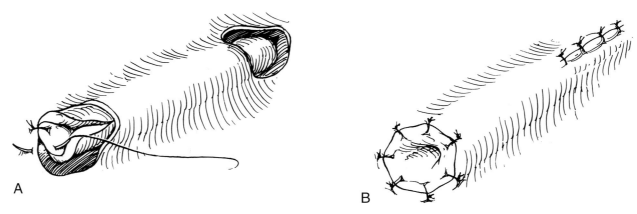

FIGURE 37-7. A, Trim the old meatus from the ureter to remove any obstructive segment and to ensure a fresh blood supply. For a small ureter, spatulate the end on the medial aspect. Anchor the tip with two absorbable sutures placed deeply into the trigonal muscle and out through the vesical mucosa. Avoid tension on the ureter. Inspect it through the old hiatus for extravesical kinks. **B,** Complete the anastomosis by carefully placing 4-0 or 5-0 synthetic absorbable sutures for a mucosa-to-mucosa coaptation. Close the upper urothelial incision vertically with the same suture material. Passing a 3.5- or 5-F infant feeding tube will detect ureteral kinks. Make additional holes in the tube and leave it indwelling as a stent to align it and avoid possibly obstructive kinks or adhesions. Suture the tube to the opposite side of the bladder near the neck with a 4-0 plain catgut suture and bring it out through a stab wound.

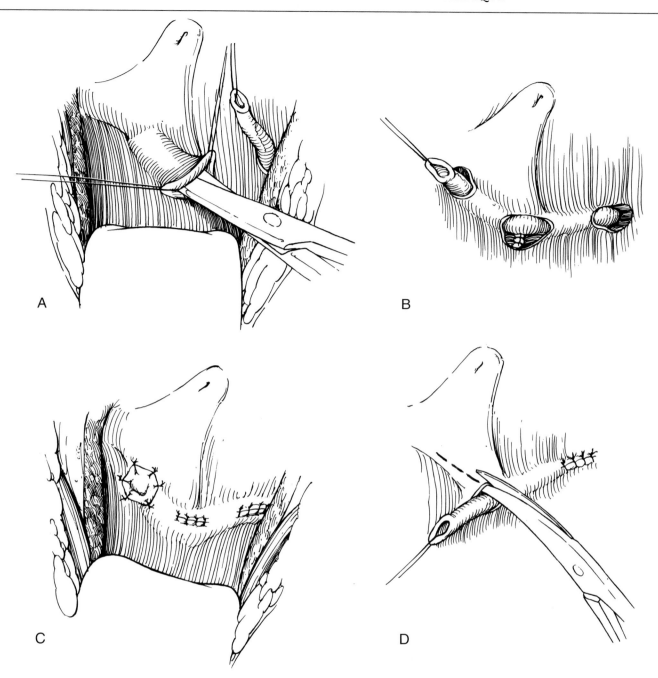

FIGURE 37-8. A, For additional ureteral length, extend the tunnel distally. **B** and **C,** Draw the ureter through the new hiatus and suture it to the margin. (If the new hiatus lies too close to the bladder neck, it will be difficult to place anastomotic sutures.) Close the two mucosal defects transversely. **D,** Alternatively, advance the meatus by incising the more distal mucosa and closing it over the ureter.

Drain the bladder: In boys, insert a 14- or 16-F Malecot catheter or use a small silicone balloon catheter. Bring the catheter through a stab wound in the bladder and body wall to exit just above the abdominal incision. In girls, the ureteral stents may be brought out through the urethra alongside a small balloon catheter. Alternatively, insert an 8- to 12-F red rubber catheter through the urethra into the open bladder, and then place a 2-0 silk suture through the tip and bring both ends through the bladder and abdominal walls. Tie them over a gauze roll for later removal.

Close the bladder in layers with a running 4-0 plain catgut suture placed in the submucosa, followed by interrupted synthetic absorbable sutures to close the muscle layer. Place a small Penrose drain in the space of Retzius and bring it out through a stab wound below the incision. Approximate the rectus muscles and fascia with 3-0 synthetic absorbable sutures. Close the subcutaneous tissue with fine plain catgut and the skin with subcuticular 4-0 or 5-0 synthetic absorbable sutures.

Postoperative care: Continue prophylactic antibiotics. At 6 weeks, obtain an intravenous urogram or sonogram, and at 12 weeks, a voiding cystogram. Monitor the urine by culture. Stop the suppressive antibiotics if reflux has ceased, but continue monitoring the urine. At 1 year, and again at 3 years, obtain a renal ultrasound study to assess renal growth and rule out obstruction.

VICTOR A. POLITANO

Commentary by

The brief descriptions and line drawings of the submucosal tunnel techniques give the surgeon an easy outline to follow for achieving good results. In reviewing the figures, it is immediately clear that mobilization of the ureter is performed in much the same way, regardless of the method used. Mobilization of the ureter must be done with care. The key to successful ureteral reimplantation is adequate mobilization of the ureter, preserving the ureteral adventitia. Stripping of the adventitia will render the ureter ischemic and necrotic. Avoid kinking, twisting, or J-hooking the ureter. When the ureter has been sutured in place, a 4- or 5-F catheter should pass to the kidney without meeting obstruction. Entering the peritoneum or perforating any viscus can be avoided with care and direct vision.

In general, I find creating the submucosal tunnel much easier by beginning beneath the mucosa at the site of the original orifice and progressing toward the site of the new hiatus. It is not necessary to have an intact tunnel and may be difficult or impossible when implanting a large ureter. The mucosa can be dissected from the muscularis laterally for the desired length and sutured over the ureter.

To stent or not to stent becomes the surgeon's choice. I personally prefer to stent for 2 or 3 days to get the patient over a period of acute edema, which may be considerable and obstructive. The stent also tends to align the ureter in good position, preventing any kinks or adhesions that may become obstructive later.

The first successful submucosal tunneling technique for correction of vesicoureteral reflux was described just over 30 years ago by myself and Wyland Leadbetter, and it certainly has withstood the test of time.

JOSEPH G. BORER

Commentary by

The authors have provided a thorough description and visual representation of the Politano-Leadbetter technique for ureteral reimplantation. I agree with the authors in this particular case, and in general regarding the use of a headlight, believing that a surgeon equipped with a headlight will be better able to consistently see the critical details of this highly successful procedure.

At initial ureteral dissection, an option different than that described by the authors is use of a pinpoint electrocautery tip with preservation of a circumferential cuff of mucosa around the ureteral meatus. I have found that if the native meatus is of relatively normal caliber and there is no preoperative suspicion of an obstructive component, then I believe that preserving this mucosal cuff simplifies the eventual anastomosis.

To facilitate dissection of the peritoneum off of the posterior aspect of the bladder, at times it may be helpful to use a lighted suction tip. You may also combine the intravesical dissection as described by the authors with an extravesical component of the dissection as has been described by others. This combined approach should further decrease the risk of entering the peritoneal cavity and potentially injuring bowel during this procedure.

One additional step to this procedure, that of making a small longitudinal incision in the caudal aspect of the neohiatus, may decrease the angle at which the ureter enters the bladder and in this way lessen the likelihood of obstruction at this site. Extending the ureter beyond the site of the native meatus, as described by the authors, is a maneuver that safely increases the length of the submucosal tunnel.

Stenting of the ureter following reimplantation via any technique is a decision of surgeon preference. I typically stent those ureters that drain a solitary kidney, a ureter that is tapered, or in the setting of complex adjunctive surgical procedure(s) such as augmentation cystoplasty.

Chapter 38

Distal Tunnel Reimplantation

Implantation is made under direct vision without blind extravesical dissection. The ureteral orifice is fixed well down on the trigone, thus providing maximal defense against reflux and an orifice that can be readily catheterized. A ureter of near normal size is required.

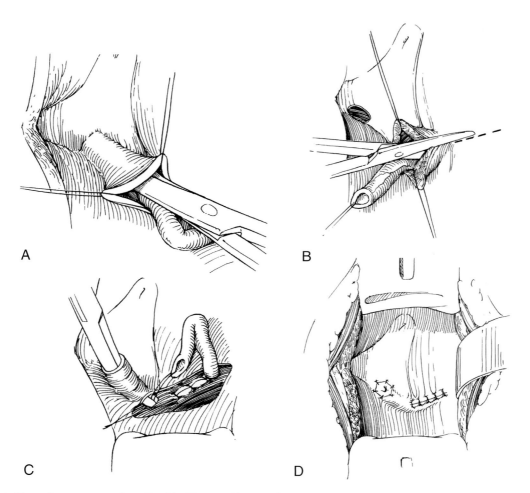

FIGURE 38-1. **A,** Free the ureter as described in Figures 37-1 to 37-5 of the Politano-Leadbetter technique (see Chapter 37). Create a suburothelial tunnel distal to a new hiatus. **B,** Incise the entire thickness of the vesical wall above the original hiatus. Take care not to deviate the bladder laterally. **C,** Close the defect behind the ureter with interrupted 4-0 synthetic absorbable sutures. **D,** Draw the ureter through the tunnel with a right-angle clamp. Trim it and anastomose it to the vesical mucosa. Do not make the tunnel too tight. (Insert a right-angle clamp to test it.) Close the original urothelial defect.

JAMES F. GLENN

Commentary by

The distal tunnel technique that Dr. Anderson and I have described and used preferentially since 1966 is an evolution of the contributions of Paquin, Politano, Lich, Gregoir, Innes Williams, and others. However, it embraces a fundamental principle of fixation of the ureteral orifice well down on the trigone, providing for maximal closure and prevention of reflux, as first stated by Tanagho. Further, the distal tunnel technique can be accomplished in almost every patient, particularly if superior displacement of the hiatus is accomplished in the manner illustrated. Next, the position of the neo-orifice on the trigone permits ready accessibility in contrast to displacement contralaterally above the trigone. Finally, as the procedure is accomplished under direct vision without blind dissection extravesically, the potential for damage to adjacent viscera or perforation of the peritoneum is obviated. Use of synthetic suture material is preferred to minimize inflammatory reaction. Indwelling ureteral stents are generally unnecessary. Urethral catheter drainage permits early ambulation and hospital discharge. Complications have been rare (2% persistent reflux, 1% stricture).

DARIUS BAGLI

Commentary by

The Glenn-Anderson ureteroneocystostomy is essentially a combination of a distal and proximal reconfiguration in situ. The distal portion is a minor ureteral advancement into a new, and slightly more distal, submucosal tunnel. The proximal portion is a repositioning of full-thickness bladder muscle under (or behind) the ureter. This latter maneuver brings new detrusor backing to the ureter, effectively adding tunnel length when the mucosa is closed over the ureter, without appreciable pulling of additional ureter into the bladder; hence the reconfiguration in situ. As stated previously, this is likely to be effective only with the nondilated ureter. Finally, although blind dissection of the ureter at its original hiatus is avoided, one should still keep in mind the possibility of peritoneum reflecting on the ureter while it is being freed from within the bladder (as one does in the Politano-Leadbetter technique), especially at the moment that the full-thickness incision of the bladder wall is being made.

Chapter 39

Transtrigonal Technique

The ureter continuing its natural course with the original hiatus unchanged makes the risk of obstruction low, but subsequent ureteral catheterization may be difficult.

Free the ureter as previously described (see Figs. 37-1 to 37-5). Assess the size of the hiatus. If it is too large, narrow it with two or three fine synthetic absorbable sutures, but be sure the ureter remains freely mobile. For more exposure, incise the superolateral margin of the hiatus with the cutting current and lift the edge with small vein retractors. This maneuver will also allow a higher, and consequently longer, tunnel.

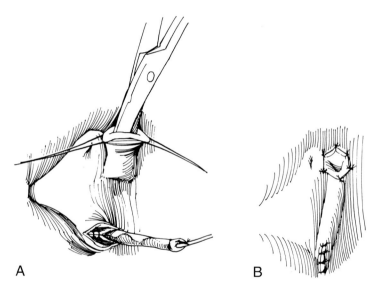

A   B

FIGURE 39-1. A, Incise the epithelium vertically just above and slightly lateral to the opposite ureteral orifice, depending on the size of the trigone. Pull up on that edge of the bladder with Allis clamps to tent the wall. Steady the bladder wall and straighten the bladder base with a moist Küttner dissector placed just lateral to the proposed orifice. Flatten this area by pulling the orifices laterally, stretching the intratrigonal area. Insert tenotomy scissors and gently open and close them to advance a tunnel across the trigone to a point approximately 1 cm above the opposite orifice, depending on the size of the ureter and on the development of the trigone. Be careful when crossing the midline with tenotomy scissors not to let the tips go too deeply into the muscle, or worse, if they are directed too much anteriorly, they can perforate the mucosa. **B,** For the first implant, choose the ureter with the lesser displacement of the orifice. Remove the tube from it. Insert a curved clamp through the tunnel, grasp the traction suture, and draw the ureter through until it lies free of tension. Trim the end of the ureter, spatulate it if it is small, and anchor it with a 4-0 chromic catgut suture through all layers of ureter and bladder. Approximate the epithelium with 5-0 synthetic absorbable sutures, and close the original hiatus with the same material. Check the course of the ureter with an infant feeding tube.

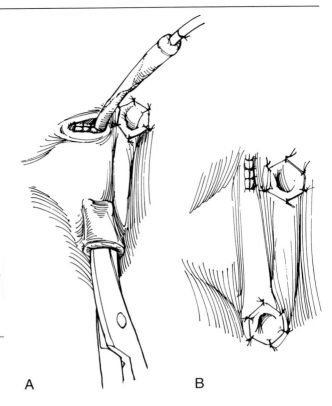

FIGURE 39-2. A, For bilateral implantation, make a separate tunnel for the second ureter from the original hiatus of the first ureter. Run it cephalad of the first tunnel to allow formation of a longer tunnel. Alternatively, bring this ureter through the original tunnel. Greater tunnel length may also be gained by incising the bladder wall in a superolateral direction. **B,** Draw this ureter through the new tunnel and suture it in place with fine absorbable sutures. Insert a 3.5- or 5-F infant feeding tube to be sure that the ureter takes a smooth, curving course. Consider tacking the tube laterally to the mucosa with a 3-0 plain catgut suture and leaving it as a stent. Close the remaining defects in the mucosa. In boys, it may be advisable to leave a small Malecot catheter in the bladder for 48 hours. It should exit from a stab wound. In girls, a Robinson catheter will suffice, held by a silk suture through the bladder dome and skin. Insert a Penrose drain, and close the bladder and wound in layers. Leave the stent in place for 48 hours. The ureter may subsequently be tailored in situ should reflux persist.

POSTOPERATIVE PROBLEMS

Bladder spasms occur after intravesical implantation, but may be reduced by giving ketorolac 0.5 mg/kg intravenously at the end of the procedure and every 6 hours for 2 days. Alternatives include a continuous epidural anesthesia.

Persistent ipsilateral reflux is usually of low grade and will resolve spontaneously. It is usually from technical failure, such as mobilizing the ureter inadequately, making the tunnel too short, or placing the orifice inappropriately. Rarely is it due to ureterovesical fistulization.

Before reimplanting a ureter, look for vesical dysfunction. The non-neurogenic neurogenic bladder syndrome of vesical-sphincter incoordination can lead to failure to correct the reflux or may result in secondary obstruction at the new orifice. Such dysfunction may also be responsible for the postoperative appearance of contralateral reflux.

Incomplete emptying can appear postoperatively, especially after bilateral extravesical implantation. Just dissecting perivesically can influence bladder function, but expect return to normal. Injury to the pelvic plexus, particularly if bilateral, may lead to bilateral hydronephrosis and renal insufficiency. To prevent nerve injury, free the distal ureter close to the ureteral adventitia and avoid dissection outside the mesoureter, especially dorsally and toward the trigone to preserve the terminal branches of the plexus.

Ureteral obstruction from angulation or constriction at the hiatus may appear after removal of the stent, causing flank pain, nausea, vomiting, ileus, and even sepsis. Rarely will percutaneous nephrostomy be required. Obstruction

that occurs soon after operation as a result of edema or from contraction of the thickened bladder wall during spasm is especially troublesome in infants younger than 3 months of age and in those with dilated ureters preoperatively. In such patients, stenting should be routine. Sepsis means obstruction and must be handled by its release.

Late ureteral obstruction is of concern if it persists longer than a few weeks and may require endoscopic manipulation or reoperation. If it occurs only when the bladder is full, it is the result of extravesical ureteral angulation and a laterally placed hiatus. Too large a hiatus may allow compression of the ureter by a paraureteral diverticulum. An ischemic ureter due to too much dissection may contract and obstruct. In any case of continued hydronephrosis, look first for persistent bladder dysfunction, as well as for residual valves and high urine output.

Extravasation, especially after tailoring, indicates early obstruction from edema, angulation, or constriction at the hiatus. Prolonged stenting is indicated. Gross hematuria is not unusual. Clots indicate inadequate intraoperative hemostasis, but bleeding rarely requires transurethral fulguration or reexploration. Check the ureteral catheters for patency. If stents are not used, consider reopening the bladder and placing stents retrogradely or install a nephrostomy tube percutaneously.

Fever may appear postoperatively if the urinary tract had not been cleared of infection. Antibiotic administration continued for 4 to 6 weeks reduces the chance of chronic infection. Later, recurrent infections are limited to the lower tract and are usually related to bladder dysfunction. Urinary retention following bilateral extravesical implantation is generally temporary.

COMPLICATIONS

Failure to correct the reflux is the most common problem, usually resulting from excessive remaining ureteral diameter or inadequate length of ureter in the tunnel. Rarely is a ureterovesical fistula the cause. Low-grade obstruction will usually resolve spontaneously under antibiotic coverage. Persistent urinary drainage is best managed by insertion of a self-retaining ureteral J stent and a urethral catheter. Realize that a vesicovaginal fistula can be overlooked in girls, although it is a rare occurrence. Ureteral obstruction may result from devascularization at the site of the ureteroneocystostomy, from kinking or torsion, or from an inadequate hiatial diameter. De novo contralateral reflux after unilateral extravesical implantation is uncommon and usually temporary. As noted, bladder dysfunction, even urinary retention, may appear, especially after bilateral extravesical implantation, but it usually will resolve spontaneously.

REOPERATION

Look first for bladder dysfunction. If it is on a functional basis, the dysfunction must be corrected by retraining before reoperation is attempted. Approach a persistently refluxing ureter transvesically. Circumscribe the meatus, and open the entire subepithelial tunnel to allow removal of the intact ureter. Mobilize the ureter above the hiatus to get more than enough length. Reimplant it with the Politano-Leadbetter or transtrigonal technique.

For an obstructed ureter, if the obstruction is limited to the meatus, an endoscopic method such as the passage of a stent, balloon dilatation, or a limited intravesical procedure is adequate. For a more extensive obstructive lesion, approach the ureter extravesically to obtain an unoperated portion for implantation, ignoring the original intravesical portion. Should that leave the ureter too short, proceed with a psoas hitch (see Chapter 58). If the ureter is still too short, resort to transureteroureterostomy (see Chapter 52). If both ureters are involved, one solution is to insert one ureter into the bladder with a psoas hitch and the other into the implanted ureter.

JOHN W. BROCK

Commentary by

When choosing a transtrigonal technique it is critical that, even though the original hiatus has been left intact, do not create any kinking as the ureter comes across the trigone. It is not unusual to have to open the posterior wall of the bladder on one side and move the ureter superiorly to create this gentle curve without kinking. When this is performed the hiatus is closed inferior to the original hiatus. The formation of the submucosal tunnel can be performed with either the Jamison scissors or a right-angle clamp. A critical technical aspect is that both surgeon and assistant provide gentle traction on the mucosa to create the countertraction necessary to develop this plane. To provide a very long tunnel take the tunnel past the orifice on the other side. It is also important that this not be taken up onto the sidewall of the bladder. As described previously, if doing a bilateral reimplantation you can put both ureters in the same tunnel. It is clearly my preference that this procedure should *not* be done in one tunnel, for the theoretic disadvantage of potentially allowing both ureters to become obstructed by the same process.

Chapter 40

Sheath Approximation Technique

Contralateral reflux occurs about 20% of the time after correction of unilateral reflux. This operation reconfigures both orifices and does so without ureteral mobilization or reimplantation.

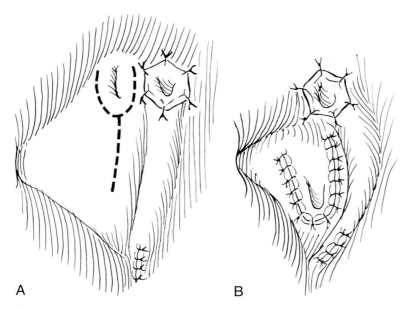

A   B

FIGURE 40-1. A, Make an incision three quarters around the ureter. Carry the incision transversely toward the location of the native contralateral ureteral orifice to expose the underlying trigone. Catch the periureteral sheath at the inferior margin of each ureter with a single nonabsorbable mattress suture. **B,** Tie the suture to draw the ureter toward the midline, thus lengthening the suburothelial tunnel.

MARC CENDRON

This technique avoids extensive dissection of the contralateral ureter in cases of unilateral vesicouretral reflux. Contralateral reflux is reported in less than 20% of cases and, in general, is of lower grade (I to III) with a high rate of spontaneous resolution. Nevertheless, the occurrence of contralateral reflux after open surgical repair is a major complication in the eyes of the parents who will, at times, perceive it as complete failure to treat reflux. Ensuring that contralateral reflux does not occur is therefore very reasonable.

Of importance is the most distal anchoring stitch, which will prevent the ureter from springing back to its original location. It will serve to prevent cephalad displacement of the ureter during bladder contraction and thus foreshortening of the submucosal tunnel. A 4-0 reabsorbable buried suture is used, anchoring the ureter to the detrusor muscle. This is an effective technique, but its long-term outcomes have not been extensively evaluated.

Commentary by

Commentary by
HOWARD SNYDER

It is important to emphasize that this advancement technique creates only a modest gain in intravesical positioning of the ureter. Accordingly, it is not very effective as a primary operation for reflux in a ureter. It can, however, be helpful to prevent postoperative reflux, as noted previously in the text, in the contralateral ureter. It is important also to emphasize that the technique is very safe. I have never seen an obstruction with this technique. If a nonabsorbable suture is used, it is important not to transgress the uroepithelium or a stone may form on the exposed nonabsorbable suture.

Chapter 41

Extravesical Trough Technique

Extravesical techniques may be simpler to perform, are effective, and ensure more comfort for the child postoperatively. They are not suitable, however, for very young infants with thin bladder walls, those with severely trabeculated neuropathic bladders, or those requiring bilateral reimplantation, who would be prone to inefficient voiding postoperatively. Care is necessary to avoid interference with the vesical nerve supply.

To prepare for the procedure, insert a balloon catheter attached to a Y-tube and a drainage bag and fill the bladder to one-third capacity. During the dissection, change the volume to aid orientation and to make separation of the detrusor muscle from the mucosa easier.

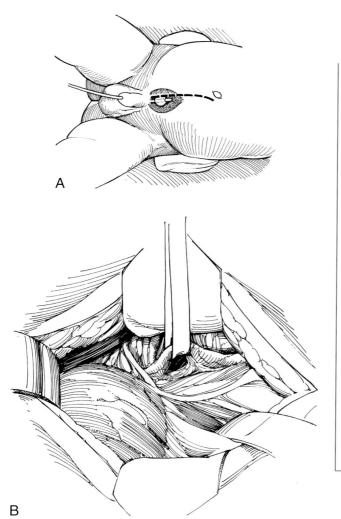

FIGURE 41-1. A, Incision: Make a lower midline incision (see Chapter 62) as shown, or better, use a lower abdominal transverse (Pfannenstiel) incision (see Chapter 63). Incise the fascia superficially over the bladder. Free the bladder and draw it cephalad with a finger on either side to expose the obliterated hypogastric (umbilical) artery on the affected side between the bladder and the pelvic sidewall. **B,** Insert a ring retractor. Dissect the white, cordlike obliterated hypogastric artery to its crossing of the ureter. Undermine it with a right-angle clamp, tie it in continuity, and divide it between the ties. Avoid dissecting toward the origin of the artery and thus entering the venous plexus there. Adjust the retractor to hold the bladder wall away from the pelvic sidewall and place a Deaver retractor to draw the bladder caudad. Follow the obliterated hypogastric artery to expose the ureter between it and the pelvic wall.

Caution: The nerves to the bladder run from the pelvic plexus in close proximity (dorsomedial) to the ureterovesical junction. Keep dissection close to the ureter. Extravesical implantation, if bilateral, is even more likely to cause urinary retention; if the dissection is limited and the electrocautery is used judiciously, the risk is small.

Place a Penrose drain around the ureter. Ligate the several perforating vessels behind it, but direct the dissection laterally to preserve as much of the adventitial vasculature as possible. Dissect the ureter toward the bladder to expose the terminal 4 to 5 cm, ligating uterine vessels as necessary.

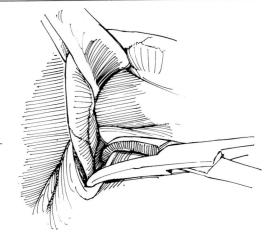

FIGURE 41-2. Lift the ureter in the Penrose drain sling. With a Schnidt clamp, separate the intramural portion of the ureter from the detrusor muscle circumferentially to reach the vesical submucosa.

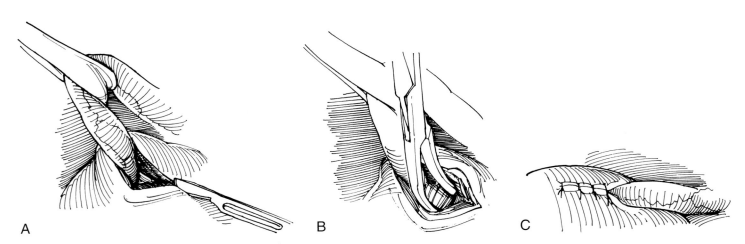

A   B   C

FIGURE 41-3. A, Divide the detrusor muscle down to the subepithelium with a #15 blade, cutting in a vertical direction for a distance of 2.5 to 3 cm from the ureter. Because this cut is made with the bladder rotated, the direction it should take may not be immediately apparent. Release the long blade of the ring retractor to let the bladder drop back; again fill the bladder, note the natural course of the ureter, and then make the cut accordingly. Place a stay suture on each side of this line to support the bladder wall.

B, Undermine the bladder muscle for a distance of 2.5 to 3 cm (five times the diameter of the ureter). Divide the muscle from the mucosa with the electrocautery, and undermine it slightly. This maneuver forms a trough and also provides lateral flaps to cover the ureter. Close any tears in the bulging submucosa with figure-of-eight 6-0 chromic sutures. Cutting a Y-shaped incision proximally can help release the flaps longitudinally. If a longer tunnel is needed, first free the ureter circumferentially at the orifice. Place paired horizontal mattress sutures lateral and medial to it. Pass these through the adventitia of the ureter near its junction with the bladder and then out through the inner surface of the detrusor muscle. Tie them to draw the end of the ureter into the bladder (i.e., "advancement"; see Chapter 42).

C, Lay the ureter into the new bed and cover it loosely, distal to proximal, with the edges of the detrusor muscle to provide backing, using interrupted 3-0 synthetic absorbable sutures. Avoid constriction of the ureter at the point of exit. Allow the bladder to fall back. Now be sure the course of the ureter is straight, without kinking or compression. Insert a Penrose drain (optional), and close the wound in layers. Drain the bladder for 3 days with a urethral catheter.

The original Gregoir technique does not require mobilization of the intramural ureter. After exposing the junction of the ureter to the bladder, make a vertical incision on the posterior bladder wall just above the ureterovesical implantation, over a length of from 3 to 5 cm, according to the size of the child. Divide the detrusor muscle to the subepithelium and undermine it slightly. Place the ureter into the groove in contact with the bladder epithelium, and close the muscle over the ureter with interrupted 4-0 chromic catgut or synthetic absorbable sutures. Start the first suture exactly at the level of the ureterovesical junction. Place a second layer with a continuous suture in the adventitia of the bladder. Avoid constriction of the ureter at the point of exit. The Lich-Gregoir reimplantation can also be performed laparoscopically (see Chapter 43).

WILLY GREGOIR

Extravesical reimplantation of the ureter can be done by a somewhat different technique. First, make a vertical incision through the detrusor muscle to the mucosa on the posterior bladder wall as near as possible to the normal line of contact between ureter and bladder. Make a very small opening in the lower angle of the incision, as shown in the figures for the external tunnel technique (see Chapter 44). Place a suture in the ureteral tip, introduce the ureter through the orifice, and secure the suture to the bladder wall, tying it externally. Proceed as described for my antireflux technique to cover the ureter in its bed. A stent is not necessary. Leave a suction drain for 24 hours; remove the indwelling bladder catheter in 4 or 5 days.

GUY BOGAERT

Just over 30 years ago, Professor Willy Gregoir published the Lich-Gregoir operation in a pediatric urologic surgery textbook. It is an excellent technique that is still a good and valid procedure today (especially when combined with some modifications and tips and tricks learned from experience). However, I am not certain if this still will be the case 10 years from now: the subostial and intraureteral injection technique with Deflux gel (dextranomer microspheres and stabilized, non-animal hyaluronic acid) can reach resolution of vesicoureteral reflux in up to 90% of cases. In addition, in the situation of ureteral duplication and certainly in the presence of a ureterocele, we prefer transtrigonal (Cohen) surgery.

The advantage of the Lich-Gregoir technique is that it is easy to perform, easy to learn, and more comfortable for the child compared with intravesical repair. It is important that the ureteral orifice not be damaged or displaced in the bladder (for future, eventual endoscopic instrumentation). Also, the bladder does not need to be opened; thus, there is no need for ureteral stenting.

However, this extravesical ureteral reimplantation technique has some pitfalls or dangers, such as possible damage to the vas deferens or ovarian tube, or damage to the ganglion pelvicum, the coordinating center for normal bladder function.

Therefore, we recommend performing extravesical ureteral surgery either unilaterally (with 3 months' interval in between the contralateral sides), or bilaterally, to implement special care for bladder-emptying problems postoperatively. It is mandatory to discuss this preoperatively with the parents and child.

We fill the bladder before surgery with a solution obtained by mixing 20 mL iso-Betadine (polyvidone-iodine, 100 mg/mL) in 80 mL sterile water and filling the bladder up to one third of the calculated bladder capacity (age plus 2 fluid ounces). This has a local disinfection effect and allows us to clearly see the refluxing ureter, which has been filled with the dark solution.

We have learned from Professor Rudi Hohenfellner and his research that the ganglion pelvicum is located 1 cm dorsal and 1 cm caudal from the ureterovesical junction, so we only dissect the cranial and ventral circumference and leave the detrusor fibers located caudal and dorsal as intact as possible. By respecting the dorsal and caudal detrusor muscle (even in simultaneous surgery) we have encountered no (long-term) bladder function problems. As well, we attempt to achieve a 4-cm detrusor tunnel for the ureter.

We use poliglecaprone 25 (Monocryl) 3-0 or 4-0 for the detrusor muscle adaptation sutures. When there is mucosal damage or a tear, we close it with a polyglactin 910 (vicryl) 6-0 suture. A transurethral catheter (silicone) is left for 3 to 5 days. Children can go home usually 1 to 2 days postoperatively.

Chapter 42

Detrusorrhaphy (Modifications of the Lich-Gregoir Technique)

Prepare the patient so the bladder volume can be manipulated during the operation. Fill the bladder one-third full.

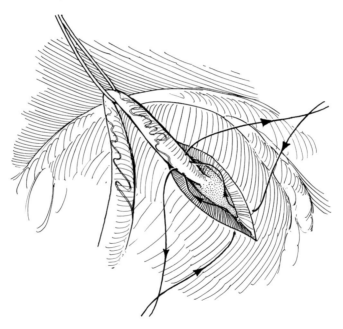

FIGURE 42-1. Though a Pfannenstiel incision, rotate the bladder to expose the ureter extravesically. Place a vessel loop around it to use for traction and allow dissection to its junction with the bladder. Preserve as much of the periureteral vasculature as possible, but free the terminal ureter of its perivesical and muscular attachments. Distend the bladder moderately. Make limited incisions through the detrusor muscle, one proximal and one distal to the attachment of the ureter. Make them in line with the normal course of the ureter. (It is easy to go off line and angulate the ureter; if in doubt, deflate the bladder for reorientation.) Start laterally to elevate the muscle, including the fibers of Waldeyer's sheath, from the mucosa to form detrusor flaps. Expose the surrounding bladder uroepithelium in a 5-cm arc about the orifice. (Take care not to dissect externally and thus denervate the detrusor muscle and avoid perforation; if the bladder mucosa is breached, drain the bladder and close the defect with a fine figure-of-eight suture before proceeding.) Traction sutures in the edges of the detrusor muscle (not shown) aid in the dissection. The degree of pouching of the epithelium may be regulated by filling and emptying the bladder.

Ureteral invagination: Use 3-0 or 4-0 synthetic absorbable sutures (not catgut, which would be absorbed too quickly). Place the suture first through the muscle of the bladder wall at the lower edge of the opening from outside in to exit at the edge of the epithelial-muscularis dissection; then pass it through the ureteral wall at the former ureterovesical junction at the 5-o'clock position. Finally, pass it distally to exit inside out near the point of entry (not shown). (This vertical mattress suture forms a vest-over-pants stitch.) Place a second suture in the same way at the 7-o'clock position on the ureter.

242

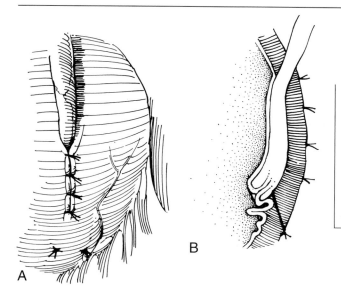

FIGURE 42-2. A and **B,** Tie the sutures to telescope the ureter into the bladder, thus forming a long subepithelial tunnel. For duplex ureters, place an extra suture between the pair. Close the hiatus loosely with running or interrupted 4-0 synthetic absorbable sutures to back up the tunnel. Neither a stent nor a drain is needed. Leave the balloon catheter in place overnight; remove it the next day. Check for incomplete emptying, especially after bilateral repair, and be prepared to start clean intermittent catheterization.

MARK ZAONTZ

Commentary by

The extravesical techniques are all similar in nature, with modifications as described. The main difference between the technique described by Lich-Gregoir and that of Hodgson is that the latter performs the extravesical technique with ureteral advancement. In Chicago, we termed this technique *detrusorrhaphy.* An important tip in doing detrusorrhaphy involves ensuring that the detrusor incision, which usually is initiated with electrocautery, is made in the same direction that the ureter is heading to avoid unnecessary angulation of the ureter. Traction on the ureter after it has been dissected down to the epithelial junction helps define the path the ureter should be taking. The initial detrusor incision is usually more lateral than one would expect.

Prior to beginning any of the extravesical techniques, it is important to place an indwelling balloon catheter and to fill the bladder roughly one third to one half of its calculated volume with sterile saline. The catheter is hooked up to a drainage bag and is clamped until the ureteral repair is completed. This allows for easier dissection of the detrusor muscle off of the underlying epithelium. Stay sutures of chromic catgut should be used liberally to retract the margins of the detrusor muscle to allow for easier dissection. Tenotomy scissors and moistened Küttner dissectors are used to mobilize the detrusor muscle off of the epithelium. Should an inadvertent rent in the epithelium occur, this readily can be closed with 6-0 chromic catgut sutures in a figure-of-eight fashion. If the ureteral hiatus is particularly close to the bladder neck, the majority of the detrusor dissection should occur in a cephalad direction, as opposed to distally toward the bladder neck. The critical portion of this procedure involves the advancement of the ureter onto the trigone toward the bladder neck with a pair of vest-over-pants sutures of 4-0 chromic catgut or polyglycolic acid. The sutures must engage the ureter in its seromuscular plane at the 5- and 7-o'clock positions, respectively, at the ureteroepithelial junction. The detrusor muscle defect is closed with a running 4-0 polyglycolic acid suture. A second layer of interrupted Lembert sutures may be used to reinforce the initial closure.

Care is taken to avoid making the exiting ureter too snug at the hiatus. No ureteral stents or drains are necessary, because there have been no reports of ureteral obstruction or urine leaks after detrusorrhaphy. The urethral catheter is left overnight and removed the following morning. The advantages of this operation include its high success rate, low morbidity, little or no hematuria, few bladder spasms, and absence of wound drains or ureteral stents. Additionally, hospital stay is usually only 1 or 2 days. Caution is advised in considering this operation for bilateral reflux. There have been numerous instances of prolonged urinary retention and the need for intermittent catheterization on a temporary basis. This has been thought to be caused by partial bladder denervation by the extravesical technique. In the past few years, research has revealed that the pelvic plexus that has to do with bladder contractility runs dorsomedial to the ureterovesical junction into the bladder. Subsequently, when doing the extravesical technique avoid dissection in this direction as well as extensive cautery in this location. This should markedly cut down on the risk of bladder denervation. In addition, minimizing the length of the dissection also helps in this regard.

Refluxing and obstructive megaureters can be corrected using the detrusorrhaphy technique as described, with the exception of disconnecting the ureter at the ureteroepithelial junction for tapering. The ureter is then intubated with either the KISS catheter or the Dow Corning cystocatheter. The stent is brought out through a separate stab wound in the bladder after passing it through the original epithelial rent. The tapered ureter is then reanastomosed to the epithelium with 5-0 chromic catgut in interrupted fashion. The advancement technique is the same as that described.

Recent work has shown clearly that we can do the extravesical technique through inguinal incisions as small as 15 to 20 mm. There is a small triangular gap within the aponeurosis of the external oblique and the transversalis fascia, which brings you right to the point of the ureterovesical junction. Using mini Deaver retractors, excellent exposure is afforded and the technique for extravesical advancement is unchanged as described. The advantage of these small incisions is decreased morbidity with rapid recovery and discharge from the hospital.

Chapter 43

Laparoscopic Extravesical Ureteroneocystostomy (Lich-Gregoir Adaptation)

Create a pneumoperitoneum and insert two 10-mm trocars, one in the left midclavicular line 5 mm above the umbilicus for the camera, and one in the midline below it for various instruments. Also insert two 5-mm trocars in the left and right midclavicular line at the level of the anterior superior spine for the dissecting instruments. Identify the obliterated hypogastric artery. Open the peritoneum over the iliac vessels and identify the ureter in the peritoneal cavity. Insert a 30-degree lens into the port on the ipsilateral side of the reimplant in the midclavicular line at the level of the umbilicus, to become the camera port. Place the second trocar on the contralateral side at the midclavicular line, 2 cm below the umbilicus. In an older child with a larger pelvis, place the contralateral working port slightly lower than the umbilicus on the midclavicular line to increase the working angle.

Open the peritoneum over the ureter and bladder below the iliac vessels and locate the ureter. To identify the correct angle for the new ureteral tunnel, fill and empty the bladder. This is important to prevent angulation and distal obstruction. Note that as the bladder fills, it expands radially out over the ureter. With the electrocautery, mark the site on the bladder wall that makes contact with the ureter lying in its normal position in the retroperitoneum with the bladder full. This will be the site of ureteral entry. Fix the bladder to the abdominal wall using a through-and-through abdominal wall stitch on a Keith needle. This elevates the posterior wall of the bladder and provides a stiff backboard to help incision of the detrusor muscle during dissection of the tunnel as it exposes the ureter behind it with its entry into the trigone. You can now visualize and orient the future tunnel.

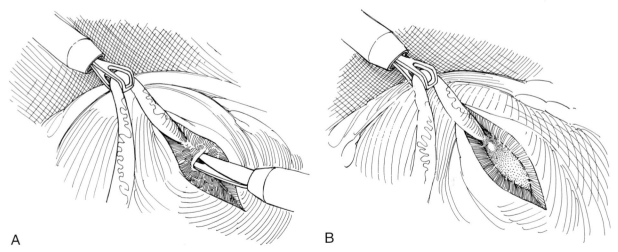

A   B

FIGURE 43-1. **A** and **B,** Incise the detrusor muscle for about 3 cm, extending from the electrocautery mark to the medial and lateral surfaces of the ureter. Be careful not to veer laterally along the bladder but stay perpendicular to ensure the correct location of the tunnel and good detrusor muscle for the closure. Complete the trough with scissors and blunt dissection to expose the vesical mucosa. Do not free the ureter circumferentially but leave it attached for 90 degrees at the 6-o'clock position; this will hold the ureter to the trigone and ensure good fixation of the ureter to the bladder, and also prevent later shortening of the tunnel should the ureter migrate.

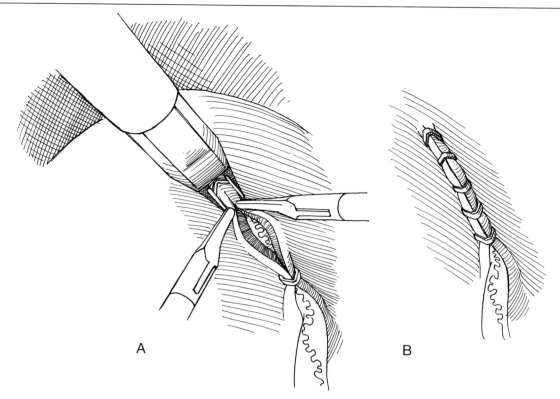

FIGURE 43-2. A, Free the ureter from its retroperitoneal attachments to elevate it into the tunnel. Grasp the ureter with 5-mm Babcock-type forceps or use an Endoloop to elevate the ureter to put tension on the periureteral tissue and allow blunt dissection of the terminal 2 or 3 cm. **B,** Close the detrusor muscle over the ureter medial to lateral with interrupted absorbable sutures. Moving the ureter in and out of the tunnel facilitates insertion of the sutures. Alternatively, use the hernia stapler to place a staple through the edges of the distal end of the incision in the detrusor muscle to contain the ureter, and then staple the rest of the incision closed.

Release the traction stitch to allow the bladder and ureter to fall back into the pelvis. The suture line should lie flat in the pelvis under the bladder. Evacuate the pneumoperitoneum and close the trocar ports.

CRAIG PETERS

Commentary by

The ultimate utility of laparoscopic antireflux surgery remains to be determined, but the techniques should be developed and assessed. Currently, robotic assistance has made this technically demanding procedure much more efficient and the methods are similar to that described. The important elements of the procedure include port positioning, ureteral exposure, tunnel creation, and tunnel closure.

Port position can include the camera port in the umbilicus rather than above, as this is more cosmetically pleasing. The working ports are both lateral and adjusted for size; smaller patients require ports above the umbilicus. The need for a fourth port is relative. It is not used in our practice with the robot, but can be useful for exposure. The hitch stitch for the bladder wall is important.

Exposure of the ureter is different for boys and girls. In the boy, the crossing vas must be swept superiorly with a transverse incision in the peritoneum at the posterior reflection onto the bladder, just near the vas. In the girl, the peritoneal incision is made anterior to the uterus and uterine ligaments. The ureter is then found inferiorly, just above its hiatus. It is cleared for about 4 cm. Care must be taken to avoid devascularizing the ureter in efforts to mobilize it.

Creating the detrusor tunnel is challenging and requires accurate orientation as described, and assessing how full the bladder is, as this will determine the functional tunnel length. The tunnel should not be too long, as it may kink the ureter. The bladder should be partially filled to judge tunnel orientation and length of about 3 cm. Lateral flaps of detrusor muscle should be mobilized to provide for space for the ureter in the tunnel. If the mucosa is violated, it is closed with a single figure-of-eight chromic suture (5-0 or 6-0).

The tunnel is then closed with interrupted absorbable sutures. It seems to be more efficient to do this from the top down (proximal to distal), as this approach holds the ureter in the tunnel while the sutures are placed.

It remains uncertain precisely why bilateral extravesical ureteroplasty for reflux causes urinary retention, but it clearly does and this can occur with laparoscopic methods as well, despite some limited optimistic reports. Nerve-sparing techniques have been discussed, but few details as to how the nerves are actually identified and spared are available. We use this technique bilaterally in a limited number of patients with careful preoperative teaching.

We close the peritoneal defect after completion and if the mucosa has been maintained intact, we do not leave a bladder catheter in unilateral cases.

Commentary by
STEVEN DOCIMO

The biggest controversy regarding this operation is whether there is a morbidity advantage over a similar operation via a Pfannenstiel or inguinal incision. The cosmetic outcome is not better, as the scars are above the bikini line, and there is nothing to suggest that the outcome is better than other procedures. This technique represented a breakthrough at the time of its original description, and the technique described is elegant. Its use has been supplanted for most by minimal incision open techniques, transvesical endoscopic techniques, and subtrigonal injection.

Chapter 44

External Tunnel Method

The external tunnel method is especially suitable for kidney transplantation. The technique may also be applied to the correction of megaureters.

Arrange a Y-connector setup with closed sterile drainage so that the bladder can be filled and drained during the procedure. Alternately, prep the urethra into the field and position the patient slightly frog-legged so a catheter (hence bladder volume) can be manipulated intraoperatively. Fill the bladder fairly full, and clamp the urethral catheter that is connected to closed sterile drainage. Place a stay suture in the bladder wall, and roll the bladder medially. Expose the ureter through a Pfannenstiel incision. (An extended inguinal incision is an alternative, passing through the posterior wall of the inguinal canal above the inferior epigastric vessels.)

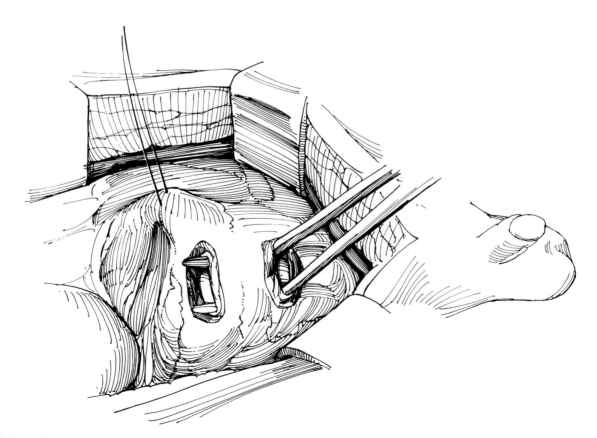

FIGURE 44-1. Make an incision 2 cm long with the scalpel through the adventitia and muscle down to the subepithelium. Make a second incision 3 cm distant. With a curved clamp, develop a tunnel between the incisions; spread the clamp to make the tunnel 2 cm wide.

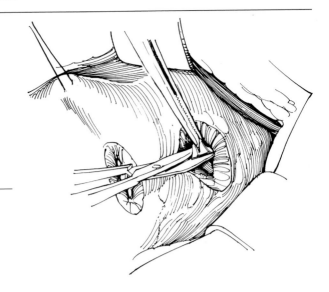

FIGURE 44-2. Grasp the epithelium through the distal incision with vascular forceps. Drain the bladder. If a small tear is made inappropriately in the mucosa, lift it with fine forceps and ligate it with a fine synthetic absorbable suture. Close large tears with a running suture. Excise a button of epithelium with Lahey scissors.

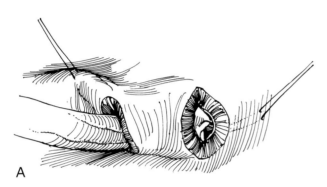
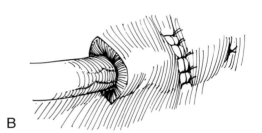

A   B

FIGURE 44-3. **A** and **B,** Draw the ureter through the tunnel and trim it to fit. Suture it to the opening in the bladder with three 4-0 synthetic absorbable sutures. Place one or two additional interrupted sutures between them. Draw the ureteral tip further into the bladder by placing a suture through the full thickness of the tip of the ureter, thread both ends on curved needles, and pass them successively from the bladder lumen out through the bladder wall 1 to 2 cm distal to the exit site of the ureter. Tie the two ends together. Close the distal bladder opening with 4-0 synthetic absorbable sutures to all layers but the epithelium. Stents and drains are not needed. Leave a balloon catheter in place for 5 days.

Intraoperative complications include perforation of the bladder mucosa while forming the tunnel. Close it with fine sutures and proceed. If the disruption is too great, make a new tunnel. Postoperatively, stenosis may occur at the ureterovesical junction and require a repeat operation. Reflux may be managed with subureteral injections (see Chapter 46). Paraureteral diverticula may be ignored.

JOHN M. BARRY

Commentary by

The unstented, parallel-incision, extravesical ureteroneocystostomy has been the standard technique for urinary tract reconstruction following kidney transplantation for 25 years in our kidney transplant program. Placement of a double-pigtail ureteral stent has been up to the transplanting surgeon. We use a suction drain in all renal transplant operations in children. It is always easier to remove a drain later than to wish you had placed one at the time of surgery. The short-term reoperation rate has remained under 2%, and the reflux rate has been less than 1%. The technique has also been used in nontransplant patients, including those who required a psoas hitch procedure.

Chapter 45

Revision Transplant Ureter

Reflux into a transplant ureter places the patient at risk for pyleonephritis and damage to the renal graft. Patients with a febrile urinary tract infection after transplantation should be evaluated with a voiding cystourethrogram. Those with lower tract dysfunction secondary to neurogenic causes such as meningomyelocele, obstruction due to posterior urethral valves, or complex ureterocele anomalies are at an increased risk for reflux after the initial surgery.

The most common reason for reflux after transplantation is a short tunnel performed using the external tunnel technique (see Chapter 44). Most patients with reflux into their transplanted kidney will never have symptoms or untoward graft consequences. Patients who are symptomatic may have the reimplant revised with attention to normalizing bladder function in patients at risk.

Preoperatively, culture the urine and give appropriate antibiotics. Urodynamic studies and appropriate bladder rehabilitation should be addressed for patients with abnormal bladder function.

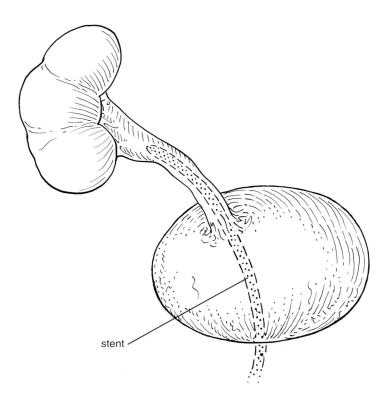

stent

FIGURE 45-1. Identify the transplant ureter orifice endoscopically. The typical location of the orifice is superior at the dome of the bladder on the patient's right side. Care should be taken to eliminate any air in the cystoscopic irrigation, which will impede vision as the air bubbles rise to the dome of the bladder. Pass an external stent into the transplant ureter for subsequent ureteral identification during the open procedure. In young children, size 3 to 4 F is appropriate and in adolescents and teenagers, size 5 F. Secure the stent to a urethral catheter.

249

FIGURE 45-2. Reposition the patient from lithotomy to supine, keeping the urethral catheter and stent sterile and exposed on the surgical field for manipulation of the bladder volume. Re-explore the previous transplant incision in the right lower quadrant using the medial one half of the incision. Identify the bladder and transplant ureter by palpation and direct vision of the stent within the transplant ureter. Pass a vessel loop around the ureter for traction. A right-angle clamp facilitates dissection of the adherent detrusor muscle to the ureter, exposing the underlying urothelium.

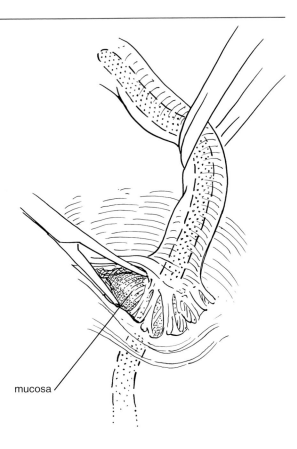

mucosa

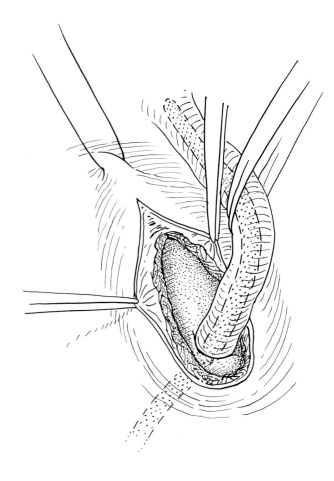

FIGURE 45-3. Working underneath the transplanted ureter, dissect the detrusor muscle off of the submucosa, blue-domed urothelium, creating a tunnel measuring 4 to 6 cm. The ureter is not detached from its previous anastomotic site to the bladder. A holding suture placed superiorly facilitates bladder traction.

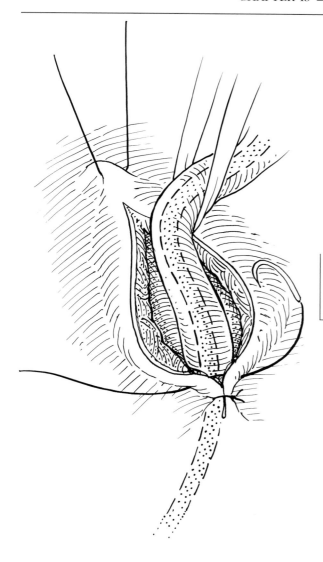

FIGURE 45-4. Place the ureter through the muscular trough in a fashion that avoids kinking or obstruction. Use 3-0 or 4-0 synthetic absorbable sutures to close the muscle layer over the ureter within the new trough.

FIGURE 45-5. Reinforce the transplanted ureter within the new muscular tunnel to prevent future reflux. Leave the externalized stent and urethral catheter for 3 to 5 days postoperatively. Continue the patient on perioperative antibiotics for 24 to 48 hours, followed by daily suppression. Use an epidural catheter for the infusion of narcotics to prevent bladder spasm and control incisional pain. Irrigate the wound, and close the fascia with 2-0 or 3-0 synthetic sutures and the skin with a fine subcuticular absorbable suture.

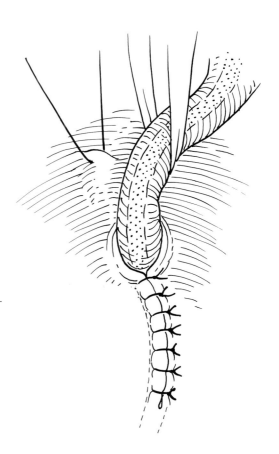

POSTOPERATIVE PROBLEMS

Bladder spasms can be avoided by an epidural catheter in the postoperative period. Transient ureteral obstruction is prevented by the externalized stent, which is removed 3 to 5 days after surgery. In the rare circumstance where the transplanted ureter is placed at the dome of the bladder and the bladder cannot be mobilized to facilitate an extravesical tunnel, the ureter can be detached and reimplanted in a more inferior location. In this case, placement of a double-J stent will facilitate ureteral healing and decrease the chance of anastomotic leak and stricture.

ANAND KRISHNAN

Commentary by

Fortunately, the incidence of symptomatic reflux in a transplant kidney is rare. In the pediatric population, in which lower urinary tract dysfunction is more common, we advocate a nonrefluxing extravesical reimplantation at the time of transplantation to minimize this problem. However, any patient regardless of age demonstrating recurrent pyelonephritis and graft reflux requires repeat reimplantation to maximize graft longevity and minimize the morbidity of recurrent infections and renal biopsies. We have found placement of an externalized ureteral stent to be invaluable in aiding dissection in a predictably scarred surgical field. We prefer to use the same incision employed for the initial transplantation. An extravesical reimplantation with a formal detrusorrhaphy is efficacious, avoids manipulation of the original ureteroneocystotomy, and has the advantage of decreased morbidity from opening the bladder. We have not found the need for an advancing stitch to fold the ureter at its attachment to the bladder mucosa. We leave the externalized stent in for 3 days postoperatively and remove it prior to discharge.

Chapter 46

Endoscopic Reflux Correction

Endoscopic ureteric injection may be the first line for correction of reflux to restore the backing at the uretero-vesical junction. It is more successful with lower grades of reflux. The reported success rate is between 70% and 85%.

Preparations available for injection are polytetrafluoro-ethylene (Teflon), polydimethyl siloxane (Macroplastique), dextranomer/hyaluronic acid copolymer (biodegradable Deflux), silicone microimplants, injectable bioglass, detach-able membranes, and bovine collagen. In children, Teflon paste carries some risk from dispersal into the lungs during a lifetime, and silicone may initiate an autoimmune reaction. In contrast, dextranomer/hyaluronic acid copolymer has an advantage in that it is biodegradable. If bovine collagen is used, it should be applied first to the child's forearm to test for sensitivity, looking for an erythematous reaction within a month.

SUBURETERIC INJECTION TECHNIQUE

Place the child in the lithotomy position and prep the genitalia. Use general anesthesia. Preoperatively, confirm sterile urine. Administer intravenous antibiotics perioperatively and obtain a urine culture. Use the smallest endoscope possible to accommodate the endoscopic needle and visualize the ureteral orifice.

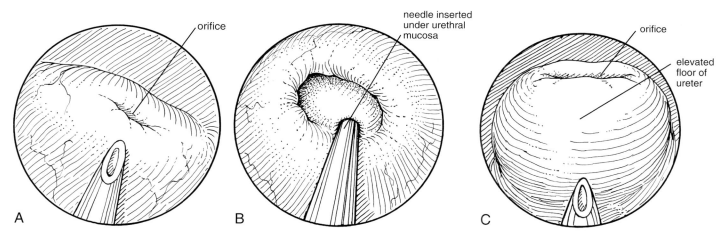

FIGURE 46-1. A, Partially fill the bladder and identify the refluxing ureteral orifice. Place the endoscopic irrigation to maximum, which will typically allow the ureteral orifice to open. **B,** Insert the needle directly into the open ureteral orifice 1 to 2 mm from the opening. Advance the needle under the urethral mucosa for 2 to 4 mm and hold it steady. **C,** Slowly inject the agent while observing the crescentic orifice created by elevation of the floor of the ureter. Use between 0.5 and 1.5 mL of the agent depending on the size of the orifice. Occasionally, one or two subsequent injections may be required, but if a third injection fails, resort to surgical repair. Do not expect added difficulty at operation. If the contralateral orifice does not reflux on voiding cystourethrography, prophylactic injection is not indicated.

ANDREW J. KIRSCH

There are many pearls for the successful endoscopic correction of vesicoureteral reflux (VUR). A significant improvement was first realized with the concept of ureteral hydrodistention and intraluminal submucosal injection, otherwise known as hydrodistention implantation technique (HIT), and further improved with injection of increased volume using two tandem intraluminal injection sites (double HIT). Hydrodistention requires a pressured stream of irrigation fluid into the ureter to define the site of injection within the ureteral submucosa. Ureteral hydrodistention will always cause the ureteral orifice to open pretreatment and should remain closed post-treatment when implantation is performed correctly.

Instrumentation is critically important. An adequately sized pediatric cystoscope with an offset lens permits direct passage of the needle in-line with the ureter without bending the needle. We have avoided the use of smaller-caliber cystoscopes (<9.5 F) that impede adequate flow for hydrodistention.

We have developed an algorithm for needle placement. The first consideration is that the needle be directed in-line with the ureteral tunnel. With hydrodistention, the needle should impinge the floor of the midureteral tunnel at the 6-o'clock position to a depth of approximately 2 to 4 mm within the submucosa. Positioning and gauging the depth of the needle is facilitated by placing the beak of the cystoscope flush with the ureteral orifice during hydrodistention. Once the needle is in place, the flow of irrigation fluid should be stopped and a small volume (<0.1 mL) is injected to confirm implant location.

The first injection site (proximal HIT) should lead to coaptation of the proximal ureteric tunnel, converting all hydrodistending ureters to minimal or no hydrodistention. By placing the needle in the submucosal plane, tracking of material cephalad within the ureteral submucosa occurs. This is the most critical aspect of implantation as the length of ureteral coaptation is maximized. The distal HIT (second injection site) is performed by placing the needle to the same depth just within the ureteral orifice and injecting slowly (while pulling the needle more superficially) until the ureteral orifice is coapted and elevated to the height of the ureteral tunnel (treated with the proximal HIT). The distal HIT should result in the complete absence of hydrodistention. The end result is a mountain-range appearance of the tunnel and orifice. If the ureteral orifice does not completely coapt with intraureteric injection, a classic subureteric Teflon injection (STING) is conducted. After each injection an attempt at ureteral hydrodistention will ensure proper technique as the ureter will remain coapted with irrigation. At least 0.8 mL of material per ureter may be needed, depending on the physical characteristics of the ureteral orifice. Anticipate 20% volume loss within 2 weeks.

Our current success after one treatment for up to grade 5 VUR is 90% of patients and 93% of ureters, rivaling open surgical repair. Successful injection has also been achieved for duplex ureters, those associated with paraureteral diverticula, after failed open or endoscopic surgery, and in patients with bladder dysfunction or deficit.

MING HSEIN WANG

VUR is a complex disease process that involves a wide spectrum of clinical presentations and outcomes. Over the years, it has been observed that there are children with reflux and urinary tract infection who do well and those who do poorly with and without intensive radiographic follow-up and treatments, prolonged prophylactic antibiotics or surgical interventions. This challenges the conventional thinking that all children with urinary tract infection and reflux must be treated medically or surgically; by the same token, it is difficult to predict which child is at risk for significant renal damage. Therefore, there is a constant search for more predictive imaging techniques and less-invasive treatment options.

Current treatments include traditional, open intravesical and extravesical ureteral reimplantation, which offers close to 100% cure rate. Both avoid the need for chronic antibiotic prophylaxis; however, patients are subjected to an open abdominal procedure, hospital stay, and time away from school. The advent of endoscopic therapy with injection of bulking agent in an attempt to reconfigure the flap-valve mechanism at the ureterovesical junction has gained popularity because the procedure is done quickly, and children are able to return to full activity the next day.

STING was first performed by Matouschek in 1981, who described the injection of polytetrafluoroethylene (PTFE) paste at the ureteral orifice to correct VUR. O'Donnell and Puri popularized the procedure with their result of 75% success rate after a single injection in 103 ureters with primary reflux. However, the use of Teflon was not approved by the FDA, due to reports of particle migration outside the genitourinary system. Since then, different injectable materials have been tried, including bovine collagen, polydimethylsiloxane (a synthetic, silicone-bulking agent), calcium hydroxyapatite (a synthetic bone material), and various autologous materials such as fat, collagen, muscle, and chondrocytes. Autologous materials share the major disadvantage of significant volume loss over time. Dextranomer/hyaluronic copolymer (Deflux) is a natural material that was recently introduced and approved by the FDA. It consists of dextranomer microspheres suspended in sodium hyaluronate solution. Over time, the dextranomer microspheres are encapsulated by fibroblasts and the injected volume is stabilized.

Recently, a committee of nine pediatric urologists published the result of a meta-analysis of 63 articles focused on endoscopic therapy for VUR. They found a resolution rate of 79% for grades I and II reflux, 72% for grade III reflux, and 65% for grade IV reflux following one injection of a bulking agent. Following one or more injections, the success rate was 85%. Notably, the Atlanta group modified the original STING technique, injecting directly into the lumen of the ureteral orifice, and reports a success rate approaching results for open reimplantation, with 100% for grade I and 90% for grade IV reflux.

At this juncture, the long-term incidence of recurrent VUR following endoscopic injection is difficult to ascertain, because most parents do not want to subject their child to repeat voiding cystourethrograms beyond the first one or two negative imaging studies. Perhaps in the absence of urinary tract infections, the significance of documenting VUR is not clinically significant.

Chapter 47

Ureteroneocystostomy with Tailoring

Megaureters may be refluxing or obstructive and can result from either primary or secondary causes. Ultrasound, intravenous urogram, and isotope renal scans all show a dilated ureter with a distal funnel shape. A voiding cystourethrogram in primary obstructed megaureter is normal.

If bilateral megaureter repair and reimplantation is required into a bladder with a small capacity, reimplantation of the better ureter combined with transureteroureterostomy may be advisable (see Chapter 52), especially because the excessive dissection required may result in voiding difficulties.

INDICATIONS FOR SURGERY

Although conservative treatment is usually appropriate, intervene if the narrow distal segment is causing significant obstruction evidenced by recurrent infection, pain, calculi, progression of hydronephrosis, hypertension, or persistent hematuria. Taper, excise, and reimplant the ureter.

Perinatally diagnosed cases should be followed with ultrasound and renal scans; those at risk will have a pelvic diameter greater than 10 mm.

SURGICAL OBJECTIVES

First, reduce the caliber of the distal ureter to improve emptying and prevent reflux. Next, protect its blood supply, and last, ensure smooth passage of the ureter, without angulation, through a hiatus into the bladder. (Use of the original hiatus reduces the chance for angulation.) If both ureters are involved and the bladder has a reduced capacity from a severely damaged wall, consider reimplanting the better ureter in combination with transureteroureterostomy, especially because of the voiding difficulties that may result from the extensive retrovesical dissection required for bilateral implantation. If reoperation becomes necessary, consider using a long tunnel reimplantation with a psoas hitch for one ureter, and then performing ureteroureterostomy for the other.

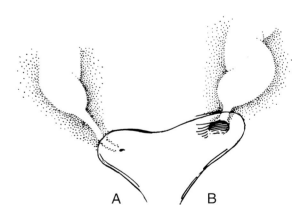 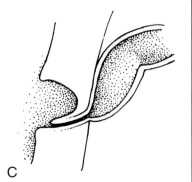

FIGURE 47-1. Identify the type of megaureter: **A,** Obstructive megaureter. **B,** Refluxing megaureter. **C,** Para-ureteral diverticulum with megaureter, a condition usually associated with massive reflux. With obstructive megaureter, the hypertrophied helically oriented muscular coats become circular at the site of the obstruction, proximal to the longitudinal bundles of the intramural segment.

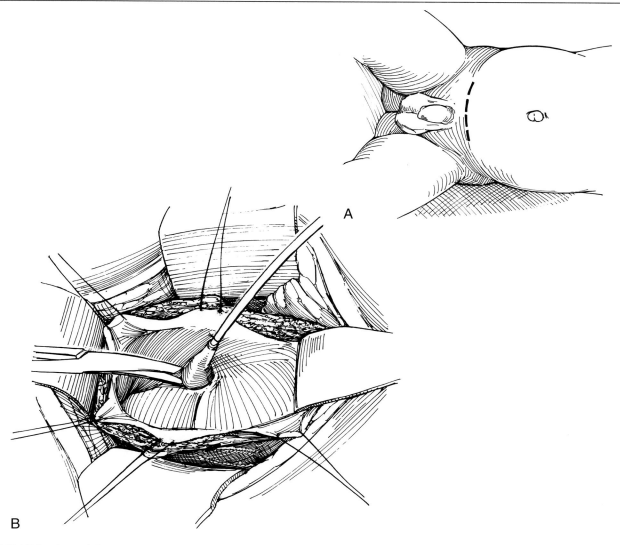

B

FIGURE 47-2. A, Incision: Lower transverse, unless there is great tortuosity requiring narrowing of the entire ureter.
B, Insert a ring retractor and open the bladder longitudinally, holding its edges with stay sutures. Insert a catheter into the affected ureter and suture it to the trigonal muscle. Dissect as much ureter as possible intravesically, as described for ureteroneocystostomy (see Chapter 36).

FIGURE 47-3. For very dilated, tortuous ureters, dissect extravesically to develop a straight length of ureter free of kinks: From outside the bladder, dissect along the hypogastric vein until the ligament representing the obliterated hypogastric artery is reached. (This route causes the least damage to the vesical nerve supply.) Divide the obliterated artery. The ureter is exposed without any further sharp dissection, because the peritoneum swings off it. Pull the ureter out of the bladder and rotate it into the paravesical field. Reclamp the catheter for traction. Cautiously free the ureter from the adjacent peritoneum, saving all the periureteral tissue by sweeping the peritoneal attachments toward the ureter, thus skeletonizing the peritoneum, not the ureter. This mobilization seldom needs to extend higher than the common iliac vessels, unless the ureter is very tortuous and so must be considerably shortened, as with prune-belly syndrome.

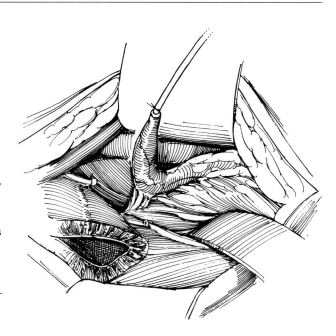

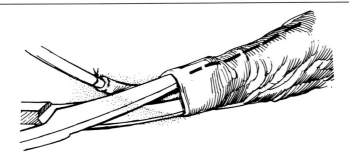

FIGURE 47-4. Dissect beneath the periureteral sheath on the lateral aspect of the ureter to allow insertion of Lahey scissors; then open the sheath, also on the lateral aspect, to expose the segment of ureter to be narrowed. Turn the sheath back, preserving the contained collateral vessels.

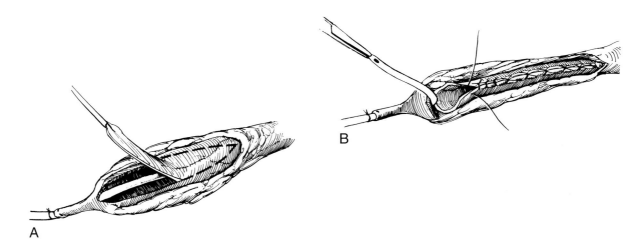

B

A

FIGURE 47-5. A, Incise the lateral aspect of the adventitia for a distance slightly longer than the length of the proposed tunnel. Preserve the periureteral tissue with its vessels. Dissect the adventitia back from approximately half the circumference of the ureter. Distend the ureter with saline, and mark the portion to be excised with a marking pen. Usually make the strip for excision approximately one third of the ureteral circumference, because some of the remaining wall will be used up in the closure. Excise the longitudinal strip of excess ureteral wall freehand with Potts scissors. Excising too much jeopardizes the blood supply and predisposes the ureter to stenosis. Leave the terminal segment as a handle. **B,** Close the proximal two-thirds to form a tapered portion of the ureter with a running locking everting stitch of 5-0 synthetic absorbable suture. Complete the closure of the distal third with interrupted sutures of the same material because the length needed is uncertain at this stage. Take care not to constrict the lumen. Check the suture line by filling the ureter with saline injection.

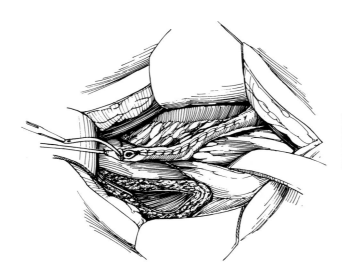

FIGURE 47-6. Close the preserved flaps of periureteral tissue that were previously around the ureter with a loose running 4-0 or 5-0 synthetic absorbable suture.

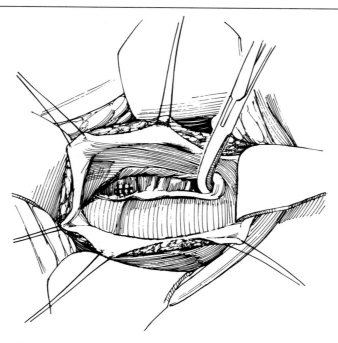

FIGURE 47-7. Return intravesically and close the original hiatus with several 4-0 or 5-0 synthetic absorbable sutures. One method of creating an intravesical tunnel is to incise the mucosa on the back wall of the bladder with a knife 1 to 2 cm distal and 3 to 4 cm proximal to the orifice to prepare a long bed in which to lay the tapered ureter. Fold back the flaps of vesical mucosa. Make a new hiatus through the muscle from inside the bladder at the proximal end of the incision, making sure that it is large enough. It is essential that the new hiatus be in the *back* wall of the bladder; if it is misplaced on the sidewall, bladder filling will angulate and obstruct the ureter. Alternatively, a tunnel can be created by dissecting submucosally, as in a standard reimplantation.

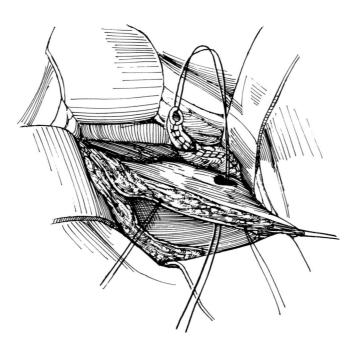

FIGURE 47-8. Draw the ureter through the new hiatus. The taper will end only a few centimeters above it, approximately at the level of the common iliac vessels. Be sure the suture line lies posteriorly when the ureter is placed in its bed. This will reduce the incidence for a fistula.

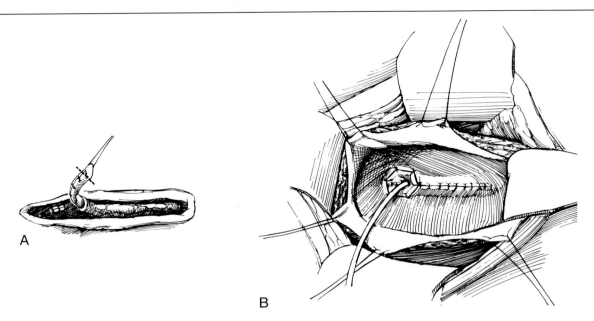

FIGURE 47-9. A, Cut the end of the ureter to an appropriate length, long enough to reach the site of the original hiatus. Place two stitches of 4-0 or 5-0 synthetic absorbable sutures through the end of the ureter, and then into the bladder wall at the end of the tunnel to include muscle and mucosa. This anchors the ureter in place with the sutured side down. **B,** Complete a mucosa-to-mucosa anastomosis of the tip. If using the open tunnel technique, close the mucosal flaps with interrupted fine stitches of 5-0 synthetic absorbable sutures. The ureter may also be implanted by the transtrigonal technique (see Chapter 39). Insert a fenestrated 5-F plastic catheter to the renal pelvis (it should pass freely) and lead it out through stab wounds. Drain the bladder with a urethral balloon catheter.

In cases in which the bladder is small relative to the size of the ureter, and especially in reoperative cases, perform a psoas hitch (see Chapter 58). Close the bladder in two layers and provide a Penrose drain to the area. Leave the stent in place for 14 days. Remove the catheter 1 day after the stent.

It is important that (1) the tunnel be long enough (five times the diameter of the revised ureter), (2) the new bed lie along the posterior wall of the bladder, (3) the hiatus not be situated laterally, (4) the tapering not extend higher than the level of the iliac vessels, (5) the new suture line lie posteriorly, and (6) the ureter not be angulated as the psoas hitch is made.

For duplex systems, mobilize the ureters in their common sheath, while preserving as much adventitia as possible. If the ureters end in a common stem, excise the obstructive segment, taper both ureters along their lateral aspects as described previously, and reimplant the two ureters together. If only one ureter is grossly dilated, excise its wall to tailor it and reimplant the two ureters. Alternatives include ureteroureterostomy with implantation of a single tapered ureter.

ALTERNATIVE TECHNIQUE: URETERAL WALL EXCISION

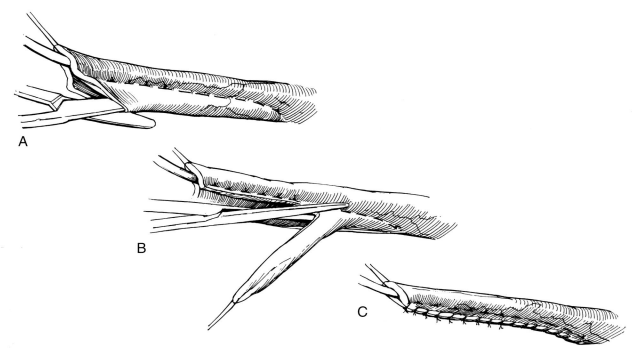

FIGURE 47-10. A, Pull the stented ureter into the bladder through the hiatus. Run a horizontal mattress stitch of 3-0 synthetic absorbable suture lateral to the stent, placing interrupted sutures distally. Cut the resulting free lumen longitudinally. **B,** Trim the edges to excise redundant ureteral wall. **C,** Run a second row of 3-0 synthetic absorbable sutures to approximate the raw edges. Proceed with implantation. Consider a psoas hitch for better support of the tunnel.

ALTERNATIVE IMPLANTATION TECHNIQUE

An extravesical implantation by a modification of the Lich-Gregoir technique (see Chapter 41) may be faster than a combined intravesical-extravesical method and may be as effective.

Through a Pfannenstiel incision, rotate the bladder to expose the ureter extravesically. Place a vessel loop around it to elevate it and allow dissection to its junction with the bladder. Preserve as much of the periureteral vasculature as possible, but free the terminal portion of its perivesical and muscular attachments. Distend the bladder moderately. Make limited incisions through the detrusor muscle, one proximal and one distal to the attachment of the ureter. Take care not to denervate the detrusor muscle. Starting laterally, elevate the muscle, including the fibers of Waldeyer's sheath, from the mucosa to form detrusor flaps. Expose the surrounding bladder submucosa in a 5-cm arc around the orifice, taking care not to perforate it. (If the bladder mucosa is breached, empty the bladder and close the defect with a fine figure-eight suture before proceeding.) Place traction sutures in the detrusor edges to aid in the dissection. The degree of pouching of the epithelium may be regulated by filling and emptying the bladder.

Select 4-0 synthetic absorbable sutures. Place the suture first through the muscle of the bladder wall at the lower edge of the opening from outside in, to exit at the edge of the mucosa-muscularis dissection, and then pass it through the ureteral muscle at the former ureterovesical junction at the 5-o'clock position. Finally, pass it distally to exit inside out near the point of entry. (This is a vertical mattress suture that forms a vest-over-pants stitch.) Place a second suture in the same way at the 7-o'clock position on the ureter.

POSTOPERATIVE MANAGEMENT

Continue low-dose antibacterial suppression for 3 months. At that time (in the absence of flank pain or sustained fever that would warrant earlier studies), obtain a voiding cysto-urethrogram or nuclear cystogram and renal bladder ultrasound. If the obstruction/reflux is cured, antibiotics may be discontinued.

POSTOPERATIVE PROBLEMS

Bladder spasms are common in infants and children, who tolerate urethral catheters poorly. Use epidural continuous infusion of bupivacaine to greatly reduce the problem. Oral diazepam and oxybutynin are also useful. Ketorolac tromethamine has proven to be an especially effective anesthetic.

Complications after tailoring procedures are more common than after simple ureteroneocystostomy but are of a similar nature. Obstruction results from angulation or from ureteral stricture. Reflux is secondary to providing too short a tunnel. Implantation in the presence of abnormal bladder function has a higher rate of failure.

Obtain an ultrasound scan 4 to 6 weeks postoperatively to assess obstruction and obtain a radionuclide cystogram to check for persistent reflux. Do not hurry to reoperate, because it may take as long as 2 years for high-grade reflux to resolve after implantation. In addition, these patients often have decreased renal function with high urine output, placing an added load on the ureterovesical transport mechanism.

Provide adjunctive measures postoperatively, such as intermittent catheterization if the bladder empties poorly or anticholinergic medication if there is poor compliance. Careful follow-up for at least 5 years to detect silent malfunction is mandatory.

W. HARDY HENDREN

Commentary by

Megaureter is not a diagnosis, but a descriptive term for a ureter that is wide and sometimes very tortuous. Megaureters can be obstructive or refluxing. In primary obstructive megaureter, the ureteral orifice looks normal endoscopically. There is a terminal segment 1 to 3 cm long that contains excess fibrous tissue and lacks muscle. Biopsy of the dilated ureter above that segment shows muscle hypertrophy. The kidney in obstructive megaureter is often better preserved than in refluxing megaureter. In megaureter secondary to massive reflux, the ureteral orifice is usually dilated and often laterally placed. In some there is a paraureteral diverticulum just above the orifice. Frequently the kidney is badly damaged in a case with massive reflux, from a combination of back pressure from the bladder during voiding and infection. A few megaureters can paradoxically have both obstruction and reflux, when the ureter ends ectopically in the bladder neck or urethra. In the resting state, the ureter is obstructed, but during micturition it can show reflux.

Not all wide ureters need to be corrected surgically. For example, in boys, endoscopic ablation of urethral valves can reduce intravesical pressures, allowing secondary megaureter to then improve spontaneously. Similarly, megaureters in association with myelodysplasia can resolve when the bladder is emptied by intermittent catheterization.

When a large ureter must be corrected surgically, dissecting the ureter free from the bladder, and then shortening, tapering, and reimplanting it to provide normal drainage without reflux are involved. The tunnel length should be about five times the diameter of the ureter to be reimplanted, just as in ordinary ureteral reimplantation. Thus, tapering the terminal ureter makes it feasible to reimplant a dilated ureter and achieve a satisfactory ratio of tunnel length to ureter diameter. Ureteral peristalsis cannot be effective when the ureter is dilated, because the walls do not coapt. Tapering the lower ureter to improve peristaltic efficiency allows the ureter to empty actively. This effect results in improvement in dilatation of the upper tract.

When the ureter is not tortuous, the operative approach can be through a transverse lower abdominal incision (see Chapter 63). This approach affords adequate exposure of the lower pelvis, as would be customary for a usual ureteral reimplantation. However, when there is great ureteral tortuosity, as is often present in prune-belly syndrome, dissection higher into the gutters may be necessary to shorten excessive length of the ureter. Here it is better to use a vertical transabdominal approach to provide greater operative exposure. The Denis Browne ring retractor is very useful in this case. By sewing a catheter into its orifice, the ureter is mobilized intravesically. The ureter is freed using that approach, as long as it proceeds easily. Then exposure is shifted paravesically to continue its mobilization upward. To locate the ureter with minimal paravesical dissection, which can cause nerve damage to the bladder, dissect along the hypogastric vein to the obliterated umbilical artery-ligament. It is divided. This allows retracting the peritoneum cephalad. The ureter lies immediately beneath the ligament. Mobilizing the ureter and bringing it upward into the paravesical field are facilitated by dissecting along the anterior wall of the ureter from below, penetrating the paravesical tissue at the level of the ligament, and then pulling the ureter through to that point. When dividing the attachments of the ureter during its mobilization, it is important that they be divided as far as feasible from the ureter. This retains as much as possible of the attached periureteral tissue for collateral blood supply. Unless the ureter is extremely elongated and tortuous, we generally mobilize it only as far as the point where it crosses the common iliac vessels.

Tapering the ureter is performed on its lateral aspect, because the main collateral blood supply is along its medial wall. Further, when the suture line for tapering is closed, it should be placed posteriorly next to the detrusor muscle when the ureter is reimplanted into the bladder. This reduces the likelihood of a fistula forming into the bladder. We formerly employed special ureteral clamps, but in recent years we have generally not used them. The ureter is distended via the catheter used in its mobilization. A ligature around the tip of the ureter retains the saline within it. The periureteral sheath is opened by dissecting carefully between the sheath and the wall of the ureter on its posterolateral aspect. The sheath is incised and laid back about half the circumference of the ureter to expose the segment to be removed; this area is identified with a skin-marking pencil. Using sharp, straight scissors, the strip of ureter is removed; it must not be too wide. Trimming the ureter excessively will result in its being made too narrow, which will jeopardize its blood supply. Some added width will be taken up in the closure, which is done with a running, locking suture to avoid reefing the closure. The ureter is filled again with saline to make certain that it is watertight. The periureteral tissue is then closed over the ureteral suture line.

It is important that the new hiatus through which the ureter will be brought be in the back wall of the bladder. It is a common error to bring the ureter through the sidewall, which will cause it to be angulated when the bladder fills. After closing the original ureteral hiatus, a bed is prepared for the ureter. This bed starts at the new hiatus, which is more cranial and more medial than the original hiatus. The bed extends downward to just above the bladder neck. Instead of making a submucosal tunnel, which is often used in ordinary ureteral reimplantation surgery, it is easier to lay back mucosal flaps before implanting the ureter. The ureter is brought through the new hiatus, taking care that there is no angulation or tension. It is laid in the bed prepared for it, with the ureteral suture line posteriorly against the bladder muscle. The ureter is trimmed to appropriate length. The two most distal sutures are placed in bladder mucosa and muscle to the 6-o'clock position of the ureter; this anchors it firmly. Remaining sutures close the mucosa of the bladder to the open end of the ureter and mucosa-to-mucosa closure covers the ureter. A small plastic drainage catheter is passed up the ureter to the kidney for 8 to 10 days while the repair heals. Contrast medium is injected before removing the catheter to make certain that there is no extravasation. After bilateral megaureter repair, catheters are removed on successive days, not simultaneously. Lower megaureter repair, when done as described, should have a complication rate almost as favorable as reimplantation of nondilated ureters, that is, less than 5%.

In some highly abnormal bladders, as in boys with urethral valves or the prune-belly syndrome, or in patients with multiple previous operations, it may be impossible to get two good ureteral reimplants into the bladder. In many such instances we have found it best to reimplant the better ureter, together with psoas hitch fixation of the bladder, with transureteroureterostomy of the contralateral ureter.

In the majority of cases, successful repair of the lower ureter will result in straightening of tortuosity of the upper ureter and gradual reduction in its caliber. There are, however, some cases in which the upper ureter needs to be repaired. This is technically easier than repair of the lower ureter. The kinked ureteropelvic junction is straightened between the upper ureter, after it is shortened, and the renal pelvis. This may be all that is required. If the upper ureter is also quite dilated, it can be trimmed in the same fashion as the lower ureter. A temporary nephrostomy is placed when the upper tract is dilated. Contrast medium is injected through the nephrostomy tube a week later to be certain that there is free passage to the bladder and no extravasation. The tube is removed.

Kalicinski (see Chapter 48) has described an infolding technique to narrow the functional lumen of the lower ureter, as illustrated. This technique was developed to lessen the risk of devascularizing the ureter while trimming it. This infolding has also been successfully used by other surgeons. It should be stated, however, that the likelihood of devascularizing the ureter by trimming should be minimal, if it is performed in the manner we have described. In more than 350 megaureter repairs in the past 28 years, ureteral fibrosis from devascularization was rarely a problem. Somehow it seems more appealing to place a trimmed ureter into a tunnel, rather than one with excessive bulk. Infolding the dilated ureter in experimental animals has been shown to result in spontaneous disappearance of the infolded segment in some cases, presumably from its devascularization from being infolded. Thus, it may be that both methods achieve a similar end after healing is completed. Like many problems in surgery, there is often more than one way to get the desired end result.

SAVA PEROVIC

Commentary by

Surgical management of megaureters is one of the most difficult problems in urologic surgery, particularly in neonates and infants. Several surgical techniques are proposed, consisting of an intravesical approach or a combined intravesical-extravesical approach. The most popular is ureteroneocystostomy with tailoring of ureters, especially when they are very wide.

During the last 20 years, we developed the detrusor-tunneling, extravesical ureteroneocystostomy technique, which we use in all cases, even for the treatment of very wide ureters. It is characterized by minimal surgical trauma and maximal preservation of all anatomic structures. A long, wide submucosal tunnel without detrusor muscle resection is created extravesically, and a markedly dilated ureter can be inserted into it without any remodeling. It is noteworthy to mention that this technique allows spontaneous ureteral accommodation, primarily because the unresected detrusor muscle makes ureteral remodeling unnecessary. Maximal shortening and straightening of the angulations of wide ureters is much more important

Continued

than reduction of ureteral lumen. The benefits of these maneuvers are a shorter route and good urinary flow because even in cases with poor ureteral peristalsis, urine drainage is achieved by hydrostatic urine pressure (i.e., gravitation). It must be noted that angulations of the upper part of the ureter are not obstructive by themselves; any remaining after surgery straighten spontaneously with patient growth. If secondary kinking of the ureteropelvic junction causes obstruction, pyeloplasty is necessary.

A satisfactory antireflux mechanism mainly depends on the relationship between the submucosal tunnel and intravesical pressure. In this technique the ratio between length of submucosal tunnel and ureteral diameter should be 3:1, but in general, a longer tunnel can be made to achieve a successful outcome. The position of the ureter on the lateral bladder wall ensures that all future endoscopic procedures can be performed with ease.

This technique is especially applicable in neonates and infants whose bladder is small and vulnerable; in such cases formation of a sufficiently large submucosal tunnel intravesically is difficult and sometimes impossible, even after ureteral remodeling. Also, the technique can be successfully used in cases with a hypertrophic detrusor muscle, in which an intravesical or a combined intravesical-extravesical approach is difficult to perform.

For successful performance of our detrusor-tunneling extravesical ureteroneocystostomy, it is important to point out some tips and tricks of this technique. The approach is through the extended inguinal oblique incision—the external aponeurosis is incised, while the external ring remains intact. The retroperitoneum is approached through the posterior wall of the inguinal canal above the inferior epigastric vessels, which remain unresected. The internal oblique and transverse muscles are incised longitudinally, except in neonates and infants in whom it is not necessary. The umbilical cord is resected and ligated only if it produces obstruction of the ureteral route. The bladder is mobilized to gain sufficient length of the submucosal tunnel and proper ureteral direction.

Formation of the detrusor tunnel starts with splitting of the detrusor muscle of the semifilled bladder on its lateral wall at two different points, up to the mucosa; their distance is determined by the predicted length of the submucosal tunnel. Bulging mucosa is gently retracted by two pairs of atraumatic forceps to achieve its straightening. At this point the bladder is emptied to minimize danger of mucosal rupture during tunnel creation. If a long tunnel is required, formation of 3 to 4 detrusor holes lessens the risk of mucosal damage. In cases where the detrusor muscle is excessively weak and trabeculated, resection of this muscle over the submucosal tunnel with wide mobilization of both edges is recommended to avoid risk of muscle perforation. In cases of a double-wide ureteral system, two separated submucosal tunnels can be created. If a long tunnel is required and the ureter is short, an additional psoas hitch technique is applied.

The ureter, which passes through the submucosal tunnel, is fixed to the neohiatus first. The submucosal tunnel is lengthened for 2 to 3 cm below the distal hole, and the anastomosis is made between the ureter and bladder mucosa with ureteral stenting. The distal part of the ureter is pulled further distally and fixed to the detrusor muscle over the anastomotic side using U sutures that prevent shortening of the tunnel and also create a valvular antireflux mechanism.

We applied this technique successfully in over 400 megaureters during a 20-year period. The most frequent indication was primary megaureter, particularly obstructive form; the most frequent cause of secondary megaureters was previous failed ureterocystotomy.

Minor surgical trauma due to an undisturbed detrusor muscle with preserved contractility over an implanted ureter and absence of urinary leakage allows short hospitalization. The method is not recommended as a one-stage procedure in bilateral cases, which is the only shortcoming. The choice between conservative and surgical treatment of megaureters presents a special problem, especially in cases in which watchful waiting is applied. However, making a decision for surgical treatment is much easier with this technique because it gives minimal surgical trauma with good long-term results.

Detrusor tunneling ureteroneocystostomy provides good results in the hands of an experienced surgeon and, in our opinion, is one of the best techniques for surgery of megaureters.

Chapter 48

Ureteral Tailoring (Folding) Technique

This technique leaves the intrinsic ureteral blood supply intact, vessels that might be transected during longitudinal excisional tailoring. It also reduces the time for postoperative stenting. However, a bulky mass of ureter does remain to be implanted.

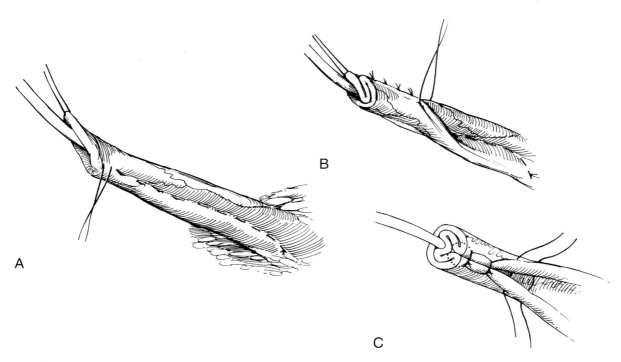

FIGURE 48-1. A, Dissect the ureter intravesically (extravesical dissection may be needed in secondary reimplantation or with very redundant ureters). Dissect the ureteral orifice and pull the ureter into the bladder through the hiatus. Trim the distal obstructing tip. Insert a 10-F infant feeding tube into the ureter, and displace the tube to the medial side with the fingers. Run a 4-0 synthetic absorbable suture down the ureter on the lateral side, away from the catheter, to reduce the effective diameter. Tie it several centimeters from the end. Continue the suturing with interrupted mattress sutures to the tip to permit trimming after placement. **B,** Fold the free margin of the ureter around the stented portion and fasten it with multiple interrupted 4-0 synthetic absorbable sutures. Enlarge the original hiatus. Proceed with implantation through it by a standard technique, avoiding twisting, tension, and constriction in the tunnel. (The transtrigonal technique has merit here; see Chapter 39.) Leave the stent for 14 days. **C,** Alternately, fold the lateral margins of the deflated ureter inward, holding them with imbricating sutures.

STEVE ZDERIC

Commentary by

This approach to ureteral tapering was first described by Kalicinski in 1977 as an alternative to the excisional tapering advocated by Hendren. As shown in the figure, the repair is carried out by removing the obstructing distal segment and then running a reabsorbable suture obliquely down the ureter in such a way as to defunctionalize the excluded ureteral lumen that is then folded over the remaining functional lumen. In addition to the use of the folding method, Kalicinski advocated that tapering be restricted to the distal ureter. His rationale for this approach was that it would result in better preservation of the ureteral blood supply, and thus minimize the chances for ischemia and subsequent stenosis. In an experimental model of this procedure, Whitmore and Ehrlich noted that fibrosis developed in the excluded ureteral remnant, and this resulted in a successful diminution of luminal diameter.

A long-term follow-up by Perdzynski and Kalicinski encompassing all patients operated on between 1978 and 1990 demonstrated a 93% success rate, with two cases of residual reflux and two cases of obstruction that required revision. Similar results have been reported in several other series, though not with this length of follow-up.

As with most surgical procedures, patient selection is essential for success, and in my view, age is a critical consideration. Given that this approach to tapering the ureter still leaves a large and bulky ureter for reimplantation into the bladder, this is a more difficult procedure to perform in the neonate with a distal ureteral obstruction. In such a setting, consideration should be given to performing a cutaneous ureterostomy that can then be taken down. Often in such a setting, a tapering is not even required at the time the ureterostomy is reversed. Such an approach allows time for the bladder to grow in size and to undergo the developmental changes in physiology that take place in the first year of life. It is important to note that in the long-term follow-up paper of Perdzynski and Kalicinski, the age range of the patients varied from 1.5 months to 14 years, but the average patient age at the time of surgery was 4 years. In addition, many of these patients presented with symptoms; 60% of the patients in this study showed poor weight gain with body weights less than the 10th percentile. Great caution should be taken in applying such a technique to an asymptomatic neonate with hydronephrosis detected in utero. However, in an older patient with a larger bladder capacity, the Kalicinski repair is a viable option, with good results reported across several series.

Part II

Operations for Ureteral Duplication

Chapter 49

Ureteroneocystostomy for Duplicated Ureters

Approach the operation knowing the degree of damage to the involved segment and whether reflux is present in the lower segment, because removal of the damaged upper pole with subtotal excision of the ureter is usually needed (see Chapter 28). However, with some function remaining in the upper pole, ureteral reimplantation, ureteroureterostomy (see Chapter 50), and ureteropyelostomy (see Chapter 51) are alternatives, depending in part on the length of the duplicated ureter.

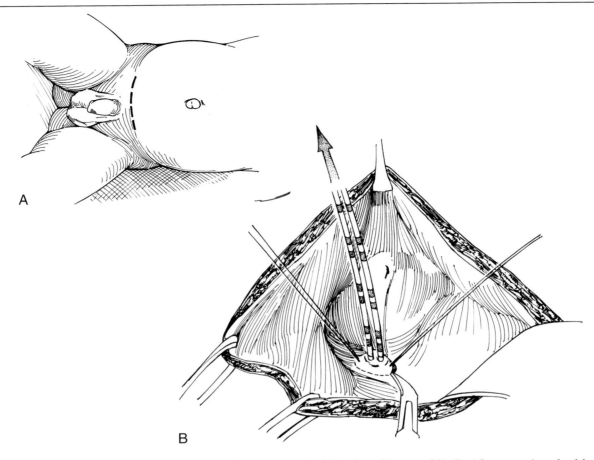

A

B

FIGURE 49-1. A, Incision: Use a lower abdominal transverse incision (see Chapter 63). **B,** After opening the bladder, place a 5-F infant feeding tube into each ureter and fix them in place with a 4-0 synthetic absorbable purse-string suture. With traction on both catheters, incise the mucosa around both orifices with a hooked knife, and then develop a periureteral plane inside the sheath with Lahey scissors. Free up the ureters well outside the bladder. Do not attempt to separate them.

FIGURE 49-2. A, Trim and discard the distal ends of the ureters. If the duplication is incomplete, trim the terminal segment of the ureter enough to expose two lumina. **B,** Perform ureteroneocystostomy with a Politano-Leadbetter, Glenn-Anderson, or Cohen technique, suturing the luminal edges to each other and to the vesical mucosa. The ureters may now lie side by side or the lower segment may be located closer to the vesical neck.

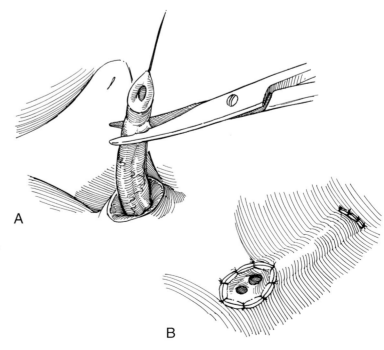

A

B

POSTOPERATIVE PROBLEMS

Complications are similar to those after ureteroneocystostomy (see Chapter 49) and include extravasation, gross hematuria, ureteral obstruction and anuria, persistent reflux, and sepsis.

JOHN W. BROCK

Commentary by

If a duplication is complete, depending on the proximity of the two orifices, the dissection is carried forth in a common sheath fashion by making a circumferential incision around the orifices. After the dissection is complete and the decision is made on the type of ureteral reimplantation to be employed, the distal limbs of the ureters are most commonly discarded. After spatulation the orifices are usually joined by an anastomatic technique to produce a single double-barreled orifice. The ureters are then reimplanted, usually with a side-by-side technique. Occasionally the orientation from the original anatomy will change. In a more unusual circumstance the orifices in a duplex system are not side by side originally and the ureters have to be dissected individually. After this is done, again the technique of spatulation and creation of a single opening with the side-by-side anastomosis is performed in exactly the same fashion as previously described.

Chapter 50

Ureteroureterostomy for Duplicated Ureters

In children with an ectopic upper-pole ureter in a duplex system, a low anastomosis of the diseased ureter to the normal mate will relieve obstruction.

With the aid of a cystoscope, transurethrally place a stent into the normal lower-pole recipient ureter.

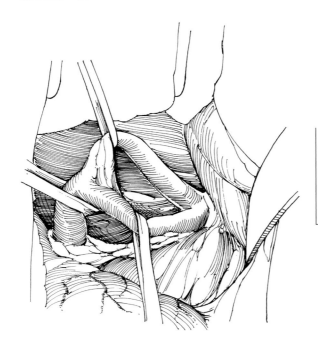

FIGURE 50-1. Incision: Through a lower abdominal transverse incision (see Chapter 63), expose the terminal portion of the double ureter extraperitoneally as far as the bladder. Separate the ureters above their common sheath at a site where they are readily accessible. Use sharp and blunt dissection, preserving the adventitia, and loop each ureter with a small Penrose drain.

FIGURE 50-2. Place a stay suture in the obstructed ureter. Clamp and divide it obliquely below the stay. Remove the distal ectopic stump as far distally as possible.

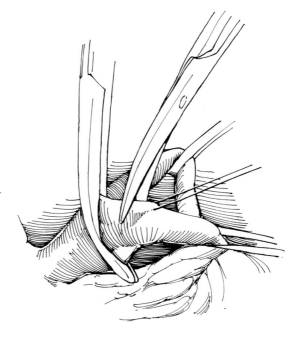

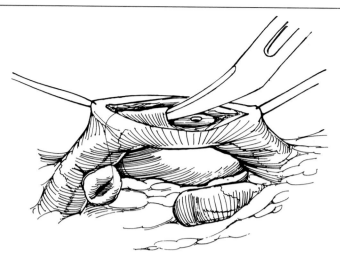

FIGURE 50-3. Place two stay sutures in the recipient ureter 1 to 2 cm apart depending on its size, and incise between them with a hooked knife.

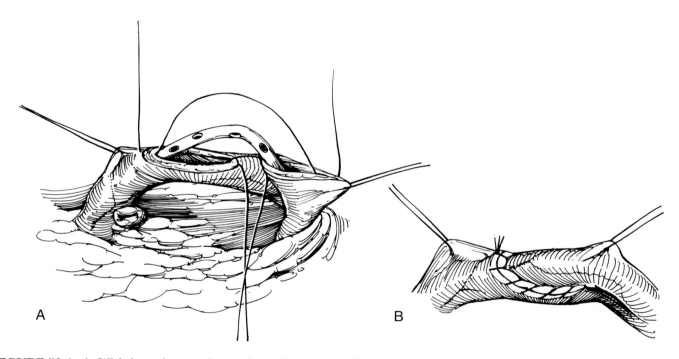

A

B

FIGURE 50-4. A, Withdraw the stenting catheter from the recipient ureter and pass it up the donor ureter. Insert a 4-0 or 5-0 synthetic absorbable suture through each end of the ureterotomy, and then pass one of them through the tip and the other through the base of the donor ureter. **B,** Tie them both, and then run one suture down the respective side from inside the ureter and the other up the near side, with an occasional lock-stitch suture. Tie each to the origin of the other. Drain accurately with a Penrose drain. Insert a catheter in the urethra to keep the bladder empty for 2 or 3 days. Secure the stent to the catheter. Remove both 3 to 5 days after surgery after urine leakage from the Penrose drain ceases.

GEORGE W. KAPLAN

In my opinion, this is a procedure that is greatly underused. It really is a simple solution to many of the difficult problems associated with the repair of abnormal duplex systems. I routinely begin the procedure with cystoscopy. A retrograde pyelogram is obtained to identify which ureter is which and a ureteral catheter (or a double-J stent) is left in situ. If a ureteral catheter is left, it is secured to a Foley catheter with 2-0 silk ties.

I then use a lower abdominal transverse (muscle-splitting) incision (see Chapter 63). On entering the retroperitoneum, the ureters are identified. The presence of a ureteral catheter or a ureteral stent clearly identifies which ureter is which. I then separate the two ureters both distally and proximally. I use this procedure for the anastomosis of an obstructed system to a nonobstructed system (usually the upper pole to the lower pole), for a refluxing to a nonrefluxing system (usually the lower pole to the upper pole), and anastomosis of one dilated ureter to another dilated ureter that will also need to be tapered and then reimplanted. In my opinion, a misconception that has crept into the literature might lead you to believe that a dilated ureter is a contraindication to this procedure. My personal experience and data strongly suggest that not only is this incorrect, but rather, that a dilated ureter is an excellent indication for such a procedure as it often obviates the need to taper the dilated ureter. The small ureteral stump that is left has not produced problems in my experience.

In the past, stents were not left in place and only a Penrose drain was left in situ. More recently, I have been leaving a stent in place, which seems to reduce the length of time that there is drainage from the anastomosis and thereby speeds postoperative recovery. Lastly, I often use interrupted sutures rather than a continuous suture for anastomosis. In reality, neither a continuous nor an interrupted anastomosis is truly watertight. For this reason, even if a stent is left in situ, a Penrose drain is also left.

LINDA M. DAIRIKI SHORTLIFFE

Because I have been using more current imaging techniques of the genitourinary system, such as MRI, I use ureteroureterostomy less, as I have found that renal function associated with renal parenchyma previously thought to be worth preserving was not found, and was instead associated with the lower pole and only appeared to have function due to partial volume appearance seen on planar images. If there is adequate polar function, however, ureteroureterostomy is useful.

I identify the ureter with the normal ureterovesical junction at the time of operation with flexible or rigid cystoscopy and fluoroscopic retrograde ureteropyelogram. I perform ureteroureterostomy with a suprapubic transverse incision while retracting the rectus fibers lateral from the midline to enter the retroperitoneum. After identifying the dilated ureter to be sutured to the normal ureter, I suture this ureter (usually the upper one) to the other one using interrupted polyglycolic acid sutures (5-0) and, depending on the size of the anastomosis, place a double-J catheter into the kidney and well into the bladder. However, if there is a previously determined, large ureteral-diameter discrepancy, I have resorted instead to a subcostal incision and plan an anastomosis of the large, dilated (usually upper-pole) ureter to the lower-pole pelvis in an ureteropyelostomy. With a tie on the distal, dilated ureteral segment I dissect it away from the normal ureter by skeletonizing the adventitial layer of the dilated ureter and maintaining all vessels. (The distal ureter can be dissected into the deep pelvis in this way.) If this ureterovesical junction is associated with an ectopic or a nonrefluxing one, rather than ligate the ureteral stump, I leave it open and tie a ureteral catheter or Penrose drain into the very distal stump with a 5-0 plain gut suture and use this as a drain. If there is any history of ureteral infection or pyonephrosis, I irrigate this stump with antibiotics for 24 to 48 hours postoperatively. If the system has vesicoureteral reflux, I do ligate the distal stump. I handle the ureter in a similar way with an ureteroureterostomy, but this procedure is less likely to need antibiotic irrigation.

Chapter 51

Ureteropyelostomy

Anastomosing the upper portion of the diseased duplicated ureter to the ipsilateral renal pelvis avoids ureteroureteral reflux.

Make an anterior subcostal extraperitoneal incision (see Chapter 9).

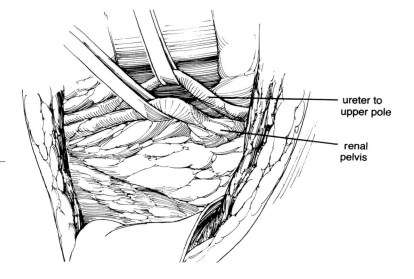

FIGURE 51-1. Expose both ureters near the renal pelvis and separate them on Penrose drains. Continue the dissection to expose the lower-pole pelvis.

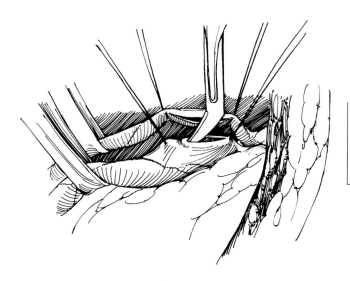

FIGURE 51-2. In the ureter to the upper pole opposite the lower-pole pelvis, place two stay sutures 2 to 3 cm apart, depending on ureteral size. Incise between them with a hooked knife. Place two stay sutures similarly in the lower-pole pelvis and incise between them.

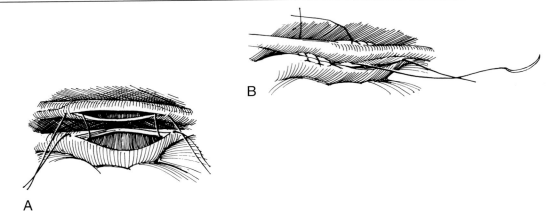

FIGURE 51-3. A, Place one 4-0 or 5-0 synthetic absorbable suture through each end of both ureteral incisions and tie them. Place a double-J stent or external stent if concerned about the anastomosis. **B,** Continue suturing down the far side with one suture and up the near side with the other, locking them occasionally. Tie each suture to the origin of the other suture. Drain the bladder with a urethral catheter for 2 or 3 days.

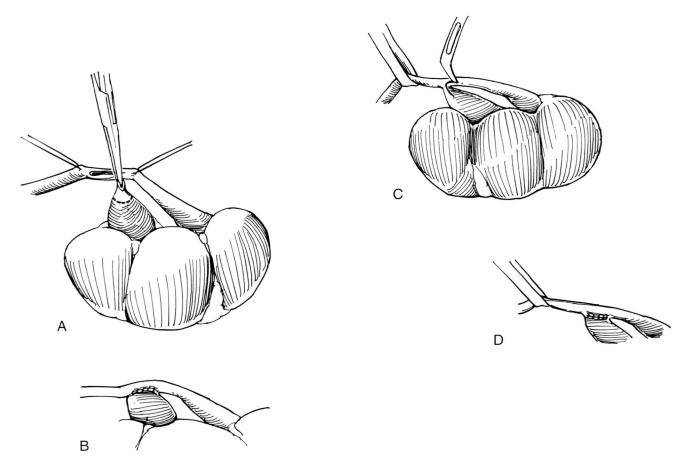

FIGURE 51-4. With *two* dilated pelvises, a similar procedure is possible: by division and anastomosis (**A** and **B**) or by making a **U**-shaped incision and connecting the limbs (**C** and **D**).

PARTIAL URETERECTOMY

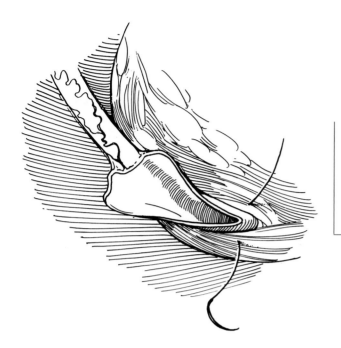

FIGURE 51-5. It is not typically necessary to resect the entire ureter of a nonfunctional duplicated system. Leave the terminal portion in place, because it shares a common wall and blood supply with its mate. After dissecting the extra ureter to within 1 or 2 cm from the bladder, divide it and incise it with scissors down the anterior wall nearly to the bladder wall. Close the short stump with 4-0 synthetic absorbable sutures. Drain the area for a few days.

DOUGLASS HUSMANN

Commentary by

There are some crucial points to keep in mind when performing an upper-pole ureteral anastomosis to the lower-pole renal pelvis. First, the key to success is based on appropriate patient selection. The upper pole of the kidney should be free from chronic infection and/or stone disease. In essence never jeopardize a functional lower-pole moiety by attempting to salvage a poorly functioning or diseased upper pole. Second, take great care to assess the anatomy of the lower-pole renal pelvis on the preoperative radiographic assessments. If the lower-pole renal pelvis is entirely intrarenal in nature, a ureteropyelostomy is possible but technically demanding and alternative procedures should be considered.

Of note are two technical points I feel are beneficial during performing this procedure: (1) At the time of the back wall anastomosis (see Fig. 51-3), place two stay stitches, one on the anterior lip of the upper-pole ureter and the other on the anterior lip of the lower-pole ureter, and then pull these stay stitches in opposite directions. This maneuver will keep the anterior ureteral walls from obscuring the surgical fields. (2) Following closure of the posterior wall, placement of a 5-F pediatric feeding tube brought out at the top of the anatamosis and removed when the last 2 to 3 stitches are placed or, alternatively, placement of a 4.8-F double-J stent into the lower-pole ureter, is helpful to prevent a technical mishap of compromising the luminal opening of your anastomosis.

The majority of times we perform this procedure we will completely transect the upper-pole ureter and remove the upper-pole distal ureteral segment as far down as we can reach, performing a partial upper-pole ureterectomy. If the segment is refluxing, we will tie off the distal ureter; if it is ectopic and obstructing, we will leave the ureter open into the retroperitoneum and place a drain in this region. In this situation, the ureteropyelostomy is then—instead of a side-to-side anastomosis—a widely spatulated, end-upper-pole ureterostomy directly into the renal pelvis.

JOHN C. POPE

Commentary by

This procedure is ideal in situations in which there is an obstructed, dilated, ectopic ureter (there is also a tremendous size discrepancy between the dilated and normal ureters) and the surgeon wishes to remain extravesical in his or her approach. In this case, it is much easier to anastomose the massively dilated ureter to the lower-pole pelvis than it is to the small, normal-caliber, lower-pole ureter. This ureter-to-pelvis anastomosis can be accomplished in a side-to-side fashion as described previously, but can also be done in an end-to-side (upper ureter to lower pelvis) fashion as well. A double-J stent can be placed across the anastomosis but is certainly not required and is left to the surgeon's personal discretion. The final question is how to handle the distal upper-pole ureter. I typically sweep the adventitia off the diseased ureter, protecting the blood supply to the lower-pole ureter, dissect the dilated ureter down as far as I can comfortably see, and then divide it. Since most of the upper-pole ureters in these cases are obstructed distally, they should be left open proximally to avoid an undrained potential space and subsequent abscess. Obviously, if the ureter refluxes or drains adequately distally, it should be ligated proximally.

Chapter 52

Transureteroureterostomy

CROSSED
URETEROURETEROSTOMY FOR
NONDUPLICATED URETERS

Ascertain by voiding cystogram that the recipient ureter does not allow reflux and is not partially obstructed. The ureters may be of unequal size. Provide antibiotic coverage.

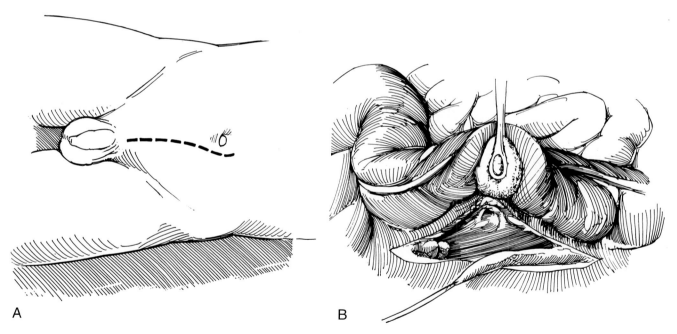

A   B

FIGURE 52-1. A, Incision: Midline transperitoneal incision (see Chapter 11). If the child has had extensive abdominal surgery, an extraperitoneal approach may be more practical. **B,** A left-to-right ureteroureterostomy is described. Hold the descending and sigmoid colon to the right and pack the small bowel into the upper abdomen. Incise the parietal peritoneum lateral to the descending colon and expose the damaged donor ureter, preserving all the adventitial tissue with its vasculature. Clamp the ureter just above the diseased portion. Place a 3-0 synthetic absorbable stay suture proximal to the clamp, divide the ureter, and ligate the distal stump with the same suture material. Free the ureter (for a distance of 9 to 12 cm in the adolescent) while preserving the adventitial vessels.

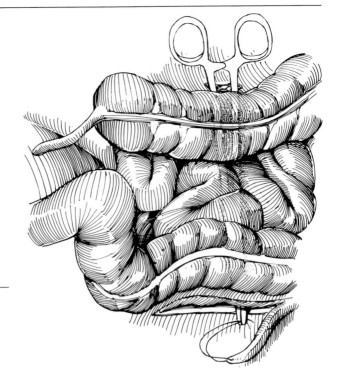

FIGURE 52-2. Make a limited incision in the posterior peritoneum over the right recipient ureter just above the pelvic brim. Make it 4 to 6 cm above the transection of the donor ureter. Expose the recipient ureter, but barely dissect it from its bed, only freeing enough to provide space for the anastomosis. Make a retroperitoneal tunnel by digital dissection, and draw the left ureter through by its stay suture. It may pass over (preferably) or under the inferior mesenteric artery, depending on the length of ureter available, but it must not be left wedged under the artery, where it may be trapped between the artery and the aorta and become obstructed from fibrosis. Be sure the ureter is not angulated and is under no tension.

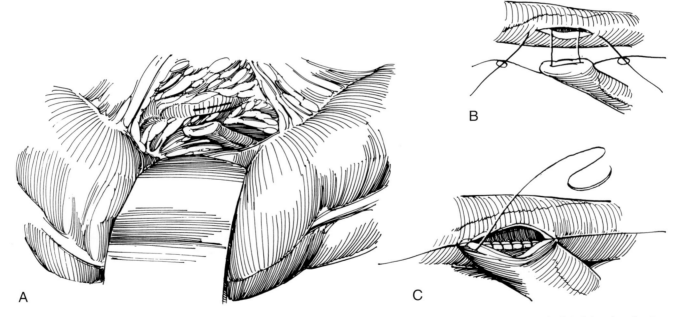

FIGURE 52-3. A, Trim the ureter obliquely to provide a 1.5-cm opening. Spatulation rarely is needed. With a hooked blade, incise the wall of the recipient ureter on its medial surface for a distance slightly longer than the spatulation. Avoid inserting the ureter into the anterior wall because of the risk of angulation. **B,** Place a 4-0 or 5-0 synthetic absorbable suture from outside in at each end of the incision in the recipient ureter and then through each extremity of the spatulation in the donor ureter from the inside out. Tie both sutures. **C,** Run the upper suture down the back wall from the inside, occasionally locking a stitch. Tie it to the lower suture. Now run the lower suture up the front wall from the outside. Consider inserting a double-J stenting catheter into the recipient ureter prior to closing it anteriorly. It is also possible to use an infant feeding tube brought out retroperitoneally through a stab wound. A second stent into the donor ureter may be inserted.

Place an omental wrap if the quality of either ureter is questionable. This usually can be done without mobilizing the omentum, merely by bringing a portion of it through the peritoneal defect. Tunnel a Penrose drain extraperitoneally from the site of the anastomosis through the body wall and skin of the flank. Close the peritoneal defects with 3-0 synthetic absorbable sutures. Drain the bladder with a suprapubic tube or urethral catheter. Close the wound. Ten days postoperatively, instill contrast medium into the stents; if you see no extravasation, remove the stents. Then remove the cystostomy tube or urethral catheter.

BARRY KOGAN

Commentary by

Though applicable only in highly selected cases, this is a very useful procedure. Examples of the indications include (1) cases of marked bilateral reflux and a bad bladder in which it is preferable to achieve one excellent ureteral reimplant and to bring the second ureter to the reimplanted one, and (2) rare cases requiring a urinary diversion in which there is a markedly and chronically dilated ureter that will serve as an end ureterostomy. The contralateral ureter can be brought to this one.

The technique described and illustrated here is excellent. The principle caveat is to preserve the blood supply, both to the ureter being crossed and the recipient ureter. The latter is particularly important as for either a reimplant or a stoma, the distal blood supply of that ureter will be severed and the distal ureter will depend entirely on the blood supply from above. The lateral ureterotomy incision and the anastomosis must be performed with meticulous attention to the recipient blood supply.

PIERRE MOURIQUAND

Commentary by

Transureteroureterostomy (TUU) is an important procedure with three major indications:

1. When both ureters are very dilated and require a reimplantation, the bladder may be too small and the trigonal space may not be sufficient to accommodate two submucosal tunnels. Performing a TUU is an option to allow only one ureteric reimplantation. In our experience, we have not found that performing a TUU and a ureteric reimplantation at the same time represents a threat for the ureteral blood supply, as long as the dissection of the recipient ureter is strictly limited as stated in this chapter.
2. A TUU might be indicated if the lower segment of one ureter is used as a catheterizable channel (Mitrofanoff).
3. When for any reason there is a shortage of ureteral tissue, a TUU might be an effective way to divert urine toward the opposite side.

As stated in this chapter, the caliber of each ureter is not a contraindication to performing this procedure. It is advisable that the retromesenteric tunnel that allows the donor ureter to cross the midline should be wide enough to avoid any urine flow impairment.

The donor ureter should not be too long and should not loop down before entering the recipient ureter. This could expose the patient to urinary tract infections, pain, and stones. We usually leave a transanastomotic double-J stent going up into the donor ureter for 10 days as well as a retromesenteric suction drain.

Chapter 53

Transureteroureterostomy with Cutaneous Stoma

This combination has contemporary use as a temporary urinary diversion in children with newly diagnosed pelvic cancer. After treatment and remission it is anticipated that diversion will be reconstructed into a continent reservoir.

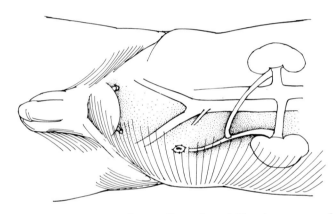

FIGURE 53-1. Approach the donor ureter retroperitoneally and mobilize it very carefully, preserving all the adventitial tissue, especially when it had been previously disturbed. Divide it distally and ligate the stump. Open the peritoneum over the recipient ureter and create a wide, straight tunnel retroperitoneally from both sides with the fingers. Pass a large clamp to retrieve the stay suture on the donor ureter. Be careful that the ureter is not trapped at the takeoff of the inferior mesenteric artery from the aorta (consider passing the ureter above or divide the vessel). Carefully mobilize the recipient ureter as high as needed (even to the renal pelvis) to reach the skin. Divide and ligate it distally. Form an end-cutaneous ureterostomy (see Chapter 87). Anastomose the donor ureter to the recipient ureter as high as is feasible by cutting the ureteral end obliquely and the recipient ureter vertically on the medial aspect. Be sure to leave the recipient ureter in its normal bed. Use everting, full-thickness 6-0 synthetic absorbable sutures. Stent both ureters if the recipient ureter is large enough, or use one stent if that ureter is normal. For stenting of transureteroureterostomies in complex reconstructions involving ureteroneocystostomy and nonrefluxing colonic anastomoses, place two 5- or 8-F infant feeding tubes, brought out retroperitoneally via stab wounds. In addition, nephrostomy drainage may be wise if the ureter has been mobilized or tapered. Place suction drain tubes from both sides.

POSTOPERATIVE PROBLEMS

Obstruction at the site of anastomosis can be detected by ultrasonography and a retrograde ureterogram. Leakage will almost always stop spontaneously. Watch for stenosis at the stoma. Ileus and pelvic abscess have been reported.

Intraperitoneal leakage can result from tension on the anastomosis and will evidence itself as ileus from urinary ascites. Diversion by percutaneous nephrostomy may be needed. Stricture of the normal ureter is rare and usually can be treated by ureteroscopic techniques.

RICHARD LYON

This description of this surgical procedure is so thorough that all I can do is reemphasize the importance of anastomoses without tension. I have found a Z-plasty ostomy site the most reliable. I do have a small criticism as to the type of drainage. The suction drain is meant for self-limiting collections of blood and exudate, and not the occasional prolonged demand for evacuation of urine from a slowly healing anastomosis. Using two Penrose drains, never just one, at each potential leak site has been the invaluable secret taught to me by John Schulte and Bill Smart, for a single drain can be collapsed by tissue pressure. An avenue outside the drains always results with two in place.

SINGLE STOMA OSTOMY

A variation of this procedure has been especially helpful in the treatment of boys with severe posterior urethral valves and bilateral hydroureteronrephrosis. The single stoma ostomy is successful if care is taken to place it in the optimum position, about halfway to the umbilicus, so that the appliance will seat well and thus years of appliance use will be well accepted. A urine density of 1.006 or less will consistently cause prepubertal years of disabling wetness. It has seemed to me important to make the decision to divert as early as possible, surely within the first year, for the child then happily accepts its benefits, and parents escape years of wet diapers and later socially disabling incontinence. Although the enlarged ureters make an open stoma not difficult to achieve, I consistently adapted the Y-V plasty and do not remember a stenosis.

Chapter 54

Calycoureterostomy

Be sure to consider all the other procedures for bridging a defect between pelvis and ureter because a calycoureteral stricture may result from this operation: autotransplantation (see Chapter 60), ileal ureter (see Chapter 55), and nephrectomy (see Chapter 29). The renal cortex over the involved calyx must be thin and have a dilated collecting system because the parenchyma tends to contract around the ureter.

An anterior subcostal incision (see Chapter 9) is usually adequate but an anterior transperitoneal incision (see Chapter 11) allows intestinal interposition if that proves necessary.

Place a ureteral catheter cystoscopically; identification of the ureter may be difficult. Proceed as for ureteropyeloplasty (see Chapter 21). In addition to thoroughly mobilizing the kidney, it is important to be able to control the renal artery if the need should arise. Identify the normal ureter distally and place a small Penrose drain around it. Continue ureteral dissection up to the scarred ureteropelvic junction (UPJ). The ureter may now be long enough after the diseased portion is resected, or an alternative procedure may be preferable. Place a fine traction suture in the ureter and a clamp just above it. Divide the ureter and ligate the stump on the pelvic side with a 2-0 synthetic absorbable suture.

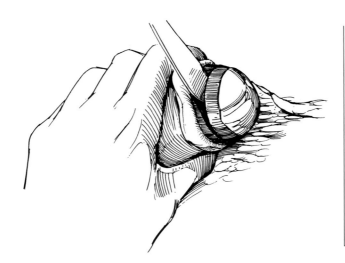

FIGURE 54-1. Incise the capsule around the lower pole of the kidney in the frontal plane and carefully peel it back. It probably will be quite adherent. Estimate the plane of the upper-pole infundibulum from the pyelogram, and bluntly divide the renal parenchyma there with the knife handle, cutting the arcuate vessels with scissors. Remove more parenchyma if necessary to expose the infundibulum of the lower calyx because excess parenchyma may contract around the ureter and constrict it. Control the bleeding with the left hand encircling the lower half of the kidney while placing figure-of-eight sutures of 4-0 synthetic absorbable material, tied by your assistant, to control the arteries. Hemostasis must be complete. Free the calyx enough to receive sutures or free the infundibulum of the calyx and cut it tangentially.

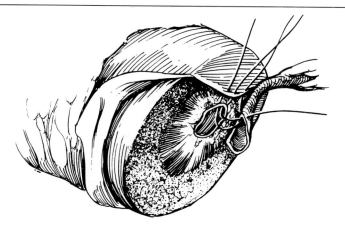

FIGURE 54-2. Spatulate the ureter on its lateral side for a distance equal to the length of the calyceal defect. Anastomosis is similar to that for pyeloplasty (see Chapter 21). Place two 4-0 synthetic absorbable sutures side by side through the capsule and then into the medial end of the calyx and out through the ureter at the notch of the spatulation. Tie them. Run one suture along the posterior edge to the opposite end, with each bite-catching capsule, ureter, and calyx. Lock an occasional stitch. Do the same with the anterior suture, here including, in order, the capsule, ureter, and calyx. Before the defect is completely closed, place a double-J stent extending down the ureter to the bladder and up into the renal pelvis. Additionally, with a curved clamp, draw a small Malecot catheter through the cortex into a middle calyx and fix it to the capsule with a 2-0 synthetic absorbable suture. Complete the ureterocalyceal anastomosis and tie the two running sutures together. Irrigate through the nephrostomy tube to be sure the closure is watertight. Place a stitch for nephropexy and drain the area well with a Penrose drain that exits retroperitoneally. Replace the perirenal fat with Gerota's fascia to encase the repair. If coverage seems inadequate, bring the omentum into the retroperitoneum and tack it about the anastomosis. Postoperatively, before removing the nephrostomy tube, withdraw the stent and check pressure and flow through the anastomosis.

DAVID A. BLOOM

Commentary by

Calycoureterostomy is arguably the *one* operation performed one operation *too* late. In some instances, such as giant hydronephrosis, in which the UPJ is quite cranial compared to the dependent lower-pole calyces, dependent drainage might be best assured by a calycoureterostomy as a first procedure rather than defaulting to a routine pyeloplasty. Most instances of calycoureterostomy, however, are performed for failed pyeloplasties. Once a pyeloplasty has failed we have found endoscopic interventions generally unrewarding except as temporizing procedures. The alternative of the Davis intubated ureterotomy is only of historical interest, in which results are validated by historical word of mouth rather than any substantive clinical series. Autotransplantation and creation of an ileal ureter are higher-magnitude procedures in general than the calycoureterostomy and I believe their use should be quite occasional.

Nephrectomy, of course, is the last resort for a failed pyeloplasty. The steps for ureterocalycostomy are well explained and illustrated in this chapter. Perhaps they could be summarized into six critical principles: (1) thorough exposure with a wide operative field, (2) identification of a healthy ureter, (3) generous guillotine lower-pole amputation to expose a wide dependent calyx, (4) complete coverage of exposed lower-pole parenchyma by capsule (we differ from the author in that we first sew the stripped-back renal capsule to the actual calyceal epithelium such that the lower-pole parenchyma is completely covered right to the calyx; only then do we separately sew the calyx to spatulated ureter), (5) secure drainage with either a nephrostent or a double-J catheter, and (6) insulation of the site of repair with fat or omentum.

EVAN KASS

Commentary by

We have used calycoureterostomy primarily when there is a UPJ obstruction with massive hydronephrosis and thin renal parenchyma. In this setting, it may not be possible to achieve dependent drainage with a primary ureteropelvic anastomosis. It is essential for the parenchyma over the most dependent calyx to be thin so that minimal if any renal tissue has to be excised. A button of tissue is excised and a primary epithelium-to-epithelium spatulated anastomosis is performed in a tension-free manner. A nephrostomy tube and stent should be used routinely and left in place for 7 to 10 days. We have sometimes used an alternative approach when there is massive hydronephrosis and the renal parenchyma collapses into a series of folds after the UPJ is opened. In this setting, we have plicated the folds with two or three 2-0 or 3-0 absorbable sutures per fold to allow the UPJ anastomosis to be placed in the most dependent position.

Calycoureterostomy may also be necessary as a salvage procedure following a failed pyeloplasty or a complex stone operation. However, here there usually is thick parenchyma over the lower pole and considerable perirenal fibrosis. It is essential to mobilize the calyx sufficiently so that the anastomosis is epithelium-to-epithelium and free of tension. A ureteral stent is mandatory and usually is left in place for 6 weeks. We find it easier to pass a double-J stent before starting the anastomosis.

Chapter 55

Ileal Ureteral Replacement

Explore all alternatives that use tissue from the urinary tract before electing to use ileum. Consider autotransplantation. Be certain that the child has adequate renal function. Because of mucosal resorption, the initial serum creatinine level should be 2.2 mg/100 mL or less. Nephrostomy drainage will already be in place.

Prepare the child as for an ileal conduit (see Chapter 89). Do not place a urethral catheter but allow the bladder to fill. If the ureter is to be excised, insert a ureteral catheter cystoscopically for identification.

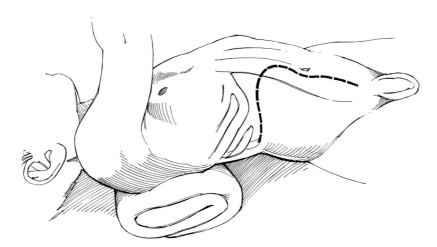

FIGURE 55-1. Position: Place the child in the lateral (flank) position with the table flexed and the shoulder and chest held at right angles to the table. Allow the upper hip to fall back as far as reasonable and place a sandbag under it.

Incision: Palpate the 12th rib and begin the skin incision over its angle. Continue semiobliquely to the midline and then vertically to the pubis. (Alternatively, use a thoracoabdominal incision to obtain greater exposure for the renal anastomosis.) For bilateral cases, a long midline incision is best. Cut through the anterior part of the latissimus dorsi muscle onto the surface of the 12th rib. Place the index finger in an opening in the lumbodorsal fascia at the tip of the rib and work posteriorly, cutting the serratus inferior posterior muscle and intercostal muscles if encountered. Divide the external and internal oblique and transversus muscles and enter the peritoneum. Divide the rectus muscle and retract it laterally while continuing the incision down the midline, opening the peritoneum further at the same time.

Incise the peritoneal attachment of the terminal ileum to the sacral promontory. Divide the lateral attachments of the ascending colon in the white line of Toldt to mobilize it to the region of the duodenum and as far medially as the great vessels, as done for retroperitoneal lymph node dissection. Let the bowel fall back. Now open the peritoneum, continuing anteriorly in the line of the incision.

FIGURE 55-2. Select a segment of ileum near the ileocecal junction, 20 to 30 cm long for an adolescent. The length will depend on the size of the child and on the length of ureter to be replaced. Choose sites of transection that will permit total mobilization of the segment of ileum by allowing cuts in the mesentery deep enough for the upper end of the loop to reach the renal area (which can be difficult) and the distal end to reach the bladder. Make certain that two major branches of the superior mesenteric artery enter the loop and take special care to preserve a good arterial supply. On the left side, a segment of descending colon can be used instead of the ileum.

Mark the bowel at each end with a stay suture. Throw a loose tie onto the distal suture as a marker to be sure that later the segment will be placed isoperistaltically. Divide the mesentery deeply between the ileocolic artery and the terminal branches of the superior mesenteric artery. Divide it also at the proximal end deeply enough for that end to reach the kidney. Apply Kocher clamps and divide the bowel, and then restore bowel continuity as described for the ileal conduit (see Chapter 89). Irrigate the loop through a catheter with a 50-mL syringe containing saline solution, followed by 1% bacitracin-neomycin solution, and finally by air. Close the mesenteric defect with 4-0 silk sutures.

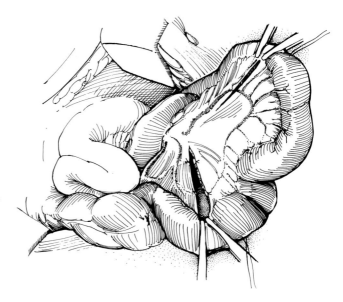

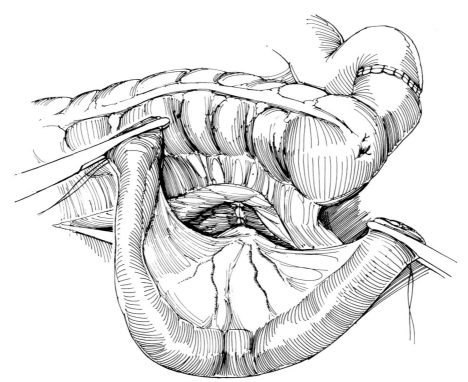

FIGURE 55-3. For replacement of the right ureter, place the ileal segment extraperitoneally by lifting the cecum forward and exposing the retroperitoneal space. Make a small opening in the mesentery of the ascending colon near the cecum and bring the ileum through it. For the left ureter, mobilize the descending colon medially by incising along the white line. Make a window in the colonic mesentery and push the isolated segment of ileum out through it so that it lies in an isoperistaltic manner in the left retroperitoneal space. Because the anastomoses to the renal pelvis and bladder are retroperitoneal, the ileum will lie behind the descending colon.

Rotate the ileum 180 degrees counterclockwise to place the knotted stay suture that marks the distal end near the bladder, assuring an isoperistaltic orientation. Carefully close the opening through the mesentery to prevent internal herniation and at the same time avoid constriction. Grasp the end of the loop again with the Kocher clamp. For unilateral ureteral substitution, close the proximal end of the loop, spatulate the ureter, and anastomose it to the ileum as described for ureteroileostomy (see Chapter 89). Connect the ureter end to side if it is dilated, even if tailoring is necessary.

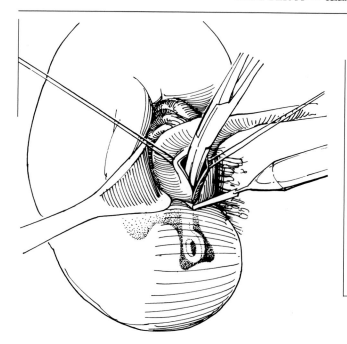

FIGURE 55-4. Pyeloileal anstomosis: For children with recurrent formation of xanthine stones, anastomosis of the pelvis to the bowel directly to allow stones to pass may be advisable. Mobilize the renal pelvis, which is often difficult after previous stone procedures. If the pelvis is obscured by scar, insert curved Randall forceps through the nephrostomy site and cut on its tip, staying away from the vascular pedicle. Leave the ureter in situ. Widely open the renal pelvis vertically. Pass Randall stone forceps through the pyelotomy into the lower-pole calyx and cut down on the forceps with the cutting current to open up the entire lower collecting system. Place 3-0 chromic catgut sutures from the capsule to the calyx to control parenchymal bleeding. Remove persisting calculi with the aid of a nephroscope. Insert a small Malecot nephrostomy tube with two wings removed through the parenchyma via a middle calyx.

FIGURE 55-5. Spatulate the ileum to form an ellipse by opening its antimesenteric border, incising it until it is large enough to fit the pelvic defect. Place a 3-0 or 4-0 chromic catgut suture through all layers of the tip of the bowel, then through the upper margin of the pelvic defect, and tie it. Run the suture down the back wall, occasionally locking a stitch. Continue the suture up the anterior wall and tie it to the end of the suture. Alternatively, use interrupted 3-0 or 4-0 chromic catgut sutures, placing the posterior row with the knots outside. Fill the pelvis through the nephrostomy tube and reinforce the anastomosis at sites of leakage. Either suture line may be reinforced with serosa-to-adventitia sutures.

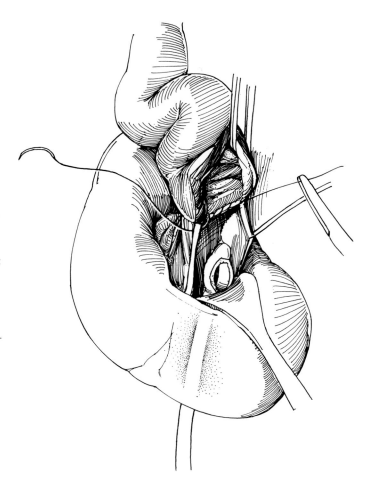

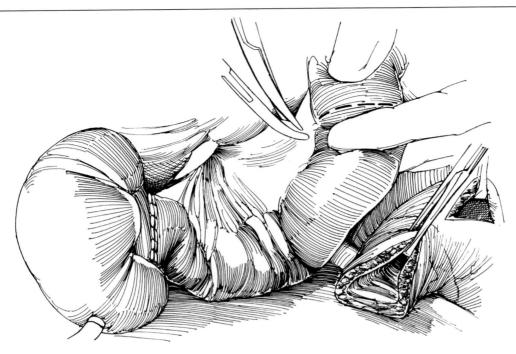

FIGURE 55-6. Mobilize the peritoneum from the upper and lateral margins of the bladder and make a short incision in the dome extraperitoneally. Insert the index finger and move the posterolateral wall of the bladder toward the psoas muscle. If the ileal loop is short, making greater vesical mobilization necessary, carry the dissection down to include the superior vesical pedicle by incising the peritoneum in the cul-de-sac. Grasp the bladder with an Allis clamp at the site of the tip of the finger over the psoas muscle and excise a small circle of bladder wall. Suture the posterior wall of the bladder to the psoas muscle with several 3-0 chromic catgut sutures. Move the ileal segment alongside to determine the length needed. Keep the loop as short as possible, but allow enough redundancy to permit formation of a nipple. (Omit the nipple if the operation is done for stone disease.) Excise the redundant portion of the ileum, first dividing its vessels close to the bowel to avoid interference with the major blood supply.

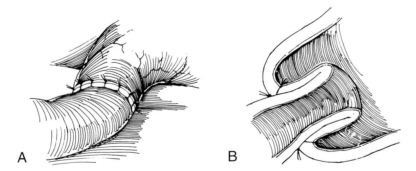

A   B

FIGURE 55-7. A, Pull several centimeters of bowel into the bladder. In children, taper the ileum and insert it in a submucosal tunnel as done for large ureters (see Chapter 47). **B,** Alternatively, turn the bowel back on itself as a cuff, and suture its mucosa to the vesical urothelium. Or perform an ileoileal intussusception. Suture the bowel to the bladder wall with interrupted 3-0 chromic catgut sutures. It may be easier to open the bladder widely and anastomose the ileum by suturing from inside the bladder. Place a Malecot cystostomy tube through a stab wound and close the bladder defect in two layers. Insert a small 5-mL silicone balloon catheter transurethrally. A stent in the ileum is probably unnecessary. Place a medium-sized Penrose drain near the pyeloileal anastomosis and bring it out through a stab wound in the posterior axillary line. Place a second drain near the vesical anastomosis and bring it out anterolaterally. Assured drainage is essential. Tack the colon laterally to the peritoneal edge to extraperitonealize the entire segment. Close the peritoneum and the wound. Finally, suture the nephrostomy and cystostomy tubes to the skin with heavy silk.

   Remove the urethral catheter on the 5th postoperative day. The cystostomy tube may be clamped on the seventh day for a trial of voiding, but there is no hurry about this. Perform a gravity nephrostogram and cystogram subsequently to check for leaks. If none are detected, remove the cystostomy and nephrostomy tubes. Remove the drains 24 hours later. Check the functional result by following the level of the serum creatinine and the anatomic result by an intravenous urogram at 6 weeks.

BILATERAL TOTAL URETERAL REPLACEMENT

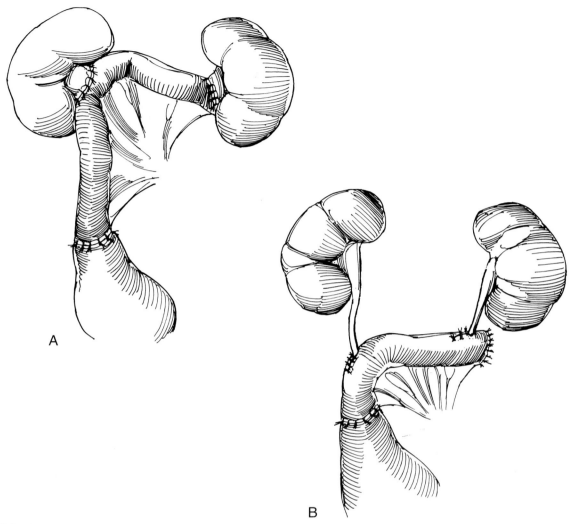

FIGURE 55-8. A, Pyeloileal anastomoses: Working anteriorly and intraperitoneally, anastomose the loop to the left pelvis end to end and connect it to the right pelvis end to side. **B,** Ureteroileal anastomoses: Bring the ureters through the posterior peritoneum near the midline and proceed intraperitoneally with anastomosis of the ureters to the loop and the loop to the bladder.

POSTOPERATIVE PROBLEMS

Anastomotic leakage with consequent urinoma or fistula can be detected by the nephrostogram, in which case, the nephrostomy is left for a longer time. Obstruction is usually due to edema or excessive production of mucus. A kink in the ileum must also be suspected. Leaving the nephrostomy tube in place allows these factors to resolve. Ischemic necrosis of the segment requires immediate reoperation.

Electrolyte imbalance is rare if preoperative renal function was adequate and the segment is short and drains well. Gross dilation of the segment with consequent hyperabsorption of electrolytes can be avoided by providing an open bladder outlet or by creating a valve at the ileovesical junction by nipple, by tapering the ileum and creating a submucosal tunnel, or by ileal intussusception. Long-term follow-up is needed to detect incipient outlet obstruction before renal damage.

DOUGLASS HUSMANN

Commentary by

It is important to stress that all possible alternative solutions need to be considered before proceeding with an ileal ureteral replacement; options include autotransplantation, transureteroureterostomy, and possible nephrectomy. We also vary in opinion from the author regarding management of the bladder neck. Specifically, the author mentions that they desire to have a wide-open bladder neck to allow ease of voiding. Since transurethral resection or Y-V plasty of the bladder neck usually results in retrograde ejaculation and fertility problems, we do not perform these bladder neck operations in children and young adults. Alternatively we would prefer to pursue intermittent catheterization as an option and will therefore work with our patients prior to surgery to verify that intermittent catheterization can be performed by the patient if inadequate bladder emptying is present postoperatively. We also differ from the authors in that we classically perform this operation in a supine position with a roll under the back or with the patient in a slightly flexed position to anteriorly displace the kidney.

Through the years one of the postoperative problems we have encountered during prolonged follow-up of these patients is the tendency to use too long a segment of ileum to perform the ileal ureter replacement. This results in a tortuous ileal ureter, which has a prolonged dwell time and leads to metabolic abnormalities, especially if a freely refluxing ileal vesical anastomosis is performed. We are therefore very meticulous in setting up the ileal segment used as the ileal ureter, verifying that it will reach the bladder without a significant amount of redundancy.

Postoperatively, once confirmation of adequate healing by radiographic studies (cystogram and nephrostograms) have been obtained we acquire baseline electrolyte values and then plug the suprapubic tube and initiate a voiding trial for a 1- to 2-week interval. During this time span the patient will measure postvoiding residual urine. If adequate bladder emptying is found we will remove the suprapubic tube. If large postvoiding residual urine or electrolyte abnormalities develop, we will begin intermittent catheterizations.

CASIMIR F. FIRLIT

Commentary by

Use of the small bowel as an interpositioned conduit from the renal pelvis to the bladder represents a creative application for the substitution of the entire ureter. Although the procedure of ileal substitution of the ureter has become less and less applicable in modern times, it nevertheless represents an operative procedure that should be retained within the urologist's armamentarium. Modern-day approaches might suggest a renal autotransplant to bridge the renal pelvis directly to the bladder in the form of a pyelovesicostomy, or, if there is enough proximal ureter, to simply bring the kidney down as an autotransplant and reimplant the ureter into the bladder. However, expertise in renal autotransplantation varies throughout the country and the world, and, in situations where that expertise is not available, the use of ileal substitution for a stenotic, fibrotic, strictured, or destroyed ureter represents a viable alternative to save functioning renal parenchyma. The illustrations in this chapter clearly present the application of this modality for both pediatric and adult urologic patients. The ileal ureter itself represents a sluggish hypoperistaltic urinary conduit; nevertheless, it does serve to salvage a kidney that has had ureteral disease and now represents an operative procedure that will salvage such a renal unit.

The ileal ureter deserves to be preserved in the surgical armamentarium for application in situations in which renal autotransplantation is not available.

Chapter 56

Ureterocele Repair

The variables that must be considered in the management of ureteroceles are duplex versus single system, function of the renal moiety subtended by the ureterocele, reflux into the remaining moieties, and whether the ureterocele is intravesical versus extravesical (ectopic into the bladder neck). Early management may decrease the rate of urinary tract infections and also reduce the need for subsequent surgical procedures.

Ultrasonography is usually adequate to delineate the relationships of the ureterocele and assess the degree of ureteral dilation. Supplement the ultrasonogram with a voiding cystourethrogram to assess the bladder and to detect reflux into the ipsilateral ureter from the lower pole, and into the contralateral ureter that then must be concomitantly reimplanted.

Start administration of antibiotic prophylaxis at the time the anomaly is detected.

Obtain a voiding cystourethrogram, using dilute contrast medium. This may not only demonstrate the ureterocele but also provide information on the size, urethral extension, and support behind it; an oblique voiding film can give important information. Finally, assess the function of the two renal moieties by radionuclide scan to determine if heminephrectomy is the more practical course.

When the child is ill, percutaneously decompress the upper tract, drain the lower tract with a catheter, or do both. Consider initial transurethral incision of the ureterocele not only as a temporizing measure but also for possible cure, especially if the ureterocele is a single system. In an ill infant, if incision proves inadequate as shown by ultrasonography and persistence of symptoms, turn to percutaneous renal drainage.

For a ureterocele with little or no upper-pole function perform nephrectomy with drainage of the distal segment (see Chapter 26). If the upper pole functions, perform ipsilateral ureteropyelostomy (see Chapter 51) or ureteroureterostomy (see Chapter 50) and reimplant the orthotopic ureter because it will reflux. If function is good, excise the ureterocele and reimplant both ureters together (see Chapter 49).

INTRAVESICAL REPAIR

If the function of the upper-pole segment warrants its salvage, excise the ureterocele and reimplant both ureters together.

SINGLE-SYSTEM URETEROCELE

Start with endoscopic puncture (see Chapter 57), which may be curative.

An extravesical ureterocele forms in the end of the upper-pole ureter of a duplex system. In three quarters of cases it has an ectopic orifice. Repair may include excision of the upper-pole moiety.

OPTIONS FOR RECONSTRUCTION OF THE EXTRAVESICAL URETEROCELE

Three approaches are available: endoscopic repair, upper-tract surgical procedures, and complete reconstruction. Definitive reconstruction is usually preferable to temporizing methods but some delay does not appear to increase the risk of complications.

For treatment based on the presence or absence of vesicoureteral reflux and renal function: If reflux is present, excise the ureterocele and reimplant the ureters; in the absence of reflux, correct only the upper-tract abnormality.

One of three approaches can be used, depending on renal function:

1. Adequate function in both segments, with reflux: Proceed with intravesical excision of the ureterocele and joint reimplantion of both ureters, as described in the section "Intravesical Repair."
2. Minimal or absent upper-pole function with a symptomatic ureterocele: Perform upper-pole heminephrectomy (see Chapter 28).
3. Functioning upper-pole segment: Perform ipsilateral ureteropyelostomy (see Chapter 51) or ureteroureterostomy (see Chapter 50). If necessary because of reflux, reimplant the orthotopic ureter.

INTRAVESICAL REPAIR

If the function of the upper-pole segment warrants salvage, excise the ureterocele and reimplant both ureters together. Clear infection with appropriate antibiotics.

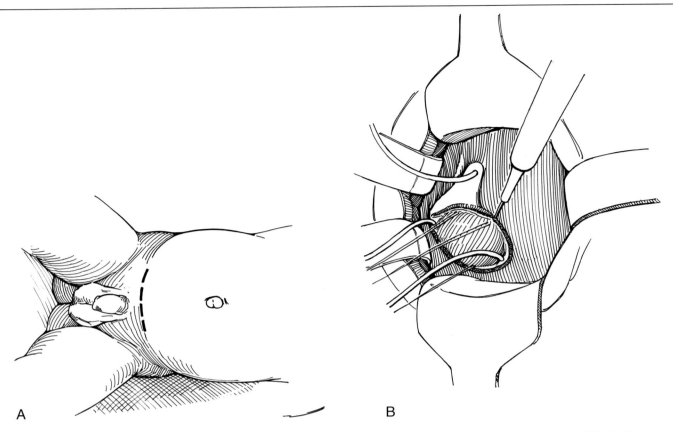

A   **B**

FIGURE 56-1. A, Position: Supine. Incision: Make a transverse lower abdominal incision (see Chapter 63). **B,** Open the bladder and intubate the orifice of the ureterocele with an infant feeding tube. Identify the orifice to the lower pole and intubate it also. Fix the tubes in place with fine sutures (not shown). Place traction sutures around the margin of the ureterocele to surround both orifices, and gather them together in one clamp. With a hooked blade or a needle electrode, incise the epithelium and subepithelium at the border of the ureterocele. Include the orifice to the lower pole.

FIGURE 56-2. Elevate the lateral border with the stay sutures, and separate the subepithelium from the underlying detrusor muscle with fine scissors. Obtain hemostasis by placing interrupted sutures around the rim of the (former) base of the ureterocele.

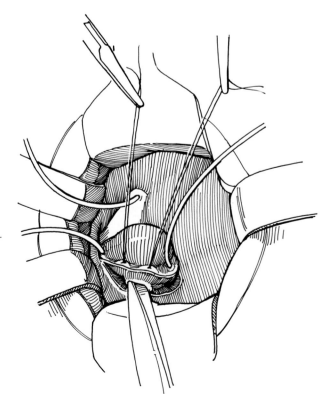

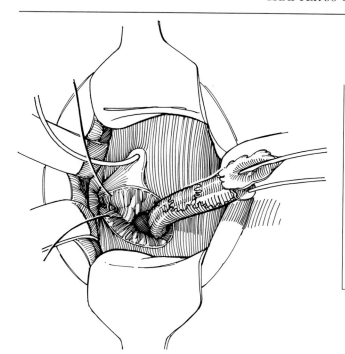

FIGURE 56-3. Dissect this combined ureteral complex through the ureteral hiatus as for ureteroneocystostomy (see Chapter 36). If the ureterocele extends into the urethra, the dissection requires great patience, because the wall of the ureterocele may blend with that of the trigone. If more exposure is needed, incise the anterior bladder wall to the level of the bladder neck, but not beyond. Moreover, be sure to remove any epithelium from the ureterocele that projects into the lumen of the urethra: It may act as an obstructive valve. Proximally, continue the dissection of both ureters in their common sheath through the ureteral hiatus. Extravesical dissection is usually not necessary. Close the defect in the detrusor muscle distal to the hiatus with 5-0 synthetic absorbable sutures.

FIGURE 56-4. Close the vesical epithelium and subepithelium over the trigone. If the ureterocele is large, reinforce the weakened detrusor muscle with transverse sutures. Remove the tubes from the double ureters. Place a stay suture through the epithelium-subepithelium above the contralateral orifice. Elevate the epithelial edge, and insinuate scissors beneath it to create a transverse tunnel that exits at the stay suture.

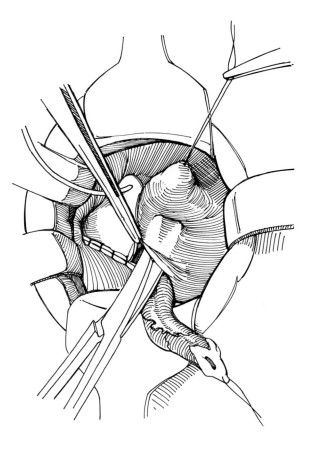

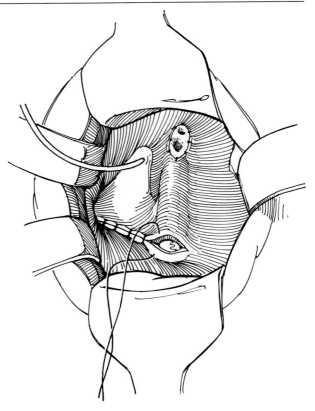

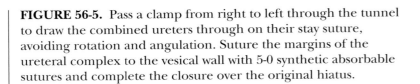

FIGURE 56-5. Pass a clamp from right to left through the tunnel to draw the combined ureters through on their stay suture, avoiding rotation and angulation. Suture the margins of the ureteral complex to the vesical wall with 5-0 synthetic absorbable sutures and complete the closure over the original hiatus.

POSTOPERATIVE PROBLEMS

Complications are similar to those after ureteroneocystostomy (see Chapter 49). Infection in a closed segment of ureter can lead to sepsis. Incontinence may result from extensive suburethral dissection and subsequently require reconstruction through a posterior sagittal transanorectal approach.

HOWARD SNYDER

Commentary by

Our thought processes about the treatment of ureteroceles have undergone a long and progressive evolution. Here is my own view based on our experience at The Children's Hospital of Philadelphia.

For a single-system ureterocele, seen more commonly in boys than in girls, we always start with endoscopic puncture of the ureterocele. In most cases, these are intravesical ureteroceles. With the technique of endoscopic puncture preserving a flap-valve mechanism of the front wall of the ureterocele, you can anticipate about a 90% success rate, without the need for any open surgery. If a single-system ureterocele were ectopic, we would still carry out endoscopic incision because, although open surgery subsequently would probably be required, the decompressed system subserving the ureterocele would then be easier to reimplant into the bladder.

With an upper-pole ureterocele in a duplex system, rarely is there enough function in the upper pole to make preservation an issue. The real problem is whether the ureter from the upper pole that subserves the ureterocele is so dilated that reimplantation would be difficult. There is now good evidence to indicate that as long as the system is decompressed and not refluxing, very poor function alone does not dictate its removal.

Associated reflux at the time a youngster is treated for a ureterocele generally drives subsequent open surgery. Rough figures are 50% of ipsilateral lower-pole reflux; 25% of contralateral systems reflux; and in about 10% of cases, reflux occurs in the ureterocele itself.

For a duplex system with an intravesical upper-pole ureterocele, we would almost always carry out endoscopic puncture, because that is very likely to be successful in leaving a flap-valve mechanism and would obviate surgery on that ureter. If surgery were needed, it would be driven by associated reflux. Once the system running to the ureterocele has been decompressed, an all-intravesical operation at the bladder level is adequate. As mentioned earlier, we no longer remove poorly functioning upper-pole units if they can be reattached satisfactorily to the bladder without obstruction or reflux. That is the value of primary endoscopic puncture.

For an ectopic ureterocele, one can anticipate finding after endoscopic puncture, a greater likelihood for an open operation at the bladder level because of the higher incidence of associated reflux. There are poor guidelines in the literature as to how to repair the bladder neck when an ectopic ureterocele is excised. We have for many years used the edge of the ureterocele to guide reconstruction, feeling that the defect created by the ureterocele reflects the potential embryologic defect in the bladder neck that could risk later incontinence. As the bladder neck is reconstructed, we continue imbricating the musculature until the mucosal edge of the resected urethra and bladder neck at the border of the ureterocele are apposed. While this requires difficult suturing with a very small, curved noncutting needle inside the bladder neck, it is technically feasible. In using this technique for more than 20 years, we have seen all children void normally after surgery and have had no urinary incontinence on our long-term follow-up.

In the rare situation of no reflux at the bladder level with a functioning upper-pole segment and sufficient extrarenal pelvis in the lower-pole system, a ureteropyelostomy would be our primary approach. However, if there is significant vesicoureteral reflux, we would apply one operation at the bladder level, as mentioned previously.

In summary, we have greatly come to depend on endoscopic puncture by the techniques we have published, followed by a one-stage open approach. This seems to be particularly appropriate when so many ureteroceles now are being seen in the newborn during evaluation of antenatal hydronephrosis. We carefully puncture to preserve a flap valve of the decompressed ureterocele, and then wait until 18 to 20 months have passed, when the elevated voiding pressures of infancy have fallen to normal. We then perform a voiding cystourethrogram, which will restage the case and permit antireflux surgery, if needed, to be done before toilet training when it is better tolerated.

Primary upper-pole partial nephrectomy, to decompress a system from above (the so-called simplified approach), might be considered in the one situation when there is an ectopic ureterocele without reflux into either the ureterocele or any other ureter at the bladder level. This is actually quite rare. In our last reported series of 44 ureteroceles, we had only one such case.

Our goal today with modern endoscopic techniques is to limit open surgery, generally restricting it to the bladder level. Our success rate at reimplanting ureters that have been decompressed serving a ureterocele has been about 90%. While not quite as good as primary reimplantation, it is good enough to be our preferred approach.

STANLEY KOGAN

Commentary by

Ureteroceles are usually diagnosed on prenatal ultrasound or during the radiologic work-up for a urinary tract infection, in which unilateral or bilateral hydronephrosis in association with a duplex collecting system and a vesical filling defect is seen. Complete or incomplete urinary retention is a less common presentation, occurring in conjunction with a bulging ureterocele prolapsed through the urinary meatus in a girl. In some instances, the diagnosis may be subtle, with an occult nonfunctioning upper-pole duplication not seen, yet the ureterocele may still be filled and obstruct the ipsilateral and contralateral ureters.

The initial evaluation begins with a sonogram and voiding cystourethrogram. Sonography is accurate in revealing the duplex anatomy and hydroureter and is exquisitely accurate in demonstrating the ureterocele as an intravesical filling defect. The voiding cystourethrogram may also demonstrate the ureterocele and give additional information regarding the size, extension, and bladder support backing the ureterocele, as well as the presence of ipsilateral or contralateral reflux, information important in subsequently planning the corrective surgical approach. Using dilute contrast material so as not to obscure the ureterocele and obtaining voiding films in the extreme oblique position are important technical aids in obtaining useful, revealing films. Finally, a functional study, such as a nuclear renal scan, is necessary to determine the functional status of all renal segments, especially the upper-pole segment attached to the ureterocele.

Review of the contemporary literature indicates that the treatment of ureteroceles is continually evolving. The goal of treatment is to prevent renal damage secondary to obstruction or reflux, and minimize the risk of urinary tract infection. First-line treatment often involves transurethral puncture of a ureterocele, a less morbid approach when compared to open surgery. Simple intravesical ureteroceles often may respond to only endoscopic incision, but postoperative reflux, infections, or persistent obstruction may eventually necessitate reoperation. Regarding the simple endoscopic incision, the surgical outcomes seem to be related to ureterocele location, the presence of a duplex collecting system, and the presence of preoperative reflux. An ectopic ureterocele location, duplex renal systems, and preoperative reflux are all independent risk factors for eventual reoperation due to the effect on trigonal anatomy after the ureterocele decompresses. Recent studies have also suggested modifications of the endoscopic incisions with fulguration of the anterior and posterior walls of the collapsed ureterocele, which decreased the incidence of de novo vesicoureteral reflux.

Continued

Primary upper-tract reconstruction as an initial procedure has its advocates as well. Upper-pole heminephrectomy as a definitive treatment is performed with hopes that the ureterocele will collapse and no lower-tract surgery will be necessary. Review of the literature indicates that the patients best served with a simplified upper-tract approach are the subset with duplex ectopic ureteroceles and nonviable or hypofunctioning renal segment without high-grade preoperative reflux. Patients with duplex-system ectopic ureteroceles only required additional surgery in 15% of patients treated with heminephrectomy, while a similar population treated with endoscopic decompression had a 64% chance of requiring an additional operation for persistent reflux. Patients with vesicoureteral reflux associated with duplex ectopic ureteroceles usually require additional surgery irrespective of whether primary upper-tract or endoscopic decompression surgery is chosen. With regard to the need for complete ureterectomy after heminephrectomy, the vast majority of patients with residual ureteral stumps do not require stump resection, though in the setting of an inadequately drained ureterocele or refluxing stump the likelihood of requiring stump removal is high.

Others indicate the benefits of lower urinary tract reconstruction as an initial procedure for poorly functioning renal moieties associated with obstructing ureteroceles. They cite that a large percentage of patients who underwent upper-tract ablative surgery ultimately require major lower-tract surgery to correct the underlying ureterocele and associated anatomic abnormalities. This risk is as high as 84% when preoperative reflux is associated with the ureterocele. Therefore the approach of ureteral tapering and reimplantation, excision of the ureterocele, and bladder neck reconstruction can be carried out while leaving the dysplastic renal moiety in situ. The theoretic risks of leaving a poorly functioning renal segment, such as infection, hypertension, and malignant potential, have never been substantiated in the literature. In long-term follow-up of patients treated in this manner, upper-tract dilation decreased or completely resolved in all patients and there was no loss of renal function.

Nonoperative intervention or expectant management may have selected roles as well. Furosemide mercapto acetyl tri glycine renal scans can be used to select patients for conservative management. One group suggested that if there was no evidence of high-grade obstruction with good preservation of renal function or if there was complete nonfunctioning of the renal moiety with or without multicystic dysplasia, patients can be selected for nonoperative management. Patients were excluded if they had ureteroceles associated with poorly functioning renal segments or if they had drainage time in excess of 30 minutes on renal scan. Patients were then followed every 6 months with ultrasound and every 18 months with voiding cystourethrogram if reflux was initially present. Indications for surgical intervention included clinical or radiologic progression of disease or breakthrough infection while on prophylaxis. Patients who eventually underwent surgical intervention due to progression of disease tended to have longer drainage time and lower-upper pole differential function on renal scan. Another group who studied patients diagnosed with ureteroceles on prenatal ultrasound excluded patients with obstruction of more than one renal moiety, bladder neck obstruction, or high-grade reflux. In this study of patients managed expectantly, hydronephrosis resolved in six patients, reflux resolved in two patients, and no patients required surgical intervention during the course of follow-up.

Currently, we approach patients from the upper end when the ureterocele is small and the collecting system is not significantly dilated, and sometimes when a chronically infected collecting system is recalcitrant to treatment. Others are approached primarily from below, excising the ureterocele and repairing the bladder muscle backing, which may be significantly thinned out at times, and doing a heminephrectomy as part of the same procedure. One surgical aid I have found useful in mobilizing the ureterocele and ipsilateral ureter, after scoring the bladder mucosa, is to develop the plane between the bladder mucosa and ureter up high, near the hiatus. This often allows a plane to be developed cleanly between the two and the underlying bladder muscle so that a rubber drain can be passed around them to elevate them as a unit, making the more difficult distal dissection easier. This approach especially facilitates dissection when the ureterocele extends into the urethra, because if it is not fully excised a residual lip may act as an obstructing valve. In these instances, the bladder neck must be carefully reconstructed.

Our preference for ureteral reimplantation has been to bring the ureter across the trigone or posterior wall of the bladder, away from the previous dissection and sutured mucosa if possible. In many instances, tapering of one or both ureters is necessary prior to reimplantation. If the upper pole is nonfunctional, the ureterocele is excised and the portion of the ipsilateral lower pole bordering the ureterocele is excised and then reconstructed over a catheter of appropriate size. If the upper pole is salvageable, the ureterocele is excised and both ureters are trimmed and tapered, preserving the blood supply through the common medial wall. When the ureter is not too dilated but is too large to reimplant without narrowing, a plication may be done rather than tapering. If the ureter is too short for adequate tunneling, as happens occasionally, a bladder psoas hitch is a useful adjunct to obtain a flat base to make an appropriately long reimplantation. Finally, special attention must be paid to the contralateral ureter in these cases. This ureter should be intubated at the onset of ureterocele surgery, as it is easy to lose sight of it in the edematous, oozing, bladder mucosa. Additionally, these ureters are often found to reflux postoperatively even when they were reflux-free preoperatively, since their normal trigonal attachments are disrupted in dissecting the ureterocele. When doubt exists regarding adequacy of their fixation and antireflux tunnel length, we do not hesitate to reimplant the contralateral ureter as well.

Chapter 57

Endoscopic Ureterocele Decompression

Assess the urinary tract by ultrasound, voiding cystography, and renal scanning. Look for bladder dysfunction, typically a high-capacity bladder with incomplete emptying.

As an emergency measure for the child who is septic, incise the ureterocele endoscopically as described in the next section.

Alternatively, decompress the upper moiety percutaneously, drain the lower moiety by urethral catheter, or do both. When incision proves inadequate as shown by ultrasonography and by persistence of symptoms, turn to percutaneous drainage of the upper moiety. For severely ill children, consider pyelostomy or ureterostomy. For azotemia secondary to bladder outlet obstruction, with or without prolapse of the ureterocele, endoscopic puncture may be required.

ENDOSCOPIC INCISION OF URETEROCELE

As treatment, endoscopic incision is an effective solution for a single-system intravesical ureterocele and may even be a permanent one. For duplex systems, incision reduces hydronephrosis and usually obviates the need for heminephrectomy, but for most children, open surgery will be required.

Intravesical Ureterocele

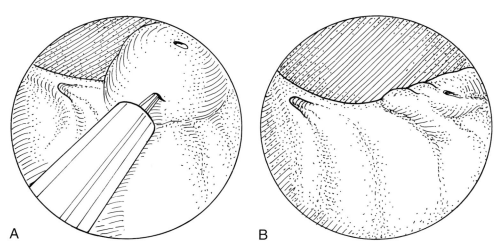

FIGURE 57-1. A, Have the bladder fairly empty to avoid obliterating the ureterocele, incise it with a cold knife or with electrocautery, or simply puncture it with an active stilet passed in a ureteral catheter through an endoscope. **B,** Make the puncture low on the front of the ureterocele wall to prevent leaving an obstructing lip of tissue; do not leave an antireflux flap valve, which is formed from the wall of the collapsed ureterocele. Such decompression at the least may obviate the need for tailoring when further surgery is performed. One complication is the onset of vesicoureteral reflux.

Ectopic Duplex Ureterocele

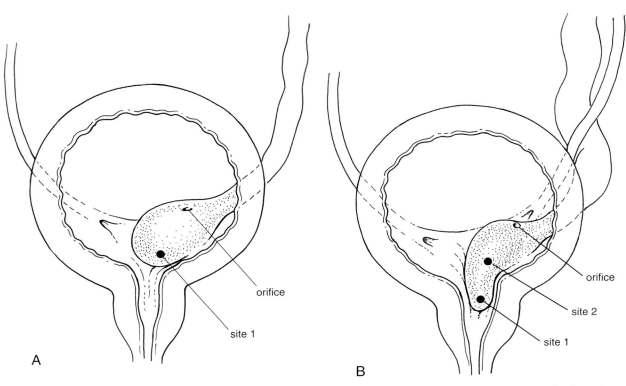

FIGURE 57-2. A, Make a single puncture (site 1) in the intravesical portion of the ectopic ureterocele, just above the posterior lip of the bladder neck (not down in the urethra), using a 3-F Bugbee electrode. Apply cutting current set high enough to ensure a clean puncture all the way through the wall of the ureterocele. Press on the flank to see that urine does efflux. About 1 case in 10, usually those with a thick-walled ureterocele, will subsequently require a second puncture. Make that puncture larger. Realize that in the more common thin-walled ureterocele, making too large a puncture may foster reflux, especially in duplex systems. **B,** If after the initial (site 1) puncture a flap of ectopic ureterocele tissue remains as a potential obstructing sail in the urethra, perform a second puncture in the proximal aspect (site 2) of the ectopic ureterocele.

DOUGLAS COPLEN

There are two important issues in the management of ureteroceles. First, obstruction is a major predisposition to infection and should be relieved. Second, concomitant reflux is common and may also be associated with recurrent urinary infections. The reflux and/or infections may be clinical indications for bladder level reconstruction. Several approaches, including endoscopic decompression, staged reconstruction, or ureterocele excision and complete reconstruction, have been used to accomplish these goals.

Ureterocele incision is a minimally invasive technique that can be performed on an outpatient basis. Incision has historically not been popular because it has often failed as a definitive procedure. Regardless of ureterocele type or position, incision or puncture effectively decompresses the ureterocele. Because of its low morbidity, endoscopic incision that attempts to avoid reflux is the foremost procedure to consider in neonates. I usually use a 3-F electrode and a pure cutting current. The thermal injury often results in a much larger opening, so avoid the temptation to make a larger incision. The older method of complete unroofing of the ureterocele should be discouraged, although this may be used as a temporizing procedure in the septic patient.

Single-system and duplex ureteroceles are entirely different clinical entities. The single system usually has excellent function, has less hydronephrosis, is almost always intravesical, and may have indeterminate obstruction on furosemide scintigraphy. Some can be managed expectantly in a fashion similar to the nonobstructed megaureter. If obstruction is present, the single-system ureterocele is best managed endoscopically with relief of obstruction without causing reflux nearly 100% of the time. Open reconstruction is rarely required in this group of patients. Once a postincision ultrasound confirms decompression, restenosis is unlikely. Repeat incision after an immediate or delayed failure is usually efficacious.

Outcomes after incision of duplex intravesical ureteroceles are also very good. This is most likely related to a more normal trigone. After incision there is sufficient detrusor support to create a flap-valve mechanism that gives a low incidence of postincision reflux. Duplex intravesical ureteroceles are much less common than ectopic ones.

When the ureterocele is ectopic, incision successfully relieves the obstruction, but it is a definitive treatment less than 50% of the time. Because the detrusor muscle is deficient the incidence of iatrogenic reflux approaches 50%. It is unlikely that this reflux will resolve. In addition, most ectopic ureteroceles are associated with vesicoureteral reflux in the other moieties that resolves less than 50% of the time. While the presence of reflux is not an absolute indication for a reimplant, ureterocele excision and bladder level reconstruction are frequently subsequently performed in these children.

Many question the benefit of incision in ectopic ureteroceles since it is a definitive procedure in a minority of patients. Most series show a reduced rate of partial nephrectomy and facilitated lower-tract reconstruction after endoscopic incision. The ureter decreases in caliber, and tapering or imbrication is rarely required if bladder level reconstruction is indicated. The indications for bladder level reconstruction decrease if it is accepted that a nonfunctioning, nondilated renal pole with no reflux can safely be left in situ.

Chapter 58

Psoas Hitch Procedure

This operation is useful in children in conjunction with urinary tract reconstruction after diversion when combined with transureteroureterostomy and primary reimplantation, and also in children with persistent reflux or obstruction after ureteroneocystostomy, or after loss of the distal ureter.

Estimate the capacity of the bladder to be sure it is sufficiently large and compliant. Provide antibiotic coverage.

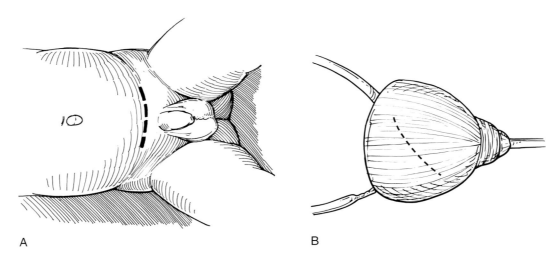

A   B

FIGURE 58-1. Position: Supine. Place the child in the frog-legged position. The supine position is better for adolescents, who are liable to get anteromedial thigh pain with paresthesia. Incision: Either a lower midline (see Chapter 62) or a lower transverse (see Chapter 63) incision (as shown) is suitable, in part depending on the position of previous incisions.

Mobilize the peritoneum medially. In boys, free the vas; in girls, the round ligament may be divided. Incise the peritoneal reflection on the dome of the bladder and close the defect with a running, plain chromic catgut suture. Take care when dissecting the peritoneum off the dome that the underlying bladder wall is not overthinned; instilling saline solution in the subperitoneal connective tissue will help this dissection. Follow the obliterated hypogastric artery down to the superior vesical pedicle. Divide the pedicle and ligate the vascular stump with a 2-0 synthetic absorbable suture. Dissect and excise the diseased segment of the ureter. Place a fine traction suture in the free end and ligate the stump with a 2-0 synthetic absorbable suture. Note: It may be necessary for mobility to divide the superior vesical pedicle on the opposite side. Alternatively, especially in secondary operations, open the peritoneum and mobilize the ureter extravesically while preserving its blood supply.

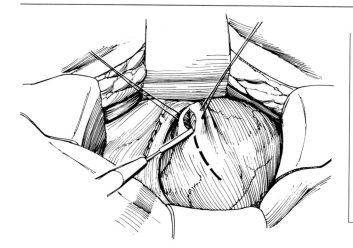

FIGURE 58-2. Place two stay sutures just above the midpoint of the anterior bladder wall and open the bladder near its equator semiobliquely between them with the cutting current (note the line of the incision in the insert in Fig. 58-1B). Direct this incision to cut across the middle of the anterior wall at the level of its maximum diameter, extending it a little more than halfway around the bladder.

When the incision is closed vertically, the anterior wall of the bladder will be elongated somewhat more than half of the maximum circumference of the bladder. The apex of the bladder can now be lifted above the iliac vessels, as high as with the Boari bladder flap (see Chapter 59).

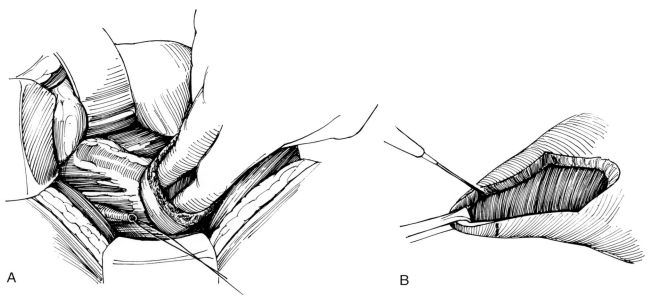

A   B

FIGURE 58-3. A, Insert one or two fingers into the fundus of the bladder and elevate it to meet the ureteral stump, thus converting the transverse incision into a vertical one. **B,** To obtain additional length, incise the margins of the elongated incision laterally.

FIGURE 58-4. If the bladder will still not reach the end of the ureter allowing for a 3-cm overlap for the anastomosis, go to the contralateral side. Dissect the peritoneum and connective tissue from the pelvic wall and from the lateral wall of the bladder to and, if necessary, including the superior vesical pedicle, which can be clamped and ligated with a 2-0 synthetic absorbable suture.

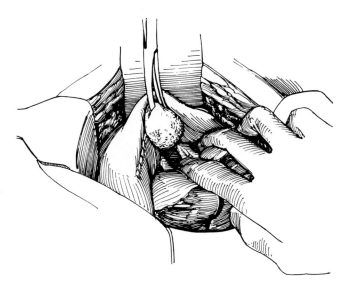

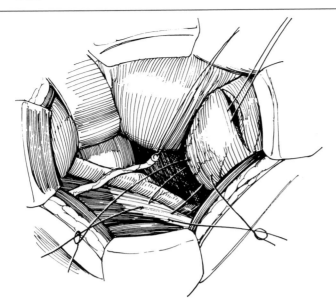

FIGURE 58-5. Insert two fingers into the bladder and hold it without tension against the tendinous portion of the psoas minor muscle to determine where the ureter should enter. Place two heavy traction sutures into the bladder wall and the tendon to stabilize the site during implantation of the ureter.

FIGURE 58-6. Ureteroneocystostomy (see Chapter 49): From within the bladder, incise the mucosa transversely at the proposed site of the new meatus. Tunnel distally under it for 3 cm with Lahey scissors. Invert the scissors and pass the tips obliquely through the bladder wall. Push the connector end of an 8 F infant feeding tube over the scissor blades and draw the tube into the bladder. Tie the ureteral traction suture to the other end of the catheter and draw the ureter into the bladder. Trim the end of the ureter obliquely and hold it with a stay suture.

An alternative method for creating the hiatus: Insert a peanut dissector into the bladder wall where the new hiatus will be formed. With the cutting current, incise the wall from the outside against the dissector. Pass a clamp though the defect and draw the ureter in to check its position, and then withdraw the ureter and create a submucosal tunnel. If greater length is required, substitute a vertical Z-plasty for the semioblique equatorial incision.

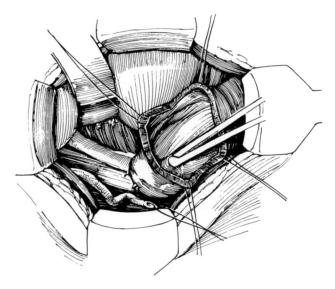

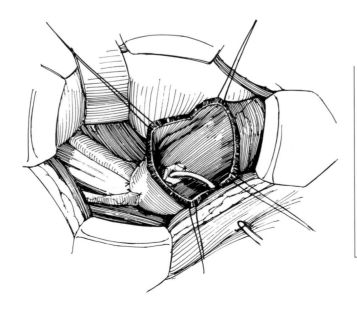

FIGURE 58-7. Place one 4-0 synthetic absorbable suture deeply into the bladder wall, and then pass it out through the tip of the ureter. Complete the anastomosis with four or five interrupted sutures that include the vesical mucosa plus half the thickness of the ureteral wall. If the bladder cannot be elevated high enough, resort to a direct (refluxing) anastomosis.

Insert an 8-F infant feeding tube to the renal pelvis as a stent, and bring the other end through the wall of the bladder and the body wall through a stab wound. Alternatively, insert a double-J stent. Suture the tube to the skin with #1 silk. Tack the ureteral adventitia to the bladder wall at the exit site with three or four interrupted 4-0 sutures.

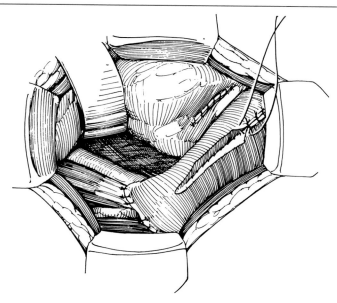

FIGURE 58-8. Elevate the bladder wall with one or two fingers and hold it against the psoas tendon 2 cm above the ureteral exit site. Place five or six 1-0 or 2-0 synthetic absorbable sutures to fasten the bladder to the psoas minor tendon, if it is present, and to the psoas muscle above and lateral to the iliac vessels. If the tendon is not developed, take deep bites in the muscle itself to anchor and prevent distraction of the ureteric reimplantation by contraction of the detrusor muscle. Take care not to include the trunk of the genitofemoral nerve. Tie the sutures loosely to avoid devitalizing the bladder wall. It is advisable to insert a suitable-size Malecot or balloon catheter into the bladder through a stab wound, especially if there is concern over healing.

If the peritoneum over the dome of the bladder has been opened, close it and check the closure. Close the bladder opening with a layer of running 3-0 plain catgut suture in the submucosa and with an interrupted layer of 2-0 synthetic absorbable suture in the muscularis and adventitia. Place a Penrose drain in the adjacent retrovesical area, and close the wound in layers. Remove the drains 2 or 3 days after drainage stops. Remove the stent in 1 week and obtain a cystogram. If that shows no extravasation, remove the suprapubic tube.

POSTOPERATIVE PROBLEMS

Prolonged urinary drainage: Obtain a cystogram. If a leak is found at the ureterovesical anastomosis, insert a double-J stent cystoscopically and place a urethral catheter to allow the fistula to heal. Obstruction to the ureter may result from constriction in the tunnel, stenosis at the ureteral orifice, or ureteral angulation during fixation of the bladder extension. Endoscopic insertion of a stent may correct the problem.

BRADLEY KROPP

Commentary by

The psoas hitch is an excellent procedure for all pediatric urologists to have in their armamentarium for reconstruction of the abnormal ureter. Fortunately, the procedure is not often required today; however, since fewer of these procedures are being performed, I think that it is important to highlight the key steps. First, it is imperative to get excellent mobilization of the peritoneum cephalad, exposing the pelvis and retroperitoneum. Second, the initial incision on the bladder must be transverse so the bladder can be elongated in a Heineke-Mikulicz fashion; therefore, if the surgeon feels intraoperatively that a psoas hitch may be required, it would be important to open the bladder in this transverse method. Third, the two tacking sutures medial and lateral to the newly chosen bladder hiatus need to be carefully and securely placed, as these will serve as the major points of stabilization of the bladder floor. Another key step would be to secure the ureteral adventitia to the extravesical portion of the hiatus, providing additional support to prevent ureteral retraction. Finally, it cannot be overemphasized that the femoral nerve is located just deep to the body of the psoas muscle; therefore, although secure "bites" of the psoas tendon and muscle need to be performed, bites that are too deep can cause permanent femoral nerve damage. Leg strength and sensation should be carefully documented pre- and postoperatively to ensure that no injury to the femoral nerve has occurred. Immediate reexploration and release of the hitch sutures should be performed to prevent permanent nerve damage.

DARIUS BAGLI

Various conditions related to trauma, extirpative surgery, reoperation, or complex reconstruction may necessitate additional mobilization of the bladder toward the ureter. Particularly in cases where ureteral length has been compromised, the psoas hitch may provide a tension-free ureterovesical anastomosis. Similarly, adequate tunnel length for reimplantation of a foreshortened ureter, or increased tunnel length requirements in the case of a widened ureter, may be facilitated by this technique.

It is particularly important to be cognizant of the genitofemoral or ilioinguinal nerves and not to mistake them for the tendon of the psoas muscle, or similarly entrap them during placement and tying of the sutures.

Since a primary function of the hitch is to prevent tension on a challenging ureterovesical anastomosis, it is logical to try to create the hitch first. The arguably more delicate tunneling and ureteral manipulation may then be carried out knowing how the bladder tissue will finally lie. Similarly, care must be taken to anticipate the configuration of the hitched bladder during filling, and avoid flexing the bladder in such a way that undue tension will be placed on the sutures in the psoas muscle during filling. Finally, if any tension exists on the hitch itself during its construction, this may increase the chance of the hitch coming apart during filling, and then transmitting immediate tension to the ureterovesical anastomosis, the very thing you aim to prevent by creating the hitch in the first place.

Chapter 59

Bladder Flap Repair

BOARI FLAP

Although a psoas hitch procedure is preferable to a flap (see Chapter 58), if more than 6 cm of additional length is required, make this bladder flap repair. Other alternatives are ureteroureterostomy (see Chapter 50), renal displacement, or renal autotransplantation (see Chapter 60). Replacement of the ureter with ileum is an alternative if an appreciable length is missing. Relative contraindications to bladder flap repair are a contracted bladder (try recycling), severe neurogenic bladder disease, and previous pelvic irradiation.

For bilateral ureteral injury, although a bladder flap may be adapted, consider ureteroureterostomy with a psoas hitch.

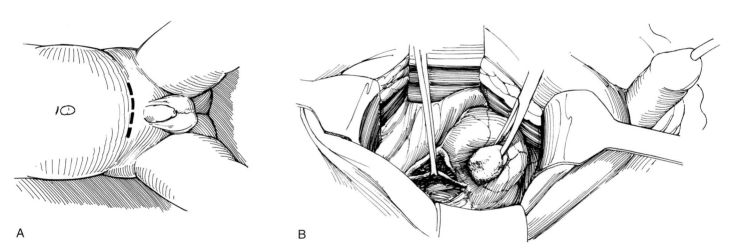

A   B

FIGURE 59-1. A, Position: Supine. Incision: (May be predetermined by the scars from previous operations that caused the destruction of the distal ureter.) Either a midline incision (see Chapter 62), which has the advantage that it may be extended upward if needed, or a transverse lower abdominal incision (see Chapter 63) is suitable. **B,** Mobilize the peritoneum medially, along with the vas deferens or round ligament, to expose the normal ureter above the defect, usually best identified at or above the level of the bifurcation of the common iliac artery. Encircle it with a Penrose drain, and then dissect it toward the bladder as far as practical.

Transperitoneal approach: For very scarred ureters, use this less desirable option to avoid dissection in the retroperitoneum with the accompanying high risk of injury to the iliac vein during the lateral mobilization of the peritoneum. Reflect the cecum or sigmoid colon medially to open the posterior peritoneum along the lateral gutter, and then dissect the ureter distally over the iliac vessels as far as the bladder.

To prepare the bladder flap, dissect the peritoneum from the posterior lateral surfaces of the bladder. Infiltrating the subperitoneal tissue with saline helps with this dissection. Isolate and divide the urachal remnant.

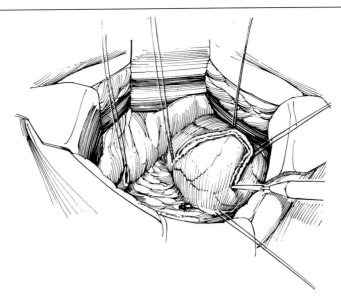

FIGURE 59-2. Excise the diseased portion of the ureter if practicable. Place a fine stay suture in the proximal, normal end for traction. Ligate the distal end. Mobilize the bladder fully, including division of both the superior and inferior vesical arteries on the opposite side. Try pulling the unopened bladder into a tube-shape onto the psoas muscle. At this point, it may be clear that a psoas hitch is all that is needed. If not, proceed with making the bladder flap. Fill the bladder and with an umbilical tape, measure the length of flap needed to extend from the posterior wall of the bladder to the proximal cut end of the ureter. Mark the outline of the flap with a marking pen.

Place two stay sutures in the fixed portion of the bladder at the proposed base of the flap. In the adolescent they must be placed at least 4 cm apart to provide a broad base. The longer the flap, the wider the base must be. Avoid incorporating scarred regions of the bladder, and handle the flap with care to avoid postoperative (obstructive) edema. Place two more stay sutures at the distance measured by the umbilical tape to mark the distal end of the flap. Site the flap transversely, or, if greater length is required, make an oblique or an S-shaped flap. Usually, on a distended bladder, 3 cm is enough length. At its distal end, make the width of the flap three times the diameter of the ureter to avoid constriction after tubularization. Now, outline the flap very superficially with weak coagulating current, which also serves to fulgurate surface vessels. Recheck the dimensions of the flap. (If a longer tube is needed, mark and cut a flap spiraled anteriorly and inferolaterally toward the contralateral bladder base.) Recheck the dimensions of the flap.

Cut across the distal end of the flap inside the stay sutures with the cutting current. Place two stay sutures in the corners of the proposed flap and cut the rest of it with the cutting current. Fulgurate bleeders as they are encountered (or clamp and ligate them with fine plain catgut ligatures). Inspect for vascularity and trim ischemic areas accordingly. Insert a 5-F infant feeding tube into the contralateral ureter.

FIGURE 59-3. The flap should now overlap the ureter by at least 3 cm to allow for a proper tunnel. If not, mobilize the ureter but leave its adventitia undisturbed because it now derives all of its blood supply from the renal pedicle. In some cases, omission of the tunnel by directly anastomosing the ureter to the bladder wall may be necessary. If the ureter is still too short, free the kidney inside Gerota's fascia and move it down to gain 4 or 5 cm in ureteral length. Avoid tension at all costs.

Dissect a subepithelial tunnel with Lahey scissors for a distance of 3 cm before bringing the tip of the scissors through the epithelium. Injection of saline subepithelially helps in formation of the tunnel. Install the broad end of an 8-F infant feeding tube (with the cap removed) on the tip of the scissors and draw the tube up through the tunnel.

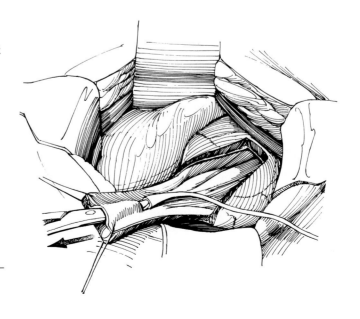

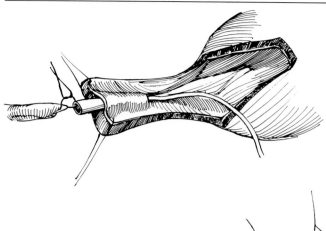

FIGURE 59-4. Attach the ureteral stay suture to the tube and draw the ureter down through the tunnel. Trim the ureter obliquely, and then spatulate it.

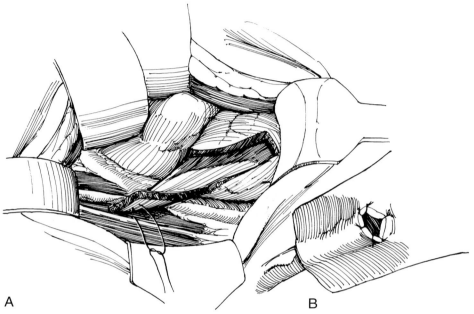

A   B

FIGURE 59-5. A, Fix the flap to the psoas minor tendon, avoiding the ilioinguinal and genitofemoral nerves. **B,** Anastomose the ureter accurately to the flap. To provide ureteral fixation, the most distal suture should include the vesical submucosa and muscularis. Complete the anastomosis with three or four more interrupted sutures to the vesical mucosa. Insert an infant feeding tube in the ureter as far as the renal pelvis. Tack it to the mucosa of the flap just distal to the anastomosis with 3-0 plain catgut. Bring the free end through a stab wound in the bladder and body wall and fix it at once to the skin with 2-0 silk. Place a Malecot or silicone balloon catheter through the opposite bladder wall, to exit via a stab wound.

FIGURE 59-6. Close the new tube and the bladder with a running 3-0 plain catgut suture. Place a second row of interrupted 3-0 plain catgut or synthetic absorbable sutures through the adventitia and muscularis, excluding the mucosa. Place a few sutures of 5-0 chromic catgut to approximate the end of the flap to the adventitia of the ureter. Hitch the bladder at the base of the tube to the psoas muscle with 3-0 chromic catgut sutures. Place Penrose drains retroperitoneally, to exit through a stab wound. (For the transperitoneal approach, close the peritoneum and drain the area extraperitoneally.) Remove the stent on the eighth postoperative day and the bladder catheter 2 days later if no drainage occurs.

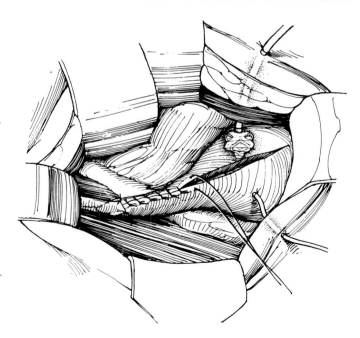

POSTOPERATIVE PROBLEMS

Injury to the opposite ureter should be considered if the patient has pain or low-grade fever. Perform intravenous urography or sonography and a stent ureterogram.

If urinary infection with a febrile reaction occurs on removal of the stent, give antibiotics. If the infection is severe and prolonged, use ultrasonography followed by percutaneous nephrostomy, because obstruction at the orifice must be bypassed. Leakage usually arises from the area of the bladder closure, not from the anastomosis. Leave the catheter indwelling until it stops. If it continues, make an intravenous urogram to locate the site. If the anastomosis is at fault, intubate it transurethrally and leave the stent in place 5 or 10 days. In a few difficult cases, an ileal ureter must be constructed or a nephrectomy done. Late stenosis from scarring can occur and requires revision or, if detected too late, nephrectomy.

ERIC KURZROCK

Commentary by

The Boari flap is a wonderful operation that should be in all urologists' armamentaria for penetrating trauma and iatrogenic ureteral injuries. As noted, the psoas hitch is almost always sufficient to reach the healthy portion of the ureter. For pediatric urologists, this operation is most often used for reimplant "cripples," or those who have had numerous ureteral surgeries. Fortunately, this is a very rare referral; usually, normal ureter can be found below the pelvic brim, allowing a simple psoas hitch. Presurgical imaging of the ureter and bladder is very important as the bladder incisions are different for a psoas hitch and a Boari flap.

In general, a transverse skin incision will not allow sufficient exposure of the mid-ureter. A Gibson or midline incision is best. A retroperitoneal approach is theoretically superior but rarely possible due to scarring from previous surgery or trauma. I do not necessarily ligate the contralateral vesical arteries. I no longer use Penrose drains for ureteral reimplantation or essentially any bladder surgery. Unlike a simple ureteral reimplant, drainage of the bladder for a few days is recommended, since the flap does not heal as fast and these patients tend to have inefficient voiding.

Chapter 60

Renal Autotransplantation

Autotransplantation is used in cases of extensive ureteral loss, severe renal trauma, and complicated renovascular disease. It avoids the mucus and electrolyte problems of the ileal ureter.

Make a long midline incision or a subcostal incision for freeing the kidney and a lower oblique extraperitoneal incision to expose the iliac artery and vein and implant kidney.

Dissect between the vena cava and aorta to pull the artery out from under the vena cava. To obtain as much length as possible, divide the renal artery as close to the aorta as possible. Similarly, divide the renal vein very close to the vena cava. Dissect the adrenal gland carefully from the kidney.

Preserve the pelvic and ureteral blood supply by avoiding the adventitia of the pelvis and ureter. Alternatively, a laparoscopic approach to detach the kidney from the artery and vena cava can be performed with the kidney delivered through the lower extraperitoneal incision for inspection prior to autotransplant.

Transfer the kidney to the iliac fossa and anastomose the renal vein to the iliac vein, and then anastomose the arteries. Restore ureteral continuity with ureteroneocystostomy, pyelovesicostomy with or without a bladder flap, or ureteroureterostomy. Provide an externalized stent to monitor renal function, being alert for vascular thrombosis and urinary extravasation.

DAVID A. HATCH

Commentary by

Renal autotransplantation is the optimal management option only in rare cases. Patients with extensive ureteral scarring, ureteral loss, or complex vascular problems may benefit from autotransplantation when the contralateral kidney is at risk for dysfunction. When the contralateral kidney has normal function, a nephrectomy may be the best option. Renal autotransplantation avoids the risks of mucus production, stone formation, infection, and stricture associated with replacement of the ureter with ileum. However, it carries its own set of potential complications, including thrombosis, stenosis, vascular leak, and urine leak.

As with kidney transplantation, adequacy of the vascular supply at the site of intended autotransplantation must be ensured prior to surgery. The iliac artery and vein are the most common vessels used in autotransplantation. In small children and those whose iliac vessels are not available, the lower aorta and vena cava may be used.

Management of urine drainage in autotransplantation can be challenging because loss of the ureter is often the indication for the surgery. In such cases, anastomosis of the renal pelvis directly to the bladder (pyelovesicostomy) or to a Boari flap may be best.

Chapter 61

Ventriculoureteral Shunt

After multiple failures from ventriculoperitoneal shunts, this shunt may be a useful alternative without the need for nephrectomy.

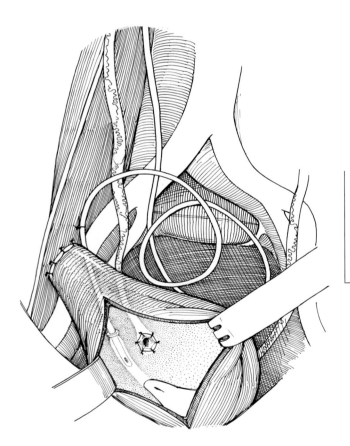

FIGURE 61-1. Divide the ureter 3 cm above the bladder. Insert the shunt tube into the ureteral stump until it is 1 cm short of the ureteral orifice. Fix both tube and ureter to the external bladder wall. Anastomose the ureter to the bladder by a combined intravesical and extravesical technique (see Chapter 37). If necessary, perform a psoas hitch (see Chapter 58). Consider a transureteroureterostomy (see Chapter 52) as an alternative.

Section 6

BLADDER

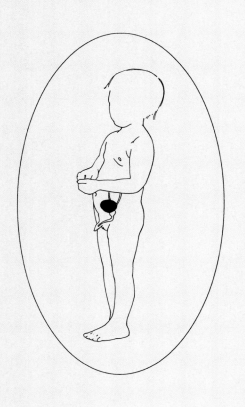

Part I

Approaches to the Bladder

Chapter 62

Lower Midline Extraperitoneal Incision

The lower midline extraperitoneal incision provides exposure of the lower ureter, bladder, and prostate. Elevating the pelvis may help in exposure in a child. An extended midline extraperitoneal incision can give simultaneous access to both upper and lower retroperitoneal organs.

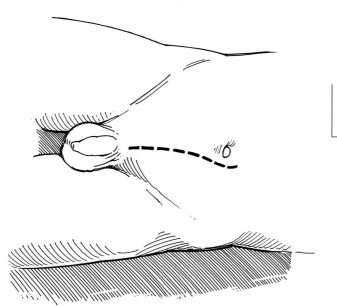

FIGURE 62-1. Incision: With the child supine and the buttocks over the kidney rest, make a midline paraumbilical incision, extending down over the symphysis pubis.

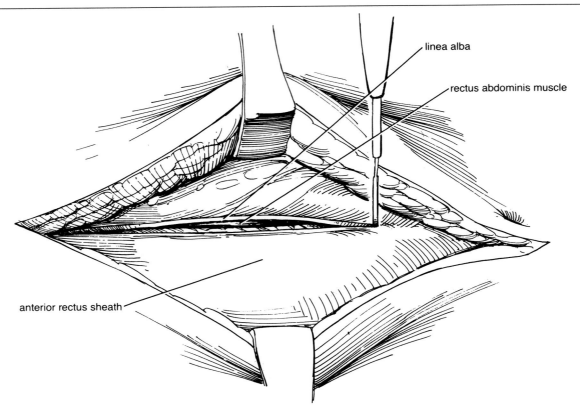

FIGURE 62-2. Incise the linea alba of the rectus fascia for a short distance. To be certain of the midline, look for the edge of the rectus muscle on one side or the other. Continue the incision well over the symphysis pubis to the insertion of the fascia. This will allow the incision to open at the lower hinge to the fullest extent.

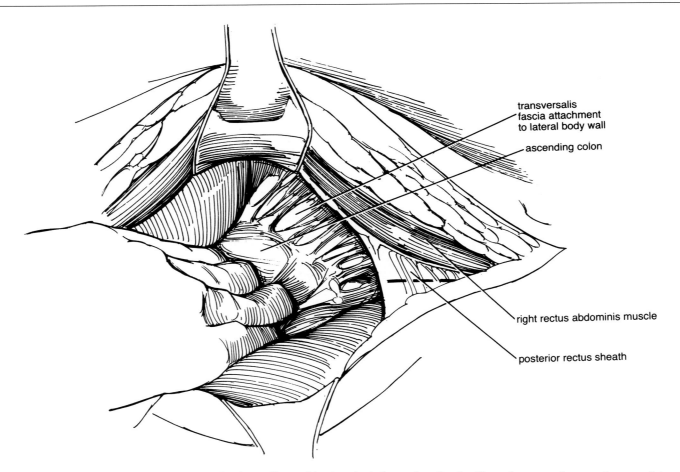

FIGURE 62-3. Retract the rectus muscles laterally and incise their investing fascia. Sharply open the contiguous thinned transversalis fascia laterally where it lies beneath the rectus muscle, to expose the retroperitoneal connective tissue.

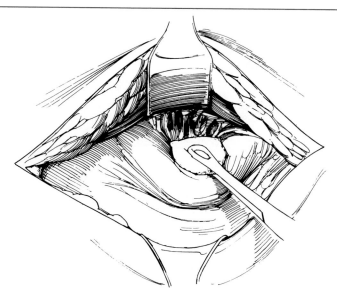

FIGURE 62-4. Dissect anterior to the retroperitoneal connective tissue inferiorly and laterally with sponge sticks, thus mobilizing the peritoneum medially, but stay deep to the inferior epigastric vessels.

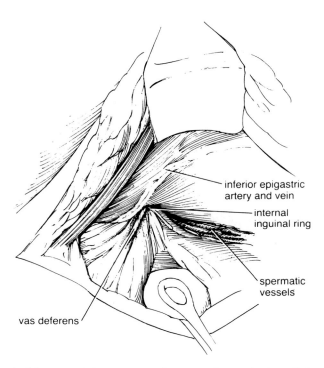

FIGURE 62-5. Follow the obliterated hypogastric artery to the superior vesical pedicle, if indicated, and follow the vas to the inguinal canal.

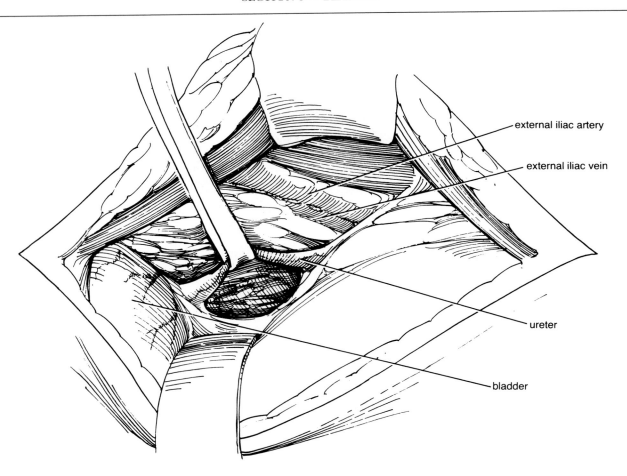

FIGURE 62-6. Identify the ureter attached to the peritoneum as it crosses the iliac vessels and encircle it with a small Penrose drain. If the urinary tract has been opened, bring a Penrose drain through a stab wound. Close the rectus fascia with a running or interrupted absorbable suture in infants or a nonabsorbable suture in adults and close the skin with a subcuticular 4-0 or 5-0 synthetic absorbable suture.

YOSHIYUKI SHIROYANAGI AND YUICHIRO YAMAZAKI

Commentary by

A major advantage of the infraumbilical midline incision with an extraperitoneal approach is the ability to extend the incision inferiorly. We have only used this incision for reconstruction of posterior urethral injuries with symphysiotomy or pubectomy.

In the case of symphysiotomy, we extend the incision to just above the base of the penis, and retropubic tissues are meticulously dissected to allow passage of a right-angle clamp behind the pubic bone.

Following the obliterated hypogastric artery allows easy identification of the ureter. To mobilize the obliterated hypogastric artery off the peritoneum, use a right-angle clamp to hug the border between the artery and peritoneum, as these structures are intimately related. The obliterated hypogastric artery is then ligated and cut, and followed proximally. The branching vessels of the obliterated hypogastric artery are carefully coagulated with bipolar electrocautery to avoid bleeding.

Commentary by MARC CAIN

I will generally open the skin to the left of the midline, using a scalpel to incise just through the dermis, and then complete the remainder of the incision using cutting current with a needle electrode. After opening the rectus fascia in the midline, the superficial transversalis fascia can be opened in the midline just above the bladder, and the lateral dissection described in Figure 62-4 can be performed by placing a finger just lateral to the bladder neck and sweeping gently in a superior fashion, which will minimize bothersome bleeding from a lateral dissection. Once the lateral space is opened, I usually trace the obliterated hypogastric artery to the ureter, and then place a handheld Deaver retractor and bluntly dissect the peritoneum superiorly along the psoas muscle to allow easy identification of the ureter and vas deferens.

If the bladder is opened I will usually use a three-layer closure to allow early (24 hours) removal of the Foley catheter. I do not routinely use postoperative drainage, but prefer closed suction drains (e.g., small, flat Jackson-Pratt drain) to minimize postoperative nursing care.

The midline abdominal incision provides excellent exposure for complicated reoperative procedures or radical cancer surgery, but for the more common extraperitoneal procedures that require just a bit more access to the superior retroperitoneal space I prefer a transverse low abdominal incision with suprafascial subcutaneous flaps raised superiorly and inferiorly with a midline vertical fascial incision. This provides a more cosmetic scar, but still allows access into the high retroperitoneal space.

Chapter 63

Lower Abdominal Transverse Incision

LOWER ABDOMINAL TRANSVERSE INCISION (PFANNENSTIEL)

The lower abdominal transverse incision is an incision useful for operations on the bladder and lower ureter, as well as other pelvic operations. An extended Pfannenstiel incision can be used for ileocytoplasty or with laparoscopic assistance.

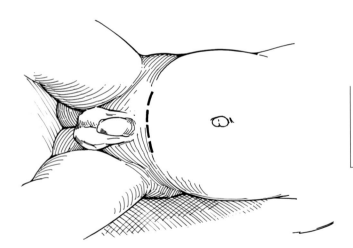

FIGURE 63-1. Incision: Make a symmetric, semilunar incision through a point one fingerbreadth above the symphysis pubis. Carry it down to the rectus sheath, but check the distance (one fingerbreadth) above the symphysis by palpation before incising the sheath.

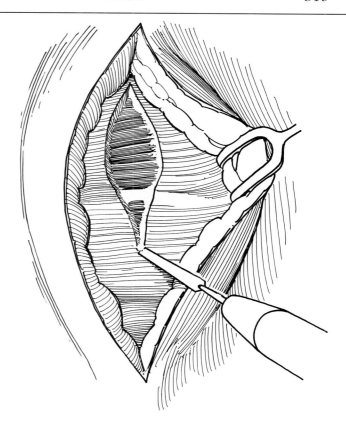

FIGURE 63-2. Incise the rectus sheath with a needle electrode in a semilunar arc to avoid the inguinal canals. Continue the incision laterally to divide some of the external and internal oblique and transversus abdominis aponeuroses and muscles at each extremity.

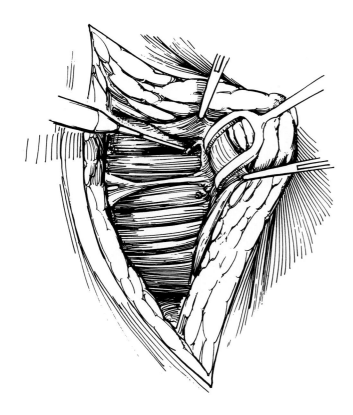

FIGURE 63-3. Grasp the upper edge of the rectus sheath with Kocher clamps, elevate it, and divide its midline attachment with the cutting current for at least 10 cm in the adolescent. Push down on the muscle with sponge sticks to free it from the sheath. Take care to avoid the two symmetric perforating branches of the inferior epigastric vessels, or coagulate and divide them.

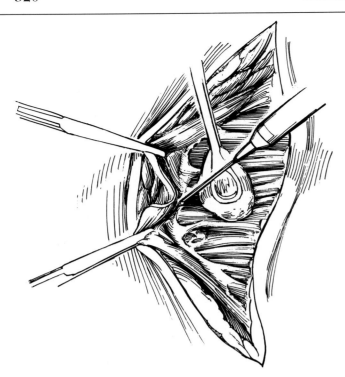

FIGURE 63-4. Free the lower flap similarly, elevating both pyramidalis muscles if they are well developed, or leave them attached to the rectus sheath.

FIGURE 63-5. Cut in the midline to enter between the rectus muscles and between the pyramidalis muscles by sharp incision of the transversalis fascia or by separation with a curved clamp until the preperitoneal and prevesical spaces are identified. The muscles may then be split with the fingers. If greater exposure is required, the tendinous insertions of the rectus muscle may be divided at the symphysis (Cherney incision), but the subsequent closure is less stable.

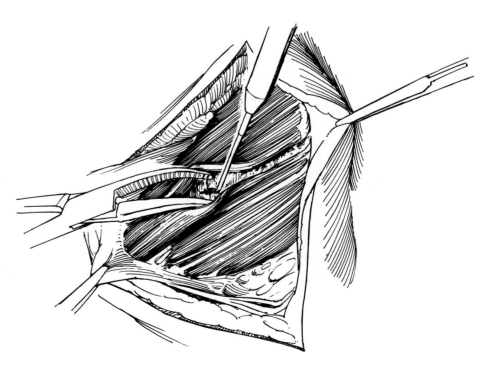

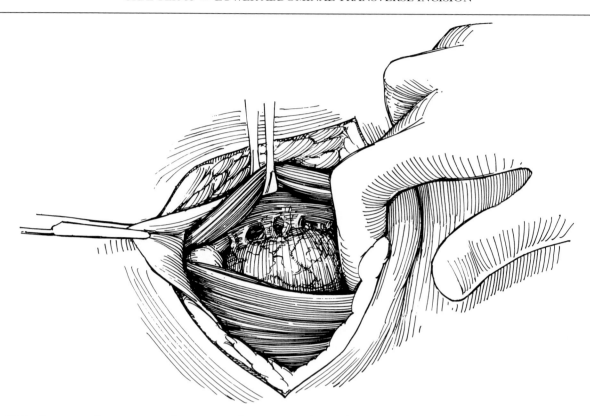

FIGURE 63-6. Separate the attenuated transversalis fascia in the midline to expose the anterior surface of the bladder and vesical neck. Closure begins with loose approximation of the rectus muscles and closure in layers of the transversus, internal, and, finally, external oblique aponeuroses.

PATRICK C. CARTWRIGHT

Commentary by

The lower abdominal transverse (Pfannenstiel) incision is highly useful in urology. Its advantages are that it is muscle-splitting, cosmetically appealing, and made along Langer's lines. It can be used for most bladder, bladder neck, and lower ureteral procedures, including ureteral reimplant, ureterocele/ectopic ureter repair, bladder neck reconstruction, bladder neck sling, lower ureterolithotomy, distal cutaneous ureterostomy, and autoaugmentation. An asymmetric Pfannenstiel incision can also be used as skin access for a vertical paramedian fascial incision to gain access to the distal ureter or the lateral perivesical space. I also prefer the Pfannenstiel incision (made slightly higher than usual) for transperitoneal exposure for bilateral, intra-abdominal testes, if the open route has been chosen over laparoscopy. While it is possible, I find this incision poorly suited for enterocystoplasty or Mitrofanoff exposure. The high or retrocecal appendix can be a huge exposure challenge via this incision. As well, if later exploration is required for complications, much wider mobilization and superior exposure is provided if the original incision was midline and can be reused.

For the standard Pfannenstiel approach, skin symmetry is ensured if the planned midline and corners are marked before incising. The corners must always swing superiorly as the incision follows Langer's lines. In children, the incision can be quite short (3 to 4 cm) and still give good intravesical exposure. It is also possible to make the skin incision just at the upper margin of the pubis; this allows it to be hidden later (for children) within pubic hair. If this is done, then the dissection through subcutaneous fat is simply angled slightly in a superior direction so that rectus fascia is encountered 1 cm above the pubis and incised at that level. In cases of reexploration via a prior Pfannenstiel incision, the choice at this point, when the fascia is reached, is whether to take the usual Pfannenstiel approach through the fascia or to dissect fat away from the anterior rectus muscle and make a linea alba midline incision. Either works equally well in my experience. In either case, if the superior dissection is carried one half to two thirds of the way from pubis to umbilicus, subsequent exposure is likely to be good. Also, exposure is best if the fascial incision is a bit more generous than the skin incision. A fixed retractor, such as a Bookwalter or Denis Browne ring retractor is very useful with this incision. I prefer the best inferior blade on the ring to be a rake with the prongs placed just anterior to the pubis.

Continued

Closure can be carried out easily in one layer in children, but will require two layers in adults. The two layers (lateral to the rectus edge) of fused lateral abdominal muscular fascia must be identified and both included in the closure if this is done in a single layer. The deeper of the two layers commonly withdraws beneath the more superficial one and must be sought out. A Penrose drain (if one is desired) may be brought out the center of the wound safely and external ureteral stents may be brought through the corners of the incision. Finally, if the fascial incision extends much more laterally than does the skin incision, any ureteral stent may need to come through fascia more medially (versus at the corner of the fascial opening) to avoid kinking as it courses between fascia and skin.

ADAM HITTELMAN

Commentary by

The lower abdominal transverse incision, or Pfannenstiel incision, as first described by Herman Johannes Pfannenstiel in 1900, provides excellent access to the lower abdomen and pelvis. Shared by general surgeons, gynecologists, and urologists, the so-called "bikini cut" is extremely versatile and has excellent cosmetic outcomes and better wound healing. It has been applied broadly across these surgical specialties and is commonly used in cesarean sections and other gynecologic and obstetric procedures and in abdominal explorations, including sigmoid resections, appendectomies, and hernia repairs. It also provides excellent access to the bladder, ureters, and prostate. In line with maintaining cosmetic benefit, it is commonly used as a portal for intact specimen extraction in laparoscopic surgeries. With puberty and the growth of pubic hair, this incision is often well concealed.

While the skin and fascia incisions are transverse, elevation of the anterior rectus fascia allows cranial and caudal exposure. Incision of the linea alba and lateral retraction of the rectus muscles avoids muscle division and further reduces postoperative pain. This approach has the reported benefit of a lower rate of incisional hernias, but recent studies describe an increased incidence of inguinal hernias. This is likely due to inadvertent injury or conformation changes of the inguinal canal when extending the incision laterally; incidence of this complication can be reduced with careful attention to incision and closure of the fascia. Neuroma formation and entrapment of the ilioinguinal or iliohypogastric nerves and resultant postoperative pain is another documented complication due to lateral extension of the incision, which can be reduced with prospective identification and preservation of these nerves. Modifications of the approach, including division of the tendinous rectus insertion as well as midline fascial incisions, can provide better exposure, although they do compromise the integrity of the closure and increase the risk of incisional hernia. If there is concern that in oncologic processes the disease has spread cranially, or if extensive pelvic dissection is required, alternative incisions should be considered.

Chapter 64

Gibson Incision

Access to the lower third of the ureter is possible through a variety of incisions. Because the ureter terminates near the midline, an approach that is as direct as the midline incision is through an oblique incision in the right or left lower quadrant—the Gibson incision. Currently, the primary role of the Gibson incision is for renal transplantation.

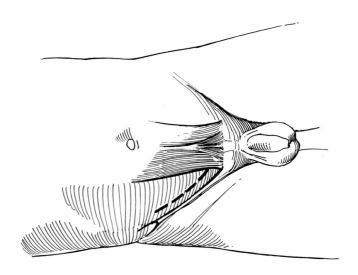

FIGURE 64-1. Position: Place the child supine in a partial Trendelenburg position. Incision: Make a hockey stick incision extending from 2 cm medial to the anterior superior iliac spine, running 0.5 cm above the inguinal fold, and ending at the border of the rectus muscle.

FIGURE 64-2. Divide the external oblique aponeurosis in the direction of its fibers.

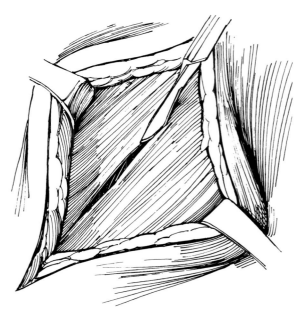

323

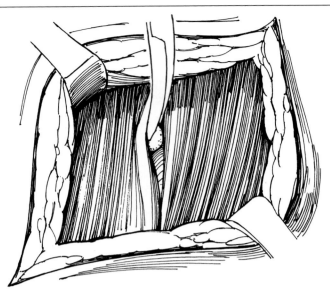

FIGURE 64-3. Separate the internal oblique muscle in the direction of its fibers, and open the transversus abdominis muscle layer. If greater exposure is required, the muscles may be divided.

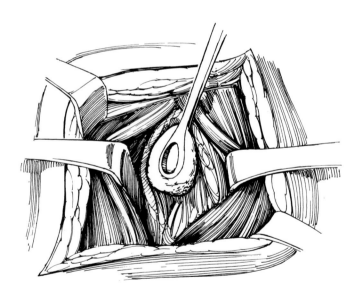

FIGURE 64-4. Draw the transversalis fascia medially (here it is a thin structure), carrying the peritoneum off of the vessels and the lateral body wall. Divide the residuum of the processus vaginalis at the internal ring (or the round ligament in girls) so that the peritoneum can be completely mobilized medially as the lateral subperitoneal spaces are opened and the iliac vessels exposed.

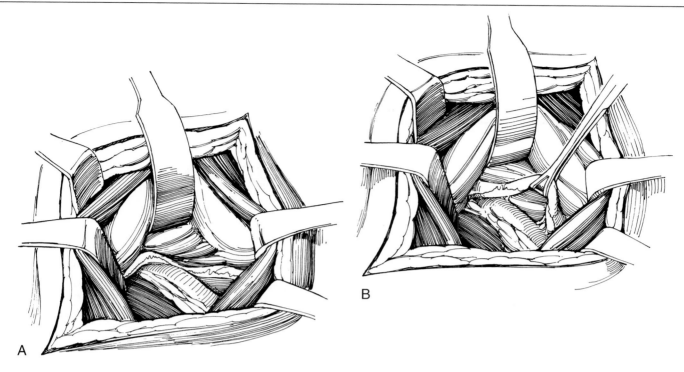

FIGURE 64-5. A, Identify the ureter against the peritoneum as it crosses the iliac vessels. **B,** Grasp the ureter in a Babcock clamp or encircle it with a Penrose drain for further dissection.

Commentary by

JULIA SPENCER BARTHOLD

The muscle-splitting Gibson incision was used in the past to approach the lower ureter, principally to remove calculi. With the advent of sophisticated ureteroscopy for calculi and laparoscopy for reconstructive procedures, such as ipsilateral ureter-oureterostomy, we rarely use this incision now. However, the extended Gibson incision with division of the muscles remains the standard for renal transplantation when the graft is to be placed extraperitoneally. The incision should be sufficiently large not only to gain vascular access but also to allow the comfortable placement of the graft. In small children this usually requires extension from the costal margin to the suprapubic area. This extended incision also permits the dissection of the vessels to above the aortic and caval bifurcations in order to place the vascular anastomosis in the most favorable position.

Commentary by
GERALD C. MINGIN

The advantage of the Gibson technique is that it allows the surgeon to extend the incision in a superior fashion up to the costal margin, providing additional exposure when necessary. This allows for easy access to the proximal ureter or kidney. In addition the technique may decrease any potential surgical complications by confining bleeding or a urine leak to the retroperitoneum. The inferior epigastric vessels rarely need to be divided.

Chapter 65

Mobilization of the Omentum

Plan to provide proper access, usually by using a midline incision, if you think an omental graft, wrap, or interposition might be needed. Tissue growth may also be stimulated because the omentum may possess an angiogenic factor and its rich lymphatic drainage absorbs debris and exudates that could form abscesses. Because of its good blood supply, it maintains its flexibility for protection of moving structures against fibrosis. Unfortunately, in children there may not be enough omentum to supply the need. A well-vascularized rectus muscle on a pedicle supplied by the inferior epigastric vessels may have to be substituted to fill large defects.

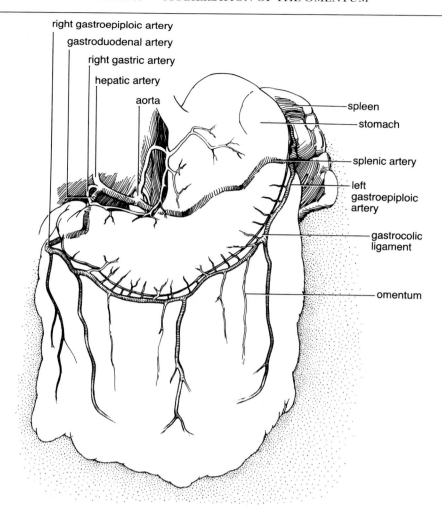

right gastroepiploic artery
gastroduodenal artery
right gastric artery
hepatic artery
aorta
spleen
stomach
splenic artery
left gastroepiploic artery
gastrocolic ligament
omentum

FIGURE 65-1. Mobilization of the omentum based on the *right* gastroepiploic vascular pedicle in a left-to-right fashion is preferred, because the right pedicle is larger and more caudal in origin than the pedicle on the left, which arises higher in the abdomen. Transilluminate the omentum. Note that the blood supply to the omentum comes from both sides. The larger right gastroepiploic artery is a branch of the gastroduodenal artery. The relatively small left gastroepiploic artery arises from terminal branching of the splenic artery. Together they form the gastroepiploic arterial arch. Because of this dual blood supply that allows division on the left, a long omental flap can be released after division of the short gastric branches to the arch.

Bear in mind important anatomic facts: (1) the larger right gastroepiploic branch of the gastroduodenal artery supplies two thirds to three quarters of the apron. Thus, for placement of the omentum into the pelvis, base it on the right gastroepiploic artery, unless it has been damaged by previous surgery; (2) in 1 case in 10, the gastroepiploic arcade from left to right is deficient, usually near the origin of the left gastroepiploic pedicle; (3) the often-illustrated arcade running across the lower margin of the apron is inconstant and of small caliber; (4) partial transverse division of the apron below the gastroepiploic arcade divides the vertical vessels and diminishes the circulation to the apron; and (5) the origin of the right artery is lower than the left, so a short apron mobilized on a full length of the gastroepiploic arcade will reach the pelvis. In one third of adolescents and adults, the lower margin of the omentum can be applied to a pelvic defect without mobilization. However, in these cases, the omentum should be separated from its natural adhesions to the transverse colon and mesocolic vessels to prevent its dislocation by postoperative abdominal distention. In another one third of cases, division of the left gastroepiploic artery is all that is needed. In the remaining cases, full mobilization on a right epiploic pedicle is required to achieve enough length.

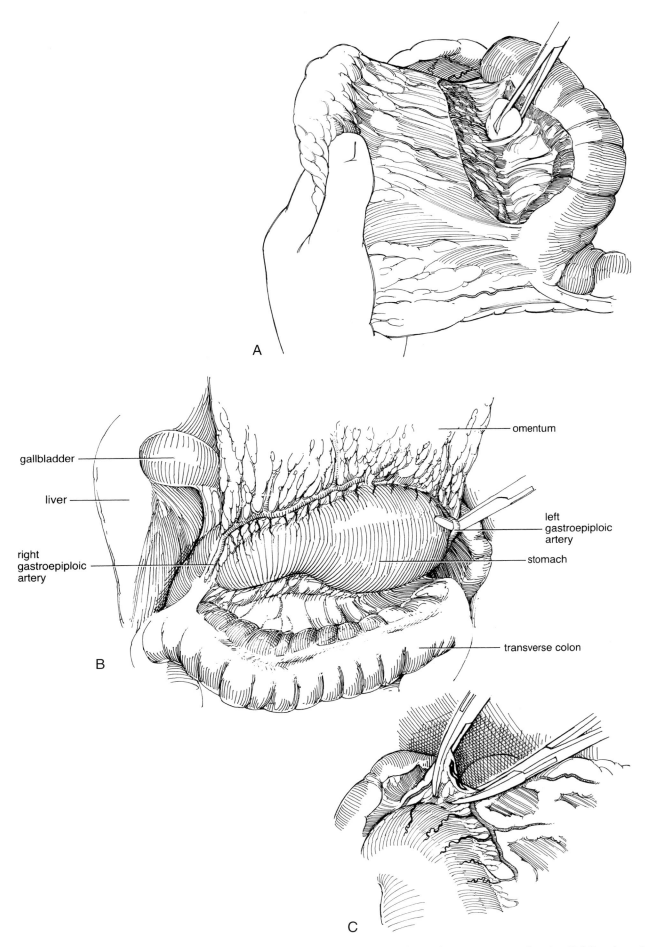

gallbladder

liver

right gastroepiploic artery

omentum

left gastroepiploic artery

stomach

transverse colon

A

B

C

FIGURE 65-2. **A,** Palpate the right gastroepiploic artery. Free the omentum from the transverse colon by dividing its relatively thin avascular connection. **B** and **C,** Trace the exposed gastroepiploic arch to the left to locate its connection with the ends of the splenic arterial branches. Divide and ligate its splenic origin. It is not necessary to divide it as high as is illustrated.

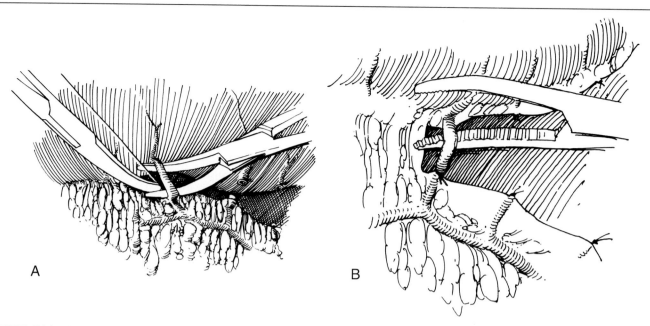

FIGURE 65-3. A, Pass a clamp through the omentum on each side of the first short gastric branch of the left gastroepiploic artery, elevate it, and draw a 4-0 synthetic absorbable suture under it (nonabsorbable sutures could foster infection and drainage in the recipient area). Tie the suture. **B**, Clamp and divide the artery close to the stomach, and then ligate the end of the vessel in the clamp. This technique of ligation avoids retraction of the proximal (omental) end that quickly produces a potentially harmful interstitial hematoma. An alternative, and safer, method is to pass and tie two sutures without clamping the vessel.

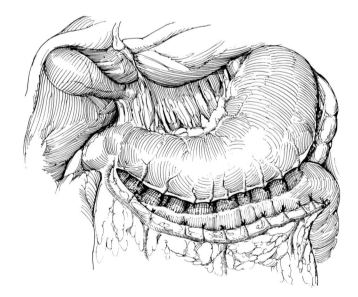

FIGURE 65-4. Continue dividing the remaining 20 or 30 branches individually to work up the gastroduodenal origin of the arch. Avoid mass ligation that will reduce the available length of the gastroepiploic arterial arch itself. An undivided branch is easily torn when the omentum is pulled into position. Preserve a 5- to 7-cm band of omentum at the right end intact to protect the vessels from avulsion.

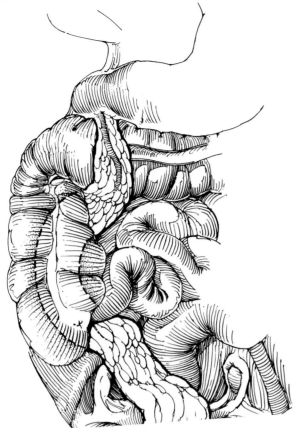

FIGURE 65-5. For use as graft or for interposition in the pelvis, mobilize the ascending colon and allow the omentum to lie behind its mesentery, in the paracolic gutter. Tack it in place with fine synthetic absorbable sutures. Perform an appendectomy, because appendicitis could jeopardize the omental pedicle. In a complicated case with an extensive graft, place a nasogastric tube into the exposed stomach. Use Penrose drains rather than suction drains, which tend to be clogged by the loose omental surface.

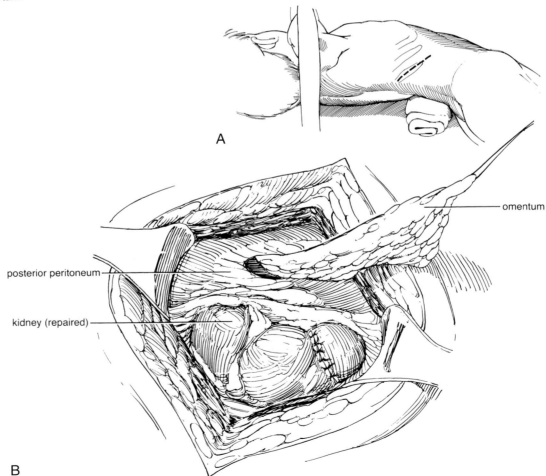

A

posterior peritoneum

kidney (repaired)

omentum

B

FIGURE 65-6. **A** and **B,** Omental wrap: For use as a wrap about the kidney or upper ureter, omental mobilization may not be necessary. It is easy to pass the omentum through a window in the colonic mesentery.

POSTOPERATIVE PROBLEMS

Infection, abscess, or persistent leakage at the site of the repair can occur as a result of technical errors that damage the blood supply during mobilization of the vascular pedicle, such as failure to make the tunnel behind the peritoneum large enough (which could compromise the omental blood supply) or failure to provide enough bulk of omentum to fill and cover. Ileus and abdominal distention can interfere with circulation to the graft. Gastric suction is important prophylactically; gastrostomy may be more humane.

RICHARD TURNER-WARWICK

Commentary by

The omental apron of children is not fully developed; consequently, it tends to be relatively short. Therefore, full mobilization of its vascular pedicle more often is required to enable it to reach the pelvis than it is in the adult. Even full mobilization may not be sufficient, so that alternative pedicled support tissue, such as the gracilis muscle or a rectus abdominis muscle supplied by the inferior epigastric vessels, may have to be used. Complex reconstructive operations in the pelvis involve (1) replacement of a deficient bulk of pelvic septal or perineal tissue; (2) vascular support of tissues compromised by previous surgery, infection, or irradiation; (3) closure of complex fistulas; and (4) preservation or restoration of the mobility of the urinary tract to allow it to perform its urodynamic function.

Proper access and planning are essential for complex reconstructive pelvic surgery—a midline abdominal wall incision is essential to enable the vascular pedicle of the omentum to be mobilized from the greater curvature of the stomach when this is necessary.

The "magic" of the omentum depends not only on its good blood supply but also on its excellent lymphatic drainage, which provides a physiologic "drain" for the macromolecular exudates and debris of an inflammatory response that otherwise can accumulate and result in abscess formation. In addition, unlike the fatty tissue of the retroperitoneal and retropubic areas, it retains its flexibility after an inflammatory response; consequently, it has a unique urodynamic value in preserving the functional mobility of urinary tract reconstructions when it is used as a supporting wrap for these.

In 30% of patients, the omental apron is long enough to reach the perineum without any mobilization of its vascular pedicle; however, it generally is advisable to separate its natural avascular adhesion to the transverse colon and mesocolic vessels to prevent its dislocation by postoperative gaseous distention of the bowel (see Fig. 65-1). In another 30% of cases, simple division of the left gastroepiploic vascular pedicle is sufficient to enable the omental apron to reach the pelvis.

When full-length mobilization of the omental pedicle is required to enable it to reach the pelvis, this should be based on the right gastroepiploic vessels (see Fig. 65-2). This is because the right gastroepiploic pedicle is larger than the left, and it directly supplies approximately three quarters of the omental apron. In addition, its origin from the gastroduodenal vessels is lower in the abdomen than that of the left gastroepiploic pedicle from the splenic vessels. Further, mobilization of the full length of a normal gastroepiploic arch from the greater curvature of the stomach enables the omentum to be redeployed in the pelvis, but whether the bulk of this is sufficient for the intended purpose depends on the actual size of the omentum apron. And, finally, the vertical branches of the gastroepiploic arch that supply the omental apron do not have the sizeable distal collateral arcade communications that are commonly illustrated in textbook diagrams; consequently, if the omentum is mobilized by horizontal incisions from the left side that transect its vertical vessels below the gastroepiploic arch, the extremity of its apron generally becomes imperfectly vascularized.

The mobilization of the full length of the main right gastroepiploic vascular pedicle of the omentum requires careful individual division of every one of its 20 to 30 branches to the stomach, using an absorbable ligature material and avoiding mass ligation, which can critically foreshorten the effective length of the gastroepiploic pedicle (see Fig. 65-3).

After full-length mobilization of the right gastroepiploic pedicle of the omentum, it generally is advisable to protect the extended route to the pelvis by mobilizing the ascending colon and laying its slender vessels behind it (see Fig. 65-4). A prophylactic appendectomy generally is advisable to avoid the possibility that the subsequent removal of the appendix as an emergency might jeopardize the omentum. Temporary gastric drainage generally is advisable after extensive mobilization of the right gastroepiploic omental pedicle from the stomach, and a temporary gastrostomy is a more humane procedure than a nasogastric tube. Because the fenestrations of a suction drain tend to become clogged by the supple mobilized omentum, a Penrose drain generally is preferable.

Postoperative problems resulting from the redeployment of the omentum are rare, provided the anatomic principles of the mobilization of its vascularization are carefully followed. It must be remembered that there is only one omentum, and its loss as a result of careless technique can be a disaster for a patient whose reconstruction partially depends on it.

A postoperative ileus lasting 1 or 2 days is not unusual after full-length mobilization of the gastroepiploic pedicle from the stomach; hence the advisability of nasogastric or temporary gastrostomy drainage. The stomach has an abundant blood supply, and deprivation of its gastroepiploic vascularization does not cause problems.

Omental adhesions in the peritoneal cavity are the natural result of the resolution of any localized intra-abdominal inflammation, but unlike direct bowel-to-bowel adhesions, they rarely cause intestinal obstruction.

SABURO TANIKAZE

Commentary by

The omental apron of children is not fully developed; for example, the lower part of the apron covers most of the intestines and more fat, and occasionally some lymph nodes are recognized at about 1 to 5 years of age. Therefore, full mobilization of its vascular pedicle, mostly dependent on right gastroepiploic vessels, is often required to enable it to reach the pelvis in young patients.

However, for surgery to the upper urinary tracts, it is easier to take a part of the omentum to the surgical fields. Although it may seldom be necessary in surgical practice, it is generally understood that adhesion of intestines beneath the wound is avoidable by covering with omentum. Omentum is effective in supporting the damaged tissue, preventing local infection as a vascular cover, or adding lymphatic drainage. For example, tucking in the omentum will be effective for drainage in resection of large exudative renal cyst. Omental coverage may be necessary in complex reconstructive operations with incorporation of intestines in the pelvis, such as augmentation of the bladder. Finally, omental incorporation is indispensable to the closure of recurrent fistulas between the urinary tract and the rectum or vagina.

A midline abdominal wall incision is essential to enable the vascular pedicle of omentum to be mobilized from the greater curvature of the stomach. The first step is to dissect the omentum from the transverse colon. Next, the full length of the main right gastroepiploic vascular pedicle of the omentum is freed with careful individual division of small branches to the stomach, using an absorbable suture or reliable electrical equipment (e.g., LigaSure) to avoid mass ligation, which can critically foreshorten the effective length of the gastroepiploic pedicle. When right gastroepiploic vessels and surrounding fatty tissue are used as a pedicle of a gastric segment to bring down as a gastrocystoplasty or gastric urinary reservoir, this meticulous ligation is required.

Chapter 66

Posterior Midline Approach to the Bladder Neck

This technique is particularly useful in the placement of an artificial sphincter (see Chapter 72) or bladder neck wrap (see Chapter 71).

FIGURE 66-1. After exposure of the anterior and lateral walls of the bladder, divide the urachus and free the fundus (dome) of the bladder from its peritoneal attachments, reflecting the peritoneum cephalad. Continue the dissection medially along that plane down the back wall of the bladder until the trigone is reached.

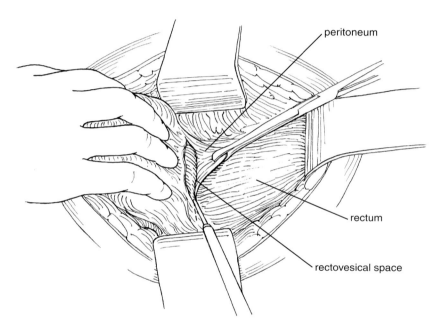

FIGURE 66-2. A sponge stick facilitates retraction of the rectum. The vas deferens can be seen entering just off the midline of the bladder. No attempt should be made to release the posterolateral attachments of the bladder.

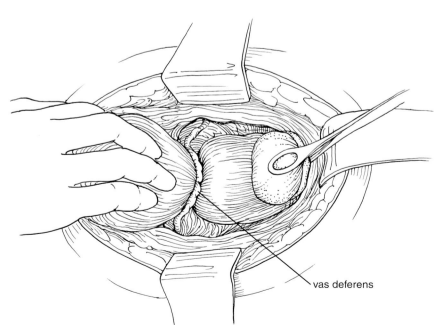

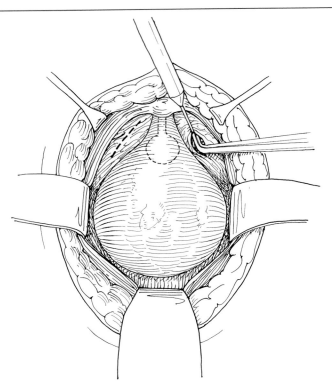

FIGURE 66-3. Once the dissection is carried inferior to the Foley balloon a right-angle clamp can be passed along each side of the bladder neck through the endopelvic fascia. With the fascia tented up by the clamp, the former is incised sufficiently with cautery to allow for the eventual placement of the sphincter cuff (or of the sling).

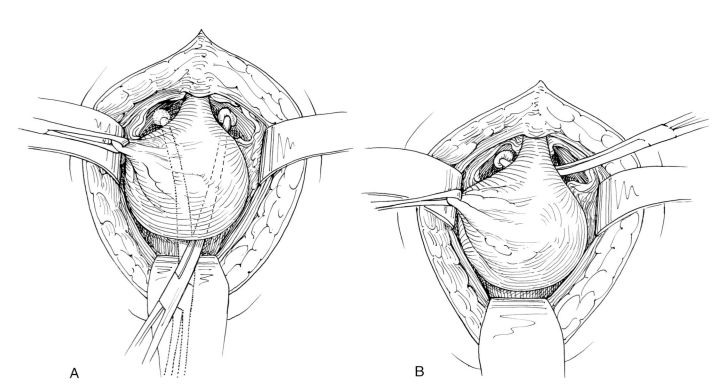

A   B

FIGURE 66-4. **A**, The endopelvic fascia is perforated inside out, thus avoiding any harm to the bladder wall, genital ducts, and rectum in males or vagina in females. **B**, A nonlatex tape or clamp is passed down one side and up the other side of the endopelvic fascia to encircle the bladder neck. An artificial sphincter or bladder neck procedure is then performed.

HENRI LOTTMAN

Commentary by

A blind dissection of the bladder neck may lead to injury of the bladder, genital ducts, and rectum in males or vagina in females; in case of an implantation of an artificial urinary sphincter, these injuries may lead to a straightforward failure or delayed rejection of the prosthesis consecutive to infection or bladder neck erosion. Also, during a blind dissection of the bladder neck, significant bleeding may occur; thus, sometimes it is necessary to open the bladder to facilitate the dissection. The posterior midline approach allows for an anatomic approach to the bladder neck, with excellent visual control of the surrounding structures, therefore minimizing the risk of erosion and bleeding. Also, it is easy and reproducible and primarily consists of separating medially the dome and posterior aspect of the bladder from the peritoneum, with no attempt to dissect the neurovascular bundles laterally. A natural plane is opened and the bladder blood and nerve supply are not compromised; as well, the use of electrocautery should be minimal during the dissection and there is no need to open the bladder except when a simultaneous bladder augmentation is needed. (If a ureteral reimplant is required, it can be performed extravesically). Only when the patient has had a previous bladder augmentation is this approach not easy, and under such circumstances, not superior to the classical blind dissection.

DUNCAN WILCOX

Commentary by

The initial separation of the peritoneum off the bladder is the most difficult. A stay stitch placed at the urachal remnant can help with countertraction. It is usually easier to start out lateral on the bladder to find the plane between the bladder and peritoneum. Once the plane has been identified and the dissection started, blunt dissection can be used quickly to move further posteriorly. When both sides have been dissected, the medial separation of peritoneum from bladder can be done with more ease. Laterally, bleeding can be encountered close to the insertion of the ureters and so care is required. This dissection is more difficult in patients with gross trabeculation, as the plane is less well defined.

A Foley catheter placed in the bladder with the balloon inflated and traction applied is a good way of identifying the location of the bladder neck. When the dissection has progressed inferior to the bladder neck, creating a space 360 degrees around the urethra is relatively straightforward. This technique has greatly simplified the placement of a sling, wrap, or sphincter cuff around the urethra.

Part II

Bladder Reconstruction

Chapter 67

Pubovaginal Sling

Test the child urodynamically to be sure that the principal cause of incontinence is an incompetent urethra, which is usually the result of multiple surgical attempts, pelvic trauma, or a neurologic defect. Be sure that leakage is not from detrusor muscle hyperactivity or only from vesicourethral malposition. Determine detrusor muscle contractility, because if it is absent, the child will require intermittent catheterization. For children with meningomyelocele with poor compliance or intractable, uninhibited contraction and incontinence, perform augmentation cystoplasty in addition to the sling procedure.

Exhaust medical approaches with alpha-adrenergic and anticholinergic medications. Caution the family about the possible need for intermittent catheterization, the persistence of detrusor muscle instability, as well as upper-tract damage and urinary tract infection.

Arrange for two surgeons for the procedure. Use a low lithotomy position; suspend the legs by the feet. Prep the lower abdomen and perineum, and in girls, prep and drape for access to the vagina. Place a balloon catheter in the bladder. One surgeon, the retropubic operator, stands on the left side of the child and the other, the perineal operator, between the child's legs.

FIGURE 67-1. Retropubic operator: Make a transverse
lower abdominal skin incision (see Chapter 63) and
expose the rectus sheath. Incise the sheath transversely
above the symphysis for 5 to 15 cm, depending on the
size of the child. Lift up both edges and separate them
from the rectus muscles superiorly and inferiorly, as is
usually done for this incision. Place a stay suture at each
end of the lower flap and cut a slightly fusiform strip of
fascia from it, the length determined by an estimation
of the distance around the urethra and through and
over the rectus muscle and fascia. The center of the strip
should be as wide as 2 cm, depending on the age of the
child, to provide broad urethral support. Cover it with
moist gauze, and put it aside. Alternatively, harvest the
strip of fascia through a midline skin incision by making
a vertical incision in the rectus fascia. It may be obtained
after the retropubic dissection.

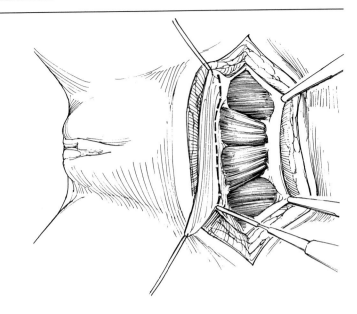

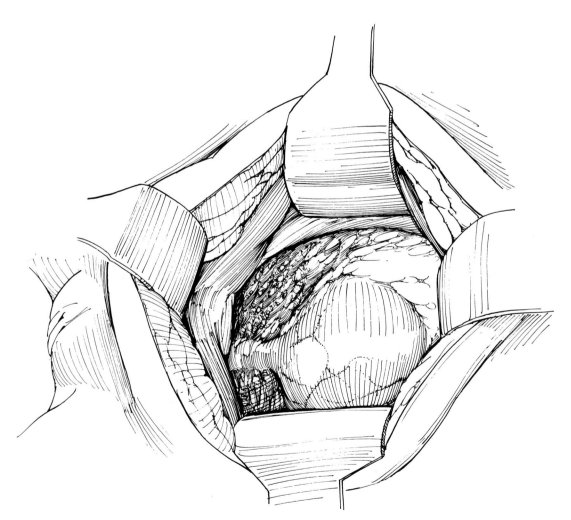

FIGURE 67-2. Bluntly and sharply, dissect the anterior bladder wall and urethra. Continue the dissection to the
endopelvic fascia of the pelvic floor. In difficult cases (e.g., after multiple procedures), detach the rectus muscles from
the symphysis for a short distance and dissect with the point of the scissors directly on the periosteum of the symphysis
pubis to its lower margin while depressing the bladder posteriorly. Opening the bladder at this point can facilitate the
dissection, but is usually not needed.

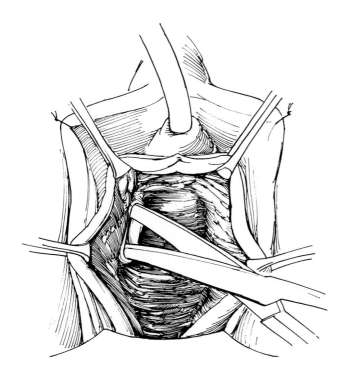

FIGURE 67-3. Perineal operator: Make a 2-cm vertical incision in the vagina, and dissect lateral to the urethra until the retropubic space is reached at the inferior margin of the pubic symphysis. Free only the vaginal epithelium, leaving the white paraurethral fascia behind. As an alternative, incise the pelvic floor and dissect with the fingers superiorly and laterally to develop the retropubic space. If not done earlier, open the bladder to help with orientation for creation of the tunnels for the sling and to allow detection of vesical injury.

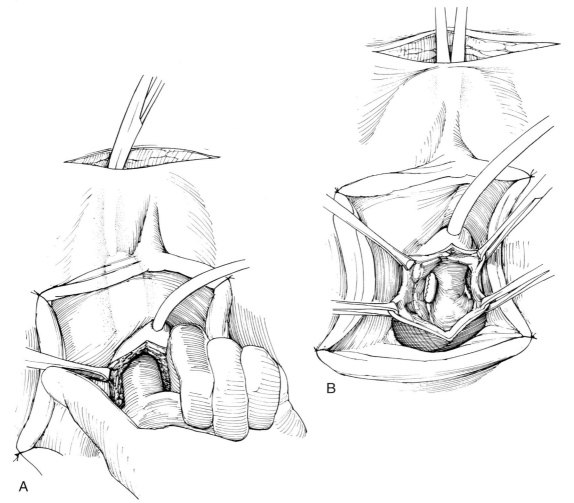

FIGURE 67-4. A and **B,** Retropubic operator: Free the urethra and insert the scissors lateral to it on both sides to make an opening in the pelvic floor at its attachment to the symphysis. Be sure to direct the points of the scissors laterally and superiorly toward the anterior superior iliac crest. Enlarge the opening in the same direction with the finger. Insert one finger of the left hand in the vagina. Grasp a curved clamp in the right hand with the concave side up and advance it down the right side from above, keeping the tip against the symphysis to avoid entering the bladder.

FIGURE 67-5. Grasp one end of the sling or its stay suture that is presented by the perineal operator and draw it retropubically into the upper wound. Spread the middle portion of the sling and tack it with an absorbable suture, smooth surface down, to the paraurethral tissues and the perineal fascia, to secure as broad a bearing as possible under the urethra. Repeat the procedure on the left side, passing the clamp down that side and drawing up the other end of the sling. Suture one end to the rectus fascia with multiple interrupted 2-0 or 3-0 nonabsorbable sutures.

Alternatively, pass a tonsil clamp through the belly of the rectus muscle on the right and draw the end of the strip through it and its fascia. On the left side, bring the other end of the strip through muscle and fascia similarly. Suture one end to the fascia with 2-0 or 3-0 nonabsorbable sutures, taking three bites in the fascial strip with the suture. Have the perineal operator close the incision in the vaginal mucosa before the retropubic operator tightens the sling. Alternatively, bring the strip through the fascia and muscle and suture one end of the strip over the other on top of the rectus fascia for added strength. Also suture the strip to the fascia at the point of exit. This allows the strip to have an ovoid shape, which keeps better tension on the urethra.

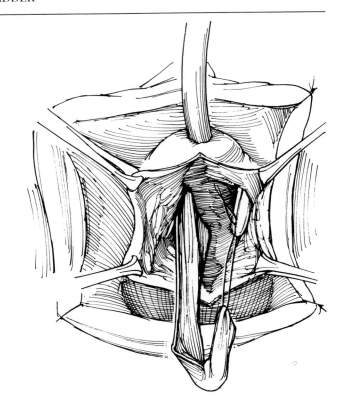

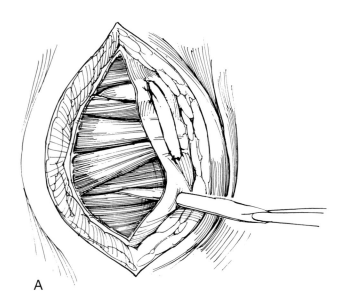

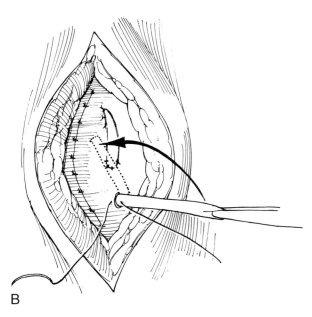

A

B

FIGURE 67-6. A, Draw on the other end of the sling until approximately 6 to 7 cm of water pressure is exerted on the urethra. This can be checked by endoscopic inspection or by profilometry. A good way to check is to insert an endoscope and increase sling tension to slightly compress the proximal urethra under the sling. **B,** Trim any excess from the sling, and suture the free end to the fascia with 2-0 or 3-0 nonabsorbable sutures. Another way to fix the sling is to place multiple sutures in each end, and then tie them together over Teflon bolsters. (Note: Obtaining correct tension requires considerable judgment because no exact criteria can be given.) Insert a catheter through the bladder wall, and close the bladder and suprapubic wound. Place a gauze or vaginal pack and then remove it with the catheter after 3 days; at this time, start intermittent catheterization if the child is unable to void.

POSTOPERATIVE PROBLEMS

Urinary retention is the greatest concern and usually results from too much tension at the urethrovesical junction. Straining to void only tightens the sling, so the child must learn to void by perineal relaxation with its associated reflex detrusor muscle contraction. The options are continued intermittent catheterization or removal of the fascial sutures (as a come-and-go procedure), placing dependence on the fibrosis that has developed. Expect one third of children to be able to void at least by 7 days, and one third within 3 months; the remainder will require longer-term intermittent catheterization. In one fourth of patients, uninhibited detrusor muscle contractions may persist postoperatively, but usually respond to anticholinergic medication.

Other problems that may be encountered are erosion of the sling into the urethra or bladder neck, obliterating the lumen or creating a fistula into the vagina, or compression of the urethra by the sling because of excessive scarring from previous procedures.

JULIAN WAN

Commentary by

The pubovaginal sling is an effective method of improving urinary continence in patients with a dysfunctional bladder neck and proximal urethra. It is particularly well suited for patients with intrinsic sphincter deficiency or those who have urethral hypermobility and who are quite active physically. Its application in children differs in several important ways. Children usually do not have hypermobility but can suffer from situations where the bladder neck or proximal urethra is wide open and dysfunctional. When present, this finding is often part of a more complex genitourinary problem such as spina bifida or other anomalies. Among otherwise normal adults the sling offers a way of improving resistance to surges in intravesical pressure while still allowing normal voiding. In children it allows a way of functionally closing off the urethra but retaining the patency of the urethra should catheterization be required.

Before the procedure, all patients should be evaluated with urodynamics. If available, fluorourodynamics should be considered, and a Valsalva leak point pressure test should be performed in addition to a cystometrogram to assess bladder compliance. All patients should be taught clean intermittent catheterization. For patients who are having the sling done as part of a more complex procedure, such as augmentation cystoplasty, this would be part of the standard preoperative preparation. Patients or their families should be able to reliably perform catheterization before the surgery. For patients who are otherwise neurologically normal they should be carefully counseled that an indeterminate period of retention may be possible.

Natural fascia is usually preferable where feasible. Synthetic materials carry a small but real risk of infection. The fascia strip does not necessarily need to be long enough to reach back up to the level as long as it clears the vagina. When tying down the crucial fascia stitch over the pledget, it is hard to know how much force to use. The knot needs to be snug and laid down squarely but not so tight that it creates ligature effect. The most common advice is to make the tension sufficient to stop easy urethral motion.

Spread out the sling against the urethra and make sure it is not twisted or folded and stays in the proper position. It may be necessary to place a fine (4-0 or 5-0) chromic suture through the sling into the periurethral tissue to help keep the sling flat and from slipping. When dissecting down through the endopelvic fascia stay close on the periosteum of the symphysis. Do not be afraid to feel the scissors or hemostat literally scrape up against the periosteum. The vaginal dissection can be trickier in children due to their smaller size. The usual vaginal speculum is sometimes too large to be of practical use. Nasal specula borrowed from our otolaryngology colleagues can be a useful addition for smaller children.

The incision to the vagina can be made easier by first infiltrating under the mucosa by injecting saline or lidocaine with epinephrine using a 26-gauge needle. An alternative to the vertical incision is to make an upside-down U-shape incision. Getting into the proper plane is an important part of the procedure. Use a sharp-tipped pair of scissors and try to get into the proper plane with the first few snips. The vaginal mucosa is often thicker than you would expect. It should be thick enough to avoid buttonholing the mucosa but not so deep as to disturb the well-vascularized muscle layers of the vagina.

Should there still be incontinence after the catheter is removed, be careful before immediately reconsidering further surgery. Allow sufficient time to pass so that the tissue edema has resolved. A deliberate, thorough reevaluation should be conducted, including repeat urodynamics.

STUART BAUER

The pubovaginal sling has proven to be a durable alternative to bladder neck reconstruction for the neurologically impaired bladder with intractable incontinence due to low bladder outlet resistance. The fascia is generally readily easy to harvest from the anterior abdominal wall but if that is insufficient there are a number of synthetic sources that seem to work as well, if not better, in some surgeons' hands.

The uncertainty involves deciding whether this procedure should be combined with bladder augmentation. Preoperatively, when bladder capacity is close to expected capacity for age ([30 + age] × 30 = expected bladder capacity in mL), detrusor muscle compliance is high throughout bladder filling (during the cystometrogram) in assessing the cause of the incontinence. The urethral resistance is low (less than 40 cm water) throughout, drops episodically, or diminishes gradually with bladder filling to below that level. In this situation, then, a stand-alone sling seems to be an ideal approach to solving the incontinence. In addition, a wide-open, low-lying bladder neck on voiding cystography is an additional parameter that sways us toward performing a fascial sling.

When the detrusor muscle pressure rises to above 20 cm water or there is overactivity with bladder filling, or the capacity is less than 50% of expected bladder capacity, then augmentation cystoplasty will be needed in addition to the sling to ensure a reservoir of adequate storage capacity and a continent individual.

The difficulty comes when the detrusor muscle changes its characteristics in response to a rise in bladder outlet resistance, by whatever means employed. It is almost impossible to predict that a "good" detrusor muscle will remain so postoperatively or that a small bladder of good compliance will not expand after bladder outlet surgery. Occluding the bladder outlet at the time a preoperative cystometrogram is done may help, but it is not always predictive. Approximately 30% to 40% of patients will need an augmentation after the sling has been inserted. In some reported series, a total of 75% to 80% of patients will need an augmentation to achieve dryness (with 30% to 40% having it done initially at the time of the sling and an additional 30% to 40% requiring it as a secondary procedure).

Another issue is how tight to make the sling to achieve continence. Part of the issue relates to whether the individual will catheterize the bladder through the urethra. If the patient has a continent, catheterizable stoma, the sling can be made as tight as possible to ensure no leakage from the urethra, but if the patient will be catheterizing the bladder through the native urethra, we generally secure the sling to the anterior abdominal wall fascia on one side and pull up tightly on the opposite side while an operative assistant tries to catheterize the bladder. If there is any difficulty, the tension is lowered somewhat and the assistant tries again. We like to create as much tension as possible but not so much tension that the patient cannot be catheterized. Once the sling is secured on both sides to the anterior abdominal wall fascia, we use Credé's maneuver on a three-quarters–filled bladder to see how much pressure is needed to produce leakage. Tension on the sling may have to be readjusted if leakage occurs fairly readily.

This technique has not resulted in any urethral erosions on a long-term basis. Our success in achieving continence has approached 75% in stand-alone slings and over 85% to 90% when performed in conjunction with an augmentation cystoplasty.

One potential issue encountered in females is making sure that the urethral meatus does not retract so much after the sling is in place that a "hypsopadiac" urethra is created, thus making it difficult for the individual to catheterize herself. The sling can be a useful adjunct in prepubertal boys but is less than ideal for postpubertal males. As a result we would caution its use in the latter.

Chapter 68

Trigonal Tubularization

Determine by urodynamic studies that the child's incontinence is due to low urethral closure pressure, usually associated with scarring and fixation of the urethra from previous operations, and that the detrusor muscle is compliant.

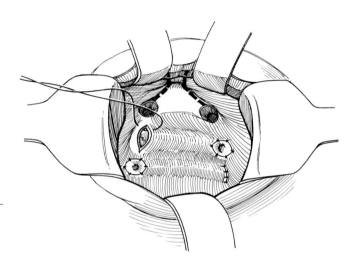

FIGURE 68-1. For exposure, proceed as described for vesical neck tubularization (see Chapter 69), but note that the more posterior aspects of the bladder and urethra need not be mobilized. Open the bladder in the midline and extend the incision into the deep urethra. Insert 5-F silicone catheters into the ureters. Mobilize the ureters extravesically, taking care to bring them under the vas or uterine vessels. Implant each ureter 3 to 4 cm more cephalad, using a tunnel technique. Transtrigonal implantation (see Chapter 39) is a good choice.

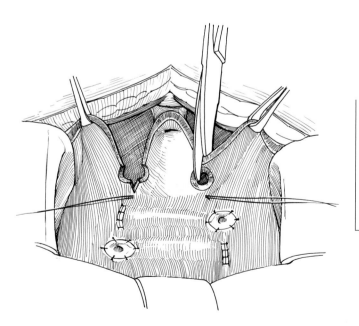

FIGURE 68-2. Place a stay suture in the anterior urethral wall at the apex of the initial cut. With curved scissors, divide the entire thickness of the urethra and bladder wall. Begin just lateral to the stay suture and continue through the site of the previous orifice and 1 to 2 cm beyond. The entire trigone must be tubularized. This leaves a posterior segment 1.5 to 2 cm wide and 4 to 5 cm long. Place an 8- or 10-F silicone catheter up through the urethra.

343

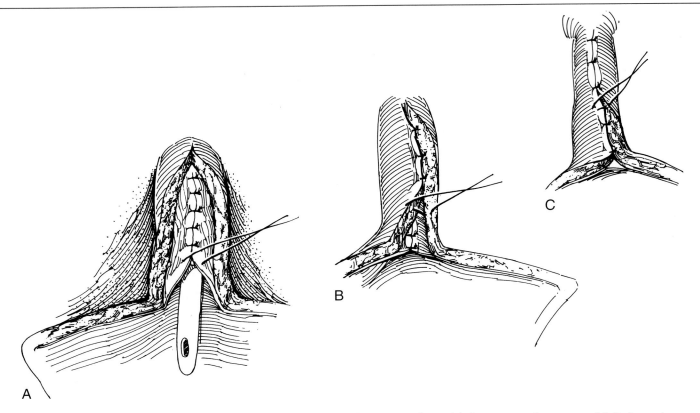

FIGURE 68-3. A, Approximate the mucosa of the edges of the neourethra with interrupted sutures of 5-0 chromic catgut, making the strip snug around the catheter. In fact, it is difficult to make it too tight. If placing the distal sutures is difficult, consider spreading the symphysis with a pediatric rib spreader. **B** and **C,** Imbricate the detrusor muscle in the neourethra by suturing one edge firmly to the undersurface of the opposite edge, and then lapping that edge back to the first side. If the resulting bladder capacity is small, consider augmentation followed by intermittent catheterization.

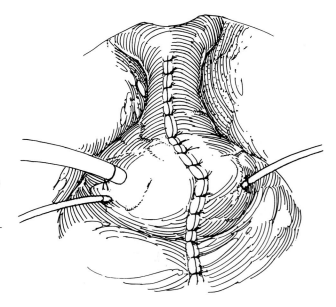

FIGURE 68-4. Draw an 18- or 20-F Malecot or balloon catheter through the bladder and body walls and fix it to the skin with a size 0 silk suture. Have the catheter in each ureter exit through a stab wound. An 8- or 10-F balloon catheter may be left as a urethral stent if desired. Close the bladder defect with a running 4-0 plain catgut submucosal suture, placing interrupted 3-0 or 4-0 chromic catgut sutures to the muscle and adventitia. Close the wound around a Penrose drain. Remove the stents in 1 week and the suprapubic tube in 2 weeks.

POSTOPERATIVE PROBLEMS

Urinary retention is rare; children who undergo this procedure seem able to void unless the bladder has been augmented. In that case, intermittent catheterization may be needed. Incontinence may persist and, if due to poor vesical compliance, requires vesical augmentation. If outlet resistance is low, a sling procedure or implantation of an artificial sphincter may be needed. Ureteral obstruction can occur as with any ureteroneocystostomy. Failure of the cystostomy site to close indicates stenosis in the new urethra.

GUY W. LEADBETTER, JR.

Commentary by

The following are some comments and tips gained from 25 years of experience with this operation: First, the procedure often is long and arduous and tests the surgeon's equanimity.

It is important to place sutures at the sites of the ureteral orifices to mark where the trigone is to be tubularized. It is essential for continence that the trigone be tubularized to make the new bladder neck.

In a child, splitting the symphyseal cartilage and spreading the symphysis with a pediatric rib spreader may give better exposure and room for suturing, but never spread an adult symphysis, as this will cause severe pain in the sacroiliac area postoperatively. Here it is better to remove a portion of symphysis if necessary. This trigonal flap method is contraindicated in adult males unless total prostatectomy has been done. Do not remove dog-ear flaps from the bladder after the urethral bladder incision has been made, as this would cause a decrease in bladder capacity. When reimplanting the ureters, it is important to be certain that they are brought out from under the vas or uterine vessels. This then allows a straight entrance into the bladder. If this is not done, the ureters will be obstructed by the vas or vessels as the bladder fills.

Ureteral and suprapubic catheters are left in place for 7 to 14 days. This allows healing to occur in a urine-free field. I believe this prevents possible fibrosis or fistula formation, which may occur if urine should leak into the reconstructed bladder neck area.

Chapter 69

Vesical Neck Tubularization

Vesical neck tubularization is applicable for male or female epispadias, short urethras, and selected cases of high urogenital sinus or urethral trauma in both boys and girls. If reflux is present, use trigonal tubularization (see Chapter 68) instead.

Clear (or suppress) bacteriuria. Panendoscopy may show a treatable bladder neck stricture or residual obstruction. Cystometrography may show treatable detrusor muscle hyperreflexia. Children with hyperactive neurogenic dysfunction are not candidates for this operation, but those with compliant bladders do well if intermittently catheterized. The wall of an atonic bladder is not suitable material for a tube, nor is that of a bladder subjected to previous cystostomies and anterior incisions.

Position the patient supine with pelvis slightly elevated. Use a modified lithotomy position for girls, and the frog-legged position for infants. After prepping and draping, insert an 8- to 16-F, 5-mL balloon catheter and half fill the bladder. Use a lower midline extraperitoneal (see Chapter 62) or lower abdominal transverse (see Chapter 63) incision.

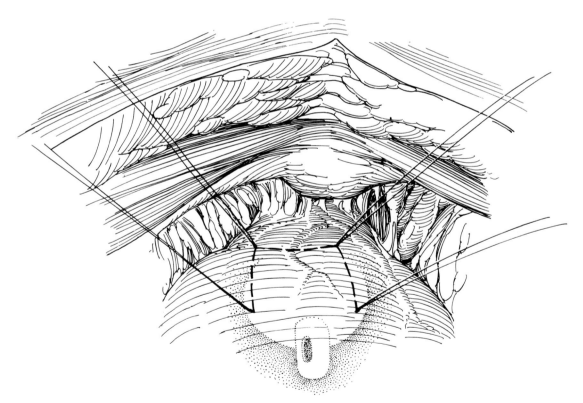

FIGURE 69-1. Reflect a limited area of the peritoneum from the anterior bladder surface. Dissect carefully in the space of Retzius to expose the proximal two thirds of the prostate in boys. In girls, expose the urethra to the level of the endopelvic fascia. In a girl who has had previous procedures, take care not to disturb the vessels on the anterior bladder wall.

Dissect laterally around the vesicourethral junction, identified by the balloon. Avoid the rectum or vagina and the neurovascular bundle. Outline a flap on the anterior surface of the bladder with four stay sutures, marking a 1-inch square beginning exactly at the internal meatus. The two distal sutures will be in the prostate (or urethra if the prostate has been removed) in boys and in the urethra in girls.

346

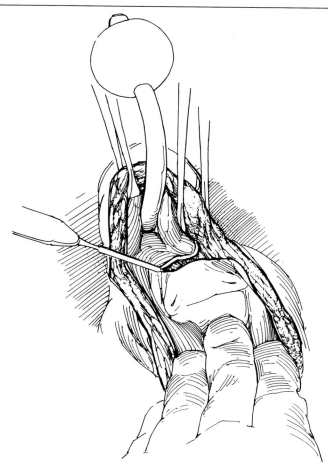

FIGURE 69-2. Make a full-thickness transverse incision across the bladder neck just below the distal sutures with the cutting current. Once inside the bladder, extend this incision laterally. Identify the trigone and ureteral orifices. Cut deeply enough at the apex of the trigone to expose the seminal vesicles and ampullae in boys, to allow the base of the bladder to slide upward for 1 or 2 cm.

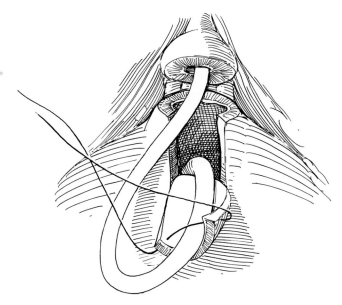

FIGURE 69-3. Make two parallel cuts running from the lower to the upper stay sutures. Reflect the flap upward. Insert a Malecot catheter through one side of the dome of the bladder as high as possible. Lead it out through a lower abdominal quadrant and anchor it to the skin with a silk suture. In boys, excise a wedge from the anterior surface of the prostate to narrow the opening. Roll the bladder flap into a tube around the balloon catheter. Suture the sides together with full-thickness stitches of 3-0 or 4-0 synthetic absorbable sutures. Be sure to catch the (retracted) middle layer of the detrusor muscle in each stitch. Start with one suture at the base of the flap and then one at the apex, and then fill in between them.

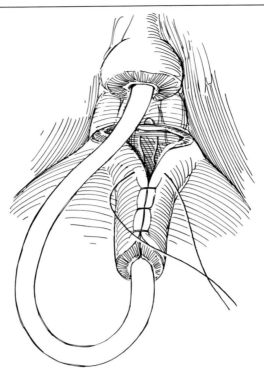

FIGURE 69-4. Attach the apex of the trigone to the base of the tube with a mattress stitch. Close the remainder of the defect in the bladder transversely.

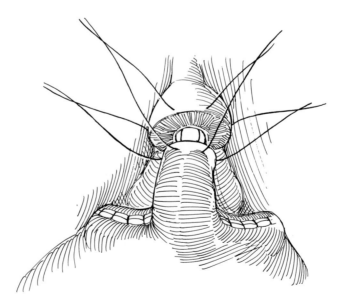

FIGURE 69-5. Anastomose the tube to the cut end of the urethra with five or six 3-0 or 4-0 synthetic absorbable sutures. First place all the sutures, and then pull them down and tie them successively. In boys, insert two 3-0 or 4-0 chromic catgut sutures into the anterior bladder wall close to the base of the tube and bring them through the lower rectus fascia. In girls, use sutures in the vaginal wall as for suprapubic vesical suspension.

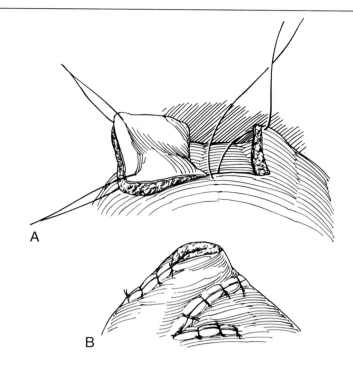

FIGURE 69-6. **A** and **B,** Alternative: Raise a transverse flap and suture it to the urethra in a corkscrew fashion (Flocks and Boldus). Place Penrose drains to the posterior suture line. Close the wound. Maintain cystostomy drainage for 3 to 4 weeks, and then test for residual urine before removing the tube.

POSTOPERATIVE PROBLEMS

Persistent incontinence can occur in children with noncompliant bladders or in those with tubes constructed from bladder wall of poor quality. A stricture can develop between the tube and the prostatic fossa, requiring internal urethrotomy. Postoperative instrumentation and catheterization may be difficult and must be done under direct vision.

Commentary by EMIL A. TANAGHO

Formation of an anterior bladder tube is a useful reconstructive procedure that enables regaining of continence in boys and girls born with epispadias. It also is beneficial in girls with a short urethra (significant hypospadias) or a high urogenital sinus with a short urethral segment, which might have to be mobilized independently of the urogenital sinus and brought down to the vaginal vestibule. The technique also can be used in cases of trauma in which the urethrovesical segment is disrupted, especially in girls, and in selected cases of flaccid neurogenic bladder.

The rationale of the procedure is to incorporate in a bladder flap the ventral condensation of circular fibers that extends above the internal meatus for approximately 1 inch on the anterior bladder wall. Normally, if this area has not been violated before by surgery or trauma, the condensation of circular fibers raised in a flap and turned around into a tube will have enough tonus to provide an occlusive effect and sphincteric function, which can replace a nonexistent or traumatized normal sphincteric segment.

Do not try to make the tube too long; it should be confined to the condensation of circular fibers in the anterior bladder wall; if this is less than an inch in length, the tube should be made shorter. It is the quality of the muscles in the tube rather than the length that is important. The tube should not be occlusive; it should be of adequate diameter to wrap easily around a 16-F catheter, although in pediatric cases we usually wrap it around a 10-F catheter. Bring the apex of the trigone to the base of the tube, and recreate the bladder neck configuration, providing for a sharp transition from the big cavity of the bladder

Continued

to the adequate lumen of the reconstructed tube. Extreme care should be taken in mobilizing the anterior bladder surface, keeping all the adventitial layers and blood vessels on it. During exposure, aim at the urethrovesical junction. Do not try to free too much of the anterior bladder wall, because this might interfere with the blood supply to the flap. Mark the flap with the bladder half distended before starting the incision to avoid losing orientation. The flap consistently looks narrower after it has been delineated and cut because of the contraction of the circular fibers in it; this is a good sign.

It is essential to handle the tissue with the utmost care to avoid devitalizing any of the critical, delicate muscle tissue. Accurate coaptation of epithelium to epithelium with full-thickness muscle-wall sutures is essential in both constructing the tube and establishing the anastomosis between the tube and the urethra. The procedure is suitable for both female and male patients. In cutting the bladder neck completely from the urethra, extreme care should be taken posteriorly not to enter the vaginal wall in girls and not to injure the seminal vesicle and vas in boys. However, a full-thickness cut into the bladder muscle wall is essential to permit the bladder to slide upward.

Closure of the rest of the bladder will leave two small dog-ear flaps; do not attempt to smooth these, because they will round themselves and become absorbed into the bladder cavity with time to provide additional capacity. If there is a midline incision in the bladder from a previous cystostomy and if conditions are favorable, a one-sided tube can be used; the site of the midline incision can be one lateral margin, and the flap can be taken more from one side. Extensive previous surgery on the anterior bladder wall will doom the operation to failure. Proper suspension and support should be provided without putting tension on the tube and on the suture line between it and the urethra. Mobilize the bladder base and trigone upward to prevent formation of a sharp posterior angle, which can be obstructive. Suprapubic drainage should be adequate for at least 3 weeks and tested for adequate voiding with minimal residual urine before removing the suprapubic tube. Temporary stenting of the reconstructed tube and site of anastomosis by urethral catheter is desirable for 10 days.

In selected patients with a flaccid neurogenic bladder, a tube also can be most effective. Its purpose is not to act as a sphincter but to provide resistance to permit continence between intermittent catheterization. Emphasis is on supporting the tube after its reconstruction to prevent it from being telescoped or crushed by the weight of the bladder above it. Thus, some kind of suspension is created using either the vaginal wall in girls or the anterior bladder wall in boys and in small girls if the vaginal wall is not appropriate for suspension.

The surgeon must be extremely aware of the major potential causes of failure of this technique: a devascularized flap leading either to contracture or sloughing and fistulization, a too-wide flap becoming funneled and absorbed into the bladder cavity, a too-narrow flap becoming a precursor for ischemia once it is wrapped into a tube around the catheter, inaccurate apposition of epithelium-to-epithelium sutures at the site of an anastomosis, and lack of proper suspension of the bladder after tube reconstruction.

Chapter 70

Intravesical Urethral Lengthening

INTRAVESICAL URETHRAL LENGTHENING (KROPP)

In a child with a poorly compliant bladder, consider simultaneous bladder augmentation, because a low-pressure reservoir is essential for continence. In older boys, consider an artificial sphincter or continent diversion as an alternative, especially because intermittent catheterization of the male urethra is usually not well accepted.

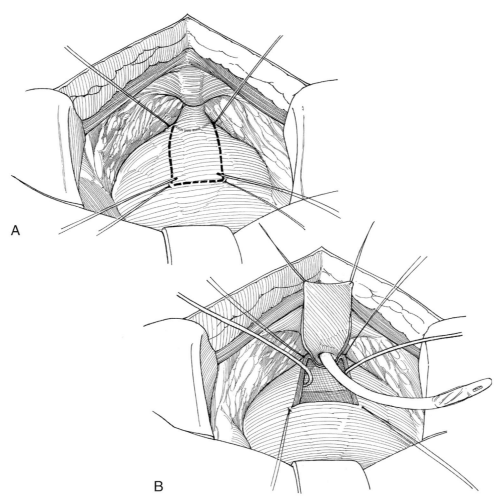

A

B

FIGURE 70-1. Insert a 24-F balloon catheter. Incision: lower midline extraperitoneal incision (see Chapter 62). Expose the bladder neck and posterior urethra. **A,** Mark a rectangular bladder flap with stay sutures with the base at the bladder neck. The length should be that required for the new urethra (4 to 6 cm) and the width should be the proposed circumference (knowing that 20 F = 2 cm). **B,** Incise the flap with the cutting current and continue the incision posteriorly around the bladder neck. (An alternative to separation of the tube from the bladder, leaving it attached only by the rectangular strip, is to preserve the outer posterolateral musculoadventitial fibers.) However, the midline posterior bladder muscle must be incised completely, to allow conversion of the bladder neck–anterior bladder flaps into a tube.

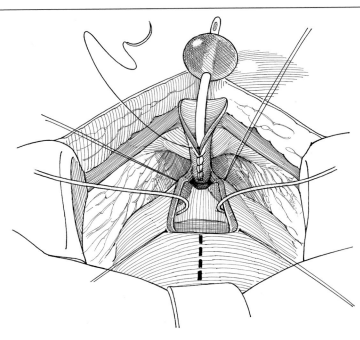

FIGURE 70-2. Roll the flap into a tube over a 20-F balloon catheter and close it, starting at the distal end, with a layer of continuous submucosal plain catgut suture and a second layer of interrupted 4-0 chromic catgut sutures.

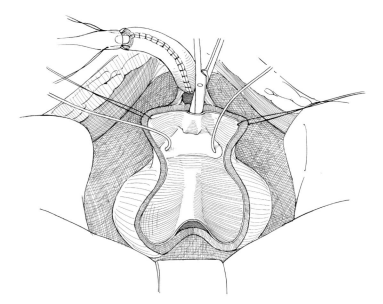

FIGURE 70-3. With scissors, make a wide tunnel beneath the vesical epithelium and over the trigonal musculature that extends between the ureteral orifices, using blunt and sharp dissection. An alternative is merely to create a channel in which to place the new urethra, and then cover it with adjacent epithelium. Insert the end of the new urethra into the flange of a Robinson catheter and insinuate it up through the tunnel. At the same time, pull the bladder down over the new tube to reach the former bladder neck.

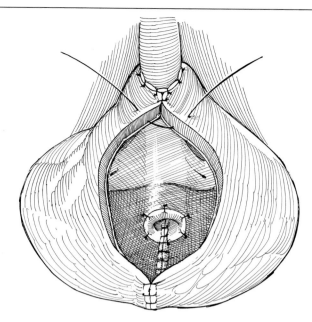

FIGURE 70-4. Bring the ureteral catheters out through stab wounds in the bladder (not shown). Secure the end of the urethral catheter (not shown) to the bladder wall in the fundus with interrupted 4-0 absorbable sutures and to the former bladder neck with similar sutures. Open the peritoneum and proceed with vesical augmentation, or close the anterior bladder wall starting distally around the urethra with a running subepithelial suture, reinforced with interrupted 4-0 sutures. Alternatively, start the closure proximally.

Postoperatively, most urine drains through the ureteral catheters. Remove the ureteral catheters in 10 to 14 days to allow the bladder neck to remain dry with the urinary diversion. If augmentation has been accomplished, irrigate the suprapubic and balloon catheters alternately with 30 to 60 mL of sterile water, and make sure that the family knows how to irrigate so that no mucus buildup can occur and cause plugging of the Foley and suprapubic catheters. In addition, instill 10 mL of acetylcysteine (Mucomyst) twice a day, and clamp both catheters for 15 minutes to keep the mucus in a more liquid state.

Between 4 and 6 weeks postoperatively remove the balloon catheter and clamp the suprapubic tube. If the patient is performing catheterization easily, remove the suprapubic tube. Advise catheterization every 2 hours for the first several days, working down over the next 3 to 4 weeks to four to six times per day.

POSTOPERATIVE PROBLEMS

The arrangement does not have a safety valve, so obstruction to catheterization can be a serious problem. It may require cystoscopic manipulation, and, in boys, a perineal urethrostomy may be necessary. Leaving the urethral stent in place for 5 to 6 weeks reduces the problem. Reflux may develop postoperatively but may not require correction if catheterization is done frequently.

KENNETH A. KROPP

Commentary by

We have recently reviewed our first 39 children with urethral lengthening followed from 42 to 163 months (median is 102.6 months). All but one were children with meningomyelocele who had failed to attain dryness on intermittent self-catheterization. All but six had a simultaneous bladder augmentation, and five of these six subsequently required augmentation. Nineteen of the 39 have not experienced any complications. Mucus has not been a problem for any after the early postoperative period. Thirty-three children (84%) have never had any difficulty with catheterization. Six children (16%) have experienced two or more episodes of difficulty, usually in the first few months. Placing a Foley catheter for 3 to 7 days solved most of these problems. With more than 50 children living in our area with urethral lengthening who catheterize themselves four to six times per day, we have not seen a single child present to our emergency room or office in the past 2 years who has had difficulty with catheterizing. Thirty-one (80%) are completely dry day and night; three have rare leakage but require no pads; three leak rarely but wear a pad for security. Only two are back in diapers because of leakage.

INTRAVESICAL URETHRAL
LENGTHENING (PIPPI SALLE)

This technique is a modification of the intravesical urethral
lengthening procedure (Kropp).

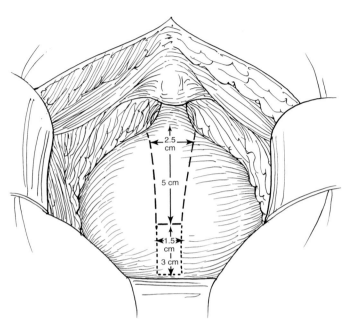

FIGURE 70-5. Insert a balloon catheter and partially fill the bladder. Make a midline lower abdominal incision or transverse
incision. Expose the bladder neck and bladder surface. Outline the anterior flap starting at the bladder neck and work
toward the dome. The dimensions of the flap should be 2.5 cm wide tapering to 1.5 cm, with the total length 8 cm.

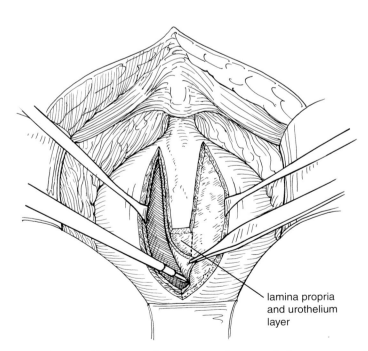

lamina propria
and urothelium
layer

FIGURE 70-6. Incise the flap with the needle electrode. Remove the muscle layer, preserving the lamina propria and
urothelium on the distal 3 cm of the flap.

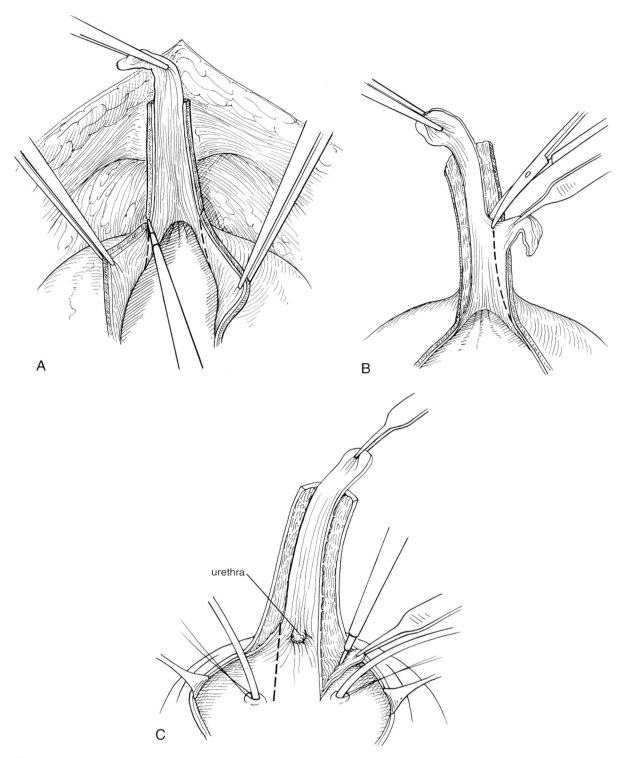

FIGURE 70-7. A, Incise the lateral aspects of the anterior flap to the bladder neck. **B,** Trim 2 to 3 mm of lamina propria and urothelium off each side of the flap, preserving the muscular layer of the bladder. **C,** This dissection should proceed on the posterior wall to just below the ureteral orifices (4 to 5 cm long to match the anterior flap), mobilizing a wedge of submucosa and urothelium on either side of the flap. If necessary, reimplant the ureters by the transtrigonal technique (see Chapter 68).

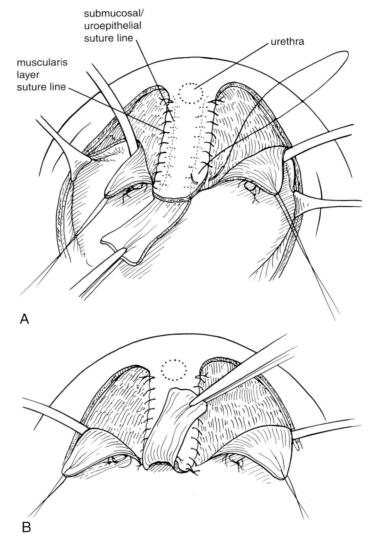

FIGURE 70-8. A and B, Insert an 8-F catheter (not shown), place the flap against the posterior bladder wall between the incisions, and run a suture on each side to approximate the submucosa uroepithelium to submucosa uroepithelium. Attach the muscularis of the flap to the exposed muscle of the bladder wall with continuous sutures. Elevate the lateral epithelial edges.

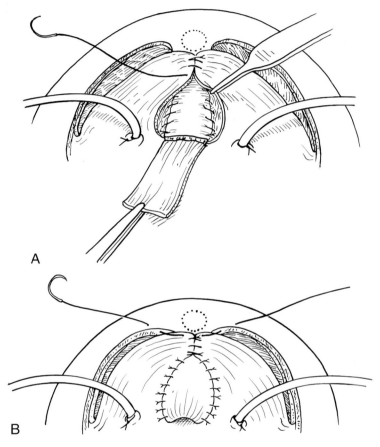

A

B

FIGURE 70-9. A and **B,** Bring the lateral epithelial edges together over the lateral defect with a continuous absorbable suture. Insert a suprapubic catheter. Augment the bladder if necessary. Stent the ureters as needed. Cover the extended urethra with the anterior submucosa uroepithelial flap. Close the bladder by starting with a short transverse suture line at the origin of the flap and continuing with a continuous suture. The feeding tube should remain for 3 weeks before beginning intermittent catheterization. If a leak does occur, it will be where the bladder neck is closed over the tube.

J. L. PIPPI SALLE

This procedure is indicated mainly for cases of either refractory neurogenic incontinence that have failed all conservative measures or in selected cases of other congenital anomalies in which the need for bladder emptying with intermittent catheterization is anticipated. As patients will not be able to spontaneously void, it is essential to provide instructions about the imperative need for diligent postoperative intermittent catheterization and have the family or caregivers support compliance with this regimen. A catheterizable stoma (i.e., Mitrofanoff, Monti-Yang, or Macedo channel) is recommended in most cases; therefore, be mindful of the importance of appropriate preoperative selection of stoma location in these patients who often have severe lower-body deformities.

IMPORTANT TECHNICAL POINTS

Several technical points must be followed to achieve optimal results:

In deformed and often obese patients the bladder neck and proximal urethra are deeply positioned, making exposure very challenging. If possible, when positioning on the table, the pelvis should be exposed by appropriate padding under the buttocks. In addition, gentle traction at the bladder dome with retractors also improves bladder neck exposure.

The fashioning of the anterior bladder wall flap should have a trapezoid shape (larger in the base) to improve blood supply and avoid ischemia of its distal aspect. The mucosal edges of the flap must be excised to result in a rectangular shape. As a result, the base of the trapezoid should have a wider denuded area of detrusor muscle to avoid overlapping suture lines when approximated at the posterior bladder wall. This maneuver prevents formation of urethrovesical fistulas and recurrence of incontinence.

Mucosal coverage of the intravesical neourethra is performed by undermining the mucosa of the bladder in the trigonal area and with the redundant tissue left at the tip of the flap.

Ureteral reimplantation can be avoided in the majority of cases, as augmentation is usually concurrently performed, resulting in low-pressure reservoirs.

Closure of the anterior bladder wall should be performed without tension over the neourethra to avoid compression and ischemia of the flap.

ADVANTAGES

The main advantages of this procedure are that the anterior and posterior walls of the constructed urethra are pliable and amenable for the injection of bulking agents in case of persistence of incontinence. Also, the constructed urethra is easily catheterizable in most cases; therefore, bladder emptying can be accomplished using both the abdominal stomal and urethral routes. This facilitates mucus evacuation and potentially diminishes stone formation in augmented bladders. In addition, it is preferable to have an alternative site for catheterization other than the abdominal stomas alone, as these can develop complications over time, posing difficulties for catheterization in retentive patients. And finally, it is interesting to note that although a flap-valve mechanism is constructed, most patients who undergo the Pippi Salle procedure appear to have a pop-off mechanism in case of delay of catheterization due to difficulty of passing through the catheter or lack of compliance by the patient.

COMPLICATIONS

Persistence of incontinence can be secondary to the development of urethrovesical fistula usually located at the base of the neourethra. Such complications occurred mainly at the beginning of our series when additional removal of mucosal edges of the flap was not performed. When this maneuver is done, it avoids overlapping of suture lines (a known factor for development of fistulas). Persistent urinary incontinence may also be secondary to impaired flap blood supply due to compression by the anterior bladder wall. This can result in a short flap-valve mechanism, which in turn leads to an incompetent mechanism to retain urine in the bladder.

Difficulty for urethral catheterization can occur in approximately 15% of patients and may be related to lack of uniformity in the suture lines of the flap. Some of these patients also have difficulty with catheterization when the bladder is overdistended; thus it is important to instruct strict adherence to a catheterization program.

Chapter 71

Bladder Neck Wraps

An alternative approach to lifting the bladder neck for the treatment of urinary incontinence is to wrap the bladder neck with rectus or detrusor muscle or rectus fascia.

RECTUS MYOFASCIAL WRAP

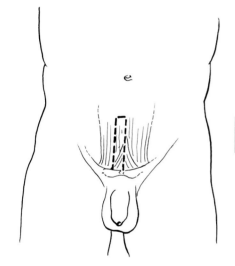

FIGURE 71-1. From the rectus abdominis and pyramidalis muscles and fascia, form a myofascial pedicle flap parallel to the midline.

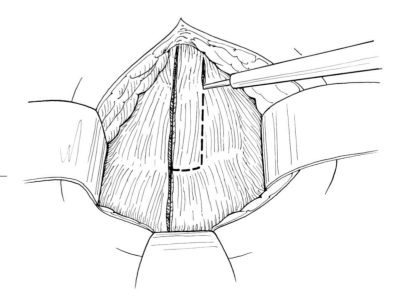

FIGURE 71-2. Make the size 2 × 8 to 10 cm in girls and 2 × 12 to 14 cm in boys. Keep the distal blood supply intact.

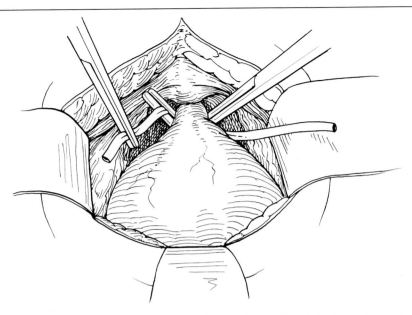

FIGURE 71-3. Expose the anterior bladder wall and neck. Incise the endopelvic fascia lateral to the bladder neck on both sides. Pass a right-angle clamp behind the bladder neck anterior to the vagina or the seminal vesicles and place a vessel loop. Dissect laterally and anteriorly around the bladder neck. Alternatively, dissect in the posterior midline of the bladder (see Chapter 66).

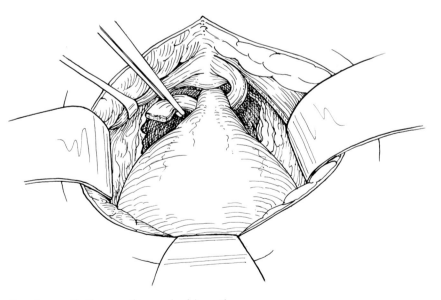

FIGURE 71-4. Pass the flap beneath the urethrovesical junction.

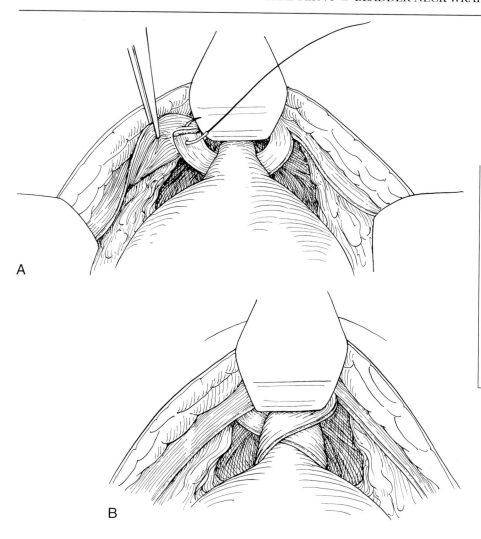

FIGURE 71-5. A, Suture the sling to the contralateral rectus sheath with a nonabsorbable suture. **B,** For greater tension, loop the sling around the urethra once as a U, or even twice (a "cinch"). Test tension by filling the bladder while increasing tension on the sling until continence is achieved. Before fixing the sling, perform augmentation cystoplasty and ureteral implantation if necessary. Leave the catheter in place for 5 to 10 days for a simple sling and for 2 to 3 weeks after augmentation. Then start intermittent catheterization.

BLADDER WALL PEDICLE WRAPAROUND SLING

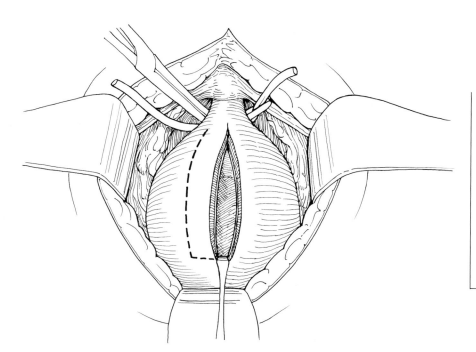

FIGURE 71-6. Expose the anterior bladder wall and bladder neck. Open the bladder in the midline to the bladder neck. Place a retractor in the dome of the bladder to stretch the bladder neck superiorly. Using a finger in the open bladder neck as a guide, pass a right-angle clamp behind the bladder neck anterior to the seminal vesicles or vagina. Replace the clamp with an umbilical tape. Mark a 1.5 × 8 cm pedicle of anterior bladder wall based on the left side of the bladder neck.

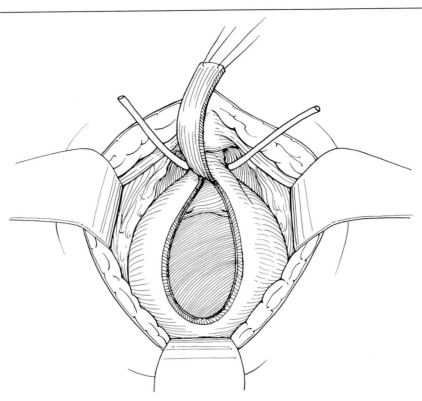

FIGURE 71-7. Denude the urothelium from the detrusor pedicle. Use stay sutures or a nonperforating clamp at the apex of the pedicle for traction.

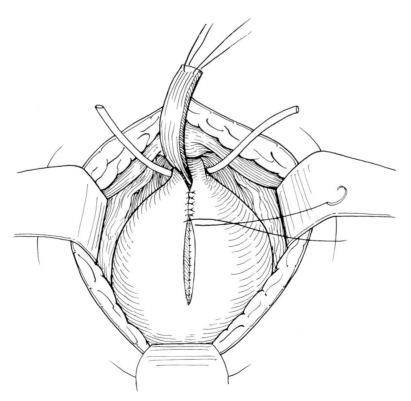

FIGURE 71-8. Close the inferior 5 cm of the bladder incision in two layers, exteriorizing the pedicle.

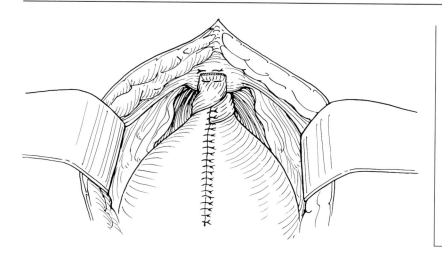

FIGURE 71-9. Pull the pedicle in clockwise fashion under and around the bladder neck. Increase tension while visualizing the bladder outlet until the bladder neck is snugly coapted. Secure the sling to the pubic symphysis and anterior fascia with two permanent horizontal mattress sutures. Pass a catheter to ensure ease of catheterization. An augmentation procedure is then performed, if necessary, and a suprapubic tube is left in place. A urethral catheter is not used postoperatively. The patient is discharged home with the suprapubic tube in place. If a cystogram 3 weeks postoperatively is normal, the patient resumes intermittent catheterization.

RECTUS FASCIAL WRAP AND BLADDER NECK TIGHTENING

FIGURE 71-10. The bladder neck is exposed and circumvented as previously described. Narrow the bladder neck by excising a diamond-shaped, full-thickness wedge and reapproximating the defect with absorbable sutures.

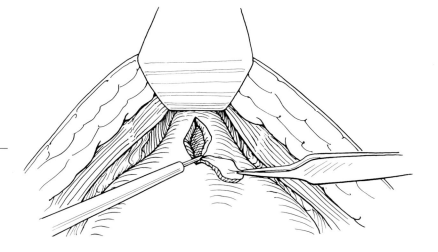

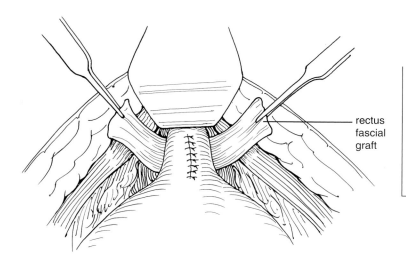

rectus fascial graft

FIGURE 71-11. Harvest the fascial graft by exposing the rectus fascia in a transverse or longitudinal direction. Mark the graft with a felt tip pen with the length being the circumference of the bladder neck plus 1 cm and the width being 1.5 cm. Dissect the graft from the rectus muscle with a combination of blunt and sharp dissection, removing any fat. Place the rectus fascial graft around the bladder neck.

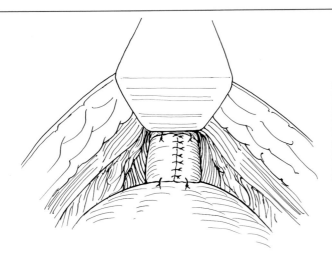

FIGURE 71-12. Sew the graft in place with interrupted 2-0 or 3-0 nonabsorbable sutures. The graft is also sewn to the bladder and urethra to keep it from rolling. Check for ease of catheterization and perform cystoscopy to ensure that there is no injury to the urethra and bladder neck. Postoperative complications are similar to those of pubovaginal slings (see Chapter 67).

ERIC KURZROCK

Commentary by

Prior to surgery, urethral function should be documented with urodynamic measurement of Valsalva leak point pressure. The urologist has to decide if the child will be catheterizing the urethra. There are two schools of thought; one is that all patients needing an augmentation should have a continent diversion, and the other is that treatment should be individualized according to the patient's needs and anatomy. In either case, numerous series have demonstrated that wraps and slings provide *complete* continence in 80% to 90% of females and only 50% of males. One distinct advantage of slings and wraps is ease of catheterization. On rare occasions, boys may have difficulty catheterizing if the bladder neck is suspended too much. If a diversion is concurrently performed, a Kropp or Pippi Salle bladder neck reconstruction will yield higher continence rates but will usually require ureteral reimplantation. I would not use these particular procedures if urethral catheterization is being considered.

Creation of the passage posterior to the bladder neck is the most daunting aspect of slings. Significant bleeding can be incurred in older males and vaginal injury is difficult to avoid. Some authors advocate posterior exposure through the peritoneum as described by Lottmann and colleagues. I do not use this approach but certainly can appreciate its value. As the vast majority of patients are undergoing concurrent bladder surgery, I guide the passage of a large right-angle clamp under the bladder neck with my left index finger in the intravesical bladder neck. I err on the side of injuring the vagina, because this is easily repaired, rather than entering the posterior bladder neck.

I prefer pulling umbilical tape through the pathway, rather than a vessel loop, as it is stronger and I can mark it with a pen for measuring the necessary length of the flap. I complete the bladder neck reconstruction and sling prior to starting the augmentation. For all of the described wraps and slings, I taper the bladder neck. Coaptation is the goal; thus, tapering is an integral aspect of the surgery. If using an anterior bladder wall wraparound sling, it is important to de-epithelialize the pedicle. In addition to sewing the pedicle to the pubic periosteum, I also sew the pedicle to the bladder and to itself. I leave an 8-F Foley catheter in the urethra postoperatively to prevent early cicatrix formation.

Chapter 72

Insertion of Artificial Sphincter

Over four fifths of both boys and girls with neuropathic incontinence may achieve continence with an artificial sphincter. In general, patients with the ability to spontaneously void prior to the procedure are able to spontaneously void after placement of an artificial sphincter. In a child with isolated epispadias the sphincter has a high rate of success, in contrast to vesical exstrophy, in which the artificial sphincter is seldom successful. Postoperative complications are more common after previous bladder neck surgery. Mechanical complications may be easily corrected. Expect that a revision will be required within 8 years. Pump erosion of the labial-scrotal folds is a special problem in children who are wheelchair-dependent. Subsequent bladder augmentation is needed in about one quarter of children. Because the sphincter is so efficient, careful follow-up is essential to catch deterioration of the upper tract.

The age of the child is important. Reserve sphincter placement for the older or postadolescent child who will not outgrow it. Consider alternatives: bladder neck reconstruction (Young-Dees-Leadbetter), anterior bladder wall flap (Tanagho), urethral lengthening and reimplantation (Kropp), fascial slings, and periurethral injection of bulking agents.

Before insertion treat urinary tract infection and give perioperative cephalosporin. Have the child shower preoperatively using organic iodine soap solution. In the operating room, prep for 10 minutes with iodophor, including the perineum and external genitalia (and the vagina in older girls). Restrict traffic and reduce room contamination to a minimum (most infections in prosthetic devices are caused by airborne *Staphylococcus epidermidis*). Spray the wound with a dilute antibiotic solution throughout the operation.

Provide a basic set of instruments, including genitourinary fine set, Scott retractor with small and large stays, baby Deaver retractor, skin hooks, Babcock clamps, Lahey clamps, large right-angle dissecting scissors, four curved and four straight mosquito clamps shod with silicone tubing, DeBakey forceps, two pairs of Cushing forceps (smooth and toothed), Hegar dilators, headlight, soft adjustable stool, selected prosthesis in three sterile packages (pump, prep package with sizer and blunt needles, and connectors), one bowl for 11.5% iothalamate meglumine (Cysto-Conray II), one bowl for dilute antibiotic solution (50,000 units bacitracin, 1 g neomycin, 300 mL saline), dilute methylene blue solution, two basins with 1500 mL of water to wash gloves, nonpenetrating towel clips, silicone sheet to block anus, 14-F, 5-mL silicone balloon catheter with syringe, lubricant and plug, scrotal supporter, 2-0 Prolene sutures for connectors, 4-0 chromic catgut with RB-1 needle, two half-inch Penrose drains, and vacuum suction and tubing. Be sure to flush all air from the components of the system.

BLADDER NECK PLACEMENT

The bladder neck is the site of application for children, who have small bulbar urethras. This position has advantages: It is more physiologic than the bulbar urethral site, is less prone to erosion, and is less irritated by intermittent catheterization. Avoid placing a cuff around a previously operated bladder neck. If placed around bowel, add extra fluid, as the wall will shrink. Use a surface-treated cuff in children with meningomyelocele or other types of neurogenic bladder.

FIGURE 72-1. Incision and approach: Make a vertical lower abdominal incision. A transverse lower abdominal incision may be a better choice for children. Insert a 5-mL balloon catheter of suitable size. If operating after previous retropubic operations or trauma, insert a rectal tube or vaginal pack to help identify the tissue planes. Open the bladder if necessary for orientation. Incise the visceral extension of the endopelvic fascia and bluntly establish a plane between the bladder neck and the underlying vagina or rectum. Push the tissue containing the neurovascular bundles laterally. Stay cephalad of the parietal endopelvic fascia and below the level of the trigone. With the thumb and index finger, palpate the catheter and trigone anteriorly and the vas deferens posteriorly. Pinch the trigone anteriorly to separate it from the vasa. Use a right-angle clamp and also scissors on the finger to dissect between the bladder neck and the ejaculatory mechanism. Pass an umbilical tape through the tract for traction to expose and allow control of any venous bleeders. Avoid clips; metal could erode into the silicone rubber of the device.

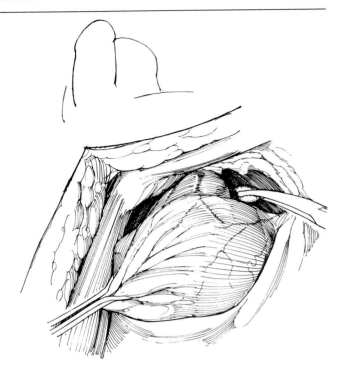

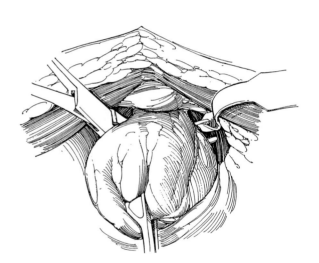

FIGURE 72-2. Remove the balloon catheter. Pass a large right-angle clamp under the bladder neck and draw the sizer tape through.

FIGURE 72-3. Hold the sizer tape against the bladder neck and measure its circumference using the markers on the tape. In boys, the caudal edge of the tape should be at the top of the prostate; in girls, the cephalad edge should lie just above the bladder neck as determined by palpation of the catheter balloon.

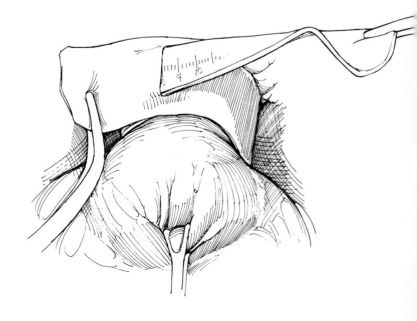

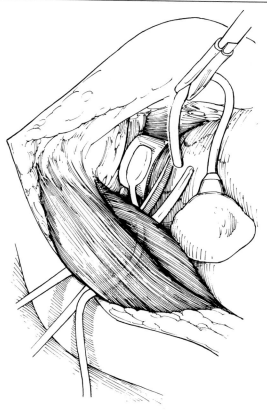

FIGURE 72-4. Replace the tape with an inflatable cuff of the correct size and snap it into place. Pass a large clamp down through the inguinal canal and draw the tubing from the cuff and reservoir through the canal. Alternatively, use the blunt tubing needle supplied and work from inside out.

FIGURE 72-5. Run a large Hegar dilator or large curved clamp down into the scrotum or labia. Insert the pump and milk it into position. Select the pressure reservoir that will just maintain continence. Although several methods have been described to determine the pressure required, none are reliable. Fill the reservoir with 18 mL of isotonic contrast medium (11.7% Cysto-Conray II) or physiologic saline and connect its tubing to the cuff tubing. Clamp both tubes with rubber-shod hemostats (one click only). Withdraw the fluid from the reservoir. If it contains less than 16 mL, the cuff size is too big and should be replaced (see Fig. 72-4). If it is the correct size, refill the reservoir with 20 mL of solution and connect the tubing with stainless steel connectors. Test for continence. Close the wound in layers without drainage. Continue parenteral antibiotics for 4 days and oral antibiotics for 2 weeks. Activate the cuff 6 to 8 weeks postoperatively. Use firm pump pressure to displace the poppet valve and thus allow the fluid to flow through the pump to fill it.

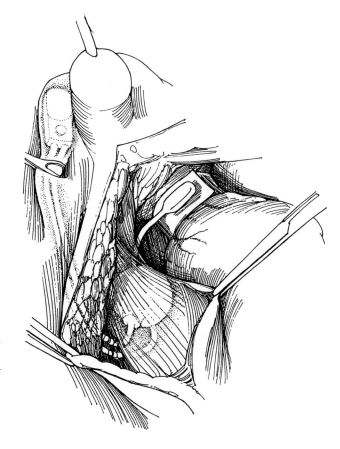

POSTOPERATIVE PROBLEMS

Persistent incontinence may result from leakage or from pressure atrophy under the cuff. If particulate matter was left in the system, pump action may be intermittent and suggest a leak. Kinks in the tubing may do the same. Incontinence may also come from reflex bladder activity or poor detrusor compliance.

Infection is the most common and the greatest hazard. Preoperatively, the urine must be cleared of bacteria because once infected, the device must be removed. For this reason, continue to maintain strict asepsis postoperatively. Culture the urine if doubt exists, or if, for any reason, catheterization is necessary. Myelomeningocele patients have a high rate of infection of the prosthesis with both gram-positive and gram-negative bacteria; they require assiduous attention to bacteriuria. Should a dental procedure be required, prophylactic coverage is essential. When the device does become infected by bacteria carried by the bloodstream, it will be at the cuff, the area of poorest vascularity. Prompt drainage and irrigation of the infected area with antibiotic solutions can occasionally save the device.

Erosion of the cuff into the urethra is heralded by burning perineal pain and swelling in the scrotum or labia about the pump. Check by cystoscopy and, if erosion is present, proceed with removal of the cuff. In an occasional case, evacuation of the purulent collection in the periurethral area, diversion of urine, and irrigation with antibiotic solutions can save the device.

Manage bladder instability with anticholinergics or enterocystoplasty.

BLADDER AUGMENTATION

Augmentation becomes necessary in one third to one half of these children as detrusor function deteriorates. Progression of vesical imbalance from the meningomyelocele may also be a factor, and placement of a cuff may influence detrusor dynamics. If detrusor overactivity is present, consider simultaneous cystoplasty, although the need for augmentation cannot be predicted by urodynamics preoperatively.

Outgrowing the sphincter can be a serious problem because removing and replacing it is technically difficult. Consider inserting the cuff postadolescence. Upsizing by loosening the sphincter in the maturing male does not restore the ability to void spontaneously (Kaefer, 1997).

RICARDO GONZÁLEZ

Commentary by

The AS800 artificial urinary sphincter (AUS) is the best model to increase outlet resistance in males, regardless of their ability to empty the bladder spontaneously, and for females capable of spontaneous voiding or who wish to catheterize urethrally. It is important to implant the AUS around a virgin bladder neck. Previous surgery in this area significantly increases the possibility of erosion. The AUS is a poor salvage measure when other bladder neck operations have failed. We found the AUS equally effective before and after puberty. As achievement of continence at a normal age is important for the psychosocial development of the child, waiting until after puberty for implantation is not advisable. When preoperative urodynamic studies suggest the need for a simultaneous augmentation, I prefer the seromuscular technique. The majority of pediatric patients undergoing AUS implantation have a neurogenic bladder; therefore, latex precautions during and after surgery are essential. Preoperatively we recommend a mechanical bowel preparation to have an empty rectum (many patients have chronic constipation). Make sure the urine is sterile and use prophylactic antibiotics appropriate for implantation of a prosthetic device.

During surgery, I do not rely on the balloon of the catheter to identify the bladder neck. This is often misleading. Instead, I first ligate the veins of Santorini's plexus and then dissect lateral and posterior to the bladder neck to identify the seminal vesicles and find the plane between the vesicles and the vasa and the bladder neck. It is important not to implant the cuff below the ejaculatory ducts to prevent interfering with ejaculation. After the dissection is completed, I fill the bladder with a methylene blue solution to make sure I have not made any inadvertent opening in the bladder.

In females, I prepare the vagina and include it in the sterile field. The use of a vaginal finger helps to guide the dissection between the vagina and the urethra. I find that packing the vagina or the rectum interferes with the dissection. I do not use the inguinal canal to bring the tubes to the subcutaneous space and routinely use the sutureless connectors provided by the manufacturer. It is important to prime and fill the system with a contrast solution approved by the manufacturer.

For the pressure balloon I use the 61 to 70 cm of water balloon filled with 22 mL of fluid exclusively and do not test for continence during the operation. With good bladder capacity and compliance and a cuff of the appropriate size, continence is almost guaranteed. Infection and erosion of the tissues in contact with the sphincter components are the most serious, though fortunately infrequent, complications.

STUART BAUER

Commentary by

The AUS has proven to be the most durable and reliable prosthetic device developed for urinary incontinence during the last 35 years. It is a well-designed, expertly manufactured, reliably efficient, anti-incontinence mechanism that can make a sustained and prolonged difference in carefully selected patients. A meta-analysis of all reported series in children over the last 11 years revealed that 80% were continent, 32% voided spontaneously, 43% required no additional surgery, 31% underwent a subsequent augmentation due to detrusor overactivity or worsening compliance, 28% needed a revision, and 19% had removal due to an erosion or infection of a component.

Using a new posterior approach to dissecting the bladder neck from surrounding tissue planes (see Chapter 66), color-coded tubing to differentiate the balloon and cuff tubing, and the Quick Connect system, insertion of the device has been made infinitely easier.

In the course of inserting the device, all components and tubings are kept to one side of the midline, preferably the side opposite the dominant hand. This makes it easier to deflate the pump so that any subsequent surgery on the bladder need not expose any portion of the prosthesis. Balloon pressure (in cm H_2O) should not exceed diastolic pressure to ensure adequate tissue perfusion. Despite a multitude of observations no one has identified a reliable preoperative urodynamic parameter that would indicate the likelihood of poor detrusor compliance or overactivity, postoperatively. Thus, careful and lifelong surveillance with renal ultrasonography, residual urine measurements in those who spontaneously void, and cystometrography are paramount to ensure long-term health of the urinary tract.

With the advent of creating a continent catheterizable stoma for ease of emptying the bladder, the AUS can be placed around the bladder neck or urethra in those individuals with intractable incontinence who cannot be catheterized easily. It also simultaneously allows for abdominal access to the bladder without the need to close off the bladder neck.

Chapter 73

Closure of Vesical Neck

Provide continent diversion or place a cystostomy at the end of the procedure. Clear the urine of infection and provide antibiotic coverage.

The most successful approach to ligate the bladder neck is to separate the urethra from the bladder through an abdominal approach. Consider externalized ureteral stents to divert the urine from the ligated bladder.

EXTRAVESICAL APPROACH WITH URETHRAL INVERSION

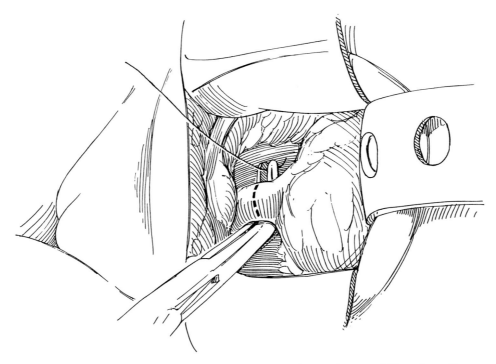

FIGURE 73-1. Through a lower transverse abdominal (see Chapter 63) or lower midline (see Chapter 62) incision, enter the retropubic space, and free the urethra by dividing the pubourethral ligaments superficial to the dorsal vein complex. Dissect the urethra distally from the prostate or vagina with the aid of a finger in the rectum or vagina, respectively. Elevate the urethra from the vagina or rectum by sharp dissection with a knife to include the adventitia. The longer the segment freed by sharp dissection, the easier the procedure. Divide the urethra and ligate both ends, leaving the proximal suture long. Consider placing omentum (see Chapter 65) between the distal urethral stump and ligated bladder.

INTRAVESICAL APPROACH WITH URETHRAL INVERSION

The simplest method to close the male or female vesical neck is to open the bladder, make a circumferential incision around the bladder neck to remove a divot of epithelium, and then close the muscularis and subepithelium with two layers of purse-string absorbable suture. More security may be obtained by inverting the urethra, as is done with the combined approach. The key to success is to be sure that all of the epithelium has been removed, so that the surfaces in contact are bare.

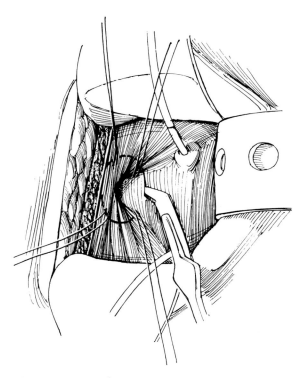

FIGURE 73-2. Open the bladder and visualize the outlet. Insert ureteral catheters for safety. Place four 3-0 synthetic absorbable traction sutures through the epithelium, closely surrounding the vesical neck. With a hooked knife, cut through the epithelium circumferentially 1 to 2 cm away from the outlet, and free up the epithelial margins with scissors.

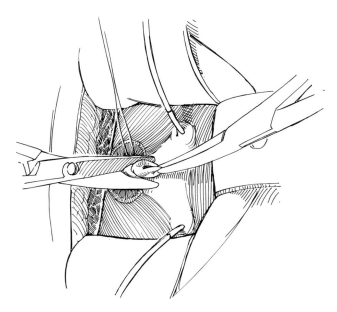

FIGURE 73-3. Trim the freed epithelium flush with the outlet, being certain that all the lining of the outlet is removed. Insert a curved clamp into the cut-off urethra, grasp the suture on the end of the proximal suture, and invert the urethra into the bladder. Trim the urethra.

FIGURE 73-4. A, Close the end of the
trimmed urethra with inverting sutures,
and tack it to the surrounding detrusor
muscle. **B,** Place a 3-0 or 4-0 synthetic
absorbable purse-string suture 1 cm from
the urethra that inverts the urethral
epithelium as the suture is tied. Place
a second circumferential suture 1 cm
outside the first and tie it. Close the
epithelium of the bladder over the
repair with interrupted 4-0 plain catgut
sutures. Insert a Malecot catheter to exit
through a stab wound. Close the bladder
and the wound. Further security may be
had by excising the urethral epithelium
perineally and obliterating that space.

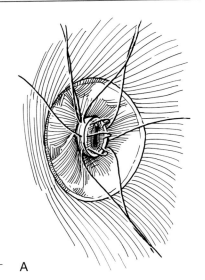
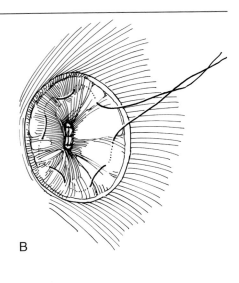

A

B

URETHRAL APPROACH

This approach avoids an abdominal incision yet inverts the
urethra into the bladder.

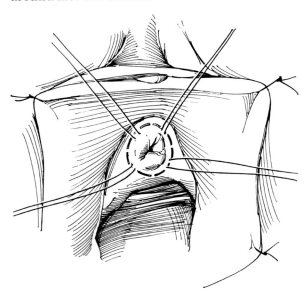

FIGURE 73-5. With the child in the dorsal lithotomy position, place
four traction sutures about the meatus that extend through the
urethral subepithelium. Incise the meatus circumferentially. Free
the urethra from the vagina and from the retropubic tissue to the
level of the bladder neck by dividing the endopelvic fascia laterally
and entering the retropubic space. It is necessary to divide the
pubourethral ligament to expose the base of the bladder.

FIGURE 73-6. Place three end-on 4-0 synthetic absorbable mattress
sutures in the urethral wall to invert the meatus. Alternatively, the
urethra may be trimmed and closed with an inverting purse-string
suture.

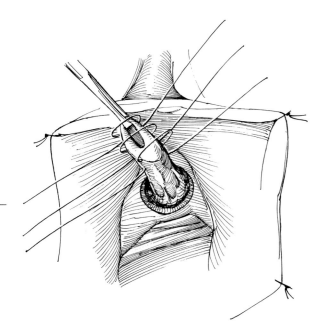

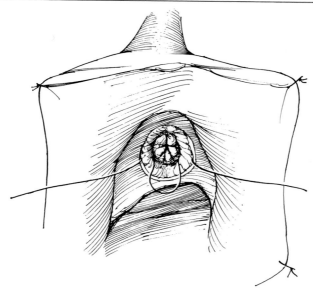

FIGURE 73-7. Approximate the periurethral fascia with several 4-0 synthetic absorbable sutures, and close the epithelium vertically with interrupted 4-0 chromic catgut sutures. Pack the vagina to reduce the chance of formation of a hematoma.

TRANSVAGINAL APPROACH

The method may be appropriate for adolescents, especially if paraplegic.

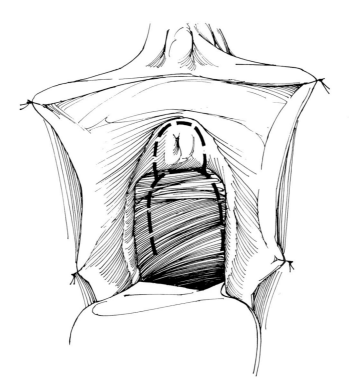

FIGURE 73-8. With the child in the dorsal lithotomy position, fix the labia laterally with stay sutures, and place a small posterior retractor in the vagina. Incise widely around the urethra, as far as the introitus, and continue the wings of the incision into the vagina beyond the bladder neck as an inverted U.

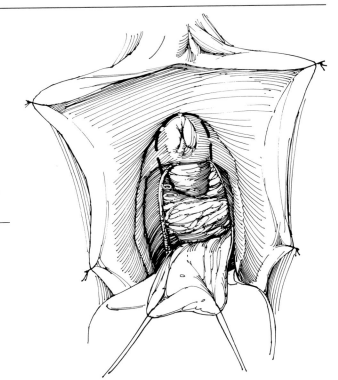

FIGURE 73-9. Free the vaginal flap from the urethra and posterior bladder neck after injecting normal saline beneath the anterior vaginal wall to help delineate the plane.

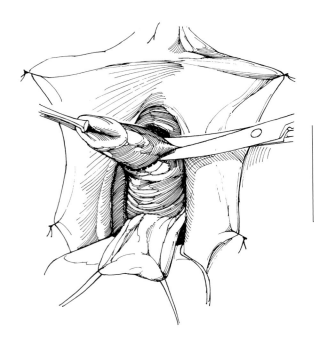

FIGURE 73-10. Continue the dissection around the urethra and bladder neck. Separate the bladder from the endopelvic fascia and from its retropubic attachments, including the pubourethral ligaments, staying close to the vesical wall. Give 5 mL of indigo carmine intravenously to identify the ureteral orifices, and then trim the urethra flush with the vesical neck.

FIGURE 73-11. Close the vesical neck with a running 3-0 plain catgut suture placed subepithelially in a vertical direction. Over this, place a running 3-0 synthetic absorbable suture.

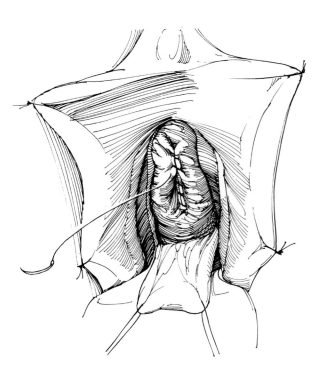

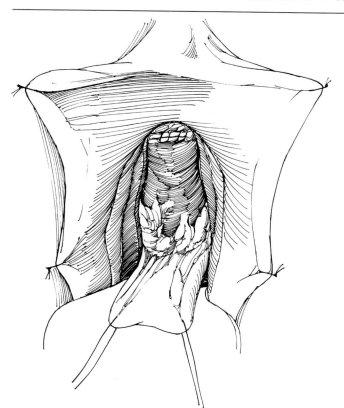

FIGURE 73-12. Reinforce this suture line with a transversely placed running 3-0 synthetic absorbable suture to the perivesical fascia and superficial layer of the bladder wall, which will move the repair behind the symphysis.

FIGURE 73-13. Bring the vaginal flap forward to cover the urethral defect, and tack it in place with four or five 3-0 synthetic absorbable subcutaneous sutures. Run a 3-0 synthetic absorbable suture with occasional lock stitches to fasten the flap to the defect. Alternatively, bring a vascularized labial fat pad into the defect before suturing the flap (see Chapter 172). Test for watertightness. Pack the vagina over strips of petroleum jelly gauze. Perform a continent diversion procedure, or install a suprapubic cystostomy.

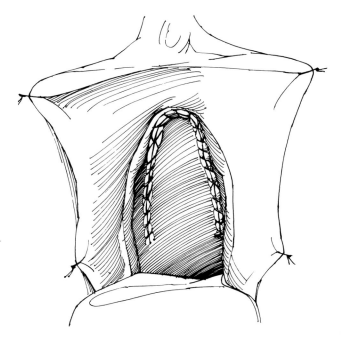

POSTOPERATIVE PROBLEMS

Leakage may appear immediately if the bladder has not been continuously decompressed. It may occur later as the sutures are resorbed and areas of injured tissue break down. Providing prolonged suprapubic drainage and ureteral stenting sometimes will allow the fistula to close.

MARC CAIN

Commentary by

This chapter provides a variety of techniques for bladder neck closure, and I would agree that the most successful and commonly used approach in the pediatric/adolescent patient is a transabdominal procedure in which the urethra and bladder can be completely separated. This in part is because most pediatric patients requiring this procedure will have some type of simultaneous continent bladder reconstruction, and/or will have had a history of multiple, prior failed continence procedures on the urethra/bladder neck, and will require careful dissection to both preserve the remaining vascular supply at the bladder neck and also avoid entering the rectum or vagina and risking a vesicovaginal fistula.

The key to a successful outcome is a multilayer closure with offset suture lines, inverting the mucosa of both the urethra and bladder neck, and interposing some type of vascularized flap to prevent a postoperative fistula. Many of these patients have had prior abdominal procedures or ventriculoperitoneal shunts, making mobilization of an omental flap either difficult or impossible. In this scenario I have preferred to use a vascularized muscle flap from the lower rectus abdominis muscle, basing the blood supply on the inferior epigastric vessels, which can be placed tension free and secured to the oversewn bladder neck.

Postoperative drainage is another important aspect in the multiply operated field, and my preference is to leave externalized ureteral stents in place for several weeks, as well as a large suprapubic catheter.

HIEP T. NGUYEN

Commentary by

Using the techniques demonstrated, bladder neck closure is an effective means of achieving urinary continence in girls in whom all other bladder neck surgeries have failed. Conceptually, this procedure is simple in nature; however, there are several intricacies in performing bladder neck closure to ensure surgical success. Regardless of the approach taken, it is important to completely expose and mobilize the urethra and bladder neck. This could be more easily done with a transvaginal approach, as previous retropubic surgery may have led to scarring and fixation of the bladder neck and proximal urethra. After complete division of the urethra, it is important to completely invert the epithelium of the urethra and bladder neck with multiple layer closure. In addition, vascularized tissue such as the omental or labial flap should be interposed between the urethral and bladder neck stump. These maneuvers will help to prevent fistula formation between the two ends. With the transvaginal approach, meticulous dissection of the bladder and interposition of vascularized tissue are required to prevent the formation of vesicovaginal fistulas.

Surgical success is not only dependent on intraoperative techniques but also on postoperative care and management. Drainage of the bladder with a suprapubic catheter is usually required for 3 to 4 weeks. Urinary diversion with ureteral stents also should be considered in cases in which multiple previous surgeries may have compromised the quality of the bladder or urethral tissue. After all the drainage tubes have been removed, it is important that the patients remain strictly compliant with intermittent catheterization. Failure to do so may lead to fistula and recurrent incontinence. Compliance with intermittent catheterization will also help to reduce the risk of stone formation, urinary tract infections, and bladder rupture.

Chapter 74

Vesical Exstrophy Primary Complete Closure

The goal of complete primary exstrophy/epispadias repair is to achieve normal bladder function. It combines the goals of staged reconstruction in a single operation—that is, bladder closure, epispadias repair, and the achievement of urinary continence. The operation preferably is done during the newborn period. However, the technique can be used in older children that have not been previously closed or have failed previous attempts at closure. Consider osteotomies especially in patients older than 48 hours, or in large-term infants with wide diastasis of the symphysis. Have blood available prior to the surgery. A renal sonogram will confirm two normal kidneys, a classic finding in bladder exstrophy. Broad-spectrum antibiotics are administered prior to the incision.

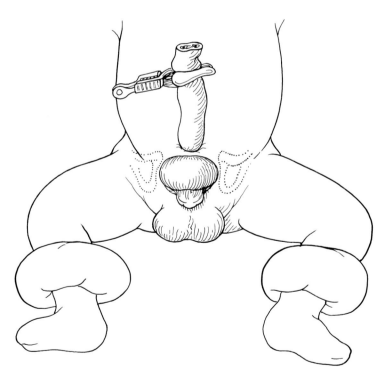

FIGURE 74-1. Begin the operation with a full body preparation from the thorax to the toes using stockings for the lower extremities. This will facilitate hip adduction in sterile fashion when bringing the pubic bones together at the completion of the procedure.

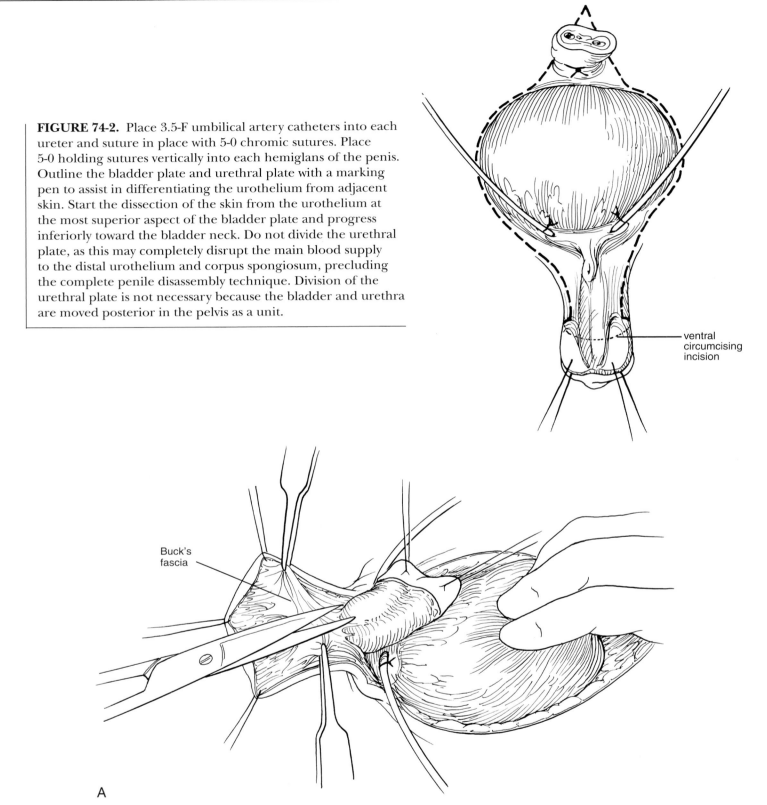

FIGURE 74-2. Place 3.5-F umbilical artery catheters into each ureter and suture in place with 5-0 chromic sutures. Place 5-0 holding sutures vertically into each hemiglans of the penis. Outline the bladder plate and urethral plate with a marking pen to assist in differentiating the urothelium from adjacent skin. Start the dissection of the skin from the urothelium at the most superior aspect of the bladder plate and progress inferiorly toward the bladder neck. Do not divide the urethral plate, as this may completely disrupt the main blood supply to the distal urothelium and corpus spongiosum, precluding the complete penile disassembly technique. Division of the urethral plate is not necessary because the bladder and urethra are moved posterior in the pelvis as a unit.

ventral circumcising incision

Buck's fascia

A

FIGURE 74-3. A and **B,** Continue dissection as a circumcising incision along the ventral aspect of the penis between Buck's fascia and the overlying tissue. Preserve the urethral plate and sharply dissect it from the anterior surface of the corporeal bodies. Buck's fascia stops at the lateral edge of the urethral plate and is best identified ventrally. Therefore, start the circumcising incision at this point and carry it laterally around the penis to the edge of the urethral plate. Continue the skin incision along the edge of the urethral plate and meet the previous incision at the bladder neck. Limit blood loss and assist in dissection by injecting surrounding tissues with 0.25% lidocaine and 1:200,000 units/mL epinephrine.

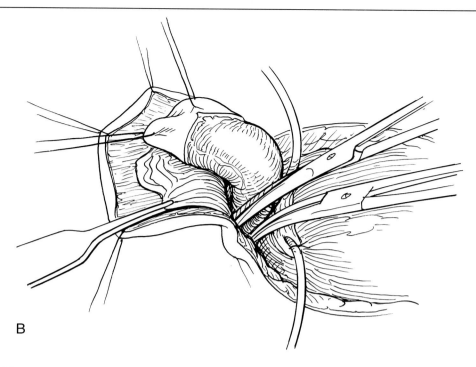

B

FIGURE 74-3, cont'd.

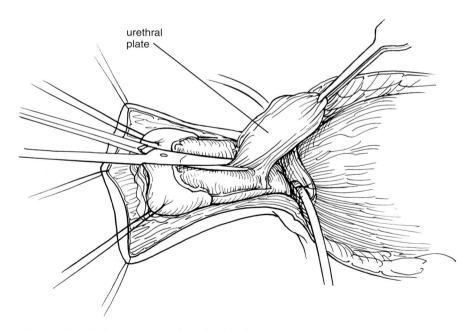

urethral
plate

FIGURE 74-4. Dissect the urethral plate proximal to the bladder neck. It is important to avoid narrowing the urethral plate that will subsequently need to be tubularized later in the operation. To preserve the blood supply, *all* spongiosal tissue *remains* with the urethral plate. Inclusion of the whole corpora spongiosa with the urethral plate gives this unit a triangular appearance. The neurovascular bundles are lateral to the lateral edge of the dorsal urethral plate and within Buck's fascia.

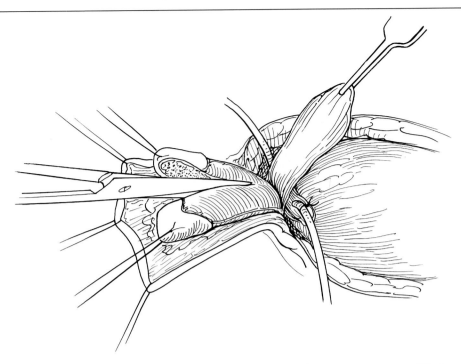

FIGURE 74-5. This dissection allows the penis to be disassembled into three components: (1) the right and (2) left corporeal bodies with the respective hemiglans, and (3) the urethral plate and the corpora spongiosa. This dissection is easiest to initiate proximal and ventral at the level of the tunica albuginea on the corpora, which is a relatively avascular plane. Bleeding usually indicates injury to the corpora spongiosa or corpora cavernosa. Create a plane between the urethral plate and corporeal bodies, and then carry dissection distal to divide the glans penis in the midline, allowing the three components to be separated, as previously described. The independent blood supply of these three components allows this separation. The hemiglans exists on a separate blood supply based on the paired neurovascular bundles. The underlying corpora spongiosa must remain with the urethral plate. The blood supply to the urethral plate is based on this corporeal tissue, which is wedge shaped after it is dissected from the adjacent corpora cavernosa.

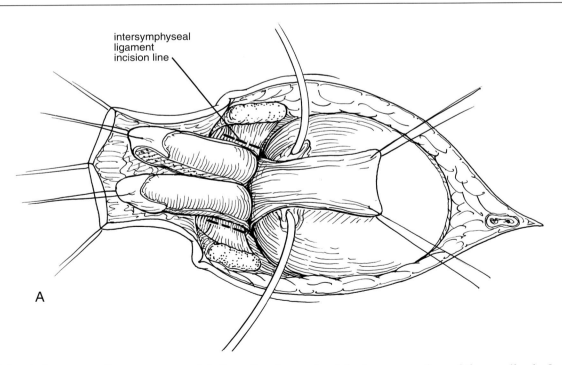

intersymphyseal
ligament
incision line

A

FIGURE 74-6. As in any penile surgery, careful dissection is required during separation of the penile shaft skin from the corporeal bodies laterally. The medial plane of dissection is the tunica albuginea of the corpora. This plane is followed proximally to the intersymphyseal ligament (anterior coalescense of the pelvic diaphragm). **A,** Intersymphyseal ligament incision line.

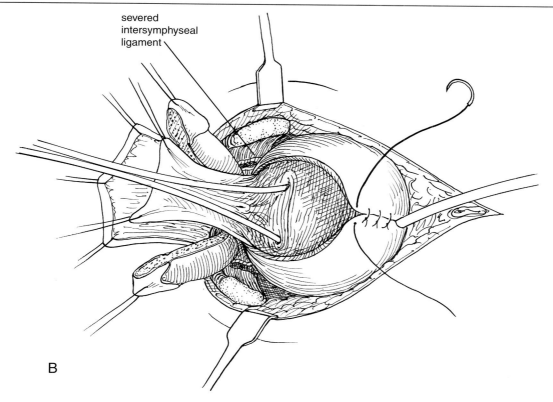

severed
intersymphyseal
ligament

B

FIGURE 74-6, cont'd. B, Severed intersymphyseal ligament.

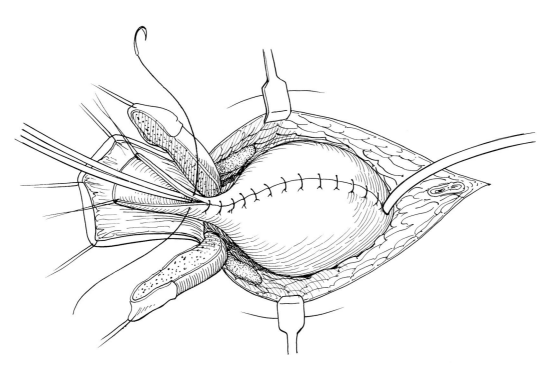

FIGURE 74-7. Now tubularize this urethral corporeal component and place it ventral to the corporeal bodies. Proximal dissection of the urethral plate from the corporeal bodies is critical to posterior placement of the bladder neck and proximal urethra. Incomplete posterior dissection of the bladder and urethral plate or inadequate division of the intersymphyseal ligament creates anterior tension along the urethral plate and prevents posterior movement of the bladder, bladder neck, and urethra in the pelvis, which increases the likelihood of dehiscence and likely jeopardizes later urinary continence.

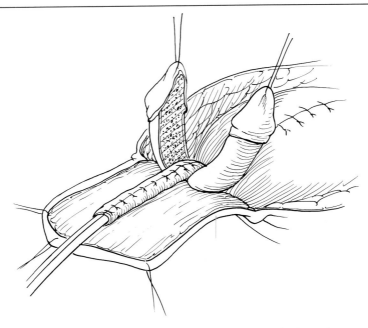

FIGURE 74-8. After the bladder and urethral plate are adequately dissected, close them as a continuous unit. Divert the urine through a suprapubic tube brought out through the umbilicus. Reapproximate the edges of the bladder plate using a three-layer closure with monofilament absorbable suture.

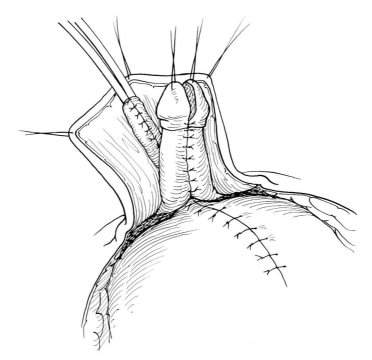

FIGURE 74-9. Tubularize the urethra using a two-layer running closure with monofilament suture. No special effort is made to narrow the bladder neck. However, there should be no step-off at the bladder neck when incision of the pelvic diaphragm is performed adequately. Bring the ureteral catheters out through the urethra.

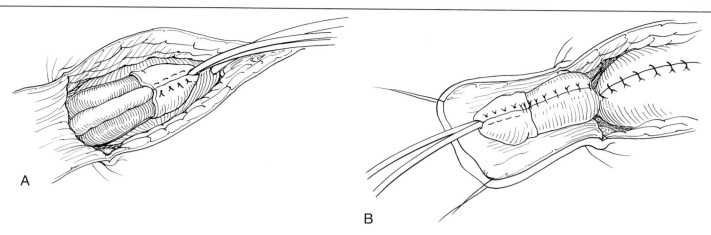

FIGURE 74-10. A, Ureteral reimplantation is not performed at primary repair because the exstrophic bladder is still immature. However, vesicoureteral reflux is assumed to exist in these patients until proven otherwise. The corporeal bodies tend to rotate medially, which assists in correcting dorsal chordee. **B,** Reapproximate the corpora with fine interrupted sutures along the dorsal aspect. Then bring up the tubularized urethra to each hemiglans ventrally to create an orthotopic meatus. Reconfigure the glans using deep interrupted mattress sutures followed by horizontal 6-0 monofilament mattress sutures to reapproximate the glans epithelium. Close the neourethra with 7-0 suture, similar to standard hypospadias repair. If necessary, perform glans tissue reduction to create a conical-appearing glans. We routinely note excess tissue at the base of the glans dorsally, which should be trimmed. The urethra may lack sufficient length to reach the glans. In this situation the urethra may be closed along the ventral aspect of the penis, creating hypospadias that may be corrected later. This represents an inherent lack of length in the urethral plate, and hypospadias results from aggressive posterior mobilization of the bladder and urethra. Redundant shaft skin is left in place ventrally in these patients to assist in later penile reconstructive procedures.

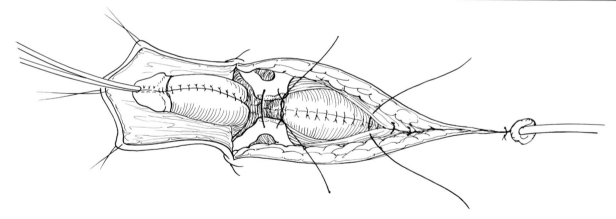

FIGURE 74-11. To reapproximate the pubic symphysis use size 0 or 1 TiCron suture placed anteriorly to help prevent suture erosion into the bladder neck. Reapproximate the rectus fascia using a running 2-0 polydioxanone (PDS) suture.

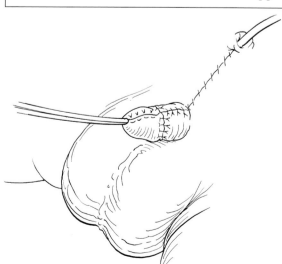

FIGURE 74-12. Reconfigure penile shaft skin using primary dorsal closure or reversed Byars flaps if needed to provide dorsal skin coverage. Reapproximate the skin covering the abdominal wall using a 5-0 absorbable monofilament suture.

FEMALE EXSTROPHY CLOSURE

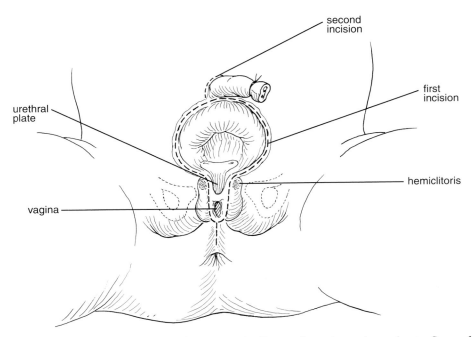

FIGURE 74-13. Principles of closure in female patients are similar to those in male patients. Several points are important. The clitoris is separated, which precludes the need to disassemble it. The perineal incision must be extended around the vagina and deep into the pelvis in a Y-V advancement. The vagina and urethral plate are considered a single unit and never separated.

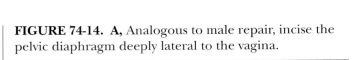

FIGURE 74-14. A, Analogous to male repair, incise the pelvic diaphragm deeply lateral to the vagina.

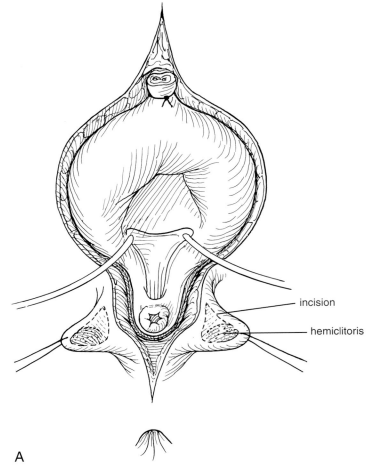

A

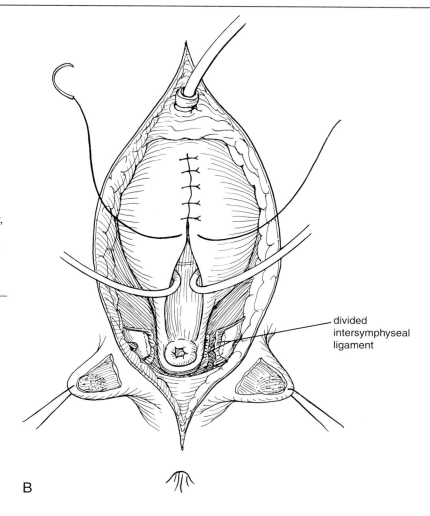

FIGURE 74-14, cont'd. **B,** Closure of the bladder, urethra, and clitoris is analogous to bladder, bladder neck, urethral, and penile repair in male patients. Secure ureteral stents with 5-0 chromic sutures and bring out through the new urethra.

divided
intersymphyseal
ligament

B

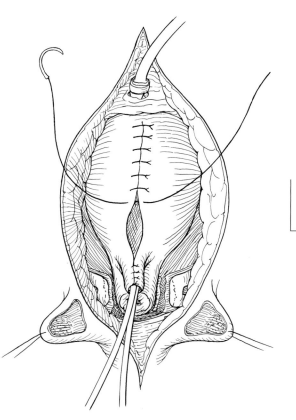

FIGURE 74-15. Close the bladder in three layers and the urethra in two, using absorbable sutures. The umbilicus is fashioned using the suprapubic cystostomy tube as an exit site.

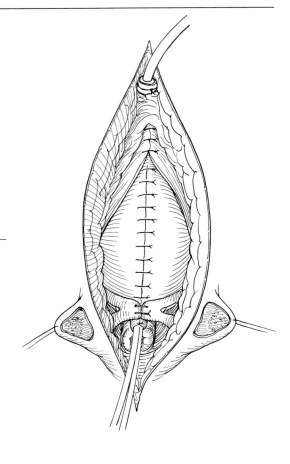

FIGURE 74-16. Reapproximate the pubic symphysis using size 0 or 1 PDS placed anteriorly to help prevent suture erosion into the bladder neck.

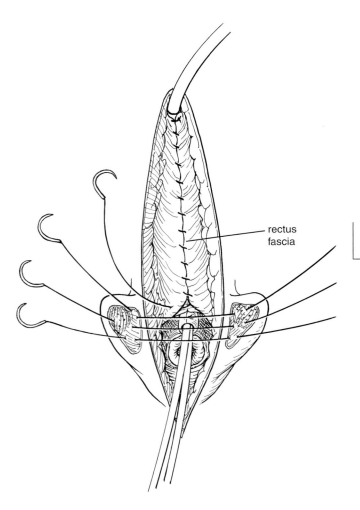

rectus
fascia

FIGURE 74-17. Reapproximate the rectus fascia using a running 2-0 PDS suture.

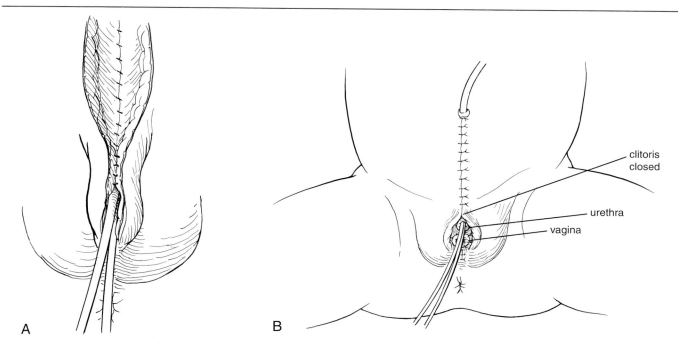

FIGURE 74-18. A and **B,** Close the skin of the abdominal wall and the reapproximation of the clitoris using 5-0 absorbable monofilament suture.

POSTOPERATIVE CARE

Patients are maintained postoperatively in Bryant's traction for 2 to 3 days and then fitted with an exstrophy splint to maintain hip adduction. Alternatively, a spica cast may be used for 3 weeks of immobilization. Ureteral catheters are brought out through the urethra and left in place. They are removed 7 to 10 days after the operation.

MICHAEL MITCHELL

Commentary by

Little has changed in the technique over the past 15 years. The most important aspect of the procedure is exposure of the pelvic diaphragm medial to the corpora and deep incision of this structure bilaterally to permit the bladder and proximal urethra to sink deep into the pelvis without "step-off" at the bladder neck. With reapproximation of the symphyseal diastasis there is no compression of the proximal urethra and good potential for sphincter function. The result is bladder cycling (filling and emptying), which is the stimulus for the pathologic bladder of the newborn exstrophy patient to change and become normal. To this point, of our complete primary repair of bladder exstrophy (CPRE) patients closed in the last 20 years, we have had to augment only *one* bladder.

The issue of osteotomy is still in debate; however, we presently tend to perform osteotomies in the newborn, as we feel the osteotomy facilitates the closure and long-term anterior support to the repair. We apply a spica cast to all CPRE patients with or without osteotomy. This enables a shortened hospitalization (our average hospitalization for newborn CPRE is 4 days postsurgery). We usually leave two 3-F umbilical artery ureteral catheters in place, which also function as urethral splints postsurgery. These are held in place with 6-0 chromic sutures through the catheter and through the bladder wall at the ureteral meatus. These catheters are brought out together through the reconstructed urethral channel and permitted to fall out; it usually takes 5 to 7 days for this to happen. A bladder tube is left in place, and this is brought out through the neoumbilicus. We have been pleased with the pigtail suprapubic 8-F tube and have been disappointed with the silastic Malecot tubes, which tend to be rather undependable in staying in the bladder.

Recently, we have been more aggressive about proximal urethral lengthening at the time of primary closure (if the size of the bladder plate permits). We have neither selected patients based on bladder plate size, nor used bladder plate size as a criteria for closure (and therefore have closed all exstrophies in the manner described, regardless of size). We feel strongly that the advantage of CPRE is the potential for early bladder cycling to permit the abnormal bladder present at birth to change and to heal. This maximizes the potential for the exstrophic bladder to function normally. Almost one third of the patients we have closed primarily have gone on to void normally and have gone through potty training with good continence and without the need for bladder neck repair. As well, bladder augmentation has been reduced from 30% to less than 5%. However, although the critical timing of closure has not been defined, it does seem that if the bladder is not permitted to cycle in the first few months of life then the potential for normalization of bladder structure and function will be limited.

DOUG CANNING

When planning closure of bladder exstrophy, our philosophy at The Children's Hospital of Philadelphia is to provide a consistent team with each member assigned a series of tasks to provide each child with as consistent a repair as possible. The complete repair of bladder exstrophy is an extensive operation requiring meticulous attention to detail for a prolonged period. If the team is changing, it is difficult to ensure that each member is experienced enough to maintain this level of performance for the entire operation. To this end, the same orthopedist and the same two experienced pediatric urologists work together on each procedure. From a practical standpoint, to assemble this team consistently precludes operating on the first days of life for most of these babies. We have found that no harm comes to the bladder if we send the infant home with his mother and father in the newborn period with a small piece of clear plastic wrap inside the diaper to protect the bladder from the diaper. With this approach, the infant bonds with his or her mother and the family. I also think this time at home provides time for the family to accept the defect and to prepare for the surgery and the postoperative care.

The infant and his or her family returns 4 to 6 weeks later to meet a well-rested, organized team. No longer do we push to do these surgeries at the end of a difficult operating day but start early in the morning with rested surgeons, nurses, and ancillary personnel. We obtain a renal sonogram and because we perform osteotomies in all of our cases, blood is available. Transfusion is required, in our experience, about half the time.

After mobilizing the bladder and dissecting the skin and dartos tissue from the corpora cavernosa on each side, the most difficult portion of the operation begins as we free the urethral plate from each corpus. Too lateral a dissection along the spongiosal tissue will enter the corpus on either side. Too medial a dissection will risk injuring the corpus spongiosum, which will result in urethral stricture. We never divide the urethral plate. Inadvertent division of the urethral plate precludes epispadias repair at the time of the initial closure. To prevent thermal injury to the corpora, we tend to use bipolar cautery with our dissection. This allows for a more predictable path of the electric current through the tissue. Precise dissection of the urethral plate and corporeal bodies is critical. Loss of the neurovascular bundle on either side will result in the potential for glans injury. Loss of spongiosal blood supply will result in meatal stenosis or urethral stricture, and loss of the blood supply of the main penile artery as a result of torque on the penis (from the springing effect of the pubis after closure in patients without osteotomy) will all result in injury to the glans, corporeal bodies, urethra, or all three.

Aggressive proximal dissection on each side of the urethra and deep incision of the intrasymphyseal ligament posterior to the urethral plate allow the bladder to achieve a posterior position within the pelvis. We use a Peña nerve stimulator to stimulate contraction of the striated muscle with the pelvic diaphragm. We believe this helps us provide a frame and target for placement of the posterior urethra adequately within the pelvic diaphragm.

After closure of the bladder and the urethral plate as a continuous unit, we often add an acellular matrix plate (AlloDerm) at the junction of the bladder neck. This is one of the most fragile portions of the dissection and it is often a site for leakage. We believe that adding the matrix helps prevent dehiscence and augments the integrity of the bladder neck, which ultimately helps to provide continence.

After closure of the urethra and placement of the urethra posterior to the corpora, we place the sutures in the pubis. These sutures are placed as horizontal mattress sutures with a needle placed through the anterior ramus of the pubic bone on the right from out to in and then from in to out. The suture is then crossed to the left from out to in at a position superior on the ramus and then from in to out at an inferior position on the left pubic ramus. In this way, the knot and then suture are exterior to the pubic ramus. This prevents erosion of the suture into the newly reconstructed urethra and bladder neck. With closure of the pubis, the urethra is posterior to the corporeal bodies. We rotate the corporeal bodies medially to reposition the neurovascular bundle to a near normal position along the dorsum of the penis. To ensure maintenance of the rotated corpora, we place a series of interrupted 5-0 or 6-0 absorbable monofilament sutures just medial to the neurovascular bundle. If we injure the neurovascular bundle on either side, the glans is at risk. To lengthen the dorsum of the penis and to provide collateral circulation, we make a horizontal incision in the midline of the corpus on each side. We close these incisions vertically to lengthen the corpus on each side. These incisions are closed across the midline to each contralateral corpus to provide a diamond-shaped reanastomosis. The urethra is reconstructed with a double layer of interrupted sutures. We have found that running suture tends to reduce the ability of the urethra itself to lengthen and increases the chance that the urethra cannot be brought beyond the midshaft of the penis or even the penoscrotal junction. This does not bother us at all, however, and we (in most cases) create a hypospadias rather than push to bring the urethra out to the tip of the glans.

The female exstrophy patient is a much simpler repair. Occasionally we mobilize the urethra and vagina as a unit and move them posteriorly to provide the closure of the urethra to a posterior position within the pelvic diaphragm. We make no attempt to close the clitoral bodies on the midline.

Postoperatively we tend to maintain the infant in modified Bryant's traction for 3 to 4 weeks in an adult-sized bed. The infant's mother can nurse the child adequately in bed. We pay close attention to the suprapubic tube and urethral stents to maintain diversion of urine that we believe is critical to a successful repair. The suprapubic tube is clamped initially for short periods. Gradually, the duration of clamping is increased. We do not remove the tube until we are sure that the infant is voiding at low pressure. If ureterectasis occurs, we do not hesitate to reimplant the ureters.

Chapter 75

Modern Staged Reconstruction for Vesical Exstrophy

Cover the vesical mucosa with plastic wrap to prevent irritation. Confirm normal kidneys by sonogram. Have blood available.

The sequence for primary vesical closure is to perform osteotomies if the baby is older than 48 hours.

The sequence for primary repair in the male is as follows: In the first stage, close the bladder posterior urethra, pubic bones, and abdominal wall and create an incontinent epispadias. The urethra is brought well onto the shaft of the penis. It is essential that this initial bladder closure be successful; failure makes subsequent attempts at reconstruction much more difficult and more prone to failure. At 6 months of age (second stage), the epispadias is repaired, under testosterone

stimulation, to increase outlet resistance and bladder capacity. In the third stage, form both antireflux and continence mechanisms by reconstructing the bladder neck.

IMMEDIATE, MODERN STAGED RECONSTRUCTION (GEARHART-JEFFS)

First Stage: Osteotomy and Vesicourethral Closure

Infants older than 1 or 2 days usually require osteotomies.

Repair in the Male Neonate

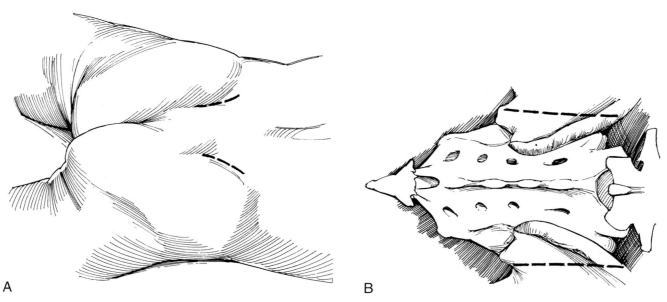

A

B

FIGURE 75-1. Prep the lower thorax to knees both anteriorly and posteriorly of the anesthetized child and place him in the supine position on sterile drapes. **A,** Make straight incisions over the skin crease at the junction of the trunk and leg bilaterally. **B,** Divide the iliac bones exactly vertically from the anterior incision. Keep the chisel close to the sacroiliac joints, but only divide the anterior table. Next make a transverse incision on the innominate bone bilaterally just above the hip joint. Perform the osteotomy and close the skin incision. An external fixator is placed at the end of the procedure in older children. Anterior osteotomies may also be needed when the pubic bones will not come together.

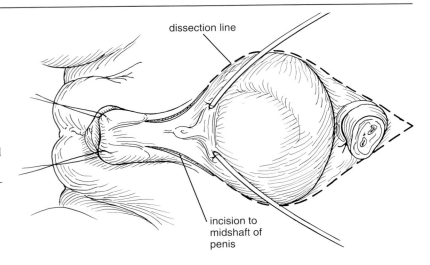

FIGURE 75-2. Remove any excess umbilical cord to avoid contamination of the wound. Place a traction suture in the glans. Mark the incision from just above the umbilicus down the junction of the bladder and paraexstrophy skin, to the level of the urethral plate and prostate.

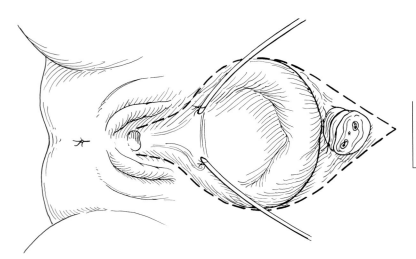

FIGURE 75-3. In girls carry the incision to the vaginal os on both sides. Anticipate closing the labia majora and clitoral hood over the completed urethroplasty.

FIGURE 75-4. Start the dissection at the umbilicus establishing a plane between the rectus fascia and the bladder. Use the urachal remnant as a handle. Ligate the umbilical vessels and allow them to fall into the pelvis. Dissect the peritoneum off the dome of the bladder to allow the bladder to be placed deep in the pelvis at the time of closure.

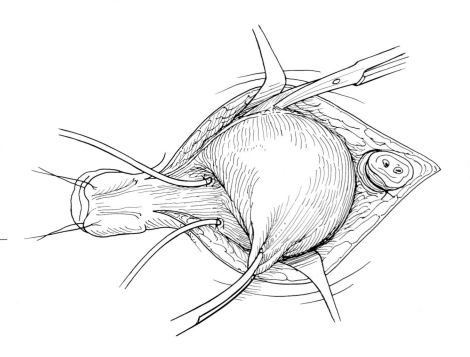

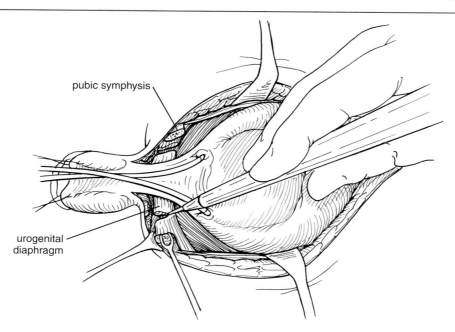

FIGURE 75-5. Continue the dissection caudally down between the bladder and rectus fascia until the urogenital diaphragm fibers are encountered bilaterally. Expose the separated pubic bone on each side. This will facilitate exposure of the urogenital diaphragm fibers between the bladder neck, posterior urethra, and pubic bone. Incise the urogenital diaphragm fibers sharply with electrocautery down to the level of the levators in their entirety. If this maneuver is not performed adequately, the posterior urethra and bladder will not be placed deeply into the pelvis. Thus, when the pubic bones are brought together, the posterior vesicoureteral unit will be brought anteriorly into an unsatisfactory position for later continence and reconstruction.

If the decision is made to transect the urethral groove, then the groove is divided distal to the veru montanum. Continuity is maintained between the thin, mucosal, non–hair-bearing skin adjacent to the posterior urethra and bladder neck and the skin and mucosa of the penile skin and glans. Flaps in the area of the thin skin are subsequently moved distally and rotated to reconstruct the urethral groove, resurfacing the penis dorsally. The corporeal bodies are not brought together at this juncture, as later Cantwell-Ransley epispadias repair will require the urethral plate to be brought beneath the corporeal bodies. If the urethral plate is left in continuity, it must be mobilized up to the level of the prostate to create as much additional urethral and penile length as possible. Further urethral lengthening can be performed at the time of epispadias repair. In the rare instance there is a good, deep urethral groove, a modified Cantwell-Ransley epispadias repair can be combined with newborn closure. We routinely do this with delayed primary repair and closure.

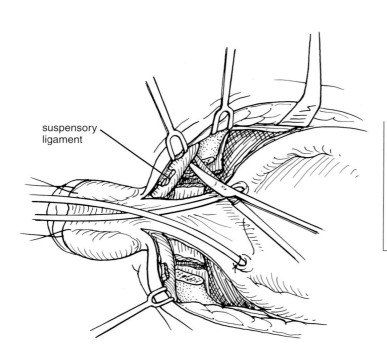

FIGURE 75-6. Free the wide band of fibers and muscular tissue representing the urogenital diaphragm and any suspensory ligaments from the corpora to the pubis bilaterally. Reluctance to free the bladder neck and urethra completely from the inferior ramus of the pubis moves the neobladder opening cephalad should any separation of the pubis occur during healing, thus increasing the chance of bladder prolapse.

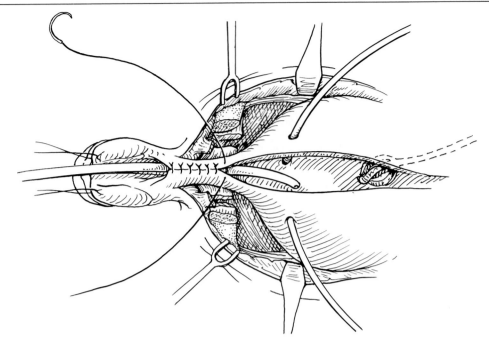

FIGURE 75-7. Close the mucosa and muscle of the bladder and posterior urethra well onto the shaft of the penis in the midline anteriorly. The size of the opening (10 to12 F) should allow enough resistance to aid in bladder adaptation and to prevent prolapse, but not enough outlet resistance to cause upper-tract changes. Drain the bladder with a suprapubic nonlatex Malecot catheter for a period of 4 weeks. If there are no problems with the stents during healing, leave them in for 2 to 3 weeks.

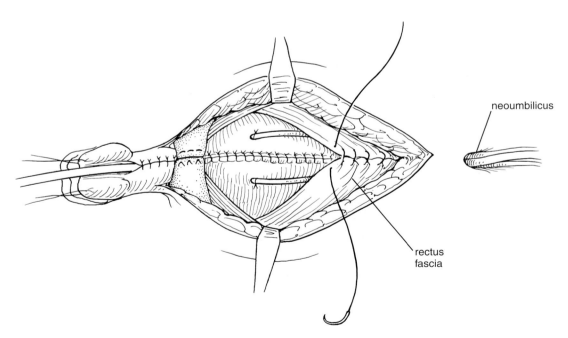

neoumbilicus

rectus
fascia

FIGURE 75-8. After the bladder and urethra have been closed and the drainage tubes placed, place pressure over the greater trochanters bilaterally, allowing the pubic bones to be approximated in the midline. Use #2 permanent horizontal mattress sutures in the pubis, tying the knots away from the neourethra. Create a V-shaped flap of abdominal skin at a point corresponding to the normal position of the umbilicus. Tack the flap to the abdominal fascia. The suprapubic tube and ureteral stents exit via this orifice.

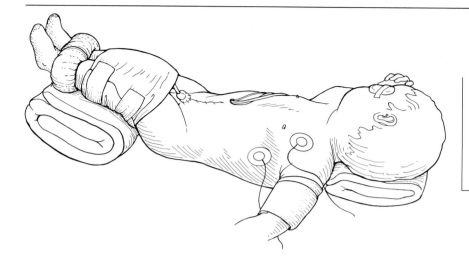

FIGURE 75-9. Multiple different dressings and devices can be used to immobilize the patient in the postoperative period. If an osteotomy is not used, modified Bryant's traction is used for a month. If osteotomy is performed, an external fixator and modified Buck's skin traction is used for 4 weeks.

MANAGEMENT AFTER PRIMARY CLOSURE

The modern staged reconstruction for vesical exstrophy (MSRE) approach converts a patient with exstrophy into one with proximal shaft epispadias and incontinence. Before removal of the suprapubic tube 4 weeks after surgery, the bladder outlet is calibrated by a urethral catheter or a urethral sound to ensure free drainage. An ultrasound examination is obtained to ascertain the status of the renal pelvises and ureters, and appropriate urinary antibiotics are administered to treat any bladder contamination that might be present after removal of the suprapubic tube. Prophylactic antibiotics should be continuous because all patients with bladder exstrophy, once closed, have vesicoureteral reflux. After the conversion from exstrophy to proximal shaft epispadias with incontinence, the bladder gradually increases in capacity as inflammatory changes in the mucosa resolve.

Should bladder outlet resistance be such that urine is retained within the bladder and reflux and ureteral dilatation develop with infected urine, it may be necessary to dilate the urethra or to begin intermittent catheterization. If bladder outlet resistance persists and infections continue, then an antireflux procedure may be required as early as 6 months to 1 year after initial closure.

In males, the second-stage epispadias (see Chapters 160 and 161) closure can proceed at 6 months of age under testosterone stimulation. As long as the patient remains infection free, bladder neck reconstruction (see Chapter 68) with antireflux surgery for persistent urinary incontinence should proceed after age 4 to 5 years.

POSTOPERATIVE PROBLEMS

Dehiscence after bladder closure, or even fascial separation, will make subsequent attempts at creating continence virtually impossible. A stricture may form at the bladder neck or in the neourethra, resulting in incomplete emptying and stone formation; if so, revision of the outlet is mandatory. It may be advisable to delay closure of the bladder neck until a time when intermittent catheterization is possible. Watch for obstruction of the upper tracts.

Long-term problems may appear after repair: For persistent incontinence after MSRE, perform augmentation cystoplasty. Urinary stones and recurrent infection are not uncommon if bladder emptying is not assured. Prolapse (vaginal, uterine, or rectal) may occur, usually around puberty; treat it by uterine suspension to the anterior sacral ligaments. Pregnancy is again possible but cesarean section is mandatory.

JULIAN S. ANSELL

Commentary by

The concept needs to be emphasized that exstrophy is a spectrum of congenital anomalies, ranging from superior vesical fistula/fissure, through continent epispadias and classic exstrophy, to the almost monstrous deformities of cloacal exstrophy. A subtitle for this procedure could be "Correction of Representative Types of the Exstrophic Spectrum/Syndrome." The second important principle needing emphasis is that in all but the least involved variations of the spectrum, closure is carried out in a series of stages, months, and years apart.

Superior vesical fissure (or fistula) is the most minor manifestation of the exstrophy complex. The bladder neck and urethra are intact, so only simple closure is needed.

Cloacal exstrophy is a form we are now seeing as often as the classic type in the Northwest United States, probably because the "cloacals" are not being given up as hopeless, but are referred for tertiary care. In these cases, the symphyses are usually more widely separated and osteotomies will probably be required.

Continued

A decision as to sex of rearing may be hastened by the need to intervene urgently to correct the omphalocele or other acute intestinal problems. Regardless of sex assignment, the ultimate genital appearance, male or female, is likely to be abnormal. Therefore, contrary to several authorities, we tend to accept the existing chromosomal and gonadal sex if in a full-term, neonatal, potential male the phallic structures are over 3.5 cm in length from pubis to midglans, even if the phallus is bifid and partially embedded in the abdominal wall or groin.

The early dominating problems are the omphalocele and intestinal obstruction due to atresia, duplication, intussusception, or some combination of these. If the intestinal problems are corrected easily, the bladder may be closed at the same setting; if not, the bladder halves can be united in the midline as part of the abdominal wall closure, and then freed at a later date and closed as for classic exstrophy. Reflux is not as common a problem in cloacal as in classic exstrophy, but in some initially and in others over time, ureteral stenosis will occur; the physician should watch for it. Bilateral, prevesical, and lower ureteral stenosis was the source of infection and sepsis and contributed significantly to the deaths of two of our neonates with cloacal exstrophy.

The short gut syndrome has been such a problem in our series that we work very hard to save a portion of the colonic plate and roll it into a tube to serve as a terminal colonic conduit and colostomy, rather than leave the child with an ileostomy. Even a short segment of colon appears to have a remarkable effect in cutting down the massive fluid loss that some of these children with ileostomies suffer.

Because the cloacal bladder is more superficially located than the classic exstrophic bladder, cloacal exstrophy is technically easier to close. However, the pubes are farther apart than the "classics" and most of them will require osteotomies to allow pubic approximation without undue tension. The bladder halves are usually generous, with plenty of room for a Young-Dees closure. The tailgut, which usually has an orifice in the colonic plate in the midline at the level of the caudal edges of the bladder halves, is extremely useful and must not be discarded. From it we have constructed urethra, vagina, and colon conduit. In some individuals it is long enough to consider as a terminal colon, which in a few of these children with functional anal muscle around the imperforate dimple might be pulled through as a rectum and anus. If you cannot figure out what to do with the tailgut at the time of the initial closure, leave it in situ attached to the bladder halves as a bladder-augmenting tube of bowel.

With a lot of support from pediatric medical and surgical colleagues, nurses, social workers, psychologists, physical therapists, and ancillary health workers, surprising results can be achieved. Of our 18 cases, 2 are truly continent and void normally with no hydronephrosis. Two others are continent with the aid of intermittent clean self-catheterization.

LOWELL R. KING

Commentary by

Bladder exstrophy remains one of the most challenging problems in urology. Closure can usually be achieved, but continence remains somewhat ethereal. In the past two decades, several principles that have evolved for the management of exstrophy have helped to standardize the treatment, and continence rates have gradually increased. Even more important, the upper tracts are now less likely to suffer hydronephrosis and deteriorate following closure (Ansell-Jeffs approach).

A consensus exists that there is an advantage to closing bladder exstrophy in the neonate. For the most part, this advantage is due to the cartilaginous nature of some of the pubic bones at birth and to the relative relaxation in the sacroiliac joints. Most prefer to use osteotomies to facilitate closure of the pelvic girdle; however, this lessens pressure on the abdominal incision after closure and makes healing *per primam* more likely. This primary closure is proving to be very important, as a much lower percentage of patients gain urinary control after secondary or tertiary bladder closures than in instances in which the bladder is successfully closed at the first operation.

Historically, approximation of the pubic symphysis over the bladder neck and urethra has never been considered important itself. However, if the distance between the pubic rami can be reduced, the bladder assumes a more normal position in the pelvis and the subsequent production of an angle between the bladder and posterior urethra may make subsequent continence more likely. If the pubic bones will not come close together after the posterior osteotomies, anterior osteotomies are needed as well. Much attention has been addressed to the short stubby penis in the boy with exstrophy after closure. An important principle is to lengthen the penis by detaching it from the pubic rami, in whole or in part, before the epispadias is repaired (Hinman, Duckett).

The kidneys can be protected after the continence procedure by ascertaining that the tubularized bladder forming the muscular portion of the neourethra is fairly uniform and approximately 10 F in caliber, as described. The upper tracts are also protected by routine antireflux implantation of the ureters into the bladder above the trigone (Leadbetter).

The development of urinary control subsequent to the procedure to provide continence takes time, often years. If the patient retains some urine in the bladder and voids intermittently, even at very short intervals, it is a good prognostic sign. When urethral resistance is adequate, the bladder will usually enlarge gradually and the intervals between voiding become longer. Many patients remain enuretic after reasonable social daytime control is achieved with time voiding. Some boys with continued incontinence after healing will gain urinary control at puberty with growth of the prostate. If a patient remains wet but unobstructed, an array of further adjuncts, ranging from an artificial urinary sphincter to bladder augmentation, are available to improve continence or bladder capacity.

When doing staged exstrophy closures between 1964 and 1980, I usually closed exstrophies the size of a 50-cent piece, or larger, and excised smaller bladder plates and performed primary ureterosigmoidostomies at 6 to 18 months of age. Of 16 primary reconstructions, two became continent while 28 of 32 with ureterosigmoidostomy did so by age 4. Additionally, three of the four who remained wet gained control with sphincter exercises.

Because the high risk of juxtaureteral colon cancer became clear, we contacted 22 of the ureterosigmoidostomy patients in 1980 and 1981, explained the risk, and offered conversion to a colonic conduit or a Kock pouch. No one accepted, although most said they would consider it later. Of special interest were eight girls in the group. They were very happy, and said they felt normal, and did not go to the toilet noticeably more often than their peers.

Of course, ureterosigmoidostomy can now be done without the cancer risk using the ileocecal segment. A nipple of ileum is intussuscepted though the ileocecal valve and stabilized. The ureters are then anastomosed to the ileal tail, and the cecal end approximated to the lower sigmoid after removal of an ellipse of sigmoid from the anastomotic site. With this arrangement, the ureters are anastomized to ileum and are in a sterile environment behind the antireflux nipple.

Later epispadias repair, with a dependent penis, is similar to that employed in a one-stage repair. The corpora are detached, rotated, and reapproximated dorsally, transposing the most proximal urethra ventrally. Since most of the ventral foreskin is needed to resurface the penis, a buccal graft is usually needed to form the penile urethra.

Although patients with exstrophy pose a surgical challenge and several operations are usually needed, the child who gains urinary control repays these efforts handsomely, as most patients with exstrophy do not have other significant congenital abnormalities and can function normally in society after successful treatment.

JOHN GEARHART

Commentary by

Bladder exstrophy remains a challenge for all pediatric urologists. Because of more accurate prenatal diagnosis, fewer of these infants are being seen in children's hospitals nationwide. Because of these issues, the United Kingdom's National Health Service has limited the care of the exstrophy-epispadias spectrum to two centers only.

Several clinical and basic science principles have improved the outcomes for these children over the last several years. These include (1) early closure in the newborn period, (2) liberal use of osteotomy if any doubt exists about the ability to bring the pubic bones into apposition at the time of closure, (3) better delineation of the abnormal pelvic anatomy, (4) early epispadias repair at 6 months of age, and (5) careful selection of patients for bladder reconstruction and doing it only in those with good overall bladder capacity of at least 100 mL.

Closure in the early newborn period has been made possible by early detection during fetal life and by allowing the parents to seek consultation with a busy exstrophy team prior to birth of the infant. This allows delivery at the same center for early closure and avoids transportation and other delays.

New data about pelvic anatomy have clearly shown both the external rotation and decrease in the actual amount of bone in the anterior bony pelvis. A paradox that exists is that the larger and better the bladder template, the wider the pubic diastasis at the time of closure. With a good bilateral pelvic osteotomy and appropriate postoperative fixation and extremity immobilization, the chance of dehiscence and bladder prolapse is markedly decreased. Recent in-depth studies of both the bony pelvis and muscular pelvic floor have shown the lack of anterior muscular pelvic support and the role of osteotomy in helping bring these pelvic tissues into a more normal anatomic position. Likewise, they have aided in helping improve the dissection of the urogenital diaphragm from the urethral plate down to the level of the levator hiatus and thus getting the posterior vesicourethral unit deep into the pelvis where the pelvic muscles can aid in the biomechanics of continence.

The epispadias repair can be done easily under testosterone stimulation at 6 months of age. The modified Cantwell-Ransley repair in our hands is safe, reliable, and helps increase bladder growth. We have avoided other methods of epispadias repair such as the penile disassembly and Kelly repair as we feel the risks with these procedures in the newborn or older infants are too high. At this juncture more penile length can be added by additional dissection of any remaining remnants of the suspensory ligaments from the pubis. Lastly, most all will require some touch-up surgery after the onset of puberty for additional penile length.

Continued

Likewise, bladder neck repair is not undertaken until the bladder has reached a sufficient capacity (100 mL ranges) and the child is ready to be involved in a vigorous postoperative voiding program. Currently in our hands, the overall continence rate with MSRE is 73% to 75% voiding and dry for 3 hours during the day and dry at night. This is slightly higher in females, who tend to get dry quicker and have a shorter interval between bladder neck reconstruction and achieving dryness. Careful management after bladder neck reconstruction requires frequent assessment of the ability to empty the bladder and upper tracts by pre- and postvoiding ultrasound for at least a year. Achieving an adequate "dry interval" comes over time as the bladder softens and regains capacity and the child learns to empty in a better fashion. Daytime urinary control usually comes up to a year or more before nighttime control is achieved. If there is failure of the bladder neck reconstruction many successful surgical options exist but bladder augmentation clearly becomes part of the solution in nearly all patients. Regardless of the type of repair chosen by the surgeon, our data clearly show that a successful, secure primary closure is the single most important parameter in achieving long-term voided continence.

Chapter 76

Plastic Correction of Exstrophy Suprapubic Defect

PLASTIC CORRECTION OF EXSTROPHY SUPRAPUBIC DEFECT (OWSLEY-HINMAN)

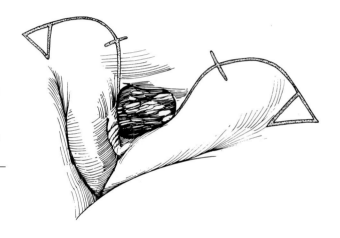

FIGURE 76-1. Preliminary skin expansion, by placing a balloon subcutaneously in the suprapubic site, may be helpful. Mark two curved incisions for rotation flaps beginning in girls just below the vaginal introitus and in boys, at the margin of the excised bladder, and ending just medial to the anterior superior iliac spine. Mark a back cut just above the inguinal crease, leaving a triangular piece of skin to be excised at the outer end of each incision.

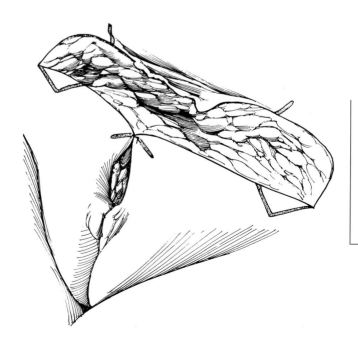

FIGURE 76-2. Elevate the skin flaps and undermine them widely. Join their tips in the midline with subcutaneous 3-0 synthetic absorbable sutures. In girls, mobilize the vagina posteriorly, and then start suturing in the midline just above the introitus. Finally, bring the bifid clitoris and its preputial hood together. Continue suturing to join the hair-bearing pubic skin in the midline using 3-0 synthetic absorbable sutures subcutaneously and interrupted 4-0 nonabsorbable sutures for the skin.

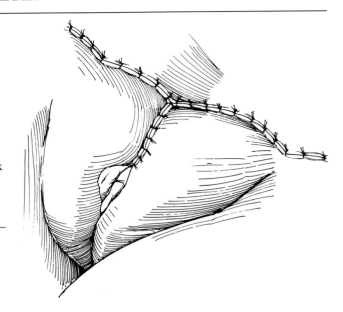

FIGURE 76-3. Approximate the skin in the superior transverse portion in the same way after an appropriate adjustment at the extremities of the incision. Insert two multiperforated drainage tubes beneath the flaps. Reinforce the abdominal wall defect by raising an aponeurotic flap from each rectus sheath and overlying skin, tissue that is supplied by the superficial circumflex iliac and inferior superficial epigastric vessels. Form such flaps by extending the lateral incisions 5 cm into the groin line to facilitate medial rotation (Arap, Giron, 1980).

CORRECTION OF SUPRAPUBIC DEFECT

A depression is left at the former site of the bladder, and the mons veneris is absent. Forming a flap will produce a more cosmetic result.

SKIN FLAP METHOD

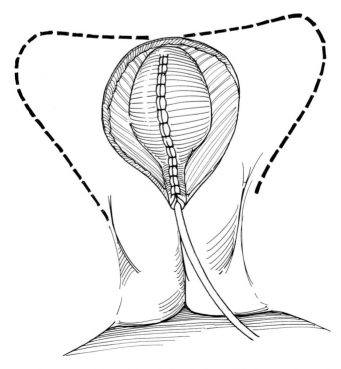

FIGURE 76-4. Mark and incise two flaps on either side of the defect with bases that arise posteriorly.

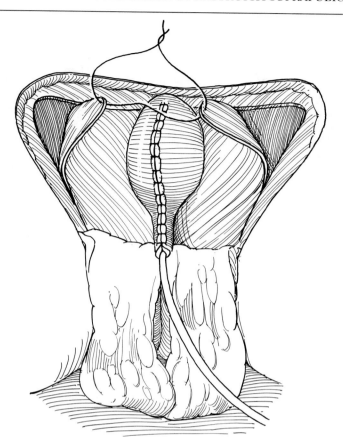

FIGURE 76-5. Incise the fascia laterally and bring the flaps together in the midline.

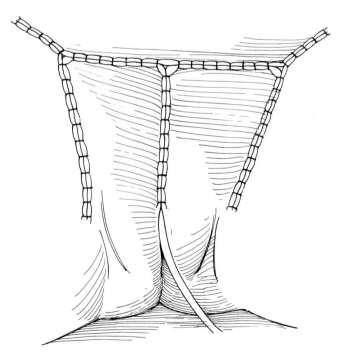

FIGURE 76-6. Close the apices and suture the skin flaps together in the midline. The main postoperative complication is necrosis of the edges of the flap, which will require wound care and healing by granulation.

MONEER HANNA

Commentary by

The external genital deformity in the female adolescent born with bladder exstrophy is that of bifid clitoris and anterior displacement of the vaginal introitus, which appears to be on the lower abdomen. The anus occupies the position of the normal vagina. The pubic hair is often bivalved by a midline hairless scar. It is possible to camouflage the deformity by uniting the clitoral halves and anterior ends of the labia to create a fourchette. When combined with excision of the pubic scars and contouring of the mons pubis the illusion is that of caudal vaginal recession. Reconstruction of the mons pubis varies from simple excision of a diamond-shaped, depressed area in the midline followed by longitudinal closure, preferably with Z-plasty, to the severely scarred pubic area, which requires rotation of a larger flap. Bilateral groin flaps fed by the superficial epigastric and superficial circumflex iliac arteries represent axial arterial flaps, which can be raised without regard to the length-to-width ratio. Incorporation of the deep fascia in these flaps enhances vascularity, and inclusion of subcutaneous fat (fascio-fatty-cutaneous flaps) provides an excellent filler for the prepubic hollow, which is a common deformity in bladder exstrophy. In some cases in which there is extensive lower abdominal scarring, tissue expanders are introduced subcutaneously and are slowly expanded over a 4-week period. The expanded skin flaps are then mobilized as bipedicle flaps to resurface the lower abdomen.

RICHARD GRADY

Commentary by

Midline correction is also a viable (and my preferred) approach to correcting the suprapubic defect with bladder exstrophy. Pippi Salle and his coworkers have described the technique with the midline closure. Midline suprapubic correction allows for easy concomitant revision of scars associated with previous exstrophy operations. It also reapproximates the labia majora and minora in an anatomically more normal position by rotating the labia medially and superiorly. It permits excellent alignment and approximation of the clitoral bodies. In my experience, vertical midline approximation results in less tension on the repair than the Owsley-Hinman correction and produces a cosmetically pleasing and anatomically normal repair. Z-plasties at the base of the repair may be required to lengthen the repair distally. This is especially useful in creating a distinct penopubic junction and adding length to the dorsal skin of the penile coverage. Finally, a vertical approximation can be carried superiorly to integrate an umbilicoplasty into the repair.

Chapter 77

Umbilicoplasty

At the time of primary closure for bladder and cloacal exstrophy an umbilicus can be fashioned by exiting the suprapubic catheter in the appropriate position. In situations in which the umbilicus is not adequate or is absent, a number of techniques are illustrated here.

SKIN DISK METHOD

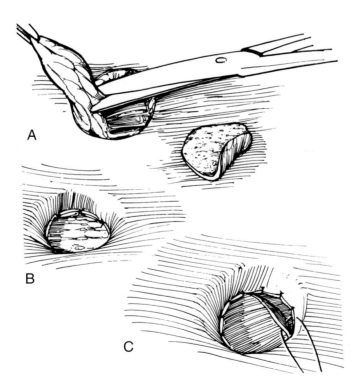

FIGURE 77-1. A, At the projected site for the umbilicus on the abdomen midway between xiphoid and pubis, mark and remove a disk of skin and subcutaneous tissue 1.5 cm in diameter. Excise deeply enough to expose the rectus fascia. Defat the skin disk. (Alternatively, obtain the disk from the shiny paraexstrophy skin around the bladder.) **B,** Suture the edges of the circular skin defect to the underlying fascia with fine monofilament sutures. **C,** Apply the disk of defatted skin and suture it in place with interrupted sutures. Apply a bolster dressing for mild compression.

UMBILICOPLASTY, BURIED SKIN TECHNIQUE

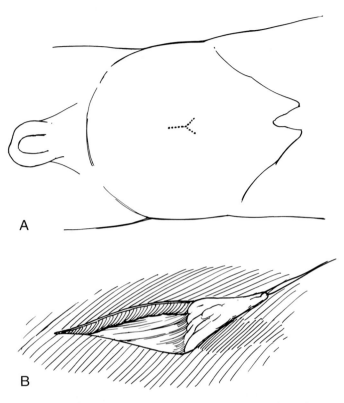

FIGURE 77-2. A, Site the umbilicus midway between xiphoid and pubis. Mark and create a Y incision with its center at the site. **B,** Elevate the V-flap and excise enough of the underlying subcutaneous tissue to expose the rectus sheath.

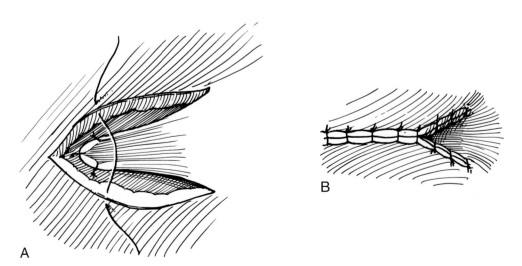

FIGURE 77-3. A, Suture the V-flap to the rectus sheath with three 3-0 synthetic absorbable sutures. **B,** Bring the edges of the Y together over the flap and suture them with two layers of sutures. Pack the wound with iodoform gauze and cover it with a transparent dressing to allow inspection. Change the gauze as necessary, but keep the pack in place for several weeks until granulation tissue has formed and epithelialization is well under way.

Commentary by
RICHARD GRADY

The quest to surgically create a consistent and anatomically normal umbilicus has led to literally dozens of techniques, including the ones described here. The Achilles heel of many of these repairs is tension on the repair, which cosmetically causes the umbilicus to vanish into a flat scar such that an initially satisfactory result disappears over time. Two other approaches to the umbilicoplasty that deserve mention include the M-plasty and the double-flap technique described by Philip Ransley.

In my hands, these approaches have produced a more effective and consistent way to produce an anatomically normal umbilicus for children who desire a neoumbilicus that has a lower likelihood of flattening over time. These approaches can also easily incorporate a Mitrofanoff stoma into the base of the repair, thus making them versatile as well as cosmetically appealing.

Commentary by
KATSUHIKO UEOKA

The constructed umbilicus tends to be smaller in diameter and shallower as time goes on, whatever method surgeons choose. So it is better to design a bigger umbilicus than expected. I prefer using a skin tube to make a constructed umbilicus deep enough. I have used the Mitchell umbilicoplasty technique in exstrophy patients whose umbilicus was created for cosmetic purposes or for an exit site of Mitrofanoff catheterizable channel with good results.

Commentary by
DUNCAN WILCOX

Creating an umbilicus can be very frustrating; at the time of operation, the umbilicus looks satisfactory, but when you want the body to heal with a scar it often appears not to, leaving an almost flat appearance.

The umbilicus usually lies at the level of the iliac crest in the midline. It is often prudent to mark this point before the operation starts, as a misplaced umbilicus is not cosmetically appealing.

The buried skin technique can give a satisfactory result. One way to create an umbilicus that sticks in is to create two rectangular skin flaps—the flaps are pointing to the midline with the vascular bases lateral. The width of the flap is the width of the future umbilicus. The apices of the two flaps are then sutured together; at this point, the apex is sutured to the underlying fascia in the midline. The two inferior sides of the flaps are sutured and then the superior sides. This acts to invert the flaps, creating the appearance of an umbilicus. This technique can work in all patients but appears most satisfactory in patients with some subcutaneous fat.

If a more complex umbilicus is required, the flaps can be created at an angle, with one sloping caudally and one sloping cranially; once the flaps are sutured together, an almost spiral appearance is created. However, the end results of these two techniques do not usually seem much different.

Chapter 78

Cloacal Repair

CLOACAL REPAIR (PEÑA)

To position, hold the child up by the heels and prep the entire lower body, because the child may need to be turned from prone to supine to prone. Locate the parts of the anal sphincter by electrostimulation, and make a transverse mark on the skin at that level.

Make an incision extending from the sacrum to the cloacal orifice.

FIGURE 78-1. Keeping exactly in the midline, divide the muscle layers including the external anal sphincter and its complex on both the anterior and posterior aspects. Use a needle tip on the electrosurgical unit. Stimulate the muscle with direct current to maintain the dissection in the midline. Divide the fine midline sagittal fascia to leave it to contain the perirectal fat. Insert two Weitlander retractors superficially, above the muscle layer. Split the coccyx in the midline to expose the levator ani muscle, which is divided in the midline to expose a yet to be identified visceral structure.

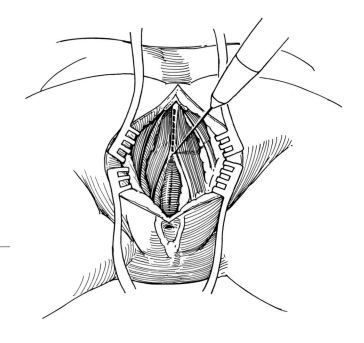

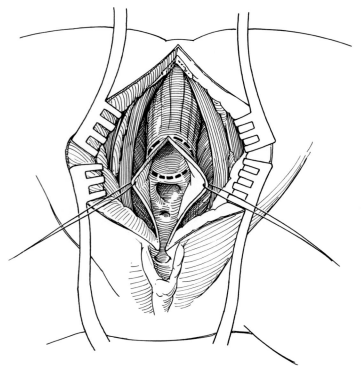

FIGURE 78-2. Open the visceral structure in the midline and hold it open with stay sutures. Within it will be found the rectum, vagina, and urethra. Dissect a plane between the rectum and vagina (the two will be densely bound together at first). Dissection will be time-consuming but is aided by injection of dilute epinephrine.

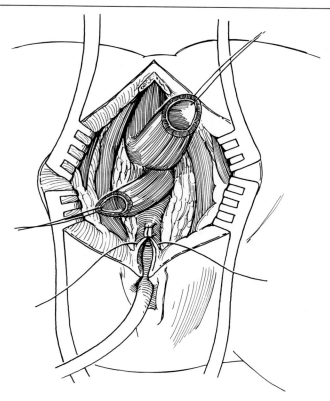

FIGURE 78-3. Separate the vagina from the urinary tract, keeping as close as possible to the heavier vaginal wall. The tissue here is extremely friable. Close the urethra using tissue from the cloacal channel.

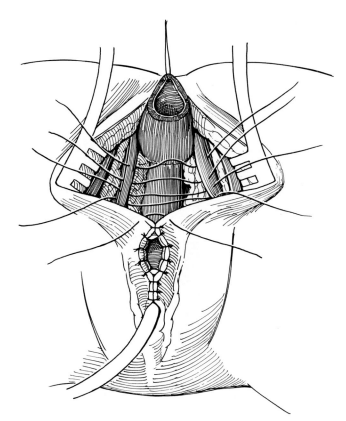

FIGURE 78-4. Suture the vagina to the perineum with interrupted synthetic absorbable sutures. With the stimulator, identify the anterior and posterior limits of the sphincter mechanisms and approximate the anterior layer with interrupted sutures.

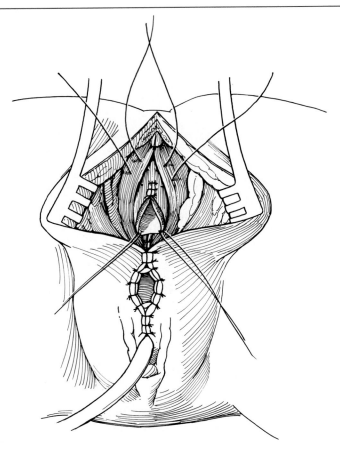

FIGURE 78-5. Because the rectum must fit between the two sphincteric layers, reduce its caliber by resecting a segment of the posterior wall and reapproximating the edges with two layers of interrupted sutures. Incorporate a bite of rectal wall in each stitch that is used to close the posterior layer of the sphincteric complex.

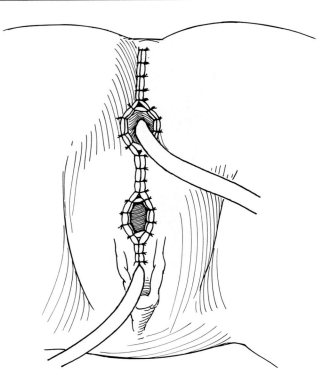

FIGURE 78-6. Fasten the rectal margin to the perineal skin with interrupted sutures and place a balloon catheter, to remain 1.5 to 2 weeks. Postoperatively, begin twice daily anal dilatations to gradually increase anal size. The vagina does not usually require dilatation, although surgery may well be needed for hematocolpos (hysterectomy, hemihysterectomy with vaginoplasty, or vaginoplasty and introitoplasty).

DUNCAN WILCOX

Prior to starting the surgical reconstruction it is advisable to perform a cystoscopy. The endoscopic examination will identify the length of the common channel and the relationship of the urethral, rectal, and vaginal openings. It will also identify how many vaginal openings there are. Often the anal cushions can be seen in the rectal fistula and care should be taken to avoid removing them during the reconstruction. This information is invaluable in planning the reconstruction and in assessing the amount of time that it will take. A short common channel of 2 cm or less is a relatively straightforward procedure; if the channel is 3.5 cm or greater then the operation can be an extremely difficult technical challenge.

The patient is placed in a prone jackknife position. The midline incision is continued until the common channel is identified. If persistent bleeding is encountered in the midline it suggests that the erectile tissue surrounding the common channel has been entered. If this is the case, then an instrument placed in the common channel can be helpful in identifying it. Once the common channel is found, the dissection is continued from distal to proximal, without disconnecting the common channel from the perineal skin. The common channel is mobilized using sharp dissection and by staying in close proximity. Once the ligamentous connections of the common channel and urethra are incised, then the further intrapelvic dissection can often be more easily completed using blunt dissection. As the dissection is continued proximally the rectum can usually be seen, except in very high lesions, entering the common channel. Rather than disconnecting the rectum now it can be helpful to continue mobilizing the whole common channel so that it can be brought down toward the perineum. This maneuver allows the difficult separation of the rectum from the common channel to be performed more easily, closer to the surface. Occasionally it is difficult to identify from outside the common channel where the rectum enters; in this situation, opening the common channel to identify the location of the various openings is helpful. Once the urethral opening is identified, a Foley catheter is placed; the presence of urine is reassuring. If the common channel is very long (4 cm or longer) when the initial identification of the common channel has been done, it is prudent to turn the patient and continue the dissection from the abdomen. Once the cloaca has been dissected off the sidewalls and is mobile, the dissection can continue prone again.

Separating the rectum from the common channel and vagina can be very difficult and is helped by multiple stay sutures and sometimes an instrument placed in the rectum or the vagina. It must be remembered that the rectum surrounds some of the lateral wall of the vagina and so the plane is usually more lateral than you might at first think. Making the first 1 to 2 cm of this dissection is the most difficult step, but then the plane becomes more easily identified. Inadvertent holes in the vagina can be repaired, but avoid overlapping suture lines. Once the rectum is dissected free, concentrate on the vagina and urethra.

In the majority of patients it is not necessary to separate the two structures, as with good mobilization the urethra and vaginal orifices can be brought down satisfactorily to the perineum. The remaining common channel can then be discarded or used to help create the fourchette. This use of the common channel will often give a superior cosmetic result, as it enables some mucosal-lined tissue to surround the urethra and vagina, which is present normally. If the vagina is too short to bring down to the perineum, the common channel is normally used to recreate the urethra. On occasion the urethra is of an adequate length and the common channel can be rotated to provide a longer posterior wall to the vagina. If these techniques do not work then a variety of options are available. The most dependent portion of the vagina may not be at the site of entry into the common channel; thus, length may be achieved by closing that opening and creating a new opening. If the vagina has been dilated by a hydrocolpos then a flap can be created and tubularized to achieve sufficient length. In very rare cases, this is still not sufficient. Peña has described a vaginal switch procedure, in which, with a bifid vagina and uterus, one uterus can be sacrificed and the bifid vagina moved so that the cervical end is brought down to the perineum. It is extremely rare if ever that a neovagina needs to be created.

With the urethra and vagina in position, ensure that a good perineal body is created before placing the rectum through the sphincter complex and creating the new anus.

At the end of the procedure a Foley catheter is left in situ. At the time of closure of colostomy a further cystoscopy is helpful in assessing the result. A further cystovaginoscopy prior to the onset of menarche is useful in deciding whether additional reconstructive surgery is required to allow for normal menstruation and sexual activity.

Chapter 79

Cloacal Exstrophy

Evaluate the patient with a multidisciplinary team made up of pediatric intensivists, general surgeons, plastic surgeons, neurosurgeons, and urologic surgeons. Stabilize the patient before any operative procedure. The exposed exstrophic hindgut and bladder plates are covered with a nonabrasive hydrophilic dressing (plastic wrap). All patients are treated empirically with intravenous antibiotics. A sonogram of the abdomen, pelvis, and spine will document expected renal and spinal abnormalities.

The procedure begins with placement of a central line for vascular access and subsequent parenteral nutrition. A total body preparation from the thorax to the toes is performed. Reconstruction begins with closure of the omphalocele. If the omphalocele cannot be closed due to increased abdominal pressure or tension, a silastic silo closure may be used as a delayed closure of the abdominal hernia. Alternatively, an alloderm graft can be used to assist in the closure.

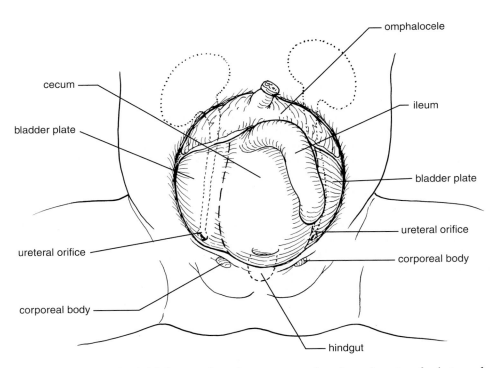

FIGURE 79-1. The primary goal of the initial procedure is to convert the cloacal exstrophy into a classic bladder exstrophy and/or attempt complete primary closure. The majority of these patients will end up with a permanent colostomy. The anatomy may vary depending on the malformation. Chromosome analysis is necessary to confirm the genotype.

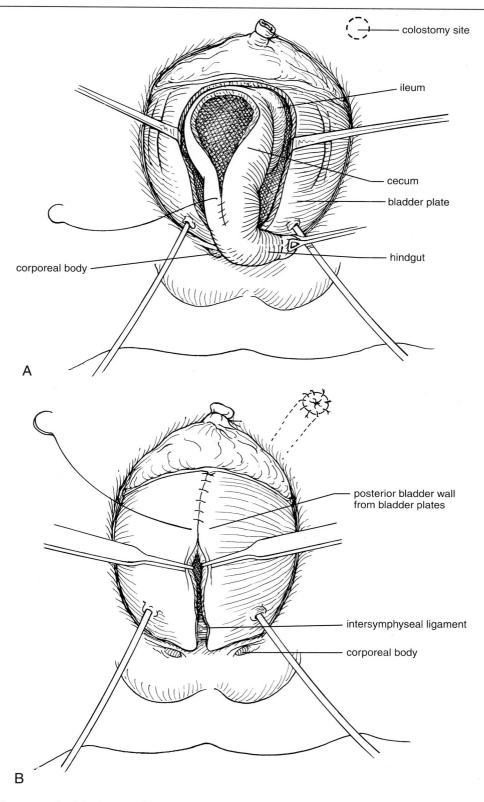

colostomy site

ileum

cecum

bladder plate

hindgut

corporeal body

A

posterior bladder wall
from bladder plates

intersymphyseal ligament

corporeal body

B

FIGURE 79-2. A, Separate the hindgut and intussuscepted ileum and cecum from the bladder plates, and then reduce and repair them. Create a colostomy. **B,** Reapproximate the bladder plates in the midline with a running 3-0 monofilament absorbable suture.

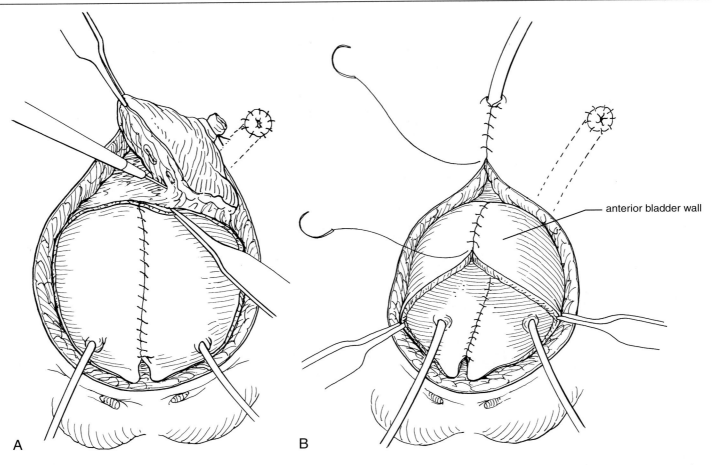

A

B

anterior bladder wall

FIGURE 79-3. A, Repair and close the omphalocele, giving the appearance of classic exstrophy. Hindgut reconstruction is individualized, and depends on patient anatomy. Options include incorporation into the gastrointestinal tract, excision if not viable, and/or conversion to a mucous fistula. The hindgut may prove useful in successive procedures, and prior planning is imperative. For example, the hindgut segment may be used in the future for anorectoplasty, bladder augmentation, or vaginal reconstruction. After conversion to a classic bladder exstrophy appearance, complete primary repair may be attempted if the patient is hemodynamically stable, the omphalocele is small, the pubic diastasis is not wide, and pulmonary function is adequate to tolerate increased abdominal pressure. Increases in intra-abdominal pressure may compromise cardiovascular status as well as the repair. If this is the case, it is prudent to stop and reconstruct the bladder in a classic exstrophy configuration for future repair. **B,** Use the complete primary exstrophy repair technique to complete the reconstruction (see Chapter 74). In the case of the male, complete penile disassembly and division of the intersymphyseal band are crucial to allow for appropriate posterior positioning of the bladder and urethra.

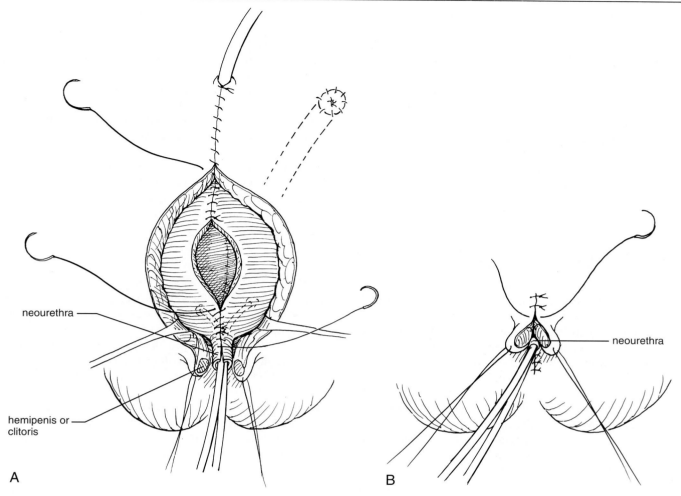

neourethra

hemipenis or
clitoris

A

neourethra

B

FIGURE 79-4. A, After the bladder and urethra are positioned within the pelvis, reconstruct the bladder, penis/clitoris, abdomen, and pelvis to approximate normal anatomy. **B,** Osteotomies will facilitate this portion of the procedure. Osteotomies are almost always necessary to assist in closure and posterior positioning of the urinary tract.

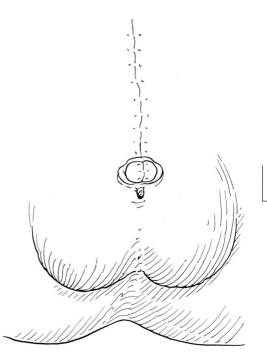

FIGURE 79-5. After complete primary closure it is not uncommon in the male for the urethra to be in a hypospadiac position.

POSTOPERATIVE CARE

Ureteral stents, a urethral catheter, and a cystotomy tube are used to provide adequate urinary drainage. Patients are immobilized with spica casts for 3 to 4 weeks. Nutritional support, pain control, and prophylactic antibiotics are continued. Ureteral stents are removed at 2 to 3 weeks postoperatively. Renal and bladder ultrasound is obtained after ureteral stent removal to monitor for hydronephrosis. The urethral catheter is removed at 3 to 4 weeks, and the suprapubic tube is removed after the patient demonstrates adequate emptying of the bladder or the family is comfortable with clean intermittent catheterization.

Additional surgery, such as orchiopexy, repair of unrecognized hernia, or hypospadias reconstruction, is performed as necessary. Colostomy reversal or pull-through may be considered at this time as well in select patients. Routine renal and bladder ultrasound is obtained every 3 months during the first postoperative year and then every 6 months for the next 2 years. Renal and bladder ultrasound is obtained annually thereafter unless there is a significant clinical change necessitating earlier or more frequent studies. Voiding cystourethrogram and videourodynamics are performed intermittently in the postoperative period to assess vesicoureteral reflux and bladder function, and when clinically indicated, as in cases of febrile urinary tract infection or progressive hydronephrosis.

Commentary by RICHARD GRADY

We have adapted the principles of the primary repair of exstrophy to cloacal exstrophy with satisfactory results. More often than not, these repair principles need to be applied in a sequential fashion over a period of weeks or months. The decision to stage the repair versus correcting the exstrophic defect in one operation depends on (1) the size of the omphalocele, (2) the child's pulmonary reserve, and (3) the physiology of the infant. If the repair is staged, the time between stages should be dictated by the speed of recovery and can be weeks to months depending on this. If at all in doubt, it is prudent to stage the reconstruction rather than risk elevated intra-abdominal pressures that could jeapordize the repair, cause internal organ ischemia, or stress the pulmonary system too much. Whenever possible, the hindgut should be removed from between the bladder plates, tubularized, and reincorporated into the gastrointestinal tract. This will reduce the need for postoperative parenteral nutrition and make fluid management easier as well, as fluid losses will be reduced by the addition of absorptive surface to the gastrointestinal tract. There is no doubt that the repair of cloacal exstrophy is one of the most complex in the field of urology; it requires a long-term commitment by surgeons familiar with the care of these patients and versatile in their surgical armamentarium.

Commentary by JOSEPH G. BORER

The initial surgical management of the patient with cloacal exstrophy is accurately described by the authors. Attention is justly given to several key steps in the process of initial surgical management of this complex entity. It is important to remove any umbilical clamps and replace them with soft umbilical "tape" or heavy silk suture in the immediate postnatal period. My preference for covering the lower abdomen including the omphalocele, if present, the exstrophied bladder and bowel, and the genitalia is a transparent adhesive dressing. This dressing will adhere to the abdominal wall surrounding these structures, and it be protective of, but not adherent to, the structures themselves.

The need for and benefit of a multidisciplinary approach to care cannot be overemphasized. Preoperative evaluation should include plain radiography of the abdomen and spine, ultrasonography of the kidney(s) and spine, and cardiac echography. Eventual imaging of the spine with magnetic resonance imaging and the bowel with fluoroscopy will also be necessary.

The authors have clearly stated the primary goal of initial surgery, that of converting lower urinary tract anatomy from cloacal exstrophy to bladder exstrophy via separation of the genitourinary and gastrointestinal tracts. Great care should be exercised if proceeding further with bladder closure and posterior urethral closure only, and particularly if proceeding to complete primary repair. The distal extent of the hindgut should be brought to the skin and a proximal protective ileostomy should be performed when presenting anatomy permits.

Temporary postoperative urinary diversion with ureteral stenting and suprapubic cystostomy tube bladder decompression (also used for future installation of contrast material at approximately 2 to 3 weeks postoperatively), with or without urethral catheterization, are of benefit in keeping the repair dry for the purpose of promoting healing in the early postoperative phase. These practices are also helpful for accurate recording of urinary output during the several-week period of immobilization following initial repair. Central venous catheter placement at the time of initial surgery and use for delivery of hyperalimentation is helpful with or without the presence of omphalocele.

Long-term care of these complex patients requires extensive and careful monitoring from several disciplines of surgical and medical expertise.

Chapter 80

Prune-Belly Syndrome: Reduction Cystoplasty, Abdominal Repair, and Umbilicoplasty

Musculoskeletal and gastrointestinal anomalies, as well as those of the genitourinary tract, including renal dysplasia, are associated with prune-belly syndrome. Cryptorchidism (with underdeveloped testes) is the rule; thus, orchiopexy should be done along with early repair of the abdominal wall and urinary tract reconstruction. Megalourethra may also need correction.

Three degrees of prune-belly syndrome are distinguished: class 1, mild—small spherical bladder, moderate megaure-

ters; class 2—megacystis, bilateral reflux, hydronephrosis, and/or unilateral renal dysplasia; class 3—as in class 2 plus severe bilateral dysplasia.

Obtain a chest x-ray to look for possible pulmonary problems from the lax abdomen and to detect possible cardiac anomaly. Assess renal function and be alert for urinary tract infections. Perform a renal scan and a voiding cystourethrogram.

ABDOMINAL REPAIR AND UMBILICOPLASTY I (MONFORT)

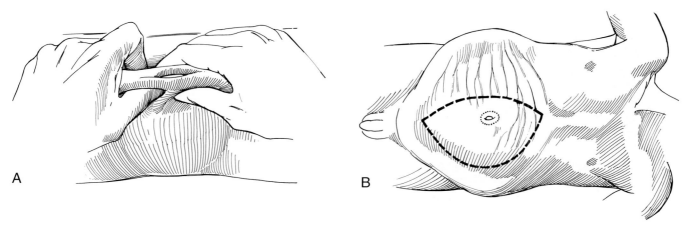

FIGURE 80-1. A, Estimate the amount of excess abdominal wall by grasping it with both hands. **B,** Mark the skin at the margin of the raised portions of the abdominal wall (dashed lines). Incise the skin and subcutaneous tissue to leave the umbilicus as an island. Start the incision near the xiphoid, following the skin marks. Leave an acute angle at either end. Incise the full thickness of the skin, and excise it, including the subcutaneous tissue, with electrocautery but leave some fat on the fascia to avoid devascularization. Hemostasis must be meticulous. Leave the umbilcus in place. The excision will leave an asymmetric defect and expose the degenerate abdominal plate that is composed of the aponeuroses of the external and internal oblique muscles, the rectus fascia, and the peritoneum.

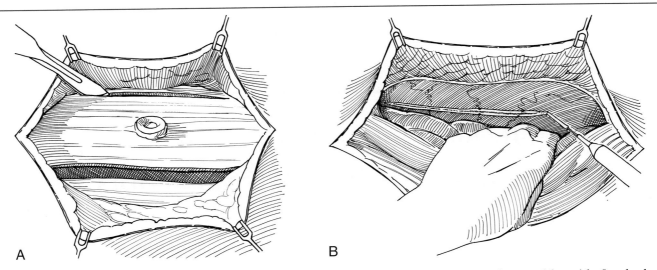

FIGURE 80-2. A, Incise the abdominal fascia and musculature lateral to the rectus muscles on either side for the length of the skin incision and enter the peritoneal cavity. The incision extends from the superior to the inferior epigastric vessels, which can now be seen from the inside. Leave these vessels intact to supply the central musculofascial plate. Now perform bilateral orchiopexy and any corrections of the urinary tract. **B,** Make a vertical incision through the peritoneum on each side in the lateral colonic gutters to lay bare a strip of the inner surfaces of the lateral abdominal wall muscles.

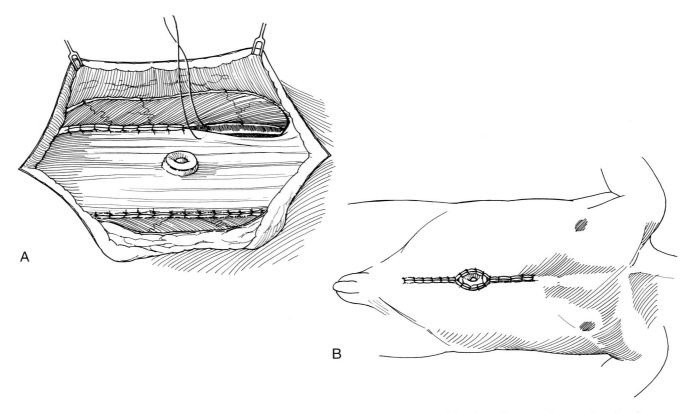

FIGURE 80-3. A, Suture the lateral margins of the central plate to the lateral body wall musculature that has been exposed by the peritoneal incisions. **B,** Trim the skin flaps to fit, provide notches for the umbilical island, and bring the flaps over the plate. Trim any excess skin and close it around the umbilical island.

ABDOMINAL REPAIR AND UMBILICOPLASTY II (EHRLICH)

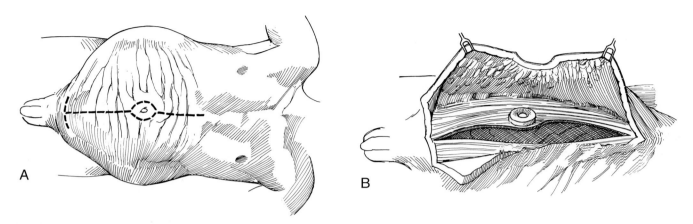

FIGURE 80-4. **A,** Make a midline incision from the xiphoid to the pubis. Proceed with orchiopexy, and any required urinary tract reconstruction. **B,** Sharply separate the skin and its subcutaneous tissue from the attenuated abdominal wall muscle and fascia on each side of the midaxillary line, leaving the umbilicus as an island on one flap. Gain hemostasis.

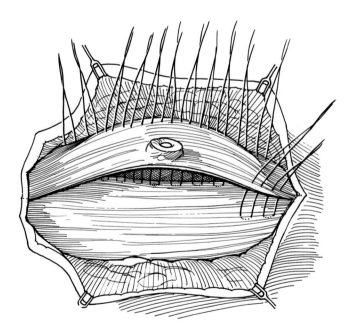

FIGURE 80-5. In a double-breasted fashion, advance one flap of fascia across the midline under the other flap, the one that has the umbilical pedicle attached. Insert a row of through-and-through polyglactin sutures to approximate the edge of the deep fascial layer to the undersurface of the overlying fascial layer. Place a second row of sutures to fasten the edge of the upper flap to the basal surface of the lower flap. Insert a few of the lower sutures through Cooper's ligament and the pubic tubercle to stabilize the lower end of the repair.

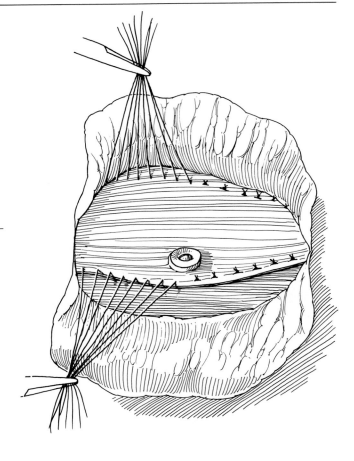

FIGURE 80-6. Hold the ends of the sutures in clamps, and then tie them successively.

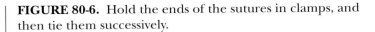

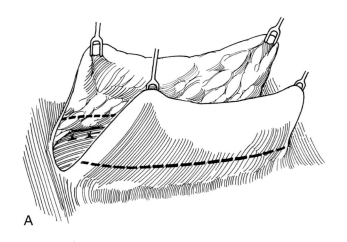

A

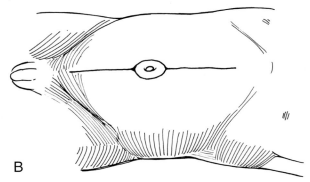

B

FIGURE 80-7. A, Excise the excess skin from the sides of the defect. Position the umbilicus in an appropriate position, trim the skin to fit around it, and fasten it with both subcutaneous and cutaneous sutures. **B,** Insert two small drains under the flaps. Close the rest of the subcutaneous tissue with interrupted chromic catgut sutures, and approximate the skin with running subcuticular 4-0 synthetic absorbable sutures.

Alternative, simplified technique: By folding the excess abdominal wall in on itself bilaterally, this method avoids opening into the abdominal cavity. Grasp the redundant skin of the abdominal wall with towel clips to determine laxity, excise the skin elliptically while preserving the umbilical island with its blood supply, and also excise the underlying fascia. Bring full-thickness folds of the fascia to the midline and hold them by first securing the bases with through-and-through running sutures, and then by abutting the apices in the midline with heavy interrupted sutures. Have the infant wear an umbilical binder for 8 to 10 weeks for support during healing.

LINDA M. DAIRIKI SHORTLIFFE

Commentary by

I have found that abdominal muscle and laxity usually permit a variation of this technique of abdominal closure, using three layers of muscle. In this case, the middle strip with the retained umbilicus is overlapped with left and right lateral fascial walls, each buttonholed for positioning of the umbilicus. Fixation is performed as described. This variation creates two layers of attenuated muscle and fascia over the central fascial panel through which the umbilical island can be pulled without difficulty, creating a full three layers in the central abdomen. This additional muscle mass improves abdominal support. It is important to place all the interrupted sutures using Keith needles prior to tying any, because tying them as you proceed makes it difficult to place subsequent sutures.

I also have found that vigorous pulmonary therapy must be encouraged postoperatively because these children will not perform adequate pulmonary toilet without assistance.

Chapter 81

Closure of Rectourethral Fistula

POSTERIOR SAGITTAL APPROACH (PEÑA)

For repair of an imperforate anus with rectourethral fistula, use the posterior sagittal approach. Consider a colostomy.

A team approach involving a pediatric surgeon is appropriate. Obtain plain films with coned views of the lumbosacral spine, and an abdominal ultrasound study looking for other urinary tract anomalies. A voiding cystourethrogram is indicated, especially if results of ultrasonography are abnormal. If abnormalities require it, intervene with a vesicostomy for significant reflux with vertebral, anal, tracheoesophageal, and renal anomalies or persistent cloaca.

Prepare the bowel (including the possibility of a colostomy) and administer antibiotics.

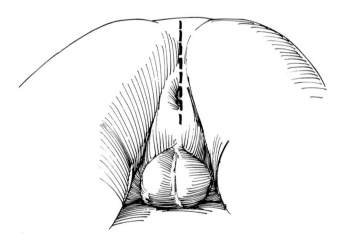

FIGURE 81-1. Position: Insert a balloon catheter into the bladder and turn the child into the prone jackknife position. Incision: Make a midline incision extending from the mid-sacrum through the center of the anal sphincter and then into the perineum beyond the site for the anus. Use an electrostimulator to identify the components of the residual pelvic and sphincteric musculature so that the incision can be made exactly in the midline.

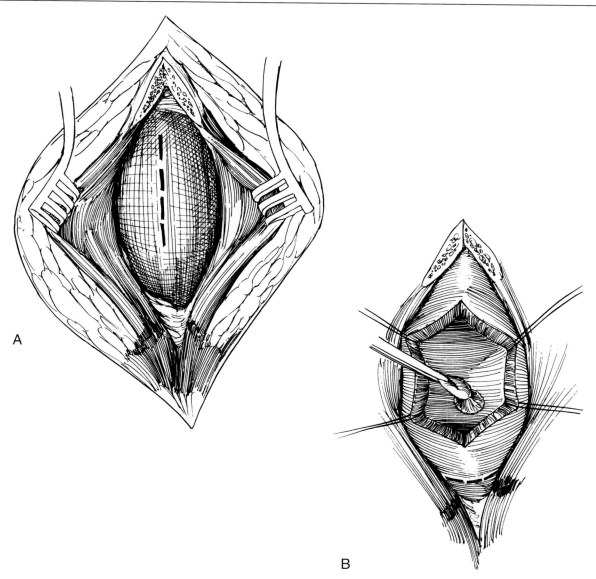

FIGURE 81-2. A, Divide the deep external sphincter into halves, and then split the coccyx. Separate the parasagittal fibers of the external sphincter and continue the incision down to the levator ani muscles and muscle complex. Open the levator muscle, allowing the rectum to bulge through the edges. Continue the incision exactly in the midline onto the longitudinal smooth muscle coat of the rectum. **B,** Place stay sutures in the rectal edges and mobilize the rectum with sharp dissection, performed as close as possible to the rectal wall to avoid nerve damage to the urinary structures. Elevate the rectal wall with 5-0 silk stitches and open it in the midline with a needlepoint cautery. Through the opening, identify the fistula site in the lowest part of the rectum.

Open the rectum further over the site of the fistula. Circumscribe the fistula and dissect it behind the prostate. It is important to dissect submucosally from the site of the fistula toward the proximal part of the rectum for at least 5 mm or so, where only a common wall separates them, to leave a layer of muscle wall over the neurovascular bundles. This avoids injuring the prostate, seminal vesicles, and vas deferens. At first the common wall is very thin, but it becomes thicker as the dissection is continued in a cephalad direction. Use multiple 6-0 silk sutures in the mucosal edge for traction. Excise the tract of the fistula into the urethra, bladder, or urogenital sinus.

Approximately 5 mm above the fistula, it will become possible to mobilize the full thickness of the bowel from the full thickness of the urethral wall. (Even though the rectum and urethra share a common wall immediately above the fistula site, the dissection will be easier.) For rectoprostatic fistulas, using traction on the sutures in the rectum, go as high as the peritoneal reflection (even opening the peritoneum, if necessary) to have enough bowel to bring down. Close the defect in the urethral (or vesical) wall with full-thickness 5-0 synthetic absorbable sutures and in the muscle with monofilament synthetic absorbable sutures. Close the defect in the rectal mucosa and muscularis similarly. It is now necessary to divide the rectum distally (dashed line) to mobilize it, so that it will reach the perineum without tension. Careful dissection is aided by making traction on silk mucosal sutures. Only a moderate amount of dissection is needed with bulbar fistulas, but for a high prostatic fistula, the dissection will be much more extensive and difficult.

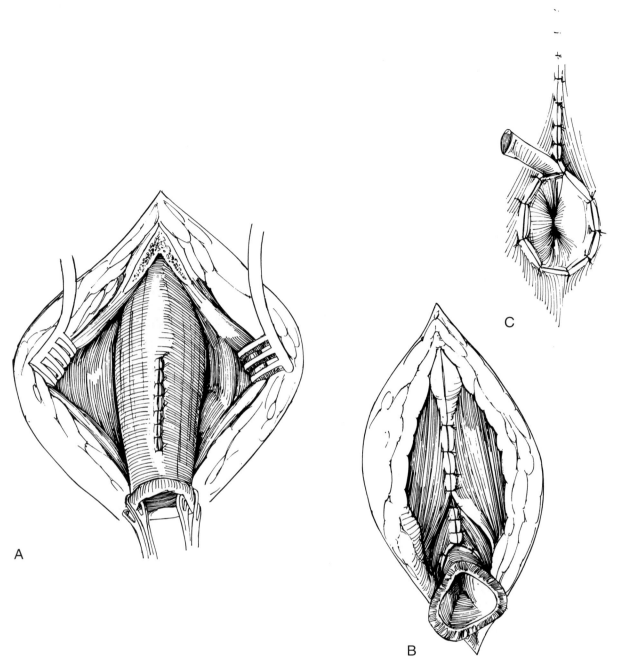

FIGURE 81-3. A, Close the rectum. It will be found dilated, so consider tailoring it by placing two layers of interrupted 5-0 monofilament synthetic absorbable sutures. **B,** Reapproximate the anterior margin of the muscle complex, as well as the margin of the external sphincter, with interrupted 5-0 synthetic absorbable sutures. Fasten both levator muscle edges with the same suture material. Pass the rectum in front and suture the remaining portion of the levator muscles together. Reapproximate the posterior edge of the muscle complex behind the rectum with stitches that include both the edge of the muscle complex and the rectal wall. Next, reapproximate, over the rectum, the posterior edge of the rectal external sphincter and the puborectalis portion of the levator muscle, and split the coccyx. Suture the muscular coat of the bowel circumferentially to the corresponding external sphincter portion of the striated muscle complex. **C,** Complete the anoplasty by trimming the mucosa to fit. Irrigate the wound well, and close the subcutaneous tissues and skin around a small Penrose drain with 5-0 nylon subcuticular sutures. Remove the drain in 3 days and the catheter in 8 days. Close the colostomy after 2 months.

POSTOPERATIVE PROBLEMS

If the fistula is not closed at this stage, construct a descending colostomy. This prevents contamination of the urinary tract, which puts these infants, who often have vesicoureteral reflux, at greater risk. Recurrent epididymitis is not rare, but it is made less frequent with prophylactic antibacterial therapy.

Hyperchloremic acidosis from colonic filling may be found after transverse colostomy, but a colostomy formed in the descending colon allows the urine to escape through the mucous fistula and avoid stagnation. Treat hyperchloremia with oral bicarbonates, looking at the same time for urethral obstruction.

ALBERTO PEÑA

Commentary by

A protective colostomy is done prior to repair. A Foley catheter is inserted into the bladder before the operation is started. A full posterior sagittal anorectoplasty is done through a midsagittal incision that runs from the middle portion of the sacrum down to and through the center of the external sphincter. In patients with rectoprostatic fistulas, try to preserve the anterior limit of the external sphincter. However, with rectobulbar fistulas, it is more convenient to continue the incision a little beyond the anterior limit of the external sphincter. Separate the parasagittal fibers of the external sphincter, and then continue deepening the incision down to the levator muscle and muscle complex. Once the levator muscle is opened, the rectum is tented with two 5-0 silk stitches and opened with the needlepoint cautery in the midline. Once the rectum is opened, identify the fistula site in the lowest part of the rectum.

The posterior sagittal approach allows a direct exposure of the anatomy of the rectum and levator ani muscle. The most conspicuous impression that we have had in our experience is that there is no way to identify the structures, such as "puborectalis," because the striated sphincteric mechanism is represented by a continuous, striated funnel-like piece of muscle. Also, there is no way to identify the "ganglia." Thus, it is necessary to mobilize the rectum with sharp dissection, performed as close as possible to the rectal wall to avoid nerve damage to the urinary structures.

Remember that the rectum and urethra share a common wall immediately above the fistula site. The best way to avoid damage to the vas deferens, seminal vesicles, and prostate is to perform a submucosal dissection from the fistula site toward the proximal part of the rectum for at least 5 mm, using multiple 6-0 silk stitches at the rectal mucosal level for traction. The reason is that immediately above the fistula, there is a common wall between the rectum and urethra that extends for approximately 5 mm. By submucosal dissection, we can guarantee that we will not damage the underlying structures. Once the dissection has reached the 5-mm distance, we can continue our dissection to full thickness, because at that point, the rectal wall and urethral wall become fully and completely separated. There are no recognizable neurovascular bundles between rectum and urethra.

Closure of the fistula site must be done by full-thickness 5-0 absorbable sutures through the urethral wall, because the separation of mucosa from muscle cannot be visualized.

A meticulous rectal dissection is then carried out while making traction on the silk sutures to gain sufficient length to be able to suture the rectum to the perineal skin without undue tension. The dissection aimed to gain rectal length usually is an easy affair when dealing with a bulbar fistula, but it sometimes entails rather complex maneuvers with rather high prostatic fistulas. The amount of circumferential dissection required to mobilize the rectum varies from case to case, so that it is not always necessary to dissect to the peritoneal reflection. In rectourethral bulbar stricture, it is unusual to see the peritoneal reflection, whereas in prostatic fistulas, frequently we must go as high as the peritoneal reflection and even open the peritoneum to be able to mobilize the peritoneum down.

The rectum usually is ectatic and distended, and frequently it is necessary to tailor it to make it fit within the muscular structures. Not every patient will need rectal tapering; the decision is made on an individual basis, depending on the size discrepancy existing between the rectum and the enclosing structures. The goal is to reconstruct the levator muscle behind the rectum and to locate the rectum within the limits of the muscle complex and external sphincter. The tapered rectum is reconstructed in two layers with 5-0 Vicryl sutures. The anterior limit of the muscle complex, as well as the limit of the external sphincter, is reapproximated with similar stitches. The same suture material is placed in both levator muscle edges, and then the rectum is passed in front of them. The remaining portion of the levator muscle is sutured together with the same suture material. The posterior edge of the muscle complex is reapproximated behind the rectum with stitches that include the muscle complex edge and the rectal wall. The anoplasty is done, and the skin is closed with subcuticular 5-0 nylon. The urethral catheter usually is left in place for 5 to 7 days.

Urinary contamination is not a problem. Approximately 80% of male patients have a rectourethral or bladder neck fistula. The opening of a colostomy during the neonatal period, with separated stomas and irrigation of the distal stoma prevents it, in our experience. As for hyperchloremic acidosis, it is true that urine may pass from the urinary tract to the rectum, and it could be absorbed in the rectum. In real practice, this situation is extremely unusual. We specifically recommend the opening of a descending colostomy. The hyperchloremic acidosis phenomenon may occur more when opening a right transverse colostomy, because then the urine sits in the rectum and has time to be reabsorbed. A descending colostomy allows the escaping of urine through the mucous fistula; therefore, we do not see hyperchloremic acidosis. Urinary tract infections only are conceivable in cases that have a defective colostomy—namely, a loop colostomy—that allows the passing of stool from the proximal into the distal colostomy.

TRANSANORECTAL REPAIR
(GECELTER)

If the fistula is small and below the peritoneal reflection, as it usually is, a colostomy is not necessary. In complicated cases, perform a colostomy some weeks before the operation. Provide bowel preparation and antibiotic coverage.

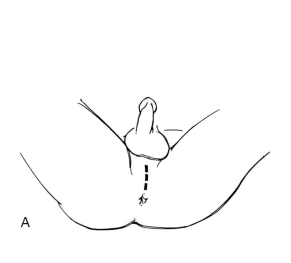

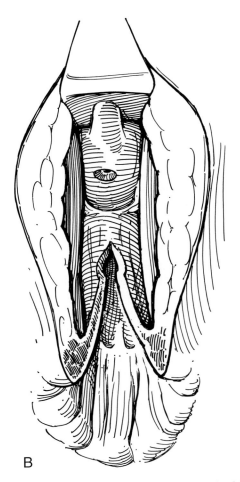

FIGURE 81-4. A, Place the child in the lithotomy position. Insert a suprapubic cystostomy. Make a vertical incision anterior to the anus. Make lateral extensions from its anterior end to expand the exposure, but avoid crossing over the ischial tuberosities. **B,** Divide both rectal sphincters exactly in the midline to avoid injury to nervous or vascular structures, and continue to open the rectum itself longitudinally. Pack the rectum with roller gauze to prevent pooling of blood and irrigant. Continue incising the rectum until the fistula is reached. Transect the fistula, and excise the scar tissue from both the rectal and the urethral walls.

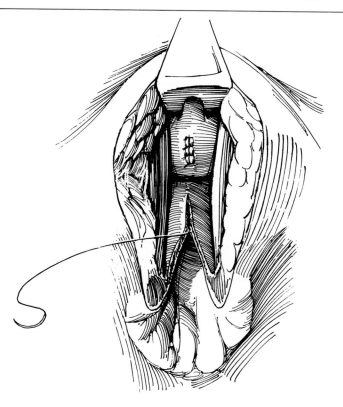

FIGURE 81-5. Close the urethral opening with a 4-0 synthetic absorbable continuous suture and a layer of 4-0 synthetic absorbable interrupted sutures. If the defect is too large, insert a skin graft. Close the rectum and anal canal in two layers: a mucosa-submucosa running 4-0 synthetic absorbable suture and interrupted sutures to the muscularis.

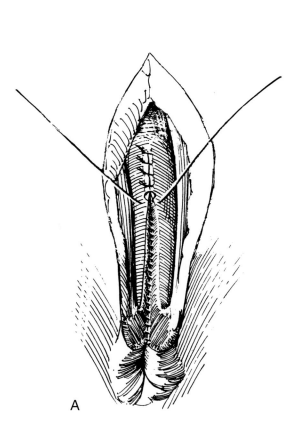

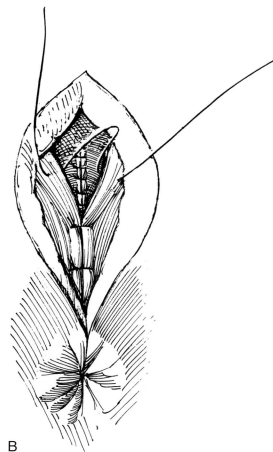

A   B

FIGURE 81-6. A, Place interrupted sutures to approximate the muscularis. **B,** Interpose any available soft tissue, and mobilize the levator ani muscles to approximate them in the midline. Place a Penrose drain, to be removed in 3 days. Continue suprapubic drainage for at least 14 days—longer if the tissues appear compromised. Obtain a voiding cystourethrogram before removing it.

Chapter 82

Excision of Urachus

PATENT URACHUS

Test for bladder outlet obstruction first.

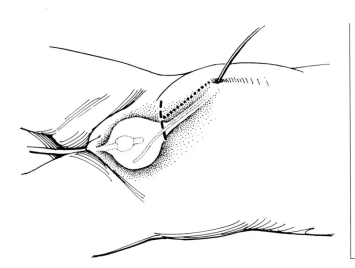

FIGURE 82-1. Position: Have the child lying supine. Insinuate a fine ureteral catheter (try different configurations of the tip) into the bladder through the urachus. Alternatively, try a stiff 3.5-F polyethylene pediatric feeding tube or even a lacrimal duct probe. If nothing will pass, mark the tract by instilling somewhat dilute methylene blue for subsequent identification. Insert a small balloon catheter through the urethra and partially fill the bladder.

Incision: Place a lower transverse incision in a skin fold well above the symphysis. In infants, because of the high position of the bladder, the incision can be placed nearer the umbilicus. A midline incision is an alternative *(dotted line)*. Dissect in the plane between the peritoneum, which lies behind the urachus, and the posterior rectus fascia anteriorly. If inflammation is present, look out for adherent loops of bowel.

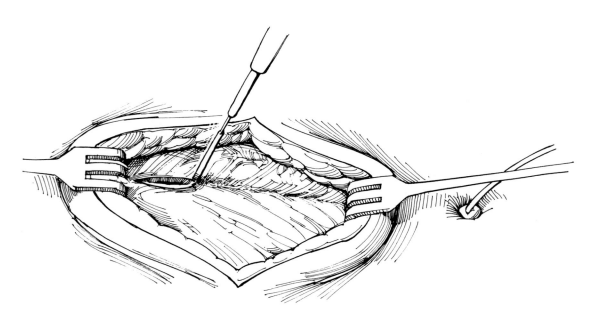

FIGURE 82-2. Divide the fascial junction between the rectus abdominis muscles. Identify the high-lying dome of the bladder extraperitoneally. Do not enter the peritoneum.

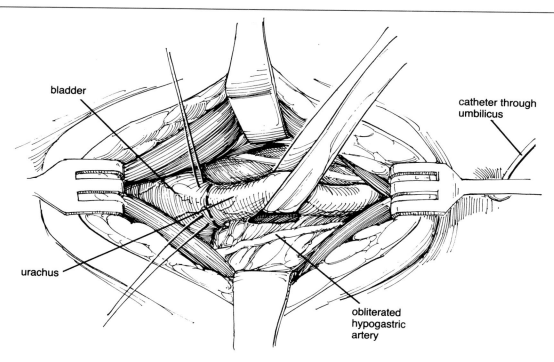

FIGURE 82-3. At the bladder dome, carefully free the connective tissue between the vesical adventitia and the peritoneum to expose the two obliterated umbilical arteries, with the urachus lying between. Bluntly dissect the urachus free at a convenient level and encircle it with a vascular tape or a Penrose drain. Continue to sharply dissect the urachus down to the bladder. Place two stay sutures in the adjacent bladder wall.

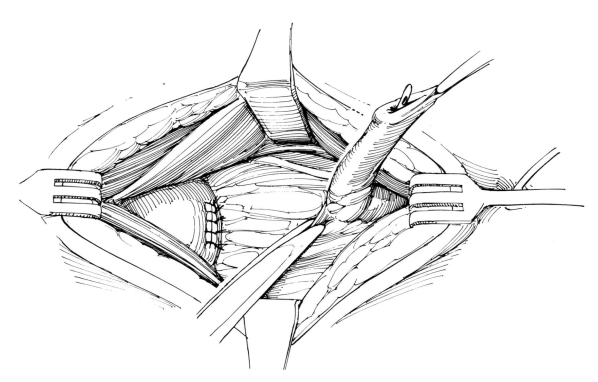

FIGURE 82-4. Divide the urachus within the bladder wall to remove a small cuff. Use progressive cuts, so that a 4-0 plain catgut continuous suture can be inserted to invert the epithelium while the area is suspended by the urachus. Add interrupted 4-0 synthetic absorbable sutures to approximate the muscularis. Elevate the upper end of the wound and dissect the urachus from the closely adherent peritoneum as far as the umbilicus. Excise the urachus along with the ends of the umbilical arteries and remove the specimen. It is not necessary to remove the last bit of the urachal stoma. Close the umbilical defect in two layers from inside, preserving as much of the umbilicus as possible for cosmetic reasons.

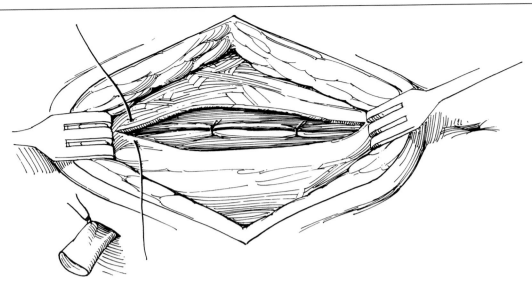

FIGURE 82-5. Place a drain through a stab wound to the bladder region. Approximate the rectus muscles loosely and close the incision in layers. Remove the drain in 3 days if the wound is dry. Leave the catheter indwelling for 7 days.

LARGE URACHAL CYST

Consider preliminary percutaneous drainage and antibiotic therapy for a large, infected urachal cyst. For excision, use the same technique described for the vesical end of the patent urachus, but first carefully dissect the bulging cyst or flabby diverticulum from the surrounding tissues and from the peritoneum behind. Take care not to injure bowel. Divide the attachment to the bladder, even excising bladder wall if needed, and close that defect. Dissect the upper end and divide it, while preserving the umbilicus. Drain the area.

URACHAL SINUS

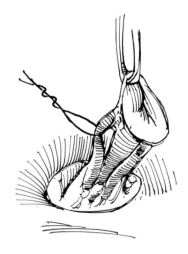

FIGURE 82-6. Incision: Make a limited circumferential incision around the opening of the sinus to preserve as much of the umbilicus as possible, although it may be necessary to remove the entire umbilicus, as shown here. (For umbilical reconstruction, see Chapter 77.) Place Allis clamps on the end of the sinus and sharply dissect the tract to its termination. Ligate the obliterated hypogastric arteries as they are encountered. Drain the area, because a sinus tract is usually infected. For urachal carcinoma, leave wide margins, especially at the upper end by excising the umbilicus.

POSTOPERATIVE PROBLEMS

Persistent urinary drainage may require replacement of a catheter to drain the bladder. Wound infection about the umbilicus is usually superficial.

ANTHONY A. CALDAMONE

Commentary by

The urachus is a vestigial structure connecting the umbilicus to the bladder. The urachus may be the source of four underlying pathologic entities: patient urachus, urachal cysts, urachal diverticulum, or alternating urachal sinus. Most of these pathologies will require surgical excision. The only exception is the patent urachus in the neonate, as some of these may close spontaneously in the absence of bladder outlet obstruction. The excision of an uninfected urachal remnant is well delineated in the text accompanying the figures. Although a transverse incision will result in excellent exposure, alternatively, a vertical midline incision along the course of the urachus may be more direct and can allow for extension to the umbilicus in a cosmetic fashion, should this be required because of difficulty in procuring the umbilical end of the urachus. Whenever possible, it is helpful to place a stent or probe through the patent urachus and into the bladder. It is advantageous to have the bladder well distended to bring the anterior bladder wall to the abdominal wall and, in doing so, pushing the peritoneum cephalad. The operation is facilitated by identifying the proper plane of dissection between the peritoneum posterior to the urachus and the posterior rectus fascia, which is anterior to the urachus. In this same plane will lie the obliterated umbilical arteries. The obliterated umbilical arteries may be ligated proximally on the bladder wall or distally at the umbilicus. It is advisable to take a small cuff of bladder wall with the urachus to prevent a residual diverticulum.

A two-layered bladder closure in the pediatric population generally will allow for a shorter period of bladder catheter drainage.

Infected urachal remnant structures, such as an infected urachal cyst and infected urachal sinus, present a more challenging dissection. In fact, it is advisable in the case of a large, infected urachal cyst, to initially drain the cyst percutaneously and allow a period for antibiotic therapy to reduce inflammation. Smaller, infected urachal cysts or urachal sinuses, however, can be managed safely with a single procedure. With these infected remnants, it may be impossible to dissect the urachus from contiguous structures. A larger portion of the bladder may need to be removed with the infected urachal cyst. Similarly, you may find it impossible to separate the infected cyst or sinus from the underlying peritoneum. Be extremely careful in identifying adherent loops of bowel that may have been involved in the inflammatory process, which can extend through the peritoneum.

TERRY W. HENSLE

Commentary by

The identification of a widely patent urachus is a relatively easy affair; however, the incomplete urachal remnant is frequently not capacious and often has areas of relative narrowing throughout its length. This makes intubation and positive identification difficult at times. At surgery the patent urachus is best intubated with a relatively stiff polyethylene pediatric feeding tube ranging from sizes 8 to 3.5 F. A smaller ureteral catheter or lacrimal duct probe can be used if the feeding tube is not successful. If intubation cannot be accomplished, the tract can be nicely outlined to help with surgical identification by injecting the umbilical portion of the duct with diluted methylene blue or canned milk.

Once the tract has been identified, a transverse suprapubic incision can be made after filling the bladder through an indwelling Foley catheter. With the bladder full, dissection is easily accomplished in a standard fashion to the dome. Once the dome is freed, the urachal remnant usually is readily identified and can be mobilized with both blunt and sharp dissection. The dissection is carried above the peritoneum to the undersurface of the umbilicus, where the urachal remnant is carefully separated from the peritoneum and divided and suture ligated. This approach alleviates the need for making a second skin incision and provides a reliable repair with a better cosmetic result than making a subumbilical incision in the skin.

Chapter 83

Introduction to Noncontinent Diversion

NEITHER URETHRA NOR URETEROVESICAL JUNCTION PRESENT

Diversion from the Bladder

A cystostomy provides direct drainage for the bladder, especially after open operations on the bladder, but for long-term drainage, the catheter may be irritating, and continuous drainage and infection may result in a small bladder. For temporary drainage, a perineal urethrostomy diverts the urine effectively from the urethra, but usually if a urethral catheter is inadvisable, a cystostomy is preferable in children. For more permanent diversion, a vesicostomy provides effective drainage at the price of poor stomal position and a tendency for stomal stenosis, infection, and stone formation.

Diversion for the Upper Tract

Percutaneous nephrostomy drainage and indwelling ureteral stents can allow relief of obstruction without formal surgical intervention, but in infants and children, the need for good drainage is imperative, and quality of the percuta-

neous drainage often is inadequate. A nephrostomy is most effective but is associated with so much infection and concomitant renal damage that it is used for more extreme circumstances and is seldom considered, even for short-term diversion. A percutaneous nephrostomy usually is better. Because the ureter and pelvis are dilated, a cutaneous ureterostomy or cutaneous pyelostomy is feasible. Cutaneous (end) ureterostomy is a simple form of urinary diversion but is more often permanent, unless done in the distal ureter. A prerequisite is a ureter dilated to at least 1 cm in diameter, thick walled and well vascularized. Be certain that a cutaneous ureterostomy is made low enough in the ureter so that it will not interfere with later reconstruction. This procedure can be appropriate for temporary diversion in infants but is seldom applicable in adolescents with normal ureters because of the high incidence of stricture from ischemia of the cutaneous portion of the nondilated ureter.

Urinary conduits formed from intestine have the advantage of relative freedom from stenosis, but late complications (especially stricture at the site of ureteral anastomosis, as well as stomal problems) have reduced their use. They largely have been replaced by forms of continent diversion, avoiding the necessity of wearing an appliance. Whether the ileum makes a better conduit than the sigmoid or the transverse colon has not been determined. Colon conduits do have the advantage of allowing formation of a nonrefluxing ureteral anastomosis.

Ureteroileostomy is a standard procedure with good short-term results, although reflux can occur with stasis. The stoma can be a problem, and a device must be worn. A transverse colon conduit is associated with few stomal problems, and the ureteral anastomosis can be made antirefluxive.

It is only after extensive pelvic irradiation, rarely seen in children, that the transverse colon conduit is preferred. It does have the additional advantage of requiring shorter lengths of ureter obtained away from the radiated field.

Long-term surveillance, no matter what form of diversion, is essential to catch dysfunction before the kidneys are irreversibly damaged. Sonograms, urine cultures, retrograde loopograms, and repeated determinations of serum electrolytes are indicated at regular intervals.

Complications

Bacteriuria is common, but symptomatic infection requiring treatment is less frequent. A normally functioning system will keep itself free of infection; the corollary is that recurrent infection suggests malfunction of the conducting structures. Pyocystis is an extreme form of infection, restricted to the totally diverted bladder, most commonly occurring in girls. Antibiotics and lavage of the bladder with saline solution with or without an antiseptic usually suffice, especially because the condition is usually self-limiting. Stomal problems begin with improperly fitting appliances. This often is associated with encrustation and stomal stenosis, the latter less often seen if skin is incorporated in the stoma. Parastomal hernia from too large a fascial defect usually requires taking the stoma down, repairing the defect, and making a new site for the stoma, preferably on the opposite side. Residual urine in the conduit may be secondary to a narrow stoma, but usually it appears later, caused by reduced peristaltic activity in the loop. Replacement of the segment may be required.

Chapter 84

Suprapubic Cystostomy

A trocar (punch) cystostomy is simple and adequate for short-term drainage.

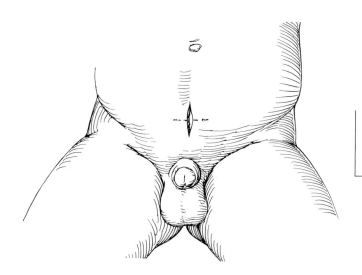

FIGURE 84-1. Position: Supine. Fill the bladder with sterile water until it is just visible or palpable suprapubically. Incision: Make a *short* vertical or transverse incision through the skin and subcutaneous layers slightly above the symphysis pubis.

FIGURE 84-2. Expose the rectus fascia in the midline by pushing back the overlying fat. Incise the fascia transversely.

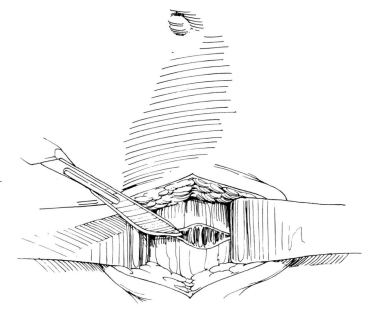

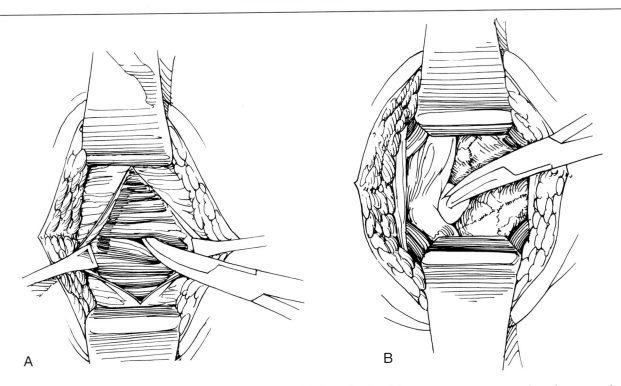

A   B

FIGURE 84-3. A, Separate the rectus muscles bluntly. Hold them back with two retractors, exposing the prevesical fat. **B,** Bluntly mobilize the peritoneal fold upward to expose a minimum of bladder surface. The vascular pattern and tissue characteristics of the bladder are usually unmistakable, but if in doubt, insert a fine needle and aspirate.

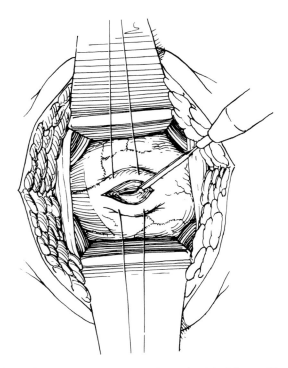

FIGURE 84-4. Place a pair of 3-0 chromic catgut stay sutures into the bladder wall or grasp it with two Allis clamps. Fulgurate obvious crossing vessels. Incise transversely between the sutures with the cutting current and enter the bladder.

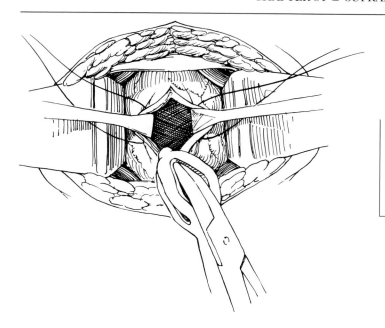

FIGURE 84-5. Reposition the Allis clamps to grasp the full thickness of the wall on both sides. Have a silicone Malecot catheter already stretched on a Mayo clamp. While urine is still running out, insert the catheter on the clamp. Withdraw the catheter slightly to be sure its tip does not touch the trigone.

FIGURE 84-6. Close the bladder snugly around the catheter with 3-0 chromic catgut sutures. If the bladder wall is thin, use mattress sutures. Tie the catheter to the bladder with the ends of one of the sutures.

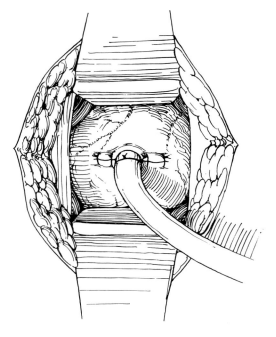

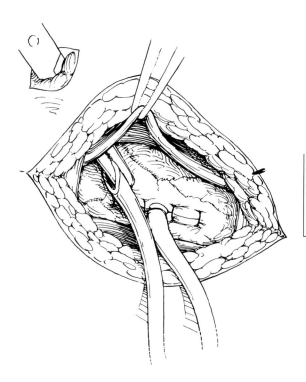

FIGURE 84-7. Make a stab wound in the skin of the abdominal wall near the incision but well above the symphysis and force a curved clamp through it to emerge beneath the rectus muscle. Trim the catheter end obliquely to facilitate pulling it through the body wall. Grasp the apex and pull the catheter out.

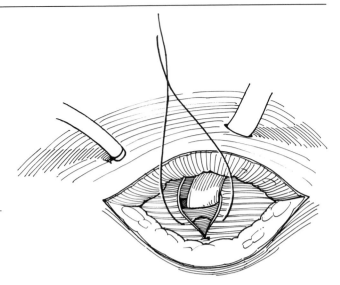

FIGURE 84-8. Close the fascia and skin around a Penrose drain with 3-0 chromic catgut sutures. Fasten the catheter to the skin with a heavy silk suture and tape it to the abdomen with waterproof tape applied over tincture of benzoin. (Check the fixation of the catheter daily.) Connect the catheter at once to sterile drainage. For a more permanent cystostomy, suture the bladder to the rectus fascia and bring the catheter through the wound.

VESICAL LITHOTOMY

Open extraction may be needed for those stones that cannot be removed instrumentally, especially in cases associated with neurogenic bladder. Proceed as for suprapubic cystostomy, but insert a Mayo clamp into the opening, aspirate the contents, and insert two fingers to make the opening somewhat larger. After removal of the stones, insert a 24-F Malecot catheter and draw it out through a stab wound in the body wall. Since infection may cause problems, drain the prevesical space with a Penrose drain that also exits through a stab wound.

POSTOPERATIVE PROBLEMS

Obstruction requires immediate irrigation. If that fails, obtain a cystogram to see if the end of the catheter is dis-placed. Urgency and pain, caused by contact of the catheter with trigone, can be distressing: retract the tube and refasten it to the skin. Inexplicable removal of the tube will happen if it is not stitched to the skin and retaped regularly with fresh tape over tincture of benzoin. Urinary infection can be delayed but not prevented by maintaining closed drainage and giving suppressive antibiotics. Peritonitis is a rare complication, secondary to puncture of the bowel during introduction of the tube.

For persistent drainage after removal of the tube, insert a urethral catheter. If the tract has epithelialized, it will not close until the surface has been denuded with a silver nitrate stick, curette, or a new wood screw.

ELLEN SHAPIRO

Commentary by

The bladder is filled in a retrograde fashion with saline if the patient is not in retention. A small incision (<2 cm in infants or toddlers) is made 1 to 2 fingerbreadths above the pubic symphysis. Holding sutures are placed in the bladder wall. The anterior bladder is opened with coagulation to avoid excess blood loss. A 10- or 12-F Malecot latex tube is preferred in those patients without latex precautions. The tube should be positioned several centimeters within the bladder, avoiding direct contact with the trigone. I prefer to bring the tube into the bladder through a separate cystotomy. Placement of a 4-0 chromic purse-string suture ensures the closure is watertight and secures the tube's position. The cystotomy is closed in two layers of 4-0 chromic suture. I do not routinely leave a Penrose drain. The course of the tube should be checked as it is brought through the fascia and the skin using a Toomey syringe to irrigate and aspirate. The suprapubic tube is doubly suture ligated to the skin with 3-0 Prolene suture. Gauze sponge dressings and Tegaderm are used to secure the tube in place. Suprapubic tubes in infants and small children are usually double diapered. The catheter, if left attached to a drainage bag, should not be taped across the hip, since hip, flexion will result in poor drainage. Long-term use of antibiotics while a tube is indwelling will often lead to funguria, which may be treated with oral fluconazole. A low dose of an anticholinergic agent will be useful for bladder spasms.

Chapter 85

Pediatric Vesicostomy

NONCONTINENT VESICOSTOMY (BLOCKSOM)

Consider placing a vesicostomy for temporary vesical diversion in (1) infants who are ill and thus reconstruction must be delayed, (2) neonates with posterior urethral valves (primary valve ablation is preferable) and severe reflux, or (3) patients (rare) with cloacal anomalies, urethral atresia, or a neurogenic bladder associated with a meningomyelocele not responsive to clean intermittent catheterization. Although vesicostomy could be useful for temporary urinary diversion in other infants who will need urinary tract rehabilitation with delayed reconstruction, realize that it reduces the amount of bladder tissue available for the final repair.

Insert a small catheter and fill the bladder until it is palpable.

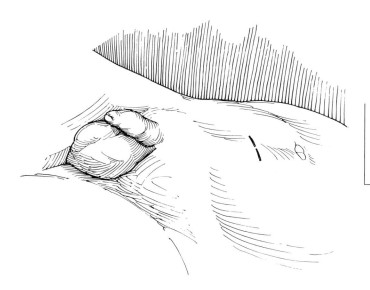

FIGURE 85-1. Incision: Make a very short transverse incision midway between the symphysis and the umbilicus. Stay at least 2 cm above the symphysis because placing an incision too low or making it too large encourages vesical prolapse. Incise the rectus fascia transversely and separate the muscles bluntly.

FIGURE 85-2. Remove small triangles from the fascia and trim some of the muscle to make an opening for the stoma.

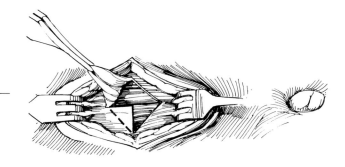

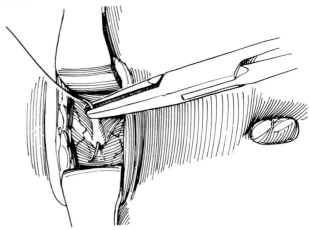

FIGURE 85-3. Expose the bladder and place several traction sutures in the anterior wall to draw it inferiorly. Dissect the peritoneum from the dome, mobilizing the bladder until the obliterated umbilical arteries and urachus are identified, marking the end of the dissection.

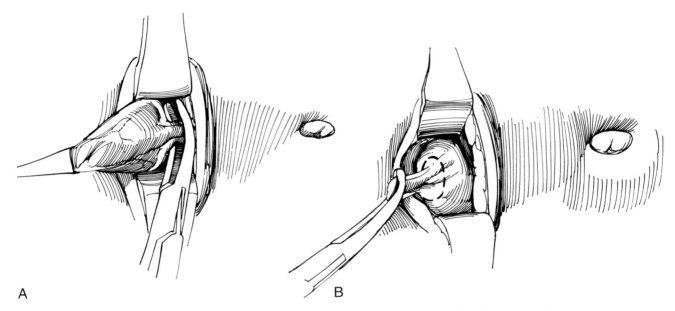

A   B

FIGURE 85-4. A, Pull the bladder into the wound until the posterior wall is level with the skin. **B,** Excise the urachus to open the bladder.

FIGURE 85-5. Suture the anterior and posterior walls of the bladder to the rectus fascia with at least six 3-0 synthetic absorbable sutures to tubularize the stoma. Close the lateral fascial defects around the outside of the bladder to achieve a 24-F lumen at the internal stoma. Too wide a stoma in a child with a normal thickness of the bladder wall promotes prolapse, but the thick bladders associated with myelomeningocele do not have this tendency. The thick-walled prune-belly bladder requires a larger stoma because of its tendency to stenose. Approximate the subcutaneous tissues.

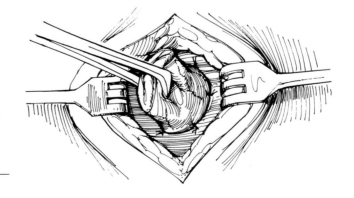

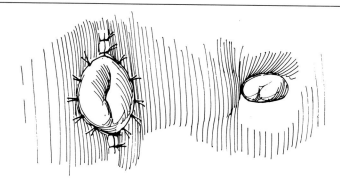

FIGURE 85-6. Suture the full thickness of the bladder to the subcuticular layer with 5-0 synthetic absorbable sutures. The stoma should not admit the fingertip but should calibrate to 24 F such that the fascial defect is narrow enough to avoid prolapse of the anterior wall of the bladder through the stoma. (In the prune belly, make the stoma larger to avoid stenosis.) Close the remainder of the incision. Apply petroleum jelly gauze and diapers.

Closure of the vesicostomy: Excise excess vesical mucosa and dissect the bladder wall free from the abdominal fascia. Close the bladder in two layers, with 5-0 plain catgut sutures for the submucosal layer and 4-0 synthetic absorbable sutures for the wall. Approximate the fascia and close the skin. Place a urethral catheter for a few days to ensure healing and prevent urine leakage into the wound.

POSTOPERATIVE PROBLEMS

Watch for inadequate decompression of the upper tracts. The trial of catheter drainage preoperatively will have shown what to expect immediately after operation. But if the ureteral orifices become obstructive from edema, inflammation, or spasm of the detrusor muscle, a percutaneous nephrostomy is necessary.

Treat dermatitis with antifungal and antibacterial agents, urinary acidification, and protective skin coatings. Prolapse of the posterior wall of the bladder results from placing the bladder incision too low and not fixing the dome. Revision is necessary: Make a new opening in the most cephalad part of the dome and narrow the fascial defect. Mucosal eversion (an esthetic problem) and squamous metaplasia are managed at the time of vesicostomy closure.

Stomal stenosis seldom is a problem because an opening of even 8 F is nonobstructive, but obstructive stenosis can occur with some thickened bladders, evidenced by residual urine, infection, and signs of back pressure on the upper tracts. Dermatitis may also narrow the lumen. Sometimes the stoma can be kept open by dilatation with an eyedropper, or later, with a 14-F catheter, but consider revision. Bladder capacity usually increases after vesicostomy.

JOHN W. DUCKETT

Commentary by

The idea of the Blocksom operation is to make a small keyhole incision and deliver the bladder through this by sweeping off the paravesical tissues as you deliver the dome out of the small opening. The opening is no more than 2 cm in diameter, admitting only the tip of the little finger. After mobilization of the bladder all the way to the dome, the obliterated hypogastric vessels are noted, marking the end of the dissection. This should allow the bladder to pouch out through the small fascial opening without any tension. The bladder is fixed to the fascia and the urachus excised. The fascia is closed around the outside of the bladder in order to provide a 24-F lumen to the internal stoma. If a stoma is made too wide, it will prolapse, particularly with the normal bladders associated with reflux. The myelomeningocele bladders are thickened and, therefore, will not tend to prolapse. In the prune-belly bladder, which is quite thick walled, the stoma needs to be made bigger than the standard 24 F, since it has a tendency toward stenosis.

MARK P. CAIN

Commentary by

A temporary cutaneous vesicostomy remains a useful and simple form of nonintubated urinary diversion for children. The most common indications for this procedure have been for children with neuropathic bladder, posterior urethral valves, and the prune-belly syndrome. The more recent focus has been away from initial vesicostomy for these conditions, introducing early intermittent catheterization for the neuropathic population and the prune-belly patient, and early endoscopic valve ablation to allow bladder cycling in the valve patient. Certainly the availability of small endoscopic instruments in most children's facilities has made transurethral procedures safe even in small or premature newborns. However, if intermittent catheterization fails to correct upper-tract dilation, especially in the patient with a neuropathic bladder, cutaneous vesicostomy will usually provide improved drainage.

From a technical perspective, the two most common complications of stomal stenosis and prolapse can be avoided by adequately mobilizing the dome of the bladder, resecting the urachal remnant to bring it out as the cutaneous stoma, and securing the bladder at the level of the fascia through a defect at least 22 to 24 F in size. We will usually calibrate the stoma on each follow-up visit with a 10- to 12-F catheter to ensure that the stoma has not contracted, and to document that there is minimal residual urine in the bladder. Occasionally, a thick-walled bladder with associated inflammation will have considerable edema, and we will have the family catheterize the vesicostomy three times a day until the upper tracts have improved. Peristomal dermatitis can occur early or late, and can cause stomal stenosis if not treated aggressively. We have had good results with a topical mixture of nystatin, zinc oxide, vitamin A and D ointment, and dibucaine.

Chapter 86

Fetal Intervention Vesicoamniotic Shunt

Vesicoamniotic shunting currently should be considered in cases of fetal lower urinary tract obstruction with oligohydramnios, in which the fetus does not have evidence of renal dysplasia. Confirmation of fetal renal function is based on improvement in fetal urine electrolyte analysis after the third of three fetal bladder urine samplings, along with improvement of sonographic imaging. Shunting and other invasive testing should be postponed until the 16th week of gestation to avoid injury to the membranes.

The procedure is performed under monitored anesthesia with local infiltration at the site of the puncture. The trocar of the chosen shunt is positioned, under ultrasound guidance, superficial to the fetal bladder. Amnioinfusion may be necessary, especially in severe cases of oligohydramnios, to create a space for the fetal bladder shunt to drain and to prevent improper placement of the amniotic coil in the myometrium or fetal membranes.

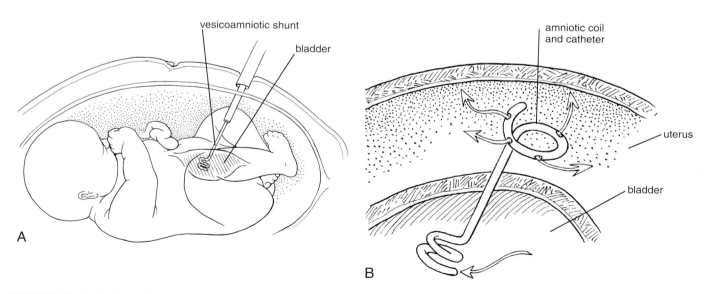

FIGURE 86-1. A, A small, maternal skin incision is made to facilitate the ease with which the trocar is correctly positioned. Use a quick and controlled motion to enter the fetal bladder, allowing urine sampling and/or placement of the double pigtail catheter. Position the trocar correctly within the vesical space to allow placement of the bladder coil. With ultrasound guidance check that the coil is positioned correctly under the straight portion of the catheter. **B,** The catheter is slowly advanced as the trocar is removed, allowing the straight portion to assume a position in the bladder wall and fetal skin and the distal curled portion to be in the fetal bladder. When the trocar is visualized at the level of fetal skin, the amniotic coil and remaining catheter are passed to assume position within the amniotic space.

COMPLICATIONS

The diagnosis of fetal-reversible fetal obstruction remains extremely difficult using sonography, MRI, and fetal urine electrolytes. Cases of prune-belly syndrome and urethral atresia with a patent urachus may inadvertently undergo fetal shunting without benefit to the infant. The fetal shunt may pierce the peritoneum, injuring bowel, vessels, and solid organs. Premature labor remains a risk for the mother and fetus.

JACK ELDER

Commentary by

One of the most controversial procedures in pediatric urology is the decision to insert a vesicoamniotic shunt in a woman carrying a fetus with suspected obstructive uropathy. Such babies without treatment generally are destined to die from pulmonary hypoplasia. The concept is that relieving the obstruction will allow the amniotic fluid to reconstitute and stimulate normal fetal lung development. Unfortunately, there are few ideal candidates, because many such fetuses are subject to early termination and, in most cases, if there is bilateral hydronephrosis and oligohydramnios, there is already significant irreversible renal dysplasia, and bladder drainage would not be helpful. Furthermore, if the treatment is successful and the baby survives, often there will be moderate or severe renal insufficiency, and dialysis and/or renal transplantation may be necessary. Some think that if the parents are older or have been trying to have a child for some time, intervention should be encouraged, whereas if the mother is young and became pregnant without difficulty, fetal intervention should be discouraged. The decision, therefore, involves many complicated medical and ethical issues, and the treatment recommendation one way or the other should be made by the perinatologist, pediatric urologist, pediatric nephrologist, and ethicist. Informed consent should include that the procedure poses a potential risk to the fetus and mother, more than one shunt may need to be placed, and placement of the shunt is considered experimental.

The ideal fetus is one with bilateral hydronephrosis, a distended bladder, oligohydramnios, and favorable urinary indices, that is, a hypotonic sodium, chloride and osmolality and a low β-2 microglobulin. In addition, as mentioned, a series of two or three fetal bladder punctures every 2 to 3 days is recommended to determine whether the bladder refills (indicative of urine production) and whether the urinary indices improve (indicative of fetal renal function). If such a procedure is performed, it is important to keep a log or registry of such cases, to help future clinicians assess whether such treatment has any benefit.

NICHOLAS M. HOLMES

Commentary by

Fetal intervention for posterior urethral valves has greatly evolved since its initial introduction in 1981 at the University of California San Francisco. The most significant improvement has been in the reduction of fetal/maternal morbidity and the use of amnioinfusion at the time of the shunt placement. It is critical to have a well-experienced fetal surgery team (i.e., a fetal ultrasonographer, maternal-fetal medicine specialist, neonatalogist, obstetric anesthesiologist, and perioperative obstetric/pediatric nursing staff) in place to facilitate a successful outcome.

Several key studies need to be obtained before considering intervention procedures:

1. Serial fetal urinary electrolytes consistent with hypotonic urine (sodium < 100 mEq/L, chloride < 90 mEq/L, osmolarity < 210 mOsm)
2. Normal appearing kidneys on ultrasound (normal echotexture, no cortical cysts)
3. Normal fetal karyotype (46 XY)

The use of the shunt is not without complications, such as shunt migration, malposition/malplacement, and blockage. If placed early in the pregnancy, the rate of shunt occlusion is quite high and serial ultrasound monitoring is a must. Repeat shunt placement may be required. At some centers, primary in utero valve ablation is performed via a fetal cystoscope/endoscope, either using laser energy or hydrostatic pressure. No one technique has proven to be superior in securing the survival of the unborn patient nor preventing the associated findings that contribute to early demise after delivery (e.g., renal failure, pulmonary hypoplasia with respiratory failure).

When counseling the families about fetal intervention, the focus of discussion should concentrate on the process, that is, it may facilitate carrying the fetus to term, however, the sequelae of posterior urethral valves may not be preventable.

Chapter 87

Cutaneous Ureterostomy, Transureteroureterostomy, and Pyelostomy

URETEROSTOMY IN SITU

Ureterostomy in situ is a simple, quick way to provide temporary upper-tract diversion. It is especially useful if direct, percutaneous renal drainage is not feasible.

Make a small incision above the anterior superior iliac spine and identify the dilated ureter through a limited mobilization of the retroperitoneum. (If in doubt, use a fine needle and syringe to aspirate the structure in question.) Make a short puncture incision in the ureter and immediately insert an infant feeding tube or a single pigtail catheter before the ureter can collapse. Pass the tube cephalad to the renal pelvis. Make a stab wound below the incision and draw the obliquely cut end of the catheter through it. Fasten the tube securely to the skin with a silk suture. After 2 weeks, replace the catheter-stent by inserting a new

catheter *immediately* after removing the initial one (you can easily lose the tract).

CUTANEOUS URETEROSTOMY

Do not consider cutaneous ureterostomy as first choice; it may complicate subsequent surgical procedures. Avoid disturbing the midportion of the ureter.

Before a ureter is brought to the skin, it should have become dilated, because the blood supply to the free end of a normal ureter is tenuous after passage through the abdominal wall. The ureter in obese adolescents sometimes will not reach the skin surface, and even if it does, it will exit so far posteriorly under the rib cage that a collecting device will not adhere.

Before operation, select and mark one or two sites on the abdomen that would accommodate a collecting device.

DISTAL-END CUTANEOUS URETEROSTOMY

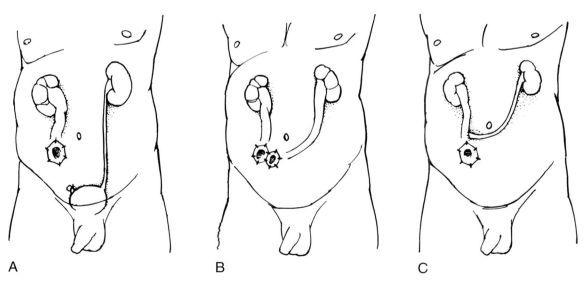

A   B   C

FIGURE 87-1. A, A ureterostomy at the distal end of the ureter, in contrast to a loop ureterostomy, may avoid a double procedure later. **B,** With a double system, and both ureters involved, consider a double stoma (see Fig. 87-5A to E). **C,** A ureteroureterostomy with a single cutaneous opening. Incision: Either a transverse lower abdominal (see Chapter 63) or a Gibson (see Chapter 64) incision is suitable. Approach the ureter extraperitoneally. (In large adolescents it may be

Continued

FIGURE 87-1, cont'd. necessary to have the ureter traverse the abdominal cavity; however, intraperitoneal disease may make an intra-abdominal approach more difficult.) Dissect extraperitoneally to reach the ureter over the sacral promontory. Free the ureter well toward the bladder, to be able to bring the proximal end to the surface after division. Mobilize the ureter very carefully, keeping well outside the adventitia to preserve as much of the blood supply coming from the upper end as possible. Free the ureter all the way to the bladder to enable it to reach the anterior abdominal wall, but do not attempt to straighten it by adventitial dissection. Clamp and divide it, and insert a stay suture in the free end. Ligate the stump.

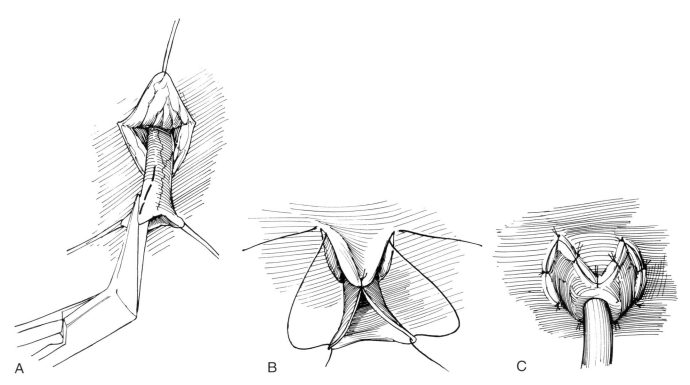

A   B   C

FIGURE 87-2. A, For connection of the ureter to the surface, incise the skin in the shape of a U or V. Make a direct tract through subcutaneous tissue, rectus sheath, and peritoneum as for ureteroileostomy (see Chapter 89), taking care to keep the body layers lined up. Draw the ureter through the opening without tension for at least 3 cm. Incise the lateral, less vascular side to spatulate it. **B,** Insert a 4-0 synthetic absorbable suture through the apex of the skin flap into the apex of the ureteral slit and tie it. Pass a similar suture through each angle of the skin incision, then through the free corners of the ureter, and tie them. **C,** Place five or six everting sutures around the circumference and tie the sutures. Then complete the attachment of the end of the ureter at the level of the skin, or better, form a little nipple so that appliances will stay on better. Stenting is not necessary.

TRANSURETEROURETEROSTOMY WITH CUTANEOUS STOMA

If the ureters are involved bilaterally, rather than forming a double stoma, bring the more dilated one to the skin and anastomose the more normal one to it by transureteroureterostomy (see Chapter 52). Bring the ureter either extraperitoneally (as shown in Figure 87-1C) or transabdominally.

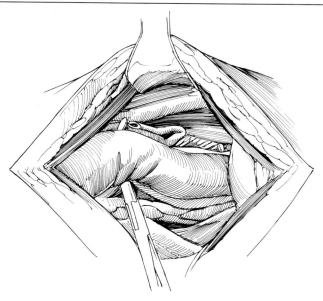

FIGURE 87-3. Incision: Make a paramedian transabdominal incision on the side opposite the proposed site of the stoma. Open the peritoneum and pack the intestines into the upper abdomen. Over the more *normal* ureter near its crossing of the iliac vessels, lift the parietal peritoneum and open it with Lahey scissors as far caudally as possible. (To expose this ureter on the left side, incise the posterior peritoneum lateral to the mesosigmoid and descending colon and retract the colon medially.) Encircle the ureter with a small Penrose drain well outside the adventitia, free it distally, and clamp it. Place a traction suture through the proximal end before cutting it and ligating the distal stump with an absorbable suture.

On the right side, open the peritoneum over the more *dilated* ureter and expose a section of it. On the *left* side, incise the posterior peritoneum lateral to the mesosigmoid and descending colon and retract the colon medially. Under vision, digitally dissect a channel from one retroperitoneal incision to the other and draw the smaller ureter through it with a curved clamp.

Dissect the larger ureter down to the bladder. Place a stay suture, divide the ureter, and ligate the stump. Continue the retroperitoneal dissection that was begun over the larger ureter around the lateral and anterior body wall to the site selected for the stoma.

Form the stoma as described previously, but dissect only through the subcutaneous tissue and muscles. Instead of entering the peritoneum, connect the stoma with the previous retroperitoneal dissection by freeing the peritoneum adjacent to it, working through its lumen. Pass a large clamp through the stoma beneath the peritoneum to grasp the stay suture on the larger ureter and bring it out through the skin. Be sure the ureter is not angulated.

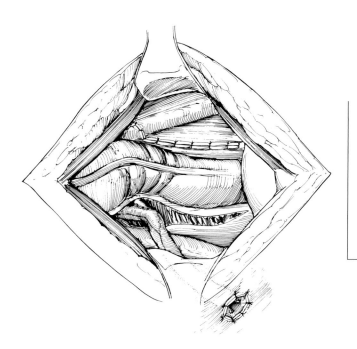

FIGURE 87-4. Trim the smaller ureter obliquely to the proper length to meet the dilated one. Make a 2-cm longitudinal incision in the dilated ureter and proceed with transureteroureterostomy by an elliptical end-to-side anastomosis with a running 5-0 absorbable suture. Consider placing stents. Bring a Penrose drain extraperitoneally from the site of the ureteroureteral anastomosis through a stab wound in the skin below the stoma. Close the incisions in the parietal peritoneum and close the abdomen. Spatulate the large protruding ureter if necessary, and then suture it to the skin as described in Figure 87-2.

SINGLE-STOMA CUTANEOUS URETEROSTOMY

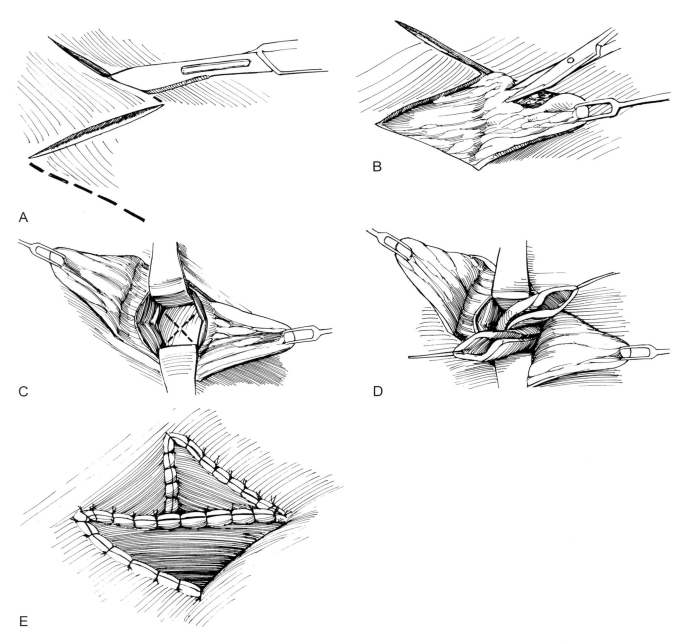

FIGURE 87-5. When both ureters are dilated, they may be brought out as a single stoma using a Z-plasty. Approach the ureters extraperitoneally. **A,** Make a Z-shaped incision in the skin in a previously selected site. **B,** Trim the subcutaneous fat from the flaps. **C,** Remove a minimum of fat to avoid inversion of skin at the site of the stoma and excise a button of anterior rectus sheath. Make an X-shaped incision in the transversalis fascia and peritoneum. **D,** Draw the ureters through the opening and trim them to length. Spatulate each ureter by incising its lateral border. **E,** Suture the flaps into the V-shapes in the ureters with 3-0 synthetic absorbable sutures. Alternative: Make a simple stoma by suturing the incised ureters together, everting them, and suturing them to the skin as shown in Fig. 87-1B).

POSTOPERATIVE PROBLEMS

Stenosis of the tip of the ureter at skin level is almost the rule because of the relative local ischemia after dissection. Try dilatation, and then intubate it with a round-tipped silicone tube. A plastic meatotomy can be done. Formal revision seldom helps because the 3 cm of extra ureteral length required is seldom available; turn to an alternate form of supravesical diversion.

Pyocystis (empyema of the bladder) occurs occasionally after diversion, especially if the bladder is denervated. Overdilate the urethra and follow with regular catheterization and irrigation for long-term relief. In girls, the urethra may be incised. If these measures are not effective, cystectomy may be necessary unless continent diversion with intermittent catheterization is not planned.

Commentary by VENKATA R. JAYANTHI

Temporary upper-tract cutaneous drainage is not commonly required. In former years, high diversions were often performed for persistent hydroureteronephrosis in posterior urethral valves but more recent data suggest that such dilation is more often due to polyuria than distal obstruction. The appropriate physiologic management of such cases is ensuring frequent bladder emptying. There may be an occasional older patient in whom bladder management with intermittent catheterization may be difficult and/or impossible and in whom transureteroureterostomy with end cutaneous ureterostomy (with an appliance for urine collection) may be needed to try to salvage renal function. This is indeed a rare situation.

Diversion is most often useful in the young infant with such massive ureteral dilation that definitive repair may be inadvisable. Temporary ureterostomy may permit decompression, reducing the risk of sepsis and potentially allowing the ureteral caliber to decrease, facilitating later reconstruction. A decision needs to be made between an end cutaneous and loop ureterostomy. My personal preference in such situations is to perform a low-loop ureterostomy. A small incision may be made at the lateral extent of what would be an extended Pfannenstiel incision and the dilated ureter easily identified. A loop of ureter may be brought out of the incision, the fascia closed under the loop, an anterior ureterotomy made, and the skin edges approximated to the ureter. The advantages of this approach include the low risk of stenosis due to the preservation of blood supply and the lack of a circumferential ureteral anastomosis. Subsequent reconstruction (ureteral reimplantation) is much easier as little dissection in the pelvis is made and the perivesical tissue is untouched. Stomal appliances are unnecessary as the urine can simply be allowed to drain into a diaper.

The advent of highly qualified interventional radiology departments and their ability to safely and easily place percutaneous nephrostomy tubes have markedly reduced the number of children who may require temporary upper-tract cutaneous diversion.

Commentary by MAX MAIZELS

Cutaneous ureterostomy remains an important procedure for select instances. Over the past 6 years I have been involved with this procedure in five instances. Reviewing specific indications for the procedure gives perspective as to the indications for its performance. Newborns who had follow-up after fetal diagnoses showed.

- Pyoureteronephrosis with the obstructed upper pole ending in an ectopic ureter. The kidney was too small to consider for percutaneous drainage. A loop ureterostomy at the level of the kidney was done.
- Massive bilateral vesicoureteral reflux and azotemia, related to atonic ureters that did provide efficient drainage to the bladder. Bilateral loop ureterostomy at the level of the kidney was done. Azotemia improved.
- Solitary functioning hydronephrotic kidney with ureter obstruction as it is ectopic to prostate. Primary reimplantation in a newborn was not performed. Loop ureterostomy was done at the level of the iliac crest. Undiversion and reimplantation was done at 1 year of age.
- Referral of management for undiversion by reimplantation of 1-year-old boy with end cutaneous ureterostomy for solitary functioning kidney with obstructed megaureter.
- Referral of undiversion management by reimplantation of a 2-year-old child with end cutaneous ureterostomy for solitary functioning kidney that had obstruction after reimplantation for ureterocele.

In such instances of performance of loop ureterostomy, my preference has been to plan a short skin incision yet mobilize the obstructed, dilated ureter widely. Wide mobilization avoids kinking the course of the ureter. Once mobilized, the layered edges of the surgical incision are fixed to the still intact and closed wall of the ureter seriatim: transversus, internal oblique, and external oblique muscles. Keeping a small skin incision with layered closure avoids wound hernia. Once the muscular layers are done, the ureter is opened longitudinally and the mucosa margin is approximated to the skin.

CUTANEOUS PYELOSTOMY

Cutaneous pyelostomy is a sometimes useful temporizing procedure in the presence of a large renal pelvis. The ureteral circulation is thus preserved for subsequent procedures.

Incision and dissection are done as described above, except that instead of actually mobilizing the proximal ureter, it is merely traced to the renal pelvis. Rotate the kidney anteromedially.

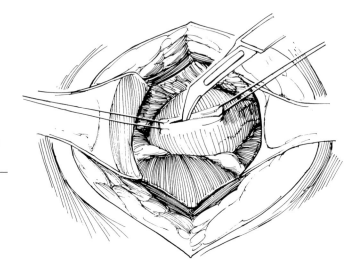

FIGURE 87-6. Place two traction sutures in the posterior surface of the dilated pelvis, well above the ureteropelvic junction. Incise the pelvis with a hooked blade for a distance of 3 cm.

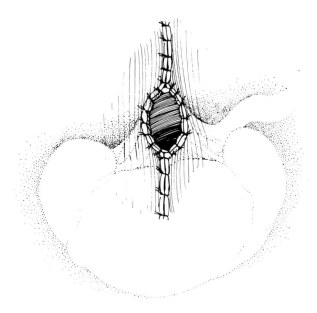

FIGURE 87-7. Place several 3-0 or 4-0 synthetic absorbable sutures between the pelvis and body wall to relieve tension. Suture the full thickness of the pelvis to the skin with interrupted sutures.

Closure of a cutaneous pyelostomy: Encircle and dissect the redundant pelvis, staying clear of the ureteropelvic junction. Trim the edges of the pelvis and close the defect with a running 4-0 synthetic absorbable suture, occasionally locking a stitch.

POSTOPERATIVE PROBLEMS

Stenosis is the most common complication and occurs if too small a portion of renal pelvis is brought out to the skin.

MIKE KEATING

The reputation of ureterostomies and pyelostomies is muddied by their creation in patients who, we now know, were unsuitable candidates for these types of diversion. Unfortunately, urothelium does not respond well to chronic exposure and ureteral anastomoses, by default, circumferentially narrow down. Diverting ureters with normal or near-normal caliber commonly results in stomal stenosis, regardless of the different skin reconfigurations meant to lessen its incidence. Most adults with obstructive uropathy, regardless of its cause, have not developed enough ureteral dilation, to avoid this sequelae. If non-continent urinary diversion is desired of a patient without ureteral dilation, other options are recommended.

The perinatal diagnosis of urinary tract anomalies should change the perception of these types of diversions. Impressively dilated ureters that result from posterior urethral valves, reflux, ectopia, or ureterocele are fairly common. Large caliber and generous vascularity undoubtedly improve their performance as cutaneous diversions in children as opposed to adults. Stomal stenosis, for example, is uncommon in my experience. What remains poorly defined is their role in the management of these different anomalies.

Contemporary pediatric urologists are able to accomplish admirable feats. For example, megaureters (some perhaps better classified as metaureters) can be tapered and reimplanted in infants and ureteroureterostomies completed between markedly distorted donor ureters and barely patent recipients in newborns. We also know that the complication rate of such challenging reconstructions increases with younger age and smaller size of the child. When a significantly dilated ureter warrants more than the temporary diversion offered by a nephrostomy tube and the benefits of reconstruction appear outweighed by its risks, there should be no embarrassment in resorting to an end ureterostomy.

End ureterostomies are a simply constructed and probably underused urinary diversion, especially in neonates and infants. The lower abdominal incision depicted offers ideal extraperitoneal exposure. The obliterated hypogastric artery can be ligated and followed posteriorly as a guide to the ureter. After being ligated and mobilized, maturation of the ureter is completed at the lateral extent of the wound. The same wound can then be extended medially at later undiversion when takedown of the ureter is a simple matter. Once mobilized, the ureter is brought medial to the rectus muscle where the bladder is exposed in Pfannenstiel-like fashion. The diversion does not burn one's bridge to later reconstruction. Instead, the decrease in ureteral caliber that occurs offers a significant technical benefit when tapering and reimplanting are done at a later age. When bilateral diversion is indicated, it is a simpler solution to divert both lower ureters rather than complete a transuretero-ureterostomy. The latter is probably best reserved for subsequent undiversion and reconstruction.

The freely draining lower stoma is easy to manage, since it requires no more than the diaper use typical for age. In contrast, the stomas of upper diversions present more of a parental challenge to urinary collection. We have found an unfolded diaper held in place by tubular mesh (body) gauze to be most effective. Standard stoma appliances are usually not a good option for either diversion, since ureterostomies and pyelostomies do not project well from the body wall.

Pyelostomies and upper ureterostomies are the best means of decompressing a hydronephrotic kidney(s) and affording maximal renal recovery. They are especially effective when the level of ureteral obstruction is variable and cannot be determined and/or renal function is poor. Any of the lower-tract pathologies cited can result in secondary upper ureteral obstructions or in ureters that are functionally obstructed and unable to effectively drain. This seems especially true of posterior urethral valves, in which markedly thickened detrusor muscle and high bladder resting pressures can retard urinary drainage, than with other causes of hydroureteronephrosis.

Historically, some groups routinely created upper diversions in most baby boys with urethral valves. While rote application seems excessive, we continue to see patients whose kidneys do not drain well after valve ablation and bladder decompression. They are ideal candidates for subsequent upper-tract diversion. The findings at flank exploration dictate whether a pyelostomy or ureterostomy is created. Both are effective. Malrotation of the kidney can make pyelostomy difficult or impossible. An upper-end ureterostomy must ensure an unobstructed path for the free drainage of urine. Kinks must be eliminated and patency confirmed. The transected end of the lower ureter is tagged to aid in its later identification.

Concerns about later undiversion and the possible need to operate on both ends of the ureter, where the vascularity to the midportion of ureter is potentially jeopardized, are unfounded. At undiversion, initial takedown and reconstruction of the cutaneous diversion, with minimal mobilization of the upper end of the lower ureter, is followed by 6 weeks of nephrostomy tube drainage. In many cases, the affected ureter(s), whose caliber is typically much smaller after being defunctionalized, regains its motility and drains effectively. When subsequent lower ureteral surgery becomes necessary, care is taken to preserve adventitial vascularity. Fortunately, this is usually generous and forgiving.

My own introduction to ureterostomies and pyelostomies was provided by Dr. John Duckett, nearly 20 years ago. At the time, he advocated cutaneous diversions for neonates with collecting system anomalies whose associated renal function could not be determined (e.g., the upper pole of a duplicated kidney). Percutaneous intervention and improved diagnostics have since eliminated this application but I would suspect that, were he still with us, this mentor would continue to hold a role for such diversions in today's armamentarium.

Chapter 88

Transverse Colon Conduit

A transverse colon conduit is suitable for long-term diversion because a nonrefluxing ureteral anastomosis is possible. However, the advent of continent diversion reduces the need for use of the colon. The tranverse colon conduit is particularly useful after pelvic irradiation.

Prepare the bowel and sterilize the urine if possible. Provide a high-calorie diet and protein supplements.

Mark the preferred stomal site with the patient in a sitting position. Instruments and postoperative problems are the same as those for ileal conduit (see Chapter 89).

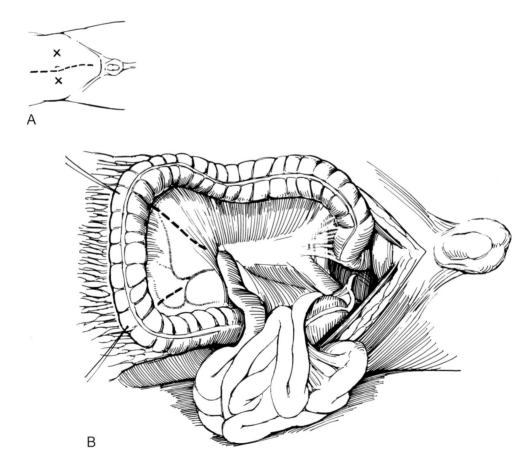

FIGURE 88-1. **A**, Incision: Make a midline incision leaving the umbilicus on the left side available for later appendicovesicostomy (see Chapter 91). **B**, Transilluminate the transverse mesocolon to choose a suitable 10- to 15-cm segment, and place stay sutures to mark it. Dissect the greater omentum from the superior surface of the transverse colon. Incise the mesocolon, making the cut longer on one side (left side shown) for increased mobility. Control the vessels.

FIGURE 88-2. Divide the colon and reanastomose it superior (or inferior) to the segment, preferably with staples. Approximate the mesentery with a few 3-0 silk sutures. Choose the portion of the conduit that looks better suited as the stomal end, and close the opposite end of the conduit. Fix it securely to the adjacent parietal peritoneum near the midline. Incise the retroperitoneum and mobilize the ureters. Lead them into the peritoneal cavity together through a suitably sited peritoneal incision. Trim the ureters obliquely to the proper length and spatulate them.

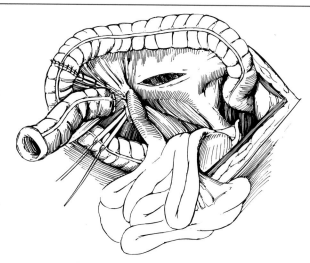

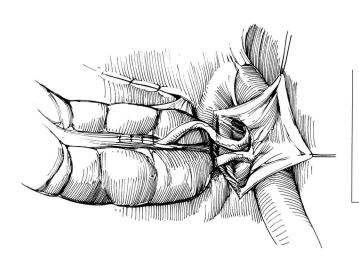

FIGURE 88-3. Incise the conduit along a tenia and anastomose the ureters directly with 4-0 chromic catgut sutures, using a submucosal tunnel technique (see Chapter 6). Place stents if the ureters are small, if they are large and aperistaltic, or if the quality of the tissue is in doubt. Bring up the inferior peritoneal flap to cover the anastomoses. Close the distal end of the conduit; use absorbable sutures to avoid formation of stones.

FIGURE 88-4. Situate the stoma in either the upper or lower quadrant, whichever provides the easiest egress for the segment. Fashion a stoma (see Chapter 89). Close the wound and place a temporary appliance.

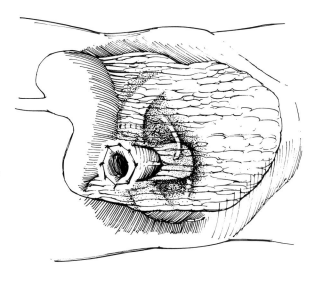

BERNARD M. CHURCHILL

Colon conduits have a distinct advantage over ileal conduits, because nonrefluxing ureteroenteric anastomosis can be fashioned. We have noticed a significant difference in the risk of upper-tract deterioration in patients undergoing colon conduits versus ileal conduits. In 82% of patients undergoing ileal conduit diversion, there was evidence of renal damage versus 22% in patients with colon conduits. This well-known risk of chronic pyelonephritis and parenchymal loss caused by freely refluxing ureteroileal anastomosis makes the nonrefluxing colon conduit a better option over the ileal conduit in patients who will require long-term cutaneous urinary diversion.

However, in this age of continent diversion, few patients will require long-term diversion. With the varied forms of continent diversion available, children may be able to undergo continent diversion and never need conduit diversion. Those who initially undergo a temporary incontinent diversion could undergo subsequent undiversion within a few years. Because the deleterious effects of ileal diversion take several years to materialize, and because undiversion usually can be performed a few years after diversion, there is no real advantage to colon conduits in most patients.

A midline incision should be made coursing around the umbilicus to the left side. This will preserve the vascularity of the umbilicus for later appendicovesicostomy. Similarly, we would not recommend performing a routine appendectomy. If undiversion is later performed, the appendix would be needed for a Mitrofanoff procedure. We now use staples for most of our bowel work. We find that even in small children, stapled anastomosis leads to good enteroenterostomies and reduces operative time. The blind end of the conduit should be closed with absorbable sutures to prevent stone formation.

Chapter 89

Ureteroileostomy (Ileal Conduit)

URETEROILEOSTOMY (BRICKER LOOP)

Have the child both sit and stand when you select a site for the stoma. Choose a plane surface of the abdomen where the skin does not roll into folds. The stoma should not be near the umbilicus (unless it is through it) or close to a prominent rectus muscle, a bony prominence, or an abdominal scar. Mark the site with a ballpoint pen or scratch it with a needle. An even better plan is to have the child wear a partially filled appliance for a day or two preoperatively to make sure the placement is optimum. The standard location for a stoma is just below the center of a line between the umbilicus and the anterior superior iliac spine. This may be too low, especially in children with myelodysplasia, in whom an umbilical stoma is easier to manage. An enterostomal therapist can be helpful, especially by counseling the child and allaying fears. Prepare the bowel.

INSTRUMENTS

Provide four Kocher clamps, curved mosquito (Providence Hospital) clamps, Kelly clamp, Adson forceps, tenotomy scissors, Balfour retractor, 5-F and 8-F infant feeding tubes, plastic rod, 4-0 silk sutures with detachable needles, 4-0 chromic catgut ureteral sutures, 3-0 synthetic absorbable sutures, and Penrose drain.

URETERAL MOBILIZATION

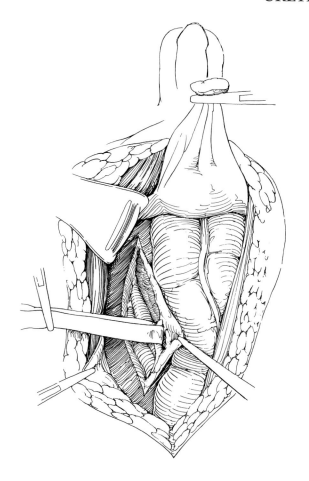

FIGURE 89-1. Position: Place the child supine. Ask the anesthetist to insert a nasogastric tube. Incision: A midline transperitoneal incision (see Chapter 11) at the base of the sigmoid mesocolon where it joins the parietal peritoneum; make a vertical incision to expose the left ureter. By dissecting medially over the left iliac vessels, the ureter can be located where it is lifted up with the peritoneum.

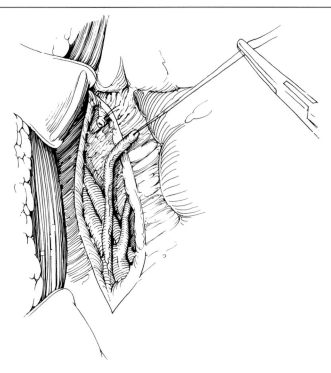

FIGURE 89-2. Free the left ureter with a right-angle clamp, followed by elevation in a Penrose drain for traction. Dissect it well into the pelvis, without disturbing its adventitial circulation. Clamp the ureter distally, place a fine traction suture on its anterior proximal surface, and divide it with a knife against the clamp. Ligate the distal stump with a 2-0 chromic catgut suture, cut long for later identification. Now dissect the ureter proximally to free about 8 cm. Repeat the procedure on the right side. Here the ureter lies retroperitoneally and just over the iliac vessels, so it is easier to find. Also less mobilization is needed on this side.

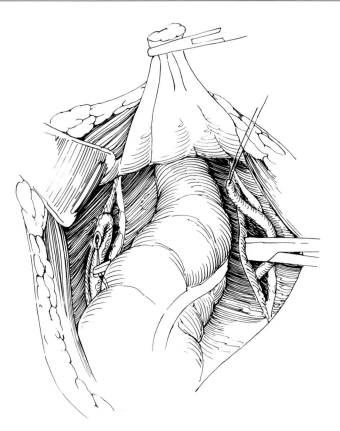

FIGURE 89-3. Using the index and middle fingers of each hand, tunnel gently between the two peritoneal openings. Stay beneath the superior hemorrhoidal vessels. Create a channel for the left ureter so that it can sweep across in a smooth arc to the right side. Pass a right-angle clamp to draw it through the channel by its stay suture. Take great care that the ureter is not angulated or twisted.

PREPARING THE LOOP

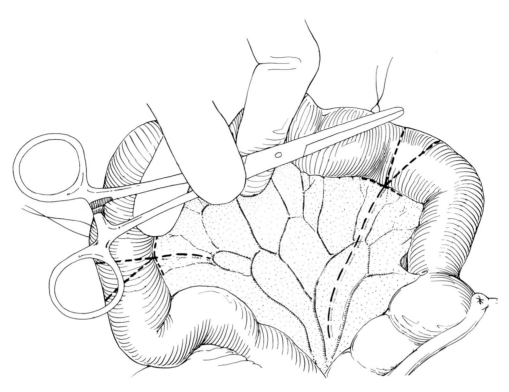

FIGURE 89-4. Select a suitable segment of ileum near the ileocecal junction by transilluminating its mesentery and visualizing the contained vessels. Usually an avascular area of mesentery is found slightly more proximally than that shown in the figure. If a suitable segment is not found here, use the more proximal ileum or jejunum or even consider a transverse colon conduit (see Chapter 88). Place a stay suture (4-0 silk with a detachable needle) in the bowel 10 to 15 cm from the ileocecal valve and beyond the ileocecal arcade, the distance depending on the size of the child. Select a loop of ileum that contains one or two distinct vascular arcades, as shown in the figure. Move the stay suture if necessary. It will mark the *distal* end of the segment so tie a knot in the end for identification, thus preventing later reversal of the loop. Measure the segment. It should be long enough to reach the skin level plus another 2 cm. In an adolescent, the length of a Kocher clamp is about right. If a Turnbull loop stoma is to be formed, obtain 8 to 10 cm more ileum. Place a second stay suture to mark the proximal end. Reexamine the loop and its arcades, moving the stay sutures as necessary to provide an adequate segment containing one, or preferably two, major vascular arcades. Hold both stay sutures in clamps.

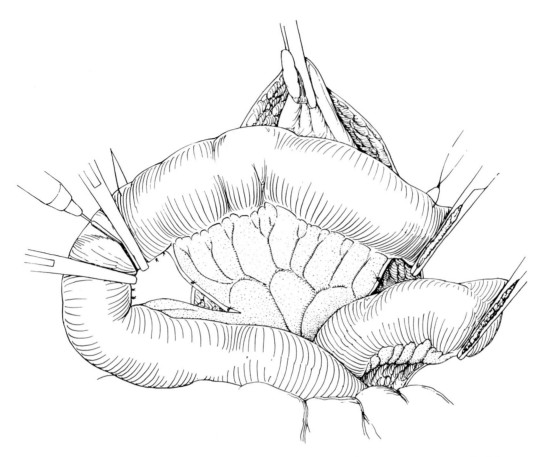

FIGURE 89-5. With a sharp #15 blade, divide the thin peritoneal layer of the mesentery on each side perpendicular to the bowel for a distance of 10 or 15 cm on the distal end and a distance of 3 cm on the proximal end. Incise the peritoneum parallel to the bowel for a short distance. With the handle of the knife, gently retract the underlying fat away from the bowel wall to expose the straight vessels running from the arcades to the wall. Insinuate a mosquito clamp under each exposed vessel; then apply the clamps in pairs very close to the bowel wall and divide between them. Immediately ligate each vessel with a 4-0 silk tie. Continue the process of sharply incising the peritoneum and clamping the vessels on the bowel margin for a distance of 1.5 cm each way from the proposed line of division.

Place Kocher clamps at 45-degree angles on the ends of the bowel that will be reanastomosed, but on the ends of the proposed loop place them at right angles. Divide the bowel with the cutting current, leaving a protruding 2-mm edge, and then fulgurate this edge. (Be sure to keep the bowel against the wound to ground it during fulguration.) Discard the excised wedges. (A sterile pan technique is not necessary because the ileal contents are essentially sterile.) Move the segment caudad and cover it with a moist laparotomy pad.

ILEOILEAL ANASTOMOSIS

Single-Layer Closed Technique

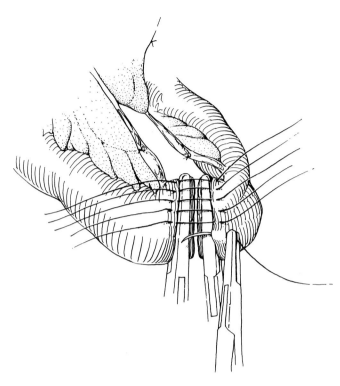

FIGURE 89-6. Hold the clamps to appose the cut ends. Place 4-0 silk detachable sutures into but not through the submucosa about 3 mm apart. See the wall blanch when the submucosa is just penetrated. (If they are placed too deep, they will catch the sutures on the opposite side and occlude the lumen.) When one side is completed, bundle the sutures into a clamp and turn the bowel over to place the sutures in the opposite side. Be certain that the sutures at the mesenteric angles are well placed; this is where leakage occurs. Again bundle the sutures in a second clamp. Slowly manipulate and withdraw the bowel clamps as your assistant gently supports the ends of the sutures.

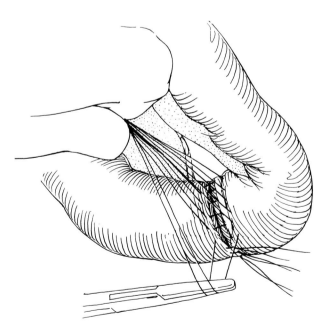

FIGURE 89-7. Tie the sutures successively, the assistant lifting them on a clamp and presenting them in pairs. Do not cinch them too tight. If the edges do not automatically invert, have your assistant hold a clamp under the suture loop and press it against the bowel edges as the knot is tied. Do not hesitate to put in extra sutures.

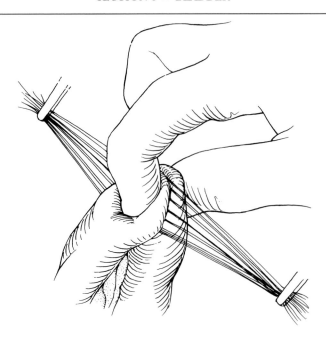

FIGURE 89-8. Check the patency of the anastomosis, first by inspection as the two bundles of uncut sutures are drawn apart, and then by palpation of the lumen with the thumb and forefinger. If in doubt, remove a few sutures and look inside, and cut any offending sutures and replace them. Cut the remaining sutures.

Single-Layer Open Technique

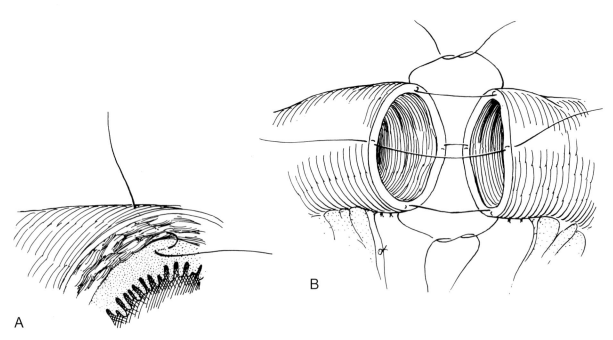

A   B

FIGURE 89-9. A and **B,** Appose the ends of the ileum with vertical mattress sutures of 3-0 silk placed in four quadrants to catch 3 mm of both the serosa and submucosa and a little mucosa. Tie these sutures and add interrupted sutures to catch the submucosa between.

Two-Layer Closure

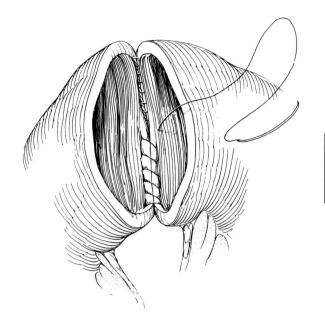

FIGURE 89-10. Approximate the posterior bowel wall with interrupted seromuscular sutures of 3-0 silk. Turn the bowel over. Place full-thickness continuous sutures of 3-0 chromic catgut to invert the mucosa of the posterior wall.

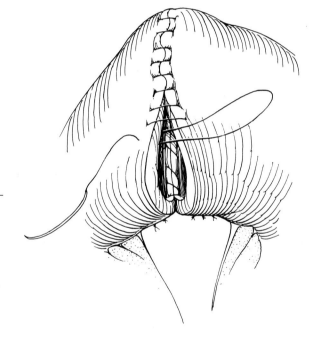

FIGURE 89-11. Continue this suture on the anterior wall and corners with a Connell stitch.

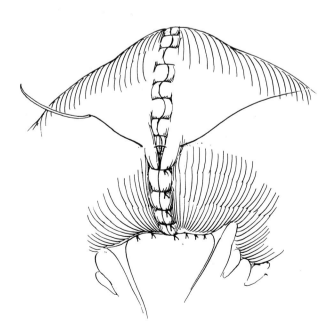

FIGURE 89-12. Complete the anastomosis with interrupted 3-0 silk sutures on the anterior seromuscular surface. For a stapling closure, proceed as described in Chapter 6.

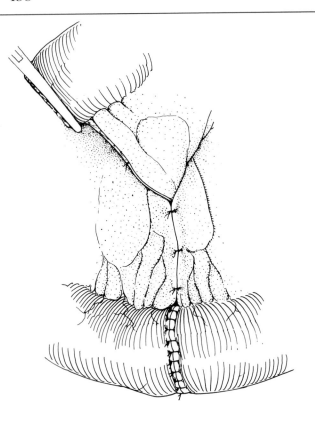

FIGURE 89-13. Close the mesentery on both sides with fine silk, taking care to incorporate only the delicate peritoneal surface. Annoying hematomas occur if a vessel is caught and breached. Test the anastomosis for patency as shown in Figure 89-8.

Formation of Stoma

It is better to form the stoma before anastomosing the ureters. Note: The stoma will not enlarge as the child grows, but may require periodic revision.

FIGURE 89-14. A, On the right side of the incision, place Kocher clamps on the fascia and peritoneum and draw them in line with the skin. Alternatively, place heavy sutures through all layers of the abdominal incision. At the stomal site marked previously, grasp the skin with a Kocher clamp, lift it, and sharply cut off the elevated mound with a knife, removing a circular piece slightly smaller than the diameter of the ileum. **B,** Grasp the subcutaneous fat with a Kocher clamp and circumscribe it with the electrosurgical blade. Take care not to angle the cut inward, which would remove a narrowing core. Avoid undermining, which is easily done because the fatty subcutaneous tissue stretches; removing too much fat allows stomal inversion.

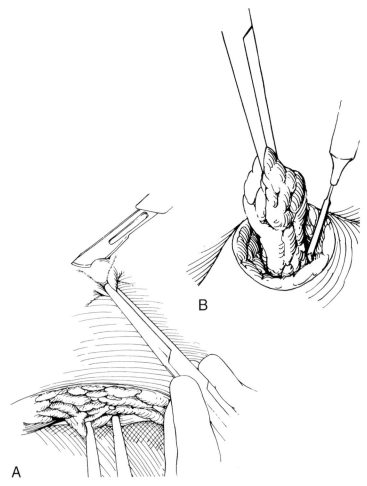

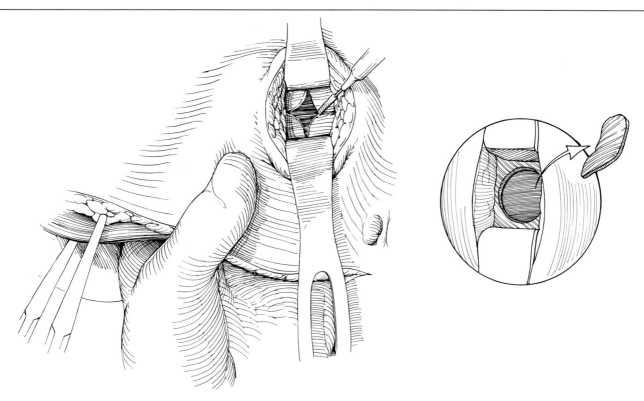

FIGURE 89-15. Incise the anterior rectus fascia with a cruciate cut with the cutting current, or preferably, remove a disc of fascia. Divide as little of the muscle as possible to avoid a parastomal hernia. Separate the rectus muscle bluntly and hold it apart with retractors to allow removal of a disc of the posterior fascial layer and peritoneum, or incise them in a cruciate fashion. Hold the left hand inside the abdomen to prevent injury to the bowel. A finger should now readily pass through all layers. Insert a Kocher clamp into the stoma, and grasp and reclamp the end of the loop as your assistant simultaneously releases it from its clamp. Draw it out, but be sure it will lie without tension 2 to 3 cm above the skin surface.

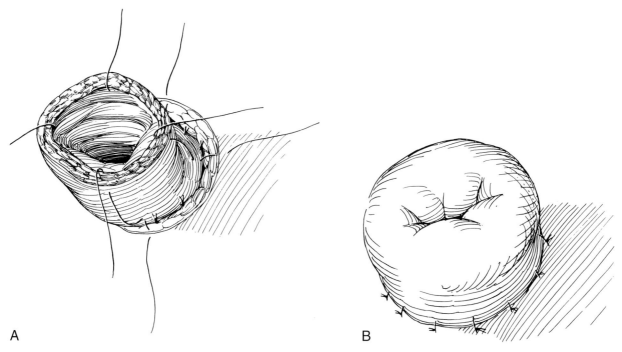

A   B

FIGURE 89-16. A and **B,** Suture the adventitia of the bowel to the fascia to prevent a parastomal hernia. Suture the opened bowel to the skin with four quadrant sutures of 3-0 synthetic absorbable material, catching the bowel well below the level of the skin to evert the stoma. Place two more sutures through skin and bowel edge between each pair of quadrant sutures. Invert these sutures so that the knots will be buried. If the loop seems too short (tension), make the stoma flush. Inside the abdomen, anchor the loop to the peritoneum and posterior rectus fascia with three 4-0 silk sutures (avoid sutures about the mesenteric border).

NIPPLE VARIATIONS

Z-Incision to Reduce Stomal Stenosis

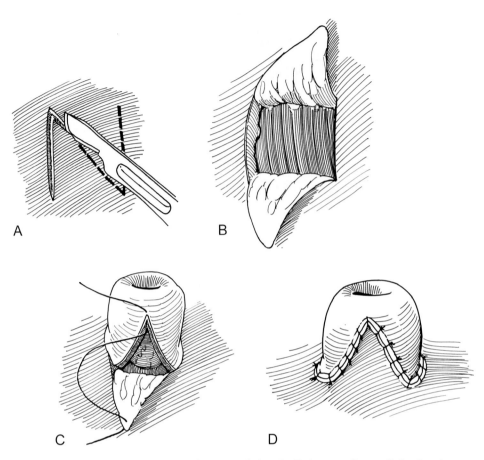

FIGURE 89-17. A, Make a Z-incision in the skin at the stomal site. **B,** Raise two flaps. **C,** Incise the mucosa and submucosa of the bowel on either side. **D,** Insert the flaps in the defects and suture them in place with 3-0 synthetic absorbable sutures.

Seromuscular Myotomy

Bring the end of the bowel through the opening in the abdomen. Make vertical incisions at the end of the segment at 3, 6, and 9 o'clock (in relation to the mesentery at 12 o'clock). Cut them deep enough to allow the mucosa to pout between the seromuscular layer. Intussuscept the end and suture the edge to the opening in the skin, catching the seromuscular layer in the suture to hold it in place.

Alternative Loop Stoma (Turnbull)

For obese adolescents with a short mesentery, provide an ileal segment that is 8 to 10 cm longer.

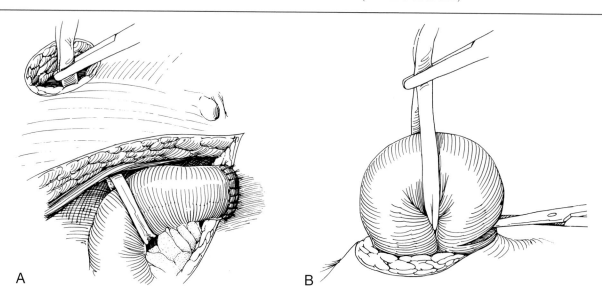

FIGURE 89-18. A, Close the distal end of the conduit as previously described for the proximal end. In these obese children, carefully undercut the mesentery of the distal end to obtain adequate mobility. Pass a clamp bluntly through the most mobile and well-vascularized part of the mesentery to loop it with a Penrose drain. **B,** Draw the bowel loop through the body wall without tension or twisting for at least several centimeters.

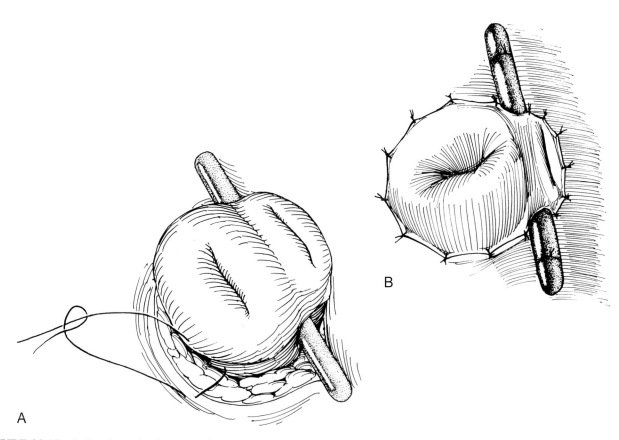

FIGURE 89-19. A, Replace the Penrose drain with a plastic rod. Open the loop transversely four fifths of the distance along the exposed bowel nearest the defunctionalized (distal) limb. Reach inside the opening with an Allis clamp and draw out the mucosa. **B,** Suture the mucosa to the subcuticular layer of skin with interrupted 4-0 synthetic absorbable sutures. Catch the seromuscular layer of the bowel to evert the stoma. The defunctionalized portion requires only superficial sutures. Fasten the rod in place with two silk sutures; it will be withdrawn 1 to 2 weeks postoperatively.

URETERAL ANASTOMOSES

Direct Anastomosis, Right (Cordonnier)

Close the left parietal peritoneal opening with 4-0 silk sutures.

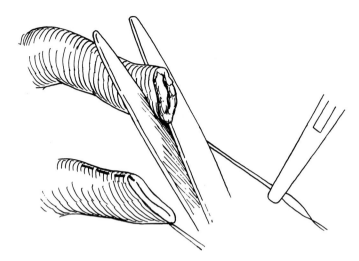

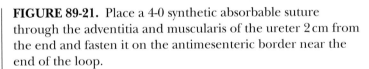

FIGURE 89-20. Cut the right ureter obliquely to freshen the end, and spatulate it *(dashes)* to provide a larger lumen for anastomosis.

FIGURE 89-21. Place a 4-0 synthetic absorbable suture through the adventitia and muscularis of the ureter 2 cm from the end and fasten it on the antimesenteric border near the end of the loop.

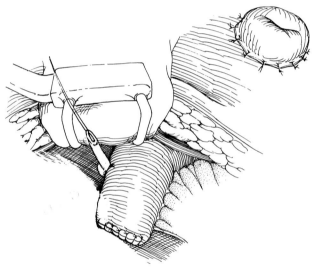

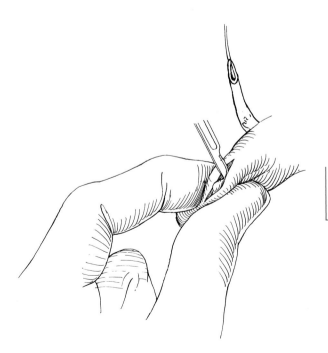

FIGURE 89-22. Pinch the bowel between the thumb and forefinger of the left hand and incise through the muscularis, exposing the fine vessels of the submucosa.

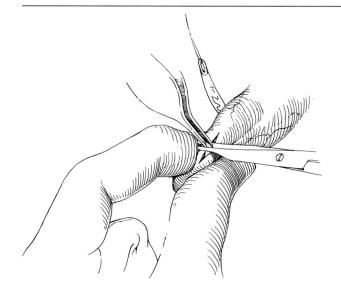

FIGURE 89-23. Grasp a bit of the extruding submucosa with smooth Adson forceps and trim it off along with the underlying mucosa with tenotomy scissors. Remove as little as possible. To check the opening, insert a mosquito clamp into the bowel lumen.

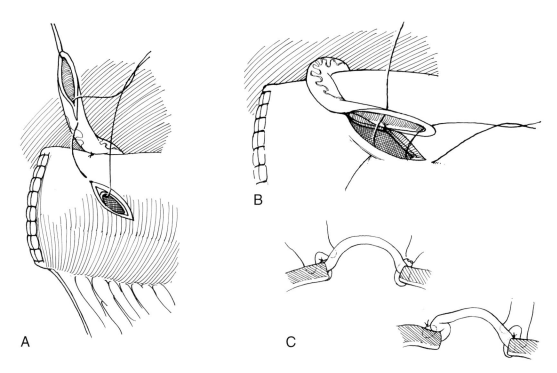

A

B

C

FIGURE 89-24. A, Place a 4-0 synthetic absorbable suture or chromic catgut through the apex of the bowel opening from outside in, and then through the apex of the ureter from inside out. Use the stay suture for manipulation; do not grasp the tissue with forceps. In each stitch incorporate a little mucosa, more muscularis, and adequate serosa. Tie the suture. **B,** Place and tie a suture similarly halfway along each side. Stents: If you are concerned about the quality of the tissues, insert a stent. However, stents can be obstructive, they take time to place, and they may come out too soon. Moreover, without them, leaks are not common. To use a stent, mount an 8-F infant feeding tube on a right-angle clamp and pass it through the ileal stoma and out through the opening in the bowel. Irrigate it clear of mucus. Take it up in a Kelly clamp and introduce it into the ureter until resistance is felt as it reaches the kidney. Irrigate again to test the position of the tip. Immediately fasten the tube to the skin with a silk suture. Later, cut the stent short to fit within the collecting bag. (An alternative is a double-J stent.) Place a fourth suture through the bowel and the tip of the ureter, which is manipulated on its stay suture. Cut the stay suture. **C,** Place three more sutures from the muscularis of the ureter to the serosa of the bowel to invert the anastomosis slightly into the bowel and provide a double layer for watertightness. Perform the same maneuvers with the left ureter. Make certain that the ureter passes beneath the colon in a smooth curve. Here, insert it 1 to 2 cm more proximally on the loop than the right, at a site where it is most easily accommodated and is not angulated. The stoma can usually be circumscribed and excised; the redundant bowel may be readily mobilized through the defect.

Trimming and Closure of the Proximal End of the Loop

Spread the loop so that it makes an easy curve from the stoma to the ureteral anstomoses. Apply a second Kocher clamp proximal to the one placed initially and trim any excess of bowel.

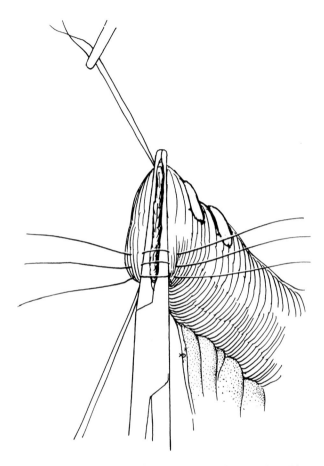

FIGURE 89-25. Insert stay sutures in the mesenteric and antimesenteric margins. Place a row of detachable 4-0 silk sutures over the clamp, passing them through the serosa and muscularis and incorporating the submucosa. Open the clamp slightly, and then withdraw it while keeping traction on the stay sutures.

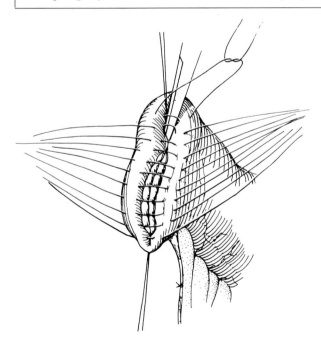

FIGURE 89-26. Tie the end sutures first, to invert the ends. It helps to have your assistant use a mosquito clamp to lift the crossing suture and at the same time depress the two edges of the bowel.

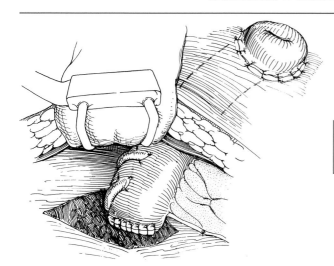

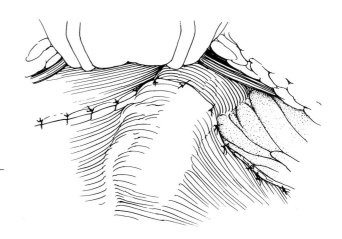

FIGURE 89-27. The loop of the proper length is shown, with the two ureters emerging from beneath it from the defect in the parietal peritoneum.

FIGURE 89-28. Pull the medial peritoneal flap over the ileal stump and ureters and fix it with interrupted 4-0 silk sutures. Continue these sutures up along the mesentery to avoid an internal hernia. Survey the conduit. If it is dusky, apply warm packs. If circulation is in doubt, excise it and start over.

CONJOINED URETER TECHNIQUES

Conjoined Side by Side

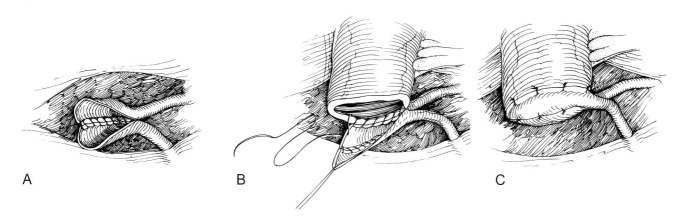

A   B   C

FIGURE 89-29. A, Leave the proximal end of the loop open. Spatulate each ureter for a distance equal to the diameter of the ileum. Join their posterior edges side by side with a fine running absorbable suture. **B,** Anastomose the joined ureters to the open bowel with two running 4-0 synthetic absorbable sutures, locking an occasional stitch. **C,** Reinforce the anastomosis with a second layer of five or six interrupted sutures. Proceed with closure of the end of the loop. If you have inserted stents, apply a collection appliance in the operating room. Drain the wound with suction drainage; remove the drains as soon as drainage stops.

Conjoined End to End (Wallace)

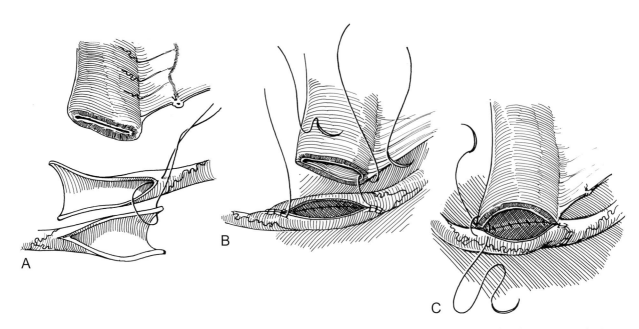

FIGURE 89-30. A, Spatulate each ureter for a distance slightly more than the diameter of the ileum. Join their posterior edges with two running 4-0 chromic catgut sutures, starting in the middle and continuing around each end. **B** and **C,** Continue the running sutures to join the back walls of the bowel with ureters. Take care to invert the angles. Then complete the closure anteriorly.

POSTOPERATIVE PROBLEMS

Anastomotic leakage is the most common and harmful postoperative complication, evidenced by decreasing output from the stoma and increased drainage. Perform a loopogram or an intravenous urogram. Look first for stomal stenosis: With a catheter, ascertain if there is residual urine in the loop; if so, leave the catheter stitched to the skin for drainage. If the drainage persists, percutaneous nephrostomy with antegrade stenting for a period of weeks may be necessary. Consider hyperalimentation.

Anuria after surgery is usually secondary to operative fluid shifts, so as the first step, challenge with mannitol. Early obstruction at the sites of anastomosis is rare. (Of course, if stents are in place and can be irrigated this need not be considered.) Place a catheter in the stoma to check for obstruction at the level of the body wall. If all fails and no urine is recovered, place percutaneous nephrostomies. Late ureteral obstruction can occur insidiously, secondary to ischemia of the terminal portion of the ureter or reaction to local urinary leakage. Balloon dilatation and endoscopic incision have a high rate of success, but open correction may be needed. Long-term stenting is an option.

Hyperchloremic acidosis, similar in consequence to ureterosigmoidostomy, may occur, but infrequently. It is usually associated with obstruction at the stoma, either from stenosis or from infrequent emptying of the drainage bag with associated back pressure. Catheterization of the conduit is immediately corrective; revision of the stoma or shortening of the loop may be needed for the long term. Jejunal conduits have greater problems with electrolyte imbalance, characterized by azotemia and hyponatremic hypochloremic acidosis; thus jejunum should be used only if other bowel is not available.

Wound infection or dehiscence is uncommon in children. Malnutrition (which should have been corrected preoperatively) can be an important factor. Disruption can be prevented by using running monofilament sutures with adequate bites of rectus fascia.

Paralytic ileus is usual and resolves quickly if gastric decompression is maintained, but intestinal obstruction may occur from herniation of the bowel into the mesenteric "trap." Continuation of decompression with a long (Baker) tube usually permits resolution, but reoperation is occasionally necessary.

Intestinal fistulas can occur from the site of the ileoileal anastomosis as a result of local ischemia from interference with the mesenteric vascular arcades. The whole segment can become necrotic if the mesentery is carelessly tacked to retroperitoneum or is subjected to too much tension. Judge the vascular supply by the color of the stomal mucosa. Leakage at the ileoileal anastomosis is usually due to tension and to rough handling of the tissue. Leakage can also occur at the suture line that closes the proximal end of the loop. Leakage from the ureteroileal anastomosis is uncommon. The source of the drainage can be determined by testing the fluid, because urine has a higher urea content than serum. Intraperitoneal absorption of urine causes the blood urea nitrogen level to rise relative to the creatinine level. Make a loopogram. If the leakage is minimal, place a double-lumen suction tube (a Malecot catheter containing an infant feeding tube connected to low suction) to allow healing. Alternatively, insert tubes percutaneously into the kidneys or place stents antegradely. If an appreciable urinoma has formed and the child is ill, reoperate and resect the anastomosis and reimplant at a new site. This is not an easy procedure, but attempts at resuturing seldom succeed. Prompt reoperation with insertion of a gastrostomy and replacement of the loop usually is required.

Redundancy of the segment is usually secondary to obstruction at the stoma or at the body wall. For correction, not only should the loop be shortened but the cause of the obstruction must be corrected.

Renal calculi may develop, although not as commonly as in adults. Chronic pyelonephritis occurs with deterioration of renal function from chronic mild obstruction and infection. Antibiotics may help, but conversion to a nonrefluxing colon conduit may be needed.

Obstruction at the ureteroileal anastomosis usually develops within the first 2 years, but may occur later. The cause is devascularization of the terminal ureter and obstruction is usually without symptoms. To avoid this complication, regular follow-up is necessary, with sonograms, scans, or intravenous pyelography, and also loopograms at regular intervals. Before reoperation, an attempt may be made at balloon dilatation of the anastomosis through a percutaneous nephrostomy tract, but this is seldom successful because of the fibrous cause of the stricture. For surgical repair, approach through a modified Gibson incision. Dissect retroperitoneally but stay away from the stoma. Incise the ureter and bowel at the site of the anastomosis and perform a Heineke-Mikulicz transverse closure. Alternatively, take an ellipse from the ureter, incise the ileum above the stricture, and suture the defects side to side. It is also possible to detach the ureter and either reanastomose it or perform ureteroureterostomy. Excess length of the loop can be resected through the stomal site by dividing the mesenteric arcades progressively as they join the bowel.

Stomal Problems

Peristomal dermatitis is common and may lead to stenosis. The cause may be (1) an improperly located or constructed stoma, (2) an appliance that does not fit, (3) poorly tolerated adhesive, (4) alkaline urine, or (5) (usually) inadequate stomal care. It starts with skin inflammation and progresses to ulceration and encrustation, finally resulting in hyperkeratosis and scarring (and leakage).

Stomal ischemia usually is temporary, but if it persists, it requires stomal revision with resection of a short segment of bowel. If the whole loop is ischemic, remove it, ligate the ureters, and place percutaneous nephrostomies. Wait

3 months, and then repeat the whole operation. Stomal stenosis occurs at the circular mucocutaneous junction. A Z-flap technique or an end-loop stoma can lessen the chance of stenosis. Everted (nipple) stomas have a lower incidence of stenosis. Stenosis usually occurs at the skin level, secondary to dermatitis, but can result from fascial angulation or ischemia of the terminal portion of the bowel. Alignment during formation and prevention (or eradication) of peristomal dermatitis are important. Surgical correction is needed if the stoma will not admit a 30-F catheter, if the residual urine is more than 10 mL, or if luminal pressure is greater than 20 cm of water.

Revision of the Stoma

The stoma can be circumscribed and excised, because the bowel is redundant and readily mobilized through the defect. Free the bowel for 10 to 12 cm through the body wall, and then dissect intraperitoneally and divide adhesions. Resect the terminal portion with its mesentery, and tack the bowel to the fascia. Form a new nipple stoma by interposing a V-flap of skin to prevent further circular contraction. Most important is obtaining improved care for the child with the help of an enterostomal therapist. Stomal prolapse results from inadequate fixation of the loop to the peritoneal-fascial layers, and the treatment is similar to that for stenosis. Parastomal hernias usually occur on the mesenteric side secondary to inadequate fixation of the conduit at the peritoneal opening. They can make fitting the appliance difficult and may lead to incarceration of the bowel. Repair them by freeing the stoma and the distal loop as done for stomal stenosis, then excising the peritoneal sac, fixing the loop internally, and closing the defect in the fascia. If this is not possible, relocate the stoma to the opposite side. Do this without opening the abdomen by passing the end of the loop from the old stoma to the new one on ring forceps.

Appliances

If it becomes impossible to keep an appliance attached because of body configuration, move the stoma up or down on the same side, place it at the umbilicus, or move it across the abdomen. Sometimes, the entire loop must be mobilized or a new conduit constructed to reach the new site.

Ureteral dilation may result from ureteral stenosis caused by a technical error, or it may appear late without obvious cause. Revision is necessary, unless the ureter is atonic, in which case a new anastomosis will not help. Renal calculi appear later, usually in alkaline urine harboring urea-splitting bacteria. Shorten the loop, increase water intake, give thiazides, add bicarbonate, and inhibit the infection with antibiotics. Pyelonephritis occurs with increasing incidence the longer diversion is present, as a result of a combination of back flow and bacteriuria. Antibacterial therapy for symptomatic attacks and attention to better drainage may help.

LOWELL R. KING

From the long description of the management of complications, the reader has gathered that an ileal loop is seldom the urinary diversion of choice in children. However, when popularized in the 1950s, the ileal loop revolutionized urology. Then, there was no treatment for incontinence or those requiring cystectomy that did not result in the need for permanent intubation with resulting infection, stones, and loss of renal function. Periodic enlargement of the stoma in a growing child mostly prevented reflux of mucus with subsequent upper-tract stones. Ileal conduits saved a lot of lives.

That having been said, when poor renal function precludes using bowel for a continent diversion, ureterostomy is a better choice provided at least one ureter is at least 1 cm in diameter when collapsed. Removal of a "cork bore" of abdominal wall at the stoma site makes ureterostomy drainage reliable, and the less dilated ureter is anastomosed to its more dilated mate so that the urine drains through a single stoma. As with an ileal conduit, stomal enlargements are usually required every 3 to 6 years as the child grows.

Alternatively, a colon conduit is also a better choice in children, as the stoma is larger and less likely to stenose. When the ureters are near normal in caliber, Leadbetter extraluminal antirefluxing anastomoses are reliable (see Fig. 88-3). Larger ureters are anastomosed to the colon conduit end to side or end to end.

When renal function is normal or near normal, a continent diversion is usually selected. Ileocecal ureterosigmoidostomy is a good choice, especially in females. The ileocecal segment is isolated, and the terminal ileum intussuscepted to make a nipple about 5 cm in length. The nipple can be stabilized without staples, which carry a stone risk, by incising full thickness the back wall of the nipple, and making a linear incision through the full thickness or the cecum opposite. The edges of the nipple incision are sewn to the edges of the cecal incision with 3-0 chromic sutures. The resulting muscular bond is very effective in preventing reflux. A medial oval of lower sigmoid is then removed, and the cecum anastomosed here, usually with running, locking, 3-0 chromic sutures. Adventitial buttressing sutures may be used if needed.

The ureters are then anastomosed to the ileal tail, avoiding the later risk of malignancy seen after conventional ureterosigmoidostomy.

Depending on bowel availability, another form of continent diversion may be elected, and the reservoir formed in whole or in part from bladder, ileum, stomach, or colon. Reasonable variations are more or less endless.

Although the ileal loop has almost had its day in children, we have learned much. Urologists are now as familiar with the abdominal cavity as general surgeons, greatly improving the results achieved after cystectomy and nephrectomy for malignancy.

STEVE SHAPIRO

Commentary by

There is not much recent experience with ileal conduits in children because of the myriad of alternative forms of urinary diversion and continent conduits and because of the many late complications of ileal conduit. However, this operation still plays a role, although it is much more limited than in the past. Kidney transplantation into an ileal conduit in cases of renal failure continues to have its advocates. In addition, the ileal conduit might serve as a temporary or permanent diversion in complex cancer cases, although other forms of diversion should also be considered.

In the early 1970s, ileal conduits were used as the primary form of urinary diversion in children. Alternatives were sought because of the many long-term complications, including renal calculi, bowel obstruction, urinary infections, and stomal problems (stenosis, prolapse, and parastomal hernias). The high incidence of long-term complications seemed independent of surgical technique and showed up in numerous large series in the late 1970s.

Antireflux implantation of the ureters has not usually been used in the construction of ileal conduits in children, although in recent years such techniques have been occasionally used in adult conduits. The concept of the short conduit and unobstructed drainage into an appliance is believed to neutralize any effect of reflux. This is in sharp contrast to the colon conduit that lends itself easily to ureteric reimplantation.

Undiversion using an ileal conduit has not been an easy task in my hands. If the conduit is constructed short, as is ideal, there is not much to work with in any reconstruction. An ileal loop that is tailored and reimplanted into the bladder will stricture in nearly all cases. If reconstruction is contemplated in the future, as much length of ureter as possible should be preserved.

Bowel anastomosis using stapling devices (GIA and TA 55) has become popular even in children. Except in infants, these anastomoses have proven reliable and they can save the time of suturing for the bowel anastomosis.

Proper placement of the stoma so that an appliance will fit is more difficult with the ileal conduit than with a colon conduit. Thus, attention preoperatively to the stoma site is of great importance.

I prefer the use of stents. For simplicity, I use 8-F pediatric feeding tubes; similarly, small pediatric single-J stents have been useful in selected cases. Urine will usually drain around these tubes even if they become obstructed (since in most cases of diversion the ureters are somewhat or largely dilated).

Because of the high incidence of late problems, long-term follow-up with periodic renal panels and ultrasound studies of the kidney and conduit is necessary on a periodic basis (e.g., every 6 months).

Part IV

Catheterizable Continent Channels

Chapter 90

Introduction to Catheterizable Channels

Access to a normal bladder, augmented bladder, or continent reservoir for intermittent catheterization may not be possible through the urethra. In this case, creating an abdominal stoma is necessary. The submucosal implantation of the appendix (see Chapter 91) provides continence and furnishes a catheterizable stoma (Mitrofanoff principle). The ureter may also be used as a conduit between the skin and the bladder when one of the renal units is nonfunctional or by performing a transureteroureterostomy. An alternative approach when the appendix is not available is an opened ileal segment closed transversely (Yang-Monti, see Chapter 92). In patients with a large, flaccid bladder a portion of the bladder may be constructed into a continent vesicostomy tube (see Chapter 93).

The Mitrofanoff principle is indicated in conjunction with closure of an incompetent vesical outlet (see Chapter 73). Because these stomas will not leak, even at high intravesical pressure, the risk of spontaneous vesical rupture is appreciable unless another route is present with a lower leak pressure. For that reason, closure of the vesical neck may not be advisable unless the child has persistent incontinence in spite of bladder neck reconstruction.

Prior to creation of a catheterizable abdominal channel the child and family must be educated in all aspects of clean intermittent catheterization. Nurse practitioners and children and their families that already have catheterizable channels are the best support resource.

Chapter 91

Appendicovesicostomy

APPENDICOVESICOSTOMY (MITROFANOFF)

Educate the patient and family about clean intermittent catheterization. Prepare the bowel and administer broad-spectrum antibiotics. Insert a balloon catheter transurethrally. If the vesical neck has been closed, depend on the suprapubic tube.

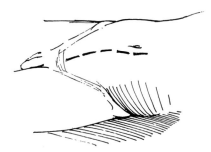

FIGURE 91-1. Incision: Use a midline abdominal (see Chapter 11), Pfannenstiel (see Chapter 63), or laparoscopic approach. Open the peritoneum. Mobilize the cecum for easy placement of the appendix without stretching of the appendiceal vessels.

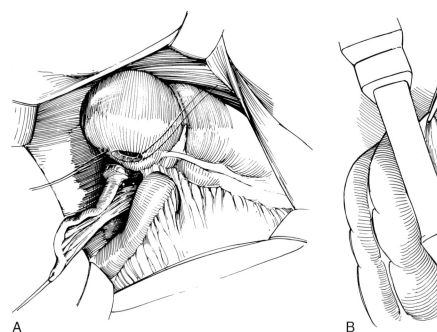

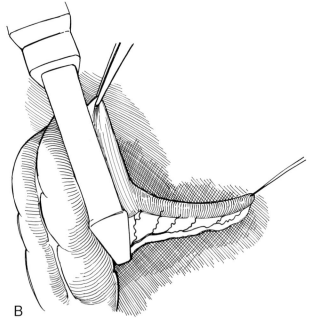

A

B

FIGURE 91-2. A, At the base of the appendix insert stay sutures and incise the wall circumferentially to take a cuff of cecum. Separate the appendiceal mesentery for a short distance from that of the cecum, preserving all of the blood supply to the appendix. Close the cecal defect left by the appendix with an inner running layer of 3-0 synthetic absorbable sutures and an outer layer of interrupted Lembert 3-0 synthetic absorbable sutures. **B,** Alternatively, secure a broad base for the appendiceal conduit by applying a stapler across the cecum a short distance from the base, taking care to preserve the vascular pedicle to the appendix. If needed, this cecal portion can be fashioned into a tube to lengthen the appendix.

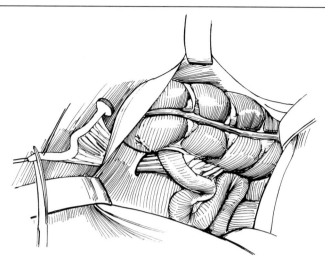

FIGURE 91-3. Extraperitonealize the appendix through a small opening in the peritoneum behind the ileocecal junction. Close the peritoneum with a running suture. Successively trim back the appendiceal tip with Mayo scissors until an adequate lumen is exposed.

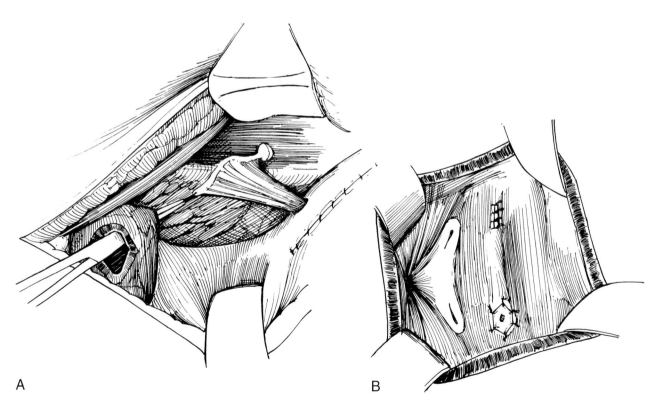

A   B

FIGURE 91-4. **A,** In the posterolateral wall of the bladder, bluntly develop a wide submucosal tunnel beginning well above the right ureteral orifice, as in the Cohen procedure (see Chapter 39), but make it longer (4 to 5 cm). **B,** Implant the appendix and its mesentery in the tunnel, stretching it so that it is not kinked. Proceed with bladder augmentation if necessary. Alternatively, use an extravesical approach as in reimplanting a ureter (see Chapters 41 and 45).

FIGURE 91-5. Pass the appendiceal base through a large opening in the abdominal muscles and a small opening in the skin sited in the edge of the future hairline in the right lower quadrant. Alternatively, it may be placed in the umbilicus. Incise a 1- × 1-cm, laterally placed V-flap on one side of the umbilicus. Make a generous opening through the abdominal wall. Raise the skin flap. Bring the end of the appendix through the skin with a Babcock clamp, without torsion of tension. Incise the antimesenteric wall of the appendix to correspond to the skin flap and place a 3-0 chromic catgut suture at the apex of flap and incision. Suture the V-flap into the appendiceal V-incision with interrupted 4-0 polyglycolic sutures. Leave a 10-F polyethylene catheter through the appendix. Hitch the bladder to the anterior abdominal wall around the opening to prevent kinking of the appendix and to compensate for its limited length. Protect the vasculature in the appendiceal mesentery.

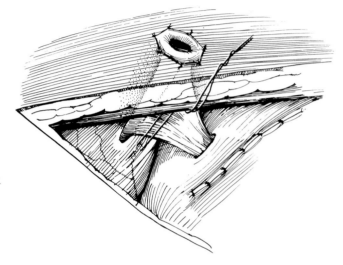

Check for ease of catheterization. For concern about the effectiveness of the new valve and assurance that it will not become kinked, fill the bladder or reservoir with water under manometric control and note the pressure at which leakage through the appendix occurs (the leak point pressure). A leak point pressure of 80 cm of water is satisfactory, but if leakage does occur at a lower pressure, consider revising antireflux measures.

In patients that have simultaneous augmentation irrigate the suprapubic tube regularly. Leave the catheter through the appendix for 3 weeks. At that time, make a cystogram through the suprapubic tube; if no leaks are detected, clamp the cystostomy and start intermittent catheterization with an 8- or 10-F catheter through the new stoma. Once an effective self-catheterization routine has been established, remove the cystostomy tube. Continue regular vigorous bladder irrigations and use ultrasonography to gauge the effectiveness of catheter drainage. Over time, the size of the catheter may be increased to 12- to 14-F.

POSTOPERATIVE PROBLEMS

Stomal stenosis is a not uncommon complication; it may be a late development that requires dilatation or surgical revision with a Y-V plasty. Triamcinolone injections at the site may inhibit recurrence. Strictures of the appendix at its vesical junction require open revision. False passages can occur during self-catheterization. Urinary fistulas may pose a problem. They can occur at the site of vesical neck closure, from a vesicovaginal fistula, or at the vesical suture line anteriorly. Vesicoureteral reflux should have been corrected at a prior stage. If it does appear after operation, perform vesical augmentation to reduce the incidence of upper-tract dilation. Mucus from the lining of the appendix will fall into the base of the bladder where it may not be evacuated during intermittent catheterization. It may result in residual urine or in frank obstruction, and it can lead to stone formation in some patients. Regular irrigation of the bladder is absolutely essential. Finally, the mucosa of the appendix may prolapse and require surgical correction.

URETEROVESICOSTOMY

The ureter may be substituted for the appendix. To use the lower end of the ureter requires a transureteroureterostomy (see Chapter 52) and an antireflux procedure performed in two stages. A ureteral conduit is especially suitable when one end of the ureter is well vascularized, as after cutaneous ureterostomy.

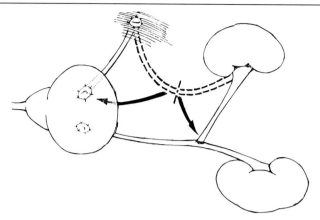

FIGURE 91-6. Divide the ureter that was implanted in the skin in its midportion. Insert the proximal end of its distal segment in the bladder or bladder substitute and the distal end of its proximal segment in the contralateral ureter, which in turn is implanted in the bladder (or augmentation) with an antireflux technique. Divide the distal end, place a rubber-shod clamp on the proximal end, and check for distal bleeding. Place one end of the ureter on the abdomen to be available for intermittent catheterization and the other end in the reservoir as a nonrefluxing valve with a tunnel of the same proportions, as for ureteroileostomy (see Chapter 89). (When the ureter is placed to exit in the perineum, the urogenital diaphragm is used for continence.) Postoperatively, discomfort on catheterization can occur, particularly when the ureter is not grossly dilated at the time of insertion.

POSTOPERATIVE PROBLEMS

Bladder calculi are not uncommon, perhaps secondary to mucus that passes down into the pouch from the appendix and is not drained by the catheter. Disruption may occur from traumatic catheterization or acute or chronic overfilling. Fistulas may occur in the early postoperative period.

PAUL MITROFANOFF

Commentary by

TIPS AND TRICKS

A larger peritoneal dissection of the right lower quadrant is necessary to place the appendix and its mesentery under the peritoneum in the best way. This dissection is easier to perform before opening the peritoneum.

I believe that the bladder should be opened for three reasons: (1) for bladder neck closure, (2) to select the best place to implant the appendix, and (3) to help accomplish the bladder hitch to the anterior abdominal wall. This hitch is useful to avoid kinking of the appendix between the abdominal muscles and bladder and also if the appendix is short.

Retaining the Foley catheter for 2 weeks should prevent a possible urethral breakdown and, of course, is necessary after bowel augmentation. No other bladder drainage is used.

As an alternative to appendicovesicostomy, I have also described a ureterovesicostomy that requires a transureteroureterostomy and an antireflux procedure performed in two stages.

PARTICULAR POINTS

If there is reflux, it requires correction in a preliminary stage, but it is usually a symptom of bladder hypertonicity that requires bladder augmentation.

Bladder neck closure is necessary in almost all cases. The bladder neck could be left open only if there is total dryness between the urethral catheterizations (and the impossibility of self-catheterization owing to an orthopedic situation). Alternatively, a urethral sling procedure may be done later if incontinence continues to be a problem.

The decision to perform an enterocystoplasty to enlarge the bladder has to be made at the first stage if the bladder is small and hypertonic, or later on if reflux or upper-tract dilation appears. This procedure seems to be necessary in about one half of neurogenic bladders retained for urinary storage.

Continued

COMPLICATIONS

Different types of complication can occur, including complications with the appendix such as stenosis of the cutaneous stoma or appendicular kink blocking catheterization. A limited reoperation is sufficient to resolve these problems. Urinary leakage by the cutaneous stoma requires a more difficult operation to lengthen the submucosal tunnel of the appendix and restore continence. However, it is essential to check if this leakage is not due to a high bladder pressure requiring an augmentation. Vesicourethral fistula, urinary infection, dilation of the upper tract, or reflux is possible. They are almost always symptoms of too small a bladder with too high a pressure. Anticholinergic drugs are usually insufficient and enterocystoplasty is necessary.

Bladder stones are promoted by the presence of the intestinal mucus. Such stones are often well tolerated and their removal is easy to perform. Prevention should be associated with an increased diuresis and catheterization with a large catheter—14-F when possible—and trying to have the child perform complete emptying at each time by siphoning. A weekly bladder wash can be useful. Most severe is the occurrence of a spontaneous rupture of an enterocystoplasty. It is probably due to too infrequent catheterizations leading to an overdistended bladder. So it is essential to teach the patients to respect a timetable with at least four catheterizations a day.

BRADLEY KROPP

Commentary by

The development and routine use of the appendicovesicostomy has added greatly to the quality of life of our neurogenic bladder patients. It has allowed them independence, freedom, and a reliable method to regularly empty their bladders. Reconstructive urology is forever indebted to Paul Mitrofanoff for sharing the principles of his procedure.

Some of the key steps in the procedure that should be emphasized are that many times the appendiceal mesentery will not reach all the way down to the bladder; therefore, often, extensive mobilization of the cecum and the root of the small intestine mesentery is required to get things to "fit." Additionally, a psoas hitch procedure can be performed to get the bladder to "reach" and provide an appropriate tunnel length for the appendix. As most of my patients are also receiving a simultaneous bowel augmentation, it is not uncommon for me to reimplant the appendix in a seromuscular trough on the bowel augmentation segment. I have found this particularly useful when the appendix is short. I also routinely request that my patients perform daily bladder washes to prevent bladder stone formation.

I believe that with the decreased number of upper-tract urinary diversions being performed today, the use of the ureter is probably limited to only a few highly select patients. However, the same principles outlined above are applied regularly with tapered and reconfigured ileum (Monti tube), which would always be my first choice if the appendix was not available for use.

One of the biggest problems that I have encountered is increased difficulty in catheterization associated with obesity as the children who have previously been reconstructed enter adolescence and adulthood. Therefore, increased emphasis on weight control to prevent complications with these stomas must be emphasized.

Chapter 92

Ileovesicostomy

ILEOVESICOSTOMY (YANG-MONTI)

When access through the urethra into the bladder is not possible, an accessory channel can be devised from transversely tubularized ileum, a technique first described by Yang in 1993 and subsequently confirmed in clinical practice by Monti. Use of the ileum is a necessity when the appendix is not available or the bladder tissue is inadequate to perform a continent vesicostomy. The availability of ileum and the durability, as well as versatility in respect to length, has led many surgeons to choose ileum as the primary source for abdominal catheterizable channels.

The Yang-Monti procedure requires only a small length of bowel, which is easy to position on its mesentery. The conduit can be readily catheterized because, after it is opened and rotated, the mucosal folds (valvulae conniventes) will now run longitudinally. Also, this conduit is continent without a leak point pressure test. An antireflux mechanism is easy to arrange without interference from the mesentery, and no staples are used, thus avoiding the risk of stone accretion. In contrast to the Mitrofanoff procedure, which uses the available appendix, bowel is always present for a redo. The tube can also be used as a continent cutaneous cecostomy for the Malone antegrade continence enema (MACE) procedure (see Chapter 94). If bladder augmentation is planned, extra small bowel may be harvested at the time of the Yang-Monti construction.

The physical principles of the tube are as follows: The length of the bowel segment determines the diameter of the tube, and the length depends on the diameter of the segment.

PREOPERATIVE INSTRUCTIONS

The patient should have a preoperative bowel cleanout and receive intravenous antibiotics to prevent intra-abdominal infection at the time of surgery. The procedure can be performed in conjunction with continent urinary diversion or augmentation cystoplasty or as an isolated procedure.

PRELIMINARY MEASUREMENTS

To determine the length needed for the short branch of the tube (usually 2.5 cm), insert a spinal needle into the abdomen at the proposed stomal site and measure the thickness of the abdominal wall. To provide valvular function, the long branch inserted into the reservoir must be at least 3 to 4 cm long. If the length required is greater than the circumference of the donor segment of intestine, place two tubes in tandem (the double-tube Monti).

Single-Tube Monti

Form the tube immediately after reanastomosis of the bowel, before constructing the reservoir, because the new tube quickly becomes edematous and hard to manage.

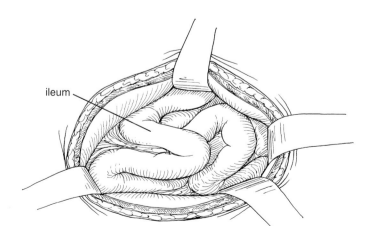

ileum

FIGURE 92-1. Expose the small intestine through a midline or Pfannenstiel incision. Use a self-containing retractor such as a Denis Browne or pediatric ring retractor to facilitate exposure.

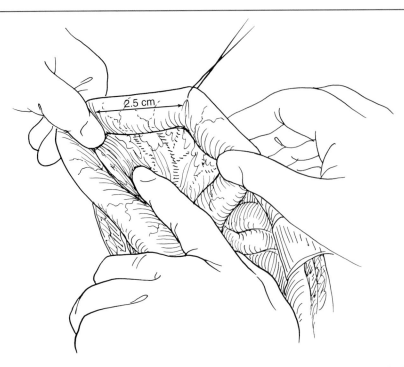

FIGURE 92-2. At least 20 cm from the ileocecal valve, isolate 2.5 cm of ileum on its mesenteric blood supply. You may isolate this segment by using a stapling device or by freehand suturing.

Note: If bowel tissue is also needed for bladder augmentation or reservoir construction, mobilize the Monti segment in continuity with the mesentery of that segment of ileum to be used for augmentation. Take more bowel initially and form the augmentation in continuity.

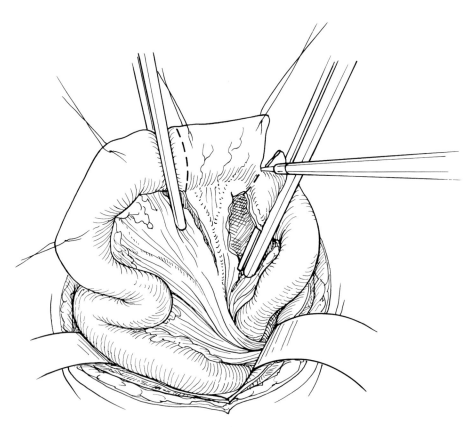

FIGURE 92-3. Use noncrushing bell clamps to facilitate isolation of the segment. Place the bowel back into continuity either with stapling devices or with handsewing of an inner layer of 4-0 absorbable suture supported by an outer layer of 4-0 silk suture. Reinforce any mesenteric holes to prevent a possible hernia.

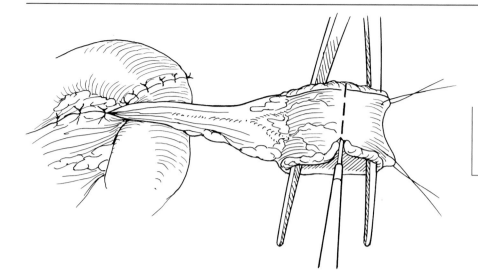

FIGURE 92-4. Prepare the isolated 2.5-cm segment of ileum with holding sutures and open halfway between the mesenteric border and antimesenteric border.

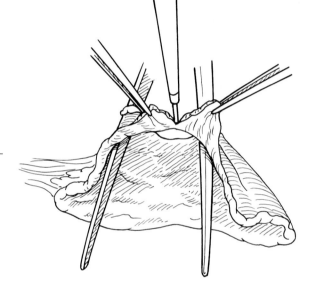

FIGURE 92-5. Use a cautery that changes the cylindrical configuration to a rectangular open plate.

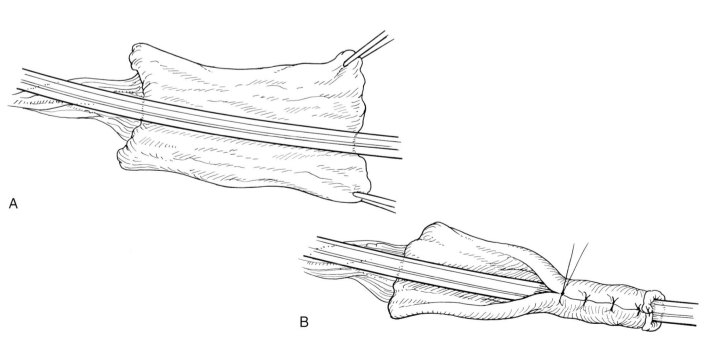

A

B

FIGURE 92-6. A and **B,** Using a 12- to 14-F catheter, form a 16- to 18-F catheterizable channel with 4-0 interrupted, long-acting absorbable sutures. Take care not to disturb the mesenteric blood supply of the catheterizable channel.

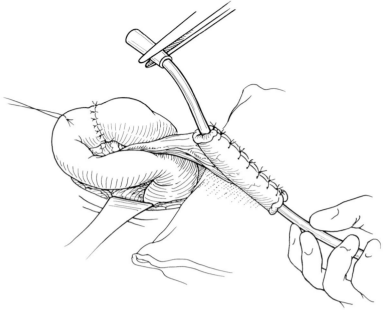

FIGURE 92-7. The completed catheterizable tube is now ready for implantation into the bladder and abdominal stoma. Orientation of the channel should not compromise the mesenteric blood supply.

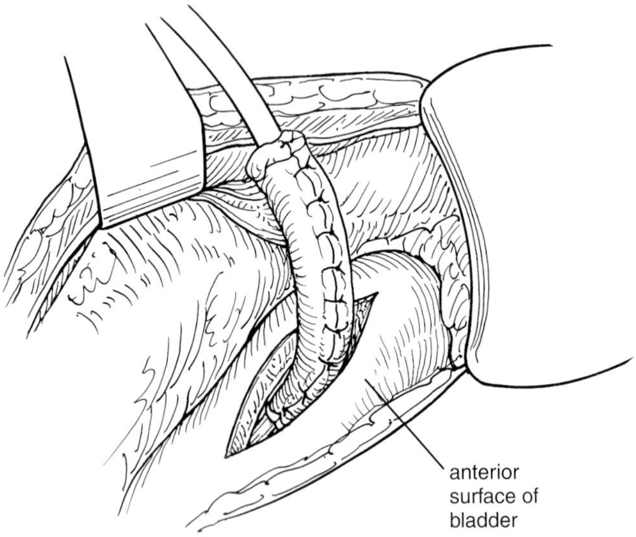

anterior surface of bladder

FIGURE 92-8. Dissect a trough on the anterior surface of the bladder in similar fashion to an extravesical ureteral reimplantation (see Chapter 43). Perform the anastomosis with 4-0 absorbable sutures and close the trough with 3-0 or 4-0 sutures, creating a flap-value continence mechanism.

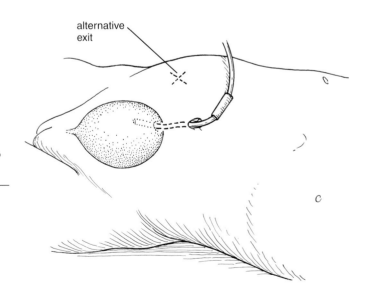

alternative exit

FIGURE 92-9. Create an abdominal stoma in similar fashion to an appendicostomy (see Chapter 71) either at the umbilicus or in the right lower quadrant. Design a skin flap to interdigitate with the catheterizable tube to prevent stenosis.

As the catheterizable channel is anastomosed to the bladder, as well as to the abdominal stoma, ease of catheterization is checked to confirm usability and prevent postoperative catheterization problems. The catheterized channel is secured to the outerlying fascia with 4-0 or 5-0 permanent suture to prevent kinking and dislodging during use. The catheter is left in place for 3 to 4 weeks postoperatively to decompress the bladder and allow the anastomotic site to heal. When bladder augmentation or continent diversion is performed at the same time, a suprapubic tube is used to facilitate urinary drainage. The catheter is removed at 3 and 4 weeks postoperatively and intermittent catheterization instituted.

Spiral Monti (Casale)

In patients with an extended distance between the bladder and the stoma site secondary to complex reconstruction or body habitus it is possible to perform a double Monti or spiral Monti. A double Monti is performed by suturing two single Monti tubes together. To avoid a circular anastomosis the spiral Monti preserves an intact bowel plate.

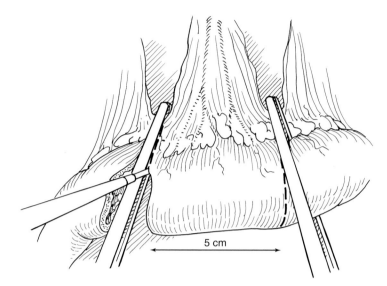

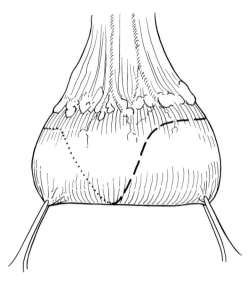

FIGURE 92-10. At least 20 cm from the ileocecal value, isolate 5 cm of the small intestine based on its mesenteric blood supply. Anastomose the remaining bowel in continuity.

FIGURE 92-11. Design the spiral Monti tube by marking the bowel approximately 0.5 cm from the mesentery, starting at each end. In the midportion of the bowel, the incision spirals around the bowel in a mirror image.

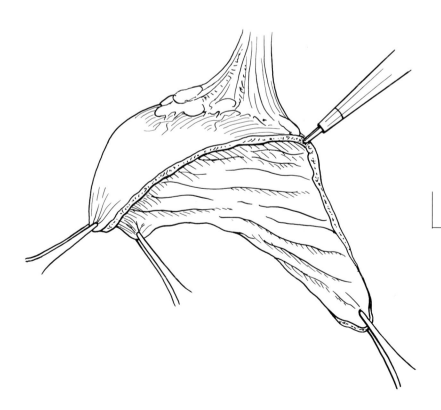

FIGURE 92-12. Use electrocautery to open the bowel along the marked spiral line.

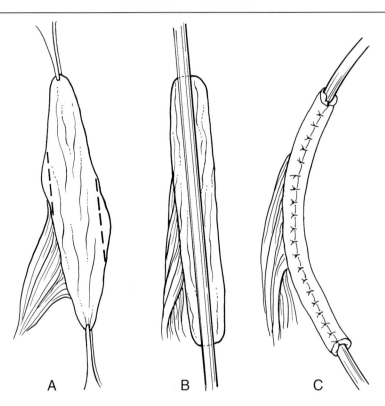

FIGURE 92-13. A, Trim the edges of the bowel at the mesenteric blood supply to facilitate a rectangular plate of small intestines. **B** and **C,** Suture the spiral Monti tube with 4-0 interrupted, long-acting absorbable sutures over a 12- to 14-F catheter to allow a channel of 16 to 18 F. Bring out the spiral Monti tube as a catheterizable channel within the umbilicus or right lower quadrant as described for the single Monti tube. Implant the remaining end into the bladder as previously described.

POSTOPERATIVE PROBLEMS

Stoma stenosis occurs in approximately 10% of patients. This can be prevented with use of skin flaps and meticulous care to preserve the blood supply to the catheterizable channel. Difficult catheterizing can also be prevented by checking the position of the catheterizable stoma during the design and securing of both the bladder and the catheterizable channel to the underlying fascia. This prevents movement and kinking of the catheter during bladder filling and emptying. Stenosis may also occur at the anastomotic site between the bladder and catheterizable channel.

Incontinence is reported in fewer than 10% of patients, and more commonly with umbilical stomas. Try medication or more frequent catheterization. If these measures fail, perform urodynamic studies to determine whether the cause is an inadequate tunnel or a malfunctioning reservoir, and then reoperate to correct the cause. Difficult catheterization may also be due to an overfilled reservoir that occludes the outlet. A safety valve is provided by an open bladder neck but if that outlet is not available, have the attendant aspirate the bladder by inserting a needle directly into the reservoir (Duckett, 1996). After decompression, the tube will usually admit a catheter. Realize that in persistently difficult cases, the catheter can be left indwelling. Periodic follow-up studies with ultrasound to assess upper-tract status and urodynamics to assess bladder compliance are indicated.

PAULO R. MONTI

Commentary by

In 1980, Paul Mitrofanoff described his technique for continent urinary diversion, using the appendix as an efferent catheterizable conduit. This procedure gained great acceptance, particularly within pediatric urology, because of its efficiency, simplicity, and use of widely known urologic principles. However, its versatility was determined by the availability of the appendix. The appendix is not always available, and this cannot be defined before surgery. Mitrofanoff himself used ureter segments as a substitute. Since then, around 14 new alternative conduits have been described, including some exotic options like the vas deferens, fallopian tube, and hypogastric artery segments. All of them have been shown to be clearly inferior to the appendix.

The new tube described in this chapter confers a new dimension to Mitrofanoff's technique, by broadening its applicability. Several studies have shown results and complications similar to those when the appendix is used. Moreover, it has freed the appendix for use in other techniques that are performed simultaneously with urinary diversions, like

MACE. More recently, the new tube has found a variety of alternative applications such as vaginal construction in cases of vaginal hypoplasia or agenesis, nonurothelial replacement of long ureteral defects, an alternative conduit for Malone's technique, continent catheterizable gastrostomy in children with cerebral palsy, and, still at the experimental stage, a replacement for the common bile duct. Although use of the ileal tube is much more recent than use of the appendix, follow-up on such cases has shown it to be a simple, reliable, versatile, and durable technique.

ANTHONY J. CASALE

Commentary by

Mitrofanoff's brilliant concept to provide extra-anatomic access to the urinary bladder through a continent abdominal wall stoma revolutionized reconstruction of the urinary tract. His procedure relied on a functional appendix to construct the channel. Unfortunately, the appendix was not always available, having been lost to appendicitis or routine excision during other surgery, and sometimes failing to develop adequate length or lumen size for catheterization. There were attempts to build channels from bladder wall with limited success. It was not until Monti noticed Yang's idea and popularized its use as a substitute for appendix that every patient was able to enjoy Dr. Mitrofanoff's contribution.

The Yang-Monti channel is simple and requires less than 2 cm of bowel, ileum is used because of the length and position of the ileal mesentery. Blood supply for the ileum is excellent and dependable. The construction can be performed in minutes and is easy to learn. The diameter of the channel can be designed by the length of bowel used in construction. The only limitation of the procedure is the length of the channel itself, which is completely determined by the circumference of the segment of bowel used. Since there is considerable variability in the circumference of bowel among patients, the length of the channel may be inadequate for larger patients with thick abdominal walls.

When the length is adequate, the Yang-Monti channel is an outstanding option with reliability rates of continence and ease of catheterization compatible with appendicovesicostomy. It has become particularly useful with the advent of MACE, which uses the appendix as a catheterizable stoma for the cecum and therefore makes it unavailable for reconstruction of the urinary tract. The Yang-Monti channel is the most common form of catheterizable urinary stoma today in centers where large numbers of children with neuropathic bowel and bladder are reconstructed.

When the length of the Yang-Monti tube is inadequate, two tubes have been sewn together end to end to create a longer channel. This has been met with mostly poor results due to difficulties passing the catheter through the anastomosis.

The spiral ileovesicostomy (Casale) tube was devised to provide a longer channel created from one section of bowel. The surgeon must be careful to make sure that the entire length of the strip of bowel to be tubularized is uniform in width so that the channel has a consistent diameter. Originally we saved the entire width of bowel but it became apparent that the bowel over the mesentery was slightly excessive. If excessively wide bowel is not narrowed either by excision or by being sutured tightly over a catheter, a pouch may develop over the mesentery and cause problems with catheterization.

The Casale ileovesicostomy requires 3.5 cm of bowel to create and produce a tube that is approximately twice the circumference of the bowel segment and usually measures 10 to 14 cm in length. The bowel is partially split in two segments for about 75% of its circumference, leaving the bowel over the mesentery and all visible bowel vessels intact. Each section is then incised at the base of the split parallel to the mesentery but on opposite sides to open the sections in opposite directions. It is this unfolding of the bowel into two strips in opposite directions that creates the important length.

We take care to use interrupted sutures for approximately 2 cm on each end of the tube so that if the channel has extra length either end can be easily trimmed. This also allows the surgeon to choose whether the mesentery lies close to the bladder or to the stoma. We take care to tack the bladder and the channel to the abdominal wall to minimize the length of the channel and prevent kinking of the channel at its anastomosis to the bladder with filling.

The results of our series are comparable to the appendicovesicostomy and Yang-Monti channels when reviewed for continence and ease of catheterization. Longer channels appeared to require more revisions at the bladder level but this finding was not statistically significant. The procedure has proven to be particularly useful in older children and adults with thick abdominal walls.

Chapter 93

Continent Vesicostomy

In the select patient with a large-capacity, low-pressure bladder a continent catheterizable channel can be formed from excess bladder tissue.

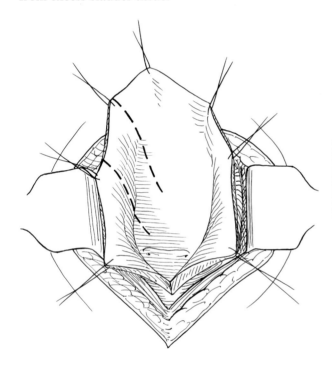

FIGURE 93-1. Open the bladder in midline for an umbilical stoma or lateral for a lower abdominal stoma. Place stay sutures to facilitate exposure. Make an incision from the lateral border to form a strip of bladder 2 cm wide. This will be the extravesical segment.

FIGURE 93-2. Mark the intravesical portion of the tube with two parallel lines. Incise along the lines and elevate the mucosa along the lateral and medial edges of the intravesical portion of the vesicostomy.

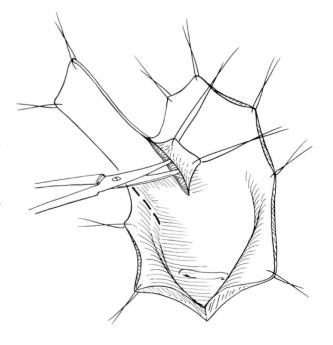

484

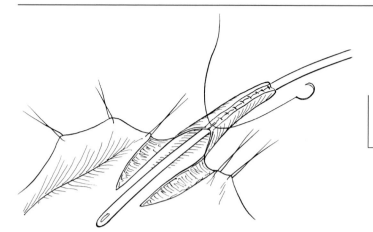

FIGURE 93-3. Close the mucosa of both the extravesical and intravesical portions with a running 5-0 or 6-0 absorbable suture over a 12- or 14-F catheter.

FIGURE 93-4. A, Approximate the lateral mucosal edges over the intravesical mucosal tube, thus creating a flap-valve continence mechanism. **B,** Close the bladder and mature the stoma to either the umbilicus or right lower quadrant. Leave the catheter in place for 3 weeks.

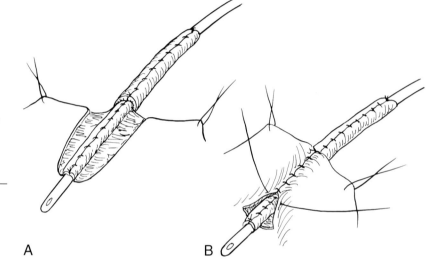

A   B

RICHARD C. RINK

Commentary by

The continent vesicostomy has a very reliable continence mechanism. It is the only catheterizable abdominal wall channel with a continence mechanism based on bladder mucosa rather than on a muscular tube. In 41 patients, none has leaked urine from the abdominal wall stoma. The procedure itself is easily performed and the channel can be reconstructed in such a way as to allow it to reach the umbilicus or either lower quadrant depending on the location of the bladder flap. Technically, the extravesical portion should be only long enough to reach the abdominal wall; that portion does not contribute to the continence mechanism. A large V skin flap is placed into the spatulated bladder tube, which is helpful in preventing stomal stenosis. The stomal construction is most easily achieved by not closing the end of the bladder tube. Do not completely mobilize the intravesical portion of the bladder mucosa, because leaving it attached prevents angulation, and thus it is easy to catheterize.

The obvious advantages of the continent vesicostomy are that a catheterizable stoma that is reliably continent and can be constructed from native bladder tissue. There is no need to violate the peritoneum or use any bowel segment. The underlying bladder pathology has not had any effect; it has been used with neurogenic and valve bladders, as well as those with exstrophy and the prune-belly syndrome, with no difference in continence or catheterizability.

There is only one disadvantage and unfortunately it is significant. We have had stomal stenosis at the skin level in 41% of our patients. This is a phenomenon similar to that seen with meatal stenosis when bladder mucosal grafts are used for hypospadias repairs. This stenosis rate is more than double that seen with appendicovesicostomies in our hands, and dramatically greater than those with Monti ileovesicostomy channels. In spite of this high stomal stenosis rate, we still have 80% of continent vesicostomies in use. We do leave a 12-F Silastic tube indwelling for 3 weeks after construction before beginning catheterization.

In summary, the continent vesicostomy is an easily performed catheterizable urinary channel using only native bladder with 100% continence rate, but stomal stenosis is not uncommon. We currently use it when the child needs only a bladder channel and no intestinal work is required. If bowel is to be used for augmentation, then we would use a Monti ileovesicostomy, reserving the appendix for those children who may need a Malone antegrade continence enema appendicocecostomy.

ANTHONY J. CASALE

The continent vesicostomy was developed to provide an alternative method of gaining extra-anatomic access to catheterize the urinary bladder when the appendix is not available, or if it is preferred to avoid intra-abdominal dissection. It was developed in the early 1990s and several of the original patients have their vesicostomies still in place and functional more than 15 years later. Some have not required any further surgery and are perfectly continent.

Of the methods designed to provide bladder catheterization via a continent abdominal wall stoma, the continent vesicostomy is the only one that can be performed without entering the peritoneal cavity. This fact saves time, avoids postoperative ileus, and does not risk adhesion formation. It is apparent that avoiding the peritoneum was valuable in patients who needed a continent stoma and were candidates for peritoneal dialysis. Since peritoneal dialysis is extremely useful in small children, most continent vesicostomies have been performed in this group.

Continent vesicostomy is the only continent catheterizable access that is constructed solely of using bladder tissue. Avoiding the use of bowel not only allows the surgeon to leave the peritoneal cavity undisturbed but it decreases the risk of infection from wound contamination and greatly simplifies and accelerates the patients' postoperative recovery. The long-term disadvantages of mucus production, stone formation, and increased risk of infection, which are associated with bowel in the urinary tract, are also avoided.

The continent vesicostomy is made from a tube created from full-thickness bladder wall and its vascularity is quite dependable. The length of the extravesical tube can be easily tailored to reach through the abdominal wall. The continence mechanism is based on a submucosal flap-valve mechanism in both the original Casale configuration and the Rink modification. The surgery is relatively simple and reliable. The continence rate has been close to 100% and the durability of the procedure is good with over 80% of the vesicostomies performed in the Indiana University series surviving after years of use.

The limiting factor in the usefulness and success of the continent vesicostomy is the high and unavoidable rate of stomal stenosis at the skin level. This became obvious early in the series and several attempts were made to avoid this complication; however, even with wide channels and deep V skin flaps interjected into the stomas, the stenosis rate is over 40%. Despite all of the advantages of this procedure, the continent vesicostomy has been relegated to a very select group of patients in whom case avoiding the peritoneal cavity is a sufficient advantage to offset the high risk of persistent stomal stenosis. The Mitrofanoff appendicovesicostomy and ileovesicostomies, such as the Yang-Monti and Casale procedures, have been more successful in providing a reliable continent catheterizable urinary stoma while requiring fewer revisions.

Commentary by

Chapter 94

Malone Antegrade Continence Enema

Fecal soiling by children with meningomyeloceles and anorectal anomalies can be avoided by regular colonic washouts using a Malone antegrade continence enema (MACE) via the implanted appendix. Untreated tap water is safe as an irrigant. The procedure can also be used for intractable constipation. The surgical technique is an adaptation of the Mitrofanoff nonrefluxing catheterizing channel.

If the appendix is not available, apply a Monti tube (see Chapter 92) or cecal or sigmoid flap. Other less desirable solutions are a Boari-style tubularized cecal tube, a defunctionalized ureter, or an ileal segment.

PREOPERATIVE INSTRUCTIONS

Prepare the bowel and give antibiotics. Mark the projected stomal site on the anterior abdominal wall; the umbilicus is usually best. Make a midline incision, especially if other procedures and an umbilical stoma are planned (see Chapter 11). Alternatively, use a Pfannenstiel or laparoscopic approach. Extract the cecum and appendix.

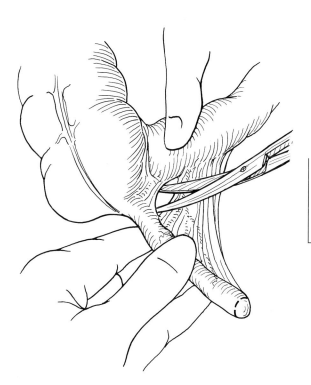

FIGURE 94-1. Mobilize the appendix and ileocecal region. Fenestrate the mesentery, taking care to preserve all of the appendiceal blood supply. Open the end of the appendix by amputation, and pass an 8- or 10-F catheter through it to make certain that the lumen is patent.

487

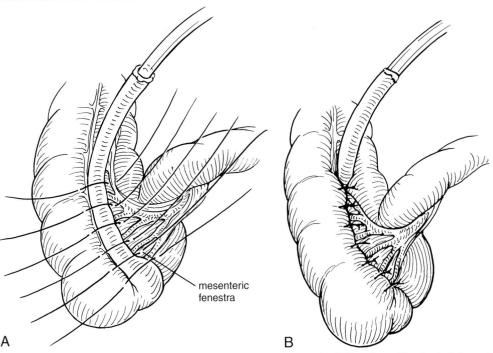

mesenteric
fenestra

A   B

FIGURE 94-2. A, Imbed the proximal half of the appendix along the tenia (Mitrofanoff principle) and close the seromuscular layers over it with permanent sutures placed through the mesenteric fenestra. Alternatively, form a 5-cm groove through the seromuscular layers of the cecal tenia libera down to the submucosa by sharp dissection. Open the mucosa at the distal end of the groove and suture the open end of the appendix to it. **B,** Bury the appendix within the groove and close the cecum over the appendix as described above. Both techniques create a flap-valve mechanism.

CUTANEOUS STOMA

Raise a broad-based triangular skin flap on the abdomen at the umbilicus (or in the right lower quadrant). Fashion the flap into a tube. Make a longitudinal antimesenteric incision in the appendix and trim any excess. Anastomose the end of the appendix to the skin tube. (This will bury the appendix and reduce discharge.) Anchor the cecum to the anterior abdominal wall with permanent sutures to ensure a straight run for catheterization. Now check to be sure that you can easily catheterize the new appendiceal tube. Leave the catheter through the appendix for 3 to 4 weeks to keep it straight during the healing process and to provide access for enemas during that time. (See also Chapter 91.)

ENEMAS

After the return of bowel function, start washout enemas through the resident catheter. Do this before discharge, usually by the third to fourth day. Start with 50 to 100 mL of tap water irrigation to fill the colon (about 5 minutes). Evacuation will occur after 10 to 30 minutes. Increase the volume by 50-mL increments every 2 to 3 days. The final volume will be determined by trial and error. The child, sitting on the toilet, can learn the 20- to 50-minute routine and repeat the enema every day or on alternate days. At 1 month, remove the catheter and teach the parent and child how to insert it into the stoma.

COMPLICATIONS

Be aware that the appendiceal stoma may stenose or perforate if improperly used. If complications occur the overwhelming majority of children and parents will request revision surgery.

LAPAROSCOPIC ANTEGRADE CONTINENCE ENEMA PROCEDURE

Give antibiotic prophylaxis but do not prep the bowel. Infiltrate a local anesthetic agent subumbilically. Make an incision large enough to allow opening of the peritoneum under direct vision. Insert a 6.5- or 10-mm trocar and insufflate the abdomen with carbon dioxide, to a pressure between 8 and 10 mmHg. Tip the patient's head down. Locate the appendix. Place a second, 5- or 10-mm trocar over the site of the appendix. With Duval forceps, bring the tip of the appendix to the skin surface and suture it to the fascia. Incise the tip longitudinally for about 1 cm, and then suture the mucosal edge to the skin. Cannulate the appendix with an 8- or 10-F silicone balloon catheter and leave it in place.

Start irrigation with 250 mL salted water (2 tsp NaCl/L) on the first postoperative day and then increase the volume up to 1 L. Leave the catheter in place for 3 to 4 weeks, and then introduce a straight catheter daily to continue with antegrade enemas.

POSTOPERATIVE COMPLICATIONS

This description of the laparoscopic antegrade continence enema procedure does not describe umbrication of the appendix into the cecal mesentery to prevent leakage. Interestingly, a number of reports suggest that simply pulling up the appendix in situ to the skin is effective without the need for a formal valve continence procedure. Nevertheless, bowel fluid can leak through the appendix in some cases. Stomal stenosis is a possible complication, occasionally requiring revision.

PADRAIG S. J. MALONE

Commentary by

The first MACE procedure was performed in the United Kingdom at the Great Ormond Street Hospital in October 1989 and a small series of 6 patients were rapidly accumulated prior to reporting the initial experience. Due to the series' success, the procedure was adopted rapidly in the United Kingdom and numerous centers reported on their experiences with the technique. The first MACE was performed in the United States by Marty Koyle, and again, with his reports of good results, the technique is now performed by most reconstructive pediatric urology centers around the world. The indications for a MACE procedure have broadened over the years; initially it was used in patients with myelomeningocele but now it can be used for any neuropathic condition, anorectal anomalies, Hirschsprung's disease, and chronic idiopathic constipation. The reported success rates with MACE washouts are dependent on the underlying condition but for neuropathic conditions and anorectal anomalies, a success rate of 85% to 95% can be expected. The technique has also been successfully adopted for adolescent and adult patients suffering from fecal incontinence. There are many studies demonstrating objective improvements in quality of life following the MACE procedure.

One of the most important aspects of MACE procedure success is patient selection. The patient and family need to be highly motivated and prepared to devote up to 1 hour per day to bowel management. There is no single recipe to washout success and most patients experiment with their washout regimen following discharge from the hospital until they find their own effective system. On occasion this can take as long as 6 months; because of this, it is vital that each patient and his or her family be counseled and supported by a nurse specialist both before and following surgery.

There is a trans-Atlantic divide in the washout regimens used. In the United States tap water alone is used in most patients but in the United Kingdom and Europe some form of stimulant enema, such as phosphate, is employed. If tap water alone does not work, try some form of stimulant enema prior to abandoning the MACE procedure.

The operative technique has been modified considerably since the original MACE. It is no longer necessary to disconnect the appendix and, if a cecal MACE is required, the in situ appendix technique described in this chapter is the procedure of choice. This can also be performed laparoscopically with imbrication as described by Professor Koyle in his commentary. The use of the split appendix or the Yang-Monti tube means that all patients can now have simultaneous Mitrofanoff and MACE conduits created if required. One of the significant problems that affected the original MACE was the length of time it would take for the washout to pass. Because of this the concept of the left colonic MACE was developed and this did seem to reduce washout times in selected patients. It is now my practice to recommend a trial of a colonoscopically placed colonic tube prior to proceeding with a definitive procedure. The tube is inserted into the descending colon using a technique identical to the insertion of a percutaneous gastrostomy and is used for 3 months. If washouts are successful, the patient then has a choice: keep the tube, exchange it for a low-profile button, or have a formal catheterizable conduit created. In my experience, we have been able to salvage some patients with this technique in whom the original cecal MACE was unsuccessful.

The main ongoing complication with the MACE remains stomal stenosis. In this chapter a tubularized skin flap is described but in my experience stenosis rates are high with these. I now routinely use two skin flaps and stenosis rates have improved (VQZ/VQC). A MACE stopper is now commercially available; this is a short silicone stopper the same size as the catheter that will be used. By leaving the stopper in the stoma for the first 6 months, the stoma is allowed to mature and, in my experience, stenosis rates are reduced still further.

There can be no doubt that the MACE works, but it is no magic cure. It takes a lot of preoperative counseling and postoperative support in a motivated family. Revisional surgery is also commonly required but most patients still contend the MACE improves their quality of life considerably. No patient should be left with fecal incontinence or have a colostomy without first being given the option of a MACE.

MARTIN A. KOYLE

The MACE has been a remarkable addition to the armamentarium of reconstructive urologic surgeons. This simple technique has benefited many children, as well as adolescents and young adults, who have suffered from intractable fecal soiling and constipation secondary to congenital structural and neurologic abnormalities. More recently, patients who are older with acquired neurologic problems have been successfully managed with the MACE.

The MACE system is usually constructed at the time of continent urinary reconstruction, when both systems require a continent stoma. The Yang-Monti ileal neoappendix has been a tremendous adjunct in the operative scenario. If the appendix is long and the patient slender, we prefer to split the appendix to use for both stomas. If the appendix, however, appears to be smaller, it should remain in situ for the MACE, and a Yang-Monti tube constructed for the Mitrofanoff stoma. We have not been satisfied trying to create a neoappendix using a cecal flap/Boari technique.

When the appendix is absent or surgically small, a neoappendix is necessary. In those patients who have a generous abdominal wall, use a Yang-Monti tube. In the more slender patient, extend the appendix by placing a 12-F Silastic catheter through the stump or the colonic wall. Grasp the colon and catheter with a series of Babcock clamps snugly applied and use a TA 55 stapler to create a second lumen without creating a flap. Cover the resulting tube by plicating it with colonic serosal wall using nonabsorbable sutures.

In double-stoma patients, the urinary stoma is usually placed in the umbilicus. The fecal stoma is placed in the right lower quadrant. There the VQZ stoma may be useful, especially in obese children, because it buries the mucosa, leaving a cosmetically pleasing result, which may reduce the incidence of stomal stenosis.

With the advent of minimally invasive surgery, we have routinely employed the laparoscope when the only procedure to be performed is the MACE. Place the laparoscope through the umbilicus, which will become the site of the stoma. Insert the working instruments under direct vision through small stab incisions, rather than using trocars, to minimize the need for closure (and to minimize scars).

Mobilize the cecum and the appendix and pass them into the umbilical site. Then open the fascia a little further to allow open formation of the imbrication, tacking the cecum to the underlying fascia, and maturing the stoma to the skin.

The laparoscope is also useful in planning a combined MACE/urologic reconstruction, especially in children who have undergone ventriculoperitoneal shunting or other abdominal surgery. Often the appendix and right colon will be fixed by adhesions in an ectopic location. Lyse the adhesions; this allows the operation to be performed through a small Pfannenstiel incision rather than one in the midline.

Many centers place tubes percutaneously rather than create stomas surgically for the MACE. For the long term, we find this to be associated with leaking around the tube as well as the cosmetic stigma of an appliance. We offer tubes or buttons to those with recurrent stomal stenosis and to those who are unsure that they want a surgical MACE.

In constipated children, the right lower quadrant cecal MACE may not give the best results. Perhaps stomas in the transverse or descending colon may provide more reliable evacuation. Like training wheels on a bicycle, we might suggest a temporary MACE in various colonic locations to choose the optimal site for the permanent stoma.

Much of the success of the MACE is patient/family dependent. In the United States, most children have done well using tap water irrigations. Still, trial and error may be necessary to achieve success. Complications, such as stomal stenosis, are frequent. The risk of multiple operations and hospitalizations becomes almost inevitable, especially when the MACE is performed along with urinary tract reconstruction. Regardless, the satisfaction of the patient and quality of life make these risks acceptable for most of these children, when compared with the options of diaper or colostomy.

Chapter 95

Colon Flap Continence Channel

Use of a colon flap for creation of a continent catheterizable antegrade enema channel is an alternative approach when the appendix is missing or has been used for urinary diversion. The bowel is prepared and broad-spectrum antibiotics administered.

LATERALLY AND MEDIALLY BASED FLAP

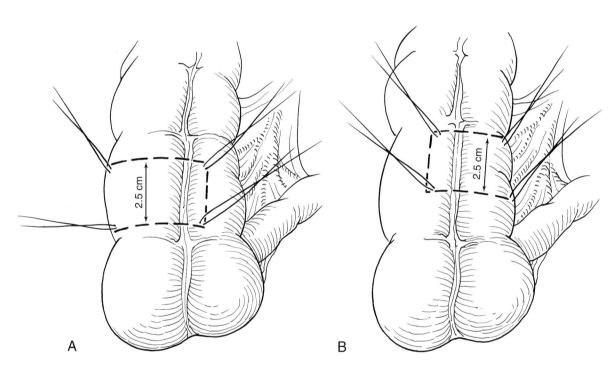

A   B

FIGURE 95-1. **A,** Mark out a lateral segment of colon lying adjacent to the umbilicus using stay sutures. Mobilize a 2.5-cm flap on the anterior aspect of the proximal sigmoid colon. **B,** Mark out a medial segment of colon above the ileocecal valve using stay sutures. Create a wide, medially based flap close to the mesentery. The end of the flap should not cross the antimesenteric zone between the free and epiploic tenia (see Fig. 95-2).

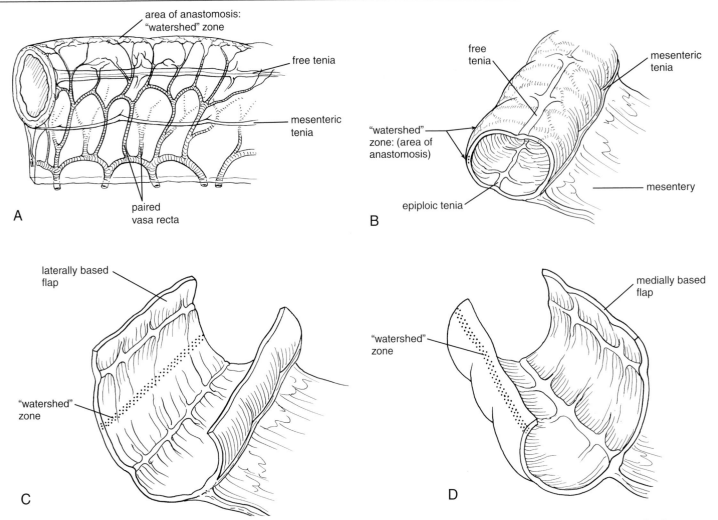

FIGURE 95-2. A, Compared to ileum, the colon has significantly fewer lateral branching arcades among terminal mesenteric arteries. Paired vasa recta arteries arise from the last series of mesenteric arcades in the human colon. The vasa recta travel between the serosa and muscularis circumferentially until reaching the antimesenteric border. **B,** There they anastomose with similar branches from the opposite side. This is the watershed zone. **C,** A laterally based flap relies on the tenuous anastomotic integrity of the antimesenteric side of the colon. **D,** A medially based flap is nourished directly from the vasa recta without crossing the anastomotic watershed zone.

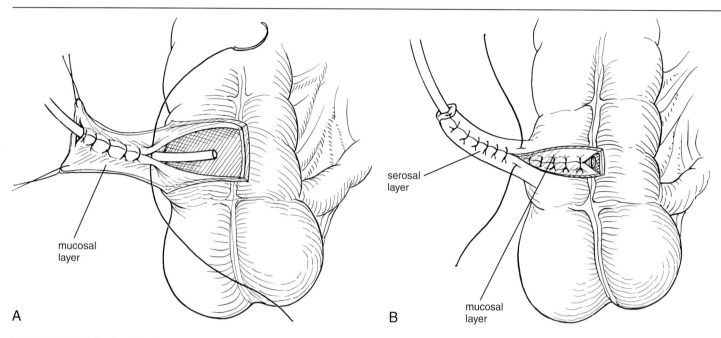

FIGURE 95-3. A, Tubularize the mucosal layer of the flap over a 12-F Mentor catheter using 4-0 long-acting absorbable sutures. **B,** Close the serosal layer over the mucosal layer ensuring a watertight closure of the colon.

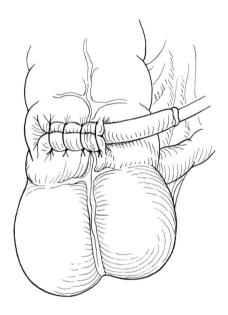

FIGURE 95-4. Fold the tube back on itself. Approximate the teniae over the tube using interrupted 3-0 silk horizontal mattress sutures. Mature the stoma to the umbilicus or right lower quadrant. Fix the colon and colon tube to the anterior abdominal fascia to prevent catheterization problems. Check the tube for ease of catheterization. Remove the catheter 3 weeks postoperatively and use the stoma on a daily basis. Begin colonic irrigation in the early postoperative period once bowel function returns.

COMPLICATIONS

Stomal stenosis and difficulty with catheterization are the two most common problems after colonic tube creation. Careful attention to preservation of blood supply and a medially based flap approach increase success.

Part V

Bladder Augmentation

Chapter 96

Introduction to Bladder Augmentation

URETHRAL AND URETEROVESICAL JUNCTIONS PRESENT

If the urethra is intact, augmentation is indicated for the small-capacity, poorly compliant bladder, whether from intrinsic disease of the detrusor muscle or from neurologic overactivity secondary to spinal cord disorders or instability. This procedure is a necessary adjunct to functional rehabilitation of the exstrophic bladder.

The upper urinary tract must be protected by antireflux mechanisms, constructed from bowel segments made by forming a flap-valve in the intestinal wall or by tunnel implantation of the ureters. Urinary reservoirs, for vesical augmentation and substitution as well as for continent urinary diversion, require adequate capacity at physiologic pressure. Detubularized bowel segments provide greater capacity at lower pressure and require shorter lengths of intestine than do intact segments. Four factors account for their superiority.

First, their configuration takes advantage of geometry: Volume increases by the square of the radius. A patch or pouch has a larger diameter than a tube. Second, they accommodate on filling more readily because, as the LaPlace's law states, the greater the radius of a container, the smaller the pressure change relative to the tension on the wall. Third, their compliance is superior to that of the tubular bowel. Last, their ability to contract is blunted because the contractile elements do not involve the entire circumference.

For these reasons, a detubularized segment will store more urine at lower pressures. The length required to achieve a desired volume may be determined from Figures 96-1 to 96-3.

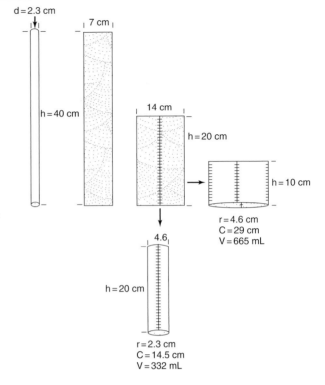

FIGURE 96-1. Small-bowel schematic: calculated capacity of a 40-cm segment opened and folded twice (665 mL) compared to folded once (332 mL).

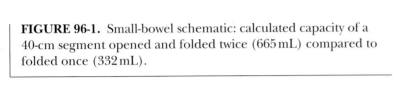

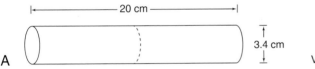

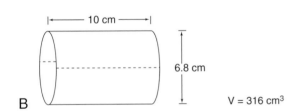

V = 158 cm³

V = 316 cm³

FIGURE 96-2. Large-bowel schematic: comparison between calculated capacity of an intact 20-cm tube (**A**) with a diameter of 3.4 cm (175 mL) and that of the same tube opened lengthwise and folded on itself (**B**) (350 mL).

FIGURE 96-3. A, A diagram of intact bowel segments with effective contraction ring. **B,** A detubularized, or folded, segment shows ineffective asynchronous contraction.

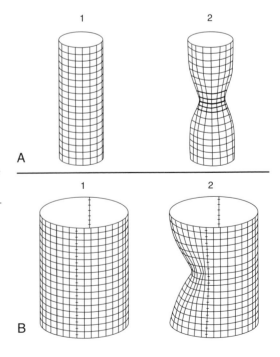

In selecting a segment, other factors to be considered, in addition to capacity and pressure, are (1) tolerable electrolyte reabsorption and loss, (2) accessibility of the segment, (3) simplicity of the procedure, (4) need for an antireflux mechanism, (5) carcinogenic risk, and (6) special requirements and age of the patient.

Selection of a particular bowel segment for bladder augmentation depends on the preference of the surgeon, as there is no objective data indicating that one region is better than another. The colon allows implantation of a normal ureter using an antireflux technique. Combining ileum with cecum based on the ileocecal artery allows formation of a mobilizable reservoir of good capacity free from mass contraction and an ileal arm to substitute for any loss of ureteral length. However, excluding the ileocecal segment from the intestinal tract in children with neurogenic bladders who rely on constipation for rectal continence may result in loose stools and fecal incontinence, as well as later vitamin deficiency. After extensive pelvic irradiation, the surgeon may have to resort to a transverse colon conduit. A segment from the stomach can be useful, especially in a child with compromised renal function in whom electrolyte reabsorption would exacerbate the problem. The stomach is elastic; half of it can provide a reservoir with a 300- to 500-mL capacity.

The objectives in any case are to make a low-pressure system that is compliant during the filling phase. This is best achieved when the tubular organization of the bowel is disrupted to protect the upper tracts from back pressure during spontaneous mass contractions, which also may induce incontinence, and to provide adequate capacity to relieve the patient of inconvenient frequent voiding or catheterization. In addition, protection from reflux must be provided and incontinence prevented.

The bladder does not need to be excised during augmentation to permit good function. In fact, excision complicates the procedure by requiring ureteral reimplantation. Attached bowel segments do act as diverticula when the communication with the bladder is restricted, but not if the bladder is bivalved and the segment is detubularized. If the ureterovesical junction is obstructive or allows reflux, reimplantation into the bladder is preferable to a ureterointestinal anastomosis.

Important Points

Take a segment that is long enough to ensure adequate capacity but not so long as to jeopardize nutrition and foster electrolyte absorption. In certain cases (e.g., irradiated bowel, cloacal exstrophy, chronic renal failure, and males in whom excess mucus could obstruct the sphincter), use of the stomach may be preferable.

Evaluation before cystoplasty includes studies of renal function to ensure at least a minimum of reserve (i.e., creatinine clearance greater than 40 mL/minute and serum creatinine level less than 2.5 mg, unless the augmentation is preparatory to renal transplantation). Urine culture provides the basis for preoperative antibiotic therapy. Sonography will define upper-tract abnormalities, and a voiding cystogram can show gross distortions of the bladder, detect reflux, and ascertain whether urine is held at the bladder neck. An existing conduit should also be evaluated radiographically, and retrograde ureterograms should be made of the ureteral stumps because these structures may prove useful in the repair.

The urethra and bladder neck should be visualized endoscopically under anesthesia to be certain that continence mechanisms are intact and that intermittent catheterization will be feasible, if required. Maximum vesical capacity can be determined at the same time. When intermittent catheterization is the goal, the bladder can be cycled using intermittent filling through a urethral catheter. Have the child do this to reveal the degree of motivation.

Urodynamic testing can document reflex activity, compliance, and sensation, with and without pharmacologic agents, and can determine the efficiency of voiding.

After augmentation, voiding dysfunction is inevitable. Resection of the bladder alters not only the sensation of filling but the ability to open the bladder neck. Substitution of bowel for detrusor muscle replaces the normal sustained detrusor contraction with the involuntary and unsustained contractions characteristic of bowel. The result is poorly coordinated voiding, often with residual urine, accompanied by infection, stone formation, nocturnal incontinence, and, if the pressure is elevated, upper-tract damage. Thus, not only must the capacity and compliance be increased by the procedure, but a balance must be established between urethral resistance and voiding pressure by altering the sphincteric mechanisms or resorting to intermittent catheterization.

Artificial sphincters can be applied after bladder augmentation or substitution and are usually necessitated by nighttime incontinence. If some of the bladder remains, place the cuff about the trigone; if not, place it around the urethra or around the emergent segment of bowel, where it appears to be well tolerated if a wide cuff is used. It is important that the reservoir be compliant and be able to store urine at low pressure. However, extra fluid must be added to the reservoir at the time of insertion of the appliance because the bowel wall will shrink. The cuff must not be obstructive, and no other causes of outlet resistance should remain. However, if incomplete emptying persists, the child may have to resort to intermittent catheterization.

UNDIVERSION

Three categories of patients are candidates for undiversion: (1) children with sufficient ureteral length to require only takedown of cutaneous ureterostomy coupled with transureteroureterostomy and reimplant, (2) those without adequate length of the ureters so that a new ileal segment must be interposed (this may be supplemented by a bladder flap and by augmentation with bowel, if needed), and (3) children with neurogenic bladders requiring excision and subtotal augmentation or substitution. Each case requires some imagination and inventiveness on the part of the surgeon.

Bladder neck reconstruction, insertion of an artificial sphincter, or construction of a continent stoma is an option for the patient with sphincteric incontinence. Young single adults most often desire undiversion. Even those patients with very poor renal function may benefit, since renal transplantation may be done later into a continent bladder.

POSTOPERATIVE PROBLEMS AFTER AUGMENTATION PROCEDURES

Select the patient for the reconstruction procedure carefully to avoid later problems. A child with marginal renal function and unsuitable bladder, ureters, or sphincters can have such problems. Most important is the capability of the child (and family) to want and care for a new system, especially the child's willingness to maintain a program of intermittent catheterization, if that should prove necessary.

Ureteral leakage is a problem if the ureter proves to be short for a tension-free anastomosis. Preoperative estimation of length is important. Intraoperatively, various techniques can be used to compensate (such as a psoas hitch, bladder flap repair, transureteroureterostomy, or, as a last resort, interposition of ileum). Reflux may arise from too short a tunnel after direct anastomosis or from failure of the constructed intestinal valve. Stricture at the site of ureterointestinal anastomosis may not appear for years.

Bladder dysfunction postoperatively leads to upper-tract damage and to incontinence. In a small bladder with poor compliance augment with adequate bowel. In a child with dyssynergia, pharmacologic manipulation and retraining may avoid complications.

Urinary infection is not a problem if the system is free of obstruction and empties satisfactorily. Bacteriuria is common and should only be treated if symptomatic.

Declining renal function results from any of these complications. Increased fluid intake will be needed postoperatively to compensate for fluid extraction by the bowel. Transient renal failure is not uncommon; in fact, a temporary rise in creatinine levels may be anticipated. Close follow-up with regular determination of serum creatinine levels is necessary. The reconstruction itself is usually not responsible for renal failure; rather, it is the progression of the underlying renal disease.

Wound infection with abscess formation is more common after colonic than after ileal operations. Enteric fistulas may result from insertion of a tube through the bowel wall. Placement of a sump drain in the retropubic space and avoidance of nonabsorbable sutures and clips help.

Inefficient evacuation of the bladder is the most common complication of cystoplasty because peristaltic contraction is unsustained during voiding and works against outlet resistance. Obstruction present before cystoplasty must be detected urodynamically and corrected. Persistent outflow obstruction can be detected by determination of residual urine by catheterization or by ultrasonography. Determine its site by voiding cystography with or without pressure flow studies. Resolution may require endoscopic incision of the bladder neck. Overdilatation of the urethra may help achieve balance in the female.

Incontinence can be a trying problem. Placement of a segment capable of mass contraction will result in incontinence, which is why detubularized segments should be used. Too small a segment will fill to its maximum capacity too fast, at which point spontaneous contractions are stimulated. Opening the segment increases the capacity and reduces the incontinence. In spite of a normal outlet and good functional capacity, nocturnal wetting still may be a problem because of the relaxation of the sphincters. Diphenoxylate hydrochloride (Lomotil) decreases bowel contractility and increases capacity but has little effect on enuresis. Timed voiding every 4 hours and intermittent catheterization may be done. If all these measures fail, consider supplementing the augmentation surgically. For the relaxed outlet, ephedrine and phenylpropanolamine may correct the problem. Otherwise, some form of continence procedure may be required.

For obstruction of the plicated ileocecal valve, try prolonged drainage, and revise the valve if necessary. Reflux can occur when the ureters are implanted in the ileum and the ileocecal valve is incompetent. Stenosis of the vesicoenteric anastomosis results in a functional diverticulum with accompanying infection and vesical irritability.

Mucus secretion is a problem usually greatest in the immediate postoperative period, because mucus production decreases with time if the bladder empties. A pouch must be irrigated completely and vigorously every 6 hours postoperatively, and the urinary flow must be carefully monitored lest the segment overfill and the anastomoses become disrupted.

Bladder calculi are common after augmentation cystoplasty, occurring in almost half of patients. The stones are usually a mixture of struvite, calcium apatite, and ammonium acid urate. Irrigation protocols delay their formation.

Renal function remains stable if the system drains effectively and the underlying renal lesion does not progress. For a child with severely impaired renal function, in whom reabsorption may tip the balance, augmentation may be considered a preliminary step to renal transplantation.

Electrolyte imbalance, with increase in chloride and hydrogen ions, can affect the bone buffers and lead to stone formation. Small bowel obstruction from adhesions may require intubation or operation. Prolonged ileus can be a problem. Neoplasms can occur, even in augmentation with ileum.

Nutritional consequences from the use of small bowel may be significant in the long term, especially deficiencies in vitamin B_{12}, methylmalonic acid, folate, and carotene.

The sites for postoperative problems and their remedies are outline in Table 96-1, but the necessity for diligent lifetime follow-up must be reiterated.

COMPLICATIONS WITH CORRECTIVE OPTIONS

TABLE 96 – 1

Location	Complication	Corrective Options
Ureter	Stricture or loss	Ureteroureterostomy
		Mobilization of kidney
		Psoas hitch; bladder flap
		Ileal ureter
		Autotransplant
	Dilation	Tailoring
Ureterovesical junction	Stricture	Reimplantation
	Reflux	Reimplantation
		Ileal nipple
		Others
Detrusor muscle	Reduced compliance	Pharmacologic agents
		Neural manipulation
		Hydrodistention
		Augmentation
		Vesicostomy
	Increased compliance	Intermittent catheterization
Outlet	Contracture	Dilatation
	Incompetence	Vesical neck repair
		Sling with intermittent catheterization
		Artificial sphincter
		Closure of neck
	Dyssynergia	Sphincterotomy
		Intermittent catheterization

Chapter 97

Ileocystoplasty

ILEOCYSTOPLASTY (GOODWIN)

Evaluate the child's general status and renal function. Determine vesical residual urine and capacity, detrusor muscle compliance, and urethral function and determine whether bladder neck reconstruction or reduction in outlet resistance is needed. Obtain an ultrasound and voiding cystourethrogram or loopogram to assess bladder size and ureteral length and configuration. A radionuclide scan helps define upper-tract function. Preoperatively, consider the feasibility of intermittent catheterization: Is the urethra patent and accessible? Teach the child how to perform self-catheterization. Especially consider the motivation of the child for reconstruction, which must be strong to warrant operation. If capacity is limited or the outlet relaxed, warn the patient and parents about the possibility of incontinence.

The ureters may be left in the bladder or may be reimplanted into the bowel via tunnels, with or without transureteroureterostomy. Implantation of the dilated ureter into the intussuscepted ileum is least desirable. In general, tunnels are preferable to nipples. Reimplant into the bladder whenever possible, although not at the risk of using ischemic ureter or reimplanting under tension.

For instruments provide an autosuture set with TA 55 (4.8 and 3.5) and end-to-end anastomosis staplers.

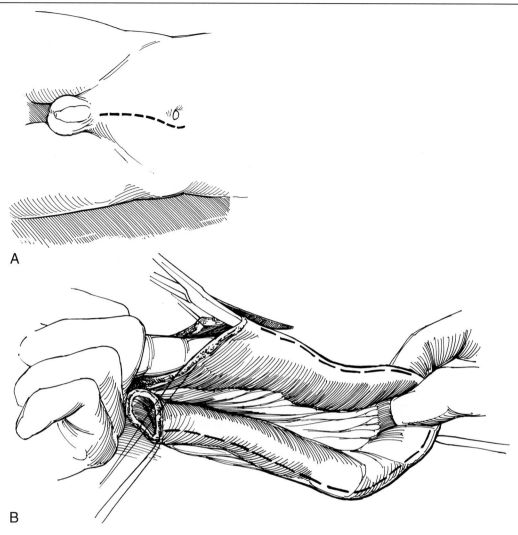

A

B

FIGURE 97-1. A, Position: Supine. Incision: Make a lower midline transperitoneal incision (see Chapter 11), standing on the left side of the patient. Check the mobility and mesenteric length of the terminal ureter. Prepare the bowel first, or open the bladder at this time. **B,** Choose a 20- to 25-cm loop of terminal ileum, leaving the last 10 to 15 cm of terminal ileum in place, as for ileal conduit (see Chapter 89). Mark the ends and the center of the loop with stay sutures. Draw the center of the loop over the dome of the bladder to be sure it will reach for the anterior part of the proposed vesical anastomosis. Divide the ileum between Kocher clamps. The mesentery, which should be well vascularized, needs to be divided for a shorter distance than for ureteroileostomy. Reapproximate the ileum (see Chapter 6). Irrigate the loop with saline solution until clear and then with 1% neomycin solution. Divide the ileal segment along its antimesenteric border with straight Mayo scissors or with cutting current. Alternatively, before opening the bowel, shape it into a loop and suture the adjacent serosal surfaces together with a running 4-0 catgut suture.

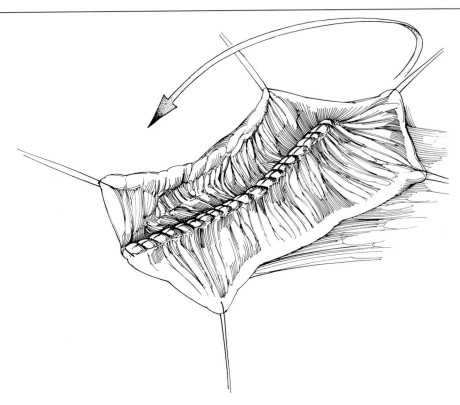

FIGURE 97-2. Suture the adjacent mucosal edges with a continuous 3-0 chromic catgut suture. Use a straight atraumatic tapered needle placed through all layers of the bowel. To prevent bunching of the suture line, tie the suture once on the outside.

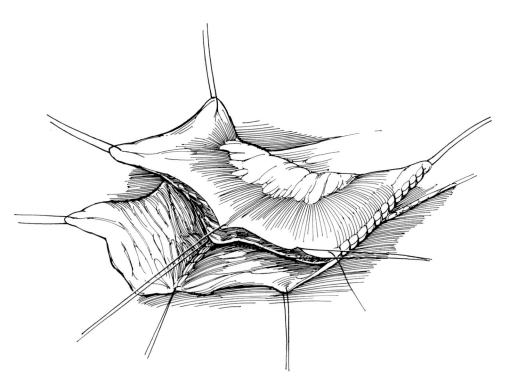

FIGURE 97-3. Fold the open end of the segment over on itself and suture it along each margin to form a cup. If a larger opening is desired for the anastomosis to the bladder, do not suture the edges together for their entire length. Watch for interference with the blood supply.

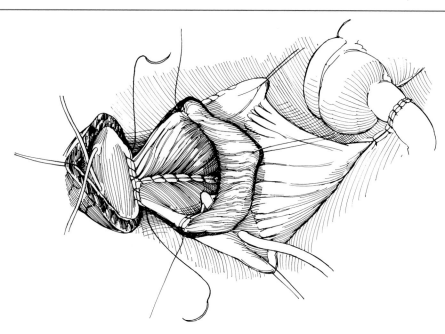

FIGURE 97-4. Grasp the bladder at the apex adjacent to the peritoneal reflection. Sharply divide the lateral peritoneal attachments as far as the superior vesical pedicle. Free the bladder anteriorly and elevate it into the wound. Open the bladder sagittally as far posteriorly as possible, using the cutting current and ligating large vessels with 4-0 catgut suture. Although a coronal incision is an alternative, a sagittal incision will suffice even for very small bladders. Insert infant feeding tube catheters to identify the ureters and place a Malecot cystostomy tube into the bladder away from the suture line. The tube should be inserted through the wall of the bladder, but if the bladder is very small, it may be placed through the augmentation as shown in the figure.

Place the posterior rim of the ileal cup adjacent to the posterior apex of the bladder incision and, starting posteriorly, run a 3-0 chromic catgut suture through all layers up each side to form a watertight closure. Tie the sutures several times during insertion to prevent gathering and take extra care where the suture lines meet. Reinforcement with 2-0 chromic catgut sutures may be helpful, especially posteriorly where tension can exist. An alternative method: Before folding the superior end of the segment on itself, start anastomosing the inferior end to the bladder, and continue the suture to the midway point of the bladder incision. Now fold the doubled ileum over and start suturing from the midline anteriorly around each side. Continue the suture to approximate the ileal edges to form the "clam" in place. An artificial sphincter may now be inserted. The chance of contamination is minimal because ileal contents are sterile.

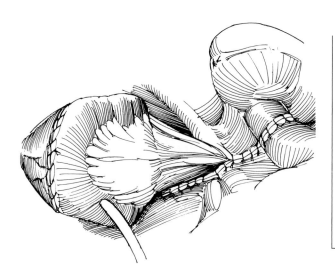

FIGURE 97-5. Remove the ureteral catheters and close the mesentery. If the peritoneum is especially redundant, incise it and wrap it around the mesentery of the augmentation to retroperitonealize the isolated bowel segment. Fix the mesentery of the segment to the posterior peritoneum to prevent an internal hernia. Free the omentum from the transverse colon and tack it posteriorly first and then wrap it around the repair to cover the suture lines. Test the augmentation by filling it with saline, and reinforce it at the site of leaks. Place one (or two, if the anastomosis is tenuous) Jackson-Pratt drain for suction. Insert a silicone balloon catheter into the bladder though the urethra for extra security during the immediate postoperative period. Close the wound in layers around the drains.

CONVERSION OF ILEAL CONDUIT

To provide a continent pouch, open the ileal conduit to be used as a patch. Reimplant the ureters by a nonreflux-ing technique into this patch. Take a new ileal segment and form an intussuscepted nipple in its distal third. Open the remainder and apply the patch to it. For extra capacity, fold the opened loop on itself twice, suture the edges, and then fold the entire plate into a cup.

HEMI-KOCK PROCEDURE

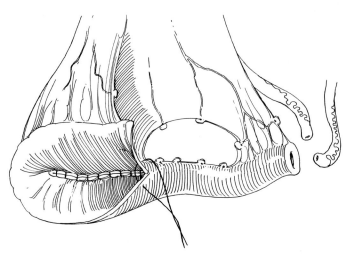

FIGURE 97-6. Follow the initial steps of ileocystoplasty as outlined previously in this chapter. Resect a loop of ileum 50 cm long, and open the distal 30 cm on the antimesenteric border.

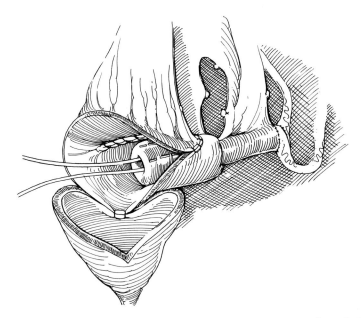

FIGURE 97-7. Fold the opened flap on itself to form a patch. Clear the mesentery from half of the more proximal segment, and intussuscept the ileum to form a nipple. Incise the full thickness of the outer wall of the nipple, denude the adjacent muscle in the pouch, and suture the two surfaces together with 3-0 synthetic absorbable sutures. Anastomose the cup to the remainder of the bladder, and implant the ureters in the end of the proximal ileum with stents. Suture the pouch to the levator ani muscles on both sides. Insert a balloon catheter through the conduit and secure it and the stents to the skin. Postoperatively, monitor urinary output from the ureteral catheters every 6 hours. If it declines, irrigate the catheters. After 2 weeks, do a cystogram at minimal pressure (15 to 20 cm water). If leakage is seen, leave both catheters in place another week and repeat the study.

EARL Y. CHENG

Numerous alternative techniques for augmentation of the neurogenic bladder have been developed over the past two decades in an attempt to avoid some of the complications associated with incorporation of an intestinal segment into the bladder. These include metabolic alterations, mucus production, infections, and stones. However, ileocystoplasty still remains the gold standard. It is imperative that the patient and family are counseled extensively preoperatively regarding some of the more dangerous complications of ileocystoplasty, including spontaneous perforation and potential for malignant transformation. They must also be extremely compliant and dedicated to lifelong intermittent catheterization.

In many cases, ileocystoplasty will be performed concomitantly with other reconstructive procedures, including a Mitrofanoff procedure, bladder neck reconstruction, and MACE procedure. To accommodate the creation of the Mitrofanoff channel, the bladder can be opened in many ways in addition to the traditional midline sagittal incision. An off-center incision can be made to allow use of the larger half of the bladder for creation of the Mitrofanoff channel. If the bladder is very small and one intends to bring the appendix out the umbilicus, a U-flap incision can be made on the dome and superior portion of the anterior bladder wall. This will allow for creation of a bladder flap that can now be flipped superiorly, with subsequent tunneling of the appendix into the base of the flap. In most cases, the tunneled appendix will now be close enough to the umbilicus for stoma maturation. The bladder can also be opened in a starlike configuration with use of one of the limbs of the star for the Mitrofanoff channel. Whatever method is used to open the bladder, the incisions need to be made adequately to eliminate any native configuration of the bladder to prevent both future contractile activity and the undesired creation of an hourglass-shaped augmentation.

Choice of the ileal segment to be used for augmentation is critical for success. The most dependent portion of the ileum is usually around 20 to 25 cm proximal to the ileocecal valve. In most cases, this segment of bowel will be dependent enough to reach the bladder. Look closely at the mesenteric vasculature of this segment of ileum to ensure a well-vascularized arcade to the ileal patch. Previous studies have demonstrated that it is difficult to predict the eventual size of the urinary reservoir that will result from an individual segment of bowel that is used for augmentation. Therefore, if anything, err on the side of taking a little more bowel as opposed to too little. Usually 20 cm of ileum is adequate in children, with an additional 5 to 10 cm in adults. The patch can be reconfigured in numerous ways, with an inverted U being the most useful. When the apex of the ileal flap will not reach the inferior aspect of the anastomosis at the bladder neck in a tension-free manner, it is important to further mobilize the mesentery proximally to gain additional length. In more difficult cases, you can also incise the peritoneal lining over the mesentery with careful skeletonization of the mesenteric vessels to gain additional length. Lastly, when other procedures are being performed concomitantly, anastomosis of the reconfigured ileal patch to the bladder plate is usually the last thing that is done prior to closure of the abdominal wall.

In the future, additional novel methods of bladder replacement such as tissue engineering of bladder tissue will likely replace ileocystoplasty as the most conventional way to augment the bladder. However, at present, ileocystoplasty remains the most reliable way to augment the neurogenic bladder with proven long-term efficacy.

Chapter 98

T-Pouch Hemi-Kock Procedure

When the appendix is absent and the bladder is too small to incorporate a catheterizable channel, a T-pouch hemi-Kock procedure is a viable option. The T-pouch hemi-Kock procedure allows simultaneous bladder augmentation and formation of an abdominal continent catheterizable stoma. The ileocecal valve is preserved.

Counsel the family and child for intermittent catheterization prior to the surgery.

Prepare the bowel and administer broad-spectrum antibiotics.

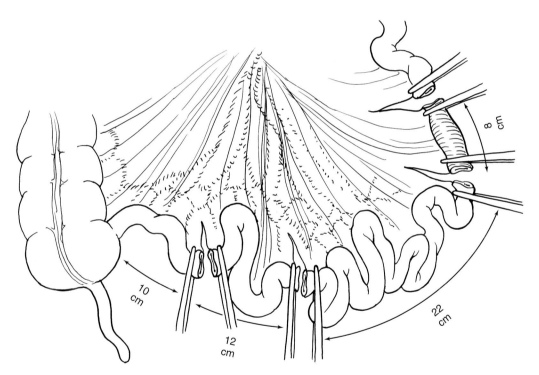

FIGURE 98-1. Isolate approximately 34 cm of terminal ileum at least 10 cm from the ileocecal valve. Use the distal 12-cm segment of ileum to form the efferent limb. Without ligating the mesenteric collaterals, remove a small segment of proximal ileum along the mesentery-bowel border to allow mobilization.

FIGURE 98-2. Place the isolated 22-cm segment (see Fig. 98-1) into an inverted **V** configuration. Adhering to the principles described for the T-pouch ileal neobladder and double T-pouch procedures, create the continence mechanism by anchoring the distal 8 cm of efferent limb into a serosal-lined ileal trough. Construct this trough by opening windows of Deaver in the efferent limb. Place small Penrose drains through each mesenteric window to help identify and facilitate suture passage.

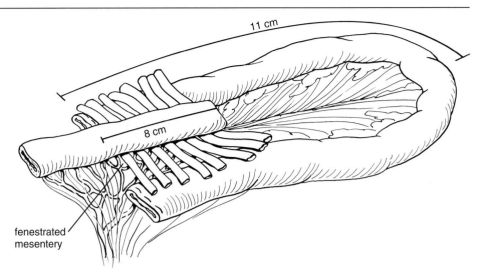

FIGURE 98-3. Anchor the distal 8 cm of efferent limb with interrupted sutures into the serosal-lined ileal trough formed by the base of the two adjacent 11-cm ileal segments.

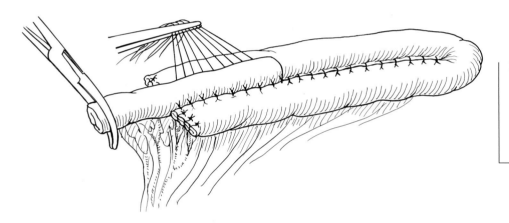

FIGURE 98-4. Taper the limb on the antimesenteric border over a 14-F catheter with 4-0 interrupted absorbable suture.

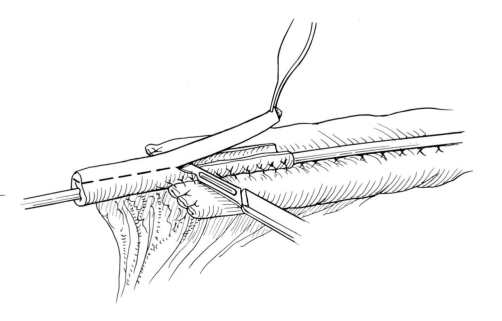

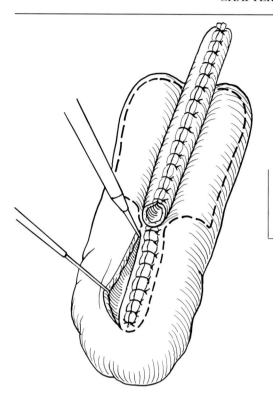

FIGURE 98-5. Starting at the apex of the V, open the bowel immediately adjacent to the medial serosal suture line. When this incision reaches the level of the efferent ostium, extend it directly lateral to the antimesenteric border of the ileum and carry it upward to the base of the ileal segment.

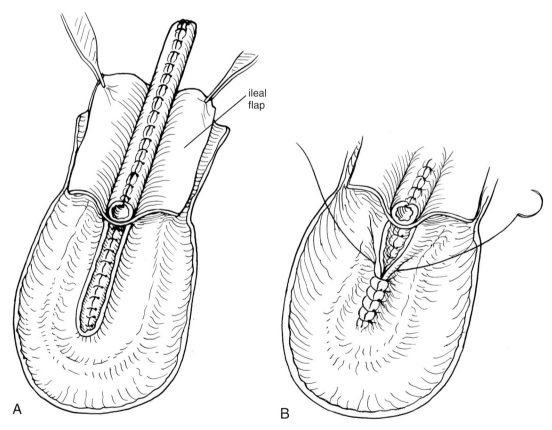

ileal flap

A   B

FIGURE 98-6. A and **B**, These incisions provide wide flaps of ileum. Bring them over the tapered limb to create the continence mechanism.

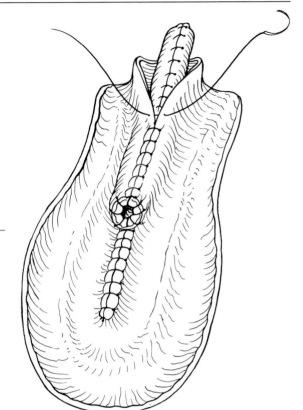

FIGURE 98-7. Use long-acting absorbable suture to close both the inside of the bowel and the serosal flap valve over the efferent limb.

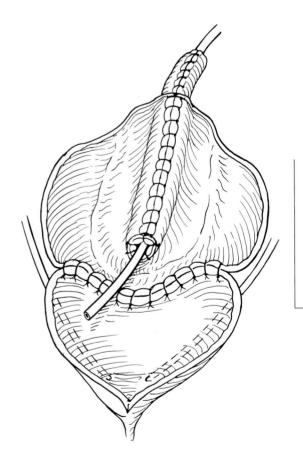

FIGURE 98-8. Rotate the hemi–T-augment and sew it onto the opened bladder. Create a stomal site at the umbilicus. Pass two horizontal mattress sutures through the anterior rectus fascia on either side of the stoma and place at the junction of the efferent limb and patch. Bring the efferent limb out of the abdominal wall foramen and fashion the sutures securely. Be sure that no redundant efferent limb is left floating intra-abdominally. The reservoir should be immediately beneath the abdominal wall. Leave a catheter in the efferent limb for 3 weeks and a suprapubic tube in the augmented bladder.

ERIC KURZROCK

Commentary by

Continent urinary diversion is one of the most fascinating procedures performed by urologists. From the complexity of the original intussuscepted Kock valve to the simplicity of a Mitrofanoff procedure, surgeons have a wealth of choices. Each efferent limb has its advantages and disadvantages. Similar to hypospadias surgery, knowing one technique is not sufficient. Urologic reconstructive surgeons should be knowledgeable and experienced in a multitude of diversions to adapt to the patient's anatomy.

A number of principles should be met when constructing the efferent limb: (1) reliable blood supply; (2) implantation, fixation, or imbrication technique to ensure smooth passage of the catheter regardless of the patient's position and fullness of the bladder (thus, no free-floating limbs); and (3) a blood supply that allows implantation, fixation, or imbrication. The hemi–T-limb is an alternative to the Yang-Monti procedure. They both have the advantage of an excellent blood supply. I use both in my practice. I prefer implantation of appendices and Monti limbs into the bladder, rather than the augment patch. When the bladder is small, I prefer the hemi–T-augment. The hemi–T-limb is also very useful as an afferent limb when a "ureteral cripple" requires augmentation. It serves as a nonrefluxing ileal ureter. Rather than an 8-cm tunnel for the efferent limb, 3 cm is adequate in preventing reflux as an afferent limb.

Chapter 99

Colocystoplasty and Sigmoidocystoplasty

COLOCYSTOPLASTY

FIGURE 99-1. Position: Place the child supine. In girls, prepare and drape the perineum so that a catheter can be inserted aseptically. Instruments and preliminaries are the same as those for ileocystoplasty.

Incision: Stand on the patient's left side. Make a lower midline transperitoneal incision (see Chapter 11) extending from the symphysis to just above the umbilicus. Alternatively, if you are confident that an ileal or sigmoid patch can be used, make a transverse skin incision combined with a vertical midline incision in the fascia, a more cosmetic but more limiting approach. Pack the small intestine in the upper abdomen. Because there is a possibility that the appendix will be needed as a cutaneous conduit, do not perform an appendectomy.

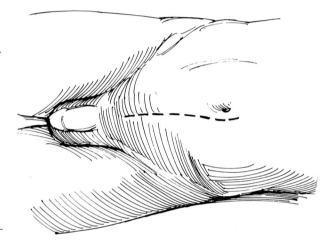

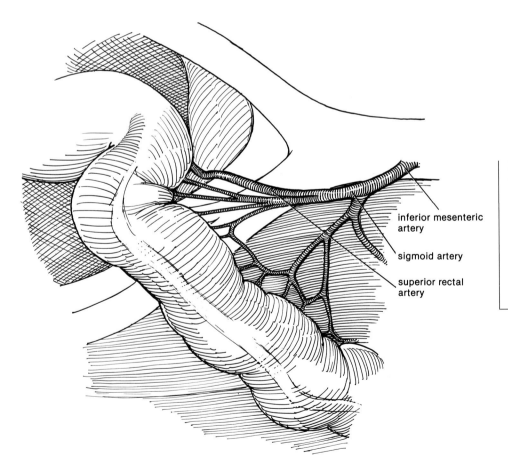

inferior mesenteric artery

sigmoid artery

superior rectal artery

FIGURE 99-2. Study the colonic vasculature for the distribution of the sigmoid artery from the inferior mesenteric artery, and select a length of sigmoid colon of at least 15 cm, preferably 20 cm or more, which is mobile and has a very broad mesentery. Be sure to take enough bowel.

512

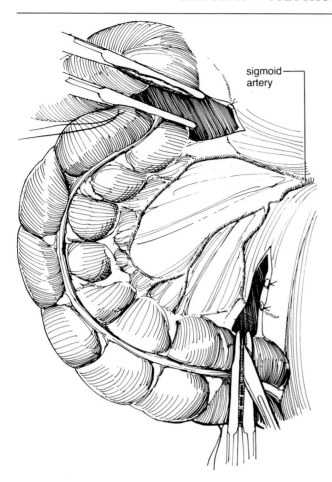

sigmoid artery

FIGURE 99-3. Separate the loop of sigmoid colon from the retroperitoneum with scissors along the white line of Toldt. Mark the selected length with a silk stay suture. Pull the loop down to be sure the bowel can be reanastomosed without tension. Divide the mesentery and the bowel between two pairs of Kocher clamps and fulgurate the exposed mucosa.

FIGURE 99-4. Reanastomose the colon in two layers with staples (see Chapter 6) or with sutures, after making sure the colon is anterior to the isolated segment. Place noncrushing intestinal clamps (Doyen clamps) 2 cm proximal to each Kocher clamp. Remove the Kocher clamps. Insert a posterior row of six or eight interrupted, inverting horizontal mattress sutures of 4-0 silk.

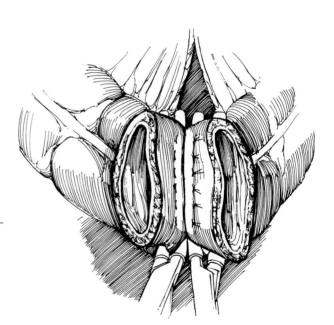

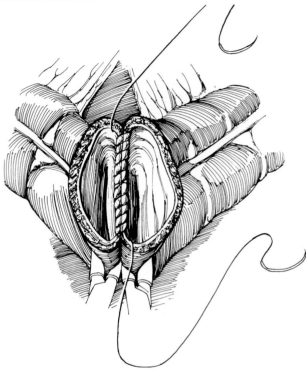

FIGURE 99-5. Start one double-armed or two single-armed 4-0 polypropylene sutures in the center posteriorly. Run the sutures in opposite directions. Take 3 mm of tissue in each bite and keep the stitches close together.

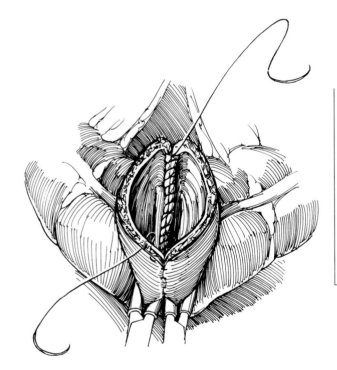

FIGURE 99-6. Tie the suture in continuity near each corner to prevent purse-stringing. Construct the corners carefully, using one suture at a time, going from mucosa to serosa on one side and serosa to mucosa on the other (half-Connell suture). Tie another incontinuity knot at each corner anteriorly. Continue with an inverting suture from each end, going in and out on one side and out and in on the other (Connell suture). Tie the sutures in the midline. Remove the Doyen clamps. As an alternative to the running 4-0 polypropylene sutures, place a layer of inverting, interrupted 4-0 silk sutures. Use of interrupted sutures in the inner layer prevents possible purse-stringing with resultant narrowing at the anastomosis.

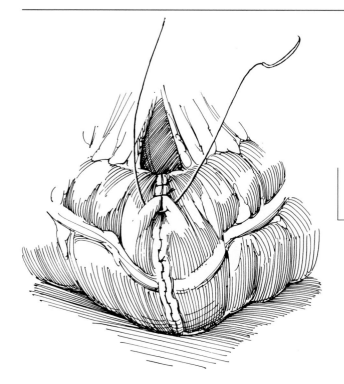

FIGURE 99-7. Place an anterior layer of interrupted, inverting sutures of 3-0 or 4-0 silk through the serosa and superficial muscularis.

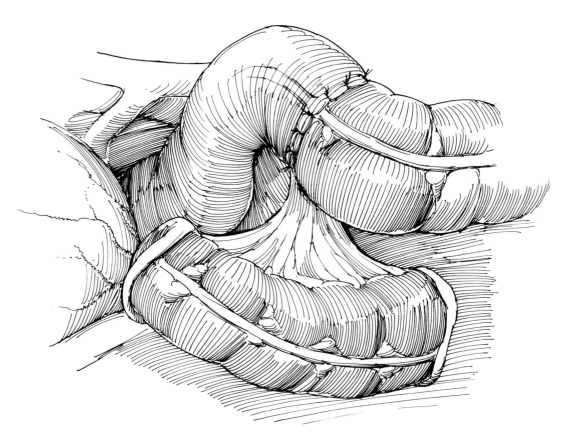

FIGURE 99-8. Close the mesocolon with a running 4-0 chromic catgut suture.

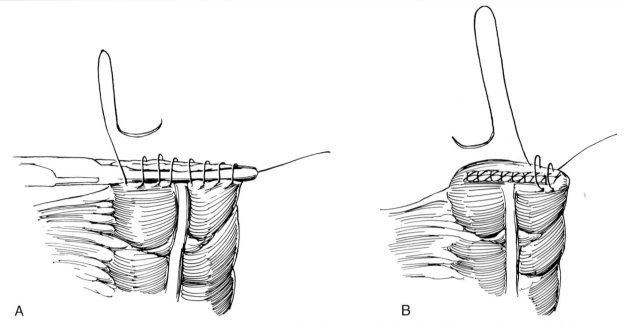

A   B

FIGURE 99-9. A, Place stay sutures at the mesenteric and antimesenteric border of the proximal end of the segment. With the Kocher clamp still on the end of the segment, place a running, inverting 3-0 chromic catgut suture to invert the mucosal edge. **B,** Remove the bowel clamp and pull the suture tight as the assistant helps invert the edge. Run the suture back to its origin and tie it. Place a second, simple running 3-0 nonabsorbable suture over this closure to ensure watertightness. Repeat the process at the distal end.

FIGURE 99-10. Open the segment along the antimesenteric border to within 1 cm of the suture line at each end. Isolate the segment with laparotomy pads and carefully cleanse it with 0.25% neomycin-soaked sponges. The sigmoid cap is now ready for placement on the bladder. If possible, dissect the peritoneum from the dome and posterior wall of the bladder.

If this cannot be done, incise the peritoneum vertically over the fundus of the bladder to expose the anterior and posterior aspects. Open the bladder between stay sutures in a sagittal plane, approaching the trigone posteriorly and the bladder neck anteriorly. The bladder opening should equal the length of the segment when it is stretched out by its stay sutures. In most cases, such as neurogenic bladder dysfunction, it usually is not necessary to resect bladder tissue. The bladder incision, however, must be extensive enough to prevent development of a diverticulum or an hourglass-type bladder. The ideal configuration after application of the cap is spheric. A transverse orientation, shown here, may fit better, but a sagittal orientation, shown in Figure 99-11, may be preferable because by orienting the bowel sagittally, tension does not develop on the mesentery with bladder filling; in fact, it may become more relaxed.

Begin the anastomosis in the midline posteriorly, running a 3-0 chromic catgut-locked suture posteriorly, including all layers of bladder and bowel.

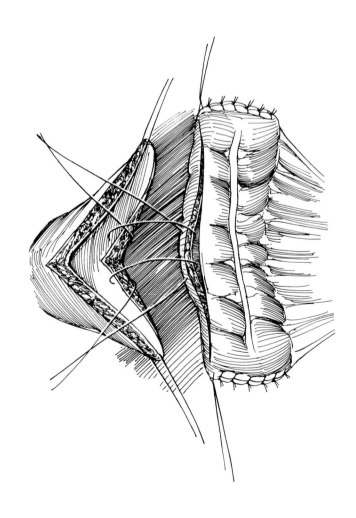

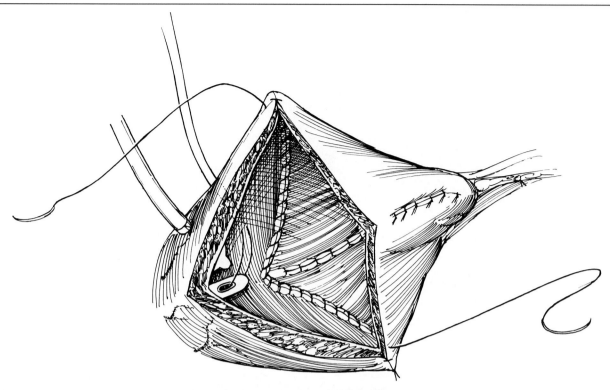

FIGURE 99-11. Run this suture from the midline posteriorly to the apex of the lateral wall or what used to be the dome of the bladder on each side. Do the same for the contralateral side. Place a second running 3-0 synthetic absorbable suture over this suture line to ensure a watertight, inverted closure. If the bladder is very small, first suture the sigmoid cap to the bladder in the sagittal plane posteriorly and anteriorly, and then close the bowel on each side as the lateral walls of the new bladder. The bladder may contract with time, leaving a rim at the bladder neck. Place a 12-F or larger single-lumen plastic catheter in the urethra and secure it with a 2-0 silk suture tied to its tip and brought through the bladder wall. Place a Malecot catheter (except in children with possible latex allergy, for whom a plastic catheter should be used) in one quadrant of the bladder, to be brought through the body wall later; avoid bringing tubes through the wall of the bowel. The size of the Malecot catheter depends on the size of the child. For smaller children, 18 F is the smallest that is acceptable; 22- to 24-F catheters are ideal because the smaller sizes more easily become plugged with mucus in the postoperative period. Fasten the tube at the bladder wall with a 3-0 plain catgut suture.

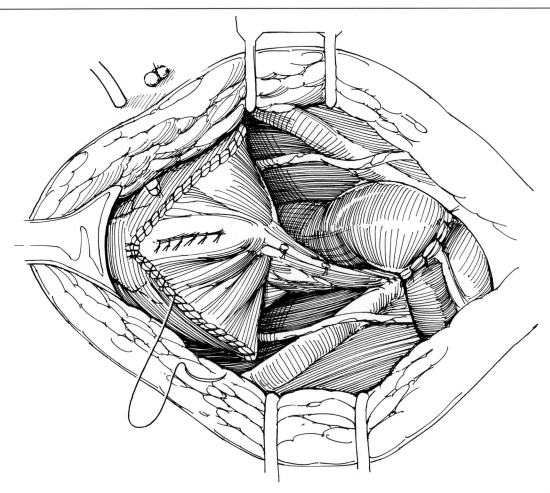

FIGURE 99-12. Close the anterior suture line in the same way as the posterior closure, except in reverse order, beginning in front and proceeding around both sides. Bring the cystostomy catheter through a stab wound in the body wall and suture it to the skin with a nonabsorbable suture. Bring the silk suture from the urethral catheter through the abdominal wall with a straight needle and secure it to a button or cotton pledget. Place a Penrose drain (0.25 inch or 0.5 inch, depending on the child's size) in the prevesical space, and bring it out through a separate stab wound. Patients with ventriculoperitoneal shunts are not drained. Insert a silicone balloon catheter transurethrally to doubly protect from mucus accumulation. Close the wound in layers, and stitch the Penrose drain to the skin.

At first, irrigate the cystostomy at least three times a day with normal (or 3N) saline to prevent mucous obstruction. Perform a cystogram in 1 week and remove the urethral catheter if the anastomoses are intact. After 1 or 2 more weeks, clamp the suprapubic tube and start the patient on self-catheterization. If you personally know that this program is being carried out in a satisfactory manner, remove the suprapubic tube after another 1 or 2 weeks, but have the child continue irrigating at the times of catheterization to remove mucus. At first the bladder will be small. Anticholinergic agents and frequent catheterization are required. For the long term, have the child use a good-size catheter (12F or greater) because mucus will plug a smaller catheter and lead to subtle retention. Even if the child voids, he or she should check for residual urine at intervals.

SIGMOIDOCYSTOPLASTY

The sigmoid is an alternative to the ascending colon used for colocystoplasty, although it is more prone to the formation of mucus.

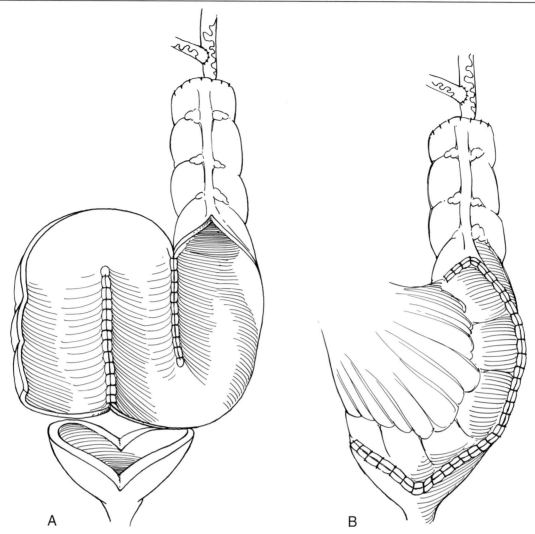

A   B

FIGURE 99-13. A, Select a 25-cm segment from the lower portion of the sigmoid colon, and check it for mobility. Incise the mesosigmoid and resect the segment. Reanastomose the colon (see Chapter 6). Irrigate the loop, and open it on the antimesenteric border, leaving the proximal few centimeters intact to receive the ureters. Form the bowel into an S shape, and suture the two sets of adjacent edges with running polyglactin sutures. Open the bladder widely in the sagittal plane. **B,** Anastomose the segment to the bladder with a running suture beginning posteriorly, tying the knots on the outside. Place a Malecot catheter (use a plastic catheter in children with meningomyelocele), and continue the suture line up the anterior wall.

POSTOPERATIVE PROBLEMS

Mucus is formed profusely at first, but after 3 to 4 weeks its secretion subsides to manageable proportions.

Colicky pain suggests intestinal obstruction; a silent abdomen suggests ileus. Adhesions may cause intestinal obstruction soon after the operation, and other causes may be an anastomotic stoma that is too narrow or herniation through an unclosed defect in the mesentery. Take lateral or upright films of the abdomen and look for gas-fluid levels proximally and for empty bowel distally.

Leakage from the bowel anastomosis can occur occasionally, caused by ischemia from resection of too much mesentery. Place a long nasogastric tube, provide hyperalimentation, and continue suction drainage. For persistence after 10 to 14 days, reoperate. Ischemia and necrosis of the segment, seen as a dusky stoma during closing, come from tension on the mesentery, from hematoma, or from inadvertent ligation of a major vessel. The bowel will remain intact for 1 or 2 weeks, but intervention is needed if recovery has not occurred by that time. Perform endoscopy on the segment to see how much is involved; if it is only the terminal few centimeters, enough ileum may be pulled out to make a new stoma. Otherwise, another segment of ileum must be attached, or a new loop must be created. Deficiency of vitamin B_{12} occurs with use of the ileocecal region for augmentation. A supplement must be given yearly.

Commentary by

MICHAEL F. MITCHELL

We have been very pleased with this form of cystoplasty as a mechanism to increase bladder volume and compliance. The same basic technique may be used for large and small bowel. The advantage of closing the ends of the bowel and the sagittal orientation is that no tension develops on the mesentery with bladder filling. If anything, the mesentery becomes more relaxed. In some circumstances a transverse orientation of the sigmoid seems to fit better and works equally well. Always take a little more than you think you will need; 15 cm is minimal. Do not cut the segment to fit the bladder. In cases in which the bladder is very small it is sometimes necessary to suture the sigmoid cap to the bladder posteriorly and anteriorly, and then bowel to bowel on each side to form the lateral walls of the new bladder. In such a case the original bladder sometimes shrinks further with time to form just a rim at the bladder neck.

There is a natural tendency as well to be timid in the sagittal incision of the bladder. This is a very important maneuver because if the incision is not generous enough the cystoplasty segment becomes nothing more than a diverticulum and the anticipated dynamic advantages of the cystoplasty may not be realized. In the same sense the antimesenteric incision in the bowel, converting the segment from a tube to a patch, is very important. In our review of over 130 cystoplasty cases, the patients who had problems were those in whom the bladder was augmented with bowel in its tubular configuration. Of the patch cystoplasty patients, less than 10% had problems with what we considered to be peristaltic contractions; most of these were believed probably to have segments that were too short.

We use only resorbable suture material on tissue that either conducts or stores urine (e.g., renal pelvis, ureter, bladder, and bladder neck). Nonresorbable material, such as silk or staples, even if used on the outside, seems ultimately to be a potential nidus for stone formation and should be avoided if possible.

Because of the initial flood of mucus, we leave two drainage tubes. The urethral catheter is removed at approximately 1 week after a cystogram has demonstrated that there are no leaks in the bladder. The patient is usually discharged with suprapubic drainage, which is continued for an additional 1 to 2 weeks. At that point the suprapubic tube is clamped and intermittent clean catheterization (ICC) is initiated. The suprapubic tube is not removed until the patient proves, beyond a shadow of a doubt, that ICC can be done effectively and regularly. The suprapubic tube is usually removed 1 to 2 weeks after the initiating of ICC. To control mucus production, which is sometimes quite significant initially, we irrigate the bladder on a three-times-a-day basis with normal (N) and sometimes 3N saline solution. Usually after several months, irrigation can be reduced to once a day and sometimes on an as-needed basis. All patients are maintained on ICC until they prove, again beyond a shadow of a doubt, that they can completely empty with voiding. Some patients catheterize once or twice a day just to be safe. Those patients who must do long-term ICC usually do best with a catheter size of 12 F or greater. Smaller catheters can lead to mucus plugs and unsuspected retention.

Finally, it sometimes takes considerable time (months) for even the augmented bladder to "stretch up" after surgery. I do not hesitate to use anticholinergic agents during this period. Patients also are sometimes distressed to find that ICC needs to be performed quite frequently, at least as often as every 2 to 3 hours initially. This requirement is usually temporary and will change gradually but requires support from a caring physician.

Commentary by

RICARDO GONZÁLEZ

The use of the sigmoid colon, with or without preservation of the intestinal mucosa, continues to be my preferred technique for bladder augmentation. However, I reconfigure it in a different manner that is analogous to the reconfiguration of the ileum originally described by Goodwin. I believe that the method of reconfiguration depicted in this chapter is responsible for the inferior urodynamic results obtained with the sigmoid colon when compared to the ileum in many series. For the augmentation I select 20 to 25 cm of sigmoid colon and leave a very broad mesentery. The continuity of the sigmoid is reestablished with a single-layer anastomosis of 3-0 or 4-0 polydioxanone suture. The bladder is widely opened in the sagittal plane. The sigmoid segment is opened along its antimesenteric border, folded as an inverted U. The posterior edges are sutured together with 3-0 Vicryl, and the posterior edge of this folded segment is sutured to the posterior edge of the cystotomy. The apex of the inverted U is then brought down to the anterior lower corner of the cystotomy. I always leave a large (20- or 22-F) suprapubic tube, which exits through the native bladder or bowel segment.

The advantages of the sigmoid include its anatomic proximity to the bladder, a lower risk of postoperative bowel obstruction, no risk of nutritional deficiencies or alteration of gastrointestinal function, and ease of implantation of a continent catheterizable channel. Clinically relevant acidosis is exceptionally rare when renal function is normal but must be addressed medically when renal function is diminished. Contraindications to the use of the sigmoid colon include previous surgery of anal or rectal atresia and known diseases of the colon. In such cases, I use the ileum.

The form of sigmoidocystoplasty with the extended proximal tail was very useful in the era of undiversion, and is almost never used at present.

Chapter 100

Gastrocystoplasty

GASTROCYSTOPLASTY (MITCHELL)

Place the child on a liquid diet for 48 hours, and 24 hours before the operation give magnesium citrate. The child may be admitted the day of surgery. Attempt to sterilize the urine and provide preventive antibiotics.

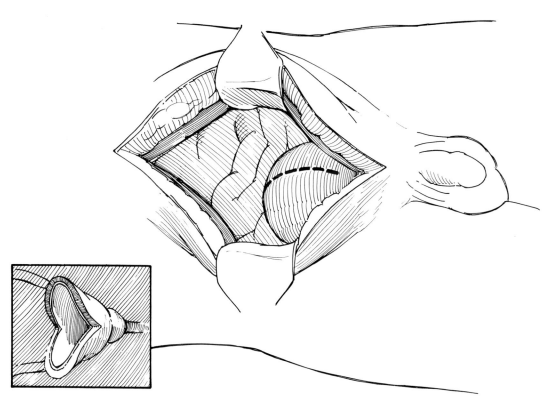

FIGURE 100-1. Insert a nasogastric tube. Incision: Make a midline transperitoneal incision (see Chapter 11) from the xiphoid to the pubis. Expose the bladder through the lower part of the incision, and open it sagittally in the midline ("bivalve"). This incision should extend from the bladder neck anteriorly to the trigone posteriorly. Control bleeding by electrocautery. Insert infant feeding tubes of suitable size into each ureter.

Preparing the bladder first reduces acid spillage, but in myelomeningocele patients with shunts, it may be better to open the bladder after the gastric patch has been prepared to avoid prolonged drainage of urine into the abdominal cavity. Place an artificial sphincter at the point, if indicated.

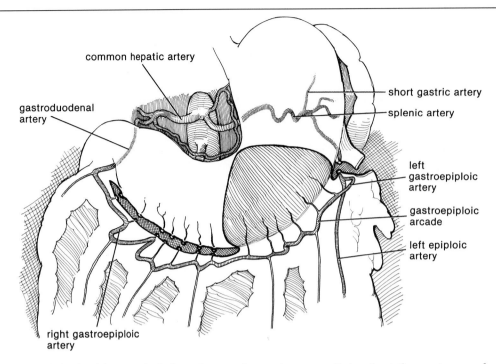

common hepatic artery

gastroduodenal
artery

short gastric artery

splenic artery

left
gastroepiploic
artery

gastroepiploic
arcade

left epiploic
artery

right gastroepiploic
artery

FIGURE 100-2. Extend the incision cephalad, and open the peritoneum. Reimplant the ureters, and prepare the bladder neck area for sphincter or sling, if indicated.

Right-sided pedicle: Draw the stomach into the wound with large Babcock clamps. Examine the right and left gastroepiploic arteries over the greater curvature of the stomach. The left gastroepiploic artery arises from terminal branching of the splenic artery. The right gastroepiploic artery is a branch of the gastroduodenal artery. Together they form the gastroepiploic arterial arch. Because the right gastroepiploic artery is subject to angulation at the gastric antrum, be sure to free the gastroepiploic vessels and check the flow after the flap is brought into the pelvis. The left gastroepiploic artery is found not infrequently to merge into the greater curvature or to taper to a small caliber, whereas the caliber of the right is more constant. For this reason, the right vessel is usually used to supply the flap.

Free the omentum from the transverse colon by dividing its relatively thin avascular connection. Incise the greater omentum 1 or 2 cm distal to the gastroepiploic artery on the right side with the electrocautery. Clamp and tie the larger vessels (see Chapter 65). Leave the vessels intact on the left, so that the omentum may descend with the patch.

Select as large a wedge as possible—one that encompasses at least a third of the stomach. Because the right gastroepiploic artery will be the base, tend to make the wedge toward the left side of the stomach to have as long a pedicle as possible. Grasp the edges of the greater curvature with Babcock clamps for traction and outline the proposed wedge with a marking pen. The length of each arm of the wedge should approximately equal the width of the patch and should approach, but not reach, the lesser curvature.

Divide the short arteries to the stomach starting at the right side of the proposed wedge and working to the right. Do this by passing a Providence Hospital clamp through the omentum on each side of the first short gastric branch, to the right of the right arm of the wedge, elevate the artery, and draw a 4-0 synthetic absorbable suture under it. Tie the suture. Clamp and divide the artery close to the stomach, and then ligate the end of the vessel in the clamp. Avoid traction on the gastroepiploic vessels to prevent arterial spasm and ischemia. Watch for duskiness or paleness indicating vascular spasm at the least. Be prepared to apply papaverine to the pedicle. This technique avoids retraction of the proximal (omental) end, which could quickly produce a potentially harmful interstitial hematoma. Continue with the remaining branches, avoiding mass ligation and any contact with the gastroepiploic arterial arch itself, to reach the gastroduodenal origin of the arch. Because an undivided branch could be torn easily when the flap is pulled into place, preserve a 5- to 7-cm band of omental vessels intact to protect the pedicle from avulsion. On the left side of the patch, the omentum is left attached to the pedicle so that it subsequently may be used to cover the repair.

Inspect the right gastroepiploic artery to be sure it has good pulsations before clamping and dividing the left gastroepiploic artery on the other side of the wedge. Again, apply papaverine hydrochloride solution to the vessels if spasm is a concern.

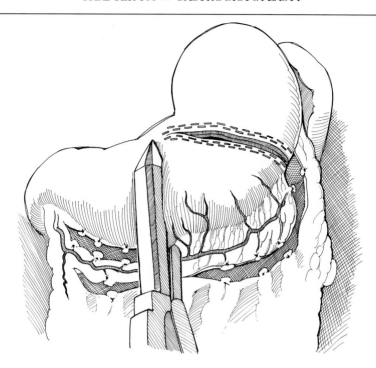

FIGURE 100-3. Bowel clamp technique: Place parallel bowel clamps on either side of the gastric wedge. Ligate the branches of the gastric vessels of the lesser curvature near the apex of the wedge to prevent significant bleeding. Pack the area with laparotomy tapes to minimize spillage. Excise the wedge, taking care not to injure the vascular pedicle. Place the wedge in a moist laparotomy tape for protection. This technique avoids cutting the staples out, but more blood is lost during reconstitution of the stomach.

Stapler technique (shown here): Insert the 70- to 90-mm gastrointestinal anastomosis stapler (GIA-90) at each of the two sites. Be careful not to damage the vascular pedicle when the instrument is placed at the right side of the wedge. Close the stapler and resect the wedge. Wrap the wedge in a moist lap tape before placing it in the pelvis; similarly, protect the pedicle itself. If the stomach has a saccular shape, instead of taking a wedge, staple off the bottom with the GIA-90 stapler. Make the pedicle as long as possible by dissecting near the gastroduodenal junction. If great length is need, divide a few more vessels distally on the patch.

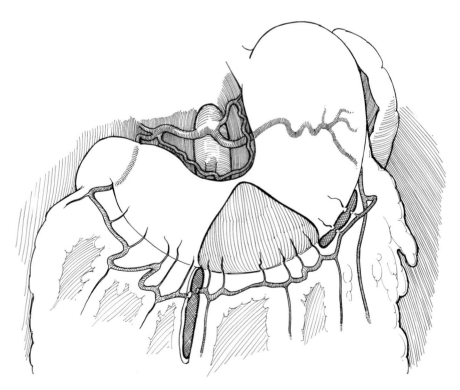

FIGURE 100-4. Left-sided pedicle: Divide the short arteries starting at the left side of the proposed wedge and continue to just distal to the origin of the left gastroepiploic artery near its origin from the splenic artery.

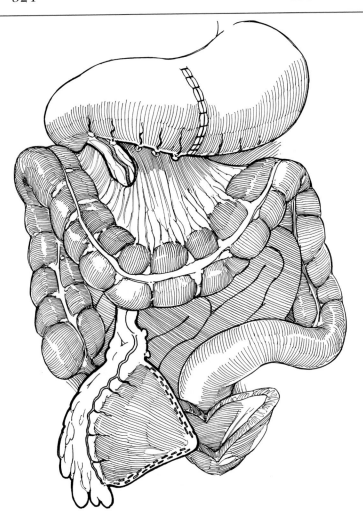

FIGURE 100-5. To close the stomach, place a posterior seromuscular row of interrupted 3-0 silk sutures, tie them, and then remove the staples, at least those on the anterior wall suture line. Place an inner through-and-through layer of running locked stitches with 3-0 synthetic absorbable suture material. Move the nasogastric tube into the antrum just proximal to the suture line.

FIGURE 100-6. Pass the flap on its pedicle under the transverse mesocolon along the root of the small intestine and through the mesentery of the small intestine *(arrow)*. Alternatively, elevate the right colon and place the entire pedicle beneath the mesentery, leaving it in the retroperitoneum. Avoid rotating the mesentery. Should the flap not reach the bladder, free more of the vessels connecting the artery to the duodenum. Recheck the pulsation in the artery of the pedicle.

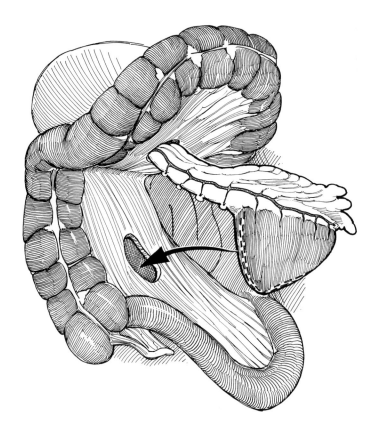

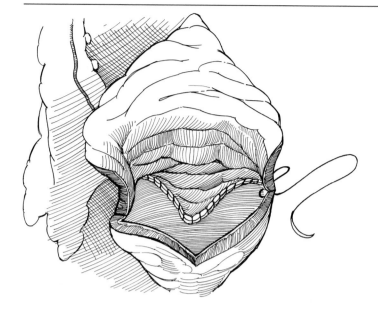

FIGURE 100-7. The former ventral side of the stomach flap will now lie anteriorly, and its apex will be fastened to the vesical neck, while the apex of the former dorsal surface extends to the trigone. Remove all of the staples on each side just before suturing that side. Run full-thickness, locked 3-0 chromic sutures from the trigone up each arm to the dome from inside the bladder. Reinforce the suture lines with a second layer of seromuscular sutures placed from the outside.

Place a Malecot catheter of a caliber adequate to handle mucus (at least 16 F) through the bladder wall (or through the patch, if necessary). Suture the exit site to the abdominal wall as for gastrostomy to prevent later intraperitoneal leakage when the tube is removed. Remove the ureteral catheters unless surgery has been performed on the ureteral orifices.

FIGURE 100-8. Insert a urethral catheter for added safety during the postoperative period and fix it transvesically on the anterior abdominal wall with a stitch through its tip and tied over a bolster.

Close the anterior portion with similar sutures (a running locked 3-0 chromic catgut suture from the inside and a running 3-0 synthetic absorbable suture from the outside). Test the suture line by filling the bladder; place additional sutures if needed. This also is a chance to see if filling disturbs the blood supply to the pedicle. Inspect the gastroepiploic artery in the pedicle again. Fix the pedicle to the posterior retroperitoneum along the root of the small bowel, or close the opened retroperitoneum over it with a running 3-0 chromic catgut suture. Place the left side of the omentum over the small bowel (and, if long enough, the anterior suture line), and use the portion from the left side that is attached to the patch to cover the posterior anastomosis. Drains are not necessary. Again, distend the bladder for a final check.

Maintain nasogastric suction until the child passes gas, and then start easily digestible liquid feedings. Check the suture lines with a cystogram. Discharge the child after 1 week with the suprapubic catheter in place, and give suppressive antibiotics. Have the child return 1 to 2 weeks later to have the tube clamped, so that either intermittent catheterization or voiding may begin. If that goes well, remove the tube 1 week later. Have the child empty the bladder every 2 hours and be awakened once at night. After another 2 weeks, empty every 4 hours. Check the results in 2 or 3 months by ultrasound and cystogram.

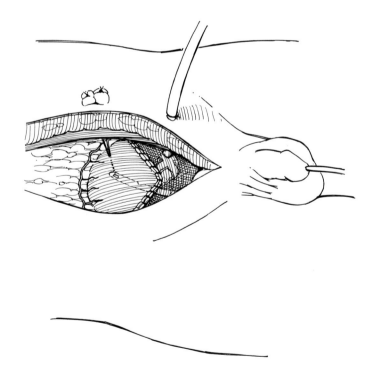

POSTOPERATIVE PROBLEMS

Penile burning with hematuria or dysuria from hyperacidic urine occurs in the majority of the children. Insensate patients such as patients with neurogenic lesions will not experience the pain in contrast to sensate patients, such as with valve or exstrophy. Treat the pain with an H_2-receptor antagonist or proton-pump inhibitor. Giving the child an antacid tablet after meals clears the penile burning quickly. Alkaline bladder irrigations are usually not needed. Check urinary pH levels regularly. Asymptomatic bacteriuria does not need treatment. Electrolyte imbalance will be detected by monthly determinations for the first 6 months. It may become severe if the child has an episode of vomiting or diarrhea with resultant salt loss and hyperchloremic acidosis. If this occurs, salt replacement is mandatory.

MICHAEL E. MITCHELL

Commentary by

There are two foci of potential vascular obstruction in the pedicle of the gastric flap. One is at the gastric antrum, where angulation can occur if the right gastroepiploic artery is used as the pedicle. To avoid this, free the gastroepiploic vessels, so that there is no possible tethering by short vessels to the gastric antrum. Always check this area after the gastric flap is brought into the pelvis. The second focus is the distal end of the gastroepiploic artery where it enters the flap. It may be necessary to divide one or two of the most proximal short vessels to the flap to prevent angulation. This will not jeopardize the blood supply to this portion of the flap and will protect the blood supply to the entire flap. Vascular spasm rarely is observed during the completion of the posterior suture line of the bladder anastomosis. Watch for change in color of the gastric mucosa. Purple color or paleness is a sign of vascular compromise. Immediately check the proximal and distal ends of the pedicle, and apply papaverine to the entire length. Spasm occurs approximately 10% of the time but never should result in loss of the flap.

Remove the staples from the wedge-shaped flap just before suturing it to the bladder. (The wedge flap is opened along the posterior staple line and anastomosed to the posterior bladder; then, the anterior staples are removed, and anterior anastomosis is completed.) This prevents needless blood loss and spillage of gastric juices. At the conclusion of the anastomosis of the gastric flap to the stomach, all staples should be removed from the flap.

The suprapubic tube usually is brought through the native bladder. However, if it is necessary to bring it through the flap, tissue adjacent to the tube should be sutured to the anterior abdominal wall, similar to a gastrostomy. This prevents needless intraperitoneal leakage with removal of the suprapubic tube.

Nasogastric suction needs to be used only 2 to 3 days postoperatively. Patients can leave the hospital 5 to 7 days after gastrocystoplasty. The suprapubic tube is removed only after complete bladder emptying (by voiding, catheterization, or other methods) has been proved. If ureteral reimplants into the flap portion of the augmented bladder are required, the posterior aspect of the suture line is first completed, and the reimplants are performed with the standard tunnel technique. If the appendiceal Mitrofanoff technique is to be considered, it can be performed after the anterior closure and in the manner described by Barry for reimplantation of the transplanted ureter into the bladder. A direct-catheterizable channel from the umbilicus through the appendix-catheterizable channel to the bladder is thereby constructed.

Hematuria or dysuria, or both, is seen in 36% of patients with gastrocystoplasty. Of these, 5% will have significant symptoms, and approximately 20% will require periodic treatment. The critical factor in these patients is serum gastrin levels. If the serum gastrin level is persistently elevated, consideration may have to be given to alternative means of augmentation. The presence of hematuria and dysuria without gastrin elevation usually is treated with H_2 blockers and, occasionally, with alkaline irrigation of the bladder.

The long-term risk of cancer developing in a gastric-augmented bladder in children and young adults may be significant (as high as 3% to 5% after 15 to 20 years). Therefore use of this form of augmentation should be reserved for only those patients in whom no other form of augmentation is available.

RICHARD C. RINK

Use of the gastric segment for bladder augmentation has made possible lower urinary tract reconstruction in many children who were not previously candidates. It has been particularly useful in the child with a paucity of bowel, such as the patient with cloacal exstrophy, or in one requiring reconstruction following pelvic irradiation, when the bowel is compromised. The other major indication for the use of stomach has been renal insufficiency with acidosis. The gastric segment will act as a chloride pump with net chloride and hydrogen ion transport into the urine to prevent further acidosis. In comparison with bowel segments, the use of gastric segments has lessened symptomatic lower urinary infections in our series. However, this may be offset by hematuria and dysuria.

Preoperatively, it is important to rule out any history of stomach abnormalities, such as ulcer disease or gastric emptying abnormalities. A severe salt-wasting nephropathy should be identified preoperatively. Children having this disorder are poor candidates because gastrocystoplasty may worsen the fluid and electrolyte abnormalities.

I would suggest caution using stomach for reconstruction in the child with normal sensation, because hematuria and dysuria have been seen in one third of our patients. This may lead to significant perineal pain in those with normal sensation and, at times, may be quite difficult to resolve. The gastric wedge taken for augmentation generally is smaller than for the gastric reservoir. Initially, we were somewhat conservative in the amount of stomach used, and this has been reflected in marginal urodynamic studies in some of the early patients in our series. I would be certain that at least one third of the stomach is used for augmentation to ensure that the most compliant, largest-capacity reservoir can be obtained. We have not seen problems with the native stomach postoperatively, because of taking larger segments. The use of the stapler to excise the wedge may prevent some gastric spillage and blood loss, but this is offset by wasting stomach tissue during excision of the staple lines. I excise the wedge between bowel clamps. It is helpful to ligate the branches of the gastric artery to the patch near the apex of the wedge to prevent blood loss. It also is helpful to back the bowel clamp off the stomach wall and run the inner layer on the back wall of the stomach closure first, because this acts as a hemostatic closure and prevents inverting a large portion of the stomach wall.

The pedicle must be secured to the posterior peritoneum to prevent its injury and to avoid an area for bowel herniation. We generally tack the omentum along the pedicle to the posterior peritoneum as it runs along the root of the small bowel. Alternatively, the entire right colon can be elevated and the pedicle placed in the retroperitoneum behind the bowel and its mesentery. We had four bowel obstructions in our initial 41 patients, and at least one involved the gastric pedicle. The wedge generally is rotated and anastomosed to the bivalved bladder, as described in the preceding technique. However, we have, at times, rotated this only 90 degrees to achieve a better "fit." This results in the gastroepiploic artery on the wedge running in an anteroposterior fashion on the bladder, rather than in its usual transverse lie. If there is tension on the pedicle when the artery reaches the bladder, length can be gained by two methods. More vessels from the gastroepiploic artery to the stomach and duodenum can be divided, or the initial short artery from the gastroepiploic artery to the wedge itself can be divided. The richly vascular plexus keeps this portion of the wedge perfused.

I do not leave ureteral stents, because urine will help buffer any early acid production. However, double drainage by urethral and suprapubic tubes is important during the initial healing phase. A Penrose drain is left in all patients, although in those with ventriculoperitoneal shunts, it is removed early.

Postoperatively, the child is placed on H_2 blockade and is maintained on this treatment for the first month. Although mucus production is reduced with stomach versus other intestinal segments, we still irrigate the bladder free of mucus every 8 hours in the hospital, and the parents are instructed to do this twice a day after discharge. Early on, "coffee-ground" urine may be present, which is concerning to the uninitiated. This will pass. When the child returns in 2 weeks, the suprapubic tube is clamped, and intermittent catheterization or spontaneous voiding is started. The catheter is removed only when it is established that the family or child can reliably catheterize, or that the child can spontaneously void to completion. Initially, catheterization may be necessary as frequently as every 2 hours, with awakening once at night to empty. The bladder would adequately stretch during the next 2 weeks to allow catheterizations every 4 hours during waking hours and avoidance of nocturnal catheterization.

With any associated viral illness resulting in vomiting, electrolyte levels must be checked to determine whether treatment of significant hypochloremic alkalosis is needed.

Chapter 101

Ureterocystoplasty

A ureterocystoplasty is an operation for bladder enlargement in a child with a noncompliant bladder and a dilated megaureter. The ureter should be associated with a nonfunctioning kidney, be dilated enough to be useful for vesical augmentation, and be long enough to allow reimplantation with tapering. Such a dilated ureter is preferable to bowel because harvesting and application are simpler and it avoids the problems of malignancy, spontaneous rupture, electrolyte imbalance, and mucus production.

Inform the parents and prepare the child for bowel substitution should the ureter prove inadequate. Start with sterile urine. Avoid nitrous oxide anesthesia, which promotes ileus and thus stresses the new pedicles.

Select a midline transperitoneal (see Chapter 11) or a lower abdominal transverse (Pfannenstiel) (see Chapter 63) incision.

If the ipsilateral kidney is to be preserved as shown, perform ureteroureterostomy (see Chapter 52) on the proximal ureteral segment and use the lower portion for the augmentation. Alternatively, taper and reimplant the proximal portion of the ureter into the bladder. If the ipsilateral kidney is functionless, remove it by dividing the renal vessels near the parenchyma and carefully dissecting the pelvis out of the hilum to preserve as much of the important ureteropelvic blood supply as possible.

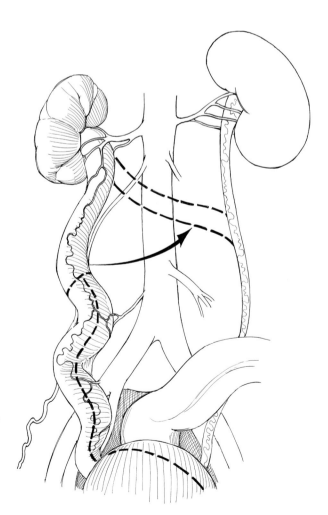

FIGURE 101-1. Dissect the ureter from the retroperitoneal tissues, keeping its segmental blood supply intact, that is, that coming from the aorta and the iliac and vesical vessels, and especially that coming from the gonadal vessels. If previous surgery has been done on the distal ureter, preserving the proximal blood supply is all the more important. Use optical magnification. Do not disturb the connections between the ureter and the bladder at the ureterovesical junction. Divide the ureter at a site that leaves enough length for end-to-side anastomosis to the contralateral ureter. Alternatively, reimplant the ureter into the bladder with a psoas hitch.

Open the ureteral segment on its anterolateral border and extend the incision through the ureterovesical junction. Stay in the coronal plane to preserve all the blood supply entering there, that is, vessels on which this segment of the ureter depends. Continue the incision on the posterior wall of the bladder, and then over the anterior wall, as for "clam" augmentation (see Chapter 96). With ureteral duplication, reimplant the ipsilateral ureter.

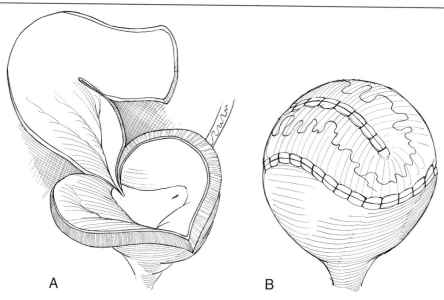

FIGURE 101-2. A, Double the ureter on itself to form a U-shaped cup. Insert a suprapubic catheter into the bladder (not shown). **B,** Apply the cup-patch to the bivalved bladder with a running locking 3-0 synthetic absorbable suture (see Chapter 96). Place a drain to the perivesical area. Connect the catheter to closed drainage; remove it in 10 to 14 days, after cystography shows that the suture line is intact.

MARK BELLINGER

Commentary by

Ureterocystoplasty is a procedure that has limited applicability and requires certain anatomic prerequisites before the procedure can be considered. When anatomy permits, this procedure is an excellent alternative to enterocystoplasty. The long-term effects of enterocystoplasty (mucus production, spontaneous rupture, malignancy) are avoided, and in most cases, the procedure can be performed via an extraperitoneal approach.

Ureterocystoplasty comes to mind primarily in cases of massive unilateral reflux, especially in neurogenic bladder or valve cases in which bladder compliance is diminished but the pop-off effect of the refluxing ureter has served well to preserve the contralateral kidney and its ureter from the development of both reflux and hydronephrosis. In these patients, it is easy to assume that reconfiguration of the refluxing megaureter will continue to provide adequate compliance once this segment is used to augment the bladder. In cases where a nonrefluxing megaureter is to be used for bladder augmentation, it is more difficult to be sure that the reconfigured ureter will provide enough volume and compliance to adequately dampen high bladder pressures and preserve the status of the contralateral kidney. This assessment must in large part be based upon clinical judgment. In all cases, preoperative preparation should include a full bowel prep, and the patient and family should accept the possibility of and sign consent for enterocystoplasty.

The most common candidates for ureterocystoplasty are patients with massive reflux into a nonfunctioning or poorly functioning kidney in whom nephrectomy is appropriate. In these patients, the kidney is removed and the ureter and perhaps part of the renal pelvis in some patients are preserved to augment the bladder. The surgical approach should be retroperitoneal unless this proves to be impossible. In most cases, a small flank incision should be used to approach the kidney and an extraperitoneal Pfannenstiel incision used to approach the bladder and distal ureter.

If nephrectomy is performed, it is important to preserve vessels passing from the renal vessels to the pelvis, and also to preserve the gonadal vessels if at all possible. As the ureter is mobilized, it is important to sweep the periureteral tissue toward the ureter to preserve as much local blood supply to the ureter as possible. Once the ureter is mobilized, the cutting current of the electrocautery is used to open the ureter longitudinally on its medial aspect, carrying the incision through the superior aspect of the ureteral orifice and across the bladder toward the contralateral ureteral orifice, bisecting the bladder. The ureter is then sewn into place using absorbable suture.

Variations on the above scenario may be used when anatomy permits, in particular considering transureteroureterostomy when renal preservation is appropriate. The bladder should be drained with a suprapubic catheter, exiting the bladder through the detrusor muscle, never through the ureter. A cystogram should be performed before catheter removal to ensure that there is no extravasation.

SAVA PEROVIC

Commentary by

Augmentation ureterocystoplasty, independently pioneered by Bellinger and Churchill, has proved to be the best choice for bladder augmentation. Indications for use of ureters for bladder augmentation are still evolving, because the number of patients with nonfunctioning or poorly functioning kidney is limited. We have used ureterocystoplasty with preservation of ipsilateral renal function. The lower part of the extremely dilated ureter is used for bladder augmentation and its upper part is anastomosed to the opposite ureter. We have developed a variant of ureterocystoplasty with preservation of kidney by dividing the megaureter and using its distal parts for bladder augmentation and its proximal parts for ureteroneocystostomy. Contrary to other authors who perform transureteroureterostomy, we prefer direct ureteral anastomosis to the bladder because extraperitoneal ureteroneocystostomy is more physiologic and avoids the transperitoneal approach, thus decreasing risk of complications.

The main disadvantage of our method is smaller ureteral surface for augmentation, however, all patients in our series had bilateral megaureters, which provides much more biomaterial for augmentation.

In patients treated with cutaneous loop ureterostomy, the distal part of the ureter was dilated preoperatively with balloon catheters to provide further enlargement.

Preservation of adequate blood supply to megaureters is crucial for a successful outcome. The ureter is divided at the level that enables good blood supply for both parts of the megaureters. Division and mobilization of the loop cutaneous ureterostomy at the stomal site is more difficult but has to be performed without jeopardizing the integrity of the blood supply to both ureteral parts.

Tubularization depends on the type of megaureters. For obstructive megaureters we leave the orifice intact to ensure better vascularization since there is minimal risk of postoperative bladder diverticulum formation. For refluxing megaureters the incision is continued through the ureterovesical junction, care is taken to prevent damage to the blood supply and creation of irregularly shaped bladder with diverticula.

Ureteroneocystostomy presents the most difficult part of the technique and depends on bladder size and wall thickness. The length of the upper part of megaureters has always been sufficient for reimplantation and there has not been a need to mobilize and fix the bladder to the psoas muscle. In the majority of our patients an extravesical detrusor tunneling procedure was performed. In the cases with thick, trabeculated bladder wall, extravesical ureteroneocystostomy is done after detrusor muscle incision. A bladder expander (conformer) is inserted intraoperatively for postoperative maintenance of volume and for adequate shaping of the augmented bladder. A filling tube is passed through the native urethra in females and through an abdominal stoma in males. The bladder expander is removed 2 weeks postoperatively. Double-J ureteral stents, which are used for ureteral implantation, are removed after 2 to 3 months.

During the last 12 years, we have performed ureterocystoplasty in 32 patients in two ways. In cases with impaired kidneys, loop cutaneous ureterostomy previously has been done to preserve and improve renal function. In other cases, bladder augmentation and ureterocystostomy were performed simultaneously. In augmentation ureterocystoplasty with both megaureters, the distal part of one is used for creation of continent vesicostomy. Ureterocystoplasty is superior to any other available technique for bladder augmentation and our variant further expands the selection of patients who may benefit from this procedure.

Chapter 102

Autoaugmentation

AUTOAUGMENTATION BY SEROMYOTOMY

Bladders with poor compliance and hyperreflexia but with only modestly reduced capacity are candidates for autoaugmentation.

Position the patient supine. Insert a two-way urodynamics catheter connected to a Y-tube with a saline filling bag held at a height of 30 cm above the bladder.

Make a transverse lower abdominal incision (see Chapter 63) or midline extraperitoneal incision (see Chapter 62). Dissect the peritoneum from the dome of the bladder.

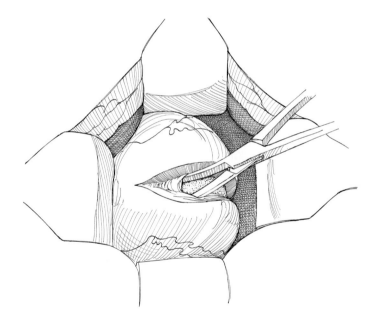

FIGURE 102-1. With the electrocautery set for coagulation, incise through three quarters of the thickness of the detrusor muscle with a vertical midline incision over the entire dome. Separate the remaining detrusor fibers with a hemostat to expose the suburothelial layer. Release the clamp on the catheter, and allow the bladder to fill. Control any leaks with fine chromic figure-of-eight sutures.

FIGURE 102-2. Grasp the edge of the detrusor muscle with two Allis clamps on each side for countertraction during the submucosal dissection. Bluntly and sharply dissect laterally in the plane between muscle and urothelium until half of the wall is peeled back. Fill and drain the bladder intermittently to aid the dissection. Excise the detrusor flaps.

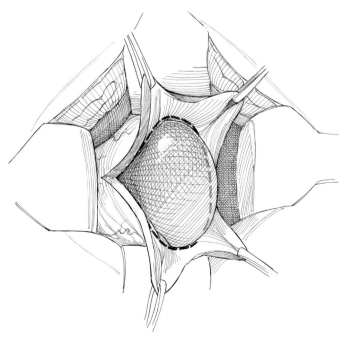

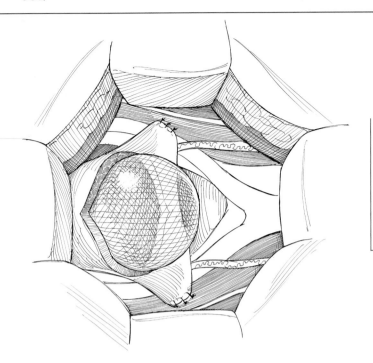

FIGURE 102-3. Hitch each of the posterior edges of the bladder to the respective psoas muscles (see Chapter 58). Drain the bladder with either a urethrally placed balloon catheter or a suprapubic tube emerging from an area of intact bladder wall. Place a Penrose drain paravesically. Perform cystography in 1 week; if no extravasation is seen, remove the catheter and have the patient resume intermittent catheterization or voiding.

LAPAROSCOPIC AUTOAUGMENTATION

Create a pneumoperitoneum of 10 mmHg. Insert one 10-mm trocar below the umbilicus, two in the right and left lower quadrants in the midaxillary line halfway between the umbilicus and the iliac crest, and a fourth in the right lower quadrant medial to the other trocar. Insert a balloon catheter, and fill the bladder with normal saline to which a vial of methylene blue has been added to help identify the mucosa. Alternatively, distend a balloon in the bladder to reduce the immediate consequences of puncture of the epithelium. Be sure to check for leaks by filling with saline after removing the balloon.

Incise the peritoneum over the dome of the bladder, and excise the perivesical fat. Clip the right and left medial umbilical ligaments to allow the bladder to fall posteriorly. Incise the serosa and muscularis with a harmonic scalpel in the sagittal plane to expose the mucosa. Dissect the muscularis from the mucosa with a ureteroscope using electrodissection and blunt dissection with the beak of the instrument. A few muscle strands may be left behind. Oversew any punctures; postoperative leakage produces harmful perivesical fibrosis. The fibrin glue Tisseal may be applied over the exposed epithelial layer to reduce leakage. Evacuate the bladder. Place a Penrose drain through one of the ports, and sew it in place. Leave the urethral catheter in place for 1 week. Perform cystography to check for leaks, and remove the catheter if the repair is intact.

PATRICK C. CARTWRIGHT

Commentary by

The surgical concept of bladder autoaugmentation is simple: create a large augmenting bulge while preserving the urothelium. This avoids the problems associated with making bowel part of the urinary tract. Although this operation continues to be modified, I believe the idea of preserving urothelium will persist.

Some points on preparation and technique must be stressed. Prepare the patient as for an enterocystoplasty because this procedure may be required if the dissection proves technically inadequate and no bulging occurs. The patient (or parents) should be counseled as to this possibility.

We now use intraoperative cystometrics to evaluate the adequacy of the autoaugmentation. After the bladder is exposed, we insert a two-channel urodynamics catheter via the urethra and generate a pressure-volume curve before dissection. New curves can then be generated as the procedure progresses to assess changes. We expect at least a 30% to 50% increase in volume at 20, 30, and 40 cm of water during filling, with shifting of the filling curve to the right (better compliance). This catheter is left in to fill and empty as needed to aid the dissection.

The dissection should not be hurried; it can be tedious, especially if the bladder is deeply trabeculated. With a fine hemostat or tenotomy scissors, the plane between urothelium and muscle is defined. Do not overspread the blades, as this tears the underlying urothelium. If a perforation does occur at the edge of the dissection, a small amount of muscle is left at this site and the dissection is continued around it. This small amount of muscle is helpful to buttress closure of the perforation.

Continued

When the procedure is nearly completed, the rim of detrusor muscle may be split in several areas down toward the bladder neck, further releasing the epithelium to bulge. We now consider the psoas hitches optional. Finally, all bleeders should be carefully controlled because blood at the surgical site induces additional fibrosis.

During the recovery period, it is important periodically to distend the autoaugmentation to avoid contraction. This can be done by filling to a predetermined volume twice daily and clamping the catheter for 30 minutes. Constant pressure may be achieved by elevating the catheter drainage tubing to 30 to 40 cm above bladder level. At 7 days, if cystography shows no leakage, the catheter is removed and intermittent catheterization is begun.

Eventual fibrosis over the autoaugmented segment is the major concern in terms of limiting the augmenting effect over time. In 25 children (mostly myelodysplastic) in whom we have done long-term follow-up, we judge overall success as good in 50%, fair in 25%, and poor in 25%. In adults, Kennelly and associates (1994) have reported uniformly good outcomes in patients with various diseases, and Stohrer and associates (1995) in Germany have demonstrated marked improvement in capacity and compliance in spinal injury patients.

Interesting variations are being investigated. Dewan and Stefanek (1994) have described covering the urothelium with a demucosalized, pedicled gastric patch. In a similar mode, Gonzalez and coworkers (1995) and Lima and associates (1995) have demucosalized sigmoid and used it as backing to buttress the repair. They report little fibrosis, and early outcomes are encouraging.

Additional experience will provide clues as to which patients respond best and which techniques give the most reliable outcome. At present, we choose autoaugmentation for patients who have poor bladder compliance but do *not* have a severe reduction in bladder capacity. If it does not provide adequate augmentation, enterocystoplasty can be pursued without difficulty.

DIX POPPAS

Commentary by

I have stopped using the autoaugmentation for surgical correction of the poorly compliant, low-volume bladder. Regardless of the technique used, the long-term satisfactory outcome in our patients has not been encouraging. The detrusorectomy approach as opposed to the detrusorotomy seems to have a longer effect before fibrosis and contracture take place. The laparoscopic autoaugmentation was preferred to the open procedure with more rapid patient recovery and the technique was easily performed. Following the autoaugmentation, it is important to place some form of a "limiter" on the catheters used for clean intermittent catheterization to prevent patients from puncturing the thin urothelial lining.

Once nonsurgical methods have been exhausted for treating the low-volume, poorly compliant bladder—including maximum drug therapy, overnight catheter drainage, and compliant clean intermittent catheterization—patient selection appears to be the most essential step for the success of autoaugmentation procedures as the clinical outcome does not look as if it is durable. Despite the morbidity and potential complications of enterocystoplasty, in the long run, it seems to be a better choice for most patients.

The surgeon will need to discuss all pros and cons with the patient and family to determine the most effective balance between the limited long-term outcome of the autoaugmentation as opposed to the definite advantages of low morbidity and limited side effects when compared to enterocystoplasty.

Current studies to provide future alternatives for this complex group of patients focus on tissue engineering, synthetic bladder augmentation, and injection therapies such as botulinum toxin (Botox). It will be several years before definitive clinical evidence will be available.

Commentary by

PADDY DEWAN

The technique described in the text does not differentiate between removal and peeling back of the detrusor muscle, which are some of the differences described in the literature. It does appear from our cases of autoaugmentation demucosalized colo- and gastrocystoplasty that, after augmentation, the native bladder does improve with time. Once the average bladder pressure has been lowered and, therefore, there is no need to remove the detrusor muscle, leaving the muscle may improve the bladder enlargement prognosis by allowing better blood supply to more of the mucosa.

The operation of autoaugmentation has been popular in Europe, even though many studies have not shown improvement in a large proportion of patients. On the contrary, our experimental studies in sheep showed that no bladder enlargement occurred; in fact, the animals in the autoaugmentation group end up with a smaller bladder than the control group.

A point to be highlighted about autoaugmentation, whether performed in isolation or as part of an operation that covers the denuded mucosa with demucosalized muscle, is that the dissection to remove the detrusor muscle is time-consuming and difficult. Perforations of the mucosa should be avoided, as they are not as simple to repair as the text suggests, and the mucosa is often fragile in these patients who have had multiple infections. Also, the marked trabeculation of the bladder can mean that the surgeon is dissecting around diverticulae, which is diffiuclt.

Careful selection of patients may give good results without the need for the use of gut or ureter. However, a longer duration of conservative methods, including anticholinergics, urethral dilatation, infection control, intermittent catheterization, desmopressin (Minirin), and Botox should be considered before embarking on this technique. A word of caution is that the use of the laparoscope does not improve the prospect of the bladder being enlarged; it merely changes the access for the procedure. Also, radiotherapy is a contraindication to the use of a procedure that includes the autoaugmentation step.

UROTHELIAL-LINED BLADDER ENLARGEMENT

Since the early 20th century, researchers have been looking for a way to replace and enlarge the bladder with techniques that produce a urothelial-lined structure. To date the most reliable way of enlarging the bladder with urothelial-lined tissue is the ureter, provided there is a ureter of sufficient volume. Reports of adequate outcomes with small ureters exist and studies have published the ability to expand the ureter for subsequent ureterocystoplasty. We have serially dilated sheep ureters and found significant bladder augmentation to be achievable, but with a multistaged procedure that is not readily reproducible in patients. However, insertion of a double-J stent was successful in allowing us to achieve a successful ureterocystoplasty in one patient. Certainly, proceeding to ureterocystoplasty early in life seems to allow for a reduction in urinary tract infections and for spontaneous voiding in those whose pathology is not neuropathic.

In our studies of bladder augmentation, we have found that the addition of demucosalized bowel or stomach to the autoaugmented bladder gives a reliable outcome for those who do not have a tiny bladder initially.

In the laboratory sheep model, stomach is the most successful material added to the autoaugmentation. The sheep colon tolerates the dissection poorly because of the sheep sigmoid colon's unusual venous drainage. Our attempts to use peritoneum as the covering layer and the use of demucosalized segments without autoaugmentation did not successfully enlarge the bladder.

Tissue engineering with muscle and mucosal growth has had limited application, and the addition of bladder epithelium as a free graft in our hands has not produced a successful outcome.

Urothelial-lined cystoplasty is a better alternative than gut mucosa, with ureter being the best option and a muscle-backed autoaugment being the next best option, while a gut mucosal–lined enlargement is needed in very small bladders with normal-sized ureters.

Part VII

Continent Urinary Diversion

Chapter 103

Introduction to Continent Urinary Diversion

Incorporation of intestine into the urinary tract can achieve a larger capacity; it is done when both the urethra and the ureterovesical junctions are present (augmentation). It can replace the entire bladder down to the urethra (substitution), it can provide a urinary conduit if both urethra and the ureterovesical junctions are gone (noncontinent diversion), or it can provide a reservoir (continent diversion).

Replacement of the bladder may be needed in a child with epispadias or exstrophy when the bladder is taken to construct a continent urethra. In general, bowel substitution is a good alternative to diversion, although nocturnal incontinence can be expected in a number of cases.

Two general types of substitution are currently in use, one formed from opened ileum and the other from some rearrangement of the cecum and terminal ileum.

The amount of bowel incorporated should be such that a capacity of 500 to 600 mL is not exceeded because larger reservoirs promote excessive electrolyte absorption and use excessive lengths of ileum with resultant diarrhea. However, the new bladder must be quite large to maintain a low pressure, because children tend to void at normal intervals. Such a child will void by abdominal straining and must arise at night to void to keep dry.

Urinary reservoirs for vesical augmentation and substitution, as well as for urinary diversion, require adequate capacity at physiologic pressure.

In selection of a reservoir, other factors to be considered in addition to capacity and pressure are (1) tolerable electrolyte resorption or loss, (2) accessibility of the segment, (3) simplicity of the procedure, (4) need for an antireflux mechanism, (5) carcinogenic risk, and (6) special requirements and age of the patient.

Selection of a particular bowel segment for bowel augmentation depends on the preference of the surgeon, because there is little objective data indicating that one region is better than another. The colon allows implantation of a normal ureter using an antireflux technique. Combining the ileum with cecum based on the ileocecal artery allows formation of a mobilizable reservoir of good capacity, free from mass contraction, and an ileal arm to substitute for any loss of ileal length. However, exclusion of the ileocecal segment from the intestinal tract in children with neurogenic bladders who rely on constipation for rectal continence may result in loose stools and fecal incontinence, as well as later vitamin deficiency. A segment from the stomach can be useful, especially in a child with compromised renal function in whom electrolyte reabsorption would exacerbate the problem. The stomach is elastic; half of it can provide a reservoir with 300- to 500-mL capacity.

The objectives in any case are to make a low-pressure, compliant system during the filling phase (best achieved when the tubular organization of the bowel is disrupted to protect the upper tracts from back pressure during spontaneous mass contraction, which may in turn induce incontinence) and to provide adequate capacity to relieve the patient of inconvenient, frequent voiding or catheterization. In addition, protection from reflux must be provided, and incontinence prevented.

NEITHER URETHRA NOR URETEROVESICAL JUNCTION PRESENT

Continent diversion requires a reservoir, an antireflux mechanism, and a stoma that will not leak but can be catheterized. Continence can be achieved by forming a conduit by ileal intussusception, plicated terminal ileum, tunneled ureter, Monti segment, or appendix. Different parts of the bowel, including the stomach, can be used as the reservoir, and selection of the antireflux mechanism depends on the site of implantation.

Detubularized bowel segments provide a greater capacity at a lower pressure and require a shorter length of intestine than do intact segments. The function of the bowel as a reservoir is determined by its geometric configuration, accommodation, compliance, and contractility. The volume in the reservoir, which rises with the square of the radius, determines the geometric capacity. Thus, folding the bowel once doubles its capacity, and folding it twice increases it four times. Accommodation follows the Laplace relation: As the viscus fills, the stress on the wall increases, which permits the pressure to remain constant. Because the bowel is viscoelastic, it demonstrates compliance as it fills. Contractility is reduced by folding, because the several components of the reservoir no longer contract synchronously.

The purpose of continent diversion is to improve the quality of life of patients who have lost a usable bladder. It may well not improve renal function or prolong survival. Ultimately, the patient must make a choice between ileal diversion and more complicated continent procedures.

Continent urinary diversion is contraindicated in (1) children who have insufficient bowel because of intestinal or mesenteric adhesions, previous resection, or disease of the bowel; (2) those who would be adversely affected by loss of bowel length, especially children with neurogenic bladders, in whom resection of the ileocecal region can produce loose stools resulting in fecal incontinence; (3) those who have had prior radiation to the intestine; and (4) those who are inadequately motivated and skilled to take care of the new system, which may require intermittent self-catheterization.

Spontaneous rupture of continent reservoirs in children can occur, especially if the conduit is leakproof. It probably occurs during overdistention in the presence of peritoneal adhesions that can induce a seromuscular tear. The parents and child must be told of the virtues of frequent emptying and the dangers of overfilling. It is advisable that the child should not only wear a medical alert bracelet that states the situation but also have access to an 18-gauge needle to allow direct vesical puncture for relief of acute retention in an emergency. Malignancy may occur in bowel interposed in the urinary tract.

Undiversion to a continent reservoir is appealing, but is not suitable for very young children (even though their parents may desire it) or for those without adequate motivation. Poor renal function is not an absolute contraindication, because undiversion not only may provide a better life but may delay the time for renal transplantation.

Preoperatively, the function of the bladder must be assessed with a voiding cystourethrogram and urodynamic assessment. A small catheter can be placed percutaneously, so that the child can fill his or her bladder to assess volume, sensation, and continence.

Other factors in selection of a segment to be considered in addition to capacity and pressure are (1) acceptable electrolyte reabsorption and loss, (2) surgical accessibility and simplicity, (3) suitability for an antireflux mechanism, (4) carcinogenic risk, and (5) special requirements and age of the child.

A definitive procedure should be done at the first attempt, preferably through a very long midline incision, including transureterostomy with stenting. Use an omental wrap to prevent adhesions, place a cuff if an incontinence device is going to be needed later, and remove all abnormal tissue except the bladder, which may be used later to form a bladder neck, for the formation of a new urethra, or for future mucosal grafts. It is advisable to take the original version completely apart and then put it together, using all your talents. The greatest error is not doing enough. For conversion from an existing conduit, take down the peritoneal adhesions and dissect the conduit from the abdominal wall. Excise the previous small bowel anastomosis, including the site of the mesenteric division. Be familiar with more than one bowel technique, so that you can adapt to the circumstances found at surgery.

Several choices are available for continent reservoirs. One constructed entirely of ileum has the advantage of avoiding use of the ileocecal region but is technically more difficult. Some form of cecoileal reservoir, despite its functional disadvantages, is the technique most often selected, especially after cystectomy, whether done for malignancy or congenital vesical abnormality. The easily constructed Indiana pouch must incorporate most of the ascending colon. However, an ileal patch can reduce the amount of colon needed. The appendix interposed for a catheterizable stoma, as is done in the Penn pouch, is an alternative to using intussuscepted or plicated ileum. Ureterosigmoidostomy, which may be an alternative in adults with short life expectancies, seldom is suitable for children.

The stoma of a continent pouch, because it will not require coverage with an appliance, may be placed in a lower position, below the belt (bikini) line, but not so low that it cannot easily be catheterized by the patient while sitting. Do not be concerned about skin folds. The umbilicus may be preferable, because that area of the abdomen is thinner, there is less chance for parastomal hernia, and the stoma is easier to catheterize, especially if the child is in a wheelchair. It may be advisable to mark the standard site as well before undertaking the operation and also warn the patient, in case a ureteroileostomy is all that can be done.

COMPLICATIONS

Select children willing and able to assume responsibility for care of the diversion and complications will be fewer. Bacteriuria is the rule after pouch diversion involving intermittent catheterization, but clinically important infections are the result of increase in bacterial population from infrequent or incomplete emptying or from refilling because of reflux. Training is necessary to teach the child how to empty to the last drop. Mucus collection requires vigorous irrigation in the immediate postoperative period but becomes less of a problem with time when daily irrigation is usually sufficient. Calculi, usually struvite stones, result from stasis, but may form on staples. It is possible to manipulate or fragment the stones through the stoma, albeit with some risk to the mechanism; direct puncture into the reservoir is an alternative. Electrolyte imbalance with hyperchloremic acidosis is especially prevalent in these children with poor renal function and requires bicarbonate supplements, at least for the first 6 to 12 months. Unfortunately, spontaneous perforation of the neobladder is not rare and is often overlooked until the child is gravely ill. Voluntary overfilling may lead to repeated ischemia at a weak point in the reconstructed bladder. Malignancy may occur.

Intussusception following abdominal or retroperitoneal surgery on the intestinal tract in children is a rare complication, and presents as prolonged ileus followed by symptoms of small bowel obstruction. The pain is not colicky, and a mass is not felt, perhaps because the site of a postoperative intussusception is high (ileoileal or jejunojejunal). Immediate reoperation is required.

Vitamin B_{12} deficiency may appear after the terminal ileum is harvested. The disorder needs to be detected by obtaining vitamin B_{12} levels at regular intervals, so that lifelong parenteral cobalamine supplement may be given if needed.

Enuresis is a common, very distressing complication, probably resulting from obtunded sensation of fullness of the bladder, combined with perineal relaxation.

Chapter 104

Ileal Cecal Colonic Reservoir

INDIANA POUCH

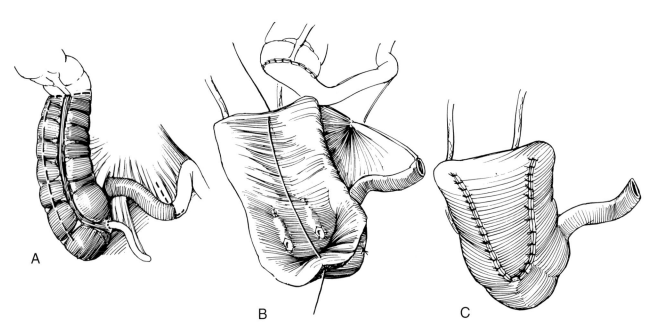

FIGURE 104-1. A, For an adolescent, take a 25-cm segment of cecum and ascending colon with 15 to 18 cm of terminal ileum. Be sure not to make the reservoir too small. If the cecum and ascending colon are short or especially narrow in diameter, take an additional 15- to 20-cm segment of ileum, open it, and place it as a patch over the open cephalad end and lateral margin of the cecum to augment the reservoir. (Alternatively, the appendix tunneled in the tenia can serve as the conduit, releasing the terminal ileum to be applied as the patch.) **B,** Split the ascending colon and cecum down the antimesenteric border to within 2 cm of the caudal tip. Proceed with appendectomy. **C,** Close the U-shaped defect by folding the distal portion of the colon into it with a running 3-0 synthetic absorbable suture to the mucosa and some of the muscularis, and a serosal Lembert stitch with occasional lock stitches, leaving the ileum to form the conduit. Anastomose the ileum to the ascending colon.

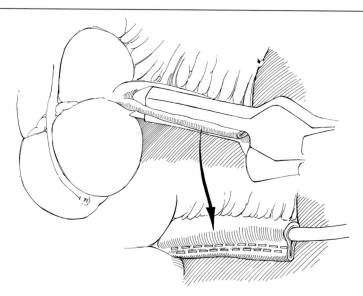

FIGURE 104-2. To form a conduit from the terminal ileum, place the GIA 90-mm stapler firmly on the antimesenteric border alongside an indwelling 14 F Robinson catheter *(arrow)*. The staple line should extend right down to the ileocecal valve. This is to create a very straight and smooth catheterizable channel. During the stapling process, make traction along the long axis of the terminal ileum to make sure the catheterizing channel is straight and free of folds. With the catheter in place, insert several interrupted sutures at the ileocecal junction to maintain the continence mechanism of the ileocecal valve, but not necessarily to "nipple" the terminal ileum into the cecum. Remove the catheter after filling the reservoir. There should be no leakage into the terminal ileum but if there is leakage, reinforce the suture line with a third layer of interrupted 3-0 silk sutures. Tunnel the ureters into the cecum through the tenia. Tack the ureters to the bowel wall outside the anastomosis and fix the adjacent cecum to the pelvic wall. Stents may be placed.

Insert a 22- or 24-F Malecot catheter as a cecostomy tube to drain the pouch for 3 weeks. Secure the pouch to the abdominal wall with 3-0 synthetic absorbable sutures so that the tube has a straight run through a stab wound. Bring the terminal ileum into the urethral remnant or, better, the umbilicus, although it may be placed in either the right or left lower quadrant. To make sure that after final positioning catheterization can be done without difficulty, repeatedly try catheterization throughout the final steps and after closing. Ease of catheterization is essential. Bring the cecostomy tube through the abdominal wall and tack the cecum to the peritoneum about it. Also bring the ureteral stents and a Penrose drain (led behind the pouch) out through stab wounds and fasten them internally to the fascia.

MICHAEL E. MITCHELL

Commentary by

The Indiana reservoir was initially developed from the Gilchrist procedure as a means of reconstructing of exstrophy in pediatric and young adult patients who previously had a cystectomy. The procedure has subsequently been successfully applied to the adult cystectomy population.

There are advantages to the procedure. It is not technically difficult to perform. The reservoir, antireflux mechanism, and continence mechanism are dependable and do not require an extensive learning curve. Furthermore, we believe the principles used are solid. Reflux is prevented by a submucosal tunnel. The reservoir is large and approaches a spherical configuration. The catheterizable channel is straight, without nipples or extensive surgical modification, to ensure ease of catheterization. No staples or nonresorbable sutures are in contact with urine in the reservoir.

Errors made in the construction of the reservoir are (1) improper selection of patients, (2) making a reservoir that is too small because not enough bowel was used (it is easy to make a reservoir too small but difficult to make one too big), and (3) making a catheterizable channel too tortuous or the plication stitches too tight so that catheterization is difficult. Repeated trial catheterization must be made throughout the final stages and after closing. Ease of catheterization is a primary objective. Proper patient selection and attention to surgical detail remain the important factors for success.

THE PENN POUCH CECOILEAL RESERVOIR (DUCKETT)

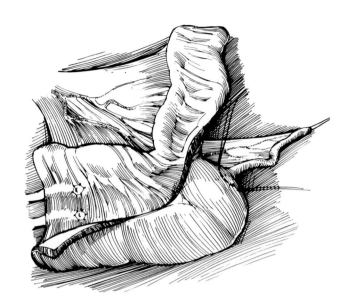

FIGURE 104-3. Prepare a cecal pouch by opening 30 cm of colon on the mesocolic tenia and 20 cm of ileum on its antimesenteric border. Fold the ileum into a U, and suture the edges with 3-0 synthetic absorbable running sutures. Insert the ileal patch into the cecal defect. Fold the distal end of the cecum to complete the pouch. If the mesoappendix is mobile and vascularized, excise the base of the appendix, taking a generous disc of cecum, while preserving the mesentery of the appendix. Close the cecal defect in two layers. Implant the ureters into the cecum by an antireflux method (see Chapter 105).

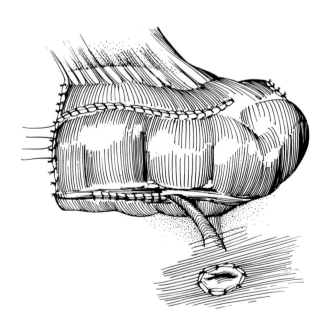

FIGURE 104-4. Rotate the appendix on its mesentery and trim its tip until an adequate lumen is reached. Calibrate it with a *bougie à boule* and continue to trim the end as necessary. Create an 8-cm trough in the most accessible tenia of the seromuscular wall of the ascending colon, laying back flaps and exposing submucosa for a width of 2 or 3 cm. The trough can be widened by grasping the bowel wall on both sides and gently pulling it open. Open the mucosa at the distal end of the groove and anastomose the opened tip of the appendix to it with interrupted 4-0 synthetic absorbable sutures. Close the lateral seromuscular flaps over the appendix with 4-0 synthetic absorbable sutures, taking care not to constrict its mesentery in the tunnel. To produce continence, 3 to 4 cm of appendix within the tunnel is sufficient. Lead the base of the appendix through the body wall in an appropriate site in the left lower quadrant, and suture it to the skin. (The actual site is not too important, as no appliance will be necessary.) Alternatively, the appendix may be shortened and placed with a V-flap in the umbilicus to hide it. Hitch the cecum and ascending colon to the retroperitoneum, so that the appendix and its mesentery are not kinked. If this procedure is used for bladder augmentation, fix the bladder to the psoas muscle so that the appendiceal mesentery does not move during bladder filling. Place a feeding tube (not such a large one that it stretches the appendix) to drain mucus from the pouch. Close the wound appropriately.

JOHN W. DUCKETT

Commentary by

The ureterocecoappendicostomy or Penn pouch uses the Mitrofanoff principle, although he did not describe this arrangement. We would, therefore, like to stake a claim to it. The Penn pouch was designed to simplify the construction of a continent urinary reservoir in patients with cancer of the bladder. Obviously, the normal anatomy must be complete—that is, the ileum, cecum, and appendix. A standard bowel prep should precede the procedure. Any refluxing implants of the ureter into the colon have been quite successfully corrected with either the Goodwin or Leadbetter techniques. The same principle applies to the placement of the appendix into the tenia. Surprisingly, the mesentery of the appendix can be engulfed in the seromuscular layer of the bowel without compression and still maintain a continent flap valve. Care must be taken to arrange the mesentery of the appendix in such a way that it is not stretched as the pouch is filled with urine. The appendicocecostomy avoids the complexity of ileal intussusception.

POSTOPERATIVE PROBLEMS FROM URINARY RESERVOIRS

Bacteriuria is inevitable in systems requiring self-catheterization, but pyelonephritis is rare. Mucus secretion is greater in reservoirs of cecum than of ileum, and will persist longer. In contrast, the ileal mucosa will atrophy. Mucus is often obstructive and requires weekly irrigations with sterile water or bicarbonate solution. Occasional obstruction during catheter drainage may be overcome by having the child cough. Stone formation is secondary to residual urine; manage it by direct-vision litholapaxy. The metabolic changes of increased serum chloride and decreased bicarbonate occur frequently. Some patients must be managed by ingestion of bicarbonate, more frequent emptying of the reservoir, and continuous drainage at night. Loss of potassium is not a problem. Renal function must be monitored. Urinary fistulas can occur around the valve in an ileocecal reservoir; they require reconstruction. A leak from an ileal pouch will usually close with continuous catheter drainage.

ALAN B. RETIK

Commentary by

Although we much prefer the Mitrofanoff, or flap-valve, principle for continence, we occasionally do not have this option and require a nipple for continence. In this situation, it is preferable to employ the Indiana rather than the Mainz pouch, because less bowel is used. This is of major importance in the myelodysplastic population. It is preferable to incise the antimesenteric portions of isolated segments of bowel with cautery rather than scissors.

When constructing an Indiana pouch, we employ staples rather than sutures. This ensures a more uniform caliber of the conduit. Babcock clamps grasp the antimesenteric portion of the ileum, which is catheterized with a 12-F red rubber catheter, and a 6-cm GIA stapler is applied to the terminal ileum. The excess bowel wall is removed by the stapler, and the remaining bowel will cover the catheter smoothly. In addition, the gastrointestinal anastomosis (GIA) stapler is used at the ileocecal junction to create a funnel-shaped segment of the terminal ileum. This area is then plicated with 3-0 silk Lembert sutures; in effect, this also plicates the ileocecal valve.

We have found the Heineke-Mikulicz principle in the formation of the Indiana pouch quite effective; for the most part, it eliminates the necessity for additional ileum as a patch. When we are converting a preexisting ileal conduit to an Indiana pouch and the capacity of the cecum is marginal, the preexisting ileum can be used to augment the colon.

No matter what technique is employed, when performing continent diversion it is extremely important to ensure at the operating table that the continence mechanism is effective and that the conduit can easily be catheterized with suitable catheters at various degrees of reservoir filling. If there is any difficulty catheterizing a conduit in the operating room, it will be that much harder afterward. Therefore, I usually test the conduit with various types of catheters that will be employed postoperatively, and I leave the conduit catheterized with an indwelling Silastic catheter, which is tied off and sutured to the skin. I leave this in for approximately 7 to 10 days.

Chapter 105

Ileal Reservoir with Ileal Catheterizable Channel

When both augmentation and suprapubic continent stoma for clean intermittent catheterization are required, the classical approach is to create an intestinal reservoir and additionally incorporate an efferent tube such as an appendix or Yang-Monti tube. A more efficient approach is a reservoir that includes a tubular continent outlet for catheterization within its design. In patients with neurogenic bowel the appendix can be left in situ for a simultaneous Malone antegrade continence enema (see Chapter 94).

Prior to surgery the patient and family should be coached on all aspects of clean intermittent catheterization. Preoperative preparation includes rigorous bowel clean out and intravenous antibiotics.

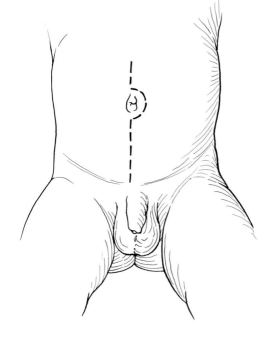

FIGURE 105-1. Position: Supine, with all pressure points padded. Incision: Make a midline incision with placement of the catheterizable efferent channel against the anterior wall of the reservoir to reinforce the effectiveness of the valve mechanism. The stoma should exit at or below the umbilicus.

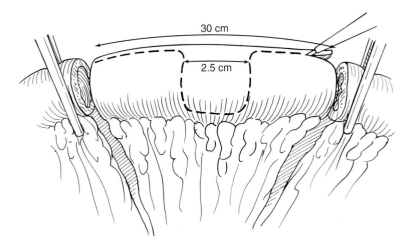

FIGURE 105-2. At a distance of more than 10 cm from the ileocecal valve, isolate 30 cm of ileum from the gastrointestinal track. Design cranially a 2.5-cm flap of the anterior wall of the ileum while opening the rest of the ileum at the antimesenteric surface.

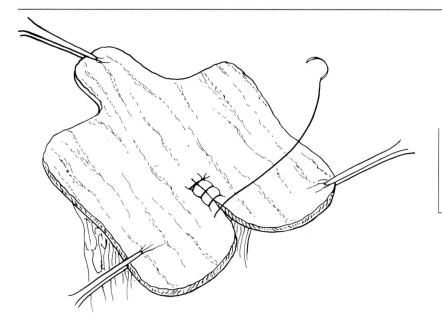

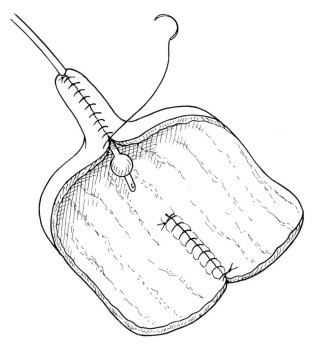

FIGURE 105-3. Place the opened ileum in an inverted-U position and anastomose the proximal borders with 3-0 long-acting absorbable sutures to obtain the posterior wall of the reservoir.

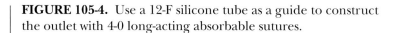

FIGURE 105-4. Use a 12-F silicone tube as a guide to construct the outlet with 4-0 long-acting absorbable sutures.

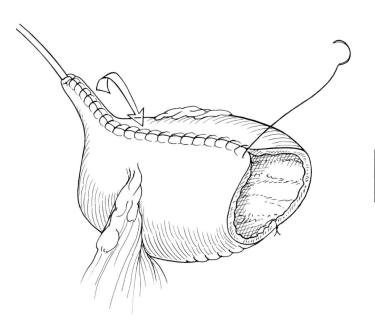

FIGURE 105-5. Applying the same principles, join the lateral borders of the ileal segment and close the anterior wall of the reservoir.

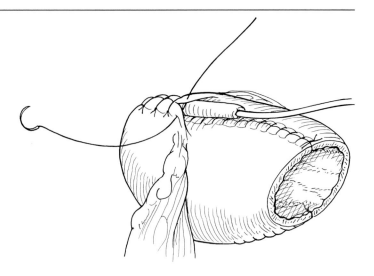

FIGURE 105-6. Embed the tube (see *arrow* in Fig. 105-5) over the seromuscular sutures at the reservoir's dome to produce the valve mechanism. Use four to five permanent Prolene 2-0 sutures to imbricate the efferent limb.

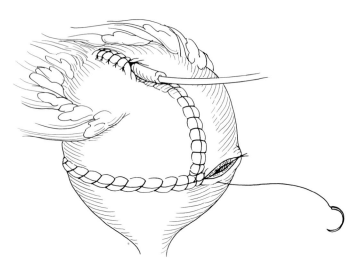

FIGURE 105-7. Use the reservoir to augment the bladder using 3-0 absorbable sutures.

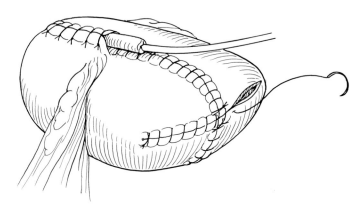

FIGURE 105-8. In the case of complete bladder substitution, harvest additional ileum, implant the ureters directly into the reservoir, or leave an afferent 10-cm nondetubularized ileal loop adjacent to the reservoir.

Isolate 30 cm of ileum for augmentations and an additional 10 cm for bladder substitutions to create an afferent loop nonrefluxing ureteral reimplantation (total of 40 cm). Open the bladder dome extensively for a wide anastomosis (augmentations).

An infraumbilical pseudoumbilical stoma is preferred in cases of bladder augmentation. Anchor the reservoir dome with permanent suture to the abdominal wall to further increase the resistance of the outlet tube against the abdominal wall. The distal part of the efferent tube should exit the valve directly toward the stomal skin without tortuosity to ease catheterization.

The same principles can be applied to the transverse colon in patients with a history of irradiation.

Leave a 12-F silicone Foley tube and cystostomy in place for 3 weeks. Parents should clean the reservoir with a saline solution daily to prevent mucus occlusion of the urinary tubes. Patients are readmitted on day 21 for self-catheterization training controlled by a stoma-specialized nurse.

POSTOPERATIVE PROBLEMS

Urinary retention due to mucus obstruction can be treated with irrigation. Difficulties with the first catheterization should be evaluated endoscopically. Typically they will resolve with additional catheter placement for 2 to 4 weeks until healing is complete. Stoma stenosis can be treated by overnight catheterization and local dilatation. Urinary leakage through the stoma should be assessed with urodynamic evaluation and may respond to injectable agents if bladder compliance is optimal.

ANTONIO MACEDO, JR.

Commentary by

The presented technique has the advantage of providing a continent catheterizable reservoir with outlet tube constructed altogether from the same bowel segment. The incorporation of appendix or a Monti tube into the reservoir is precluded thus making the procedure faster, simpler, and (theoretically) having less morbidity. The first case operated by us was done in June 1998 and, so far, 115 patients have been operated on in São Paulo. Augmentation and bladder substitution (rhabdomyosarcoma cases) with ileum and transverse colon (previous irradiation) have been performed with satisfactory results. (We reported later on the same principle of outlet channel to create left colon channels in severe fecal incontinence for MACE procedure with excellent results.)

Some lessons we have learned from experience follow:

1. The 2.5- to 3-cm–width flap from the anterior wall of the intestine can be brought through the posterior wall up to the mesentery to produce a longer flap and consequently a tube that can easily reach the skin, even in obese patients.
2. The valve-embedding mechanism of the tube is based on the serous-lined tunnel principle or a Nissen-like valve. We have proved in an experimental model that angulation of the tube against the anterior wall of the reservoir is more important than extension of imbrication to promote resistance. We therefore recommend that the anterior wall of the reservoir should be fixed to the inferior abdominal wall by sutures. The embedding sutures of the tube should include only seromuscular layers with nonabsorbable material (Prolene 2-0 or 3-0 sutures).
3. In some cases, overcontinence was found in extremely filled reservoirs not allowing introduction of a catheter through the stoma. In cases of augmentation, do not force but rather catheterize through the urethra and limit the interval between catheterizations to 4 to 5 hours.

Chapter 106

Ureterosigmoidostomy

After loss of the bladder, techniques for urinary storage should be directed not only at providing continence but also at preserving renal function and maintaining normal electrolyte balance. Ideally, the child should be freed from appliances, should be able to empty urine voluntarily, and should remain continent. Either place a substitute bladder or devise a reservoir for intermittent catheterization. Options include reservoirs formed from ileum, cecum, sigmoid colon, or stomach that include antireflux and continence mechanisms. Ureterosigmoidostomy is the oldest (and certainly the technically easiest) method of continent diversion. Despite its limitations (electrolyte imbalance, potential for upper-tract damage, and association with adenocarcinoma near the ureteral anastomosis), it still has a place in certain cases.

The Boyce-Vest operation is an alternative that may produce better long-term results at the cost of a permanent colostomy. Here the base of the closed exstrophic bladder is simply anastomosed to the adjacent bowel wall.

Determine if the anal sphincteric mechanism is intact digitally by anal stimulation, and also by having the child hold warm water for a couple of hours. Perform an intravenous urogram or computed tomography (CT) urogram to be sure there is no ureteral dilation (a contraindication to this operation). Provide both mechanical and antibacterial bowel preparation. This procedure is most successful in achieving urinary continence when done in children who have attained fecal continence.

Place the child on a liquid diet for 24 hours, and prepare the bowel with polyethylene glycol-electrolyte solution (GoLYTELY). Provide two cleansing enemas with neomycin solution the day before the operation. Give cephalosporin intravenously 6 hours preoperatively and continue for 72 hours. It may be advisable to install a central venous line.

CLOSED TECHNIQUE FOR URETEROSIGMOID ANASTOMOSIS

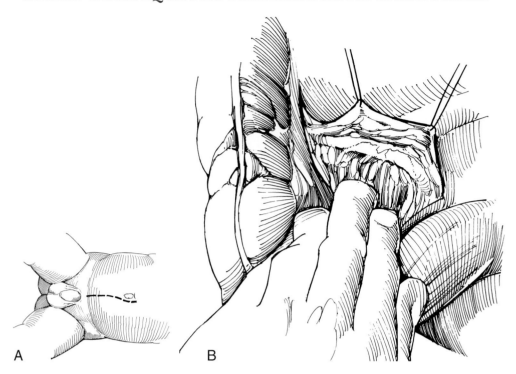

A   B

FIGURE 106-1. Position: Supine, in slight Trendelenberg position. Insert a large Malecot rectal tube and tape it near the anus with waterproof tape applied over tincture of benzoin. For a straight rectal tube, cut extra holes and suture it para-anally. If right-handed, stand on the right side of the patient.

A, Incision: Make a midline transabdominal incision. In exstrophy patients, the incision must be placed well off the midline over one belly of rectus muscle. Excise the bladder first, leaving the transected ureters to drain freely. Have a nasogastric tube inserted and palpate it in the stomach. Free any adhesions. Pack the small bowel in the upper part of the abdominal cavity. Determine the sites of the incisions in the parietal peritoneum. Move the rectosigmoid junction to the right and incise the parietal peritoneum where it touches the tenia to be sure that the anastomosis can be retroperitonealized.

B, Elevate the left peritoneal flap and expose the left ureter. Carefully mobilize it sharply and bluntly from its bed, preserving all of the adventitial vessels. Watch for vessels entering laterally below the pelvic brim and medially above it; clamp, cut, and ligate them. Continue releasing the ureter to as close to the bladder as possible to provide a long ureter for a low anastomosis. Place a 4-0 silk stay suture in the ureter; clamp it distal to the suture with a right-angle clamp, and divide and ligate it. If the ureter is small, it may be ligated just proximal to the site of division to allow it to dilate before anastomosis. Repeat the procedure on the right side by moving the sigmoid colon to the left. Incise the adjacent peritoneum at the site of contact with the colon; here the retroperitoneal incision can be made somewhat more medially. Expose and free the right ureter as was done on the left.

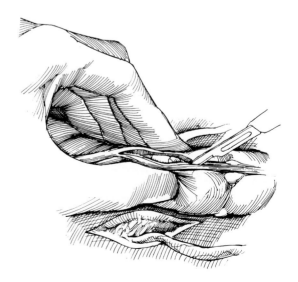

FIGURE 106-2. With the left thumb and forefinger, grasp the sigmoid colon at its junction with the rectum to elevate the tenia. Incise the peritoneal coat and muscularis for 5 to 6 cm with a long-handled #15 blade scalpel until the white submucosa is expressed.

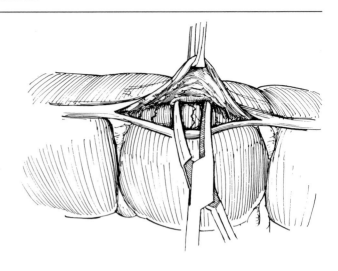

FIGURE 106-3. Separate the muscle from the submucosa with a curved mosquito clamp for at least 1 cm on either side of the incision to provide muscular flaps to cover the anastomosis.

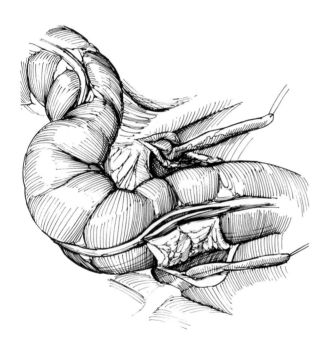

FIGURE 106-4. Tack the medial flap of the posterior peritoneum adjacent to the bowel incision on the right to the serosa with 4-0 or 5-0 synthetic absorbable sutures.

FIGURE 106-5. Hold up a bit of the submucosa in fine forceps and excise the elevated tip to leave a 3-mm opening into the bowel. Mucus will exude; if not, insert the tip of a small clamp to be sure the bowel has been entered. The opening will enlarge surprisingly during the anastomotic procedure.

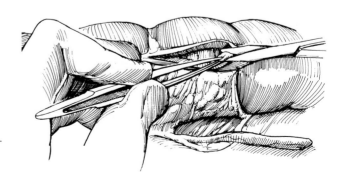

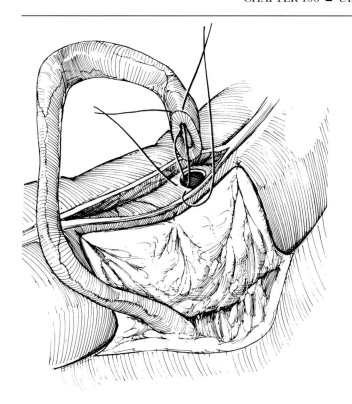

FIGURE 106-6. Trim the ureter to the proper length to avoid kinking. Spatulate it and replace the stay suture. Place a 4-0 or 5-0 synthetic absorbable suture through the mucosa and submucosa of the bowel from outside in, and then through the apex of the ureteral cut from the inside out. Place a second suture next to the first, and tie both of them.

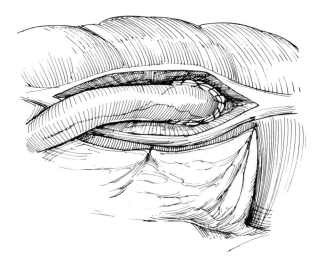

FIGURE 106-7. Run one suture down each side, locking a stitch occasionally, and tie them together at the tip.

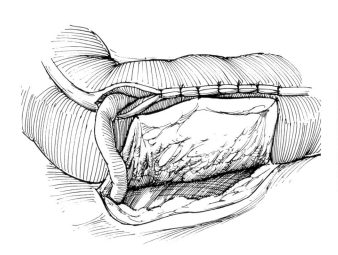

FIGURE 106-8. Approximate the seromuscular layer over the anastomosis with interrupted 3-0, 4-0, or 5-0 synthetic absorbable sutures, taking care not to constrict the site of ureteral exit (leave the hiatus twice the diameter of the ureter). Bring the area of closure to the lateral flap of peritoneum and suture it in place with 4-0 silk sutures.

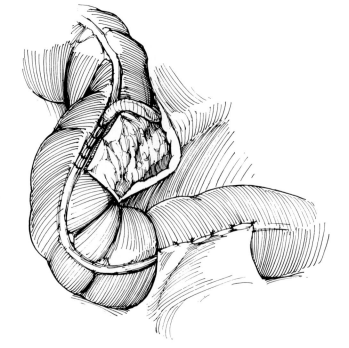

FIGURE 106-9. Repeat the procedure on the left side. Stents usually are not indicated. Close without drainage.

CLOSED TECHNIQUE FOR URETERAL IMPLANTATION (KELALIS MODIFICATION)

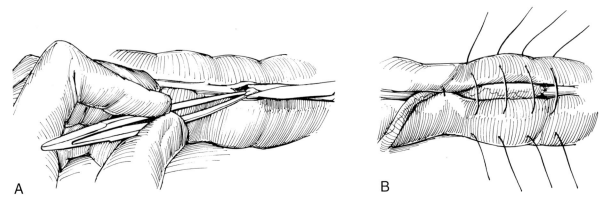

A   B

FIGURE 106-10. A, As described in Figure 88-3, spatulate the ureter. Incise through the muscular coat of the colon for 1 or 2 cm, just enough to expose the submucosa. Pick it up in Adson forceps and remove a very small button of mucosa and submucosa with fine scissors. **B,** Anastomose the mucosa of the ureter to the mucosa at the opening in the bowel using interrupted 4-0 or 5-0 synthetic absorbable sutures in a watertight fashion. Incorporate the anastomosis into the bowel by placing a series of 4-0 nonabsorbable sutures over the ureter. Insert the stitch laterally and exit about 1 cm from the tenia, and then enter on the other side 1 cm from the tenia and exit laterally. Tie the sutures successively from the distal end, making sure that the ureter is not constricted.

TRANSCOLONIC URETEROINTESTINAL ANASTOMOSIS (GOODWIN)

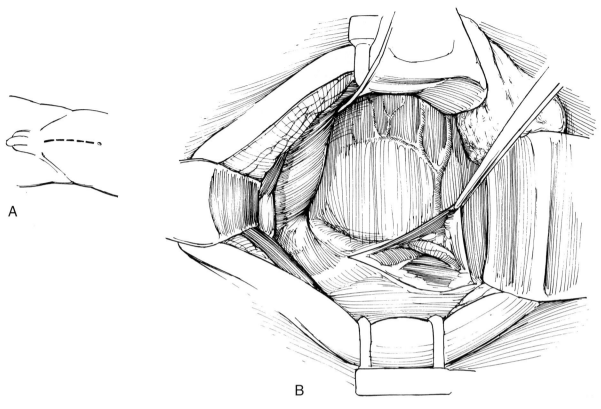

FIGURE 106-11. **A,** Incision: Lower midline. **B,** Retract the sigmoid colon to the left, and incise the peritoneum over the right ureter, just below the crossing of the iliac vessels (where it is most easily identified), and continue the incision to as low a point as possible.

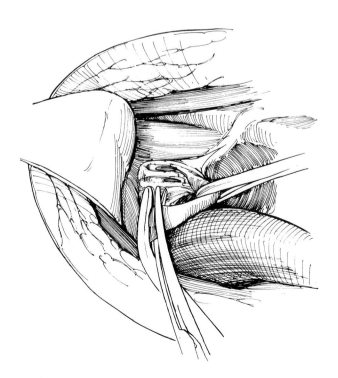

FIGURE 106-12. Free the right ureter sharply from its bed from the level of the sacral promontory, a distance of 10 to 12 cm toward the bladder, taking care to preserve the vessels in the adventitia. A small branch from the iliac artery is commonly encountered; keep it intact. Dissection of the ureter above its crossing of the iliac artery may jeopardize its circulation. Clamp the ureter distally with a right-angle clamp if it has not already been freed. Place a 4-0 silk stay suture just proximal to the clamp. Divide the ureter between, and ligate the stump with a 4-0 synthetic absorbable suture. Release the left ureter similarly.

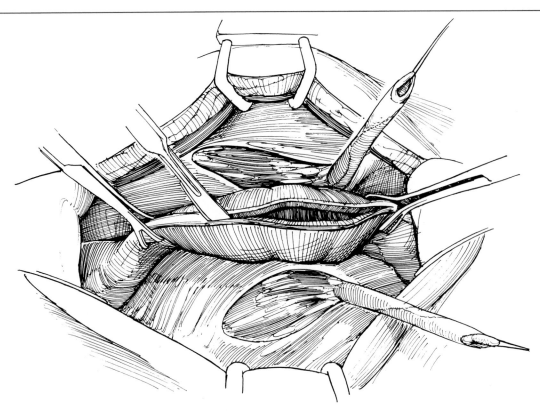

FIGURE 106-13. Grasp the rectosigmoid and pull it out of the pelvis to permit positioning of the ureterocolic anastomosis as low as possible. Incise the bowel along the exposed tenia coli as low as feasible for a distance of 10 to 12 cm, cutting through the wall into the lumen. Stay sutures may be helpful.

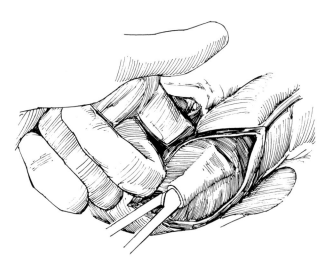

FIGURE 106-14. Insinuate the left index finger under the bowel, inserting it retroperitoneally into the defect used to expose the left ureter. Evert the posterior wall of the bowel through the colotomy. Make a 1-cm transverse incision through the bowel mucosa and submucosa against the fingertip near the distal end of the exposed bowel wall. Alternatively, remove a button of mucosa and submucosa. Place a stay suture and infiltrate the submucosa proximally with saline. Gently introduce a small curved clamp or iris scissors between the mucosal layer and the thin muscularis to make a tunnel 3 to 4 cm long, very similar to that made for ureteroneocystostomy. Alternatively, split the mucosa, lay the ureter in the trough, and cover it.

Rotate the fine curved clamp so that the tip is directed posteriorly. Press it against the finger outside and push it through the right lateral bowel wall into the retroperitoneal space. Avoid the vessels palpable in the mesentery. Spread the jaws of the clamp to make an adequate opening for the ureter in the muscularis. Pass the tip of the clamp retroperitoneally to the right, out through the peritoneal defect.

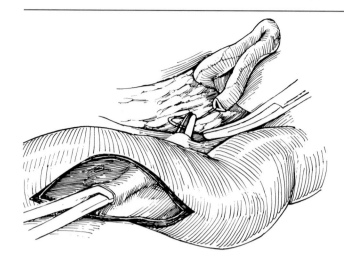

FIGURE 106-15. Grasp the stay suture on the right ureter and draw the ureter into the bowel without tension. Repeat these maneuvers for the left ureter so that it will enter the bowel alongside the right one. Alternatively, make two tunnels.

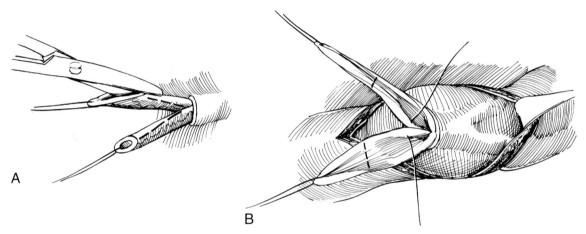

FIGURE 106-16. A, Trim excess ureteral length, and spatulate the ureters up to their point of entrance into the rectosigmoid while there is no traction on the stay suture. **B,** Suture the two ureters together along their medial edges for a distance of 2 cm with several interrupted 4-0 synthetic absorbable sutures. Use the stay suture, not forceps, for manipulation.

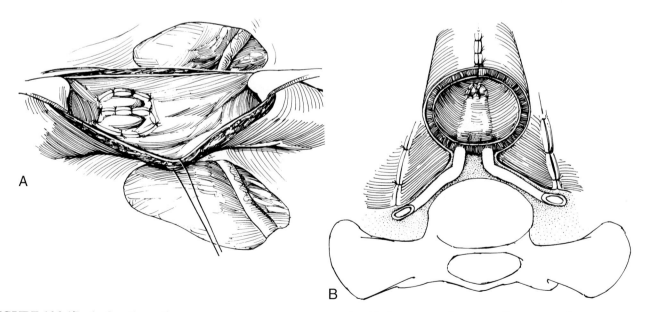

FIGURE 106-17. A, Continue the mucosa-to-mucosa anastomosis with interrupted sutures. Do not use forceps. **B,** Cross-sectional view.

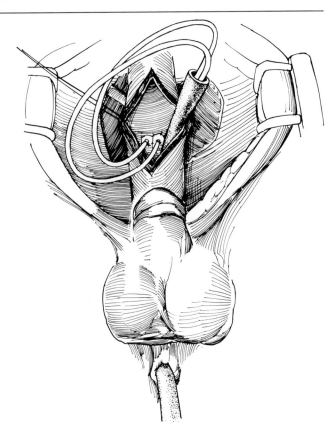

FIGURE 106-18. Stenting catheters (8-F infant feeding tubes, single-J catheters, double-J catheters, or an open-ended stent) may be placed. Cut the distal end of the left one obliquely for later identification. Suture each stent to the posterior wall of the bowel with a fine chromic catgut suture. If a rectal tube was not placed initially, pass one out the anus from above. Insert the stenting catheters into its flanged end and draw them out of the anus within the rectal tube.

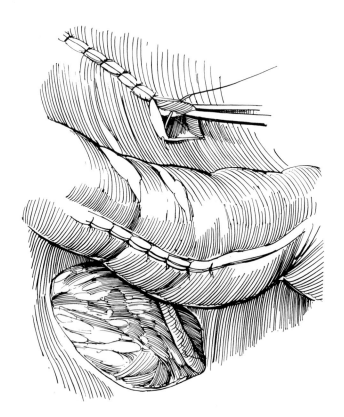

FIGURE 106-19. Close the colostomy in two layers with continuous 4-0 chromic catgut sutures for the inner layer and interrupted 4-0 synthetic absorbable sutures for the outer serosal and muscularis layers, and reapproximate the edges of the retroperitoneal openings. At the end of the operation, suture the rectal tube adjacent to the anus and tape the stents to the inside of the thigh with waterproof tape applied over tincture of benzoin. Postoperatively, check their security daily. Perform a stentogram at 7 days; if the tract is intact, remove the stents. A contrast enema probably is not needed prior to the 10th day. If no extravasation is seen, remove the rectal tube. Continue prophylactic antibiotics postoperatively for a month and watch for electrolyte disturbances.

POSTOPERATIVE PROBLEMS

Oliguria and anuria are usually secondary to intraoperative dehydration and hypotension. Give a bolus of mannitol intravenously. Perform ultrasonography to detect bilateral hydronephrosis; if present, place percutaneous nephrostomies at once before anastomotic leakage occurs. Urine leakage will be heralded by fever and signs of peritonitis. Immediate reoperation is mandatory, although small leaks have been known to close spontaneously if the rectum is well drained. A pelvic abscess may develop after the first 5 or 10 days and requires drainage. Perform an ultrasound study (or a CT scan) to detect it.

Peritonitis, formerly a frequent complication and cause of death, now seldom occurs if the bowel is well prepared, suitable broad-spectrum antibiotics have been given, and the anastomoses have been extraperitonealized. When there are recurrent urinary tract infections, look for ureteral obstruction or reflux as the cause. To detect reflux, give an enema with water-soluble contrast medium (not barium). Obstruction at the anastomotic site can be avoided by using a meticulous mucosa-to-mucosa technique. However, because of the possibility of late stenosis, urograms should be made at least yearly to allow reoperation at the first evidence of upper-tract dysfunction. Significant hyperchloremic acidosis usually occurs only in children with existent or developing renal impairment. It can be prevented by starting a low-chloride diet with added sodium and potassium as bicarbonate or citrate. Titrate the dose to keep the serum bicarbonate level nearly normal. Treat such a decompensated child with a rectal tube, fluids, and additional sodium and potassium bicarbonate. Frequent evacuation, and retention of a rectal tube at night, will reduce absorption and also avoid the not unusual nocturnal incontinence.

Adenocarcinoma occurs at the site of anastomosis in 5% of cases, after an average interval of 25 years. On the fifth anniversary, start to screen the stools every 3 months for occult blood, and perform colonoscopy yearly. Should the ureterosigmoidostomy have to be converted to a ureteroileostomy or to a pouch, be sure to excise the potentially active terminal ureter and an adjacent cuff of colon.

RAIMUND STEIN

Commentary by

Rectal reservoirs are the oldest functioning form of continent urinary diversion. Many modifications have been made over the last century, the latest being the rectosigmoid pouch. This specific type of rectal reservoir achieves lower pressures by detubularization and spherical reconfiguration.

Patient selection for this type of diversion includes identifying potential risks for postoperative stress incontinence. One test supplies a 300-mL tap water enema, which should be kept for 2 to 3 hours during normal daily activities, and overnight for a minimum of 4 to 6 hours to allow a sufficient amount of undisturbed sleep.

I agree with Goodwin that an antireflux ureteral implantation technique is required. In nondilated, nonfibrotic ureters, this is achieved by a sufficiently long submucosal tunnel. To ensure that there is no kinking of the ureter during implantation, no stent is inserted until all suturing is done. This maneuver allows the surgeon to observe whether urine drainage remains undisturbed. The stricture rate for nondilated and nonfibrotic ureters ranges between 3% and 7%. However, in most children with indications for a rectosigmoid pouch—that is, in those with bladder exstrophy with no suitable plate for primary bladder closure, or after failed primary bladder closure, and in children who live in an area with difficulties of obtaining medical supplies—a normal ureter is a rare finding. In most cases, the ureters are dilated or show some degree of fibrosis. In these cases, a simple submucosal tunnel has a high risk for complications. If the ureters are long enough, we perform a serosa-lined extramural tunnel according to the technique of Abol-Enein. Using this technique, the diameter of the tunnel can be adapted to the diameter of the ureter and a tunnel length of 4 to 6 cm can be achieved. We also use this technique for ureteral reimplantation because of potential stenosis. If the ureter is too short to achieve a sufficiently long tunnel, an ileal intussusception nipple (as used for the Mainz pouch I technique) is attached to the rectosigmoid pouch with two rows of staples. The ureters are then implanted into the ileum according to the Nesbit or Wallace technique. Another advantage of interposing an ileal segment between the ureters and the colon seems to be the reduction of risk for secondary malignancies. However, this has only been shown in an animal model and has not been proven in humans.

Long-term follow-up is essential. Stenosis of the ureters occurs mostly within the first 5 years. Thus, regular renal ultrasound is mandatory. In case of necessity of ureteral reimplantation or conversion into another form of urinary diversion, excision of the ureteral stumps is mandatory. One of our own bladder exstrophy patients, who was converted to conduit diversion, developed carcinoma at the ureteral implantation site and died due to metastatic disease. Similar cases are published in the literature.

The acid–base equilibrium including electrolytes must be checked on a regular basis. Over long-term follow-up, we could demonstrate that these patients have a higher risk of osteoporosis if the acid–base equilibrium is not balanced. Approximately 50% to 60% of our patients have to use alkalizing oral agents to prevent clinical acidosis.

Continued

Secondary malignancies are the most important late complications. Tumors develop almost always at the ureteral implantation site. In patients with bladder exstrophy, we observed adenomas after 14 to 29 years (median age of 24 years) in 13.5% of the patients and adenocarcinomas after 24 to 38 years (median age of 30 years) in 10.8% at the ureter implantation site. In all cases the sigmoid colon was resected together with the mesenteric lymph nodes. Continent cutaneous diversion was performed in two patients; one patient with impaired renal function had an ileal conduit. Two patients died from metastatic disease. In patients with urinary diversion for treatment of a benign disease, the minimal latency for tumor development was more than 10 years. When diversion was performed for a malignant disease, minimal latency for secondary malignancies was 5 years. Therefore, annual endoscopy starting 10 years after surgery is absolutely mandatory in patients with a benign disease; in the remaining patients, endoscopy should start 5 years after the operation. Patient selection regarding compliance is also strongly recommended. Sigmoidoscopy should be performed by an experienced endoscopist, who knows exactly where to look for tumors and what a normal ureter ostium looks like. If the operator is unfamiliar with this kind of diversion, he may inadvertently resect the entire ureteral implantation site. If the adenocarcinoma is detected at an early stage, curative surgery including conversion into a continent reservoir is possible.

Section 7

TESTES AND GROIN

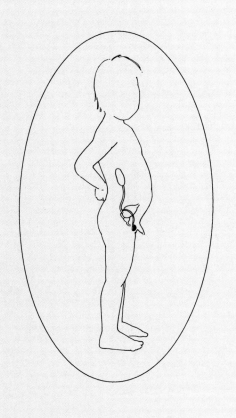

Part I

Testes Reconstruction

Chapter 107

Testis Biopsy

In boys, testis biopsy is better performed under general anesthesia. Local anesthesia (cord block) may be suitable for older adolescents.

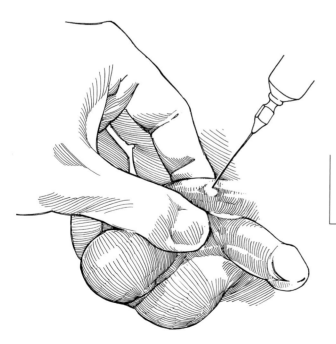

FIGURE 107-1. Provide sedation. Infiltrate about the cord with 1% lidocaine without epinephrine when the boy has been sedated and is cooperative. Avoid puncturing the vas; inject beside it.

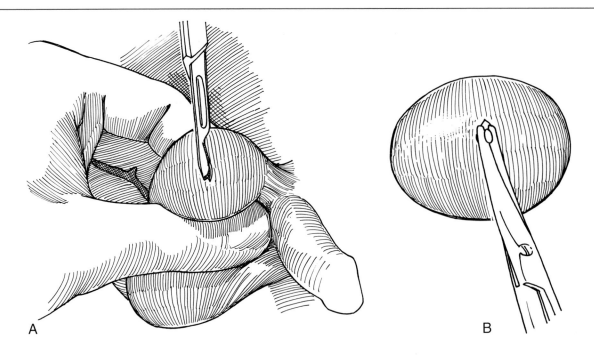

FIGURE 107-2. A, Grasp the testis in the fingers of the left hand, and press it up against the stretched scrotal skin. Infiltrate the skin and the dartos layer with 1% lidocaine without epinephrine. Do not inject the tunica albuginea. Incise transversely through the skin, dartos muscle, and tunica vaginalis; these layers will retract as the scrotum is squeezed. Make a short transverse incision in the tunica albuginea in the direction of the underlying small vessels. Because the testis itself may not be fully anesthetized, cut sharply and quickly with a #15 blade for a distance of 5 or 6 mm to allow extrusion of a bead-sized portion of testicular tubules. **B,** Excise the extruded tubules with the belly of a small curved scissors or a fresh scalpel, and pass the biopsy specimen on the scissors or scalpel directly into Bouin's solution (not formalin). Do not relax the grip on the scrotum.

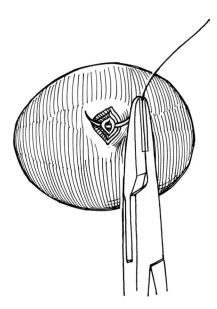

FIGURE 107-3. Close the tunica albuginea with a running 5-0 plain absorbable suture. Observe for hemostasis. Release the grasp on the scrotum.

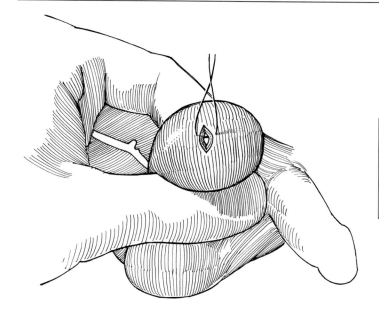

FIGURE 107-4. Approximate the skin together with the dartos layer with several stitches of 5-0 absorbable suture. Repeat the procedure on the other side, if indicated. In adolescents, apply a nonadherent dressing and a large padded scrotal suspensory. In children, simply apply collodion to the incision.

POSTOPERATIVE PROBLEMS

A hematocele can appear if the tunica albuginea is not closed over a subtunical vessel. Note: With cryptorchidism, biopsy will not detect a preinvasive phase of an adult germ cell tumor.

JULIA BARTHOLD SPENCER

General anesthesia is routine for open testicular biopsy in boys, although local infiltration of 0.25% plain bupivacaine is useful for postoperative pain control. When performing wedge biopsy, keep in mind that the areas of the testis least likely to contain major superficial arterial branches are the medial and lateral aspects of the superior pole; avoid the lower pole, particularly at its anterior aspect. I use 6-0 Monocryl suture for closure of the tunica albuginea and Dermabond adhesive for wound closure after approximation of the skin.

Needle aspiration biopsy should be considered in boys with leukemia when analysis of the testis is indicated, as it has low morbidity and appears to be similar in accuracy to open biopsy. Testicular biopsy in boys with cryptorchidism may provide some prognostic information regarding fertility potential, but limited sensitivity and specificity do not warrant its use in routine clinical settings.

HSI-YANG WU

I prefer to incise the tunica albuginea vertically, just below the epididymis, and to undermine the edges with a knife blade to free up the tubules. Regardless of which direction the biopsy is taken, the point is to avoid injuring the vessels supplying the seminiferous tubules. There have been concerns raised about the possibility of injuring the testis during biopsy. The 11-year follow-up of 112 prepubertal cryptorchid patients biopsied at the Children's Hospital of Philadelphia found no evidence of antisperm antibodies and no increased incidence of testicular microlithiasis after puberty was completed, suggesting that the procedure is safe.

Commentary by

Commentary by

Chapter 108

Inguinal Orchiopexy (Open Technique)

ORCHIOPEXY

Orchiopexy may be performed as early as 6 months of age. By that time, spontaneous testicular descent for palpable testes is unlikely and the boy is sufficiently developed to undergo anesthesia and operation. For nonpalpable testes spontaneous descent rarely occurs after 6 months and the surgery can be safely performed at that age. Furthermore, at 6 months of age the distance from the nonpalpable abdominal testes to the scrotum is less than in an older child, facilitating tension-free, testicular artery–sparing orchiopexy. Because thermal damage to the germ cells begins very early, before the end of the second year, treat cryptorchidism before these irreversible changes occur.

Orchiopexy can usually be performed as an outpatient procedure, unless a cardiopulmonary condition is present. Allow solid food up to 8 hours, formula up to 6 hours, and clear liquids up to 4 hours before surgery. Operations on infants require magnification and special technique, particularly if the testis is in a high position. Further, recognize the need for other than standard orchiopexy before dissecting the testis from its bed and losing the alternative option for one- (see Chapter 112) and two-stage (see Chapter 111) orchiopexy.

The inguinal region in infants differs somewhat from that in adults in ways that are important for surgery at this age. The superficial fascia is much thicker, resembling the aponeurosis of the external oblique muscle, which in turn is relatively thin, with delicate medial and lateral crura. The inguinal canal runs more transversely. The cremaster muscle is very well developed with fibers that blend with those of the internal oblique muscle. Before the boy reaches 2 years of age, the bladder extends well into the abdomen and can be injured during medial exposure of the spermatic cord.

A palpable, undescended testis will usually be found in the superficial inguinal pouch or close to the internal ring. If the descended testis is enlarged, consider previous contralateral intrascrotal torsion with testicular atrophy; perform scrotal exploration to locate the remnant.

A nonpalpable testis usually lies in the peritoneal cavity just within the internal ring. Several approaches are available: inguinal (see Chapter 110), laparoscopic (see Chapter 115), low ligation (see Chapter 112), staged Fowler-Stephens (see Chapter 111), or microvascular (see Chapter 114) orchiopexy.

In a boy with bilateral nonpalpable testis confirm that a disorder of sexual development does not exist such as congenital adrenal hyperplasia by karyotype. At the time of surgery, obtain parental consent for orchiectomy and insertion of a prosthesis should the testes prove to be rudimentary. They may be exchanged later for a larger size around the time of puberty after exogenous testosterone stimulation (see Chapter 121). For an algorithm for the open approach to the nonpalpable testis, see Figure 108-1.

Choose a laparoscopic or an open technique.

If cryptorchidism is detected postpubertally, perform an orchiectomy. However, after 50 years of age, the risk from surgery becomes greater than the risk of cancer.

OPEN INGUINAL ORCHIOPEXY

In addition to initiating general anesthesia, have the anesthesiologist provide a caudal block at the beginning of the procedure to reduce anesthetic requirements and block pain during recovery.

POSTOPERATIVE PROBLEMS

Inadequate testis position has an incidence as high as 10% as the result of incomplete retroperitoneal dissection; it can usually be corrected by a second operation. Late retraction of the testis occurs in a few cases.

Apparent atrophy is related to the degree of development of the testis, but the most serious complication is devascularization of the testis during dissection of the cord, which is avoided by the use of loupes, fine instruments, and sequential dissection. For an atrophic testis, orchiectomy may eventually be advisable because of the increased chance for cancer.

Accidental division of the vas can occur. Microvascular repair, either immediately or postpubertally, may correct the problem. This complication occurs more frequently in nonpalpable cases. Postoperative scrotal swelling is usually a sign of edema rather than infection or hematoma. Immediate progressive scrotal enlargement suggests uncontrolled bleeding and requires exploration. Avoid needle aspiration; it is seldom diagnostic and is harmful if the swelling should be due to herniation of bowel through the peritoneal defect.

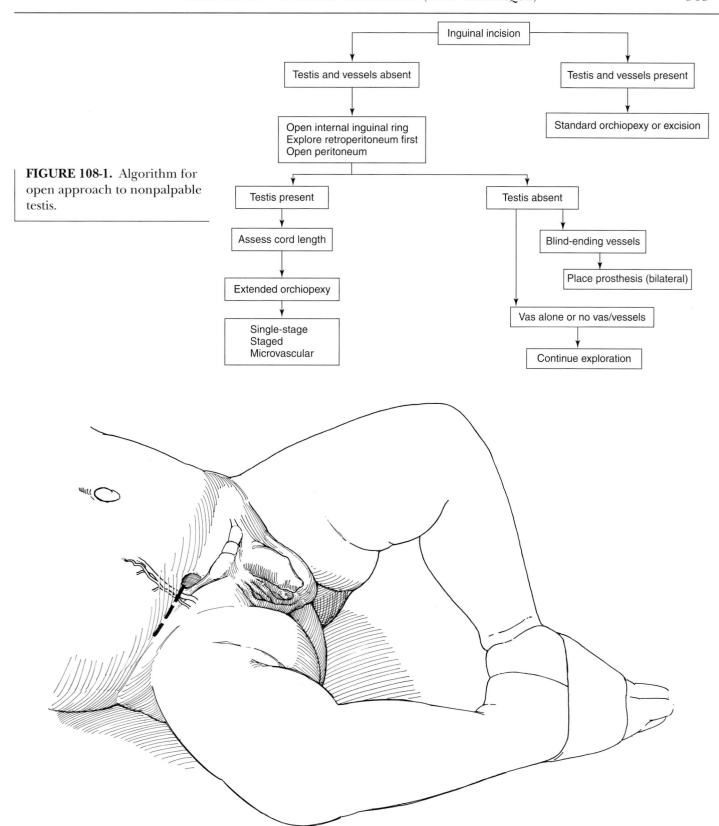

FIGURE 108-1. Algorithm for open approach to nonpalpable testis.

FIGURE 108-2. Position: Place the child supine with the knees bent and the soles of the feet approximated to separate the upper legs. Prep and drape widely in case abdominal exploration will be required. Incision: Make a 3.5-cm transverse incision in the natural inguinal skin fold, extending from the edge of the rectus muscle to a point medial to the anterior superior iliac spine. Avoid an oblique incision, which would not follow Langer's lines. If the testis was not palpable, consider making the incision somewhat higher. Divide Camper's and Scarpa's fascias and expose the external oblique fascia laterally as far as the inguinal ligament to identify the shelving edge, as well as inferiorly to reveal the external ring. Take care not to injure a testis hidden in the superficial inguinal pouch. Depress the protruding processus vaginalis to define the external ring.

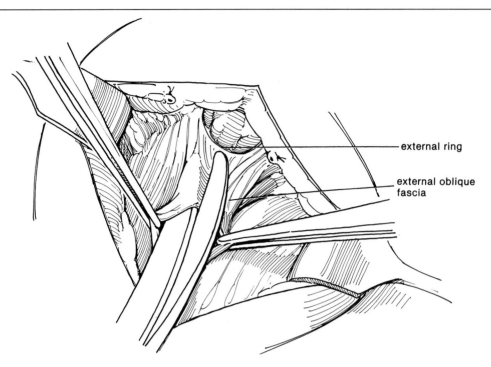

FIGURE 108-3. Sharply incise the external oblique fascia from above. Use a knife or scissors to cut between the fibers that terminate at the external ring. Avoid the underlying ilioinguinal nerve with its medial and lateral branches. Free the fascia from the conjoined muscle and the cremasteric fibers beneath it. Look for the ilioinguinal nerve and gently free it from the fascia. Separate the internal oblique muscle with scissors or a fine clamp to expose the floor of the canal.

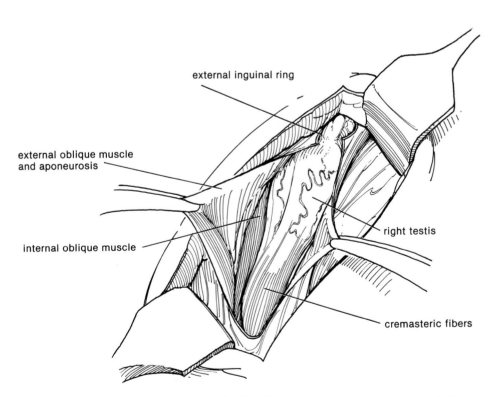

FIGURE 108-4. Identify the testis within the tunica vaginalis. Pick up the overlying cremasteric fibers on either side with a fine smooth forceps. Sharply and bluntly peel them down and off the cord. Keep clear of the external spermatic artery and vein, branches of the inferior epigastric vessels. Let these vessels drop to the floor of the canal. Keep close to the tunica vaginalis to be able to locate the communicating processus vaginalis. Excise the gubernacular attachments, freeing the testis so that its only attachment is the spermatic cord.

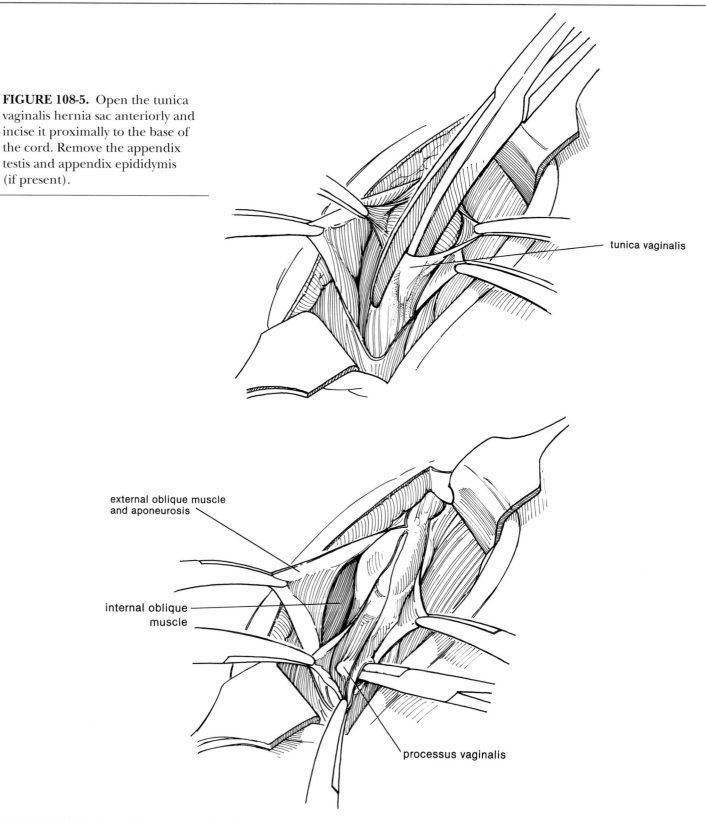

FIGURE 108-5. Open the tunica vaginalis hernia sac anteriorly and incise it proximally to the base of the cord. Remove the appendix testis and appendix epididymis (if present).

tunica vaginalis

external oblique muscle and aponeurosis

internal oblique muscle

processus vaginalis

FIGURE 108-6. Once it is apparent that the cord will become long enough when developed, grasp the edges of the tunica vaginalis near the internal ring with fine forceps, and insinuate fine scissors or a small straight hemostat between the peritoneal lining of the hernia canal and the vessels and vas. The tunica vaginalis may appear to surround the cord. It is easiest to separate it from the vessels and vas just below the internal ring. Dissect from both the medial and lateral sides. As the separation progresses, divide the free edges of the sac to obtain better exposure for the dissection, especially for the separation of the cord structures from the peritoneum. Finally, divide the posterior and lateral connections of the internal spermatic (transversalis) fascia to allow the cord to move medially.

If the cord remains too short, consider bringing the testis directly into the scrotum with the Prentiss maneuver, which bypasses the obliquity of the inguinal canal.

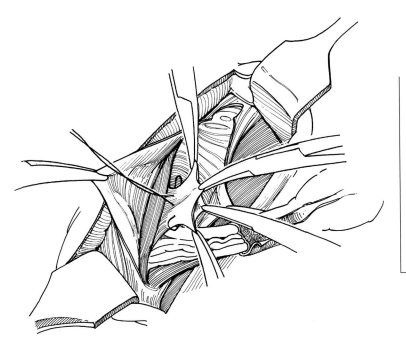

FIGURE 108-7. Place mosquito clamps on its edges, and complete the division of the sac. Close the peritoneal opening with a 4-0 silk purse-string suture, or with the usually small hernia sac, suture-ligation is enough. It may be preferable to postpone this step and close the opening after upward mobilization has been completed, for if closure is done too early, the subsequent retraction needed for the retroperitoneal dissection can tear out the repair. If the peritoneum does tear, oversew the opening into the peritoneal cavity with a fine continuous suture.

FIGURE 108-8. Inspect the testis for size and anomalies. Gauge the length of the cord by pulling the testis over the symphysis. If it is too short, meticulously free the remainder of the tunica vaginalis and the cremasteric fibers from it.

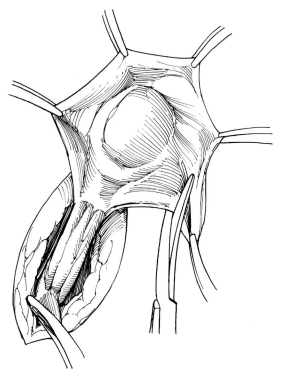

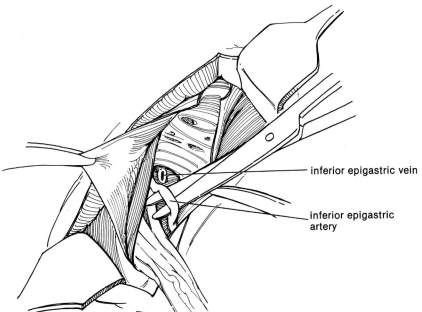

inferior epigastric vein

inferior epigastric artery

FIGURE 108-9. If necessary, open the internal ring by dividing the internal oblique muscles and more of the lateral spermatic fascia. Free the cord well retroperitoneally, and, with a peanut dissector, mobilize it medially, up toward the kidney as necessary. To avoid atrophy, dissect as little as possible about the vessels, vas, and cord structures, particularly in infants. Testes found in the superficial inguinal pouch need minimal dissection of the cord.

FIGURE 108-10. If the testis is found at or above the internal ring, first lengthen the inguinal incision: Elevate the skin at the upper end and open the lateral aspect of the internal ring by dividing the transversalis fascia. Place narrow Deaver retractors. With a Küttner dissector, bluntly develop the retroperitoneal space. Now incise the external oblique fascia in the line of the incision and split the internal oblique and transversalis fascias. Look for the vas or spermatic vessels adherent to the peritoneum under the subserosal fascia, and trace the vas to its proximal end (either to a testis or to a blind ending). If the cord, after thorough dissection and transposition, is still too short, consider an alternative procedure (see Chapter 111 or 112).

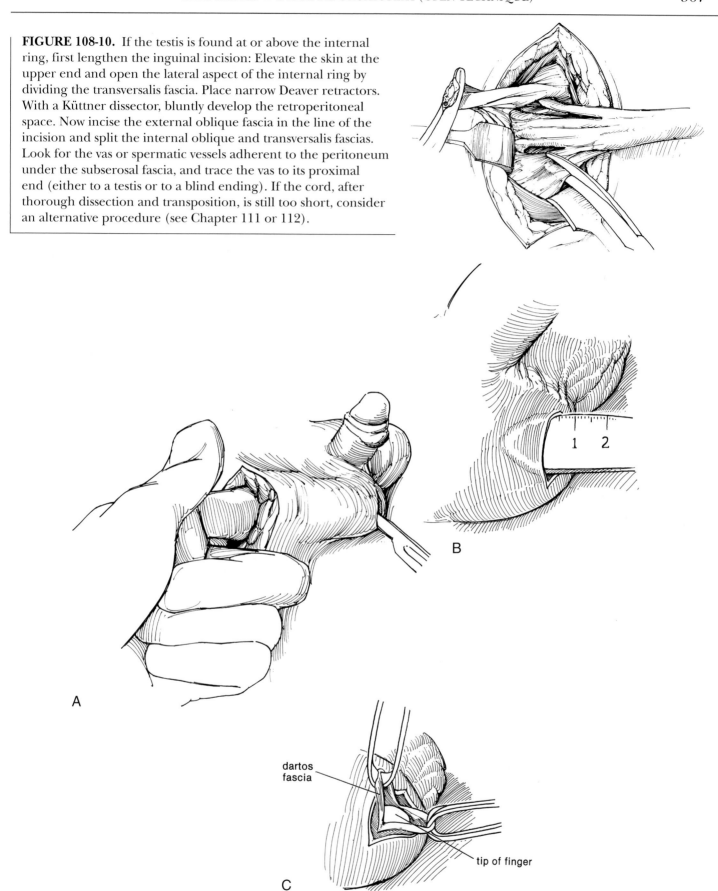

FIGURE 108-11. Dartos pouch technique for fixation of the testis in the scrotum. **A,** Pass the index finger into the scrotum along the usual course of testicular descent. Make a 2-cm incision with the scalpel through the scrotal skin. **B,** Develop a pocket for the testis from below by freeing the skin from the dartos fascia bluntly with a small clamp or scissors, for a distance of 1 to 2 cm. **C,** Make a small opening in the dartos fascia while it is tensioned over the finger. Spread this incision with a clamp and grasp the fascial edges with small Allis clamps.

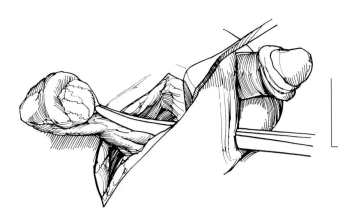

FIGURE 108-12. Draw the testis out through the scrotal incision, by passing a clamp from below against the index finger in the wound and grasping the edge of the tunica albuginea. Take care not to rotate the cord.

FIGURE 108-13. A, Close the dartos fascia behind the testis. **B,** Tuck the testis back into the subcutaneous pouch, close the skin with 5-0 absorbable interrupted sutures, and seal it with collodion.

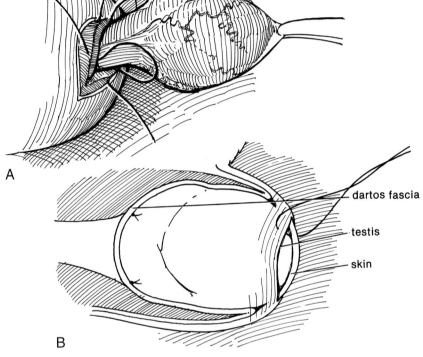

A

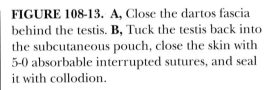

dartos fascia

testis

skin

B

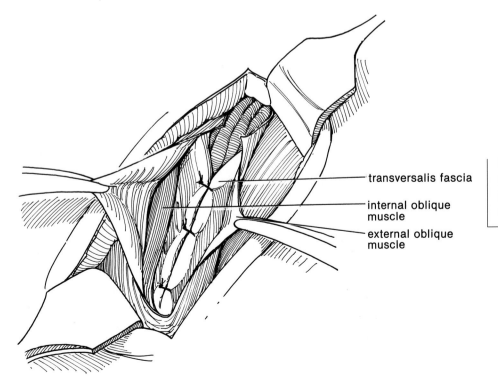

transversalis fascia

internal oblique muscle

external oblique muscle

FIGURE 108-14. Reapproximate the transversalis fascia over the cord, thereby displacing the internal ring downward.

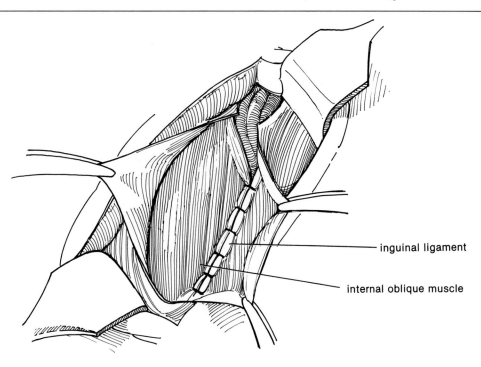

FIGURE 108-15. Suture the internal oblique muscle to the shelving edge of the inguinal ligament over the cord with 3-0 or 4-0 synthetic absorbable sutures.

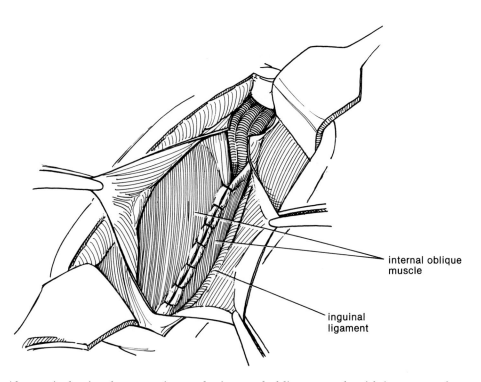

FIGURE 108-16. Alternatively, simply approximate the internal oblique muscle with interrupted sutures.

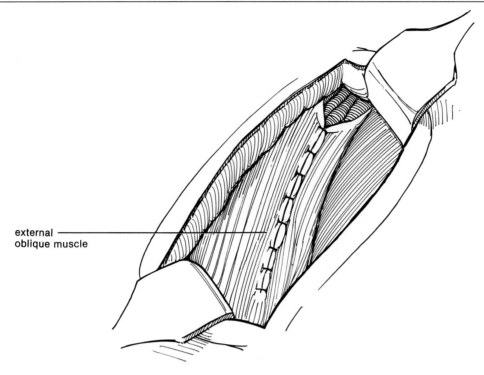

external
oblique muscle

FIGURE 108-17. Close the external oblique muscle with interrupted sutures from cephalad to caudad to create a new external ring. Do not make the ring too tight. Reapproximate Scarpa's fascia; close the skin with a running 4-0 or 5-0 synthetic absorbable suture placed subcuticularly, and seal the skin with flexible collodion.

A hydrocele may form later from proliferation of remnants of the tunica vaginalis. If small it can be ignored; if large it requires transscrotal repair (see Chapter 123). Testicular extrusion secondary to ischemia of the overlying scrotal skin is uncommon. Bladder injury has been reported from gross ligation of the hernia sac.

Commentary by JOHN R. WOODARD

I was told by one of his former residents that Dr. Robert E. Gross, the renowned pediatric surgeon and former surgeon-in-chief at the Boston Children's Hospital, considered orchiopexy to be his favorite operation. It is easy for me to see why this might have been a true story. As is elegantly described and illustrated by the author and illustrator, the procedure is an anatomically precise sequence of maneuvers that, when applied to properly selected patients, almost always leads to a successful result.

That is, the orchiopexy operation as it is described here should produce a scrotal testis in almost every young boy having an easily palpable testis at the start. In boys having a nonpalpable testis, we routinely perform laparoscopic examination, and for the truly intra-abdominal testis, would be prepared to select a technique other than this standard inguinal orchiopexy.

Precision is the key to success in orchiopexy. Each of the tissues and anatomic structures labeled in these diagrams should be easily identifiable in each case. In my experience, there are three important maneuvers that serve to add length to the cord and prevent subsequent testicular retraction: (1) complete transection of the cremaster muscle fibers, (2) good separation of the cord structures from the peritoneum just above the internal ring to accomplish high ligation of the hernia sac, and (3) incision or division of all the lateral spermatic fascia to allow medial advancement of the cord. All patients undergoing orchiopexy require all three of these maneuvers. Further retroperitoneal dissection or transection of the inferior epigastric vessels adds only small amounts of additional cord length and only occasionally is necessary. Also, dissection of the fascia (and collaterals) between the testicular vessels and the vas deferens rarely is necessary and should be avoided in most cases.

A caudal block at the beginning or end of the procedure allows the child to awaken without pain and appears to minimize postoperative nausea and vomiting. We employ this in most cases.

JOHN HUSTON

Commentary by

The authors recommend orchiopexy as early as 9 months of age, as spontaneous descent thereafter is unlikely. In my own experience spontaneous descent is extremely rare after 3 months of age, and I usually perform orchiopexy at about 6 months of age. The neonatal germ cell transforms into a type A spermatogonium between 3 and 12 months of age. This is now recognized as the essential step in germ cell development that is deranged in undescended testes, leading to an inadequate pool for spermatogenesis and subsequent infertility in adult life. In addition, it probably leaves some neonatal gonocytes within the testes, which may mutate and produce testicular tumors postpuberty. The effect of thermal damage on the germ cells begins from the first year of life in my opinion, and hence my recommendation for early orchiopexy, sometimes as soon as 3 months of age, but usually at about 6 months. This is based on the premise that correction of the thermal problem by placement of the testes within the scrotum will prevent germ cell abnormality and/or reverse any early germ cell anomalies that have occurred prior to orchiopexy.

Preliminary results from around the world do support the concept that early orchiopexy will provide better long-term results, although the definitive studies are yet to be described.

SABURO TANIKAZE

Commentary by

Because of the high incidence of undescended testis, standard inguinal orchiopexy is frequently performed at many hospitals. The key point is to have full knowledge of the anatomy around the inguinal area. The first step is to open the inguinal canal, dissect the external oblique fascia laterally, and identify the external ring. Next, open the canal from the ring, because it is easier to identify in this direction. The testis is identified and pulled out and surrounding fibrous tissue including the cremaster muscle is completely dissected up to the internal inguinal ring after division of the gubernacular attachments.

The second step is separation of the processus vaginalis, and this maneuver is the most difficult barrier for the trainee. For safe dissection, the assistant pulls down the testis and the operator opens sharply the processus anteriorly and laterally, and separates the posterior wall bluntly by scissors' tip, and then dissects up the processus to the internal ring and ligates it. To avoid tearing the thin membrane of the sac, the operator should remember that the processus straddles the spermatic cord in a saddle shape.

The third important step is more careful dissection of the lateral fibrous spermatic fascia of the cord in the retroperitoneal space. By this full dissection almost all testes can be brought down into the bottom of the scrotum, and it is not necessary to divide the inferior epigastric vessels.

For impalpable testes, there has been much debate over which is the first procedure—groin surgery or laparoscopy. Even for impalpable testes conventional inguinal orchiopexy is able to successfully bring down 40% of testes; an additional 40% are testicular nubbins that are removed. We prefer to do the inguinal exploration first, and if there is high testis peeping around the internal inguinal ring and it seems to be difficult to bring down by conventional maneuver, the skin incision is extended and high dissection in the retroperitoneal space is done. If nothing is found around the inguinal area or lower abdominal cavity, laparoscopic surgery is performed as a secondary procedure.

When the intra-abdominal testis is found by laparoscopic exploration, the testicular vessels are mobilized extensively and the testis can be brought down to the scrotum. Alternatively, the vessels are clipped and the testis is brought down to the scrotum about 1 year later as a staged Fowler-Stephens procedure.

Chapter 109

Scrotal Orchiopexy

The standard orchiopexy involves two incisions and follows three principles: (1) the stripping of the cremasteric fibers and internal spermatic fascia, (2) high ligation of the processus vaginalis (hernia sac), and (3) tension-free placement of the testis in the scrotum, often with a "straightening" of the cord using the Prentiss maneuver. Laparoscopy is useful for nonpalpable testes; however, more than 80% of testes are palpable, the bulk of which are located distal to the external inguinal ring.

The surgery is performed on an outpatient basis. After general anesthesia the location of the testis is confirmed by repeat examination. A caudal or local wound block is administered.

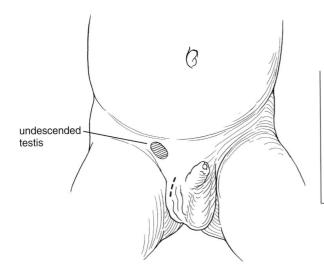

FIGURE 109-1. Incision: Make a skin incision in a cephalad scrotal skin crease. Create a dartos pouch through this incision before testicular mobilization. Have your assistant isolate the undescended testicle in a stable position, then use blunt and sharp dissection of the subcutaneous tissues to approach the testicle. The loose skin and short distance from the external ring to the scrotum facilitate easy mobilization of the skin incision to the inguinal region for dissection without opening the inguinal canal.

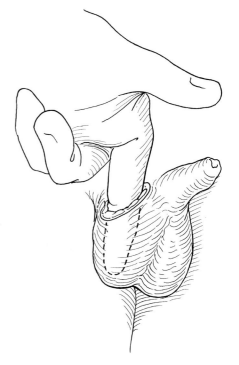

FIGURE 109-2. Release the gubernacular attachments to enable identification of the testicle within the cremasteric fibers, a patent processus vaginalis, and the cord structures. Create a dartos pouch by blunt dissection in caudal fashion just underneath the skin. During subsequent dissection protect the ilioinguinal nerve when it is clearly present (it is not routinely identified) before proceeding further.

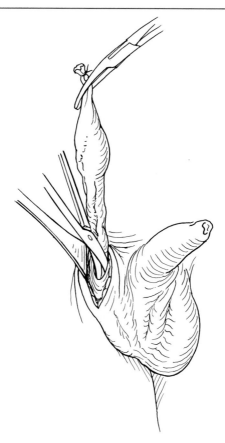

FIGURE 109-3. Carefully separate the cremasteric fibers and hernia sac from the cord structures. Under traction divide the hernia sac between hemostats and suture ligate it. When additional cord length is required, dissect further through this incision by opening the external ring and canal as necessary. When further cord length is needed, make a standard inguinal incision to allow for retroperitoneal dissection (see Chapter 108). In patients with a trapped testis the technique enables early identification of the testis and accompanying cord structures. Careful dissection cranially and en bloc fascia dissection may be required to obtain sufficient length.

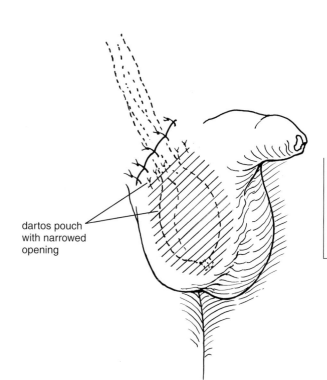

dartos pouch
with narrowed
opening

FIGURE 109-4. Relocate the testis into the dartos pouch, and narrow the pouch neck with simple interrupted absorbable suture to prevent ascent. Close the skin using a simple running subcuticular suture confirming that the testicle is residing in the dependent scrotum. Apply a collodion dressing. In neonates bathing and full activity are allowed 24 to 48 hours after surgery.

ANTHONY A. CALDAMONE

Bianchi and Squire were the first to report the prescrotal approach to an undescended testis. Other reports by Jawad, Lais and Ferro, and Caruso confirmed the applicability of this approach to the palpable undescended testis. The advantage of this approach, of course, is that it requires a single incision placed in a cosmetically perfect location. It is indeed virtually impossible to tell that a child had surgery after this type of orchiopexy. It is important to know as well that the complication rates and success rates compare quite favorably with the standard inguinal approach.

Patient selection is critical. In the very young patient, however, this approach can be used with virtually any palpable undescended testis because the scrotal crease incision allows easy access to the inguinal canal. In the older child, however, I tend to reserve this approach for those testes that can be milked to the scrotal verge. The essential step in this procedure is immobilizing the testis in the scrotal crease incision by the assistant. Once this is accomplished the dissection plane should be on the tunica vaginalis and the spermatic cord, eliminating cremasteric fibers and fascial bands to the spermatic cord. Isolation to the external inguinal ring is easy and requires very little retraction. This approach has also been used for redo orchiopexies. In those cases where the testis is located high in the inguinal canal and you might anticipate the need for a Prentiss maneuver or a retroperitoneal dissection to obtain sufficient length for scrotal placement, proceed directly with an inguinal approach.

Prescrotal orchiopexy has a high success rate with a low complication rate. Hydrocele and hernia can successfully be repaired simultaneously when using this approach. This approach should be considered when performing an orchiopexy with a patient with a palpable and mobile undescended testis. Adequately high ligation of the patent processus vaginalis has been ensured in those very few cases in which a secondary inguinal incision was made for further immobilization of the spermatic cord.

Chapter 110

Orchiopexy for Abdominal Testes

In practice, if laparoscopy has not been performed to locate the testis prior to the incision, proceed to open the peritoneum at the internal ring. If the testis is immediately identifiable and mobile, proceed with the orchiopexy. If the testis is identified high in the abdomen, the incision is closed and the LaRoque maneuver performed.

If the testis has not been localized laparoscopically, an open approach can be used to identify the presence of a retained testis followed by orchiopexy. Three approaches can be used: (1) midline transperitoneal, (2) midline extraperitoneal, or (3) extended inguinal approach (LaRoque maneuver). The midline approaches are generally reserved for known, high intra-abdominal testes as in prune-belly syndrome. In cases in which the external oblique muscle has been opened in standard fashion from the external ring,

superior and lateral toward the internal ring, and the peritoneum is opened at the internal ring without identification of either a mobile testis or testicular structures, the fascia may be closed. The same skin incision is lengthened and the fascia opened 3 cm superior for access directly into the peritoneum (LaRoque incision, which is a modification of Bevan's original groin operation for the undescended testicle).

For bilateral cases, make bilateral skin-crease lower-quadrant incisions and explore each groin. Usually, extensive retroperitoneal dissection through these incisions allows the testis to be placed in the scrotum. If the testes are not found, complete the middle of the incision and open the peritoneum, essential for adequate visualization of the internal spermatic vessels and those of the cord if a long-loop orchiopexy is planned.

TRANSPERITONEAL APPROACH

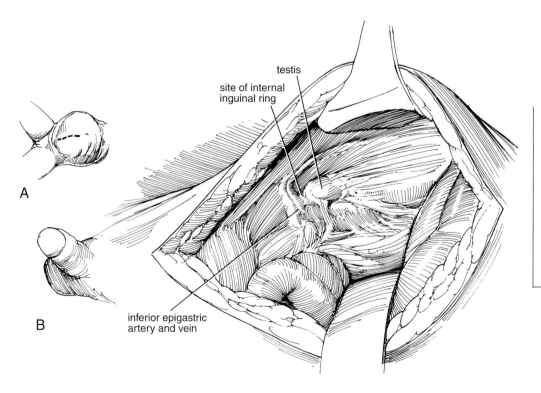

FIGURE 110-1. **A,** Make a midline incision in the lower abdomen from pubis to umbilicus. **B,** Separate the rectus and underlying areolar tissue. Open the peritoneum and pack the intestines aside. The testis is often found lying intraperitoneally, usually behind the bladder and often on a short mesentery.

FIGURE 110-2. Incise the peritoneum obliquely, and sharply free the vessels from the retroperitoneal tissue under direct vision.

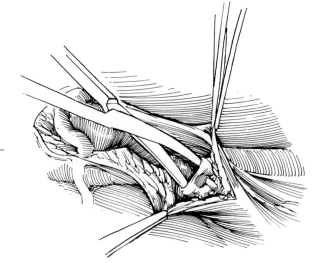

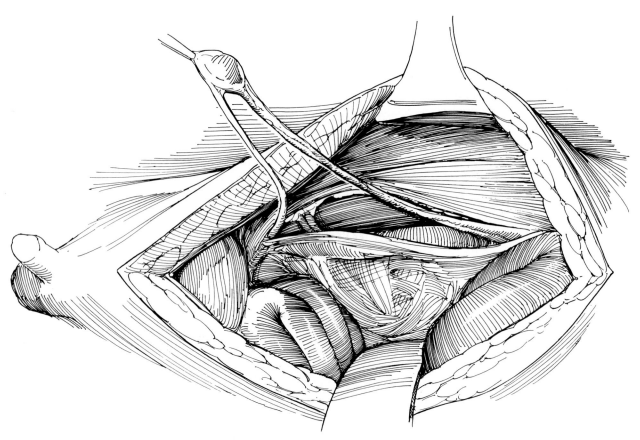

FIGURE 110-3. Sharply free the vas behind the bladder, leaving 1 cm of peritoneum on either side (not shown in the figure), until sufficient length is achieved to place the testis in the scrotum. Invert the scrotum through the external ring, as is done in palpating for a hernia, and place a curved clamp against the fingertip from above. In boys with prune-belly syndrome, the ring is relatively large. Push the clamp through the transversalis fascia and the conjoined tendon as the finger is withdrawn; then dilate the canal and scrotum with the clamp and finger as necessary to form a passage for the testis. Incise the scrotum over the finger. Place a suture in the tissue adjacent to the testis, and lead the testis through the canal to the bottom of the scrotum.

    Fix the testis in a dartos pouch by incising the scrotal skin and developing a pocket between the skin and dartos muscle by blunt dissection. Make a small nick in the dartos muscle, and introduce a curved clamp into the inguinal canal to grasp the suture and bring the testis into the scrotum with a little traction. Anchor the testis by closing the dartos muscle behind it with long-acting absorbable suture.

EXTRAPERITONEAL APPROACH

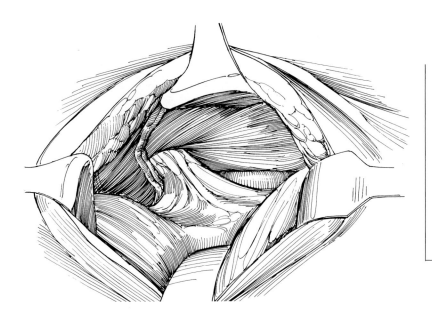

FIGURE 110-4. Make a lower abdominal midline incision from pubis to umbilicus. Separate the rectus muscles and bluntly reflect the peritoneal envelope medially. Look first in the internal inguinal ring to pick up the cord structures. If found, bluntly free them along with the testis from the canal, bring them into the retroperitoneum, and divide the gubernaculum. The inferior epigastric vessels may prevent this maneuver; if they do, divide and ligate them. The internal inguinal ring may be too tight; divide it posteriorly and repair it later.

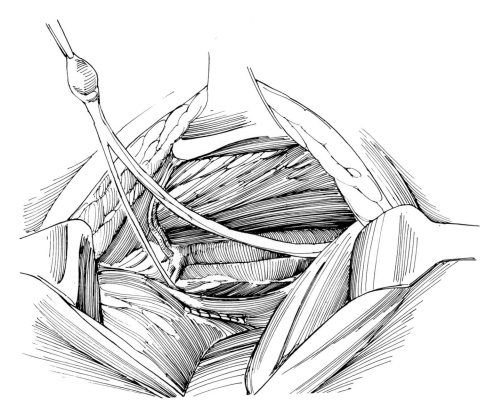

FIGURE 110-5. If the testis is not found near the internal ring, examine the posterior surface of the peritoneum within which the testis is attached. Start by locating the vas deferens behind the bladder and follow it into the canal to the testis, which is concealed because it is intraperitoneal. The blind-ending vas and epididymis may be appreciably separated from the testis.

If the vas ends blindly or in a rudimentary epididymis, identify the spermatic vessels and follow them. If they too terminate blindly, the diagnosis is an absent (vanishing) testis.

If the testis is found retroperitoneally, incise the peritoneum around it and close the peritoneal defect. A pedicled flap of peritoneum, inferior to the testis, can be left attached to the testis and placed in the scrotum with it (not shown). This flap can supplement the blood supply and is necessary if a Fowler-Stephens orchiopexy is done. Encircle the testis with a small Penrose drain for traction, and bluntly and sharply free the vas down to the area of the prostate and the vascular bundle up to the level of the kidney.

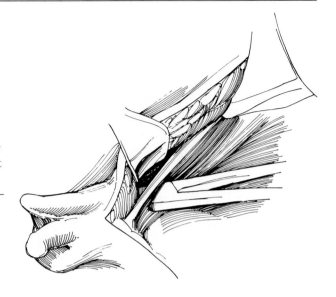

FIGURE 110-6. Make an adequate opening through the transversalis fascia and the tendinous end of the rectus muscle immediately superior to the pubis above the ipsilateral side of the scrotum. Create a scrotal pouch bluntly and install the testis in the scrotum over the dartos muscle (see Chapter 108), taking care not to twist the cord. Close the abdominal wall without drainage.

EXTENDED INGUINAL APPROACH

If the nonpalpable testis was not localized by laparoscopy, start with a standard orchiopexy incision, with the expectation that the testis is located in a relatively low position, but do not extend the opening in the internal oblique muscle into the external ring. Expose the internal ring, and pull on the processus vaginalis at its point of exit to bring the intra-abdominal testis into view. Open the anterior surface of the hernia sac and look for a long, looping vas deferens or an attenuated epididymis with a testis attached. A blind-ending vas and epididymis can be found in the inguinal canal, detached from the testes and outside the hernia sac.

If the testis is not discovered, open the external oblique muscle and retract the internal oblique muscle at the medial edge of the internal ring and open the peritoneum. Look for the vas behind the bladder near the obliterated hypogastric vessels, and trace it along with the spermatic vessels to their end, often in a nubbin that denotes anorchia. The vas should be resected for pathologic examination. If a testis is found, place a fine traction suture in the tunica albuginea at the lower pole and pull on it to assess vessel length. If it appears that enough length could be gained by high dissection of the vessels, proceed accordingly with a traditional orchiopexy. If traction shows that the vessels are too short, proceed with a two-stage Fowler-Stephens or one-stage low ligation orchiopexy (see Chapters 111 or 112).

LAROQUE INCISION

Alternatively, lengthen the skin incision, close the external oblique muscle, and create a new incision in the fascia 3 cm superior for access into the peritoneum at a higher point. Under loop magnification, the peritoneum is incised lateral to the spermatic vessels, all the way to the lower pole of the kidney. Use Army-Navy or small Deaver retractors and a capable assistant to aid exposure. Proceed with primary intra-abdominal orchiopexy, avoiding the need for the Fowler-Stephens procedure or low ligation orchiopexy.

STANLEY J. KOGAN

Commentary by

The initial problem for the surgeon is to confirm whether an impalpable testis is present in the abdomen or inguinal canal or is absent. A plethora of imaging modalities now exist, including ultrasound, CT, MRI, and diagnostic laparoscopy at the time of definitive surgical treatment. Each has its advantages and disadvantages, but allow for excellent preoperative planning of the surgical approach. When testes are impalpable, studies indicate that approximately 40% will be in the abdomen, one third in the inguinal canal, and one third will be absent.

At surgery, laparoscopy may be initiated first both to identify and exclude an absent testis ("vanishing testis"), identify a hypoplastic/atrophic testis, and localize a testis high in the pelvis or above, well away from the internal inguinal ring. Laparoscopic repair may then follow, based on the laparoscopic findings. An alternative approach is to start from below by making an initial scrotal incision, as the pathologic findings associated with the majority of impalpable testes can be localized in this manner.

When an open surgical approach is used, I prefer an extended inguinal incision, opening the internal inguinal ring and peritoneum widely. Bilateral abdominal undescended testes are best treated through a midline transperitoneal approach, since higher mobilization is possible and the blood supply from the top to the bottom is better visualized, especially in the older child. In either instance, placing a traction suture through the lower pole is the next critical maneuver, assessing potential spermatic cord length and mobility. Further mobilization may then be done retroperitoneally (while visualizing the blood supply from each side of the peritoneum), or intraperitoneally by mobilizing the spermatic vessels along their entire length through a posterior peritoneal incision.

When the testis is especially high and the initial "traction suture maneuver" indicates especially short internal spermatic vessels, these approaches may be insufficient. Early decision for deliberate transection of these vessels (Fowler-Stephens orchiopexy) is essential before mobilization of the lower collateral blood supply that is derived from the vasal vessels and other pelvic collaterals. Feasibility of orchiopexy by testicular vessel transection must be determined early in the dissection after stretching the pedicle and applying an atraumatic bulldog clamp to the internal spermatic vessels to confirm adequacy of the collateral blood supply, lest subsequent testicular atrophy occurs. If the collateral blood supply is inadequate after 1 to 2 minutes of internal vessel occlusion, the internal spermatic vessels should not be cut.

At times all these maneuvers will still not allow for optimum scrotal testis placement. Two additional surgical maneuvers may make the difference: vas mobilization and creation of a more direct path for the mobilized testis into the scrotum rather than following the natural route through the inguinal canal. I seldom find that substantial vas deferens mobilization off the posterior peritoneum and bladder is necessary. However, in exceptional cases it may make the difference between a tensioned and tension-free testis placement in the scrotum. Leaving a wide (1 cm on each side) strip of adjacent peritoneum and tissue is important to ensure that the vas deferens and collateral blood supply are not harmed. Directing the testis through a new straight path created above the pubic tubercle rather than following the longer course through the internal inguinal ring and inguinal canal may also add 1 to 2 cm of length, which is critical in some cases.

The technique of scrotal testis fixation is also important, especially when initially there is a high testis. I use a nonabsorbable Prolene suture passed superficially through the lower pole of the testis and externally through a gauze fixation pledget which is left for 3 to 4 weeks, unless testis retraction occurs during the immediate postoperative period.

It is important also to consider the longer-term aspects when performing these surgeries. Many of these testes have diminished germ cell complements and are associated with a high frequency of subfertility in adulthood, especially in bilateral cases. Furthermore, additional subsequent insults potentially resulting in worsened fertility (subsequent testis torsion, varicocele, testis loss from tumor or trauma) may occur subsequently. For these reasons, I perform testicular biopsy at the time of orchiopexy, as the germ cell status of the testis correlates well with ultimate sperm-producing capabilities, and knowledge of the function of the undescended testis may affect decisions regarding treatment when subsequent testicular conditions occur.

Presently it is reasonable to say that virtually *any* testis can be descended satisfactorily now using the innovative surgical techniques that exist. Choice of procedure and use of exacting technique significantly influence the surgical outcome.

MING-HSIEN WANG

The exact mechanism of testicular descent remains elusive. Ongoing basic and clinical research over the years has given us some insights into this complex process. Certain observations in the embryo have been consistent. As the mesonephros involutes at 7 to 8 weeks of gestation, a ridge of tissue—the cranial gonadal mesentery—persists, attaching the testis to the diaphragm and kidney. Caudally, the testis is attached to the future scrotum by the gubernaculum. The process of descent can be divided into two phases: (1) gubernacular growth and regression, and (2) transinguinal descent. Embryologic studies have shown that shortly before birth, androgens cause an involution of the cranial suspensory ligament, allowing the thickening gubernaculum to retain the testis in the inguinal region while the embryo grows. A subsequent increase in intra-abdominal pressure and elongation of the processus vaginalis pull the testis into the scrotum. Any genetic and hormonal defects occurring during these two phases can easily disrupt the normal process of descent.

It is also known that an intact hypothalamic-pituitary-gonadal axis is important for testicular descent to occur. This corresponds to our clinical experience that an increased incidence of cryptorchidism is observed in patients with disorders in androgen metabolism such as 5α-reductase deficiency, androgen insensitivity, and hypogonadotropic hypogonadism. A recent study noted that boys with cryptorchidism have higher serum follicle-stimulating hormone (FSH) compared to age-matched controls. The hormonal contribution is also supported by the fact that some inguinal undescended testes respond to human chorionic gonadotropin (hCG) and gonadotropin-releasing hormone (GnRH) stimulation.

Recent molecular studies further elucidate the genetic basis of testicular descent. Insulin-like peptide 3 (INSL3) was discovered as a novel gene product of the Leydig cells in 1993. Since then, it has been shown to be a major secretory hormone

Continued

Commentary by

of the testis in all mammalian species. INSL3 knockout mice demonstrate cryptorchidism, with otherwise normal phenotypic genitalia. Recent studies measuring cord blood INSL3 in boys with cryptorchidism showed an increased luteinizing hormone (LH) to INSL3 ratio in boys with cryptorchidism. Estrogens or environmental endocrine disruptors have been suspected of inducing a down-regulation of INSL3 expression. In laboratory studies involving diethylstilbestrol-treated pregnant mice, all newborn male mice were cryptorchid, with a significant decrease in INSL3 mRNA in their testes. This correlates with clinical findings of an increased incidence of cryptorchidism and other genital abnormalities in offspring of women were who treated with diethylstilbestrol as a hormonal support during pregnancy.

Another candidate gene that has been studied extensively and implicated in the pathogenesis of cryptorchidism is the *Hoxa-10* gene. *Hoxa-10* is a highly conserved gene within the homeobox (Hox) gene family. These genes play a critical role in anteroposterior positioning of the developing embryo. Experiments have shown that *Hoxa-10* is expressed exclusively in the gubernaculum and the kidney. A detailed study of *Hoxa-10* gene knockout mice showed a high incidence of bilateral cryptorchidism with normal virilized genitalia. Additional studies on *Hoxa-10* will give us a better understanding of its role in testicular descent.

Cryptorchidism and testicular descent with its associated disease in adults, that is, infertility and malignancy, remain to be an intriguing subject for urologists. With recent advancement in the Human Genome Project, there is hope that future studies will give us a better understanding and grasp of this complex developmental process.

Chapter 111

High Ligation Orchiopexy

HIGH LIGATION ORCHIOPEXY (FOWLER-STEPHENS)

The long-loop vas associated with an impalpable testis that lies in the inguinal canal is a specific abnormality that occurs in roughly 10% of maldescended testes. It is unilateral in most instances and the testis is nearly normal in size, with the epididymis somewhat unraveled at its junction with the vas deferens.

This procedure was developed for a high-lying testis having so short a main vascular cord that it cannot be placed directly in the scrotum. Instead, it uses the secondary vascular loops that accompany the congenitally long vas.

On examination, the testis is impalpable or gliding within the inguinal canal. The loop of the vas lies on the pubic bone and may be palpable in thin boys. The true anatomy is realized during careful clinical examination under anesthesia prior to operation: The testis may be expressed along the canal to become palpable in the external ring and a loop of vas on the pubis may also be palpable. Surgical exposure of the inguinal canal displays the testis, the patent processus vaginalis, and the loop of vas with rudimentary gubernaculum attached to the vas and tissues of the pubis, findings that make this operation especially indicated.

The long-loop vas with the undescended testis lies at the internal ring. The vasal artery (VA) runs in a long recurrent course with several anastomotic branches. The main trunk of the internal spermatic artery (ISA) branches into the testicular artery (TA) and the VA near the lower pole of the testis. The VA then runs a course that follows the looping vas and so provides several anastomotic arterial branches. In the technique described, the ISA and vein are divided, making the testis reliant on the connecting anastomotic branches that track across the loop. These must be protected.

The ideal candidate for this operation is a boy with a testis detected at the external ring or in the inguinal canal that possesses a long loop of vas deferens emerging from the external ring. It is not useful for testes situated higher in the abdomen with the usual short vas.

A separate first stage for vessel ligation is required only if the testis or the loop of vas deferens cannot be located by clinical examination. Such a stage may be done readily by a laparoscopic technique (see Chapter 115), which not only determines the presence and location of the testis, the course of the vas deferens, and the feasibility of the procedure, but also allows clipping or fulgurating of the appropriate spermatic vessels. Alternatively, an open approach can be used as a first stage, entering through a short abdominal incision to allow identification of the internal spermatic vessels and their ligation as high as possible.

OPEN SURGICAL TECHNIQUE

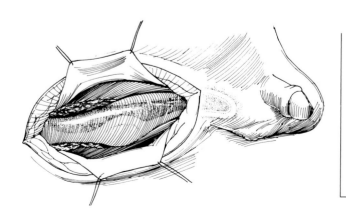

FIGURE 111-1. Make an incision in the inguinal crease. Identify the special anatomic circumstances applicable for this technique. You must plan ahead for the Fowler-Stephens orchiopexy; do not mobilize the posterior wall of the hernia sac proximal to the testis and epididymis or disturb the floor of the inguinal canal or the epigastric vessels. Expose the processus vaginalis as for a standard orchiopexy. Dilate the internal inguinal ring or, if greater retroperitoneal exposure is needed, incise the internal oblique muscle. Loupe magnification is essential.

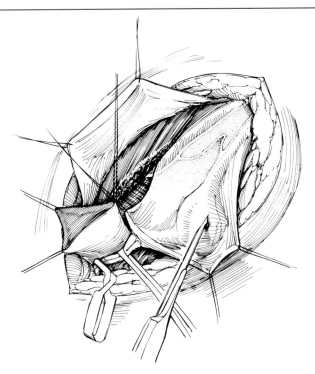

FIGURE 111-2. Open the hernia sac, identify the epididymis, and note the course of the vas with its several vascular arcades looping down the posteromedial wall of the sac below the testis. Place a traction suture superficially in the testicular capsule; traction on the testis now will determine whether it has a long mesentery and can be brought into the scrotum by standard methods or it has a short one that will require division of some of the internal spermatic vessels. Dissect the sac well up inside the internal ring to the point where the vas turns medially. At the same time, keep the broad tongue of peritoneum, which lies more distally, attached medially and posteriorly to the vas. If necessary, inject saline under the peritoneum of the processus to aid dissection, then transect it, and close the peritoneum with a 4-0 nonabsorbable purse-string suture. Carefully separate the internal spermatic vessels from the vas and its accompanying vessels where they converge on the internal inguinal ring, and also from the loose collateral arcades on the posterior wall of the processus vaginalis.

Bleeding test if the spermatic artery has not been clipped at a first stage: Compress the internal spermatic artery (ISA) and veins with a bulldog clamp cranial to the testis. Make a 3-mm longitudinal incision in the testis between the faintly visible vessels in the tunica albuginea and expect brisk bleeding. If bleeding persists for 5 minutes, collateral circulation is adequate, and high ligation of the ISA is safe. Let the cut caudal end of the vasal artery (VA) bleed for further confirmation: Place a bulldog clamp at point 1 of the arcade. If bleeding continues, it is safe to divide this branch, thus further mobilizing the testis. If greater length is needed, repeat the procedure at point 2. Now ligate the ISA and close the incision in the tunica with a fine suture. Alternatively, if the bleeding stops almost immediately, consider anastomosis of the inferior epigastric vessels to the internal spermatic vessels to maintain viability after division of the spermatic artery.

Transilluminate the cord structures to identify the vascular anastomotic arcades between the vas and the spermatic vessels alongside the testis and epididymis. This is best seen through the back wall of the hernia sac, a view enhanced by the accompanying venae comitantes. These anastomotic arcades are important to the blood supply, so divide only the arcade (or arcades) that are necessary to allow straightening of the loop of vas and placement of the testis in the scrotum without tension. Before dividing a major arcade, gently compress the vessel and note whether that impedes bleeding from the tunical opening: Continuous bleeding shows that it is safe to divide the arcade, whereas arrest indicates that the vessel is not expendable.

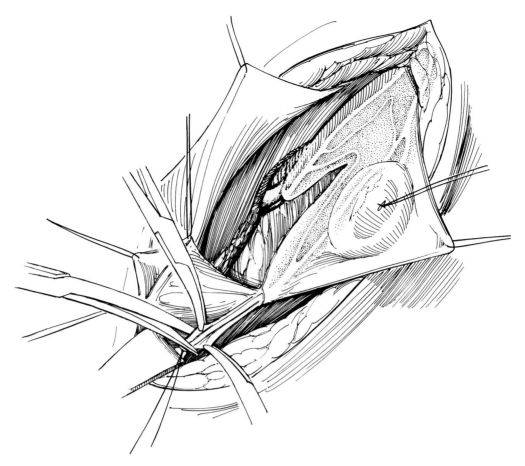

FIGURE 111-3. Close the tunica with a single fine suture, clamp and divide the pedicle above the bulldog clamp, and ligate it doubly. Grasp the areolar tissue adjacent to the artery and temporarily release the bulldog clamp. Look for free bright bleeding from the distal cut end, indicating that the collateral circulation is adequate. Ligate this end of the artery. Divide only as many of these small arcades as needed to free the testis enough for rotation on the descending limb of the loop of the vas and its main vessels.

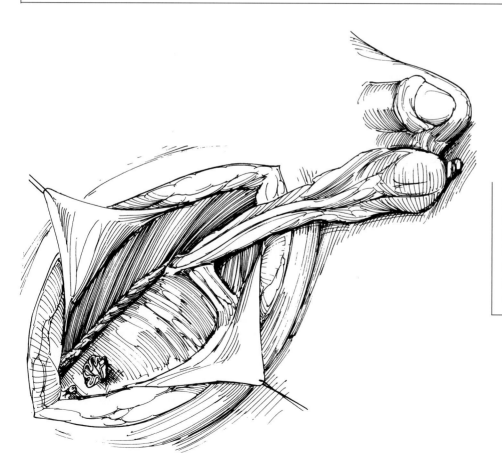

FIGURE 111-4. Turn the testis into the scrotum. For additional tension-free length, open the transversalis fascia up to the epigastric vessels. Develop a space under the vessels and pass the testis and its vessels through it. Continue as for a standard orchiopexy (see Chapter 108).

POSTOPERATIVE PROBLEMS

Testicular atrophy is the major complication. The cause may be loss of collaterals from failure to incorporate an adequate strip of peritoneum medial to and accompanying the vas, from injury to the VA, or from ligation of the spermatic vessels too close to the testis so that the arcades cannot function. The irregular pattern of local blood supply contributes to the problem. Injury to the vas or testis is also possible.

F. DOUGLAS STEPHENS

Commentary by

ETIOLOGIC CONSIDERATIONS

The etiology of this anomalous condition (and possibly other unilateral, palpable undescended or superficial ectopic testes) may not be due to hormonal deficiencies. Instead, a range of "deformations" has been described that result from physical compression on developing external genitalia and gubernaculum by the overlying foot, or feet. These deformations from focal compression include some forms of torsion of the penis and hypospadias, anomalies of testicular descent, sacral defects, and some types of "imperforate" anus.

Focal compression may arrest the emergence of the testis from the canal by pressure atrophy of the gubernatorial attachment to the testis though sparing a rudiment of the adjoining vas long loop.

The gubernaculum plays a key role in the embryogenesis of the descent of the testis. It is a definite jellylike condensation of mesenchyme attached to the lower pole of the testis and adjacent epididymis and vas deferens. It lies at first in the abdomen, close to the internal inguinal ring. Its distal end condenses and occupies the locality of the inguinal canal around which the muscles of the abdominal wall develop. At 15 weeks, the fetal testis is located at the internal ring of the canal and the processus vaginalis grows with the proximal part of the canalicular gubernaculum, while the distal part forms a core attached to the epididymis. Around this core, the mesenchyme gives rise to the cremaster muscle.

By 25 weeks, the caudal end of the gubernaculum swells, bulges through the internal ring, and migrates across the pubis and beyond into the scrotum. The fetal testis within the gubernaculum is normally fully descended by 35 weeks. Then the gubernaculum is absorbed except for an attachment at the bottom of the scrotum.

It is feasible that this jellylike structure, at any stage of development and migration, may be compressed by even gentle external focal pressure of the overlying foot.

From the 7th to the 8th week of embryonic development, the lower limbs, which up to this time are rigid structures, become mobile in the hip and knee joints. The hips abduct and flex, the knees flex, and the soles of the feet appose and overlie the developing genitalia. As the limbs elongate, the feet cross over one another and the heels overlie the puboperineum and are at risk of compressing the underlying genitalia.

Normally the limbs are free to move in the fluid-filled amniotic capsule. If, however, the amniotic membrane is tight on the ankles, the deeply situated heel may press on the inguinopubic region. In the example of the long-loop vas and cryptic testis, the focal pressure of the folded ankles and feet impairs the enlargement of the gubernaculum, thus impairing the emergence of the testis yet permitting the exit of the less bulky loop of vas and processus vaginalis.

This theory of gubernacular dysfunction due to external physical factors may apply to many forms of undescended testis, whether the testis lies ectopically, or is of the retractile type. Usually, supporting evidence of compression can be found elsewhere in these infants, such as minor deformities of the legs, feet, toes, ankles, hips, or elsewhere.

I consider that compression deformities of the genitalia, including some types of unilateral partially descended testis, are common, that not all such anomalies are due to defective hormonal control, and that such anomalies are unlikely to occur in other members of the family.

ANATOMIC CONSIDERATIONS

The anatomy of the blood vessels both outside and inside the tunica albuginea governs the steps in the operation that entail the division of the internal spermatic (testicular) vessels.

Blood vessels outside the tunica albuginea: The ISA anastomoses by one or several terminal branches with the VA near the lower pole of the testis and close to the hilum. A single, very short TA arises from the junction of these vessels, bypasses the hilum, and penetrates the tunica albuginea at the lower pole of the testis.

Blood vessels inside the tunica albuginea: Immediately beneath the tunica, the TA commonly divides into two separate branches that course longitudinally toward the upper pole, giving off end arteries, which dip into and supply the tubules in the individual septal compartments of the testis. Sometimes the vessel remains single and sometimes the two branches at first run close together. These vessels are accompanied by veins that can be seen, if carefully scrutinized, as blue streaks under the tunica.

Precautions to preserve the blood supply to the testis: Transect the internal spermatic vascular bundle cranial to the internal ring of the inguinal canal and higher than the point of deviation of the vas deferens. In this way, the main TA is divided before giving off delicate anastomosing connections to the vasal vessels. One or more of these cross connections, which may best be seen through the back wall of the hernia sac, may need to be divided under vision to free and turn down the testis from the descending limb of the loop of the vas and its main vessels. Venae comitantes enhance the visibility of these small channels.

Incise the tunica for the bleeding test longitudinally and toward the upper pole. Select a site for the incision between the main visible vessels in the tunica vasculosa or an area of nonvisible vascularity. Meticulous positioning and suturing curtail the extent of infarction that may follow an incision in the tunica vasculosa that inadvertently divides a main trunk and its septal end arteries.

Though not strictly a long-loop vas problem, division of the testicular vessels with orchiopexy can be applied to abdominal testes of the triad (prune-belly) syndrome. In this condition, however, the vas deferens is sometimes atretic in some part of its course, and hence failure of the bleeding test would indicate a lack of supply to the testis from the artery of the vas.

JOHN HUSTON

Commentary by

This chapter describes the use of the Fowler-Stephens procedure with division of the TA or ISA, allowing the testis to be brought to the scrotum on the blood supply of the artery to the vas. The authors here describe an open inguinal Fowler-Stephens procedure, very similar to the way in which I was actually taught by Robert Fowler and Douglas Stephens when I was a resident. In recent years, however, I have not found the need to do a Fowler-Stephens division of the ISA for a testis located at the external ring or within the inguinal canal. It is usually necessary, in my opinion, for intra-abdominal testes, which I would identify laparoscopically in the first instance. If I were unable to deliver the intra-abdominal testis to the contralateral internal inguinal ring (because the testicular vessels are too short to reach the scrotum), I would then do a laparoscopic ligation of the testicular vessels high up in the retroperitoneum just before the testicular vessels disappear behind the colon. This ensures that the ligation is well away from the collaterals joining the testicular vessels to the artery to the vas.

Although many authors have described doing a Fowler-Stephens operation laparoscopically, and all in one procedure, it would be my usual approach to ligate the vessels laparoscopically at a first operation and then return 6 months later and perform the second stage of the Fowler-Stephens operation laparoscopically. This would include wide mobilization of the testes and adjacent peritoneum and bringing the testes down to the scrotum through the inguinal region medial to the inferior epigastric vessels, similar to the Prentiss maneuver that was done previously at open operation. In my own hands, my success rate for intra-abdominal testes using the Fowler-Stephens approach in two stages has achieved approximately a 90% success and 10% atrophy rate.

Chapter 112

Low Ligation Orchiopexy

LOW LIGATION ORCHIOPEXY
(KOFF)

The technique of orchiopexy using low spermatic vessel ligation is performed as an outpatient procedure via a standard inguinal skin-crease incision (see Chapter 108).

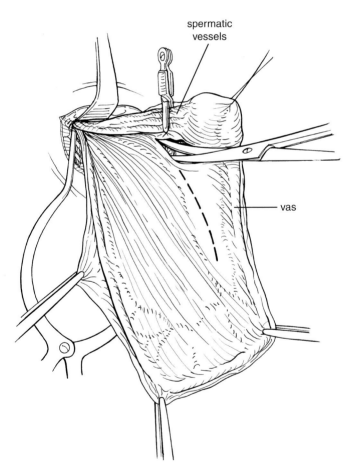

FIGURE 112-1. Access the inguinal canal by incising the external oblique fascia to a level above the internal ring. Enlarge the internal inguinal ring by retraction or when necessary by superolateral incision of the internal oblique muscle, permitting visualization of the testis within the peritoneum or protruding through the ring within a hernial sac.

When the testis is not visible, place the patient in the Trendelenburg position and open the peritoneum. Identify the testis and place a stay suture in the medial aspect of the upper pole to avoid collateral vessels. With traction on the testis and the accompanying fold of peritoneum, identify the visord collateral vessels.

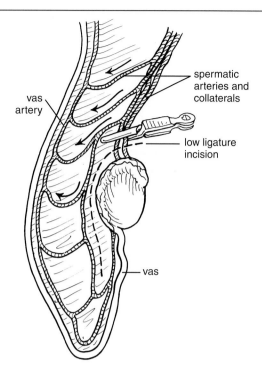

FIGURE 112-2. A decision to transect the spermatic vessels must be made early in the procedure before any manipulation of the vas or vessels, or separation of the hernial sac (patent processus) from the spermatic cord. After identifying the vascular anatomy, mark the site of transection of the spermatic vessels as close to the testis as possible without compromising any collateral vessels. Also mark the location of the extension of this incision, which will extend into a relatively avascular plane between the ascending and descending limbs of the long vas loop to allow their separation.

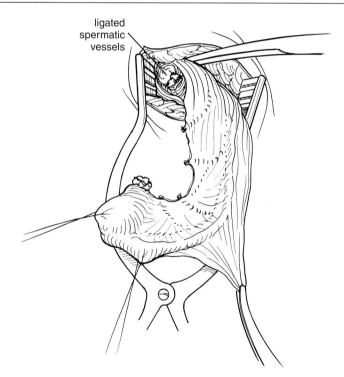

FIGURE 112-3. Before performing ligation and incision, both sides of the peritoneal fold covering these sites must be carefully incised. Ligate the spermatic vessels proximally to allow back-bleeding from the distal stump serving as an indicator of continued collateral blood flow. Incise between the two vas limbs, allowing the vas loop to be unfolded and the testis to be rotated down toward the scrotum. Divide any remaining lateral peritoneal or adventitial attachments, carefully ensuring that a continuous 1-cm–wide strip of peritoneum remains as an attached and undisturbed covering over the vas, accompanying vessels, and collaterals from their intra-abdominal location to the testis. This covering helps to preserve vascular integrity and blood flow. Separate any remaining tissue between the vasal limbs until the testis rotates down to and reaches the scrotum without tension.

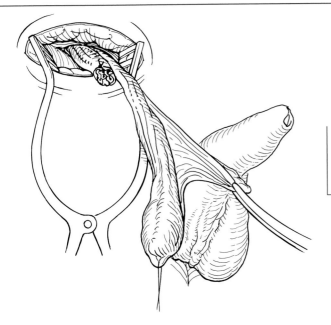

FIGURE 112-4. Close the peritoneum, leaving a small aperture for the peritoneal strip covering the vas and vessels to emerge without angulation or compression. Continued back-bleeding confirms that closure is not causing vascular compromise.

FIGURE 112-5. Narrow the canal after placing the testis in the scrotum using a standard dartos pouch technique.

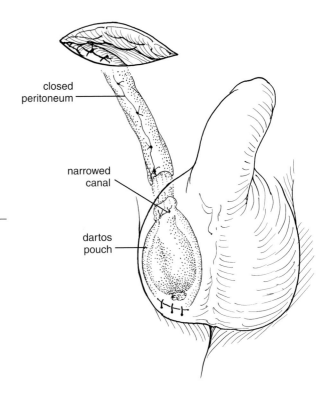

closed peritoneum

narrowed canal

dartos pouch

COMPLICATIONS

Testicular atrophy may occur if the testicle cannot survive on the artery to the vas deferens and the collateral circulation from the testicular artery.

STEPHEN KOFF

Commentary by

Low ligation orchiopexy is predicated on the robust collateralization that exists between the spermatic and vasal arteries occurring along and beneath the outer anterior margin of the testis opposite the epididymis. Traction or fixation sutures must therefore be placed medially and well away from these collaterals to ensure viability. The keys to the procedure are (1) ensuring adequate exposure and optical magnification to visualize all the vascular arcades that run in the folds of peritoneum (as many of these as possible should be preserved); (2) precise identification and incision of the avascular plane, which separates the vasal limbs if a vas loop exists or separates the vas from the testis if there is no loop; (3) dissection within the internal ring to reduce tension by further mobilizing the vas and its overlying peritoneum; and (4) avoiding the temptation to hypermobilize the testis by dissecting too close to the tail of the epididymis.

Chapter 113

Redo Orchiopexy

Review the previous operative report and caution the family about the possibility of orchiectomy and also about the indications for and contraindications to a prosthesis.

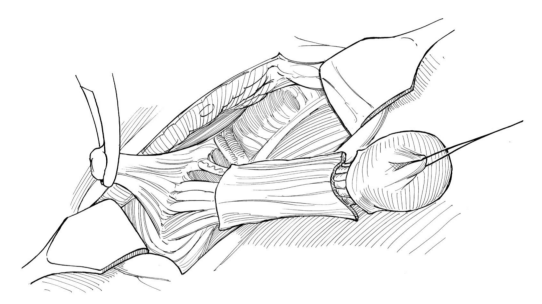

FIGURE 113-1. Reenter the previous incision, extending it slightly at each end. The testis is probably found near the external inguinal ring and the pubic tubercle. Bluntly dissect the fatty subcutaneous tissue that lies over the cord structures to expose the lower pole of the testis. Place a suture in the scar tissue in the middle of the testis. With traction, dissect on both sides behind the testis with a right-angle clamp and scissors. Dissection along the floor on the transversalis fascia can be initiated bluntly; isolate and divide the medial and lateral attachments sharply. As the dissection of the cord reaches the level of the external ring, preserve a plate of external oblique fascia that adheres to the cord structures by incising the fascia on either side. Expose the fibers of the internal oblique muscle and safely transect the external oblique fascia by connecting these lateral incisions, leaving a protective strip of fascia 1 to 2 cm wide attached to the cord. At the level of the internal ring, open the internal oblique fibers and identify the vas deferens, the spermatic vessels, and the previously ligated sac. With traction on the testis, expose the anterior aspect of the peritoneum. Open it away from the vessels and dissect, usually in fresh tissue planes, under the posterior peritoneum behind the vas deferens and spermatic vessels, as is done for an initial orchiopexy. Gather the peritoneal edges in a clamp. With the aid of Deaver retractors, dissect retroperitoneally by dividing attachments to the endopelvic fascia until enough length is obtained. Division of the lateral spermatic fascia and the inferior epigastric vessels may also be needed. Suture the peritoneal opening closed at a high level. Place the testis in a dartos pouch, or hold it with a button on the skin if scarring is excessive. Place two or three sutures from the transversalis fascia to the inguinal ligament to reconstruct the floor of the canal, thus forming a new internal ring next to the pubic tubercle, at the same time protecting the vessels and the vas. Close the internal oblique musculature with mattress sutures, and suture the external oblique muscle together. Instill 0.25 mL/kg of a 0.25% bupivacaine solution into the wound before closure to reduce pain. Perform a caudal block if it was not done at the beginning of the procedure.

HOWARD SNYDER

Commentary by

The approach I developed is intended to avoid jeopardizing the vas and vessels, as they often lie adherent to the undersurface of the external oblique fascia. Accordingly, the dissection is carried in the subcutaneous fat distally until the testis can be elevated. Dissection is then carried back up parallel to the cord structures to the pubic tubercle. At the pubic tubercle, a strip of the fascia of the external oblique muscle is outlined and incised medially and laterally to the adherent vas and vessels beneath. This helps to protect them. Posteriorly, the plane of dissection is usually easier on the transversalis fascia, the floor of the inguinal canal. If there is adherence posteriorly, the transversalis fascia is taken en bloc with the vas and vessels. The dissection is carried laterally with the strip of external oblique fascia until the internal oblique musculature is seen lateral to the internal ring. At that point, the incisions of the external oblique fascia are joined and the peritoneum is exposed. We try to open the peritoneum above where the processus vaginalis was tied off. This step enables the peritoneum to be separated from the vas and vessels in the retroperitoneum in a free plane where previous dissection has not taken place. At this point, the block of tissue adherent to vas and vessels is completely mobilized; if any further length of the vas and vessels is needed to achieve a good scrotal position for the testis, a retroperitoneal mobilization similar to what is done in a standard orchiopexy is carried upward until the testis can be placed adequately in the scrotum. If the transversalis fascia has been opened it is repaired, usually creating a new internal ring at the pubic tubercle.

HSI-YANG WU

Commentary by

The key to redo orchiopexy is dissecting in virgin territory. Preservation of a strip of external oblique fascia above the vas and vessels, and occasionally a strip of transversalis fascia underneath, minimizes the risk of injury to the testis. I do not use a traction suture on the testis, since there is usually enough scar tissue around the testis to use as a handle. A scrotal approach to redo orchiopexy can be successful if the previous mobilization was sufficient and the testis has healed in a distal location. Otherwise, a careful inguinal, peritoneal, and retroperitoneal dissection as described usually allows for proper scrotal positioning of the testis even in a reoperative situation.

Chapter 114

Microvascular Orchiopexy

In children with genetic syndromes or known high intra-abdominal testes, or in a child that has previously lost a high testis by a more traditional procedure (see Chapters 108, 110, 111, 112, and 114), consider microvascular orchiopexy.

For instruments, provide a complete microvascular setup: an operating microscope with foot pedal controls, three-power loupes, and 10-0 or 11-0 nylon sutures on BV-6 or ST-7 needles (Figs. 114-1 to 114-3).

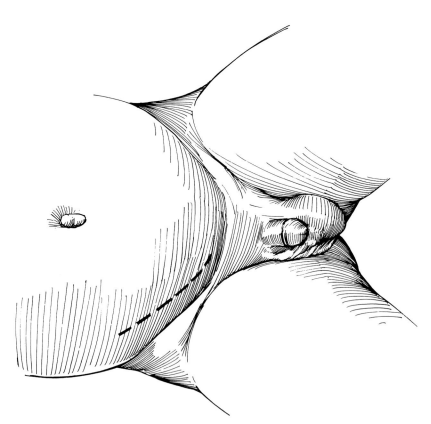

FIGURE 114-1. Place the child on a heating blanket, using a table extension to provide space for the surgeon's knees. Make a generous inguinal incision in the skin crease. Extend it well laterally to permit abdominal access (see Chapter 110).

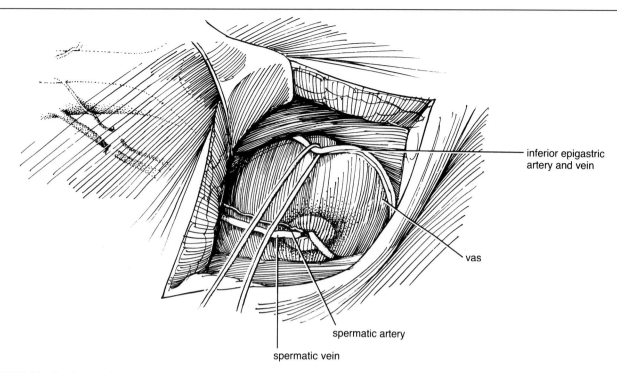

inferior epigastric
artery and vein

vas

spermatic artery

spermatic vein

FIGURE 114-2. Open the external oblique muscle and identify the gubernaculum and the processus vaginalis. Displace the ilioinguinal nerve laterally and follow the processus vaginalis to the internal ring. Watch out for a long-loop vas. Open the peritoneum at the internal ring. Locate the testis and place a traction suture in it. Expose the spermatic vessels. Move the testis out of the abdominal cavity into the retroperitoneal space and carefully dissect the peritoneum from its vascular pedicle. Close the peritoneum.

Using loupes, bluntly dissect retroperitoneally, following the vessels to near their communication with the vena cava or renal vein and aorta. Tag them with untied sutures so that the artery and vein can be individually identified later. Ensure that the dissection of the vessels extends beyond the confluence of the pampiniform plexus, forming a single vein. Preserve the vasal vessels in a large patch of peritoneum as the vas is freed into the pelvis. If the vas is too short, pass the testis under the lateral umbilical ligament (the obliterated umbilical artery).

Expose the inferior epigastric artery and its two venae comitantes by dissection through the internal oblique muscle aponeurosis and behind the transversus abdominis muscle. Divide all muscular branches. Hold them in a vessel loop. Assess them for size and flow. Ligate all of the side branches as far as possible from the main vessel because one of them may be of suitable size to be used for the anastomosis. Place a noncrushing microvascular clamp on the proximal ends and divide them high beneath the rectus muscle.

Under magnification, clear the adventitia from the artery and the larger vein, and cut them back to undamaged intima. (Preserve the other epigastric vein as a spare.) Regularly apply heparin-saline solution (10 U/mL) to the cut ends. Ligate or fulgurate their muscular branches with bipolar diathermy.

Prepare a dartos pouch. Now ligate the spermatic vessels high and divide them distal to the ligature. Check for backbleeding. Place the testis in the pouch. Close the peritoneal defect in the anterior part of the peritoneal cavity.

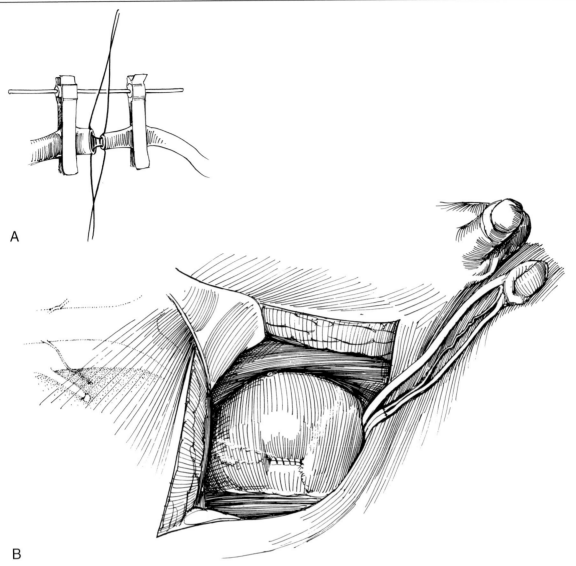

A

B

FIGURE 114-3. A, Bring the spermatic and the epigastric arteries into the microscopic field and place them in a microvascular clamp. Irrigate the ends of the vessels continuously with heparin-saline solution. Perform vascular anastomosis with 10-0 or 11-0 nylon sutures. Make the arterial anastomosis first. Expect a considerable disparity in size between the arteries; an oblique or a spatulated anastomosis may compensate for the difference. Keep ischemia time to less than 1 hour. Repeat the anastomotic procedure for the veins. If that is not feasible, ligate them and depend on collateral circulation. On release of the clamps, administer heparin in half of the full dose for the child's size.
B, Observe the anastomosis for 20 minutes to be sure occlusion will not occur. If thrombosis does result, resect and redo the anastomosis. Biopsy the testis (see Chapter 107) and look for fresh bleeding from that incision. Fix the testis in the scrotum and close the inguinal wound carefully to avoid obstructing the vessels. Follow with intravenous dextran of low molecular weight, 500 mL/24 hours for 3 days.

ADRIAN M. BIANCHI

Commentary by

The majority of palpable testes can be brought to the scrotum without tension by a minimally invasive "transscrotum" orchiopexy. For the more difficult testis, the addition of a conventional inguinal approach may provide further vessel length. The reliability of microvascular anastomosis for vessels smaller than 1 mm in diameter has removed the problem of the short vascular pedicle, so that the high inguinal and intra-abdominal testis now can be safely transferred to the scrotum with a full blood supply. Concern regarding testicular vessel size in the infant under 2 years of age is unfounded. Indeed, the genitalia and the testicular vascular pedicle are particularly well developed, possibly consequent to the heavy hormonal stimulation during the pregnancy. Recent experimental work in rats has demonstrated the absolute importance of a full blood supply and, particularly, sufficient venous drainage from the testis, in preserving spermatogenesis. It is therefore no longer logical, and is indeed self-defeating, to advocate techniques that rely on the vasal and other collaterals, following division of the main vascular pedicle, because the severe chronic ischemic injury to spermatogenic tissue or testicular venous congestion, or both, renders any surviving testis virtually sterile.

The child with an impalpable testis first should have a laparoscopy to locate and assess the testis, its vessels, and the vas. The child and parents are then counseled regarding the indications for microvascular orchiopexy. Only one testis should be transferred at any one session. There are no special anesthetic requirements, except those that are routine for a safe 3-hour procedure. No anticoagulant or other adjuvant therapy is necessary. However, cut vessel ends are constantly washed with a heparin-saline solution (10 U/mL) during the anastomoses. An operating room microscope is essential and should preferably be equipped with a foot pedal control for focus, zoom, and X-Y coupling.

The child is placed supine on a heating blanket on the operating table, and the bladder is emptied by manual suprapubic compression. The surgeon and assistant position themselves comfortably, and the microscope is adjusted for position and focus. A laterally extended skin-crease groin incision is deepened through the fibers of the external oblique muscle to identify the gubernacular structures and the processus vaginalis. The ilioinguinal nerve is displaced sideways and the processus vaginalis followed backward to the internal inguinal ring, where the inferior epigastric vessels are easily located. Care should be taken to avoid injury to a long-loop vas. The peritoneum is opened, and the testis is delivered out of the abdomen. The peritoneum is closed, and further careful blunt dissection of vessels and vas occurs extraperitoneally. Vessel dissection is taken high, toward the origin of the artery and beyond the confluence of the pampiniform plexus, to form a single testicular vein. One or two venous communications passing to the perinephric tissues are divided with sufficient length for additional venous anastomoses, if required. Vasal dissection is undertaken with due care to preserve the vasal collaterals. In the event of a short vas, additional length may be obtained by passing the testis beneath the obliterated umbilical artery. The testis with intact vas and vascular pedicle is then placed to one side. The inferior epigastric artery and its two venae comitantes are followed high beneath the rectus abdominis muscle, dividing all muscular branches, to provide a long donor pedicle and a better arterial diameter match to the much smaller testicular artery. The inferior epigastric vessels are clamped proximally with graded microvascular clamps and then divided. Under magnification with the operating microscope, the artery and the larger vein are carefully cleared of adventitia. The vessel ends are cleanly cut back in circular or spatulate fashion to undamaged intima. A wide circular (venous) anastomosis and a long, wide oblique (arterial) anastomosis are planned. The remaining inferior epigastric vein is preserved for a possible additional venous anastomosis or for vein donation, should a reverse interposition step-down graft be required for the difficult arterial anastomosis because of a marked mismatch in vessel diameter.

The testicular vessels are ligated high and divided. The testis is transferred through a prepared track to exit through a scrotal incision. Cooling with ice packs may be used but is not essential. Testicular perfusion definitively is contraindicated for fear of intimal damage. The testicular artery and vein are prepared under magnification with the operating microscope and the ends cut to match the inferior epigastric vessels. The testicular vein, at a diameter of 1.4 mm, is a reasonable match to the inferior epigastric vein, at 0.8 to 1 mm. However, there is a marked mismatch in the arterial wall thickness and the luminal diameter between the testicular artery, at 0.5 to 0.8 mm, and the inferior epigastric artery, at 1 to 1.2 mm. In the event of more than one testicular artery, the diameter may be further reduced to approximately 0.3 mm. Only one arterial anastomosis is required, and the interposition of a reversed venous step-down graft is helpful in these circumstances.

One arterial anastomosis and one venous anastomosis usually are required. Interrupted sutures of 10-0 monofilament nylon on a 3.75-mm, 75-pm needle (Ethilon W2870, or similar suture) are used to accurately appose the intimal surfaces. Vessel ends are washed constantly with a heparin-saline solution (10 U/mL). The venous anastomosis is completed first, and the microvascular clamps are removed to relieve any venous congestion from an inadequate venous collateral circulation. On completion of the arterial anastomosis, the testis becomes revascularized.

Continued

Anastomotic patency lasting longer than 20 minutes usually is associated with a good long-term outcome. Vessel thrombosis will occur within 5 minutes and is an indication of an imperfect anastomosis, for which the only management is resection and reanastomosis. A testicular biopsy is taken. Incision of the tunica albuginea will show active arterial bleeding from a pink testis of normal appearance. The testis is placed in a subdartos pouch in the ipsilateral scrotum. All wounds are closed in layers (including subcuticular skin closure) with absorbable materials. No postoperative monitoring is necessary, or indeed possible, in the young infant. The child is mobilized and allowed home within 24 to 36 hours. Successful microvascular orchiopexy is associated with an uncomplicated postoperative course and an expectation of a scrotal testis of normal consistency and mobility thereafter.

At the Royal Manchester Children's Hospital between 1981 and 1992, 49 testes in 41 boys between 2 and 15 years of age were transferred to the scrotum by microvascular techniques. Eight children had a bilateral transfer, and 31 had a unilateral orchiopexy, some for a single residual testis after loss of the contralateral organ. There has been no mortality and virtually no morbidity. A total of 45 testes is present in the scrotum, providing excellent cosmesis and "genital normality." The psychologic relief for the child, and particularly for the parents, has been noticeable. Indeed, those with bilateral intraabdominal testes insisted on the same procedure for the opposite side. No patients would accept orchiectomy as an option, even in full knowledge of potential malignancy in later life. Four testes have atrophied, either because of anastomotic failure or inherent abnormality. A few more than 50% of testes have shown varying numbers of spermatogonia, the remainder showing Sertoli cells only. There was no instance of in situ neoplasia. Most children in the series underwent the operation in the younger age group and still have not reached puberty. All testes in pubertal and postpubertal children have demonstrated good hormonal output and have grown to approximately 75% of expected volume for age. Postpubertal children are counseled regarding the malignancy risk and are taught the self-examination technique. Perhaps the most important indication for orchiopexy is the correction of an obvious genital anomaly. The provision of "normal genitalia" has a definite impact on the development of a normal psyche in the growing child and provides major relief for the parents. Enhanced spermatogenesis and reduced morbidity (torsion, hernia, and possibly malignancy) are also of major relevance.

Experience has shown that microvascular orchiopexy is a reliable and safe procedure. It is a further option in the successful transfer of the high inguinal and intra-abdominal testis to the scrotum. Whereas the child's age and the vessel diameter are no barrier, the skill of the surgeon most certainly requires laboratory and clinical development, if consistently high success rates are to be achieved. Techniques relying on vasal collaterals are associated with high atrophy rates and induce virtual sterility in surviving testes. Currently, there can be little reason for testicular transfer to the scrotum on anything less than a full blood supply.

Although microvascular orchiopexy is now a proven technique, its value in the management of the high testis on a short vascular pedicle requires long-term evaluation with reference to the development of the patient's psyche, his fertility, and the incidence of malignancy.

Chapter 115

Laparoscopic Orchiopexy Techniques

Laparoscopy falls into four categories: It (1) can be a definitive diagnostic as well as therapeutic procedure in cases of cryptorchidism, (2) may be used for gonadectomy in children with disorders of sex development and/or with a dysplastic testis, (3) is an appropriate route for the first stage of a staged orchiopexy (see Chapter 111), and (4) may be the preferable technique for orchiopexy for the high intra-abdominal testes especially in syndromic children.

The advantages of a laparoscopic approach are several: minimal incision, optimal exposure and magnification, preservation of the perivascular tissue, high mobilization of the vessels, creation of a new ring under direct visualization, and avoidance of traction. For example, with a testis lying above the inguinal canal, the vessels can be freed retroperitoneally, preparatory to an orchiopexy, that then may be done either openly or laparoscopically. If the vessels are short, a new canal may be made through which to bring the testis directly into the scrotum (the Prentiss maneuver). Or the vessels may be clipped at a high level, as in the first stage of a Fowler-Stephens orchiopexy (see Chapter 111).

Caution the parents that although the operation will be done through three small incisions, it is still a surgical procedure because bleeding and bowel injury can be serious complications. Warn them also that the procedure may not be completed as planned and an open operation may be necessary after all.

LAPAROSCOPIC TECHNIQUE IN CHILDREN

A laparoscopic approach in children is different from that in adults because the distance between the anterior abdominal wall and the great vessels is shorter, and thus the organs lie closer to the surface.

If adhesions are anticipated, prepare the bowel both mechanically and with antibiotics. It is sensible to have a standby table of laparotomy instruments ready for complications.

Use general anesthesia in children because carbon dioxide intraperitoneally causes pain, and any motion by the child is hazardous. Moreover, muscle relaxation is important because the chance for injury to intra-abdominal structures is increased in the small intraperitoneal space. Placement of an endotracheal tube is recommended to ensure absence of movement and to allow mechanical assistance to respiration as the intra-abdominal pressure rises. Be aware that in long cases, hypercarbia from absorbed carbon dioxide may become a problem.

After induction of anesthesia but before creation of a pneumoperitoneum, palpate the abdomen and inguinal area again seeking a gonadal organ that has been missed. If one is felt, it may be less expensive to explore the groin openly. This can be done rapidly, with minimal risk, and provides full information. It also may constitute the initial step of orchiopexy. Then, if no testis or nubbin is found, proceed with laparoscopy. Alternatively, make an umbilical puncture and explore with a small scope. If no testis is found, merely withdraw the instrument. But if an abdominal testis is seen, add another trocar and proceed with orchiopexy. Other uses for the laparoscope are the completion of a previously unsuccessful open orchiopexy; correction of bilateral cryptorchidism; and exploration when hypertrophy suggests maldevelopment of the contralateral testis.

INSERTION OF TROCARS

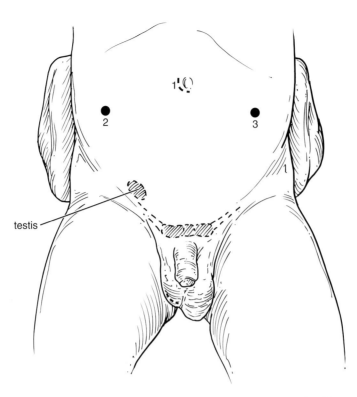

testis

FIGURE 115-1. Place the boy supine and induce anesthesia. Check again for a palpable testis: one in five may now be palpable. Insert a balloon catheter into the bladder and drain it. (Its extrapelvic position in infants make it vulnerable to injury.) Consider placing a nasogastric tube; a distended stomach may depress the omentum into the route of the trocars. Once the child is relaxed, again examine for a testis in the distal canal, a position that would allow performance of a standard orchiopexy. If the testis is high but palpable, either proceed with laparoscopic orchiopexy or limit the laparoscopic procedure to the dissection of the intra-abdominal vessels and vas preparatory to an open operation.

Insert a rolled towel under the lower back to create lordosis. Tip the table into a 30-degree Trendelenburg position to move the intestines out of the pelvis. After introduction of the laparoscope, return to a 30-degree tilt for the operation. It can also be helpful to rotate the table 30 degrees laterally toward the surgeon to raise the involved testis above the intestine. Prep the genitalia and the entire abdomen in case laparotomy will be required. Choose between a closed Veress and an open Hassan technique. Test all equipment before starting.

Veress technique: If right-handed, stand on the left side of the child. Palpate the sacral promontory and the aorta. Make a curved incision with a #15 blade in the lower edge of the umbilicus, one that penetrates the linea alba where the body wall is thinnest.

In infants less than 1 year of age, because the umbilical fascia may be very thin, do not place the incision too close to the umbilicus proper, which could foster loss of the pneumoperitoneum. It may be better to insert the needle above the umbilicus to avoid the as-yet-undescended bladder. Remember that the distance from the anterior abdominal wall to the great vessels is very short; be careful not to pass instruments too deeply.

The Veress needle has two parts: a sharp beveled sheath to pass through the body wall and a blunt obturator that springs forward to fend off the intestine. Check the mechanism and patency. Start the flow of carbon dioxide and determine the passive resistance to flow. Infiltrate the site with a local anesthetic. Elevate the fascia with towel clips. Hold the Veress needle vertically and press it firmly through the incision at a 30-degree angle directed toward the hollow of the sacrum. Feel it pass first through the fascia and then through the peritoneum.

Check the position of the needle by aspiration with a syringe; there should be no return of blood or bowel contents. Apply the saline test: inject 10 mL of saline irrigating solution; it should not be possible to aspirate it. (Return by aspiration would indicate preperitoneal placement.) Alternatively or additionally, place a drop of saline in the hub of the needle; normally it will disappear. Swing the needle through 360 degrees. Check intraperitoneal pressure to be sure it is less than 12 mmHg and that it shifts with respiration.

Anatomic detail is seen more clearly in children because of the small amount of preperitoneal fat. This characteristic also reduces the chance for preperitoneal placement of the tip of the trocar during insertion, but because the peritoneum is more loosely attached, this space is more susceptible to emphysema. Also, the weak adherence of the peritoneum to the abdominal wall makes the intraperitoneal introduction of large cannulas difficult. An instrument may have to be inserted through a smaller port to assist entry of the large port.

FIGURE 115-1, cont'd. Hassan technique: Make an infraumbilical incision and insert two stay sutures on either side. Incise the peritoneum and palpate the underside of the abdominal wall with a finger to be sure it is clear of adherent bowel or omentum. Insert the obturator of the cannula. Move the outer conical sheath forward and push it tightly in the fascial opening; then secure it to the sheath. Draw the stay sutures up and fix them to the struts on the sheath of the cannula to produce a tight seal. Remove the obturator.

Begin insufflation with carbon dioxide at a rate of 1 L/minute. If the flow remains low with high pressure, the needle tip lies preperitoneally; reposition it. Continue filling until the pressure in a typical relaxed child reaches 8 mmHg, realizing that relaxation is achieved at different rates.

Insertion of sheath and trocar (site 1): Incise the fascia of the linea alba with a #11 blade. Identify the peritoneum, open it, and insert a 5-mm sheath (this is large enough for infants) with its contained, short pyramidal trocar. Point the trocar at the sacral promontory while pressing on the upper abdomen, and insert it into the abdominal cavity. Keep the index finger extended on the instrument to prevent the tip from going too deeply. When gas is heard escaping, quickly remove the trocar from the sheath to let the valve in the sheath close the channel. Connect the carbon dioxide supply and set the flow control on the insufflator to provide a pressure of 5 to 6 mmHg above baseline. Inflate until the abdomen becomes tympanitic.

Insertion of the telescope: Insert a 5-mm laparoscope and attach a full-beam video camera to the eyepiece. Monitor the area on the screen placed at the foot of the table. First check to be certain no intra-abdominal structures were injured during insertion. Then systematically inspect the pertinent organs in the peritoneal cavity.

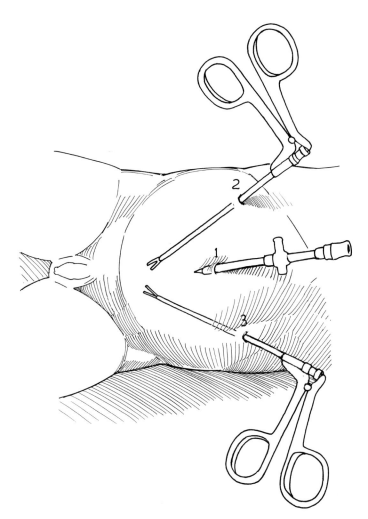

FIGURE 115-2. Insertion of working ports: Rotate the lens to bring the anterior abdominal wall above the bladder into view. While the abdominal wall is transilluminated from within, insert two 5-mm working ports, one at each McBurney's point (sites 2 and 3). (Place them higher in infants, to provide adequate working distance at the umbilical level.) Insert these ports by elevating the body wall with towel clips and then rotating the trocar to aid penetration. Avoid traversing the inferior epigastric vessels, which are visible by transillumination.

General precaution: To avoid injury to abdominal structures, be sure to keep the inner ends of all instruments in view; do not leave them unattended.

NORMAL LAPAROSCOPIC LANDMARKS

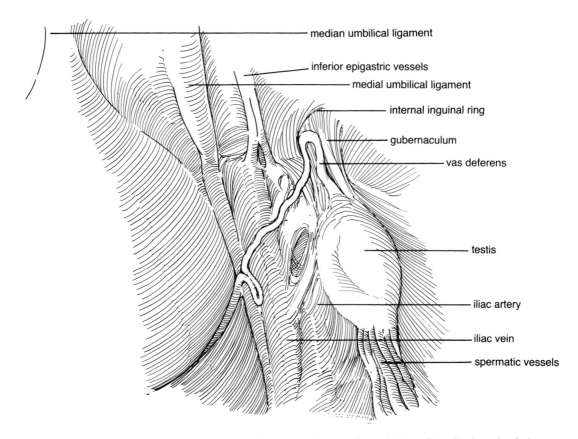

median umbilical ligament

inferior epigastric vessels

medial umbilical ligament

internal inguinal ring

gubernaculum

vas deferens

testis

iliac artery

iliac vein

spermatic vessels

FIGURE 115-3. Inspect the peritoneal cavity, especially the underlying bowel. Visualize the inguinal ring contralateral to the affected testis, with its vessels and vas. Now visualize the ring on the cryptorchid side. Look for the vas where it crosses the medial umbilical ligament. Traction on the scrotum may make the vessels more obvious.

   Landmarks: The median umbilical ligament (the urachal remnant) runs from the bladder dome to the umbilicus. Lateral to it, find the medial umbilical ligament (the obliterated umbilical artery) extending from the hypogastric artery to the umbilicus. Identify the internal inguinal ring, the gubernaculum, the vas deferens (it may end blindly), and the gonadal vessels that normally run into the internal inguinal ring but may be atretic or absent. (If visualization and identification are problems, check the carbon dioxide insufflator for better insufflation.)

EXPLORATION FOR THE UNILATERAL NONPALPABLE TESTIS

Look for one of seven possibilities:

1. The spermatic cord passes through the internal inguinal ring. This indicates the presence of a testis or remnant in the area of the groin. Press on the external ring to see if the testis can be pushed back into the abdomen. If it responds, perform either a standard or a laparoscopic orchiopexy. A standard orchiopexy can be facilitated by laparoscopically mobilizing the spermatic vessels to the level of the kidney.

2. The testis is found just above the internal ring, but with a short processus vaginalis. Here too, either type of orchiopexy is feasible.

3. No testis is found, but the cord structures disappear into the canal. Use a grasper to pull on these structures to expose a testicular remnant in the groin. If there is still a question, consider inguinal exploration through a small incision.

4. A testis with adnexae and a long looping vas is found lying well above the internal ring. This is best managed by a staged Fowler-Stephens orchiopexy (see the section, "Laparoscopic Two-Stage Orchiopexy [Fowler-Stephens]"). As the first stage, clip or fulgurate the spermatic vessels now.

5. No testis is found. Look for blind-ending spermatic vessels as proof of testicular absence (the "vanishing testis").

6. If an atrophic or dysmorphic testis is found, remove it either laparoscopically or through a muscle-splitting incision in the lower quadrant.
7. If only a blind-ending vas is found at the internal ring but the vessels cannot be identified, indicating that a testis is present, search the entire retroperitoneum to the lower pole of the kidney, even if this requires reflection of the colon.

To summarize, inspect the normal side for orientation. If cord structures enter the canal, follow them with the laparoscope to reach the testis. If none is found, place a second 5-mm port on the same side, and with grasping forceps search for the testis intra-abdominally in the paracolic gutter at the base of the colonic mesentery. If a dysplastic gonad is found, biopsy, resect, and remove the remnant.

Instruments for exploration include a 5-mm laparoscope with attached video camera and a 5-mm biopsy forceps. For orchiopexy, have available two 5-mm working ports.

SINGLE-STAGE LAPAROSCOPIC ORCHIOPEXY

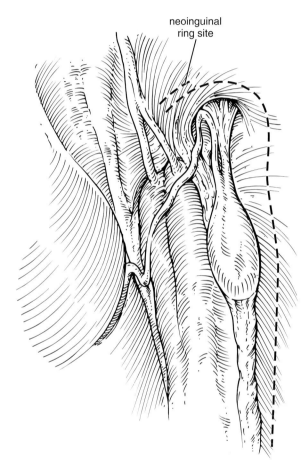

neoinguinal ring site

FIGURE 115-4. Stand on the side opposite that of the abnormal testis, with your assistant across from you. Inspect the pelvic peritoneal cavity with a 30-degree lens. Locate the medial umbilical ligament (urachal remnant) and the sigmoid colon. Move the colon medially for proximal access to the spermatic vessels. Formal colonic mobilization is not needed, because once the peritoneum has been incised, the colon becomes displaced medially.

Identify the intra-abdominal testes. Grasp the gubernaculum and pull the testes over to reach the contralateral internal inguinal ring. If it reaches, it probably can be placed in the ipsilateral scrotum. If the vessels are too short, proceed with their division as described in Fig. 115-5, setting up for a two-stage procedure.

Incise the peritoneum starting around the internal ring distally up to the gubernaculum and bordering the testis laterally *(long dashed line)*.

To provide a large peritoneal covering that encompasses the vas deferens and the testicular blood supply, mobilize a flap of peritoneum that extends laterally 1 cm from the spermatic vessels toward the lower pole of the kidney and ventrally 1 cm from the vas deferens extending from the internal ring into the pelvis. Releasing the peritoneal attachments under the spermatic vessels will allow mobilization of the testes. During the dissection, watch out for the ureter, which runs over, then lies medial to, the iliac vessels.

For the site of the new inguinal canal, make a short incision in the peritoneum *(short dashed line)* between the bladder and the medial umbilical ligament, just lateral to the median umbilical ligament, to the site of the new canal.

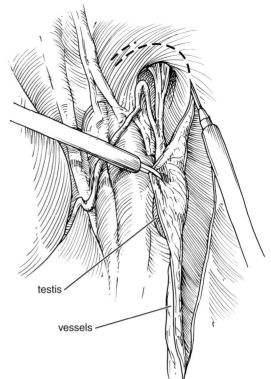

FIGURE 115-5. Start dissection of the gubernaculum distally as far as possible to preserve all collateral vessels. Release the gubernacular attachment typically from within the open internal ring. Check the mobility of the testes for placement into the scrotum by again seeing if it will reach the contralateral ring. If more mobility is necessary, continue to raise the testis on the flap of peritoneum, leaving a broad isthmus of peritoneum on the vas.

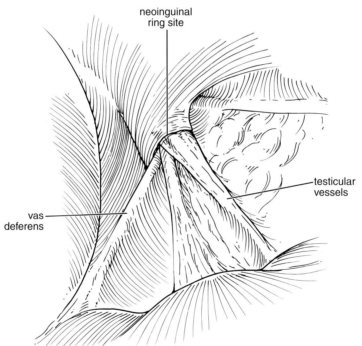

FIGURE 115-6. Make a 2-cm external incision in the scrotum (see Fig. 115-9). Form a new inguinal canal medial to the medial umbilical ligament by passing a clamp, an Amplatz dilator, or a radially dilating trocar from above through the peritoneal incision, then along the ventral surface of the symphysis, and out though the scrotal incision (the Prentiss maneuver). Lead a clamp or cannula back from below to pass out through the scrotal incision. Grasp the testis and draw it into the scrotum (this may be done through the cannula, if one is used). Have your assistant keep pressure over the canal to conserve carbon dioxide although the gas will be retained once the testis is in place. With traction on the testis, divide any remaining retroperitoneal attachments from above.

Fix the testis beneath the dartos muscle with fine synthetic absorbable sutures (see Chapter 108). Do not place a fixation suture into the testis itself, which could impair fertility.

Close the scrotal wound with subcuticular synthetic absorbable sutures. Replace the parietal peritoneum over the area of the patent processus vaginalis. Inspect the vas and associated structures for torsion and the operative area for bleeding. Aspirate most of the carbon dioxide to reduce peritoneal irritation, and remove the instrument sheaths in order. Finally, before removing the visualizing port, inspect for bleeding at a pressure of 6 mmHg. Close the skin with subcuticular sutures. Discharge the child on recovery from the anesthetic. Complications are rare.

LAPAROSCOPIC TWO-STAGE ORCHIOPEXY (FOWLER-STEPHENS)

If the testis is found associated with a long, looping vas deferens or lacks mobility within the abdomen, proceed with this first stage of a two-stage laparoscopic orchiopexy. Each stage may be done as an outpatient procedure.

First Stage: Laparoscopic Vessel Ligation

Position the patient as for one-stage laparascopic orchiopexy and gain laparascopic access.

Pull on the testis to help decide whether the vessels are short and will require clipping, as a first stage, or whether to proceed at once with laparoscopic orchiopexy. If no testis is located, use graspers to move the abdominal organs and thus reach the lower pole of the kidney to search in that area. If a dysgenic testis is found, remove it.

Divide the vessels as high as possible. Several methods are available: The least secure is to insert an electrode, elevate and fulgurate the vessels with unipolar or bipolar current, and then divide them. Clipping is, however, preferable. Separate the cord into bundles, and then pass a 10-mm clip applier and clip the vessels as high as possible. Apply a second set of clips so that the vessels may be divided between them at the second stage.

Remove the instrument sheath, evacuate the carbon dioxide to a level of 6 mmHg, and inspect the area for venous bleeding. Remove the visualizing port. Close the 10-mm port opening with a 4-0 silk arterial suture to approximate both peritoneum and fascia. Close the skin with subcuticular sutures and sterile strips.

Second Stage: Placement of the Testis

After 6 months, on a come-and-go basis, place the child supine. Insert a rolled towel under the lower back to create lordosis, and tip the table into a 10-degree head-down position to allow the intestine to drop out of the pelvis. After induction of anesthesia, shift the child to a 30-degree head-down position for placement of the initial port. After inserting both ports, tilt the table laterally 30 degrees to raise the involved testis above the intestines.

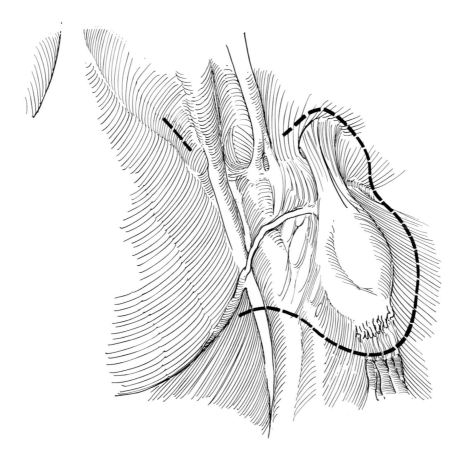

FIGURE 115-7. Incise the peritoneum starting around the internal ring distally up to the gubernaculum and bordering the testis laterally *(long dashed line)*. To provide a large peritoneal covering that encompasses the vas deferens and the collateral blood supply, take a generous triangular flap of peritoneum that extends laterally 1 cm from the spermatic vessels toward the kidney. Bring the incision medially at the site of the previous spermatic vessel ligation, preserving the collateral blood supply. Distally at the site of the internal ring the peritoneal incision should be ventrally 1 cm from the vas deferens, extending from the internal ring into the pelvis. Bluntly mobilize the spermatic vessels to the site of fulguration, and free the vas deferens.

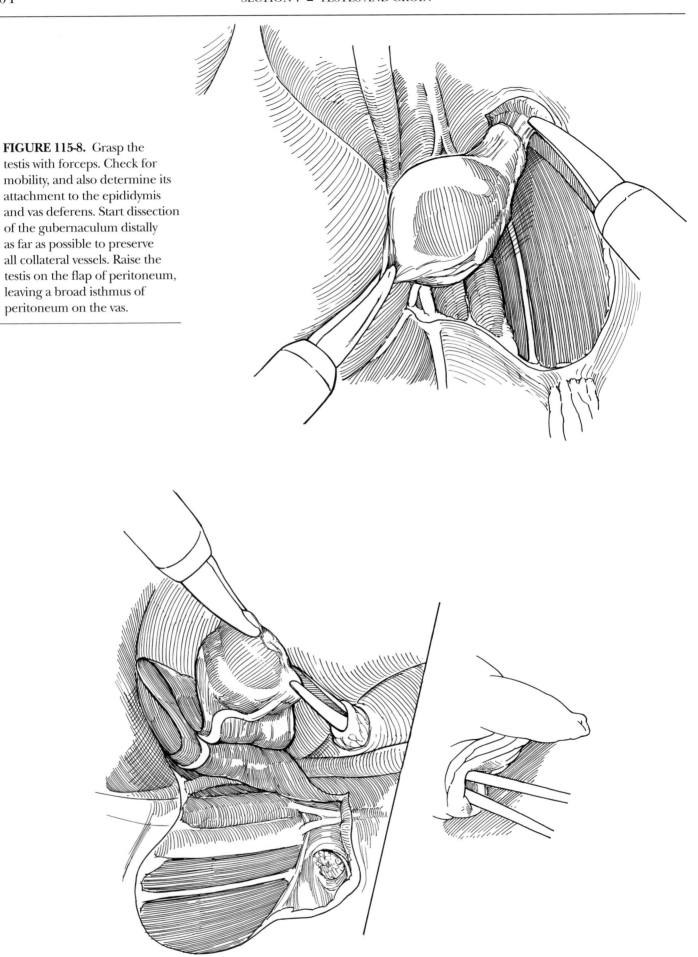

FIGURE 115-8. Grasp the testis with forceps. Check for mobility, and also determine its attachment to the epididymis and vas deferens. Start dissection of the gubernaculum distally as far as possible to preserve all collateral vessels. Raise the testis on the flap of peritoneum, leaving a broad isthmus of peritoneum on the vas.

FIGURE 115-9. Place the testes into the scrotum as described in Figure 115-5.

POSTOPERATIVE PROBLEMS

Problems during Any Laparoscopic Procedure

Most complications occur at the time of the initial insertion of the trocar, or during insufflation.

Preperitoneal emphysema makes identification of landmarks difficult. Emphysema of the omentum causes it to obstruct the view. Too high an insufflation pressure causes tension pneumoperitoneum, a harmful event that can be missed in obese children. Puncture of the abdominal aorta or other major vessel is made obvious by a vigorous spurt of blood: Leave the sheath in place for tamponade and for a guide to the site of injury, and proceed with emergency laparotomy. Recognize injury to the inferior epigastric vessels by blood dripping into the pelvis. Cauterize the route of these vessels or enlarge the incision to transfix them with sutures above and below the puncture site. For injury to the bowel from the trocar or sheath, open the abdomen and repair the bowel. It is seldom necessary to resect the bowel or divert the fecal stream. A puncture wound of the bladder can usually be sutured laparoscopically, or closed by a suture passed through a small suprapubic incision. For ureteral injury, especially if caused by electrocoagulation, stent the ureter.

Problems from Laparoscopic Procedures on the Testis

Postoperative bleeding rarely occurs if the site of operation and the trocar sites have been closely inspected at low pressure at the end of the procedure. An incisional hernia, or dehiscence through a large port site, can occur if the fascia was not closed. Suspect bowel injury if nausea and vomiting and ileus appear. Institute nasogastric suction and, if improvement does not follow, explore the site.

Testicular retraction is the most common problem after orchiopexy. The cause is usually inadequate initial mobilization of the testis or failure to route the cord by a direct route (the Prentiss maneuver). After the boy has fully recovered, reoperate through the groin. Dissect inferiorly, and then mobilize the spermatic cord en bloc (see Chapter 113), leaving the densely scarred tissue in place. Dissect into normal retroperitoneum where it may be possible to lengthen the cord. Other complications include hematoma, transection of the vas deferens (requiring microsurgical vasovasostomy later), and a missed direct or indirect inguinal hernia. Testicular atrophy may result, either from actual division of the spermatic artery or, more often, by persistent vasospasm from excessive tension during fixation.

GUY BOGAERT

Commentary by

Looking back to 1991 when laparoscopy had started to become part of the normal, routine pediatric urology practice, I was extremely fortunate to work with a mentor, Barry Kogan, who was one of the pioneers experimenting with the limitations of laparoscopic surgery for abdominal testis. We still perform the same tricks as we used to in the early days.

However, I remember well that John Duckett tempered my overenthusiasm to perform laparoscopy in every child with a nonpalpable testis. He stated, correctly, that in most cases the cause and the definitive treatment in the situation of a nonpalpable testis can be found and solved by an initial inguinal exploration. From this inguinal incision, you can indeed remove an atrophic testis or a blind-ending vas deferens, or, in some situations, luxate the intra-abdominal testis into the groin and mobilize the testis into the scrotum. Now we perform laparoscopy only in situations of an empty groin and an absent vas deferens and vessels. For laparoscopic therapeutic procedures, usually three ports are standard. Do not be afraid to switch the camera to one of the site ports; sometimes it may be handier to view the site differently or to have access from the midline.

When a child younger than 10 years old has a normal descended contralateral testis and an intra-abdominal testis, we will initially try, after dissecting the testicular vessels as far as possible, to mobilize this testis directly to the paravesical space (ventral of the symphysis) toward the scrotum (Prentiss maneuver). If this is possible, a subdartos pouch is created and a long Faure clamp is introduced from the scrotum over the symphysis into the abdomen (be aware that the intra-abdominal pressure—and your view—can drop, as the carbon dioxide will leak from now on) and the testis is handed over from a laparoscopic clamp. The testis is then fixed into the subdartos pouch from "outside." However, if the vessels are insufficiently long, we ligate or coagulate the testicular vessels above the testis as high as possible (to allow the collateral blood supply) and mobilize the testis toward the scrotum as we just described: a one-stage Fowler-Stephens technique. The reason is obvious: The paternity chance in unilateral cryptorchidism is the same as in bilateral normal descended testes. In addition, testicular (exocrine) quality of an intra-abdominal testis is never very favorable. There is improved outcome of the Fowler-Stephens technique, even in the single stage, by performing it laparoscopically: The excellent view for dissecting the vas deferens and respecting these vessels, together with the correct angled view, contributes to the improved success in testicular survival. There is almost no benefit between a one-stage and a two-stage Fowler-Stephens orchiopexy.

When a boy younger than 10 years old has a normal descended testis and a contralateral intra-abdominal testis, this testis should be removed. It is obvious that the most effective way to remove an intra-abdominal testis is with laparoscopy.

STEVEN DOCIMO

First, we would not recommend a rolled towel to create lordosis. This will move the great vessels closer to the anterior abdominal wall, as well as decrease working space. We prefer an open technique through a small incision using a radially dilating trocar for initial access, which nearly obviates the risk of great vessel injury. The working ports can be 3 mm in infants and small children, giving a superior cosmetic result with no disadvantages with instrumentation. The exception is in the case in which clips will be used on the spermatic vessels, requiring one 5-mm trocar. The testis will not reach the contra-lateral ring prior to dissection in most cases, so this should not be used as the indication for a staged Fowler-Stephens pro-cedure. Instead, the appearance of short, taut vessels with a testis more than 2 cm from the ring is an indicator of inadequate length for primary orchiopexy. The dissection is carried out with the aim of maintaining the distal triangle of peritoneum between the vessels and vas. The peritoneum over the proximal vessels can be divided, giving quite a bit of added length. This is often easier after the testis has been delivered into the scrotum. We would tend to create the neocanal medial to the inferior epigastric vessels, but lateral to the medial umbilical ligament to avoid bladder injury.

Part II

Testis Exclusion

Chapter 116

Simple Orchiectomy

Simple orchiectomy is rarely indicated in the pediatric urologic patient. Indications include a nonviable testis from either torsion or trauma and removal of a gonad in a patient with a disorder of sex development for an increased potential for malignancy.

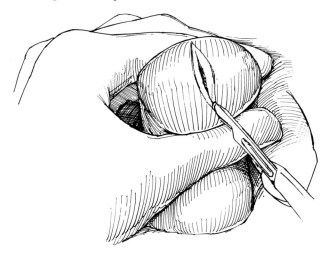

FIGURE 116-1. Position: Supine. Stand on the boy's right side, pull the testis down to relax the cremaster muscle, and grasp the cord with the left hand at the top of the scrotum, placing the thumb in front and the index finger behind it. With the needle approaching the index finger, infiltrate the cord with 1% lidocaine solution without epinephrine through a 2.5-inch, 25-gauge needle. Grasp the testis with the fingers and thumb to stretch the skin over the testis. Make a transverse incision in the scrotum to avoid the scrotal vessels. For bilateral excision, make a vertical incision in the scrotal raphe. Incise the dartos muscle and cremasteric layers onto the bluish tunica vaginalis. Control bleeding vessels with the electrocautery held in the other hand. Push the scrotal layers away with sponge dissection and deliver the testis within the tunica vaginalis into the wound. Alternatively, open the tunica vaginalis before delivering the testis.

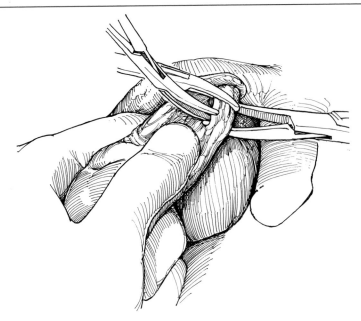

FIGURE 116-2. Draw the testis down to expose the epididymis and cord. Bluntly dissect the spermatic vessels from the vas deferens and from each other. Divide and ligate the vas with 3-0 synthetic absorbable suture. In adolescents, clamp each group individually, and ligate them with the same type of suture. It may be wise to use a suture-ligature for the spermatic artery, because this vessel retracts after division and loss of the ligature results in major (hidden) retroperitoneal bleeding. Should this occur, quickly extend the incision to expose the cord in the retroperitoneal space via the inguinal canal. In children, individual ligation is not necessary; the entire cord may be clamped, especially with torsion and the cord suture-ligated. Before closing, coagulate any bleeders in the dartos muscle and subcutaneous tissue to avoid a distressing scrotal hematoma. Close the dartos layer with a running synthetic absorbable suture and bring the skin together with the subcutaneous tissue with interrupted 4-0 or 5-0 synthetic absorbable sutures or with a fine subcuticular running suture, with or without a Penrose drain pulled back into the scrotum. A fluff pressure dressing does not stop significant oozing.

POSTOPERATIVE PROBLEMS

Continued oozing with formation of a scrotal hematoma is the most common complication and is the result of incomplete hemostasis in the several loose layers of the scrotum.

Placement of a drain before closure avoids formation of a hematoma but should not be necessary if good technique is followed. Drain a hematoma only if it becomes distressingly large or infected.

H. GIL RUSHTON

Commentary by

Testicular torsion would be the primary indication for simple orchiectomy in the pediatric population. Always perform a contralateral simple orchidopexy in these cases. In this setting, the surgeon will frequently encounter significant thickening of the scrotal wall and venous oozing as a result of scrotal edema and hyperemia.

Leaving an adequate stump of the spermatic vessels extending beyond the edge of the clamp will reduce the risk of bleeding associated with slippage of the ligature. I would only recommend spermatic cord block as the primary form of anesthesia in a postpubertal adolescent, because younger children generally are not cooperative enough to perform this procedure under local anesthesia.

HUBERT S. SWANA

Commentary by

In children, simple orchiectomy is reserved primarily for cases of testicular torsion. Fixation of the contralateral testis with permanent sutures is mandatory. An incision through the median raphe provides an excellent cosmetic outcome and allows for easy access to both testicles. However, a medium raphe incision does violate the neuroinnervation of the scrotum, which would support the use of two transverse incisions.

In testicular torsion of long duration the surgeon frequently encounters impressive scrotal wall edema and venous bleeding. With careful attention to hemostasis throughout the case, drains are rarely needed. When ligating the vascular pedicle, care should be taken to allow an adequate "stump" of vessels beyond the clamp so that you can securely place the ligature. In the setting of acute testicular torsion it is rare to find a child or adolescent that can tolerate the procedure with local anesthesia alone.

Chapter 117

Laparoscopic Orchiectomy

Laparoscopic orchiectomy is recommended for removal of a small intra-abdominal testis in a postpubertal patient in whom orchiopexy is not appropriate. It may also be useful for excision of discordant gonads in disorders of sex development.

Follow the techniques and insertion of the laparoscopic sheaths as described in Chapter 115. Through a small sub- umbilical incision, open the peritoneum and insert an initial camera port via either the Hassan or Veress technique. Place two additional 3- or 5-mm working ports, depending on the side of the abnormal testes.

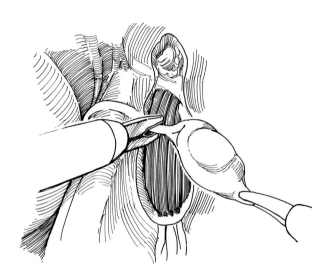

FIGURE 117-1. Locate the small testis endoscopically among the sites suggested in Figure 115-1. It will usually lie along the course of normal descent. Grasp and incise the peritoneum over the upper pole of the testis to identify it, and begin blunt dissection. Fulgurate the (usually small) spermatic vessels. For larger vessels, after making a window, put tension on them with a 5-mm grasper, and then doubly clip them. Dissect the testis from its bed along with a short length of vas deferens. Pull on the gubernaculum and fulgurate it. Clip the vas on the distal side and divide it. Usually the testis is small or atrophic so that it can be withdrawn through the sheath or removed after enlarging one of the accessory ports. Alternatively, place the testis in a specimen retrieval bag, and draw the mouth of the bag to the sheath of the trocar at the anterior abdominal wall. Withdraw the sheath, clamp the bag, and draw the testis through the puncture site. Now inspect the bed before withdrawing the trocar, and then close the site. Alternatively, first locate the testis endoscopically. Then make a small, localized incision over it, and excise the testis using clamps, sutures, and scissors.

Commentary by
RONALD SUTHERLAND

In the infant, the spermatic vessels and vas deferens can usually be cauterized using the hook electrode or endoscissors, and the testis or discordant gonad removed easily through a 5-mm port. In the older male, however, the vessels and vas should be clipped and divided prior to removal of the testis. If the testis is "peeping" into the inguinal canal, make a small groin incision to remove the testis.

Commentary by
H. GIL RUSHTON

The laparoscopic removal of the testis is indicated in the case of an atrophic or hypoplastic undescended intra-abdominal testis when orchiopexy is not considered more appropriate, particularly in the postpubertal adolescent. Other less common indications would include the removal of abnormal premalignant gonads found in some intersex states, such as testicular feminization and mixed gonadal dysgenesis. If laparoscopic examination demonstrates that the testis has actually migrated into the inguinal canal, a small groin incision can be made to remove the testis.

Chapter 118

Radical Orchiectomy

Perform scrotal ultrasound. Obtain serum for markers: alpha-fetoprotein (AFP) and human chorionic gonadotropin. After removal of the testis, repeat the measurement of the serum markers, obtain a chest film, and perform abdominal and thoracic computed tomography (CT) to stage the disease at that time. Determine the pathologic type of tumor and treat accordingly. For an infant with a yolk sac tumor, radical orchiectomy is adequate primary therapy; reserve irradiation and chemotherapy for residual tumor. For boys with stage I, IIa, or IIb seminomas and normal AFP levels, apply radiation therapy postoperatively; for boys with bulky or disseminated seminoma or other germ cell tumors, treat according to stage.

Organ-sparing techniques for tumor in a solitary testis if the preoperative testosterone levels are normal, or for bilateral tumors, are as follows:

Method 1 (Steiner, 2003): For small tumors 25 mm or less in diameter and distant from the rete in boys with normal plasma levels of luteinizing hormone and testosterone, stage the tumor and localize it with ultrasound. Occlude the spermatic vessels and cool the testis. Resect the tumor, taking biopsies of the adjacent tissue.

Method 2: Percutaneously apply high-intensity focused ultrasound to destroy the tumor while preserving the surrounding parenchyma. Then irradiate the testis (20 Gy) to obliterate intraepithelial neoplasia.

RADICAL ORCHIECTOMY

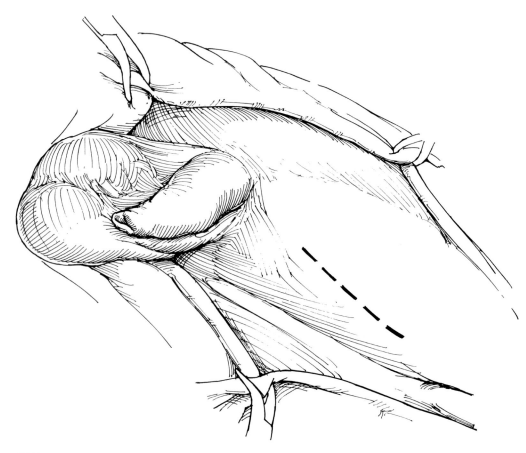

FIGURE 118-1. Prep and drape the lower abdomen and genitalia. Incise the skin above and parallel to the inguinal ligament, as for inguinal hernia repair. Divide the subcutaneous fat and ligate the several veins with 3-0 synthetic absorbable sutures as encountered.

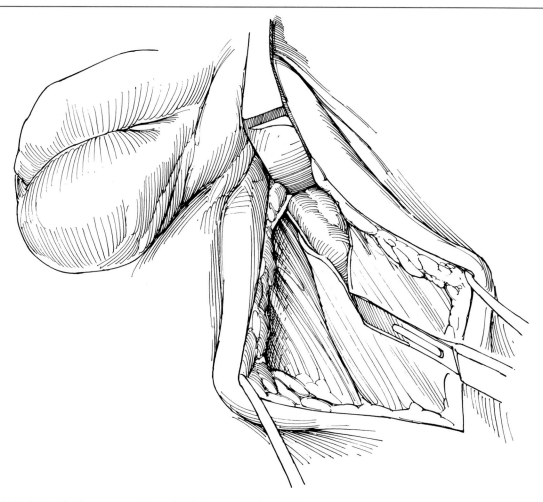

FIGURE 118-2. Identify the external inguinal ring, and sharply incise the external oblique fascia. Take care to avoid the ilioinguinal nerve lying just beneath it.

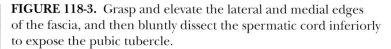

FIGURE 118-3. Grasp and elevate the lateral and medial edges of the fascia, and then bluntly dissect the spermatic cord inferiorly to expose the pubic tubercle.

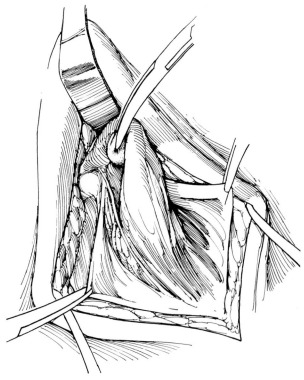

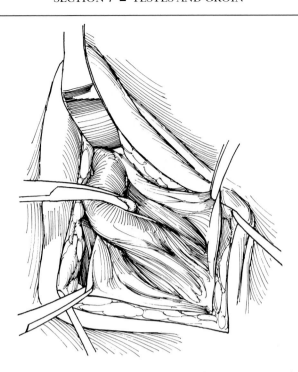

FIGURE 118-4. Repeat the dissection medially, elevating the medial fascial edge so that all of the cord structures, including the cremaster muscle, can be surrounded with a Penrose drain.

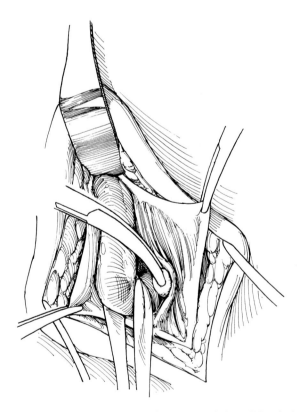

FIGURE 118-5. Lift the Penrose drain and free the cord to the internal ring. Watch for a perforating cremasteric vessel, which must be ligated. Follow the vas medially to separate it from the vessels, and clamp and divide it between nonabsorbable ligatures.

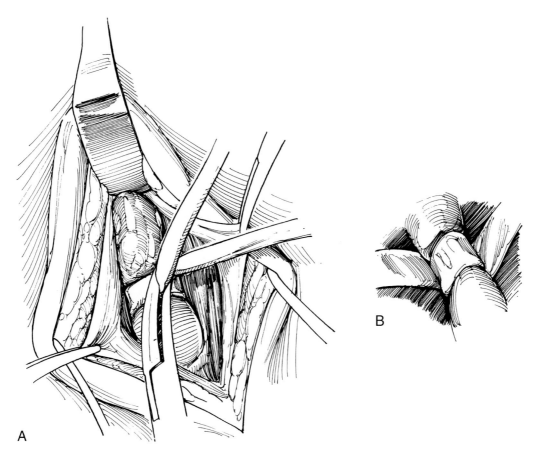

FIGURE 118-6. **A** and **B,** To prevent escape of malignant cells into the bloodstream during manipulation, place a small latex catheter around the cord below the ring as a tourniquet.

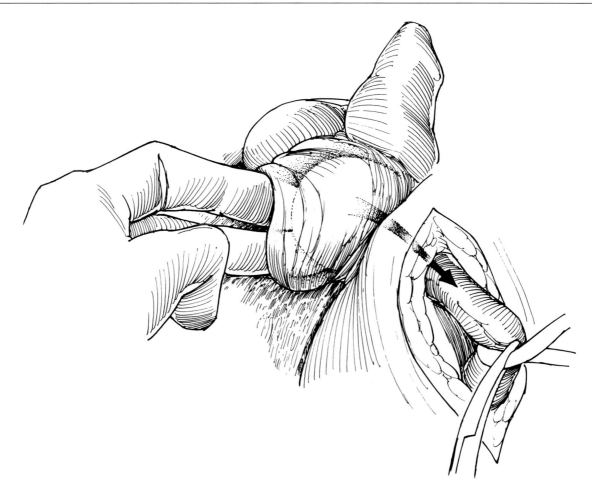

FIGURE 118-7. Stretch the neck of the scrotum and push the testicle upward. For large tumors, Scarpa's fascia may require further division, but avoid extension of the incision distally over the symphysis.

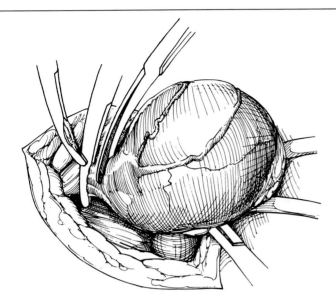

FIGURE 118-8. Clamp and divide the gubernacular attachments and ligate them.

FIGURE 118-9. Biopsy: If at this point there are any doubts about the diagnosis, place the testis on a sterile towel, where the tunica vaginalis may be opened. Inspect the testis directly; rarely will biopsy with frozen section be necessary. However, this can be done without risk of spread if the testis is draped out of the field for the biopsy and the surgeon changes towels, gloves, and instruments after removing the testis. Open the internal oblique muscle at the internal ring for 2 or 3 cm and dissect the vas and spermatic vessels as far as feasible through this incision.

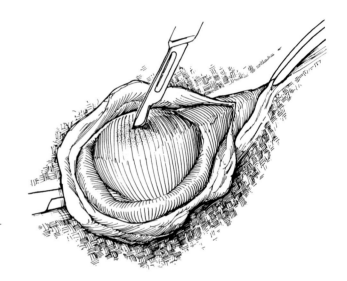

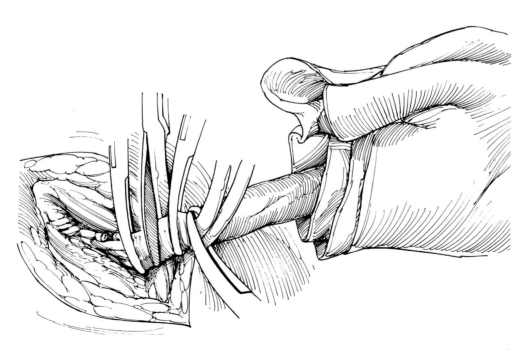

FIGURE 118-10. Doubly clamp, divide, and doubly ligate the cord at the internal ring above the tourniquet, using 2-0 or 3-0 nonabsorbable sutures. Cut the ends of the sutures sufficiently long to allow identification later at node dissection. The cord should now lie retroperitoneally so that the end can be reached readily later. Observe for hemostasis and irrigate the wound. Should the proximal ligature slip, the cord will retract above the canal. Immediately open the external and internal oblique layers in the line of the incision, and grasp and religate the free end of the cord.

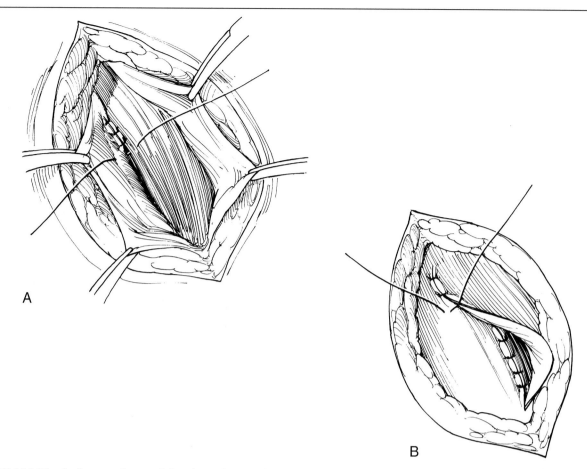

FIGURE 118-11. A, Suture the conjoined tendon to the shelving edge of the inguinal ligament. **B,** Imbricate the external oblique fascia with 3-0 synthetic absorbable sutures. Close the subcutaneous tissue with fine synthetic absorbable sutures and run a 4-0 synthetic absorbable suture subcuticularly. Do not place drains. Use fluffs to compress the empty scrotum, or, if it is large, suture it up to the lower abdomen over a gauze roll. Concomitant placement of a testicular prosthesis is not advisable; moreover, the child and the parents may prefer a scrotum free of all foreign masses.

ORGAN-SPARING SURGERY FOR TUMOR

In contrast to those in adults, a third of testicular masses in children are not malignant. Orchiectomy may produce psychological harm, and cause physical harm as well should the remaining testis be lost due to trauma or tumor. After preoperative assessment of tumor markers, evaluation by scrotal ultrasonography, and examination intraoperatively by frozen section, consider organ-sparing surgery (Weissbach, 1995; Valla, 2001; Steiner, 2003) as an alternative to orchiectomy for small tumors less than 2.5 mm in diameter, for bilateral malignant germ cell tumors, for a tumor in a solitary testis, and for non–germ cell tumors, whether unilateral or bilateral (Bartsch, 2003). At the operating table, expose the spermatic cord at the inguinal ring and place a latex-tube tourniquet around it to prevent tumor cells from escaping into the circulation. Expose the testis on a lap tape. Incise the tumor. Often the diagnosis of a benign lesion is clear. If it is not, send tissue for frozen-section diagnosis. If reported malignant, either excise the lesion (tumor enucleation) and check the margins by frozen section or divide the cord proximal to the tourniquet and remove the testis. Discard the lap tape.

POSTOPERATIVE PROBLEMS

Hemorrhage can be a major complication caused by not separately controlling the vas and vessels or inadequately ligating the cord. An expanding hematoma or evidence of retroperitoneal bleeding warrants reopening and extending the inguinal incision to reach the retracted vessels.

JONATHAN ROSS

Commentary by

Inguinal orchiectomy for testicular cancer is a well-established operation. However, some technical points are important to keep in mind. While there is little evidence to support the practice, early control of the spermatic cord seems prudent and is a standard part of the procedure. Since the cremasteric fibers arise from the internal oblique muscle and attach to the musculofascial layers distally, dissection of the cord and testicle is most easily accomplished by opening the cremasteric sheath in a longitudinal direction on the anterior surface of the cord. The cord is then circumscribed, excluding the cremasteric fibers. In this plane, dissection of the cord and testis can be accomplished easily and dissection of the cord above the internal ring is facilitated. Ligation of the cord above the internal ring makes excision of the intraperitoneal cord easier at any future retroperitoneal lymph node dissection. Dissection within the cremasteric sheath also precludes the need to repair the floor of the inguinal canal at the end of the procedure. The closure consists of simple reapproximation of the external oblique aponeurosis, Scarpa's fascia, and skin.

With regard to testis-sparing surgery, the most important consideration is the appropriate setting for this approach. Most testis tumors in postpubertal males are malignant, and testis-sparing surgery should be considered only when the combination of ultrasonographic findings and tumor markers suggests a benign lesion such as an epidermoid cyst. However, in prepubertal patients most tumors are benign, particularly in the setting of a normal AFP level. When interpreting the AFP level it is important to remember that "elevated" levels are normal in the first months of life, starting in the tens of thousands in the newborn, and do not start dropping to normal "adult" levels until approximately 8 months of age. Therefore, testis-sparing surgery should be considered in any prepubertal patient with a normal, age-adjusted AFP level. An inguinal approach with frozen-section analysis as described is appropriate. In this population, testis-sparing surgery may be undertaken regardless of the size of the tumor. Even tumors that seem to nearly replace the testis can be enucleated with normal testicular volume at follow-up.

FERNANDO FERRER

Commentary by

While some controversy exists in the literature, perhaps due to observations of center-specific series, the tests of the Prepubertal Tumor Registry and the Surveillance Epidemiology and End Results (SEER) data suggests that yolk sac tumors followed by teratoma are the most common prepubertal tumors.

Data suggest that upward of 38% of prepubertal tumors are benign; thus, appropriately, a significant emphasis has been placed on testis-sparing surgery. The techniques described herein are uniformly accepted, but it is important to note that a recent review suggests that violations of acceptable surgical technique are commonplace. Hence, operators should be mindful of the potential malignant diagnosis and adhere to meticulous technique.

AFP levels are elevated in normal infants up to 10 to 12 months of age, which limits the value of this study in young children. However, in children less than 1 year of age, the median AFP is still significantly greater in children with yolk sac tumors and it can still be useful.

Teratomas appear to be uniformly benign in prepubertal children and amenable to partial orchiectomy. This is not the case for postpubertal children or those displaying pubertal changes microscopically. These children should undergo orchiectomy.

Chapter 119

Reduction of Testicular Torsion

First, differentiate extravaginal torsion from intravaginal torsion.

Extravaginal torsion: The neonate presents with a firm, nontransilluminating scrotal mass with a bluish cast. It is often painless. Doppler ultrasonography usually shows no signals of vascular return. Manual detorsion is not applicable. Because surgical salvage is usually unsuccessful, remove the testis. Contralateral orchiopexy can be performed at the time of orchiectomy; however, the evidence-based rationale remains controversial.

Intravaginal torsion most commonly occurs in adolescent boys between the ages of 12 and 18. The onset is acute, usually associated with scrotal pain that is moderate to severe. Treat it as an emergency. In equivocal cases, in those with gradual onset of mild to moderate pain over days, perform a clinical examination, with or without blocking the cord, and look for the displacement of the lower pole of the epididymis away from the lower pole of the testis (the anomaly that permits torsion). If in doubt, order a color Doppler ultrasound examination, which is highly sensitive for obstructed blood flow. But do not delay treatment if these studies are not immediately available. For salvage, correction must be done within 6 to 8 hours.

MANUAL DETORSION OF INTRAVAGINAL TORSION

In adolescent boys (who will have intravaginal torsion), consider manual detorsion. Create a local cord block (Fig. 107-1). The older the boy, the greater the chance of achieving an effective block. Place local anesthetic in and around the cord, easily identified as it courses over the symphysis. Injection into the cord itself will make it balloon under the fingers. Always withdraw before injecting. The block is successful if the scrotum can be grasped firmly without causing pain. Grasp the testis lightly and draw it distally. With torsion of 360 degrees or less, it may "snap" as it becomes detorsed. Otherwise, first attempt detorsion by outward rotation because two out of three cases will have torsed inwardly. On the left, rotate the testis counterclockwise, and clockwise on the right. If there is resistance, try rotation in the opposite direction. Success is when you feel a sudden release and the testis literally snaps into place. It is ensured when the testicle finally lies in the bottom of the relaxed scrotum, freely mobile without tension. If this is not achieved, proceed with surgical detorsion as soon as possible.

If detorsion was successful without question, proceed with the definitive surgical procedure of scrotal fixation, usually within the next 24 hours. The hope is that the testis has retained some blood supply. Although the possibility of salvage is high, warn the parents of possible loss of the testis.

SCROTAL FIXATION OF THE TESTIS

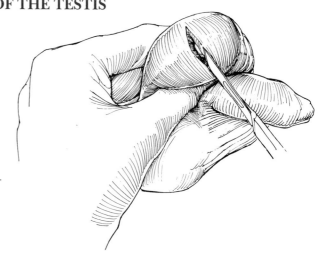

FIGURE 119-1. A caudal, ilioinguinal, or cord block will decrease postoperative pain. Prep the entire genital area. Incision: Grasp the scrotum with the thumb and index finger of the nondominant hand and press the testis forward against the skin. Make a short anterolateral incision through the skin and then through the dartos fascia, which may be found edematous.

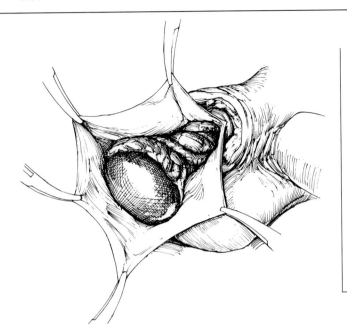

FIGURE 119-2. Extend the incision onto the tunica vaginalis, now possibly darkened from contained bloody serum. Open the tunica vaginalis and evacuate accumulated hydrocele fluid. Extrude the testis, untwist the cord if any torsion persists, and then wrap the testis in warm saline sponges.

Nonviable testis: Check the color of the testis. If it remains dark and was associated with sanguineous hydrocele fluid, make a short incision in the tunica albuginea. Wait 10 minutes. If no active bleeding is seen, the testis is not viable. Palpate and inspect the contralateral testis. If that testis is normal, proceed with an orchiectomy (see Chapter 116) on the affected side by dividing the cord structures between clamps and ligating with 2-0 chromic catgut sutures, including a transfixing stitch. If the quality of the contralateral testis is in doubt, leave the affected testis for its hormonal function.

FIGURE 119-3. Viable testis: If the testis is judged to be viable, trim excess tunica vaginalis and obtain hemostasis along the edge with careful fulguration. (When fulgurating, keep the testis grounded against the wound, not extended on the cord, or use bipolar electrocautery.)

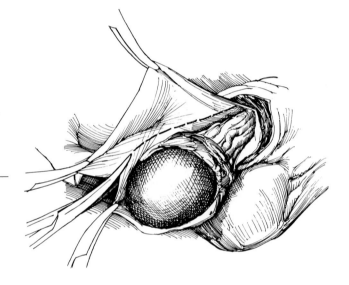

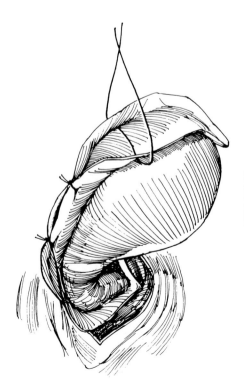

FIGURE 119-4. Place two or three interrupted 3-0 synthetic absorbable sutures in the cut edges of the tunica vaginalis, approximating them behind the testis to eliminate the potential for formation of a hydrocele.

FIGURE 119-5. Dartos pouch: Place the testis in a dartos pouch. Make an incision on the cephalad aspect of the scrotum. Incise the parietal tunica vaginalis and extrude the testis until the cord is invested only by the visceral portion of the tunica. Close the divergence of the tunica vaginalis, fixing it to the internal spermatic fascia covering the cord. Create a scrotal pouch manually between the dartos muscle and the external spermatic fascia. Suture the cut edge of the external spermatic fascia to the tunica vaginalis covering the cord. Close the dartos fascia, incorporating that portion of the tunica vaginalis covering the cord. Alternatively, taking care not to penetrate the tunica albuginea, invert the scrotal septum with a finger, and fix the tunica albuginea to the dartos layer and septum in three places, two laterally and one inferiorly, with interrupted mattress 3-0 nonabsorbable sutures.

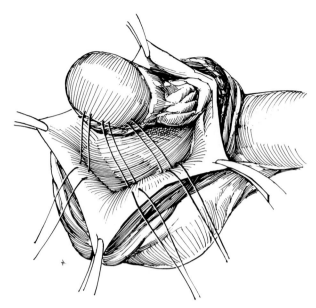

In all cases, open the contralateral scrotal sac and fix that testis also. Close the dartos layer with a figure-eight absorbable suture, and approximate the skin with a 4-0 or 5-0 absorbable subcuticular suture. Place a dry dressing with scrotal support. Inform the parents of the odds for salvage.

POSTOPERATIVE PROBLEMS

Hematoma is rare. Retorsion can occur, for which suture absorption may be a factor. After release of the torsion, reperfusion may cause apoptotic injury to the contralateral testis; warn the parents of possible loss of testicular function.

Fertility may also be affected if an ischemic testis is left in place. Should an ischemic testis become purulent, usually after several weeks, it must be removed.

In antenatal torsion the contralateral testis may also have a hydrocele. Exploration through the groin will take care of the patent processus vaginalis.

RICHARD P. LYON

Commentary by

Several important points regarding reduction of testicular torsion are as follows:

1. The younger the child, the more likely that the torsion will appear painless; therefore, in this age group, the swollen scrotum by itself indicates that surgery is required.
2. In the newborn, the torsion is not necessarily extravaginal, but the need for operation bilaterally is clear.
3. The teenager and adult usually present with intermittent scrotal pain, not always with swelling. Here, the diagnosis may be made by a scrotal examination that detects the displacement of the epididymis away from the lower pole of the testis; a bare lower testis is diagnostic.
4. At operation, orchiectomy is indicated only if the necrosis has reached the stage of purulence. Contralateral orchiopexy is mandatory, whether the anatomy is normal or not.

In the emergency room, try to manually detorse the testis. The older the child, the greater the likelihood of being able to obtain an effective cord block, which should be tried first. Carefully grasp the swollen testis and place the cord on tension. This may be enough for derotation to occur by itself. Otherwise, rotate counterclockwise on the left, clockwise on the right, which will be correct 75% of the time. If there is resistance, try the opposite direction. You will have no doubt that you are successful when you feel a sudden release—the testis literally snaps into place.

Proceed to the operating room and fix the testis in the scrotum, with a high possibility of successful salvage. Make a transverse scrotal incision and incise the distended tunicae. Clear fluid is favorable; blood-tinged fluid suggests tissue necrosis. Surprisingly, often the testis has rotated not 360 but 720 degrees. Usually the testis is found mottled brown to black, but I have learned to leave it in place and hope for at least partial salvage, at a small risk of later orchiectomy.

Use two absorbable sutures to attach the tunica albuginea. It is wise to place two small Penrose drains fixed to the skin. Through a similar contralateral scrotal incision, examine the opposite testis. Half the time it will also present with a high epididymis, the classic bell-clapper deformity. In any case, fix it with two or three nonabsorbable sutures.

Postoperative problems: Should the testis become purulent, a rare event that takes several weeks to develop, resort to orchiectomy. Tell the parents of the salvage attempt; they will accept this later orchiectomy with appreciation of your efforts.

CLAIRE BRETT

I propose that when considering surgical care for the newborn, we must analyze pre- and postoperative care as well as intraoperative management. Significant morbidity is associated with both inadequate preoperative assessment and postoperative supportive care. The infant is in many ways, and the newborn is in particular, a distinct species, and variability and unpredictability characterize his or her clinical performance. Developmental factors related to cardiorespiratory, renal, hepatic, and neurologic immaturities are also of paramount importance when discussing the newborn.

There is data from the last 50 years relevant to what has been called an increased risk of "anesthesia in the newborn." The first report of increased anesthetic mortality in younger-aged patients was published by Beecher and Todd in 1954, who compared children younger than 10 years old with adults. In 1961, another report noted that the incidence of cardiac arrest was 16.2/10,000 in children 1 year old or less, and 6/10,000 in children less than 1 year old. Over the next 40 years, many other investigators have documented that critical events such as cardiac arrest, bradycardia, and respiratory events are all higher in newborns and young infants than in older children and adults. However, even though the morbidity associated with anesthesia is higher for infants, the incidence of critical events is remarkably low.

Recently, Jeff Morray, in conjunction with the Committee on Professional Liability of the American Society of Anesthesiologists (ASA) and the American Academy of Pediatrics, examined the incidence of cardiac arrest associated with anesthesia in a multicenter study, which included 63 sites, most of which were university affiliated (Pediatric Perioperative Cardiac Arrest [POCA] Registry). Over a span of 3 years he identified 150 out of 289 cardiac arrests that were anesthesia related. All 39 deaths in this group of 289 were associated with severe underlying disease. Of note, over half of the cardiac arrests that occurred in healthy children (ASA 1 and 2) were medication related, that is, usually a halothane overdose or some mismanagement with respect to medication was associated with the cardiac arrest. But the only predictors of mortality secondary to the arrest were ASA status and emergency surgery. These cases were different from the cases of malpractice. These are different from those from closed claims cases. The POCA registry is self-reporting format and the entry criteria include cardiac compressions, excluding other critical events such as those related to ventilation or intubation problems. Notice that, as in earlier studies, the rate of this event was higher in the younger infants, but, overall, the incidence was low ($1.4 \pm 0.45/10,000$/year). Of these patients, 43% were less than 5 months old and 55% were less than 1 year old. The low incidence occurred in tertiary care centers with pediatric anesthesiologists, not community hospitals without pediatric-trained anesthesiologists.

In short, the surgeon must tell the anesthesiologist whether he or she needs to go forward and operate on a patient. Choose a pediatric anesthesiologist who takes care of newborns, if one is available, as the infant will then have a lower chance of having a poor anesthetic outcome. From an anesthesiologist's perspective, Charlie Cote said, "We are left with the best clinical judgment about an individual patient undergoing a specific procedure for a specific duration of time by a specific surgeon, and we are stuck with doing that every day in the operating room."

During the first week of life, a newborn becomes much more stable with respect to glucose, calcium, liver function, and temperature. These may seem like relatively minor issues, but for the first week of life, these metabolic problems are common in sick newborns and can be associated with significant morbidity if not adequately and promptly recognized and treated. In general, such metabolic problems are not encountered in the normal newborn that readily establishes feeds. On the other hand, a newborn headed to the operating room may need to rely on intravenous therapy. A normal 1-week-old infant is much different from a 1-hour-old newborn. Glucose is not a major problem for most normal newborns who are appropriate-for-gestational age, who are not septic, and who are eating. Certainly after 1 week metabolic problems such as hypercalcemia and hypoglycemia have subsided, and body temperature regulation has stabilized. The newborn's answer to everything is apnea: if they are cold, if they are hypoglycemic, if they are hypocalcemic, they stop breathing. Thus, the surgeon should meticulously analyze the entire perioperative site (pre- and postoperative) to ensure expert care for a newborn. In particular, after anesthesia and surgery, a newborn may be particularly fragile, especially if pain medications or mechanical ventilation are required.

Other issues to consider:

- The transitional circulation is a potential source of morbidity during the first days to weeks of life, depending on the particular patient.
- Transition from hemoglobin F to A occurs over the first 3 or 4 months and physiologic anemia is most significant at 2 to 3 months of age.
- Cardiovascular (beyond the transitional circulation) and renal adaptation continues well past 1 year of age.
- Transepidermal water loss is a major problem for premature infants. It is not a problem for term babies.

Some morbidities are "hidden" in newborns. For example, a patient with an interrupted aortic arch may appear healthy at birth, as long as the ductus arteriosus is patent. At 2 to 3 weeks of age, such an infant may come into the emergency room after a cardiovascular collapse, as flow through the ductus decreases. For the first several weeks, if not months, of life, there could be congenital anomalies, that is, hidden mortality and morbidity, that may not be apparent at birth. Again, if a newborn is subjected to surgery and anesthesia he or she requires meticulous preoperative assessment and postoperative supportive care by experts in neonatal medicine and surgery.

GEORGE KAPLAN

Commentary by

Extravaginal torsion is a problem that is seen almost exclusively in the neonate. It occurs because for the first 4 to 6 weeks of life, there are loose attachments between the tunica vaginalis and the dartos muscle that allow extravaginal torsion to occur. Testicular salvage is rarely successful in this group, but exploration is still preferable for two reasons: (1) occasionally tumor is the genesis for the torsion, and (2) it affords the opportunity for contralateral orchiopexy, even though the evidence for its necessity is somewhat controversial.

Intravaginal torsion can occur at any age. It should be treated as an emergency. It is my opinion that a classic history of sudden onset of pain, especially associated with nausea and vomiting, should be treated immediately without delay for imaging. I have no objection to a trial of manual detorsion, but I would caution that relief of pain does not necessarily indicate total untwisting of the spermatic cord. Hence, even if there is what is felt to be a successful detorsion of the cord, the patient should be taken promptly to the operating room so that the testis can be fixed in place.

If the patient presents more than 8 hours from the onset of symptoms, I then prefer to obtain an ultrasound examination first to ascertain whether torsion exists. If there is adequate flow, torsion is very unlikely and I will usually treat the patient medically. It is important to recognize that at times there is intermittent torsion and an ultrasound examination may indicate flow at the moment, but subsequently there can be torsion with decreased flow. Usually, if this occurs, there is increased pain at the time of changes in flow.

Because experimental studies have shown that the best fixation of the testis occurs when the tunica albuginea is adjacent to the dartos muscle so that firm scar can occur, I fully concur that the tunica vaginalis should be brought behind the testis and sutured to itself as shown in Figure 119-4. I then usually tack the tunica albuginea to the dartos muscle with a couple of interrupted absorbable sutures to hold the testis in place while the scar is forming. Although recurrence of torsion has been reported, most of those recurrences seem to have occurred in an era when two or three absorbable sutures between the tunica albuginea and the tunica vaginalis were used to tack the testis in place. Once again, experimental studies have shown that this is inadequate, as the only scar that forms is at the point of suture rather than against the entire surface of the testis.

ALAN B. RETIK

Commentary by

Salvage for an in utero or neonatal torsion is very rare. Presentation in the newborn period is usually a firm, nontender mass of varying size, depending on the duration of the torsion. These are invariably extravaginal torsions, although we have seen an occasional intravaginal torsion. Surgery was not recommended in the past because of the uniform nonviability of the testicle. However, we have observed bilateral neonatal torsions, several of which occurred within weeks of the presenting torsion. We therefore recommend immediate surgery. If the diagnosis is straightforward, the approach can be through the scrotum.

If there is any question as to the diagnosis, or if the scrotum is very inflamed, a groin approach is recommended. The torsed organ is almost always nonviable and should be removed. The contralateral testicle is sutured to the septum with three 5-0 nonabsorbable sutures. Torsion of the testis in the older child and adolescent is fairly common.

Acute scrotal pain and swelling in these age groups should be regarded as a torsion of the testis and these boys should be seen promptly. Most often the diagnosis is obvious and the child should be taken immediately to the operating room. If there is a question as to the diagnosis, a Doppler ultrasound is indicated. The surgical approach is through the scrotum. If the testicle is obviously nonviable, it should be removed. If the organ is questionably viable, it should be retained and sutured as described previously with 4-0 nonabsorbable sutures. Fixation of the contralateral organ is done in a similar fashion.

Chapter 120

Repair of Testicular Injury

Ultrasound is useful to confirm the diagnosis. Explore the scrotum through a transverse incision. Rule out a history of a ruptured testicular tumor, which would necessitate an inguinal exploration.

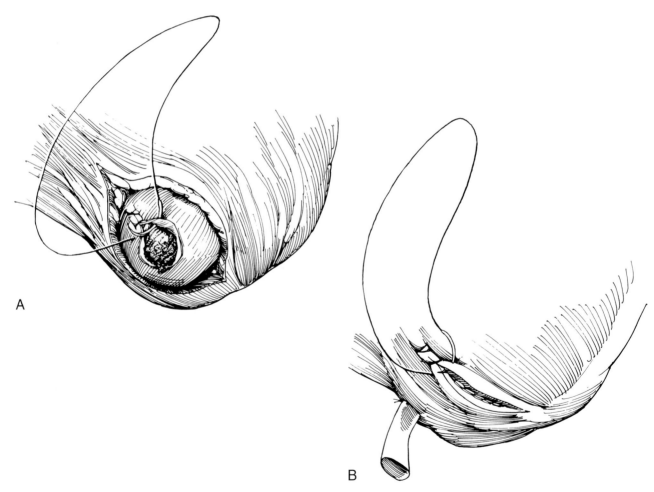

FIGURE 120-1. A, Debride necrotic seminiferous tubules until viable tissue. Close the tunica albuginea with a running 4-0 chromic stitch. **B,** Consider placing a small Penrose drain to exit through a stab wound, before closing the scrotum in layers.

DAVID C. S. GOUGH

Commentary by

An avulsion injury is rare, and when I have seen it in children, it has been related to a pedestrian being crushed by a motor vehicle.

In children, the length of the penile skin tube out of which the penis has been avulsed is relatively short, and its vascularity, in my experience, is not compromised; therefore, reconstruction can take place with debrided local tissue. Other injuries in the area, to the pelvis in particular, usually make it necessary for the bladder to be drained by an 8- or 10-F balloon catheter.

Where there has been a loss of scrotal tissue, which is exceptionally rare in children, I would not disagree with the subcutaneous burying of the testicle, should the whole scrotum be missing. The size of the testicle and scrotum in small children has been a factor in my experience, and we have never had to do such a procedure, relying on local tissue and careful debridement for reconstruction.

Suture material for repair is not critical, and lately we have used 6-0 or 7-0 polydioxanone suture. Broad-spectrum antibiotic coverage and closed-suction wound drainage have been used when significant dead space is likely to be encountered.

Rupture of the testis occurs in childhood, usually secondary to kicks. Immediate exploration, debridement, suture repair of the tunica albuginea, and careful hemostasis with bipolar diathermy usually allow control to such an extent that drainage is not required.

Commentary by
JAMES M. BETTS

Color-flow Doppler ultrasound is invaluable in the evaluation of these injuries. The surgical approach to either hemiscrotal compartments or to both sides is more easily performed through a midline vertical incision in the scrotal line raphe rather than through a transverse incision. I use Vicryl or polydioxanone suture for closing.

Chapter 121

Insertion of Testicular Prosthesis

Testicular prostheses are typically placed for bilateral anorchia although unilateral anorchia in adolescence is also an indication. Be certain that the parents and teenager understand the value of a prosthesis and of the possibility of operative complications.

For bilateral anorchia, testicular prosthesis placement is facilitated by exogenous testosterone supplementation. This will masculinize the scrotum, allowing the scrotal sac to stretch and accommodate the prosthesis.

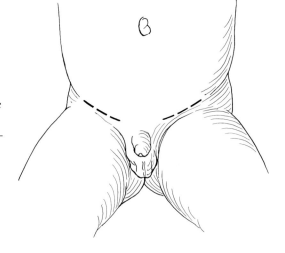

FIGURE 121-1. Insertion as an independent procedure: Make a transverse inguinal incision. (For bilateral implantation, use two separate incisions.)

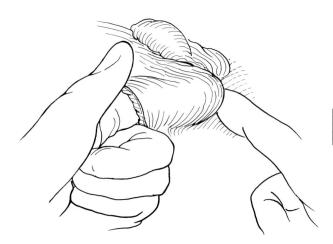

FIGURE 121-2. Stretch the scrotal sac vigorously with the index finger, taking care not to tear it.

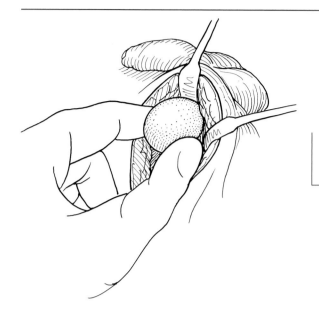

FIGURE 121-3. Select the size of prosthesis that is normal or slightly large for the size of the adolescent. In babies with bilateral anorchia it can be replaced with a more suitable size later when the boy is grown.

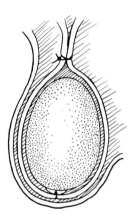

FIGURE 121-4. Place a purse-string suture to close the scrotal neck, taking care not to pierce the capsule of the prosthesis with the needle.

Insertion during orchiopexy: Select a prosthesis of a size suitable for the age of the child. It can be replaced with a larger size later, although this is seldom requested. Digitally enlarge the scrotal sac and insert the prosthesis. Place a purse-string or figure-eight synthetic absorbable suture to close the neck of the scrotum.

COMPLICATIONS

Infection will require removal of the prosthesis. Necrosis of the stretched skin over a prosthesis that is too large can occur. A scrotal hematoma is rare.

HUBERT S. SWANA

Commentary by

Meticulous attention to sterile technique and gentle tissue handling will help avoid infection and bleeding in most cases. In cases of unilateral prosthesis placement I tend to encourage patients and parents to wait until the child reaches puberty. This way only one surgery is needed for an appropriately sized implant.

In patients that require larger prosthesis, dilatation of the scrotal neck is sometimes challenging. I find the use of Hegar dilators to be most helpful in these cases.

It is important to ensure that the prosthesis is properly oriented and secure in the most dependent position in the scrotum. This helps to prevent troublesome implant migration. Newer prostheses are designed to allow placement of an anchoring suture in the bottom of the implant. Make sure that this suture is not placed "too deep," such that it puckers or pierces the scrotal skin.

Part III

Groin Reconstruction

Chapter 122

Inguinal Hernia Repair

Children may be born with a communicating hydrocele, in which the peritoneum has not been sealed off at its continuation with the tunica vaginalis, or a persistent processus vaginalis. Most can be ignored because they seldom persist longer than 18 months before the connection closes spontaneously. Operation is needed only for those few with a persistent open canal and a hernia.

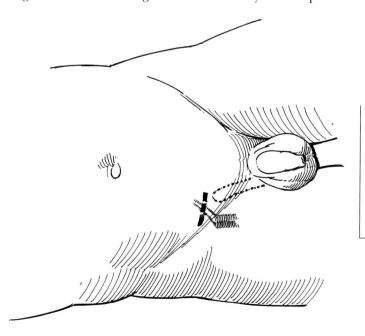

FIGURE 122-1. Position: Supine. Incision: Stretch the skin, and make a 2- to 3-cm transverse incision in the prominent fold above the external ring. Carry it through Camper's and Scarpa's fascias, directly into the external oblique aponeurosis. Identify the external ring by following the spermatic cord proximally until the vessels and vas can no longer be felt. Loupe magnification is essential in infants.

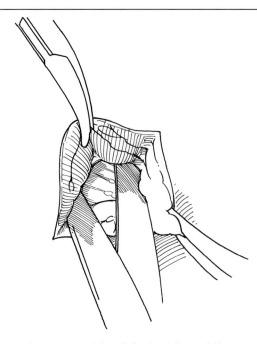

FIGURE 122-2. Grasp the subcutaneous fat on one side of the incision while your assistant holds the other side, and separate the fat from Scarpa's fascia with fine scissors. Typically, the vessels can be avoided by retraction; however, if necessary, coagulate or ligate. (In infants, Scarpa's fascia is relatively dense and may be mistaken for the aponeurosis of the external oblique muscle.)

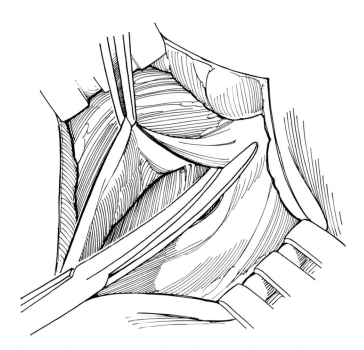

FIGURE 122-3. Lift Scarpa's fascia with fine forceps and divide it in the line of the incision. Separate the fatty layer beneath Scarpa's fascia with scissors to expose the loose tissue over the external oblique aponeurosis. Have your assistant retract the lower edges of the incision. Expose the external ring (external oblique aponeurosis, external spermatic fascia, and shelving edge) by dissection with scissors.

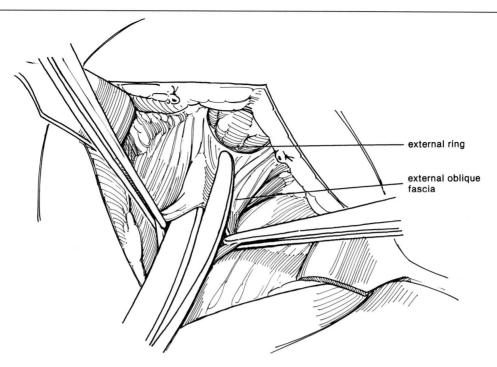

external ring

external oblique
fascia

FIGURE 122-4. Elevate the edge of the external ring with scissors to avoid the ilioinguinal nerve and divide the external oblique aponeurosis in the direction of its fibers. Alternatively, open the aponeurosis starting above the external ring with a knife.

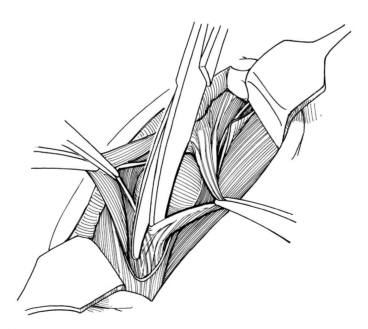

FIGURE 122-5. Grasp one side of the cremaster muscle as your assistant elevates the other side, and incise it generously to reveal the internal spermatic fascia.

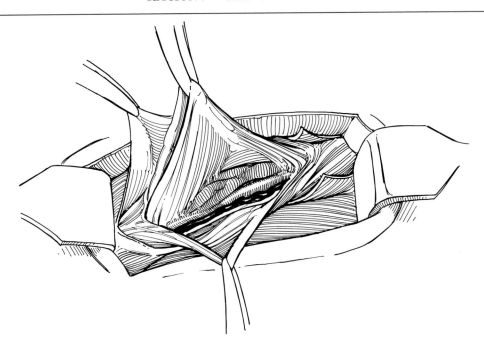

FIGURE 122-6. Spread the internal spermatic fascia to expose the hernia sac. Do not disturb the vas deferens and spermatic vessels lying laterally and posteriorly. By placing the anterior and lateral surfaces of the sac on tension, dissect the sac from the spermatic vessels using a fine clamp or scissors. Once the sac is free from the posteriorly located vas and vessels, a peanut dissector or finger can tease off the remainder of the posterior sac from below the level of the internal ring.

At this point, consider looking for a contralateral occult hernia by instilling carbon dioxide at less than 20 cm of water into the peritoneal cavity through the opening in the hernia sac and palpating the contralateral groin. Or consider performing laparoscopic inspection of the contralateral ring though the sac.

FIGURE 122-7. Suture-ligate the sac with a fine synthetic absorbable suture. It is not necessary to trim the remainder of the sac unless you need pathologic confirmation. Ascertain that the testis is in scrotal position. Approximate the external oblique aponeurosis with fine interrupted synthetic absorbable sutures, taking care not to encroach on the external ring, and then join Scarpa's fascia with a few sutures. Close the skin with a fine running subcuticular suture. Consider local infiltration of the incision with a long-acting anesthetic solution if a caudal nerve block was not performed at the beginning of the procedure.

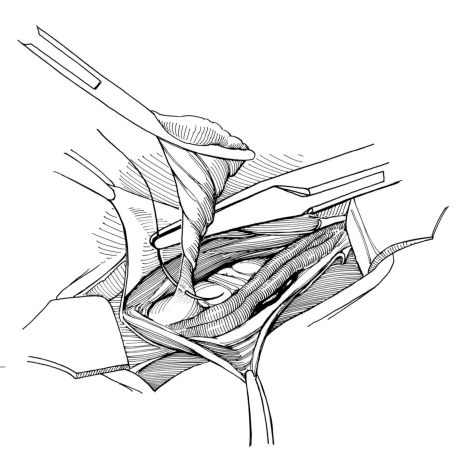

JOHN PARK

Commentary by

Once the Scarpa's fascia is incised, the anatomic landmarks—the shelving edge of the inguinal ligament and the external inguinal ring—must be identified to maintain the proper orientation during subsequent dissection. If the landmarks are not readily visible, then the dissection may be either too superficial or too medial, especially in obese patients. In infants, the inguinal canal is quite short, and the hernia repair may be performed without formally opening the canal. In most cases, however, opening the canal a short distance through the external ring provides a reliable exposure to the cord structures as well as the internal ring. It is less likely to injure the ilioinguinal nerve by incising the aponeurosis of the external oblique muscle from lateral to medial toward the external ring, where the nerve often crosses over the cord. Once the cremasteric muscle fibers are spread to expose the cord underneath, the hernia sac is found anteromedial to the cord structures. In separating the sac from the cord, it is useful to open the sac when it is very large; this minimizes confusion and provides a better cord orientation. If the sac is very large or thickened, the internal contents must be examined via direct visualization in case there is a sliding hernia with either bladder or bowel. The distal sac does not need to be removed completely. In children, a formal repair of the floor of the canal is typically unnecessary. During the restoration of the inguinal canal, care must be taken to avoid ilioinguinal nerve entrapment and cord constriction at the external ring.

Although the inguinal hernia repair is one of the most commonly performed procedures in pediatric urology, a successful outcome is achieved by strict adherence to sound surgical and anatomic principles.

MICHAEL DISANDRO

Commentary by

To avoid becoming "lost" in the groin, the location of the inguinal incision and the exposure of the external oblique fascia are paramount for a successful inguinal hernia repair. The skin incision should be made one third of the way between the pubic tubercle and the anterior superior iliac spine. This will place you just proximal to the external ring, which is exactly where you want to make your incision in the external oblique fascia. Prior to making this incision, the external oblique fascia should be completely exposed; this is best accomplished by placing scissors just lateral to the fascia and opening the scissors perpendicular to the fascial fibers, thus creating an open space between the external oblique fascia and the sidewall. You will then be able to clearly see the external ring and the proximal fascial fibers and thus be certain you are in the right place.

If the patient has a clinical hydrocele (as opposed to a clinical hernia), it is best to pick up the hydrocele sac with DeBakey forceps and with your other hand use another set of DeBakey forceps; with the forceps partially closed, gently peel the posterior cord (vessels and vas deferens) off the sac. If you are ever confused as to the exact anatomy, simply let everything go, and start again by regrabbing the hydrocele sac. Often this maneuver alone will allow you to see the sac much more clearly. The hydrocele sac should be able to be completely freed without ever having to mobilize the spermatic cord, without having to open the sac, and without having to cut any cremasteric muscle fibers. If the patient has a clinical hernia, however, it is best to open the hernia sac anteriorly. As soon as the hernia sac is opened, a clamp should be placed at the apex of the sac to avoid the sac tearing proximally into the abdomen. Scissors can then be used to create a plane between the posterior hernia sac and underlying cord structures. This is best done by placing the closed scissors between the sac and the cord structures, opening them to create a small plane, rotating them 90 degrees, and opening them further to develop the plane. At this point, once the contents of the hernia sac are taken care of, contralateral hernioscopy can be performed. With proper technique, contralateral hernioscopy can be performed in 2 to 3 minutes.

First, an 8 F feeding tube is placed through the opening of the sac into the abdomen, and the abdomen is insufflated through the tube. Next, an arthroscopic scope with a 70-degree lens is placed alongside the feeding tube. Without looking at the monitor, and instead looking at the light transilluminated through the patient's skin from the scope, the scope is pushed in up against the patient's abdominal wall and across to the contralateral inguinal canal. It is best not to go straight across, but to aim for the umbilicus and then, once past the midline, come back down to the contralateral inguinal canal. Then simply rotate the scope so the lens is facing the internal ring and look up at the monitor, and you should have clear visualization of the ring.

When there are abdominal contents within the hernia sac, even if it is not incarcerated, sometimes it is difficult to reduce the hernia through the small proximal opening. When this occurs, placing a Senn retractor into the opening of the sac and gently retracting anteriorly will usually allow the contents of the sac to slip back into the abdomen without having to manipulate the abdominal contents too much. Even with this maneuver, sometimes omentum still will not cooperate, and, in this situation, it is usually best to perform an omentectomy rather than to risk tearing an omental vessel trying to force the omentum back into the abdomen.

Chapter 123

Correction of Hydrocele

NONCOMMUNICATING HYDROCELE

Adolescents and teenagers may develop a hydrocele, the result of collecting serous (peritoneal) fluid inside the tunica vaginalis after the processus has closed.

The sac may be obliterated by an eversion technique—the Lord procedure—which is simple and successful for a large, offending noncommunicating hydrocele, but not for a communicating hydrocele.

LORD PROCEDURE

For instruments provide at least eight small Allis forceps, a Wietlander retractor, and 4-0 synthetic absorbable and 4-0 chromic catgut sutures on half-circle needles.

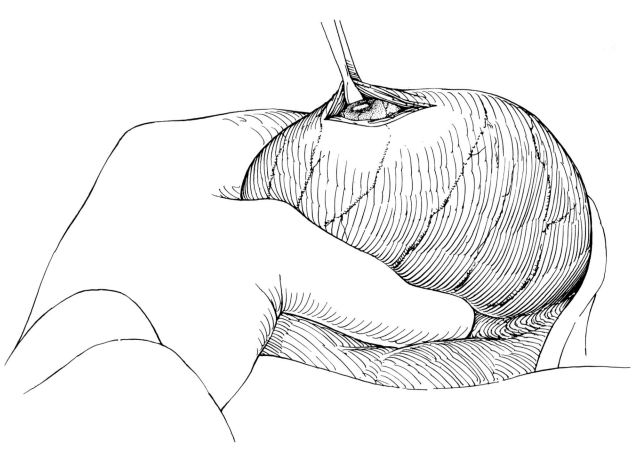

FIGURE 123-1. With the boy supine, anesthetized, and prepped, stand on his right side if you are right-handed. Infiltrate the cord structures at the base of the scrotum with 1% lidocaine (optional). Grasp the hydrocele in the left hand. Press it firmly against the scrotal skin to stretch the skin and dartos muscle and to compress the scrotal vessels. Make a 2-cm incision in the skin between the visible vessels and then through the dartos muscle down to the surface of the tunica vaginalis. The initial incision includes the thin dartos layer. Fulgurate the fine vessels as they are exposed.

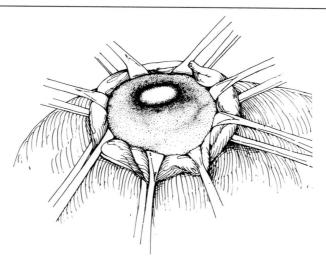

FIGURE 123-2. Pick up the full thickness of all the incised tissue layers on each side with three or four small Allis forceps, each one catching the skin *and* the tissue immediately adjacent to the tunica vaginalis. By keeping the tissues under tension with the left hand, the Allis forceps can be placed to evert and compress the cut edge, thus controlling any bleeding and, most important, preventing dissection among the easily irritated layers of the scrotum. With the knife handle, separate the dartos layer from the tunica vaginalis to form a pouch large enough to hold the testis. Release the grasp on the scrotum.

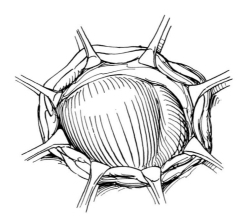

FIGURE 123-3. Hold the suction tip nearby. Incise the tunica vaginalis, and aspirate the fluid. Expand the opening with scissors, and squeeze the testis out. Inspect and palpate it.

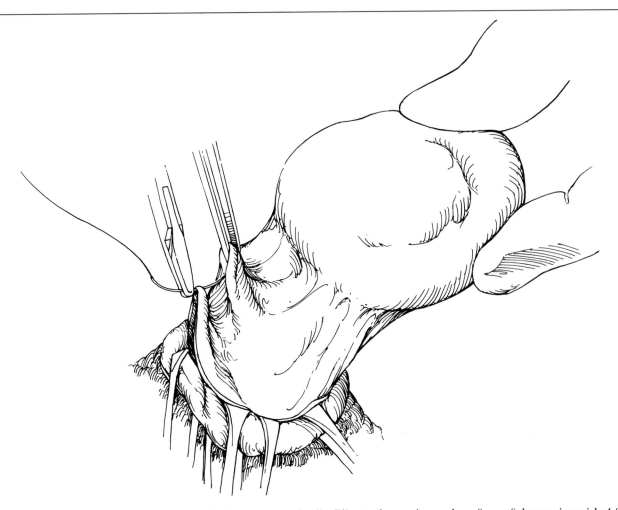

FIGURE 123-4. Lift the testis up to stretch the tunica vaginalis. Plicate the peritoneal surface of the tunica with 4-0 synthetic absorbable sutures. Do this by picking up the edge of the tunica with the needle and then taking a small bite of the shiny surface held up successively by fine-toothed forceps every centimeter, until the junction with the testis is reached. Tie this suture, or alternatively, place all the plicating sutures before tying them.

FIGURE 123-5. Repeat plication sutures at intervals around the circumference of the testis, placing from six to eight sutures in all. With the aid of a flat malleable retractor, replace the testis in the scrotum by squeezing it into the new pouch created beneath the dartos layer.

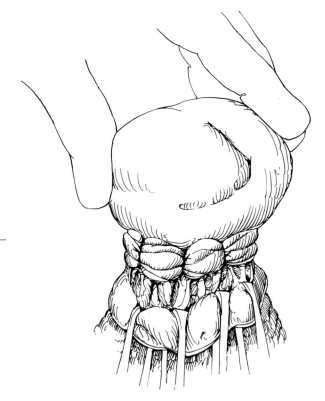

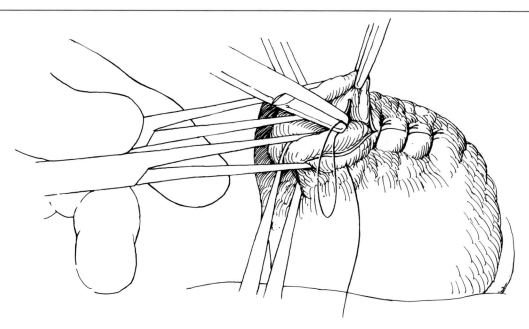

FIGURE 123-6. Remove the Allis forceps in pairs from the dartos muscle while rotating the next pair to allow placement of interrupted sutures of 4-0 chromic catgut. These include full-thickness skin, dartos muscle, and all the areolar tissue. Placing a towel clip on each end of the wound for traction helps with eversion. The subcutaneous space is now obliterated. Place a sheet of treated gauze and several 4 × 4 sponges over the incision. Apply a suspensory in older boys. No drainage is necessary if the subcutaneous fascial space was not violated.

POSTOPERATIVE PROBLEMS

Hematoma formation is rare if the entire thickness of the scrotal wall was included first in the Allis forceps and then in the sutures at closure.

Recurrence of the hydrocele is likewise rare because the operation leaves no dead space for a seroma around which the peritoneal lining can grow.

Commentary by JASON WILSON

In the patient with persisting hydrocele beyond 2 years of age and younger than adulthood, an inguinal approach is used in anticipation of performing high ligation of a patent processus vaginalis. It is not uncommon to encounter a "tongue" of peritoneum (funicular process) and an apparent obliteration of the patent processus per se. In this case, we routinely perform high ligation, as the space can enlarge, becoming an inguinal hernia. These cases often present the challenge of effectively draining the fluid that has remained distally, unable to be reabsorbed. The tunica vaginalis can be easily identified and opened widely through the inguinal incision. It is not necessary to completely deliver the testis in an attempt to widely excise the excess tunica, as reaccumulation of fluid after this maneuver is uncommon. The risk of contralateral asynchronous hydrocele is probably around 3% and does not warrant routine contralateral exploration.

The young adult with a recently discovered hydrocele has been generally approached with an inguinal incision, as you may expect to encounter a small communication that requires high ligation. To date, an age above which you may use the scrotal approach has not been determined, though history is a very good indication of whether there may be a communication present. When in doubt, it is prudent to use the inguinal approach. Excising excess tunica can cause unnecessary blood loss and may increase risk of injury to the vas deferens. A plicating procedure (Lord) may be performed with braided, absorbable suture if necessary for hemostasis and prevention of recurrence.

The rare case of abdominoscrotal hydrocele is worthy of an entire chapter. This entity can be diagnosed by physical examination, and then an inguinal approach with delivery of the testis is employed. A high scrotal approach is indicated if the examination imparts 100% confidence that there is no chance of encountering a communication. Alternatively, you may begin with a high scrotal incision, probe the proximal aspect of the visceral tunica, and make a small inguinal incision if a communication is discovered. Another advantage to the inguinal approach is the ability to close the internal ring, as it may be widened with the very large abdominoscrotal hydrocele. The inguinal approach can be used safely for any hydrocele encountered in childhood.

NICHOLAS M. HOLMES

Commentary by

This is an effective technique for the noncommunicating hydrocele or for the redo scrotal hydrocele due to the ablation of the potential space for recollection of serous fluid. It is imperative that a persistent patent processus vaginalis is not present for this approach to be successful. If the hydrocele is not reducible on physical examination or the parents do not report variable changes in the size of the scrotal sac, this reinforces the diagnosis of a noncommunicating hydrocele.

The plication sutures can be any absorbable suture, but our preference is to use Monocryl (poliglecaprone 25) over chromic catgut, as it has less of an inflammatory tissue reaction. The edges of the incised hydrocele sac may require cauterization. Persistent bleeding on this surface may contribute to possible recurrence. If the hydrocele sac is quite large or has areas of loculation, a persistent bulky scrotal mass may result afterward. This may give a less than ideal cosmetic appearance. Other techniques such as a radical excision of the hydrocele sac or Jaboulay bottleneck procedure may be appropriate.

Chapter 124

Introduction to Varicocele Ligation

Palpate the spermatic cord while the patient is erect and doing a Valsalva maneuver. The Doppler probe can help provide confirmation. Proceed to varicocele ligation in adolescents if testicular atrophy exists or if the varicocele causes pain or is excessive in size.

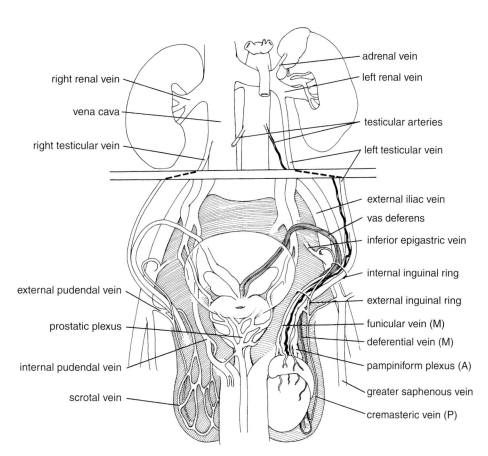

FIGURE 124-1. The veins draining the testis, epididymis, and vas deferens connect with deep and superficial venous networks. The deep venous network has three components: the testicular vein and the pampiniform plexus *(labeled* A *for anterior set)*, the funicular and deferential veins *(labeled* M *for middle set)*, and the cremasteric veins *(labeled* P *for posterior set)*.

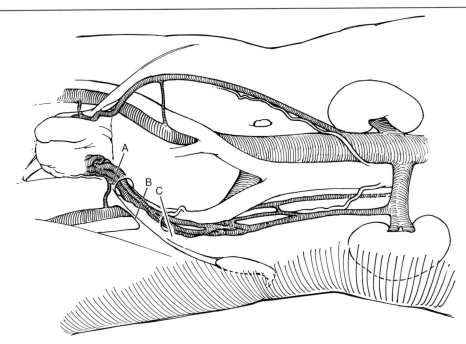

FIGURE 124-2. Three approaches are currently used: A subinguinal approach (Marmar) (A); an inguinal approach (Ivanissevich) (B), in which the spermatic artery is spared; and an abdominal approach (Palomo) (C), in which the artery may be included in the ligation.

Chapter 125

Subinguinal Varicocelectomy

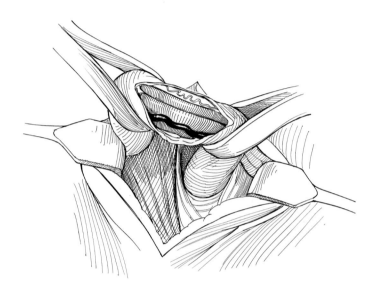

FIGURE 125-1. Spermatic cord identified within the subinguinal canal.

Identify the external ring digitally and make a 2- to 3-cm transverse incision directly over the external ring. Continue the incision through the subcutaneous layer and Scarpa's fascia, aided by small retractors. Identify the external inguinal ring and the spermatic cord. Inject long-acting local anesthetic under the cremasteric fascia with a fine needle to anesthetize the cord, and inject it also at a higher level through the canal, guided by a fingertip in the ring. Grasp the cord with a Babcock clamp, draw it slowly out of the wound, and encircle it with two Penrose drains. Keep the distal one tight to stabilize the cord, but leave the proximal one loose to maintain the superficial blood supply. Alternatively, place a tongue depressor under the cord. Clip or tie any dilated posterior cremasteric veins. Open the external spermatic fascia. With the aid of a 2.5× optical loupe or an operating microscope set at 6× to 10× magnification, identify the spermatic veins as part of the pampiniform plexus and dissect them free in groups. Displace the vas deferens and artery, but ligate the veins that accompany them if they are larger than 2 mm.

Apply the operating Doppler probe to identify and avoid the spermatic artery. Preserve the lymphatics. Spray the area with 2 to 3 mL of 30 mg/mL papaverine hydrochoride to relieve vascular spasm. Tie the veins in groups with 2-0 or 3-0 silk suture. Close Scarpa's fascia and the skin with a 4-0 running subcuticular suture.

The mini-incision, microsurgical subinguinal varicocelectomy is an alternative technique that also ensures complete venous ligation. As is done for the subinguinal approach, make a 2- to 3-cm inguinal incision in the skin and the external oblique fascia over the external ring, and dissect and encircle the cord. Then draw the testis out of the wound. Identify and ligate the external spermatic and gubernacular veins, along with any other veins accompanying the gubernaculum. Return the testis to the scrotum, and dissect the veins from the cord itself. Use an operating microscope to ensure ligation of all the small veins except those accompanying the vas deferens. Spare the spermatic artery and adjacent lymphatics.

DIX POPPAS

Commentary by

The subinguinal approach to the surgical correction of the varicocele is the most effective and least invasive approach, in my opinion. In my practice, the subinguinal microsurgical varicocelectomy, described by Goldstein, has proven to be the most effective and least invasive approach. As well, it has the lowest postsurgical hydrocele rate. Using the subinguinal approach, it is possible to perform the procedure using less than a general anesthesia. I used the laparoscopic technique for several years and found that when compared to the subinguinal microsurgical approach the laparoscopic technique required excessive operative time and was associated with attendant complications. Furthermore, isolating and preserving the testicular artery was not always easy and had a higher postsurgical hydrocele rate.

With regard to the inguinal approach, it should be considered for redo varicocele repairs as well as for the rare case requiring a subinguinal varicocelectomy. It should also be considered for finding many small veins surrounding the testicular artery. In the latter case, recognizing this early and moving to an inguinal approach may improve success. Extending the subinguinal incision and opening through the external ring is often all that is needed to get to an area of the cord that contains larger but fewer veins. During the subinguinal repair, in addition to identifying and saving the testicular artery and the vas deferens and its blood supply, it is important to save several of the lymphatic vessels to prevent postsurgical hydroceles.

STUART S. HOWARDS

Commentary by

The technique describe previously is a very reasonable approach to varicocelectomy. We use a slightly different method. We place one Penrose drain under the cord. We routinely spray the cord with lidocaine, thus reserving papaverine, which is more expensive, for those situations in which we can neither visualize a pulsating spermatic artery nor identify it with a micro-Doppler probe. We routinely use a microscope but feel that it is not necessary to remove the testis from the scrotum as recommended by Goldstein. It should be mentioned that although every effort should be made to preserve the artery, testicular atrophy is extremely unusual even if the artery is sacrificed unless there has been previous inguinal or scrotal surgery.

Chapter 126

Abdominal and Inguinal Approaches to Varicocele Ligation

Palpate the spermatic cord while the boy is doing a Valsalva maneuver while standing. Doppler sonography can provide confirmation and accurately measure testicular size. Proceed to varicocelectomy if testicular asymmetry is noted.

Provide a basic set of instruments: a headlamp; three-power loupes; Sims, Wietlander, and narrow Deaver retractors; vascular forceps; tenotomy scissors; and peanut dissectors.

A varicocele may be managed open with an abdominal approach (Palomo), an inguinal approach (Ivanissevich), or a subinguinal approach.

ABDOMINAL APPROACH (PALOMO)

With this approach, adequate collateral will remain should the artery be compromised. It is easily done on these typically slender boys.

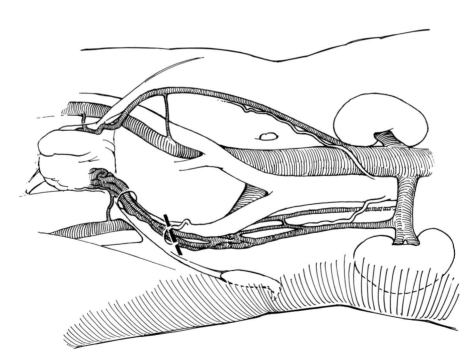

FIGURE 126-1. Position: Place the boy supine with a footplate to allow shifting to the reverse Trendelenburg position to fill the veins. If the boy is old enough, use local anesthesia. Incision: Make a short semioblique incision through the skin and subcutaneous tissue over the site of the internal inguinal ring. Insert a Wietlander retractor. The heavy dashed line indicates the site for transection of the veins.

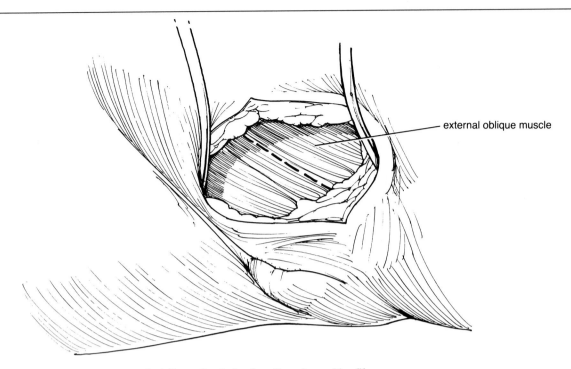

external oblique muscle

FIGURE 126-2. Incise the external oblique fascia in the direction of its fibers.

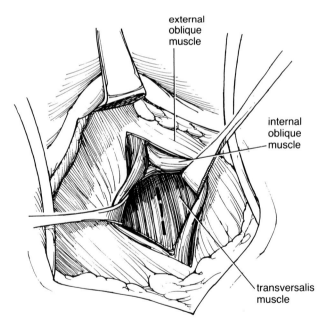

external
oblique
muscle

internal
oblique
muscle

transversalis
muscle

FIGURE 126-3. Separate the internal oblique muscle bluntly by inserting a curved clamp. Incise the transversalis fascia.

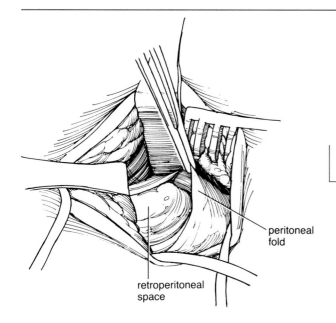

FIGURE 126-4. Enter the retroperitoneal space 3 to 5 cm above and medial to the inguinal ligament.

peritoneal
fold

retroperitoneal
space

FIGURE 126-5. Push the peritoneum medially with the peanut dissector, exposing the spermatic vessels as they rise to join the vas. Pulling on the testis at this point may be helpful in locating the vessels. A retractor placed medially could hide the spermatic veins on the posterior peritoneum.

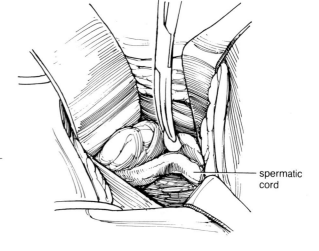

spermatic
cord

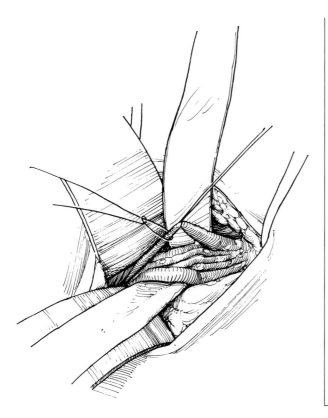

FIGURE 126-6. Place a curved clamp or drain behind the vessels to elevate them into the wound. With loupe magnification, use sharp and blunt dissection to isolate all (usually three) of the flabby veins from the adjacent artery and lymphatic vessels. If the artery is not apparent, skeletonize the cord by bluntly stripping the spermatic fascia. Drip papaverine solution onto the cord to allow the artery to dilate and become visibly pulsatile. Inadvertent ligation is rarely harmful because adequate circulation comes from vessels to the distal cord structures. The veins also may be made more obvious by dripping papaverine solution on the spermatic artery to increase the circulation to and from the testis. Placing the patient in the reverse Trendelenburg position may fill the veins and help identification.

Perform intraoperative venography if identification of all collaterals is in doubt, especially in adolescents. To do this, ligate the largest vein proximally. Tent it up and instill contrast medium distally through a 25-gauge butterfly needle, and expose a film.

Ligate each vein with two silk ties and divide between. However, complete transection of all vessels at this level does not risk testicular viability, because the vasal and cremasteric vessels remain intact. Do not resect a segment that would require unnecessary pathologic examination. Irrigate the wound and close each layer of the body wall. Infiltrate the subcutaneous tissue with 0.25% mepivacaine for prolonged regional anesthesia. Place a subcuticular 4-0 synthetic absorbable suture to close the skin. Apply support for the scrotum.

INGUINAL APPROACH (IVANISSEVICH)

This approach allows management of the internal spermatic veins where they come off the cord structures at the level of the internal inguinal ring. It is easier, especially in the more obese youth, and requires less assistance.

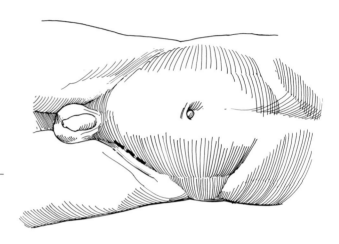

FIGURE 126-7. Position: Place the boy supine. Incision: Make a 4-cm incision two fingerbreadths above the symphysis pubis in line with the lateral aspect of the scrotum beginning above the palpable external ring, extending obliquely along the course of the canal. Divide and ligate the superficial epigastric vessels that cross the lower end of the incision.

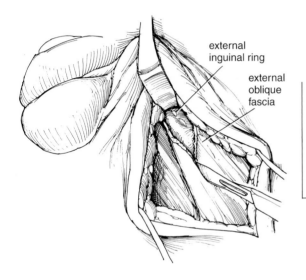

FIGURE 126-8. Divide Scarpa's fascia and bluntly clear the connective tissue overlying the external oblique fascia and external ring. Insert a self-retaining retractor. Incise the fascia in the line of its fibers, beginning at the external ring and extending above the internal ring. Avoid the ilioinguinal nerve beneath. Pick the cord up between thumb and forefinger to palpate the vas and artery. Elevate the spermatic fascia with clamps to allow separation of the cord by blunt dissection.

FIGURE 126-9. Pass a curved clamp under the cord near the pubic tubercle and draw a Penrose drain or vessel loop through for traction to allow mobilization of the cord.

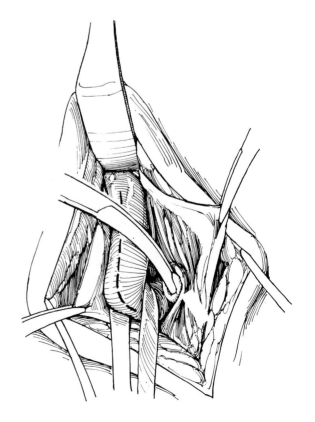

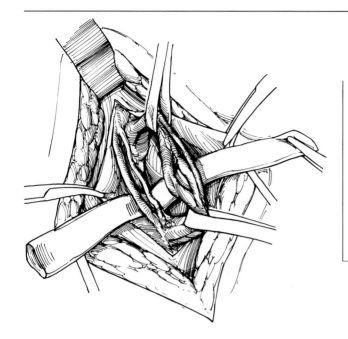

FIGURE 126-10. Hold the cord in the wound by fastening the ends of the drain to the drapes on each side. Open the cremasteric fascia. Sweep the underlying vas back out of the field. Aided by three-power loupes and microvascular forceps, dissect the spermatic fascia from each of the (usually) three branches of the spermatic vein from each other and from the more tortuous artery and the lymphatics for 2 to 3 cm in both directions. Papaverine dripped onto the cord will help visualize the artery and the veins. Look for and ligate the cremasteric vein that runs from the spermatic cord to the pudendal vein at the external ring.

FIGURE 126-11. Doubly clamp each vein in succession and ligate each end with 4-0 silk ties. Place the child in reverse Trendelenburg position to be sure no veins are overlooked. Remove the Penrose drain.

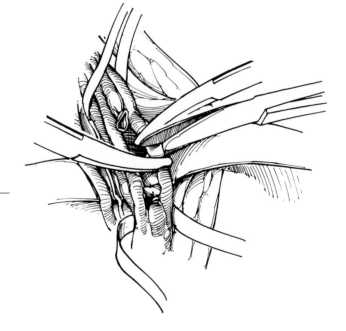

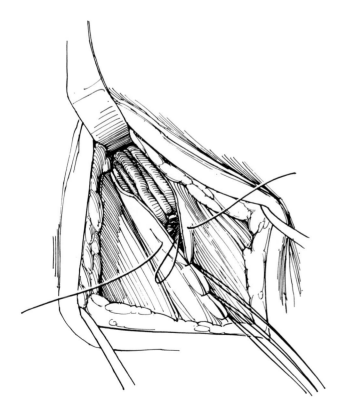

FIGURE 126-12. Close the external oblique fascia with interrupted 4-0 synthetic absorbable sutures, starting laterally and using the tied sutures for elevation of the edge. At the external ring, hold the cord down with a peanut dissector while placing the last stitch. Close Scarpa's fascia with a few fine sutures and close the skin subcuticularly. Apply support for the scrotum. Advise the boy to avoid activities that cause pain.

POSTOPERATIVE PROBLEMS

Damage to the artery can occur with subsequent testicular atrophy. It is less likely to occur with the retroperitoneal approach. The same is true for injury to the vas deferens, which should immediately be repaired. Persistence of the varicocele is not rare, due to missing a vein or because the varicocele was caused by actual venous obstruction from the so-called "nutcracker" phenomenon. It is very rare after ligation of the entire cord (as in the original Palomo procedure).

A. BARRY BELMAN

Commentary by

Varicoceles in adolescents are present as frequently as in adults (15%). However, the indications for surgery differ because in the adult population, infertility is the usual complaint. In adolescents, presentation usually follows a visit to the primary physician, with the varicocele noted when the patient is examined upright. Rarely does the patient have any complaints referable to the findings, and generally, he is unaware of the varicocele's presence even though it is usually quite large (grade II–III or III). Our indications for recommending surgical intervention remain a significant (>20%) decrease in left testicular size. However, occasionally, both testes are much smaller than would be expected for the level of pubertal development and both may grow after vein ligation.

Testes may be measured using a standard orchidometer or sonographically (the latter adds cost to the evaluation that may not be justifiable). Hormonal levels are not affected by the presence of a varicocele. However, follicle-stimulating hormone and luteinizing hormone levels may rise higher than normal in response to gonadotropin-releasing hormone stimulation in men with varicoceles. This has been used diagnostically to substantiate an adverse effect from the abnormality. However, long-term results as to its significance have not been demonstrated.

Spermatic venous ligation is recommended on the presumption that fertility will be negatively influenced in the future by the varicocele. Growth of the testis in 80% of these boys postoperatively suggests that the varicocele was indeed detrimental. Unfortunately, no long-term controlled study exists comparing two groups of adolescents to determine if surgery improves fertility.

Sparing lymphatics is important, as postoperative hydroceles remain one of the most common complications. With lymphatic preservation and ligation of the remainder of the vessels (artery included), success is close to 100%.

EVAN KASS

Commentary by

We have used the Palomo approach as our preferred method for varicocele ligation in a teenager with a varicocele. We make no attempt to identify or preserve the artery because almost invariably there are venous collaterals intimately attached to the artery that, if not ligated, result in varicocele persistence. The use of papaverine or intraoperative venograms, in our experience, did not reduce persistence of the varicocele postoperatively. In our experience, artery ligation has never resulted in testicular atrophy. We do attempt to preserve lymphatics to reduce the frequency of hydrocele formation. When patients have had prior inguinal surgery we recommend radiographic venous occlusion, or use the operating microscope to ensure identification and preservation of the artery.

In the Ivanissevich approach, it is essential for the artery to be preserved. Therefore, if choosing this approach, it is of critical importance to use the operating microscope. Loop magnification is not enough to enable identification and preservation of the artery while facilitating ligation of all venous collaterals. The success rate for the Palomo operation with artery ligation and for the microscopic Ivanissevich procedure with artery preservation should approach 98% to 99%. The success rate for techniques that preserve the artery but do not employ the operating microscope is only 85%.

Chapter 127

Laparascopic Varicocelectomy

Because of greater visualization, the laparoscopic approach has fewer negative outcomes, and hence may be considered cost effective.

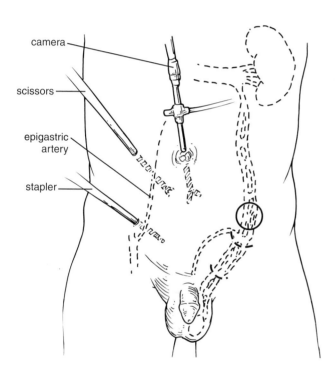

FIGURE 127-1. Place a 5- or 10-mm video port just below the umbilicus, a 5-mm port in the suprapubic area, and a 5-mm port in the contralateral side midway between the umbilicus and the anterior superior iliac spine. Stand on the right (the side opposite the varicocele), and manipulate the midline and left instruments. The assistant, holding the laparoscope, will view a mirror image of the procedure on the monitor at the foot of the table. Rotate the table to elevate the affected side, and initiate a 30-degree Trendelenburg position.

FIGURE 127-2. Identify the internal ring by following the vas deferens. Move the sigmoid colon medially; it may be necessary to free it. Compress the scrotum, and observe the filling of the spermatic veins. Try to identify the spermatic artery before arterial spasm is caused by manipulation of the vessels. Grasp the peritoneum approximately 5 cm proximal to the internal ring and slightly lateral to the spermatic vessels with grasping forceps passed through the midline port, and expose the vessels through a short T incision using laparoscopic scissors passed through the ipsilateral port. Using a straight grasping instrument in combination with the curved dissector, free the vessels from the retroperitoneal connective tissue and the psoas muscle.

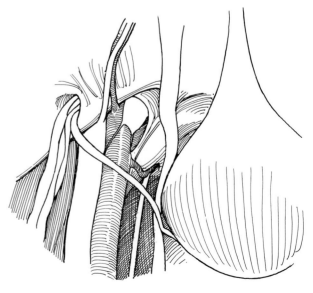

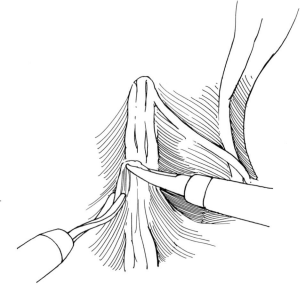

FIGURE 127-3. With two graspers, dissect the veins into multiple bundles while separating the spermatic artery from them. Traction on the testis helps identify the vessels. Avoid electrocoagulation near the delicate pedicle. Elevate the bundle, and push the spermatic artery out of the way with a dissector. Vasospasm may make identification difficult; it can be reduced by dripping papaverine or lidocaine through an aspirator-irrigator. Isolate the spermatic veins.

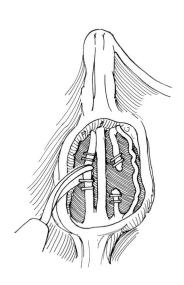

FIGURE 127-4. Place two 5-mm titanium endoclips proximally and two distally on each of the veins. Cut the veins between the paired clips with endoscissors. Smaller veins still may be present about the artery. Tease them away, and clip or fulgurate them with a fine electrosurgical probe or an Nd:YAG contact laser probe. Divide them with scissors. Inspect the area to be sure of hemostasis, and check the result of ligation by again compressing the scrotum. Place the boy flat and in a reverse Trendelenburg position. Again look for any oozing, and aspirate any blood or irrigant that may have collected. Remove all but one port, and open the valve to allow the carbon dioxide to issue from the abdomen. Place a single synthetic absorbable suture in the fascia below the umbilicus at the site of the 10-mm insertion site, and seal the skin incisions with sterile adhesive strips. The large varicoceles of adolescents may resolve slowly postoperatively, and the pampiniform plexus may remain palpable.

KENNETH GLASSBERG

Commentary by

Laparoscopic varicocelectomy is usually described as an en masse ligation of the internal spermatic cord, well above its confluence with the vas deferens. It also can be done as an en masse ligation after isolating and preserving the internal spermatic artery, or as a lymphatic-sparing procedure with or without preserving the internal spermatic artery. As an en masse ligation, it simulates an open Palomo repair and, therefore, should have the same high incidence (>20%) of postoperative hydroceles, which usually appear more than 9 months following surgery. As the magnification offered by laparoscopy is almost that used in a microscopic varicocelectomy, lymphatics can be clearly visualized and preserved, greatly reducing the incidence of postoperative delayed hydroceles, the size of the hydroceles that do develop, and the number of cases (<2%) that will require subsequent hydrocelectomy.

We choose to preserve the artery in cases where there has been previous ipsilateral groin surgery and where there is already a possibility of arterial damage, as in previous failed inguinal varicocelectomy or inguinal hernias. We have been successful, only saving the artery 80% of the time. Barqawi and coworkers (2002) have done en masse ligation in this scenario without compromising the testicle.

We started out doing laparoscopic varicocelectomies approximately 10 years ago but initially reserved the procedure predominantly for bilateral varicocelectomy, where it has its greatest advantage. We were so happy with the approach that it became our primary repair for unilateral cases as well. In addition, we find it easy to teach residents. The vessels can be safely handled with small Maryland graspers; other types of graspers will rip the veins. Any contact made by an instrument with the artery will likely cause arterial pulsation to stop, making identification of the artery at that point almost impossible. We find that LigaSure is very useful for ligating vessels.

Section 8

PENIS, URETHRA, AND GENITALIA

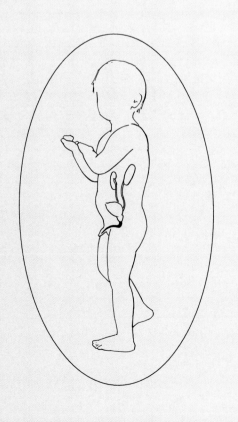

Chapter 128

Introduction to Hypospadias Repair

GOALS

Hypospadias is defined by the three major anatomic defects: (1) the abnormal location of the urethral meatus, (2) penile curvature, and (3) abnormalities of the foreskin.

The objective in treating patients with hypospadias is to reconstruct a straight penis for normal coitus and place the new urethral meatus on the terminal aspect of the glans to allow a forward-directed stream. There are five basic steps for a successful hypospadias outcome: (1) orthoplasty (straightening), (2) urethroplasty, (3) meatoplasty and glanuloplasty, (4) scrotoplasty, and (5) skin coverage. These various elements of surgical technique can be applied either sequentially or in various combinations to achieve a surgical success.

MEATAL ABNORMALITIES

Hypospadias is characterized by an abnormality in location and configuration of the urethral meatus. The urethral meatus may be ventrally placed just below a blind dimple at the normal meatal opening on the glans or so far back in the perineum that it appears as a "vaginal" hypospadias. Most patients present with the meatus somewhere between these extremes. The meatus is encountered in a variety of configurations in form, diameter, elasticity, and rigidity. It can be fissured in both transverse and longitudinal directions or can be covered with delicate skin. In the case of the megameatus intact prepuce the distal urethra is enlarged, tapering to a normal caliber in the penile shaft. Often, there is an orifice of a periurethral duct located distal to the meatus that courses dorsal to the urethral channel for a short distance. It is blind ending and does not communicate in any way with the urinary stream. The periurethral duct corresponds with Guérin's sinus or Morgagni's lacunae. Unless these ducts are inadvertently closed, leading to a blind-ending epithelial pouch, they are of no clinical consequence.

SKIN AND SCROTAL ABNORMALITIES

The skin of the penis is radically changed as a result of the disturbance in the formation of the urethra. Distal to the meatus, there is often a paucity of ventral skin that may contribute to penile curvature. The frenulum is always absent in hypospadias. Vestiges of a frenulum are sometimes found inserting on either side of the open navicular fossa.

The skin proximal to the urethral meatus may be extremely thin, so much so that a catheter or probe passed proximally is readily apparent through a tissue-paper thickness of skin. When it is present, it abrogates the use of perimeatal skin flaps in repairs.

The urethral plate extending from the hypospadiac meatus to the glanular groove may be well developed. Even with a meatus quite proximal on the shaft, this normal urethral plate is quite elastic and typically nontethering. Artificial erection demonstrates no ventral curvature in these situations. A normal urethral plate may be incorporated into the surgical repair. However, if the urethral plate is underdeveloped, it will act as a tethering fibrous band that bends the penis ventrally during artificial erection. When this fibrous chordee tissue is divided, the penis will frequently straighten.

Normally, the genital tubercle should develop in a cranial position above the two genital swellings. The penis may be caught between the two scrotal halves and become engulfed with fusion of the penoscrotal area. The boundary between the penis and the scrotum may be formed by two oblique raphes that extend from the very proximal meatus to the dorsal side of the penis.

PENILE CURVATURE

The curvature of the penis is caused by deficiency of the normal structures most commonly on the ventral side of the penis. It has been labeled chordee; however, this term implies a strand of connective tissue stretched like a cord between the meatus and glans, which is rarely found in practice. Penile curvature can be from skin deficiency, a dartos fascial deficiency, a true fibrous chordee with tethering of the ventral shaft, or deficiency of the corpora cavernosa on the concave side of the penis.

There are occasional reports of other penile anomalies that represent variations of the embryologic defect causing hypospadias. They can be characterized as a defect in the course of the urethra such as congenital urethral fistula and a group characterized by curvature of the penis without hypospadias or so-called chordee without hypospadias.

HYPOSPADIAS SURGEONS

Success is directly related to the experience of the surgeon. For a successful result in hypospadias repair, the penile tissues must be handled with great care. Experience in mobilizing and rotating skin flaps is needed, as are the minutia involved in plastic surgical techniques. It is not enough to review pictures and follow descriptions; training in the techniques is essential. Knowledge of a few methods is not enough, because the one used must be the best for the individual situation of the child. A pediatric urology fellowship is the appropriate place to become competent in hypospadias surgery.

PREOPERATIVE EVALUATION

Because hypospadias is an isolated anomaly, the entire genitourinary tract does not require evaluation. The absence of one gonad, perineal hypospadias, severe chordee, or a bifid scrotum suggests a disorder of sex development and requires genotypic evaluation. If both gonads are not palpable, consider the possibility of congenital adrenal hyperplasia in a phenotypic female.

AGE FOR OPERATION

Select a time between 6 and 9 months for surgery. At this age the infants are easiest to manage, are not walking, and remain in diapers. Babies appear to have fewer bladder spasms and require smaller doses of pain medication. They do not seem to remember the surgery as teenagers and adults. Parenteral testosterone may be administered to increase the size of the penis and especially the size and vascularity of the prepuce should it be needed for proximal and perineal hypospadias repair. Give 25 to 50 mg intramuscularly, repeated once or twice at 3-week intervals before operation. Expect somewhat more bleeding as a result.

OUTPATIENT REPAIR

An uncomplicated hypospadias operation can be done without hospital admission. Have the parents and child visit you sometime before the date of surgery for history taking and examination, as well as for instructions in feeding and preoperative care. The surgeon and nurse should give considerable support to the parents because of their need to know what to expect. At this visit you can explain the procedure, hand out suitable booklets describing details, and obtain informed consent. Review the postoperative catheter care and medications.

PROPHYLACTIC ANTIBIOTICS

Prophylactic antibiotics are not essential except for salvage repairs, although administration intraoperatively of a systemic antibiotic may be wise. If antibiotic coverage is needed, begin immediately and continue postoperatively until the catheter is removed.

MAGNIFICATION

As a pediatric urologist, you should have your own 2.5- or 3.5-power loupes or commercial magnifying visor. An operative microscope with a stand placed at the end of the table and covered from the field can be very helpful, especially if the assistant has matching eyepieces. Use microsurgical instruments and sutures, for as confidence is gained, magnification becomes a boon, not a hindrance.

NERVE BLOCK

Caudal nerve block is a good alternative to or a supplement for local anesthesia (see Chapter 5). Performed by an anesthesiologist at the start of the operation, it has become the standard of care.

Local nerve block is an alternative. At the beginning of the operation, place a penile nerve block with 3 to 4mL of 0.5% long-lasting bupivacaine mixed with 1% quick-acting lidocaine (see Fig. 6-63). Inject it at the base of each crus just below the notch of the symphysis, or vertically in the midline deep to the notch of the symphysis, with a 1.5-inch 22-gauge needle. When placed at the beginning of an operation it will reduce the amount of general anesthesia required and will provide anesthesia that will last well into the postoperative period.

HEMOSTASIS

For hemostasis use a solution of 1:100,000 epinephrine in 1% lidocaine and inject it through a 27-gauge needle within the glans and the area of abortive spongiosum. Wait 7 minutes for it to act. This vasoconstrictor will reduce the bleeding during the dissection but if the operation is prolonged beyond 90 minutes, rebound vasodilation can be expected. Remember that halothane anesthesia sensitizes the heart to catecholamines, thus promoting arrhythmias. Avoid electrocoagulation as much as possible; if it is necessary, use a monopolar or cautery to only the forceps unit set at a low current.Moreover, once the skin flaps are applied, bleeding seems to stop, and a pressure dressing will usually assure hemostasis. On rare occasions the tourniquet used for artificial erection can facilitate hemostasis.

ARTIFICIAL ERECTION

Saline induced erection: Place a broad rubber band or small red rubber catheter around the base of the penis and secure it with a hemostat. Introduce a 25-gauge butterfly needle through the glans into a corpus cavernosum or directly into the corpus cavernosum. Gently distend the penis with injectable normal saline solution; avoid overdistention. Maintain

the erection during evaluation of the chordee. After the chordee has been corrected, create a second erection to check penile alignment.

SUTURING

Absorbable sutures are best for the skin and subcutaneous tissues because anesthesia is not required for their removal. Alternatively, use fine sutures of 6-0 polydioxanone, although Vicryl or Dexon-S may occasionally be suitable. Polyglycolic acid sutures are not as good as polyglactic sutures; they last too long and thus may promote fistulas. Place sutures subcuticularly to avoid sinuses caused by epithelium growing in along the suture track (this occurs more frequently with braided sutures).

LOCAL URINARY DIVERSION IN CHILDREN

Diversion of urine away from the suture lines has always been a problem in children because any indwelling tube, particularly one terminating in a balloon, induces bladder spasms that force urine around it into the repair. This disrupts the suture line and leads to formation of fistulas. Besides, the lumen of a balloon catheter is small compared to that of a straight catheter, especially a plastic one.

Many techniques have been tried to minimize these problems with diversion. The simplest method for infants, one that combines stenting with drainage, is to insert a fine silicone tube, such as 6-F peritoneal shunt tubing or neurosurgical tubing with its wandlike end, into the bladder through the urethra and fasten the end to the glans in one or two places with nonabsorbable sutures. Alternately, place a 6-F Kendall catheter of soft Silastic, with a Luer Lock at the end, to prevent internal migration and to allow irrigation (Fig. 128-1). Whatever intubation system is used in infants, collect the urine in a double diaper. For older boys use a urethral balloon catheter; tape it to the abdomen so that it cannot disturb the ventral glans repair. Drainage should be continued for 4 to 7 days for distal and penile shaft repairs and 7 to 10 days for more severe hypospadias repairs.

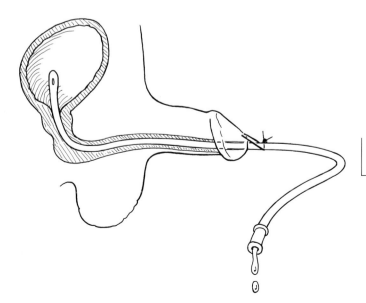

FIGURE 128-1. Urinary drainage for hypospadias reconstruction.

DRESSINGS

Apply a dressing to immobilize the area, to reduce edema, and to prevent the formation of a hematoma. Use transparent and permeable absorbent plastic film (Tegaderm or Op-Site) applied over Telfa or tincture of benzoin. Let the catheter drain into an outer diaper. The dressing may be removed in 2 to 3 days after a few warm baths at home. Once the dressing has been removed use petroleum jelly on the diaper to keep the repaired penis from sticking, typically for 4 to 5 days.

SETUP FOR OPERATION

Select instruments designed for delicate handling of tissues. A reasonable list would include loupe magnification; genitourinary fine and microsurgery sets; microsurgical knife (Weck); toothed and nontoothed forceps (Adson); fine Allis clamps; two pairs of Bishop-Harmon forceps or 0.5 platform forceps; jeweler's forceps; sharp small tenotomy scissors, iris scissors, microtip Castroviejo scissors; microtip Castroviejo needle holders; four small two-prong and two small one-prong skin hooks; plastic scissors and plastic needle holders; a peanut dissector; and a ring retractor (Scott) and hooks.

Also have available bougies á boule; 5- and 8-F infant feeding tubes; rubber bands; a marking pen; a 25-gauge butterfly needle and syringe and a hand-held Bovie, or an ophthalmic electrocautery.

Have fine sutures of appropriate sizes and types at hand but unopened: synthetic absorbable suture, nonabsorbable suture (e.g., Prolene on a C-1 tapered needle for glans traction, 7-0 polydioxanone suture for urethral anastomosis, and 6-0 or 7-0 chromic catgut suture) for the skin.

SELECTION OF THE OPERATIVE TECHNIQUE

After anesthesia is induced, a caudal nerve block administered, and the field prepared for surgery, the quality of the urethra and supporting spongiosum is assessed. Several procedures are available for the repair of hypospadias depending on quality of the preputial flap (see Chapter 129) or, in cases when local skin is not available, the use of free graft such as bladder (see Chapter 130), buccal (see Chapter 131), or preputial skin grafts (see Chapter 132) is considered. Mild and moderate penile curvature can be corrected by dorsal midline (see Chapter 133) or lateral (see Chapter 134) placement of sutures in the tunica albuginea. For severe curvature requiring resection of the urethral plate and not responsive to dorsal plication, dermal grafting is warranted (see Chapter 135).

The shape of the glans is useful for determining the appropriate operative technique. With a flattened glans, the urethral plate usually is normal and may be preserved for subsequent tubularization or application of an onlay flap with the glans supporting the repair (see Chapter 136). In contrast, a cone-shaped glans usually is accompanied by a fibrous urethral plate requiring division, followed by a transverse island flap and a tunneled glanuloplasty or two-stage repair. Skin coverage depends on leaving the dorsal skin intact and recreating the incision from a circumcision, along with a ventral midline seam (see Chapter 137).

SPECIFIC OPERATIONS

An algorithm is presented for the reconstruction of hypospadias (Fig. 128-2). A tried and true approach is to start each repair by preserving the urethral plate, dissecting the

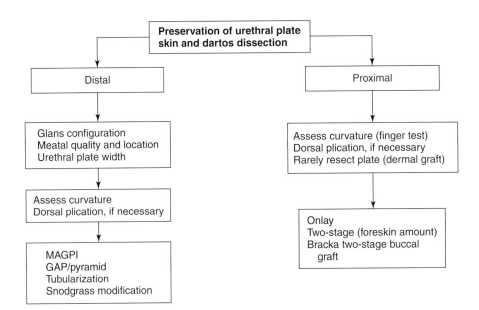

FIGURE 128-2. Algorithm for hypospadias repair.

skin to the penile scrotal junction, and assessing for the presence of penile curvature. If curvature is not present or is mild to moderate and amenable to dorsal plications (see Chapter 133) then a one-stage approach is typically successful. The specific repair is now dependent on the meatal configuration and the surgeon's preference.

Patents with a coronal mobile meatus and a web of tissue within the glans can be treated with the meatoplasty and glanuloplasty procedure (MAGPI repair) (see Chapter 138). Patients with a fish mouth meatus and glanular or distal meatus can be treated with the glans approximation procedure (GAP) (see Chapter 139). The hypospadiac variant of megameatus intact prepuce is amenable to the pyramid procedure (see Chapter 140). With their abundant dorsal vasculature, island flaps (see Chapter 143) laid on as patches have become increasingly popular as the poorer vascularization associated with the Mathieu/flip-flap procedures (see Chapter 141) has been recognized. Urethral advancement with the ability to place the new urethral meatus in a normal position within the remodeled glans favors the balanic groove technique (see Chapter 142).

For penile shaft and more severe hypospadias the onlay island flap has been tested over time (see Chapter 143). In patients with a healthy urethral plate, primary tubularization (see Chapter 144) alone or in combination with incision of the urethral plate (Snodgrass modification) (see Chapter 145) is gaining widespread popularity.

In patients with severe hypospadias requiring resection of the urethral plate, one-stage procedures, the tranverse tubularized island flap (see Chapter 146), or the specialized onlay urethroplasty with parameatal foreskin flap (see Chapter 147) is an alternative. Free tube grafts also have their use in more severe cases (see Chapter 148). For severe hypospadias a planned two-stage approach (see Chapter 149) for primary repairs is an acceptable alternative to a one-stage repair with a high complication rate. Repair of penoscrotal transposition (see Chapter 151) is typically done in a second stage. The special circumstance of foreskin preservation is requested by more and more families. This technique can be performed safely in patients with minimal penile curvature (see Chapter 152).

POSTOPERATIVE PROBLEMS

Bladder spasms not only cause the child to move about in response to pain, but also force urine through the repair. Give analgesics and antispasmodics, such as oxybutynin (Ditropan). Give stool softeners and a suitable diet because the antispasmodic regimen may result in constipation and lead to straining and urine leakage.

Bleeding is an infrequent problem. A compressive sandwich dressing will resolve the problem in all but the rare patient.

In selected cases, give a broad-spectrum antibiotic such as trimethoprim-sulfameth-oxazole (Septra) or a cephalosporin, and continue it for a few days after the tubing has been removed. Should postoperative erections in older boys become a problem, use amyl nitrate ampules or diazepam sedation to reduce them.

Remove the catheter at the agreed-on postoperative day. Continue bathing the child twice a day 7 to 10 days after the catheter is out to reduce swelling and facilitate healing. See the patient 6 weeks and 1 year after the repair. Reevaluate after potty training and at puberty to confirm patient satisfaction and the absence of fistula, stenosis, diverticulum, recurrent chordee, and cosmetic issues.

COMPLICATIONS

Complications occur after 10% to 20% of hypospadias operations. These include meatal retraction; urethrocutaneous fistula formation; meatal stenosis; urethral stricture; development of a diverticulum (sometimes with hair, followed by stones); and persistent chordee. Of these, strictures (see Chapter 150), fistulae (see Chapter 153), and urethral diverticuli (see Chapter 154) account for most of the late problems. Manage these complications for at least 6 months from the time of the initial surgery.

OUTCOMES

Results today cosmetically and functionally are better than those in the past. The use of a one-stage hypospadias repair at an early age with a low complication rate encourages our current positive outlook for this condition. Curvature correction with the aid of an artificial erection is extremely important for assuring satisfactory sexual function. With the placement of the urinary meatus at the tip of the glans, the infertility potential has been improved unless the patient has other coexisting testicular problems. Evidence shows that the neourethra grows with the child, and subsequent repairs are seldom necessary.

Early hypospadias repair with minimal hospitalization helps to avoid separation anxiety and castration fears. We can now counsel parents confidently that there is an excellent outlook for a good cosmetic, functional, and emotional result in boys with all degrees of hypospadias.

PRACTICAL CONCLUSIONS

1. Hypospadias should be repaired within the first year of life, preferably at 4 to 6 months of age. Pain control and catheters seem better tolerated and the baby's lack of mobility simplifies postoperative care.
2. A terminal slitlike meatus should be the goal with or without preservation of the foreskin depending on parental preference.
3. Preservation of the urethral plate creates the best possible chance to recreate normal urethral anatomy by incorporating the abortive spongiosum into the repair.
4. Midline dorsal plication is safe and effective for the correction of penile curvature in the majority of patients. (Placing more than two rows of sutures is a sign that another technique such as dermal grafting is indicated.)

5. In the small percentage of patients that require resection of the urethral plate a two-stage approach is generally warranted.

6. Vascularized pedicle onlay flaps are successful in primary and redo hypospadias surgery.

7. De-epithelialized vascular flaps should be used as a second layer for all urethroplasties.

8. Patients with a paucity of skin are best managed with the Bracka two-stage buccal repair.

9. Coronal fistulas require a redo glansplasty.

10. Surgical volume correlates with successful outcomes.

Commentary by NORMAN B. HODGSON

GENERAL COMMENTS

The essence of hypospadias repair is adapting the available tissues to the needs of the child. This has been expressed in a seemingly endless variety of ways in which there is a common thread: In most of the depictions and descriptions, the focus is on the cuticular layer. That has always limited the perception of the choices. From my perspective, the emphasis should be on the quality of the dartos muscle and the attendant blood vessels. I know that is hard to depict, but it is the determining factor in outcome expectancy and it defines the choice of operation (there now are approximately 220 different techniques).

Imagine the frustration of Ormond Culp with his watershed of cases. The tissues had been manipulated, large chromic sutures had been used with resultant scarring, the chordee was still there, there were holes around and about, the instrumentation was gross, and latex was the material for drainage. In his gentle, offbeat manner, he was able to dissuade the uninitiated from attacking the formidable. As consulting editor for *The Journal of Urology* in the 1960s, he was responsible for delaying the introduction of one-stage repairs until Bill Scott came to Milwaukee for a visit and was shown a group of children. The delay was for the best, because those were the formative years.

The learning curve of tissue management always will demand sufficient case material for growth. This dictates that not everyone will do these procedures; rather, one surgeon per million patients will tend to, and should, do them all.

Hypospadiac disability continues to occur but in sharply declining numbers. Thankfully, most of the repairs are done in some variation of a single-stage procedure. Most children are handled as outpatients or with brief hospitalizations. The overall cost of management has been sharply reduced. All in all, the management of the problem has become a success story in hands across the world. Still, the writings and subtle variations continue to surface. Tissue glues and other sealants are used by some surgeons. The variations in the raphe, the redundancy of the dimples, the arching of the axial vessels, the density of the prepuce, the elasticity of the dartos muscle and the skin, the configuration and size of the glans, and the fibrosis of chordee all challenge the intellect and hands of the operator. It must be frustrating to the uninitiated and uninterpretable to the disinterested.

ONE-STAGE HYPOSPADIAS REPAIRS

Fortunately, knowledge regarding ONE-STAGE repairs is well disseminated so that the appropriate choices and nuances that seemed subtle now can achieve an appropriate focus. The concept that the child selects his own operation is quite true, because the combination of chordee and preputial distribution predicts the choices and eventual outcome. The quality of the tissue, as witnessed through the dartos muscle, limits the choices and defines the character of the healing process.

I start with an incision tracing the raphe as it splits into its diversion to the preputial hood. I then carry it back toward the coronal margin, as suggested by Firlit, to provide for Firlit flaps, which may be swung onto the ventrum for covering. The tissues are valuable but not universally applicable, so they may or may not come into play in the final closure. This incision then allows mobilization of the shaft skin and visualization of the dysplastic bifurcated corpus spongiosum. At this juncture, an artificial erection demonstrates the components of the chordee. Does this involve glans tilt, fibrous dysplasia of the spongiosum, or, indeed, corporeal disproportion? All of these can be elements in the presentation of curvature and disfigurement. Resolution of chordee proceeds.

Having accomplished that, the release of the glans wings can then guide the surgeon toward the repair.

The surgeon is obligated on the ventrum to remove thin cutis lateral of the midline and not join the urethral meatus to the tip of the glans. These tissues are dysplastic and will not serve the repair well. Their dartos tissues are thin or nonexistent, and attempting to sew these will only add frustration. At this point, the best procedure for the child can be determined. The initial appraisal will rule in or out the glandular reconstruction procedure, such as the Arap or Zaontz (notice that is an A-to-Z alphabetical order) for it has been described repeatedly by a number of different surgeons and is only occasionally (i.e., rarely) of value. The child must present with just the right amount of tissue to allow the tubularization to proceed. The covering tissues ordinarily will have to come from elsewhere, and even with the tiny sutures now available may well experience impaired healing. These procedures are relatively straightforward in their presentation, but because of their simplicity, will be more commonly chosen than they should be.

Similarly, the Mathieu procedure demands an excellent dartos layer for covering of the suture line, and this is not as commonly present as one would hope. When it is sparse, supplemental denuded rotational flaps can be brought from either side but this might create problems in glans closure or bulk. Thus, the natural attention is directed toward the two-faced preputial flap. Its transposition to the ventrum depends on the vessel supply and distribution, which can be defined by trans-illumination. It can be developed on the ventrum with preputial extension with meatal continuity (Broadbent), by mobilized patch (Hinderer, Orandi), or from a fully mobilized flap on the dorsum. If a hinged flap is rotated at the ventrum by a transverse incision of the prepuce at the coronal margin (Hodgson IV, Asopa), the tissues fall to the ventrum, and the strip selected may come from the inner face, the verge, or the first part of the outer face. Choice is made according to the thickness of the tissue and the width of the strip needed. This can be isolated by incision or excision to provide the necessary dartos healing surface.

An axial incision can be made down into the prepuce to select a tangential flap, if the tissues so align (Hodgson XX). Lastly, its double pedicle creates ventral problems (ventral tissue abundance) that may be hard to resolve.

In my multiple writings, I chose a series of numbers to outline these choices, but they reflect mainly the options of the two-faced flap.

Suture choice will depend on the individual surgeon, and each has its proponents, but all of the suture is fine at 6-0, 7-0, and 8-0. Subcuticular inverted knots for skin closure with no sutures penetrating the skin are now in vogue.

Currently, I accomplish urinary diversion with a Firlit-Kluge tube, which is remarkably well tolerated by the bladder and less prone to produce bladder spasms. In our setting, urine continues to be collected in a double diaper.

Buccal flaps seem to have an advantage over bladder epithelium or free skin grafts. On the other hand, preputial tissue continues to be the first choice.

A mobilized inner face flap (Duckett) is available for the longer defects but has been used less commonly in recent years.

There is an abundance of choices that follow these same principles, all going to the same end. Most young surgeons have these options in their armamentarium, so it will be fascinating to see which ones they ultimately select.

E. DURHAM SMITH

Commentary by

More than 300 operative techniques for the repair of hypospadias have been described, and any author clearly has a selection problem to be able to describe appropriate techniques in a short chapter. In this chapter, Dr. Hinman handles this well by not urging any particular technique; rather, he provides the essential points of surgical technique common to all repairs. Details of the construction of the neourethra are found in subsequent chapters.

Accordingly, this commentary focuses mainly on two areas: chordee correction and the selection of operative techniques appropriate to the clinical situation.

CHORDEE

The assessment of chordee and its total correction are far more important than the actual site of the urethral orifice, which changes after chordee is corrected, a point made in the text. Also stressed is that the major cause of chordee is adherency of ventral skin to underlying structures. The old concept that chordee was a central white fibrous band distal to the orifice defied experience, in that most of us could never find it! Two points should be stressed. First, the whole shaft of the penis should be exposed by a 38-degree circumferential cut of prepuce and penile skin, freeing all skin back to the base of the penis or beyond. This is because most of the chordee structures are proximal to the orifice, not distal to it. Second, the surgeon needs to deal with each element of the chordee in a progressive seriatim manner—free all skin first; in most cases, this is all that is required. Recheck for chordee by artificial erection or simply by placing traction with the fingers on the lateral shaft of the penis. If there is still chordee, dissect fibrous tissue from the corporeal tunica (a vascular exercise) or in the intercorporeal groove. If chordee persists, the urethra itself may require release from its distal site to a more proximal position. Finally, although not performed until a later step of the repair, the ventral deficiency of skin is made up by transference of dorsal preputial and penile skin to the ventral side.

Continued

The text suggests that in severe chordee without hypospadias, the urethra may need to be transected. Years ago, when the importance of skin tethering was not appreciated, transection was commonly performed. In recent years, I have not found this necessary on a single occasion, although it may be required in rare cases.

SELECTION OF TECHNIQUE

The inevitable argument of one-stage versus two-stage repairs continues. No one could argue that, given the right circumstances, the completion of a repair in one stage is preferable to submitting the child to two operations. However, the key to the debate is "the right circumstances." Unfortunately, an attitude has been fostered, especially in the United States, often with evangelistic zeal, that one-stage repair is sacrosanct and must be attempted at all times, whereas two-stage repair is reactionary, conservative, and out of context with modern surgical techniques. The result is a plethora of techniques of increasing complexity to bridge the gap in efforts to complete the repair in one stage, including long pedicle tubes, and free bladder and buccal mucosal grafts. These techniques are more difficult to perform and potentially carry more surgical hazards. They are dexterously performed with elegant results in certain centers of excellence where the volume of cases is large and the surgeons have immense experience. But it is quite a different matter to advocate such repairs for the larger bulk of surgeons, who may see fewer than 15 patients with hypospadias a year. It is simply not possible to develop the necessary operative skills for such complex procedures on such a clinical volume. The bad results of such a policy are all too plain to see as one travels the world to many centers. A failed one-stage repair is not necessarily a minor complication but often a complex problem requiring a complete redo, perhaps in multiple stages.

For the surgeon of moderate or small experience, a technique is required that is simple in concept, easy to execute, and absolutely reliable in results. These objectives are achievable by certain types of two-stage repairs. Furthermore, the acceptance of the two-stage concept also simplifies the operative choices; in fact, the technique I describe here can, if necessary, be a "universal" operation, applicable to any clinical situation. Only one technique is required to be learned, and expertise thus can be maintained, even with a small clinical volume. Having to perform two relatively uncomplicated operations, each requiring less than 45 minutes in the operating room, is a small price to pay for a constantly predictable result, especially because one or both stages can be done on an outpatient basis. Compare this with the multiple hours of complex operation required to construct mucosal free grafts or pedicle tubes, the surgical hazards of blood supply to such tubes, the presence of an anastomosis, the complexity of instrumentation, and so forth, all in an effort to save one stage. For these reasons, I applaud the author's statement that a one-stage procedure is best but a staged procedure is better than being forced to redo.

This is not to say that one-stage repairs should never be done. I do one-stage repairs; however, the guidelines of choice are not dictated by prejudice but by specific clinical features. One, as mentioned, is the experience of the surgeon. Another is the extent of the chordee, and a third, not mentioned in the text of this chapter, is the shape of the glans and depth of the central ventral groove. The significance of the latter is that a wide, splayed glans with a deep groove is an optimum precursor of a flip-flap repair, because it permits the closure of the glans tissue over the tube; conversely, a narrow, cone-shaped glans with a shallow groove makes this difficult and is likely to result in a stricture.

I have no serious disagreement with the author's recommendations regarding selection of technique, except for the choice of pedicle island tubes for those with marked chordee. Pedicle tubes in Duckett's hands are superb, but in *principle*, transferred tubes (either on a pedicle or as free grafts) involve the complexity of an anastomosis, a more precarious blood supply than a Duplay tube constructed of penile and preputial skin already in situ, and no anastomosis, as in my technique.

RECOMMENDATIONS

My recommendations are simple:

1. An orifice in the coronal groove or more distal in the glans and minimal chordee—one-stage MAGPI repair.
2. An orifice on the distal shaft or coronal groove with skin-tethering chordee only, and a wide, splayed glans with a deep central groove—one-stage flip-flap repair.
3. A distal orifice with marked chordee and/or cone-shaped narrow glans, all with more proximal orifices either before or after release of chordee—two-stage Smith repair.

The literature does not support the Denis Browne repair or its modifications, scrotal repairs, pedicle tubes in nonexpert hands, and all free grafts. Free grafts have the highest rate of fistula formation and stricture of all repairs.

HYPOSPADIAS DISABILITY

Comment is appropriate for the repair of hypospadias disability, that is, failed repairs with fistulas, residual chordee, strictures, deformed shape, skin shortage, and so forth. I support the general concepts of the last paragraph in this chapter. In practice, I find it best to lay the whole repair open back to healthy urethra, and start with a two-stage repair again. It often is said that it may be impossible to construct a tube from existing penile and preputial skin, because previous repairs have created gross deficiency of these tissues. For that reason, intervening grafts, such as bladder mucosa, are recommended. In more than 500 repairs as of 1994, and many scores of cases since, including many people with hypospadias disability, I have not once found such a skin deficiency that precluded a Duplay tube, nor has a free graft ever been necessary. There nearly always is some skin laterally or distally that can be mobilized and grafted to the glans as a first stage, but if it cannot, ventral skin always can be found by releasing skin from the dorsum, even to the extent of releasing the whole dorsal surface to the base of the penis. A large dorsal defect is easily closed by a Wolfe free skin graft from the inner thigh, which heals well on the penis. With ample skin now available on the ventral surface, a normal tube in situ can be constructed at a second stage. A free graft on the dorsal surface, unrelated to urine flow, is quite a different matter from a free graft within the urinary tract.

COMMENTATOR'S TWO-STAGE REPAIR

The present text includes reference to an important part of this repair, namely, the overlap technique of denuded skin closed as an intermediate layer. With this technique, of 303 cases done before 1978, fistulas occurred in 2.3%, and of 200 cases since, the fistula rate was 1% (Smith, 1984). From 1984 until my retirement, many additional cases were performed with the same incidence of fistulas.

OTHER COMMENTS

The recommended age for operation is supported (Smith, 1983), although I prefer the later second window at 2 to 3 years. Fundamental to age and more important than any particular recommended age is the amount of parental and house staff support. Given good parents, well-informed and unflappable, supported by a pediatric milieu in the hospital, the so-called stress of hospitalization is minimal at any age; however, the converse also is true.

For control of postoperative pain, we routinely use caudal injection and find it more effective than regional block. A fine-artery hemostat applied to the tip of the penis for stabilization of the penis actually is less traumatic than a suture; the latter often cuts out and leaves more sac than that from the hemostat.

I agree that a penile tourniquet is not necessary, but in the early stages of training the young surgeon, it is a help to be working in a bloodless field.

A COMMENT ABOUT CATHETER DRAINAGE

A per-urethral stent that does not reach the bladder is useful, as recommended, but I found some children have pain on voiding. We have standardized the use of a suprapubic stab cystostomy, which is easy to insert and almost never produces bladder spasms. It has no balloon, and it is easy to remove at the bedside. We prefer the Bonnano or Stamey catheter. Bladder spasms are lessened by (1) strapping the catheter firmly to the abdomen so that it cannot move in or out (child-proof), (2) low-pressure suction, and (3) acidifying the urine with vitamin C. We do not use any catheter for the first stage of a two-stage repair but routinely use a stab cystostomy for the second stage or for a one-stage flip-flap reconstruction. Both stages can be done on an outpatient basis, certainly for the first stage, but for the second stage with the catheter in place, most parents prefer to leave the child in the hospital. We have not used perineal urethrostomy for more than 15 years.

The text has a long series of techniques for fistula repair. One cannot quarrel with this, except that it obscures the importance of three points: (1) urethral mucosa must be closed separately as one layer, (2) a wide overlap technique of skin closure (my technique, as is used in the second stage of urethral reconstruction) for at least 1 cm proximal and distal to the fistula must be used, and (3) checking for urethral stenosis must be done.

Chapter 129

Vascularized Pedicle Flaps

Vascularized pedicle flaps have the advantage of a reliable blood supply. They can be used to augment the urethra in onlay fashion or replace the urethra in tube fashion. De-epithelialized flaps are the norm for separating the suture line on the urethroplasty from the overlying skin, thereby preventing fistula.

ANATOMY OF THE PREPUTIAL BLOOD SUPPLY

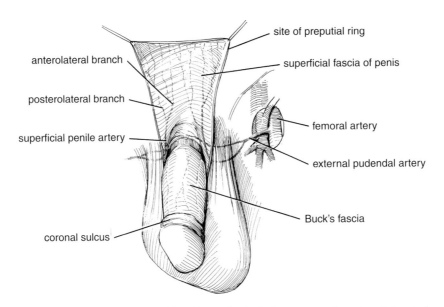

FIGURE 129-1. The superficial penile arteries, arising from the inferior external pudendal arteries, divide into anterolateral and posterolateral branches that supply the prepuce. The anterolateral and posterolateral branches have some variation but can be reliably dissected from the underlying penile skin to create a vascularized preputial pedicle flap.

PREPUTIAL ISLAND FLAP

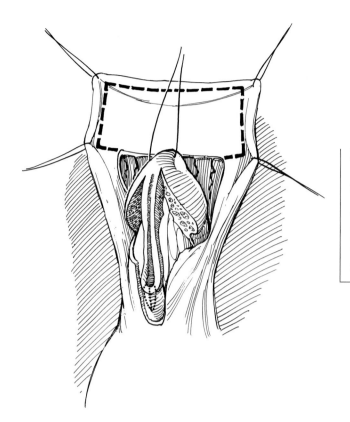

FIGURE 129-2. Place four traction sutures in the opened prepuce to fan out the ventral surface. Mark the skin for the flap *(dashed lines)*, making it larger than necessary. Incise along the marks. Develop a plane well down to the base of the penis between the flap and the dorsal skin to form a substantial pedicle. Dissecting to the base of the penis will eliminate the penile torsion from the flap. Take great care not to devascularize the flap while raising it.

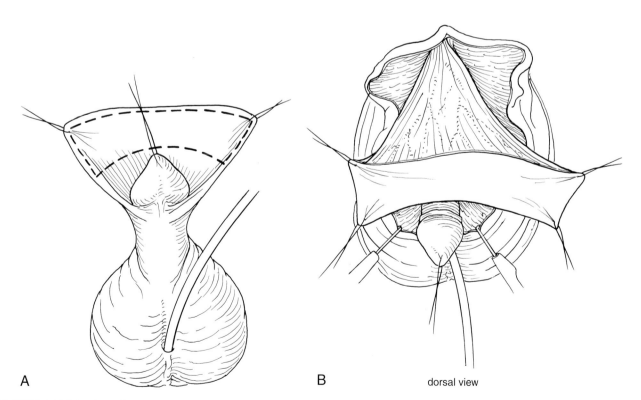

A   B   dorsal view

FIGURE 129-3. A and **B,** In severe hypospadias the inner prepuce can be outlined in the shape of a horseshoe to create a long flap necessary to bridge the urethral defect.

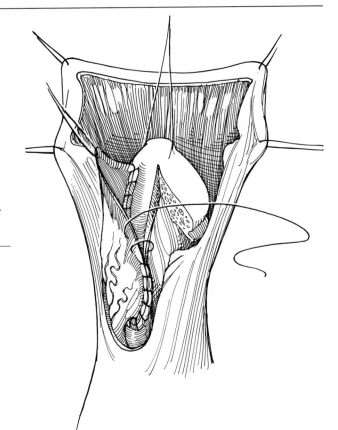

FIGURE 129-4. The flap can be rotated on the ventral aspect of the penis and used in an onlay fashion after trimming to size.

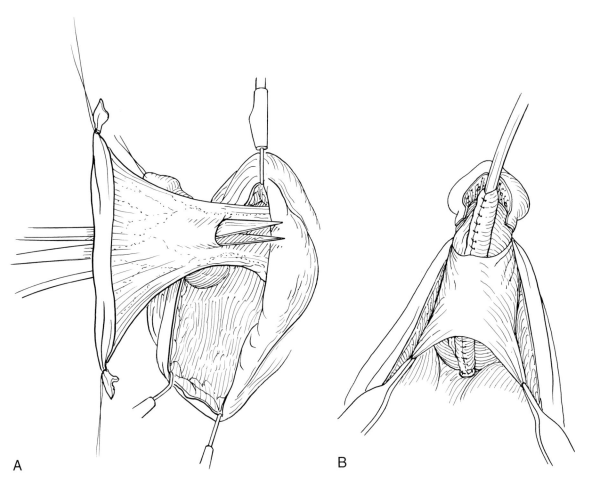

A

B

FIGURE 129-5. A, The flap may also be brought ventrally through a buttonhole. **B,** Either way, the flap may be used as a secondary layer to cover the anastomosis after removing the epithelium. Split prepuce vascularized flap.

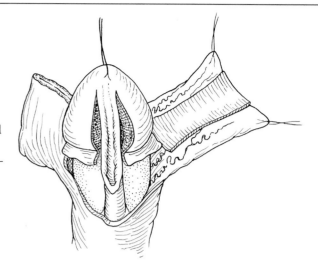

FIGURE 129-6. Half of the prepuce can be reserved for a vascularized onlay island flap and the other half for a de-epithelialized flap for secondary coverage.

TUBED TRANSVERSE PREPUTIAL ISLAND FLAP

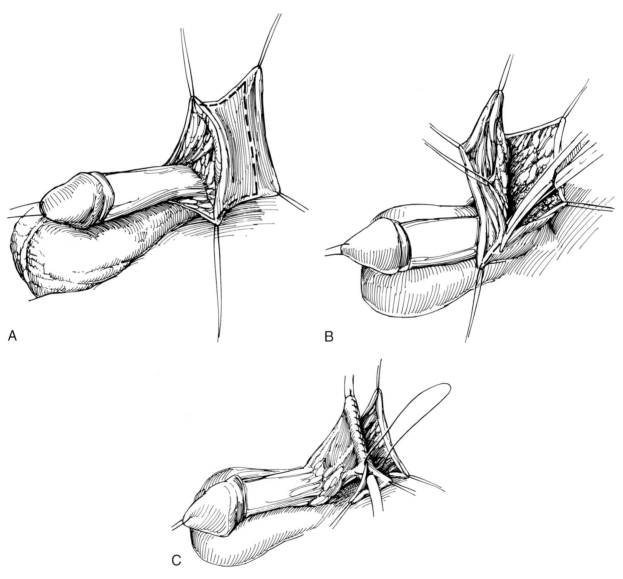

FIGURE 129-7. A, Place four fine traction sutures to fan out the ventral surface of the prepuce. Mark the skin for the neourethra to provide the needed length to bridge the gap and a width of 1.2 to 1.5 cm. Incise along the marks, just into the subcutaneous tissue. **B,** Develop a plane well down to the base of the penis between the flap and the outer prepuce to form a substantial pedicle. The vasculature of the pedicle usually is obvious, but take great care not to devascularize the flap. **C,** Roll the flap over an 8-F catheter, and approximate the edges with a running subcuticular 6-0 or 7-0 long-acting absorbable suture. Place interrupted sutures at the ends to allow trimming. Examine the ends of the flap for ischemia, and trim them appropriately. Test the caliber with a 12-F bougie à boule.

TUNICA VAGINALIS URETHROPLASTY COVERAGE

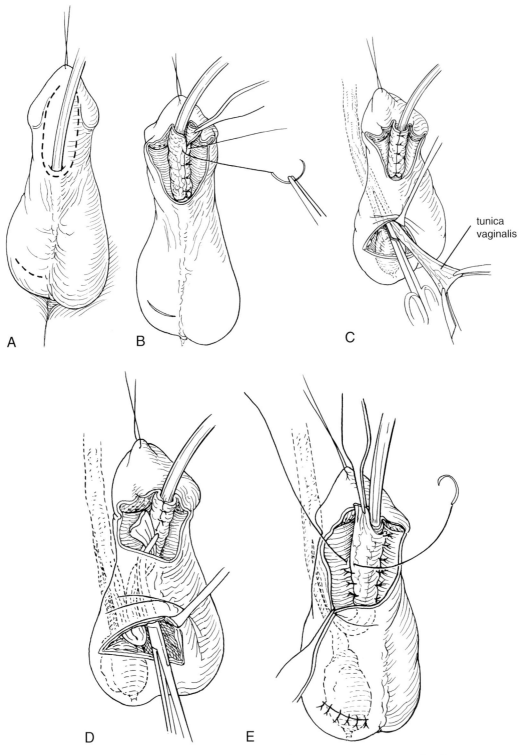

FIGURE 129-8. In complex or redo hypospadias repair, often using a two-stage approach, there may not be available subcutaneous tissue to cover the urethroplasty. Tunica vaginalis is an alternative option readily available to prevent fistula by covering the suture line. **A,** Outline the urethroplasty in a second-stage hypospadias repair. Mark a high scrotal incision. **B,** Complete the urethroplasty with interrupted sutures. Mobilize the glans wings for subsequent glansplasty. **C,** Mobilize the tunica vaginalis from either the right or left testicle. If necessary, tack the testicle in a dependent position within the scrotum. **D,** Use a clamp to pass the tunica from its position next to the testicle to the penile shaft. **E,** Use fine absorbable sutures to attach the tunica vaginalis to either side of the urethroplasty, covering the midline suture line. Close the scrotal skin with interrupted dissolvable sutures.

MONEER HANNA

Commentary by

The pedicle of the island flap, be it tube or onlay, should be mobilized sufficiently so that it does not twist the penis and create a rotational deformity. The end of the island should reach up to the glans penis without any tension. Excess tissue should be trimmed, as there is hardly any advantage to packing extra subcutaneous tissue, or in preserving excess skin for future use. This excess skin rarely proves to be useful should a revision be required at a later date, and only serves to produce a baggy, bulky, unsightly appearance.

If a tubed preputial island flap is contemplated (currently an uncommon procedure), the circumferential anastomosis has in our experience an innate tendency to stricture. Stenosis of the proximal anastomosis to the native urethra can be minimized by spatulating the anastomosis.

The dartos or tunica vaginalis flap provides excellent support and is routinely used to waterproof the suture line. This has resulted in a significant decrease in the urethral fistula rate in my hypospadias repairs. The tunica vaginalis is particularly useful in adolescent salvage urethroplasties, where the quality of the tissue is suboptimal.

DOUG CANNING

Commentary by

Vascularized pedicle flaps provide a versatile tool for the reconstructive pediatric urologist. We use these flaps as urethral patches in cases of fistula or stricture or to replace entire sections of a damaged urethra in cases of redo hypospadias repair. We also use them to provide skin coverage when the ventral penile shaft skin is short or to provide a dartos layer following a tubularized incised repair. We feel free to split the flap or cut it transversely to provide a combination of urethra and dartos layer or urethra and skin coverage. Moreover, we have rotated the tubularized flap in any direction to provide length or width. Because the blood supply is nearly constant, we cut the flap into nearly any shape required to provide good cosmesis or the appropriate length or width when reconstructing the urethra.

The important step when harvesting a vascular preputial island flap is to split the ventral penile shaft skin of the penis to the penoscrotal junction including the underlying dartos tissue to provide the ability to flatten the shaft skin completely. After incising the ventral skin, the traction sutures outlining the proposed flap improve the exposure of the plane between the inner proximal penile shaft skin and the vascular pedicle. With this exposure, the dissection begins just distal to the penopubic junction and proceeds distally to the inner prepuce. The improved view of the dorsal blood supply of the flap provides access to a more consistent plane while separating the vascular pedicle from the dorsal penile shaft skin. We have even harvested distal penile shaft skin after previous hypospadias repair and, in some cases, even after a previous dorsal preputial flap has been harvested.

Because we routinely buttonhole the pedicle rather than rotate it to one side or the other, the blood supply to the flap does not need to be mobilized as far proximally; therefore, the risk of flap injury is lessened. We have not found that a horseshoe-shaped flap is required in most cases since the pedicle flap itself can be taken on a bias (in a diagonal) to provide an additional centimeter or two of length over what would have been achieved if the flap was rolled as a rectangle rather than a diamond. We then rotate the diamond-shaped edges into the spatulated proximal urethra on the proximal shaft and into the distal urethral meatus on the glans.

When we use the tunica vaginalis for coverage of a reconstructed urethra, we frequently take two flaps, one from each hemiscrotum to provide a double layer of tissue. This reduces the risk of creating torsion from the tension of the left or the right tunica vaginalis flap on the distal urethra.

When reconstructing the urethra, whether during an onlay island flap, an onlay, or a forelay tube preputial vascular flap, I used interrupted subcuticular sutures rather than a running suture, as I believe this reduces the risk of rotation of the flap or shortening of the flap.

Chapter 130

Bladder Epithelial Grafts

The bladder can provide large grafts, which are certainly conditioned to cope with urine, but for harvesting they do need a second incision and require opening and closing the bladder. Their major disadvantage is that the meatus of the new urethra is of poor quality and tends to prolapse. This limitation can be overcome by patching a free skin graft on the distal end.

Contraindications to harvesting a bladder graft are a thickened noncompliant bladder secondary to neurogenic lesions, recurrent urinary tract infections, previous vesicostomy, or bladder exstrophy. Check the urine preoperatively to be sure that it is sterile. (In peripubertal boys, prophylactically give a broad-spectrum antibiotic.) Carry the correction of the hypospadias as far as possible before obtaining the graft.

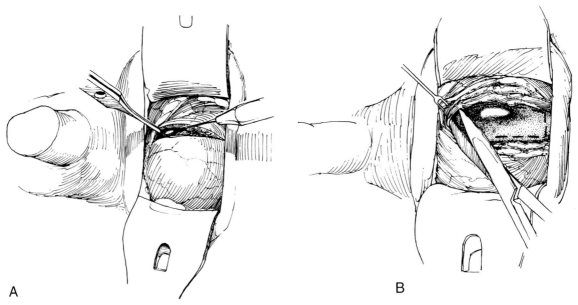

A

B

FIGURE 130-1. A, Insert a urethral catheter and fill the bladder with saline solution. Make a transverse lower abdominal (see Chapter 63) incision through the skin and superficial fascia and retract the rectus muscles with a self-retaining retractor. Expose the surface of the bladder.

B, Mark the proposed graft on the mucosa with a skin-marking pen before the bladder is opened. Carefully incise the muscle of the exposed surface of the bladder, keeping in the lamina propria, and peel the muscle from it until the thin underlying urothelium bulges out like a blue-domed cyst. Use scissors and a peanut dissector to expose an area adequate for the graft. Make the outline for the graft wide to allow for loss during suturing. Place traction sutures at the four corners. Incise the mucosa along the marks and excise it with fine scissors or scalpel. Stay in the plane of the lamina propria. Peel the muscle from the detrusor muscle with fine scissors; peanut dissectors help in exposing an area big enough for the graft. Make the bladder graft 10% longer and 20% wider than the required French size (the circumference in mm) you need for the neourethra. Realize that in contrast to skin grafts, urothelium will not shrink appreciably with placement.

For the terminal patch that will form the meatus, obtain a 1- × 2-cm full-thickness skin graft from the prepuce and clear it of subcutaneous tissue. Suture it to the end of the bladder graft to form one long graft, and then trim the skin portion to the proper overall length. Roll the combined graft around a silicone tube of appropriate size (usually 12 to 14F) and close it as a tube with an inverted running locked 7-0 synthetic absorbable suture. Switch to interrupted sutures when closing the distal skin-graft end so that it may be trimmed subsequently to the proper length at the meatus. Have the scrub nurse keep the tube moist during placement.

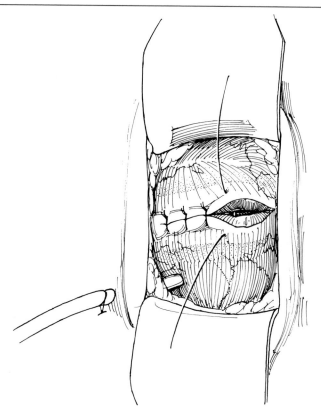

FIGURE 130-2. Your assistant can be closing the bladder with a running plain catgut suture without attempting mucosal approximation, as you apply the graft. Insert a Malecot catheter into the bladder. Cut the connector end of the tubing obliquely and draw it out through a stab wound in the body wall with a clamp. Alternatively, insert a silicone suprapubic tube, to be irrigated daily to assure patency. Stent the graft with a multifenestrated silicone stent that extends past the anastomosis but distal to the external sphincter. Suture it to the glans.

Complications include proximal and distal strictures from contraction of part or all of the graft and diverticula, especially with bladder grafts. Fistulas are uncommon, but protruding bladder epithelium may be a problem, which can be prevented by stretching and then trimming the graft at the meatus, before suturing.

QIANG FU

Commentary by

It is a challenge to reconstruct severe urethral defects in hypospadias. Bladder epithelial grafts are an excellent substitute material for this application. According to the classic method, it is necessary to incise a large piece of bladder mucosa to create a substitution tube urethra. We now prefer composite bladder mucosa that is onlayed to the preserved urethral plate.

Two parallel incisions (0.8 to 1 cm apart) are made, starting at the corona and extending just proximal to the hypospadiac meatus. The urethral plate is not dissected from the corpora cavernosa. An 8- to 12-F perforated silicone rubber tube is then advanced into the urethra 1 cm proximal to the hypospadiac meatus. Distally, the catheter is secured to the glans penis with 3-0 nonabsorbable suture. The bladder mucosal graft is then anastomosed to the urethral plate with a running suture of absorbable 6-0 material. Following this, a two-layer closure is achieved avoiding superimposed suture lines. The new meatus is located at the corona. Although the placement of the distal meatus at the corona is not perfect it does have two advantages: (1) the meatus of the neourethra is large and therefore urethral strictures are rare, especially for cases of failed hypospadias, and (2) this avoids the initial high rate of meatal prolapse with bladder mucosa grafts previously reported.

Bladder mucosa grafts have been especially useful in complex redo or severe hypospadias. After correction of chordee, skin is transferred from the dorsum to the ventrum. In the second stage the transferred skin is used as a urethral plate template to accept the bladder mucosa onlay free flap.

We prefer not to insert the urethral stent into the bladder, thereby avoiding bladder spasm that can cause urine leakage into the repair as well as secretions. This can lead to local infection resulting in a fistula.

To avoid superimposed suture lines we recommend Z closure for the skin.

Chapter 131

Buccal Mucosal Graft

Epithelium from the oral cavity has advantages over a free graft of either skin or bladder epithelium. It is thicker and easier to tailor and it is more easily immobilized. It also has much less propensity to shrink, especially compared to skin, and its thickness militates against its ballooning into a diverticulum after placement. It also tolerates exposure to urine better than skin. It may be obtained with no visible scar and with little postoperative distress. An additional advantage is that it has a thinner lamina propria, which encourages imbibition or diffusion of nutrients as well as inosculation or entry of new vessels.

Before harvesting the graft, be sure you have a well-vascularized site prepared to receive it.

The graft may be obtained either from the inner cheek or from the inner surface of the upper or lower lip. The cheek is preferred not only because it allows harvesting a larger graft, but also because it can be closed primarily and therefore causes less discomfort. Moreover, closure of too large a defect in the lip may distort the vermilion border. The mouth cannot be sterilized, so the graft will hold bacteria, but this is not clinically important.

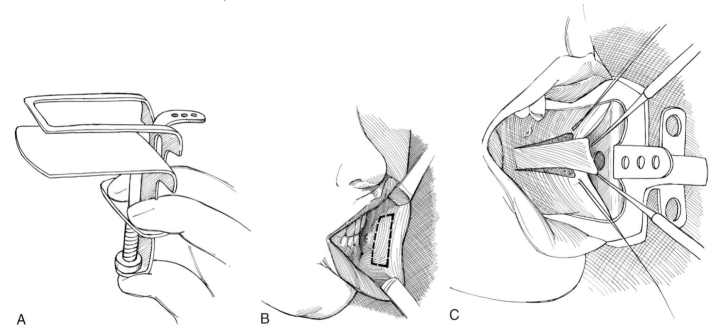

FIGURE 131-1. **A,** Have the anesthesiologist intubate the child with an endotracheal tube. A nasotracheal tube is not necessary because the endotracheal tube can be placed on the opposite side of the mouth where it will be out of the way. Insert a dental retractor such as a Steinhauser mucosal retractor. In smaller children an assistant can expose with Army-Navy retractors. **B,** Identify and avoid the opening of the parotid (Stensen's) duct, which lies below the second and third molars, inferior to the vestibular fold. Inject a solution of 1:100,000 epinephrine in 1% lidocaine beneath the mucosa to facilitate dissection and reduce bleeding. Sponge the surface dry, and then measure and mark a rectangular block for the graft with a marking pen. In contrast to a bladder mucosal graft, a buccal graft can be harvested almost on a one-to-one ratio with the defect to be filled, but make it 10% larger than the defect in anticipation of loss with suturing.
C, Cheek: Here a wider graft than the lip may be marked, extending from near the orifice of the parotid duct to the inferior vestibular fold. Such a graft probably needs not to be much larger than the defect, and seldom longer than 5 to 6 cm because two strips may be sutured together end to end for a longer graft or side to side to make a wider one. If more tissue is needed in order to form a tube, obtain grafts simultaneously from both cheeks, or even from both lips.

Measure and mark the proposed graft(s) on the cheek. Place four fine sutures at the marked corners of the graft to help elevate the edges during the dissection and avoid traumatizing the epithelium with forceps. Inject 0.5% xylocaine diluted with 1:200,000 epinephrine under the graft to make harvesting easier and to provide hemostasis. Incise the

FIGURE 131-1, cont'd. margins with a #15 blade. Using blunt hooks for manipulation, dissect with knife and scissors just beneath the (thick) epithelium to avoid obtaining too thick a graft. Stay superficial to the buccinator muscle to avoid the buccal neurovascular bundle that lies in that muscle and the facial nerve that runs beneath it. This layer should not be entered. Caution: Watch out for the parotid (Stensen's) duct by leaving the graft attached at both ends and then cutting it free when the dissection is complete. Obtain immediate hemostasis with pinpoint electrocautery and local pressure. Bleeding postoperatively may be controlled by internal pressure and external ice packs. Close the wound with a running, locking 4-0 chromic catgut suture. If needed, grafts may be obtained simultaneously from both lips or both cheeks.

Dip the graft in half-strength organic iodide solution and pin it with the inside up on a board with 25-gauge needles. For the cheek graft, trim all remaining fat (and muscle) with iris scissors to foster quick imbibition. Be sure to keep the graft moist with the warm solution. The lip graft is thicker and consequently stiffer. If it is too thick, try to remove some of the excess submucosal tissue with curved scissors or a knife, although this may be difficult. Buccal grafts do not leave a sticky protruding meatus, so a meatal skin patch is not needed.

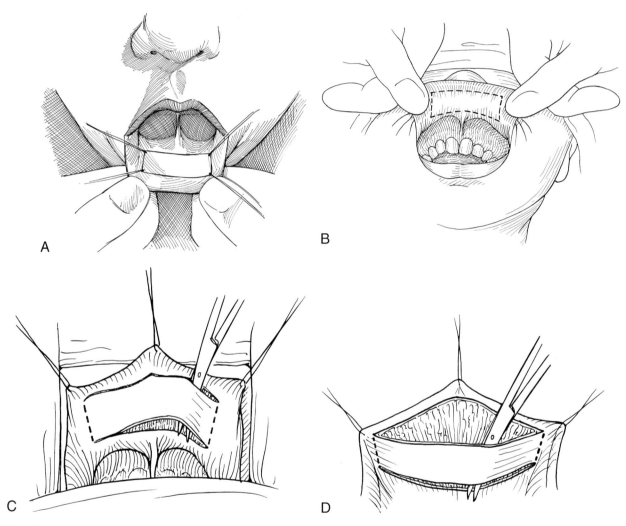

FIGURE 131-2. A, Upper or lower lip: Mark a graft up to 4 cm long and 1.3 cm wide. (Caution: If a graft is to be obtained from the lip, excision of too wide a graft can cause inversion of the vermilion border. Instead, cut two narrower grafts and suture them side by side.) **B,** In this case the upper lip graft site is marked. **C,** Inject 0.5% xylocaine diluted with 1:200,000 epinephrine under the graft to make harvesting easier and to provide hemostasis. Incise the margins with a #15 blade or ophthalmologic knife. Use an iris scissors to dissect the epidermis and lamina propria of the lip buccal graft. **D,** Keep the edges of the graft intact until the dissection is complete, which will aid in staying in the correct plane. For the defect in the lip, merely apply an antibiotic ointment twice a day until healing is complete. Infection is a rare complication.

COMPLICATIONS

The buccal neurovascular bundle can be injured by dissecting into the buccinator muscle, but damage to the facial nerve is highly unlikely because it lies deep to the buccinator. Lip contractor is rare and only occurs if the graft site is too large.

Chapter 132

Preputial Skin Graft

Free preputial skin flaps can be used as urethral replacement alone or in combinaton with bladder or buccal mucosa grafts. To harvest the graft unfold the dorsal prepuce and place four stay sutures in the inner prepuce at least 1.4 cm apart and at a distance that is 10% longer than the length needed to replace the urethra, since 75% circumferential shrinkage of the graft is expected.

COMPLICATIONS

Graft shrinkage with skin is inevitable and needs to be accounted for in graft design. Likewise, too large a graft will result in a bladder diverticulum.

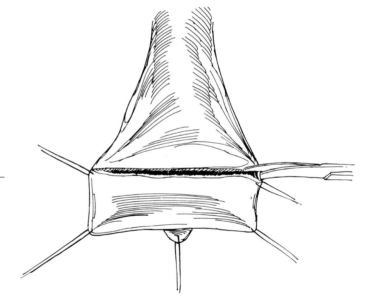

FIGURE 132-1. Cut the graft and defat it over the finger or on a plastic board using 25-gauge needles to provide tension.

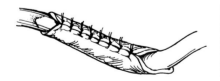

FIGURE 132-2. Attach the full-thickness, fat-free graft, skin surface inside, to a suitable-size catheter at a site that will allow the end of the catheter to lie in the bladder. Use interrupted 6-0 or 7-0 synthetic absorbable sutures. Cut both ends of the graft obliquely to prevent stenosis at the anastomotic site.

Chapter 133

Penile Curvature

RELEASE OF DARTOS AND BUCK'S FASCIAS (DEVINE)

Create an artificial erection to determine the degree of curvature. Place a broad rubber band or small red rubber catheter around the base of the penis and secure it with a hemostat. Introduce a 25-gauge butterfly needle through the glans into a corpus cavernosum or directly into the corpus cavernosum. Gently distend the penis with injectable normal saline solution; avoid overdistention. Maintain the erection during evaluation of the chordee. After the chordee has been corrected, create a second erection to check penile alignment.

Make an incision around the shaft at the site of the circumcision scar, and dissect the shaft skin back to the base of the penis.

Elevate the dysgenetic dartos and Buck's fascias that are concentrated on either side of the corpus spongiosum. In rare cases, the corpus spongiosum and urethra may have to be mobilized to resect all the fibrous tissue. Repeat the erection. If ventral curvature remains, proceed to midline dorsal plication (Baskin).

DORSAL MIDLINE PLICATION (BASKIN)

This technique should be used for mild to moderate curvature, without decreasing penile length.

Dissect the skin and subcutaneous tissue aggressively from the ventrum of the corpora proximally about the penoscrotal junction to release any tethering tissue responsible for the curvature. Check by artificial erection to see if the penis is now straight, or to locate the site of persistent curvature requiring correction.

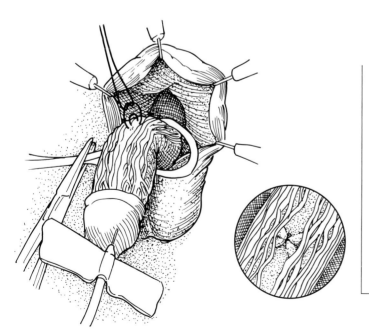

FIGURE 133-1. Place two 5-0 polypropylene sutures at the observed point of maximal curvature. Insert them side by side in the midline through Buck's fascia and then 1 to 2 mm into the corporeal tissue as inverted sutures so that the knot is buried *(inset)*. Do not mobilize or incise Buck's fascia.

Repeat the erection for confirmation. If curvature persists, as is often found in the moderate and severe cases, place another row of plication sutures. If more than two rows are necessary, select an alternative approach, such as applying a ventral graft of dermis or a patch of synthetic material. In postpubertal patients, placing 2-0 TiCron sutures in the midline at the point of maximal curvature can successfully correct the curvature. For additional coverage, loosely approximate Buck's fascia over the repair.

LAURENCE BASKIN

Commentary by

Histologic analysis of human fetal specimens has led to modifications in surgical techniques in hypospadias surgery. The basic surgical principle that the nerves should not be disturbed has allowed for translation of anatomic studies to clinical practice.

The documentation that the neuroinnervation is absent at the 12-o'clock position on the dorsal aspect of the penis and the tunica albuginea thickest at this point has led to the correction of penile curvature by dorsal midline plication. The technique is minimal and does not burn any bridges.

Another 10 years will be necessary to document that dorsal midline plication will withstand penile growth from androgen stimulation at puberty. Presently, there are no signs of recurrent curvature in the first patients that had the procedure.

At first the technique was applied a bit liberally. Presently, I employ the finger test to determine if the curved penis is amenable to dorsal midline plication. After complete takedown of the subcutaneous tissue to the penoscrotal junction, if the curvature does not correct under artificial erection with gentle pressure using your thumb and index finger, then resection of the urethral plate and ventral grafting are recommended. I would also advocate placing one row of two sutures with a maximum of three sutures in the rare circumstance. As illustrated in Figure 133-1, care should be taken to bury the knot and cover the permanent suture with subcutaneous suture.

Chapter 134

Dorsal Tunica Albuginea Plication (TAP Procedure) and Elliptical Excision Technique

DORSAL TUNICA ALBUGINEA PLICATION (TAP PROCEDURE) (DUCKETT)

For boys with an abnormal urethral plate and associated corpus spongiosum, or a short urethra, divide the urethral plate and resect down to the corporeal body. The preferred technique is dorsal midline plication (see Chapter 133); however, dorsal tunica albuginea plication remains a viable option. If the curvature is severe, proceed to dermal graft (see Chapter 135).

Insert a 5-0 Prolene traction suture vertically in the glans. Inject a solution of 1:100,000 epinephrine in 1% lidocaine along the proposed lines of incision to minimize bleeding. Make a circumferential incision 5 mm proximal to the corona to allow the penile shaft skin to drop back. Preserve the urethral plate. Dissect in a plane superficial to Buck's fascia to keep the vascular pedicle intact to the hooded prepuce.

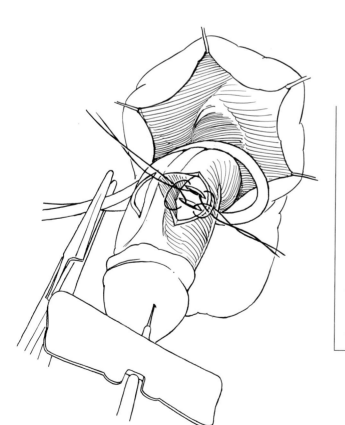

FIGURE 134-1. Perform artificial erection. Assess the quality of the urethral plate. It is usually adequate, so it may not require division. If penile curvature (due to corporeal disproportion) is significant after taking down the skin and dartos fascia, plication is necessary. If the urethral plate and associated spongiosum are abnormal or if the urethra is short, divide the plate and resect back to healthy spongiosum. Under artificial erection, determine the point of maximum bend. Elevate Buck's fascia at 10 and 2 o'clock on either side of the midline to avoid damage to the neurovascular bundle. Make parallel incisions through the tunica albuginea 4 to 6 mm apart and about 8 mm in length. Approximate the outer edges with inverted permanent sutures (5-0 polypropylene in infants). Repeat the erection to confirm that the penis is straight. Proceed with construction of the urethra.

DORSAL ELLIPTICAL EXCISION
TECHNIQUE FOR CHORDEE
(NESBIT)

With the penis erect, measure the length on the ventrum and dorsum with a tape. The difference in length determines the number and width of the ellipses to be removed. Most often, excision of only one ellipse on each side is required. For lateral curvature, site the incisions appropriately.

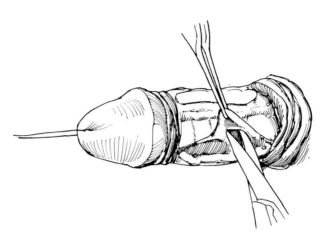

FIGURE 134-2. Make a circumcising incision 5 to 8 mm from the coronal sulcus. (If the prepuce is present, excise it to prevent postoperative edema.) Apply a tourniquet, produce artificial erection, and note the site and degree of curvature. Incise Colles' fascia longitudinally. Mobilize the dorsal neurovascular structures from each side dorsomedially along with Buck's fascia. The bundle may be elevated with a vessel loop.

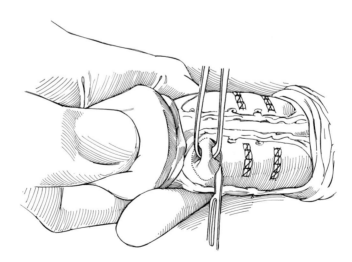

FIGURE 134-3. Grasp the tunica albuginea with Allis clamps to determine the amount of straightening needed. Excise the elevated ellipses in the clamps. Alternatively, mark 1-cm ellipses in the tunica propria on each side with a marking pen. Incise and remove the ellipses. If possible, keep the depth of the excision superficial to the endothelial layer. With corporeal disproportion, the tissue removed may be used as a graft for the opposite corpus cavernosum. After each ellipse is removed, approximate the edges of the defect with two or three interrupted 5-0 polydioxanone sutures, inverted to bury the knots. These sutures may be followed by a running suture of the same material to assure a smooth surface. Test for straightness by artificial erection. Excise additional ellipses if necessary. Be sure the erection is symmetric. Apply penile block and dress the penis. The palpable ridges from the sutures will subside but the permanent sutures may be felt.

ROSS DECTOR

Commentary by

Chordee correction can be accomplished by a variety of techniques. Chordee in the majority of boys with hypospadias and corporeal disproportion is quite nicely corrected by techniques that effectively shorten the dorsal aspect of the corpora cavernosa. The principle of each of these techniques is similar; the differences lie in the approach to the tunica albuginea of the corpora cavernosa.

In Duckett's tunica albuginea plication (TAP procedure) a longitudinal incision is made in the Buck's fascia dorsolaterally. This avoids the neurovascular bundles and allows access to the tunica albuginea. After the adjacent Buck's fascia is elevated, two parallel incisions at right angles to the long axis of the penis are made in the tunica albuginea in each corpus cavernosum. The lateral aspect of each incision is sutured to its mate with buried absorbable sutures. This effectively shortens the dorsal length of the corpora cavernosa. In most cases of hypospadias a single plication in each corpus cavernosum is all that is required.

I usually employ a slightly different approach to the dorsolateral aspect of the corpora cavernosa in boys with hypospadias. As Buck's fascia adjacent to corpus spongiosum has already been cleanly dissected off of the ventral corpora cavernosa earlier in the procedure, I start my dissection at that point. Establishing a plane between Buck's fascia—with its encased neurovascular bundles and the underlying tunica albuginea of the corpora cavernosa—is straightforward at this location. This dissection proceeds from ventrolateral around to the dorsal aspect of each corpus cavernosum. The entire neurovascular complex within Buck's fascia can then be elevated with vessel loops, and precise incisions into the tunica albuginea can be made to perform either a TAP procedure or a Nesbit plication.

When doing a formal Nesbit procedure, I inscribe mirror-image, elliptically shaped areas on the tunica albuginea on the dorsolateral aspect of each corpus cavernosum with a marking pen. The tunica albuginea is then opened using a microsurgical knife down to, but not through, the level of the tunica vasculosa. The tunica albuginea is excised without injury to the underlying erectile tissue and the defect is closed with absorbable interrupted sutures to create a linear incision oriented at right angles to the long axis of the penis. I tend to perform a Nesbit procedure with tunical excision in adolescents.

I frequently use a simple modified Nesbit procedure to correct chordee in infants and children. After the above exposure to the dorsal tunica albuginea, I make incisions parallel to the long axis of the penis into the tunica albuginea on either side of the midline. When a single absorbable suture entering and exiting at each end of these longitudinally oriented incisions is tied, the incision is closed in a Heineke-Mikulicz fashion, effectively shortening the dorsal corpora cavernosa. This technique can be nicely employed with short incisions into the tunica albuginea. I will preferentially make two incisions as opposed to one longer one when faced with more significant chordee.

Chapter 135

Dermal Graft

Dermal graft for penile straightening is indicated if the penis is not amenable to the dorsal midline plication technique. Practically, this is a minority of patients with hypospadias. After extensive dissection along Buck's fascia to the penile scrotal junction and attempts at dorsal plication are unsuccessful, the next maneuver in the correction of severe penile curvature is resection of the urethral plate and aggressive removal of all ventral tethering tissue.

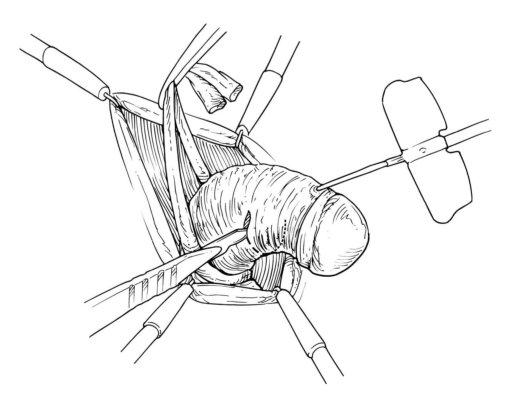

FIGURE 135-1. If artificial erection continues to show significant curvature, incise the corpora cavernosa on the ventrum at the point of maximum curvature in a semicircle. The tourniquet from the artificial erection accommodates hemostasis.

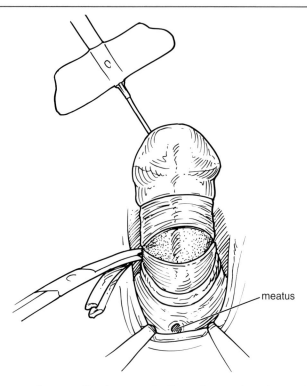

FIGURE 135-2. This incision exposes the erectile tissue and allows the penis to be straightened, lengthening the ventral aspect.

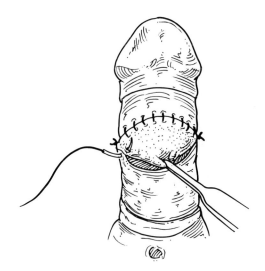

FIGURE 135-3. Trim the dermal graft, which has been previously harvested, to the size of the ventral defect. Use 6-0 absorbable sutures in running fashion to secure dermal graft to the ventral aspect of the penis. Subsequently, use a two-stage procedure to cover the ventral aspect of the penis in preparation for a second-stage urethroplasty.

DERMAL GRAFT HARVEST

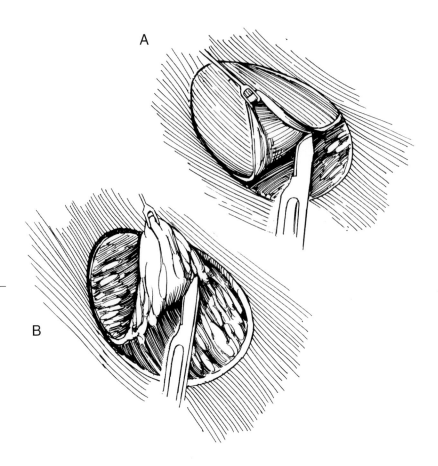

FIGURE 135-4. Mark an ellipse of skin within the inguinal crease over the iliac crest beyond the future hairline. **A,** Remove the epidermis freehand and discard it. **B,** Excise an ellipse of dermis. Close the donor site in two layers.

RONALD SUTHERLAND

Commentary by

In 1974, Devine and Horton described using dermis to correct the defect left after excision of Peyronie's plaque. Since then, dermis has become a popular and successful method to correct severe penile curvature from a variety of causes. Proximal hypospadias with severe ventral curvature in a patient with a small penis may be best corrected with a ventral dermal graft inlay rather than a dorsal plication procedure to avoid further shortening of the penis.

Perform the Gittes artificial erection test after degloving the penis and dissecting away the thickened, fibrous tissue attached to the urethra around the penoscrotal junction. This maneuver will often relieve a significant amount of the proximal ventral curvature. After the Gittes test, decide whether to perform a dorsal plication or a ventral dermal graft inlay, but avoid doing both. The dermal graft inlay alone is usually adequate to correct the most severe cases of curvature.

Obtain the dermal graft first before incising the penis to cut down on tourniquet time. A good location to retrieve the dermal graft is in the thigh fold over the adductor magnus tendon. Using a marking pen, tattoo a diamond-shaped area in the thigh fold with a 2:1 width-height ratio. Initially excise the inked epidermis off the dermis with a #15 blade being careful not to excise any dermis. Using needle-tip electrocautery on cutting current, remove the quadrangular patch of dermis. Drape the dermal graft on your forefinger to excise the subcutaneous fat, being careful to not buttonhole the graft. If there is any defect in the graft, close with a 6-0 monofilament suture to prevent bleeding once the tourniquet is released. Close the thigh wound in layers to allow the defect to heal with a minimum scar.

A 180-degree transverse incision in the corporeal bodies at the point of maximum curvature will normally spring open the penis sufficient to correct the curvature. Avoid incision into the spongiosum. In the ventral midline, the tunical edges will need to be released from the vertical tunical septum (I-beam) both proximally and distally to maximally straighten the penis.

Lay the graft onto the corporeal defect and trim it to size. Attach the graft with four anchoring 6-0 monofilament absorbable sutures and then a running suture of the same to close the remainder. Repeat the artificial erection and secure any leaks. If there is still curvature a second dermal graft can be inserted; however, this is rarely necessary except in cases where the penis is very short. If there is residual curvature it is usually along the distal shaft and can be easily corrected with a single dorsal plication. Byars' flaps are useful to cover the graft and penile shaft in preparation for a second-stage urethroplasty.

One obvious drawback from this procedure is that it precludes a one-stage hypospadias repair in most cases. It is inadvisable to place a reconstructed urethral graft or flap over the dermal graft.

Chapter 136

Glansplasty

Glansplasty is critical to the functional and cosmetic outcome of hypospadias surgery. Just as there are many different operations to correct hypospadias, a number of different approaches to recreating the glans are available.

ADVANCEMENT TECHNIQUE

This advancement technique is indicated as part of the meatoplasty and glanuloplasty (MAGPI) repair in which the urethra is mobile and glans supple.

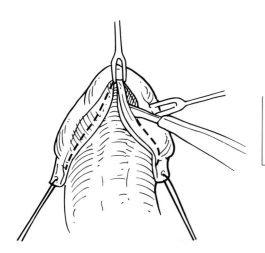

FIGURE 136-1. Lift the proximal edge of the meatus with a skin hook or traction suture, pulling it toward the tip of the glans to form an inverted V as the glans wings are pulled together. Excise the excess skin on the medial margins of these wings to expose glans tissue in preparation for a glansplasty.

FIGURE 136-2. Approximate the deep glans tissue with one or two 6-0 synthetic absorbable sutures. To close the glans, insert buried subcutaneous sutures to ensure a firm approximation and to avoid tension that would lead to a retrusive meatus. Suture the two edges thus formed together in the midline with vertical 6-0 synthetic absorbable mattress sutures. The glans closure is best done over a catheter to ensure that stenosis is not created.

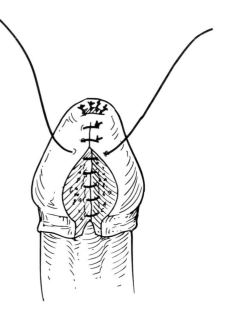

GLANS WINGS

Glans wings are indicated for the onlay and tubularization techniques. The glans has a flattened appearance.

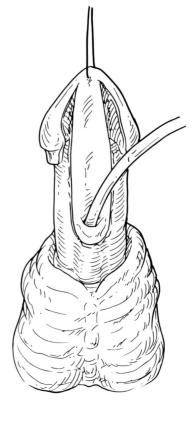

FIGURE 136-3. Begin the glansplasty by marking two parallel incisions along the urethral plate. Using the fresh scalpel or fine knife develop glans wings on each side to the urethral plate. Stay in the plane between the corporeal body and glans stroma.

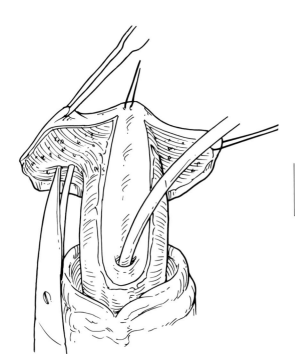

FIGURE 136-4. Mobilize the glans wings to 90 degrees in respect to the urethral plate. Do not devascularize either the glans wings or urethral plate.

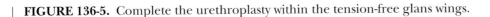

FIGURE 136-5. Complete the urethroplasty within the tension-free glans wings.

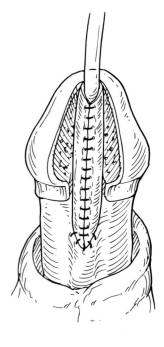

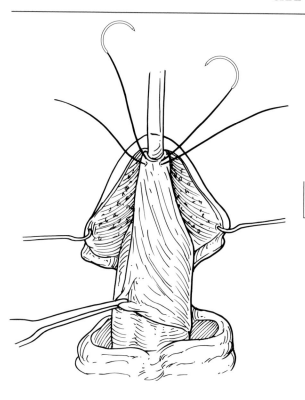

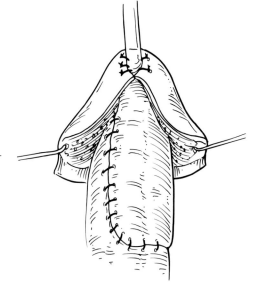

FIGURE 136-6. Cover the urethroplasty with a de-epithelialized island flap.

FIGURE 136-7. Mature the meatus 2 to 3 cm with interrupted 7-0 or 6-0 absorbable sutures on each side.

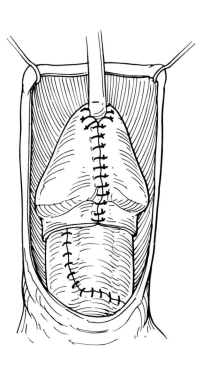

FIGURE 136-8. Close the glans in one or two interrupted layers with long-acting absorbable suture. Carefully line up the coronal margin.

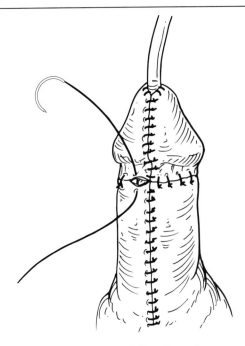

FIGURE 136-9. Complete the repair by approximating the Firlit skin collar.

TUNNEL TECHNIQUE

The tunnel technique is indicated for complete tube grafts.
The glans has a conical or normal appearance.

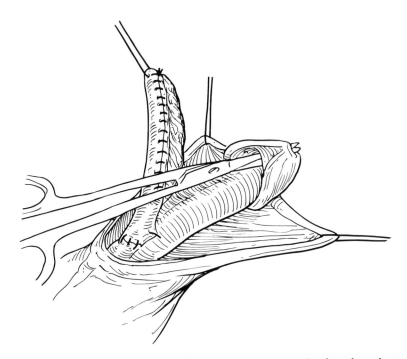

FIGURE 136-10. Insert fine plastic scissors flat against the corpora cavernosa in the plane between the cap of the glans and the corpora and snip a path to the tip of the glans. Remove a large plug of glans, 0.2 × 1.5 cm, and reach inside the meatus to excise excess glanular tissue. Provide a wide channel, at least 16 F in caliber. Make a V-shaped incision at the tip. Check the caliber with a metal sound.

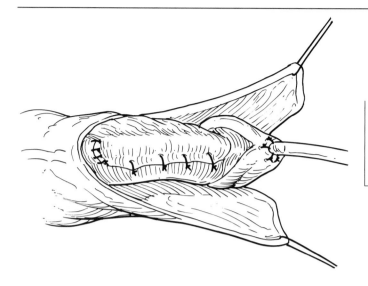

FIGURE 136-11. Pull the tubed flap through the channel keeping the suture line against the corporeal bodies. Pull it out straight to eliminate redundant tissue and trim the excess length. Suture the tubed flap to the new meatus with interrupted 7-0 chromic catgut sutures.

BALANIC GROOVE

The balanic groove allows recession of the urethra within the glans. It is indicated when glans configuration will not allow adequate mobilization to support a classic glans wing repair.

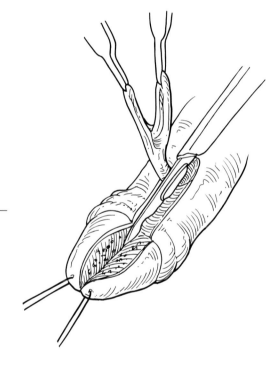

FIGURE 136-12. Sharply incise the glans ventrally from the meatus to the glans tip to form a deep groove for the new urethra. Leave the spongy tissue in place. Insert a feeding tube or catheter, typically 8 F, in preparation for the urethroplasty.

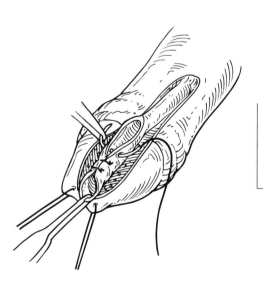

FIGURE 136-13. Suture the dorsal lip of the neourethra to the dorsal rim of the incision in the glans. Suture the edges of the proximal flap to the edges of the glanular flap on both sides with a running 7-0 polyglactin suture to form the neourethra. A second layer of de-epithelialized dartos fascia can be used to cover the urethroplasty to prevent fistula formation (not shown).

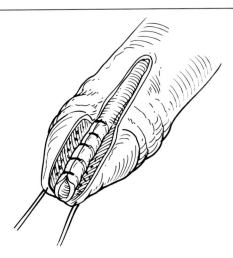

FIGURE 136-14. Fasten the two halves of the glans together over the neourethra with subepithelial mattress sutures of 6-0 polyglactin. Close the glans epithelium with interrupted vertical mattress sutures. Suture the ventral lip of the new meatus to the glans with 7-0 polyglactin and complete the formation of the meatus by joining the flap to the apex of the glans with the same suture material.

FIGURE 136-15. Bring the subcutaneous tissue together in the midline with an interrupted suture to provide a second layer. Trim and fit the remainder of the skin; use only the preputial skin that is needed for coverage and excise the rest.

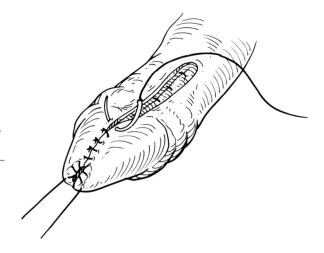

JOHN REDMAN

Commentary by

The balanic groove technique for glansplasty, as originally described by Professor Barcat, is an elegant technique, which results in a normal-appearing glans with an elliptical meatus at the tip of the penis. To properly perform the technique, there must be strict attention to detail and a meticulous dissection.

I use ×3.5 loupe magnification. With the balanic groove technique, glans wings, per se, are not elevated; only a deep midline groove is made. The initial maneuver is to outline the glabrous epithelium of the urethral plate with a skin marker. A rubber band tourniquet is employed to ensure a completely bloodless field. I use a 2- × 10-mm rubber band and leave the tourniquet in place until the glansplasty is completed, regardless of the time required for the repair. The glanular epithelium only is incised and the urethral plate is then carefully elevated proximal to the coronal margin. If the meatus is balanic or coronal, a catheter placed in the distal urethra aids in delineating the diaphanous urethra and obviates inadvertent entries into the lumen.

It will be noted that in most cases, the urethral plate does not extend to the tip of the glans. Therefore, it is important to make a 2- to 3-mm incision in the midline distal to the site of the elevated plate and then to excise the resultant triangles of epithelium. This maneuver will provide for the ultimate elliptical shape of the meatus and also simultaneously bring the meatus to the tip of the glans. The groove itself is made deeply in the midline, without any excision of spongy tissue. If necessary, to achieve a deeper groove because of a thin ventral glans, the septum between the corporeal bodies may be incised without entering either corporus. A key to properly creating the groove is the use of a miniature self-retaining retractor, the Agrikola retractor. Not only is the retractor an adjunct to the formation of the groove, it is most helpful in providing retraction during the completion of the glanular portion of the urethroplasty itself.

The glans closure begins with horizontal mattress sutures of 6-0 polyglactin (usually two sutures) placed just beneath the epithelium. At the level of the corona, I place a single suture to approximate the remaining spongy tissue of the glans and then continue it as a running suture proximally to approximate the contiguous divergent corpus spongiosum over the proximal portion of the urethroplasty (Y-to-I wrap). The maneuver provides a thick covering over the urethroplasty and obviates a dartos muscle interposition. The procedure is concluded by approximating the glanular epithelium and inner leaf of the prepuce with interrupted 7-0 polyglactin suture. Prior to closure of the glanular epithelium, it is helpful to excise any bulging epithelium along the margins of the approximated glans. This may be done by expressing the tissue between the blades of fine dissecting scissors and then cutting.

Chapter 137

Skin Coverage

MUCOSAL COLLAR (FIRLIT)

During a normal circumcision approximately 5 mm of skin is left below the coronal margin. In hypospadias surgery the goal is to obtain a final cosmetic appearance similar to a circumcised child. By bringing a collar of mucosa around the shaft, this result can be obtained.

BYARS' FLAP

The goal of skin coverage in hypospadias repair is to resurface the shaft with nonhair-bearing penile skin. The standard technique is to transfer a flap of dorsal skin (Byars' flap) to the ventrum and recreate a midline seam.

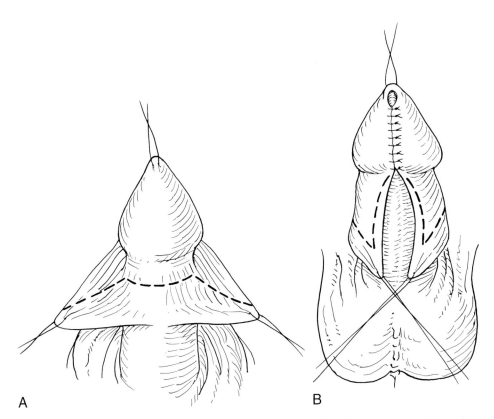

FIGURE 137-1. A, Make an incision 5 mm below the coronal margin on the dorsal aspect of the phallus in chevron fashion. **B,** Bring the incision line around the ventral aspect of the hypospadiac phallus, preserving a collar of prepuce. (In distal hypospadias the incision is brought directly across the coronal margin. In more severe hypospadias the urethral plate is preserved for the urethroplasty.)

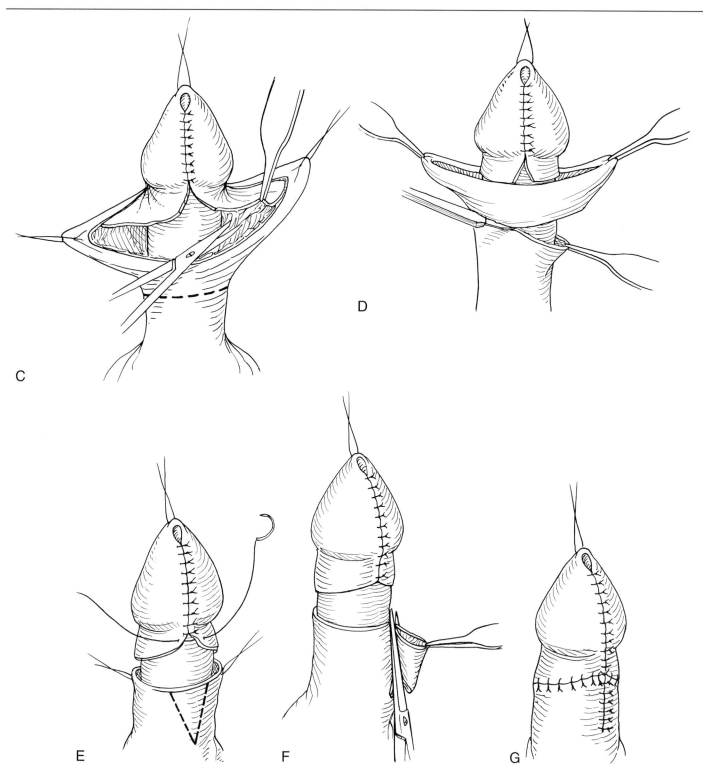

FIGURE 137-1, cont'd. C, Trim the collar after completing the urethroplasty and secondary coverage. **D,** Remove excess skin from the shaft of the penis. **E,** Since the diameter of the remaining penile skin is greater than the diameter of the mucosal collar, outline a small wedge of skin for removal. **F,** Trim the dog-ear of skin. **G,** The completed repair with the mucosal collar.

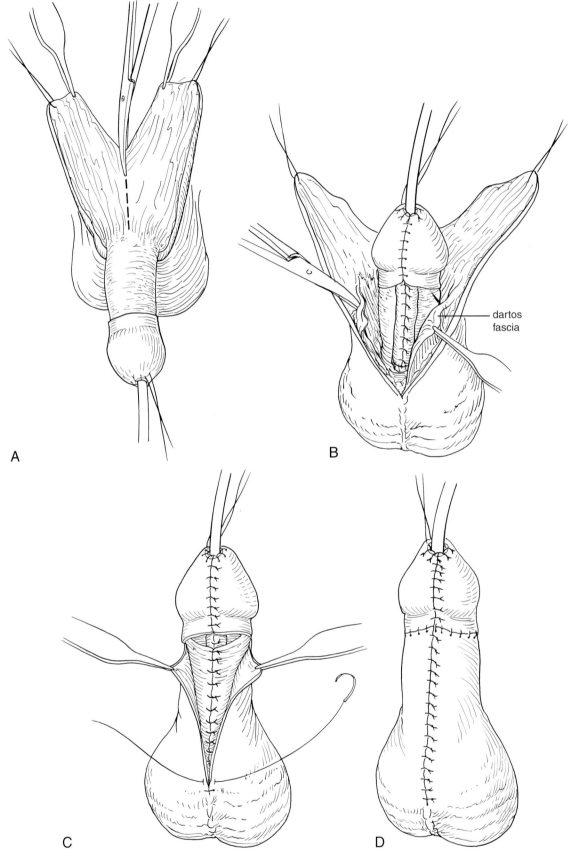

FIGURE 137-2. A, After the penis has been straightened and the urethroplasty completed, make a midline incision in the dorsal preputial flap. **B,** Transfer the Byars' flaps from the dorsal aspect of the penis to the ventral surface. Mobilize subcutaneous tissue for secondary coverage of the urethroplasty if not formally done as a de-epithelialized vascular flap (see Chapter 129). **C,** Cover the urethroplasty with subcutaneous tissue. Trim excess skin, mainly the inner prepuce, cobra eyes, and any devascularized skin. **D,** Completed repair with midline seam and mucosal collar.

MICHAEL KEATING

Commentary by

As the art and science of hypospadiology continue to evolve, genital reconstructions are aimed at achieving cosmetic normalcy. Skin reconfiguration is a crucial factor to this end that is sometimes (painfully so) nearly as challenging as completion of the urethroplasty itself. Urologic surgeons must be as dogged in their attention to detail with this aspect of the repair as with the urethral construction that precedes it.

Firlit's collar can and should be applied to nearly every hypospadias variant. The technique allows preservation of the ventral corona and results in a glanular appearance having a normal stepped-off transition with the adjoining shaft skin. When the maneuver is not employed, the ventral shaft skin must be, by default, anastomosed directly to glanular tissue. This results in a ventral glans having an abnormal appearance that blends in confluence with the shaft and lacks a corona.

One can preserve a fairly generous subcoronal collar (1 to 1.5 cm) to aid in ventral skin coverage. With most cases of hypospadias, the abnormal insertions of the hooded prepuce extend distally onto the glans adjacent to the urethral plate. The lines of skin incision follow these insertions, whose remnants are ultimately trimmed back to healthy glanular tissue, regardless of whether the plate is employed in the urethroplasty or not. Tissue mobility (as demonstrated with holding stitches that can reenact the collar technique) allows for the midline approximation of the collar and glans above most urethroplasties. It is surprising how often the mucosal collar can be employed, even with hypospadias variants whose preputial insertions initially seem too laterally displaced from the urethral plate to allow for a midline reapproximation of the glans and collar.

Byars' flaps, initiated with a dorsal midline incision to the level of the corona, allow for the ventrolateral transfer of penile shaft skin. In some cases, especially distal hypospadias variants, this allows for the ventral approximation of healthy shaft skin in the midline. Tension should be avoided; otherwise, a change in caliber between the shaft and distal collar results, giving a "lollipop" appearance. One of the drawbacks of perimeatal-based flap urethroplasties is the significant defects that result from their mobilization and that usually obviate midline closures. In other instances, a midline approximation cannot be completed because of inelastic ventral skin or when significant defects have resulted from the correction of chordee and excision of dysgenetic skin. When midline closure is not an option, the preputial wings are brought ventrally to cover the shaft. There they can be interdigitated as Z-plasties or the healthier of the two flaps can be unfurled and used to cover the skin defect.

Preputial configuration becomes a factor when choosing the best method for skin coverage when midline skin closure is not an option. Byars' flaps are ideal for variants whose prepuce has the more common "double knuckle" or "cobra eyes" appearance that can be separated in the midline to create two generous flaps. In contrast, the prepuce of some hypospadias presents with a single midline "knuckle" beyond which the prepuce is often foreshortened and somewhat deficient. We have found the buttonhole technique preferable for these cases. Here, a cruciate incision is made in the knuckle at the level of the corona and the penis is brought through the defect. After removing the darts that result from the incision, the edges of the buttonhole are matured to the corona. The prepuce is then unfurled proximally to cover the penile shaft with a U-shaped closure. With proper tailoring of excess on the sides of the repair, the cosmetic appearance is surprisingly good.

Chapter 138

Meatoplasty and Glanuloplasty (MAGPI Repair)

The meatal advancement and glanuloplasty (MAGPI) repair is an operation for distal hypospadias without chordee, with the meatus at the corona. By reshaping the glans and advancing the urethra the meatus can be relocated to a terminal position within the glans. It is especially suitable for a broad, flat glans with a dorsal web of tissue within the glans.

Typically, the dorsal web of tissue within the glans deflects the urine exiting from a coronal or slightly subcoronal meatus. Repair corrects a hooded prepuce and a coronal meatus, in addition to eliminating any associated glanular tilt.

Avoid cases with thin or rigid ventral parameatal skin, or with a meatus too high on the shaft or one too wide. For the MAGPI procedure to be applicable the skin proximal to the meatus should be mobile enough to allow the urethra to advance to a terminal position. For a wide-mouth, flat, fixed meatus that cannot be moved into the glanular groove, a primary tube repair such as the GAP procedure (see Chapter 139) is more appropriate. For a thin urethral plate without the dorsal web of tissue a primary tube with incision of the urethral plate is indicated.

Perform the operation as an outpatient procedure, under general anesthesia.

Insert a vertical traction suture and, for hemostasis, infiltrate around the corona and dorsal web of glandular tissue with 1% lidocaine solution, containing 1:100,000 epinephrine.

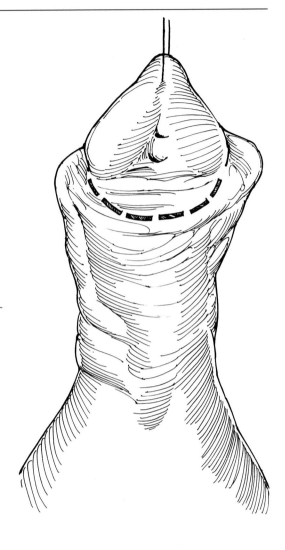

FIGURE 138-1. Place a stay suture (not shown) in the glans ventrally and in each glans wing to assist the dissection, and later to allow rearrangement of the tissues for the best fit. Incise the ventral skin transversely 0.8 cm from the coronal sulcus and meatus.

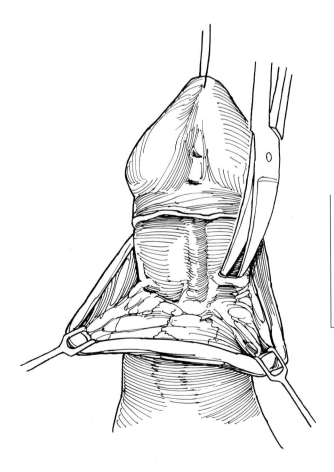

FIGURE 138-2. Dissect the skin of the ventral shaft proximally as a sleeve, taking care not to injure the urethral wall. (It is especially delicate here.) Free the skin proximally as a sleeve to the penoscrotal junction, especially if torsion is present. Clear all tethering tissue from the corpora. Create an artificial erection to be sure that the penis is straight. For residual curvature (usually due to corporeal disproportion) a midline dorsal plication can be performed (see Chapter 133).

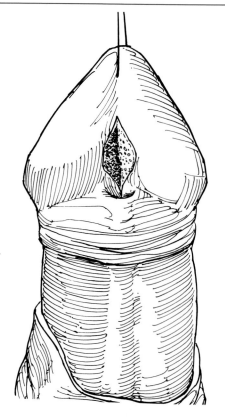

FIGURE 138-3. Starting inside the dorsal edge of the meatus, make a generous vertical incision that extends to the distal end of the glanular groove. The proximal cut results in a V that widens the dorsal meatal margin even when meatal stenosis is initially present (Heineke-Mikulicz principle). Consider excising wedges from each side of the glans to reduce prominent meatal lips.

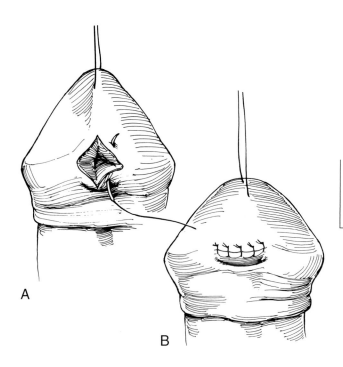

A

B

FIGURE 138-4. **A** and **B,** Suture the edges of the meatal V to the groove in the glans with fine absorbable sutures such as a Heineke-Mikulicz transverse closure. This advances the meatus and flattens the groove.

FIGURE 138-5. Lift the proximal edge of the meatus with a skin hook or traction suture, pulling it toward the tip of the glans to form an inverted V as the glans wings are pulled together. Excise the excess skin and glans tissue on the medial margins of these wings to expose glans tissue in preparation for a glansplasty.

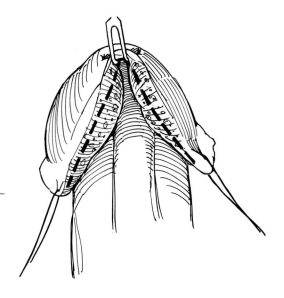

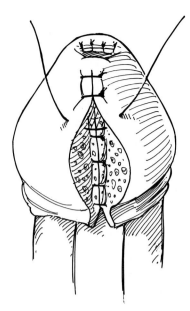

FIGURE 138-6. Approximate the deep glans tissue with one or two 6-0 synthetic absorbable sutures. To close the glans, insert buried subcutaneous sutures to ensure a firm approximation, and to avoid tension that would lead to a retrusive meatus. Suture the two edges thus formed together in the midline with vertical 6-0 synthetic absorbable mattress sutures.

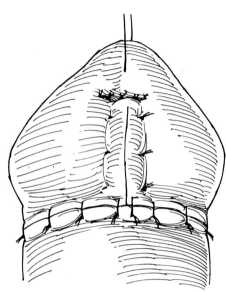

FIGURE 138-7. Align the median raphe and trim the excess preputial skin lying proximal to the wrinkled portion. Suture the edges with 7-0 chromic catgut sutures or with fine subcuticular sutures. Trim the skin edges to improve appearance.

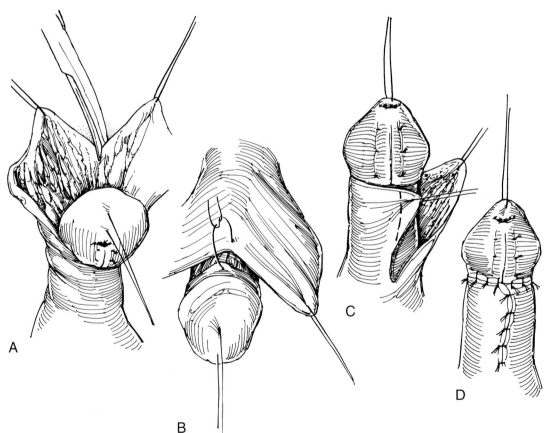

FIGURE 138-8. If the ventral skin is deficient: **A** and **B,** Split the preputial skin dorsally. **C** and **D,** Bring the edges together ventrally as Byars' flaps (see Chapter 137). Trim the flaps to preserve symmetry. It is not necessary to insert a catheter or a stent in babies less than 1 year of age. During toilet training there is an increased risk of postoperative urinary retention, which can be prevented by a temporary feeding tube secured with a plastic adhesive dressing for 48 hours.

JOHN W. DUCKETT

Commentary by

The MAGPI procedure for hypospadias has been one of the more difficult techniques to describe and to teach. Despite its simplicity, there is a gestalt about the concept that has been difficult to describe in specific terms. Hypospadias comes in such variable configurations that specific indications for the MAGPI repair are difficult to enumerate.

Since the majority (70%) of hypospadias cases have an anteriorly placed meatus, mostly subcoronal, the MAGPI procedure has a definite place in a large percentage of these. However, for a wide-mouth, flat, fixed meatus that cannot be moved into the glanular groove, a Mathieu procedure or an island onlay flap may be more appropriate. In addition, the concept of "stretching" a MAGPI repair has very limited applicability, amenable only to the very mobile distal urethra.

The glanuloplasty portion of the procedure is modified for each individual case. There is always trimming of the skin edges after the wings of the glans are approximated to make a more cosmetically normal-appearing configuration. Instructions for the beginning incision are intended to leave excess skin that will be trimmed at the end of the procedure. It is, therefore, inappropriate to design an incision proximal to the meatus in such a way that perfect reapproximation at the end is ensured. We now use holding stitches of 6-0 chromic catgut in the ventral glans and on each glans wing to move the structures and determine the appropriate configuration. Mobilization of the glans wings with further sharp dissection has not been necessary in most cases.

Maintenance of a normal urinary stream pattern with a MAGPI procedure has been confirmed by studies in Toronto.

When the technique was first published, we urged that it be learned by observing others who have mastered the technique. I still think this is an appropriate lesson, as it is very difficult to depict its variability in an atlas.

EDMOND T. GONZALES

Commentary by

Before the MAGPI procedure was described, boys with a proximal glanular or coronal meatus and no chordee were advised to forego any surgery, or to have a circumcision at most. The MAGPI procedure emphasized the importance of the meatus, both in regard to overall cosmesis and direction of urinary flow.

Unfortunately, the MAGPI repair was seen as a "simple" procedure, and at the time of its introduction, many surgeons who did not do the usual major hypospadias repairs felt comfortable doing MAGPI procedures. Given the complexity of the hypospadias anomaly, some patients thought to be suitable candidates for a MAGPI repair were found during the procedure to be better managed by a more complex operation. Not all results were good, and many reports of meatal retraction or coronal fistulas were noted. The failure of some surgeons to adhere to the technical principles of the procedure resulted too often in poor results.

With the development of better techniques for tubularization of the urethral plate, the MAGPI principle was adhered to less often. Indeed, I find that I use the technique less and less now. Current techniques for meatoplasty and glansplasty afford a more normally positioned meatus with a vertical slit than I believe can be achieved with a classical MAGPI repair. That being said, it is important to recognize that this technique challenged all of us committed to hypospadias surgery to recognize the importance of the meatus if we were ever going to achieve a near-normal penile appearance after hypospadias repair.

Chapter 139

Glans Approximation Procedure

Use the glans approximation procedure (GAP) for repair of selected cases of glanular and coronal hypospadias when the meatus is large and situated near the coronal sulcus. It is especially useful in boys with a wide and deep glanular groove or fish-mouth meatus. Recognize the GAP repair as a modification of the Thiersch-Duplay tube repair (see Chapter 144); the original operation may be more suitable in cases that do not match these criteria.

If a ridge is present in the glanular groove, incise it longitudinally and close the resulting defect transversely (Heineke-Mikulicz). This slightly advances the dorsal side of the meatus and suturing it forms a smooth urethral plate.

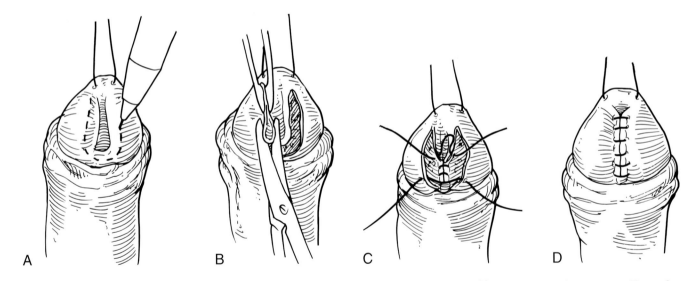

FIGURE 139-1. A, Mark the glans wings with a horseshoe-shaped incision (a deep U), encircling the meatus. Keep the marks 12 to 14 mm apart to ensure an adequate terminal urethra. **B,** With tenotomy scissors, excise the U-shaped band of epithelium on the glans that is covered by the marks. **C,** Tubularize the terminal urethra over a stent, placing two layers of fine running sutures subcuticularly. With a third layer of sutures, close the subcutaneous layer. Leave the stent as a drip tube. **D,** Approximate the glans flaps with fine interrupted sutures. If necessary, bring a portion of the prepuce around to cover the defect. Calibrate the urethra to be sure the size is 10 to 12 F. Create a mucosal collar from the prepuce for an improved cosmetic effect and approximate the skin with a midline seam. Apply a bio-occlusive dressing.

MARK ZAONTZ

Commentary by

The GAP procedure was originally intended for that specific circumstance in which the hypospadiac appearance revealed a deep and wide glanular groove. This ideally allowed for simple incision and closure of the glans with highly reproducible results. A few minor modifications over the years have been employed in my practice. These include closure of the neourethra with a double-running-layer subcuticular closure using 7-0 polyglycolic acid suture. When needed on occasion, a third layer of interrupted 7-0 polyglycolic acid Lembert sutures was employed as necessary.

In the past, if there was a transverse cleft separating the hypospadiac meatus from the glans groove, a Heineke-Mikulicz procedure was used to smooth out the posterior urethral plate. At present, I only incise the cleft longitudinally and leave the posterior urethral plate nice and flat, allowing it to heal by secondary intent. Finally, if I note any tension whatsoever on the neourethral closure I would never hesitate to deepen the glans incision as done in the Thiersch-Duplay technique to allow for a tension-free closure.

BARRY KOGAN

Commentary by

There are innumerable published and unpublished hypospadias repairs. This attests to the fact that no one repair is optimal for all circumstances. Regarding distal hypospadias in particular, it is only in recent years that repairs have been consistently performed. In general, the lesion is not associated with abnormalities of urinary or sexual function. Thus, the problem is primarily one of appearance and the psychological ramifications. Only in recent years have the approaches had high enough success rates and low enough morbidity to make these repairs commonplace.

The GAP procedure itself is only feasible for those patients with the very specific anatomic configuration of a deep glanular groove. However, the concept behind the procedure is the forebearer of many modern repairs. Indeed, when modified with an incision in the urethral plate, it can be used for the great majority of distal and many other repairs.

Although the GAP repair as described can be used as an outpatient procedure and without catheter drainage in children under 18 months, we have modified it slightly in recent years to reduce the occurrence of a fistula. As illustrated, the procedure has two overlapping suture lines. This cannot be prevented, but it is nearly always possible to develop a flap of subcutaneous tissue, either from dorsal foreskin or ventral penile tissue, to create an interposing layer. Although fistulas were uncommon previously, with this modification they should be exceedingly rare.

Chapter 140

Pyramid Procedure for Repair of the Megameatus: Intact Prepuce Hypospadias Variant

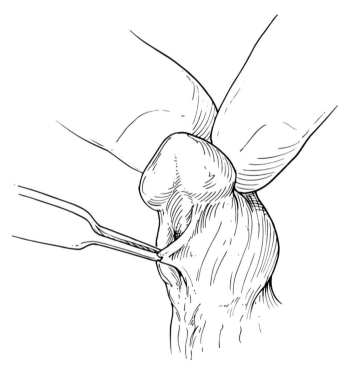

FIGURE 140-1. An intact prepuce conceals a large meatus, and a deep cleft forms the glanular groove. Techniques such as the MAGPI, Mathieu, or Snodgrass modification do not correct the abnormal meatus in this rare variant. The pyramid procedure exposes and excises the excess tissue forming the terminal urethra and then reconstitutes a meatus of the proper size (tube repair) and brings it to the tip of the penis.

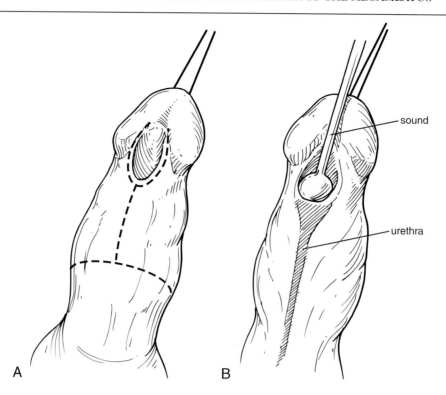

FIGURE 140-2. **A** and **B,** Place a 5-0 polypropylene traction suture on the tip of the glans and then one on each side of the base of the meatus, and one on its ventral margin to define the megameatus and the base of the pyramid. Traction here can cause injury to the urethra during mobilization. Infiltrate beneath the proposed line of incision and the glans itself with lidocaine-epinephrine solution to reduce pain and bleeding. An elastic tourniquet may help reduce bleeding.

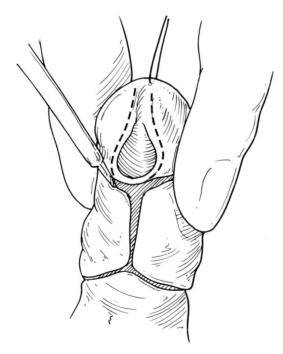

FIGURE 140-3. Mark a tennis-racket incision just medial to the glanular groove and continue it around the edge of the megameatus at the base of the traction sutures.

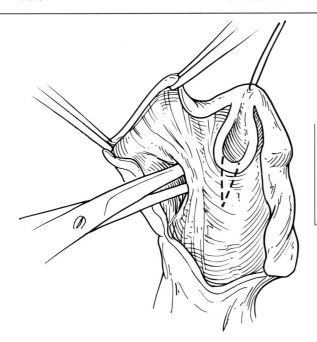

FIGURE 140-4. Incise along the mark. Using iris scissors, mobilize the urethral cone (pyramid) proximally until it becomes normal in size. Develop glans wings on either side by deepening the edges of the glanular groove laterally. Leave the distal urethral plate wide (12 to 15 mm) and intact dorsally. Tailor the widened distal urethra by removing a small wedge from the excess ventral urethral tissue.

FIGURE 140-5. Tubularize the urethra and glans strip by approximating the edges with a continuous 7-0 synthetic absorbable suture to provide a neourethra of normal caliber.

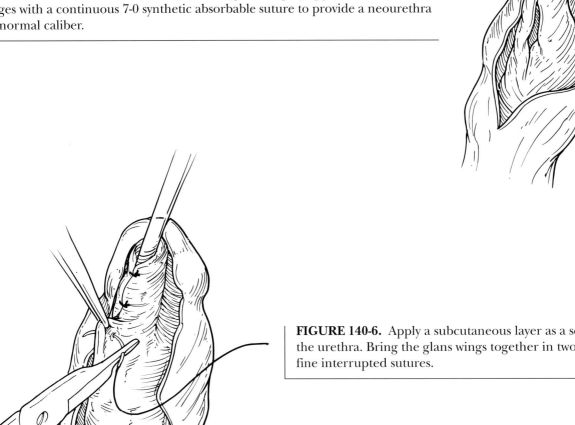

FIGURE 140-6. Apply a subcutaneous layer as a second layer over the urethra. Bring the glans wings together in two layers with fine interrupted sutures.

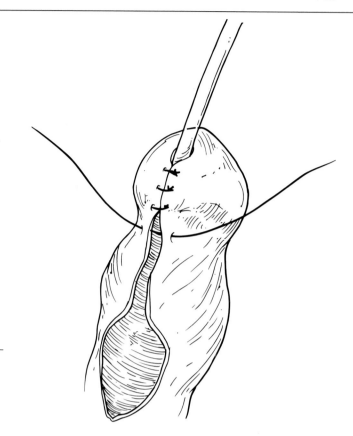

FIGURE 140-7. Close the skin with 7-0 interrupted chromic catgut mattress sutures. Check the caliber of the urethra gently with a 10- or 12-F bougie à boule, and observe the caliber of the stream by pressing over the bladder. The repair can be followed with a circumcision if that is the wish of the parents, although the particular merit of this procedure is that it preserves the prepuce.

Circumcision: Make two circumferential incisions in the skin of the shaft, the first 6 to 8 mm from the coronal edge with the prepuce retracted and the other at a similar level without retraction. Excise the prepuce and approximate the sleeve with a fine running chromic suture. Insert a 6-F silicone tube into the bladder and fix it to the glans with 5-0 polypropylene on a tapered needle, for drainage into a diaper. Place a gauze wrap to be removed by the parents in 2 days. Remove the stent in 5 to 7 days.

MIKE A. KEATING

Commentary by

The moniker "pyramid" was given to this procedure to describe its end-on dissection of the widened glans cleft and distal urethra that accompanies the megameatus intact prepuce (MIP) hypospadias variant. Historically, the MIP presented one of the most challenging hypospadias to correct. The exaggerated urethral plate that accompanies the anomaly poses a barrier to the tissue transfers of the ventral glans and urethra required of the MAGPI repair (see Chapter 138). It also presents a difficult match to the tailoring and lateral anastomoses of perimeatal-base flaps. Finally, subsequent techniques that tubularize the urethral plate alone, such as at the tubularized incised plate (Snodgrass modification), do not address the widened urethra in their closures. The differences in caliber that result between the relative urethral narrowing across the glans and uncorrected dilated urethra proximal to the repair could, in theory, lead to pressure differentials that predispose to fistula formation. Distal hypospadias variants that are not true MIPs but present with a wide urethral plate and generous urethra should be tapered for the same reasons. Simple ventral tubularizations like the Snodgrass modification should be modified accordingly.

The MIP might be better classified as a form of distal megalourethra, in which obstruction is felt to be the cause. The excavation of the distal glans and corpora (at times impressive) that accompanies the anomaly, its intact prepuce, and the absence of chordee differ greatly from generic hypospadias, in which an endocrinopathy is implicated. MIPs represent 2% to 3% of all hypospadias and often go unrecognized until after a circumcision is completed. It can be mistaken for an iatrogenic injury and serves to emphasize the need, before circumcision, to fully retract the prepuce and assess the glans and urethra. Absence of the prepuce is not a problem for the repair.

It is unnecessary to deglove the penis with MIP variants, as chordee is not an issue. Mobilizing the plate and distal urethra can be challenging. It is not uncommon for these to project far laterally into the surrounding corporeal tissue, thinning out the glans wings. Tacking sutures on the glans at the corners of the "base" of the pyramid can aid in the proximal dissection to normal caliber urethra at its apex. Care should be taken to avoid excessively thinning out the spongiosum of the glans wings during the lateral dissections. There is usually so much redundancy to the urethral plate that any unhealthy urethral tissue, perhaps compromised by an inadvertent urethrotomy, can be excised with the ventral tapering required of the repair.

One of the weaknesses of the pyramid procedure and other similar repairs that tubularize the urethral plate are their midline closures and overlapping suture lines. Once the urethral cone is mobilized, one helpful modification is to taper the plate and urethra with a lateral wedge and excision of redundancy. This allows for an offset lateral urethral closure well away from the overlying glans closure. A buttressing layer of coverage is instrumental to minimizing fistulas, the most common complication with the pyramid procedure (2% to 3%). Most MIPs are accompanied by a ventral collection of excess shaft skin that overlies the dilated distal urethra (similar to that seen with megalourethra). This provides an ideal source of subcutaneous tissue that can be easily mobilized as a vascularized flap to blanket the repair.

Despite its challenges, the MIP's clefted glans and well-developed plate are well suited to in situ tubularization. The pyramid procedure offers an ideal solution for this unusual hypospadias variant.

Chapter 141

Perimeatal-Based Flap Repair

For distal hypospadias with at most slight chordee, the Mathieu procedure is suitable. Glanular tilt and limited distal curvature may be corrected by dorsal midline plication (see Chapter 133), if care is taken to preserve the dorsal nerves. The glanular urethral groove (urethral plate) is used as the roof of the distal urethra and a meatal-based random flap as the floor. The prepuce is also preserved. If the perimeatal skin is very thin, consider a vascularized graft or tube repair.

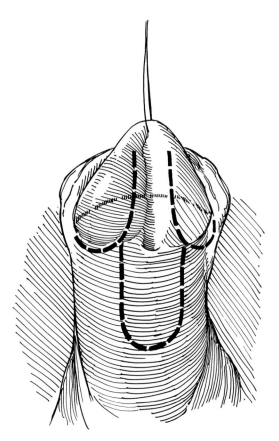

FIGURE 141-1. Insert a 5-0 Prolene monofilament suture swaged on a fine tapered needle vertically in the glans for traction. Mark lines 0.6 to 0.8 cm apart for a V-shaped glans flap on both sides of the glanular groove. Continue marking for a proximal urethral flap. Add a circumferential penile incision 0.8 cm proximal to the glans. Infiltrate the subcutaneous tissue with 1:100,000 epinephrine in 1% lidocaine. Insert a small infant feeding tube to protect the urethra. Incise along the marks, taking care not to interfere with the blood supply to the base. Incise the prepuce circumferentially 1 cm away from the glans to deglove the shaft. Use this opportunity to excise any ventral tissue producing chordee and correct any residual curvature with plication suture.

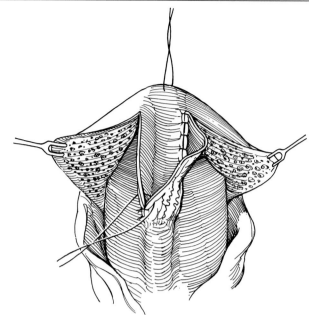

FIGURE 141-2. Place a tourniquet around the base of the penis. Develop the lateral portions of the glans as wings. Raise the flap from the shaft, while preserving its subcutaneous tissue and its blood supply. Trim the flap as needed to avoid creating a patulous pocket. Fold the flap up over the groove in the glans, and, using loupes, suture it on both sides with interrupted or running 6-0 synthetic absorbable sutures. Bring in subcutaneous tissue as a second layer for cover if possible. Tack the subcutaneous tissue of the flap to the deep tissue of the glans. Test for a watertight suture line by instilling saline under pressure. Correct leaks with additional sutures.

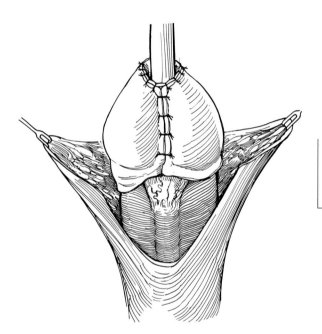

FIGURE 141-3. Approximate the glans flaps in the midline with fine interrupted sutures (be sure to undermine the flaps to avoid tension). Keeping a large catheter in the meatus while suturing helps prevent meatal stenosis.

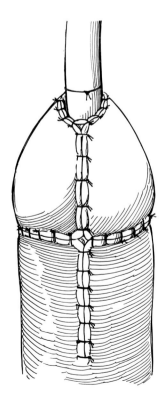

FIGURE 141-4. Split the shaft skin and pass it around as Byars' flaps. A portion of one of these flaps may be de-epithelialized to provide an extra layer of cover for the repair. Attach the neourethra to the lateral glans flaps with interrupted sutures. Trim excess skin. Close the circumcision defect, and then close the ventral defect with several interrupted subcutaneous stitches, followed by a running fine suture with several interrupted sutures added for security. For an alternative closure, use a buttonhole technique. Try not to have the suture lines meet at the base of the glans as drawn in the figure.

Finally, calibrate the urethra with a curved sound corresponding to the size of the normal urethra for the child's age. Test for a watertight suture line by instilling saline under slight pressure, and correct all leaks with added sutures. Pass an 8-F silicone catheter into the bladder, and tether it to the penis by a traction suture. Alternatively, merely drain the bladder after instilling 2% xylocaine jelly, and remove the catheter. Provide a second penile nerve block with bupivacaine. Place a plastic dressing and have the dressing removed at home in 5 to 7 days.

CHARLES E. HORTON

Commentary by

The flip-flap operation gives excellent cosmetic and functional results for distal hypospadias with chordee. It cannot be used if the midline glans flap will not reach into the existing urethral meatus without causing chordee. This factor limits the procedure to cases of distal hypospadias, but these constitute 90% of all hypospadias cases.

In the past, many techniques were described to try to bring the meatus to the tip of the glans, but the high rate of meatal stenosis due to the circumferential suture line at the tip of the glans caused most to be abandoned. The principle of interposing a midline glans flap into the circular anastomosis at the tip of the penis has obviated the meatal stenosis problem, and by bringing the lateral wings of the glans beneath the distal urethra, the abnormally shaped glans can be contoured into a more desirable conical, normal shape. Because the patient desires a normal-appearing penis, all excess skin is discarded at this operation. The prepuce is used to cover the ventral surface of the penis and is contoured appropriately at the initial operation.

Following the reconstruction of the urethra, the anastomosis is tested retrogradely with a Christmas tree–tipped syringe. Any leaks are repaired so that a watertight urethra is ensured. The use of a loupe or an operating room microscope has added greatly to the development of an atraumatic, meticulous technique that has improved healing. Complications from this operation are rare; in a series of 56 patients, a complication rate of 6% was encountered. Dressing with Opsite directly applied to the wound allows visualization through the clear material in the immediate postoperative phase. Elevation of the pelvic area and cold compresses for the first 24 hours help reduce pain and swelling. We try to avoid a catheter through the repair, as traction inferiorly on the catheter may cause dehiscence of the glans flaps. Suprapubic Cystocath diversion, a small feeding tube (8 or 10 F) through the repair, or a urethral stent with the patient's voiding through the stent and repair is most often employed. Skin sutures of 6-0 chromic catgut dissolve spontaneously, thereby obviating the necessity for postoperative removal.

MARC CENDRON

Commentary by

The Mathieu procedure first described in 1932 is an adaptation of Louis Ombredanne's "sac" technique. Popularized in the 1970s, it had been the standard repair for distal hypospadias (coronal and subcoronal) until the introduction of the tubularized incised plate repair described by Snodgrass. A technically straightforward procedure, this Mathieu or flip-flap repair gives good functional results and adequate cosmetic appearance, the main drawback being the rounded, unslit-like shape of the meatus. The technique is not applicable in two specific cases: in patients with a small glans with little or no urethral groove and in patients who are found to have very thin skin coverage over the distal urethra. In the first instance, recessing the urethra in the glans and reconstructing the glans will be nearly impossible, and in the latter instance a skin flap will be of poor quality. This technique should therefore be limited to distal hypospadias. Stretching the indications will only lead to complications such as fistula formation or outright breakdown of the repair.

Every attempt should be made to dissect out as much subcutaneous tissue as possible with the skin flap so as to ensure an adequate blood supply. A compromised flap will perform like a free graft and, over time, will contract, thus causing distal urethral narrowing.

After dissecting out the urethral plate and developing glans wings, the parameatal-based skin flap should be sewed to the urethral plate using subcuticular stitches. Watertightness is tested at this point prior to covering the reconstructed distal urethra with a subcutaneous layer of tissue. Coverage of the urethra may also be achieved by bringing the corpus spongiosum over the repair, thus providing an additional blood supply to the flap. Care is given not to reconstruct the glans too tightly, as distal urethral stenosis may ensue. Reconstruction over an 8-F catheter, which will then be replaced by a 6-F tube, may prevent stenosis.

Stenting of the repair with a small Silastic tube for 3 to 5 days has always been my practice, as urinary retention is always possible. While it is a rare occurrence, placing a stent several hours after the repair in a child with urinary retention is never fun and may require an additional anesthetic.

Chapter 142

Balanitic Groove Hypospadias Repair

The Barcat procedure, a modification of the Mathieu urethroplasty, advances the meatus to the tip by mobilizing the urethral plate from the groove in the glans distal to the meatus. The plate is formed into a tube by supplementing it with a ventral flap from the shaft. The neourethra can then be inserted deep into the incised glans.

This operation is suitable for children with hypospadias with good quality ventral skin. Its original indication was for distal hypospadias although the indication has been extended to proximal repairs.

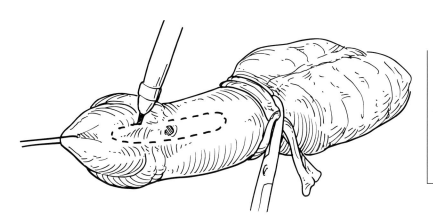

FIGURE 142-1. Measure the distance from the proximal lip of the meatus to the end of the glans. Hemostasis may be obtained by the use of a tourniquet or injection of 1% lidocaine and 1:100,000 epinephrine. Outline a flap that is 1 to 1.4 cm wider than the urethra itself, ending 3 to 5 mm proximal to the corona. Incise and elevate the flap.

FIGURE 142-2. Outline a flap around the glanular groove to mark the urethral plate and incise along the mark.

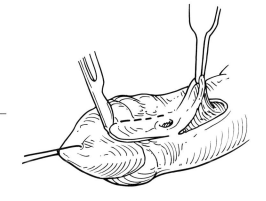

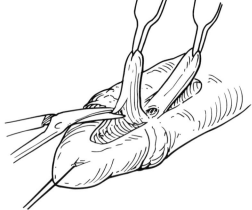

FIGURE 142-3. Elevate the flap of urethral plate that was incised in Figure 142-2. Use a thumb and finger technique to evert the glans wings, thus making the plate bulge away from the underlying glans. This keeps the dorsal aspect of the urethral plate from being made too thin.

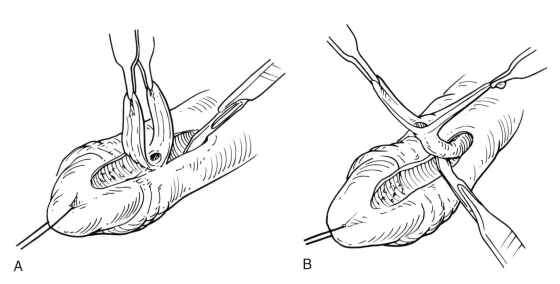

A

B

FIGURE 142-4. **A** and **B,** Extend the dissection around the meatus to mobilize the urethra. Here, be careful not to tear the fragile urethra, made clear by the presence of the catheter.

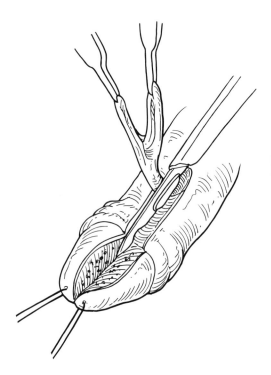

FIGURE 142-5. Sharply incise the glans ventrally from the meatus to the glans tip to form a deep groove for the new urethra. Leave the spongy tissue in place. Insert a feeding tube or catheter, typically 8 F, in preparation for the urethroplasty.

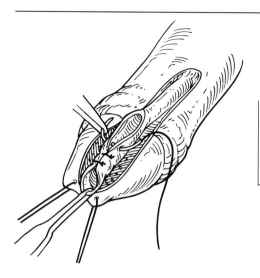

FIGURE 142-6. Suture the dorsal lip of the neourethra to the dorsal rim of the incision in the glans. Suture the edges of the proximal flap to the edges of the glanular flap on both sides with a running 7-0 polyglactin suture to form the neourethra. A second layer of de-epithelialized dartos fascia can be used to cover the urethroplasty to prevent fistula formation (not shown).

FIGURE 142-7. Fasten the two halves of the glans together over the neourethra with subepithelial mattress sutures of 6-0 polyglactin. Close the glans epithelium with interrupted vertical mattress sutures. Suture the ventral lip of the new meatus to the glans with 7-0 polyglactin and complete the formation of the meatus by joining the flap to the apex of the glans with the same suture material.

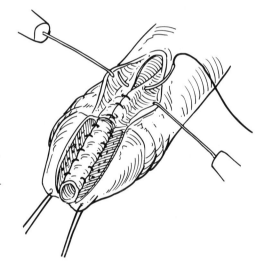

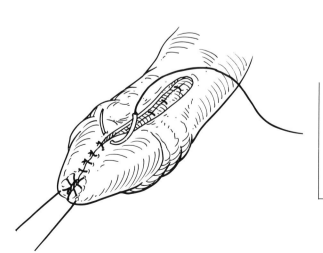

FIGURE 142-8. Bring the subcutaneous tissue together in the midline with an interrupted suture to provide a second layer. Trim and fit the remainder of the skin; use only the preputial skin that is needed for coverage and excise the rest. Replace the catheter by gently inserting a stent or feeding tube into the bladder. Apply a light pressure dressing, to remain along with the catheter for 5 to 7 days.

JOHN REDMAN

I have now used the Barcat balanic groove technique exclusively for hypospadias repairs; my experience now exceeds 20 years. I remain enthusiastic with the principles so elegantly enunciated by Professor Barcat in the late 1960s. However, the techniques, which provide for a completely normal appearance to the glans and meatus, have not been widely embraced by the urologic community. The operation is technically demanding and requires strict attention to detail. I believe that the technique has a place in our armamentarium, if used in appropriately selected cases. Although the balanic groove techniques are thought of strictly in association with a flip flap of ventral penile skin to effect a urethroplasty, the techniques may also be used with a free preputial skin graft in a very similar manner.

In my original publications, the associated fistula rate was relatively high, as it was in Barcat's series. However, no attention was given to covering the urethroplasty proximal to the corona, relying only on the skin closure for coverage. Since incorporating a Y-to-I wrap of the contiguous divergent corpus spongiosum over the urethroplasty, the fistula rate has been greatly reduced. I use the balanic groove technique in all hypospadias repairs but am now very selective in choosing those candidates for the formation of a flip flap. I now reserve flip flaps only for boys with balanic or coronal hypospadias and then only select those patients in whom I am assured that there will not be any compromise of the skin available for a ventral penile skin closure. If a wide Firlit collar can be made and there is no associated penile curvature, which may result in a significant proximal regression of shaft skin, I will generally choose a flip flap.

Important technical considerations are these. I use ×3.5 loupe magnification. With the balanitic groove technique, glans wings, per se, are not elevated; only a deep midline groove is made. The initial maneuver is to first outline the glabrous epithelium of the urethral plate with a skin marker. A rubber band tourniquet is employed to ensure a completely bloodless field. I use a 2- × 10-mm rubber band and leave the tourniquet in place until the glansplasty is completed, regardless of the time required for the repair. The glanular epithelium only is incised and the urethral plate is then carefully elevated proximal to the coronal margin. If the meatus is balanitic or coronal, a catheter placed in the distal urethra aids in delineating the diaphanous urethra and obviates inadvertent entries into the lumen.

It will be noted that in most cases, the urethral plate does not extend to the tip of the glans. Therefore, it is important to make a 2- to 3-mm incision in the midline distal to the site of the elevated plate and then excise the resultant triangles of epithelium. This maneuver will provide for the ultimate elliptical shape of the meatus and also simultaneously bring the meatus to the tip of the glans. The groove itself is made deeply in the midline without any excision of spongy tissue. If necessary, to achieve a deeper groove because of a thin ventral glans, the septum between the corporeal bodies may be incised without entering either corpus. A key to properly creating the groove is the use of a miniature self-retaining retractor (e.g., Agrikola retractor). Not only is the retractor an adjunct to the formation of the groove, it is most helpful in providing retraction during the completion of the glanular portion of the urethroplasty itself. The urethroplasty is accomplished over a 10-F red rubber catheter.

The glans closure begins with horizontal mattress sutures of 6-0 polyglactin (usually two sutures) placed just beneath the epithelium. At the level of the corona, I place a single suture to approximate the remaining spongy tissue of the glans and then continue it as a running suture proximally to approximate the contiguous divergent corpus spongiosum over the proximal portion of the urethroplasty (Y-to-I wrap). This maneuver provides a thick covering over the urethroplasty and obviates a dartos interposition. The procedure is concluded by approximating the glanular epithelium and inner leaf of the prepuce with interrupted 7-0 polyglactin sutures. Prior to closure of the glanular epithelium, it is helpful to excise any bulging epithelium along the margins of the approximated glans. This may be done by expressing the tissue between the blades of fine dissecting scissors and then cutting. If an onlay graft is chosen, I simply harvest an appropriate-sized segment from the inner leaf of the prepuce and suture it to the dorsal urethral plate, just as I would do with a flip flap.

Urinary diversion is by means of an 8-F infant feeding tube secured by the traction suture in the tip of the glans and by the silk tape used in the light, compressing penile dressing. Both are removed in 2 days. I am frequently asked: "Is meatal stenosis or a distal urethral stricture a concern?" Urethral and meatal stenosis has seldom occurred, probably because the urethra is constructed over a 10-F catheter and the deep balanic groove allows for a capacious bed for the urethra.

STEVE KOFF

The Barcat technique is versatile; it lets the surgeon position the meatus at the tip of the penis regardless of the shape of the glans or the location and depth of the glans groove.

The most challenging part of the procedure involves mobilization of the urethral plate and urethra, as depicted in Figures 142-2, 142-3, and 142-4B. The distal incisions used to mobilize the urethral plate must be sufficiently deep to develop the full thickness of the plate including the spongy tissue under it, by extending the dissection down to the tunica albuginea, which is recognized by its grayish-white color. Once this plane is reached, proximal mobilization of the urethral plate and urethra proceed easily.

The most important part of the procedure to prevent fistula formation is shown in Figure 142-7, and involves covering the neourethra within the penile shaft with a second layer of tissue derived from the deep full-thickness lateral incisions (see Fig. 142-3) and extending it down to the tunica albuginea. The resulting subcutaneous-spongy tissue closure begins with approximation of the glans wings at the junction of the glans and penile shaft and proceeds proximally as a running 6-0 polydioxanone suture. I have never needed to use de-epithelialized dartos tissue for urethral coverage, as the suture lines are not overlapping.

Cosmetic perfection with glansplasty depends on making a deep incision into the glans extending distally from the urethral plate past the distalmost tip of the glans so that the center of the new meatus will be correctly positioned at the center of the tip of the penis. Figure 142-5 illustrates this incision. Correct positioning of the meatus in the midline is aided by using a single midline holding suture to precisely mark the midline at the beginning of the procedure.

Chapter 143

Transverse Preputial Onlay Island Flap

TRANSVERSE PREPUTIAL ONLAY ISLAND FLAP (DUCKETT)

If you can preserve the urethral plate while correcting minimal or moderate chordee, use this simpler onlay procedure in preference to forming a new urethral segment. With a small prepuce, this procedure has the advantage of using only a portion of it, leaving the rest to resurface the shaft.

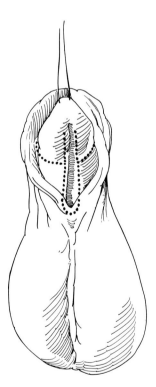

FIGURE 143-1. With a tapered needle, insert a stay suture transversely in the glans dorsal to the tip. Infiltrate the ventral perimeatal tissues with 1 or 2 mL of epinephrine-lidocaine solution and wait 7 minutes. Don a magnifying loupe or adjust the operating microscope. Mark and then incise the circumference of the coronal sulcus 5 mm proximal to the glans. Continue the incision proximally around the margin of, but not beneath, the urethral plate. Including the meatus releases the tethering skin and superficial fascia, which will usually release the chordee. If not, resort to dorsal midline plication (see Chapter 133).

712

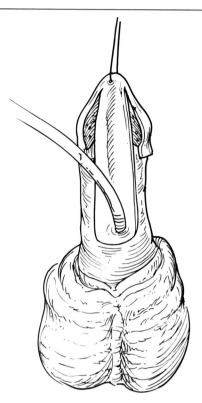

FIGURE 144-2. Dissect along the corporeal body to separate the glans wings from the distal portion of the urethral plate. Test for chordee with artificial erection; apply dorsal plications (see Chapter 133) as needed to achieve a straight phallus.

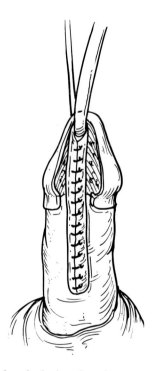

FIGURE 144-3. If the plate is adequate in width tubularize the plate over a 6- or 8-F Silastic stent with 7-0 absorbable sutures. Do not close the distal end too tightly; stenosis will result. It is advisable to leave the neomeatus oval in shape. If the plate is too narrow proceed to a preputial onlay island flap (see Chapter 143) or perform the Snodgrass modification (see Chapter 145).

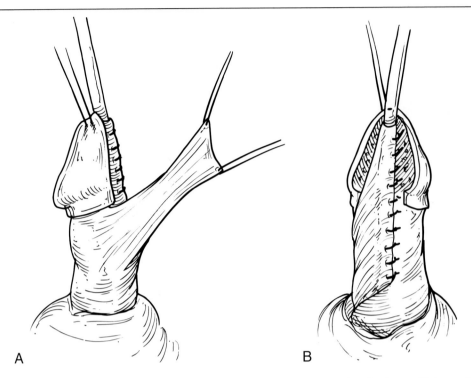

A   B

FIGURE 144-4. A, Dissect a vascularized patch of dorsal subcutanous tissue. **B,** Apply the pedicle graft to cover the entire suture line.

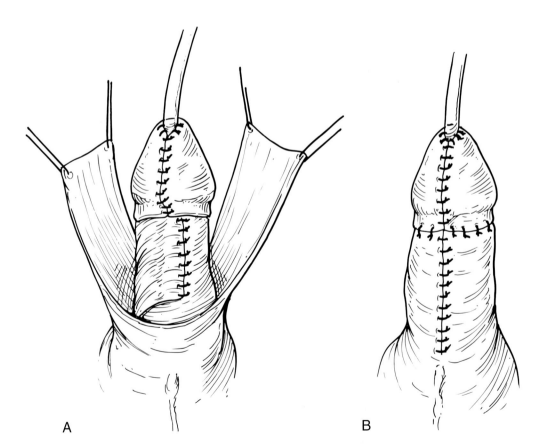

A   B

FIGURE 144-5. A, Close the glans wings and mucosal collar in the midline. Split the prepuce, and swing the distal portions around each side to cover the ventral defect. **B,** Use interrupted subcuticular sutures to close the skin defect. Secure the stent for postoperative drainage for 5 to 10 days.

EVAN KASS

Commentary by

For most patients, the Snodgrass modification will not be necessary. However, for patients without a deep urethral groove in the glans, incision of the urethral plate has provided better results than the onlay island flap in our hands. We close the urethral plate with two layers of running 7-0 absorbable sutures and cover this anastomosis with a third layer of vascularized tissue mobilized from the inner layer of the prepuce. We routinely use a silicone stent with multiple side holes, which is left in place for 4 to 7 days and is allowed to drip freely into a diaper. We have preferred to use a vessel loop tourniquet placed at the base of the penis, and released periodically, for managing bleeding during surgery rather than epinephrine infiltration.

ROSS DECTOR

Commentary by

The tubularized plate urethroplasty is a time-tested procedure for distal hypospadias. The key to performing the Thiersch-Duplay procedure is ensuring that the urethral plate is of sufficient width to allow for formation of a neourethra of adequate circumference. If the plate is too narrow to create a neourethra of adequate caliber, an onlay flap can be applied or, alternatively, the plate can be hinged (Snodgrass procedure).

Some elements of the procedure that deserve emphasis include details of the glanular incisions creating the surgical urethral plate.

After infiltration with lidocaine-epinephrine solution into the ventral glans, the incision through the glanular substance needs to go to the level of the tunica albuginea of the corpus cavernosum. Dissection at this plane facilitates glans mobilization and, in addition, small pieces of glanular substance and tissue at the lateral aspect of the urethral plate can be excised so that the subsequent glans closure over the neourethra can be performed without undue compression of the neourethra.

Coverage of the entire repair out to the ventral tip of the neourethra with a vascularized pedicle of dorsal subcutaneous tissue is critical to reduce the risk of fistula formation. Use of the subcutaneous pedicle is extrapolated from the concept of de-epithelialized skin coverage to reduce fistula formation originally described by Durham Smith and later promoted by Barry Belman. Harvesting the flap takes only a minute or two and its use almost totally eliminates fistula formation. I suture the flap using 7-0 Vicryl down to the corpus cavernosum on either side of the neourethra to ensure complete coverage of the underlying suture line.

Adequate closure of the glans in the ventral midline is critical to prevent glans separation and meatal retrusion. I use one or two 6-0 Vicryl sutures into the glans substance well below the level of the skin to be sure there is good glanular substance approximation before undertaking the superficial closure of the glans skin and mucosal collars.

Chapter 145

Incision of the Urethral Plate (Snodgrass Modification)

If the urethral plate is too narrow for primary tubularization an incision in the midline of the plate to the level of the
corporeal body will allow the urethral plate tissue to spring
open for subsequent tubularization.

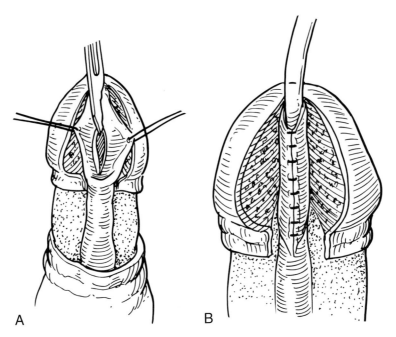

A

B

FIGURE 145-1. A, After chordee is corrected and the glans wing mobilized, make an incision in the midline through the
entire thickness and length of the urethral plate down to corporeal tissue. Even a narrow flat plate is suitable; it does not
predispose to a narrower neourethra but be certain that the incision is deep enough to allow primary closure. Separate
the plate in the midline dorsally so that re-epithelialization of this raw surface over a stent can provide the needed caliber
for the new urethra. **B,** Tubularize the plate over a 6- or 8-F stent with 7-0 absorbable sutures in two layers. Interrupted or
running suture in a subcuticular fashion will turn in the epithelial edge. Use a second layer to incorporate the preserved
periurethral vascularized tissue. Do not close the distal end too tightly leaving the neomeatus oval in shape to prevent
stenosis.

MODIFICATIONS

Despite excellent results with re-epithelialization of the raw incised urethral plate, some have felt the need to apply a graft of inner preputial skin or buccal mucosa to the open surface in a single-stage repair.

WARREN SNODGRASS

Commentary by

The previous edition of this atlas illustrated fibrotic "chordee" tissues from presumably dysplastic corpus spongiosum, once widely believed to extend fanlike from the proximal meatus to the glans, tethering the penis. Since then, three concepts have revolutionized hypospadias surgery: the urethral plate is made up of distinct, well-vascularized tissues (not fibrous scar) that should have formed the urethra; this plate only rarely contributes to ventral curvature; and dorsal incision widens the plate and heals without stricture, enabling urethroplasty without supplemental skin flaps. Tubularized incised plate (TIP) urethroplasty is based on these observations.

Key steps in TIP repair are emphasized in the text and illustrations. Deep incision of a flat or slightly cleft plate widens it to create a normal-caliber neourethra without adding skin flaps. Animal studies and extensive clinical experience show this relaxing incision heals without stricture, and for that reason grafting the defect is not necessary. Other precautions, including taking care to not close the neourethra too far distally, using subepithelial stitches to invert edges during tubularization of the plate, interposing barrier layers over the neourethra, and securely approximating the glans wings, are shared with other hypospadias repair techniques. Nevertheless, clinical studies indicate attention to these details reduces complications.

In that regard, Figure 145-1B shows tubularization of the plate further distally than I would advise. The most distal stitch should be approximately at the midglans, which is about 3 mm from the end of the plate. I suspect some do sew the tube further as suggested in the illustration, wanting to be certain the neomeatus is correctly positioned while believing it necessary to join the end of the tubularized plate to the glans wings. Instead, I close the urethral plate, taking care to leave the end widely oval, and then approximate the glans wings independently over the tubularized plate without specifically sewing glans and neomeatus together.

Complication rates following TIP are no greater than those of other currently used techniques, while cosmetic outcomes have been judged superior to those from flap repairs. The operation was first described for distal hypospadias, but today is also commonly used for proximal repairs when there is not ventral curvature leading the surgeon to transect the plate. TIP is also an option for reoperations if the urethral plate is not grossly scarred.

EDMOND T. GONZALES

Commentary by

Dr. Warren Snodgrass's contribution to hypospadias surgery has been recognized and accepted worldwide. This simple and straightforward technique allows many children with a narrow urethral plate, who previously would have had a more complex preputial or advancement flap, to be repaired by primary tubularization of the plate. Initial concerns that the deep incision in the urethral plate would heal by primary fibrosis with stricture formation rather than re-epithelialization have not been sustained, although a few long-term reports of functional flow rates performed after surgery exist.

The relative ease of this procedure has encouraged its use in much more proximal defects. Whether this extension of the principle is justified will await these reports of long-term follow-up, especially data regarding flow rates. To be sure, onlay preputial flaps have a long and successful history. In my own hands, if I incise the entire urethral plate in a patient with a proximal shaft meatus, I generally perform a dorsal inlay graft of inner preputial skin to provide a surface of new epithelium rather than depend entirely on primary re-epithelialization of the urethral caliber.

Chapter 146

Transverse Tubularized Preputial Island Flap

Historically, the tubularized transverse preputial island flap evolved from the great hypospadiologists, such as Duckett, Standoli, Asopa, and Hodgson. Use of the inner prepuce to reconstruct the urethra was necessary to bridge the gap from the resected urethral plate lost during the correction of chordee. The onlay preputial flap (see Chapter 143) is simpler than the tubularized form and less liable to complications. Realization that the urethral plate is rarely the cause of chordee has relegated the complete tube repair to hypospadias with severe curvature.

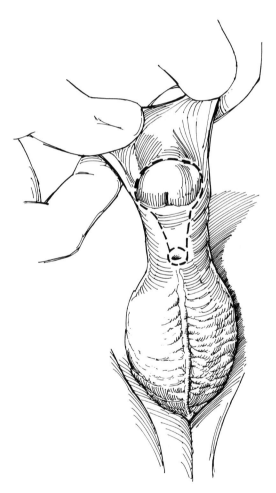

FIGURE 146-1. Place a stay suture on a tapered needle in the glans transversely. Insert an 8-F infant feeding tube through the urethra to confirm that a utricle will not hinder subsequent stent passage. If a utricle is present, passing a 5-F feeding tube into the utricle first will block the entrance, allowing a 6-F stent to now pass into the bladder. Infiltrate the ventral meatal area with 1 or 2 mL of epinephrine-lidocaine solution and wait 7 minutes.

Using a magnifying loupe, mark and incise the skin of the coronal sulcus circumferentially 5 mm from the glans. Extend the incision down the shaft and around the meatus. Leave a generous cuff of ventral tissue. Release the chordee, mobilizing it from the urethra as needed. It may be necessary to dissect around the lateral aspects of the shaft and distally under the glans. Test by artificial erection. Trim the meatus if it is of poor quality. Dissect the dorsal penile skin from Buck's fascia in the avascular plane.

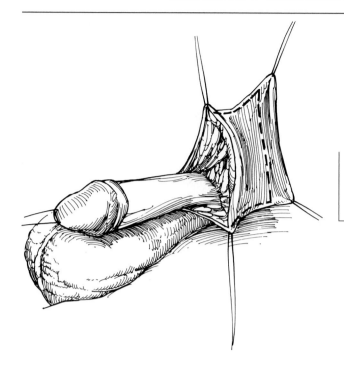

FIGURE 146-2. Place four fine traction sutures to fan out the inner surface of the prepuce. Mark the skin for the neourethra to provide for 3 to 4 cm in length and 1.2 to 1.5 cm in width. Incise along the marks just into the subcutaneous tissue.

FIGURE 146-3. Develop a plane well down to the base of the penis between the new inner flap and the dorsal skin to form a substantial pedicle. Take great care not to devascularize the flap.

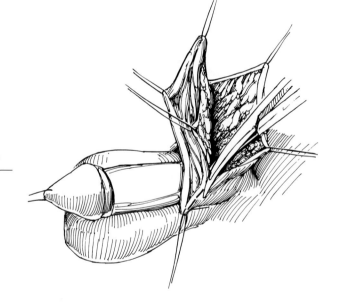

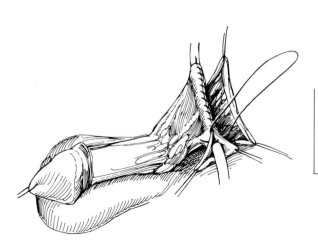

FIGURE 146-4. Roll the flap over a 10- or 12-F catheter and approximate it with a running subcuticular 7-0 or 6-0 chromic catgut suture. A second layer may be applied. At the ends, place interrupted sutures to allow trimming. Replace the catheter with a 6-F silicone catheter or infant feeding tube, passed into the bladder.

FIGURE 146-5. Rotate the flap around its base so that the right side is proximal. Trim and spatulate the distal end of the urethra. Suture the new tube to the urethra so that the suture line of the flap lies deep, against the corpora. Use interrupted 6-0 synthetic absorbable sutures placed with the knots outside.

Insert fine plastic scissors flat against the corpora cavernosa in the plane between the cap of the glans and the corpora and snip a path to the tip of the glans. Remove a large plug of glans, 0.2 × 1.5 cm, and reach inside the meatus to excise excess glanular tissue. Provide a wide channel, at least 16 F in caliber. Make a V-shaped incision at the tip. Check the caliber with a metal sound.

Alternatively and preferably, split the glans (see Chapter 136) before inserting the urethra into the groove. Close the wings with two layers of interrupted sutures.

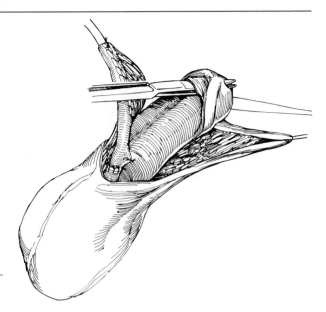

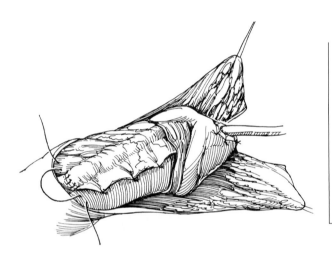

FIGURE 146-6. Pull the tubed flap through the channel or split glans, keeping the suture line against the corporeal bodies. Pull it out straight to eliminate redundant tissue and trim the excess length. Suture the tubed flap to the new meatus with interrupted 7-0 chromic catgut sutures. Fix the tube proximally along the shaft to prevent kinking of the anastomosis. Place a 6-F infant feeding tube as a stent, such that, in infants, the end lies just within the bladder. If possible, cover the anastomosis with a layer of subcutaneous tissue. Drape the pedicle over the ventrum and tuck and tack it in place so that it covers the whole repair. Be careful when placing the sutures not to interfere with the blood supply.

FIGURE 146-7. Divide the prepuce dorsally and suture it ventrally with fine chromic catgut sutures. Excise the lateral triangles to fit. Check the position of the stent, suture it to the glans, and cut it short. Dress the penis with an adhesive elastic dressing. Remove the stent in 10 to 14 days.

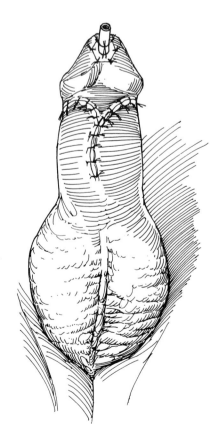

Commentary by
JOHN W. DUCKETT

Clearly, the most important elements for a successful hypospadias outcome are delicate tissue handling, familiarity with mobilizing skin flaps, and compulsive attention to detail characteristic of plastic surgical principles. It is worthwhile to apprentice yourself to a urologist who is doing these complex hypospadias reconstructions before being tempted to proceed, using only these diagrams and simplified steps. There is indeed a learning curve that can be most discouraging.

DOUG CANNING

Commentary by

We use the island tube only in boys with severe hypospadias. This amounts to about 6% or 7% of the repairs at The Children's Hospital of Philadelphia. In some of these severe cases, a large prostatic utricle is present. A large utricle will sometimes prevent easy catheter placement, as the catheter commonly enters the utricle preferentially rather than passing into the bladder neck. If the catheter is difficult to place, in addition to the technique noted in the text, we sometimes place a #1 suture wire into a 6-F Silastic catheter and bend the end of the tube upward. In this way, the tip of the catheter can then be directed anteriorly into the urethra away from the prostatic utricle and successfully placed within the bladder.

I deglove the penis with a ventral incision to the penoscrotal junction on all hypospadias operations in which I intend to use a dorsal flap. In my experience, this mobilization allows for flattening of the penile shaft skin and facilitates identification of the vascular pedicle proximally. The important step when harvesting a vascular preputial island flap is to split the ventral shaft skin of the penis to the penoscrotal junction, including the underlying dartos tissue, to provide the ability to flatten the shaft skin completely. After incising the ventral skin, tension on the traction sutures outlining the proposed flap improves the exposure of the plane between the inner proximal penile shaft skin and the vascular pedicle. With this exposure, the dissection to separate the pedicle of the flap from the shaft skin begins just distal to the penopubic junction and proceeds distally to the inner prepuce. The improved view of the dorsal blood supply of the flap provides better access to a more consistent plane when separating the vascular pedicle than from the dorsal penile shaft skin. I believe this approach reduces the risk of devascularization of the pedicle and makes a tedious dissection more rapid and consistent.

After mobilizing the pedicle of the flap, we generally buttonhole the pedicle, which if carefully performed, does not jeopardize the blood supply and allows easy passage of the pedicle from the dorsum to the ventrum of the penis for use of the preputial skin as a tube. After aggressively spatulating the native urethra, rather than rolling the flap over an 8-F tube to create the neourethra, we prefer to sew the medial edge of the flap to Buck's fascia along the ventral midline of the penile shaft. This line of interrupted subcuticular sutures begins at the native urethra and continues all the way to the glans. The flap is then aggressively trimmed and rolled in situ over an 8-F tube. A second suture line closes the tube with interrupted sutures taken from the lateral edge of the flap into Buck's fascia just adjacent to the first set of sutures. In this way, the suture line is consistently along the dorsum of the penis and the tube is secure with little risk of twisting. This technique allows the surgeon to tailor the tube during the reconstruction to provide a consistent size proximally to distally. This promotes laminar flow through the urethra and reduces the risk of fistula and diverticulum, both of which are more common when urethral flow is turbulent.

We no longer tunnel the tube through the glans, but prefer to incise the glans on the midline. We sometimes remove a segment of glanular tissue from either side to provide for adequate entry of the reconstructed neourethra through the glans. The adjacent dartos tissue accompanying the flap is used as a second layer.

If a postoperative fistula occurs, we do not address it for at least 6 months. In our experience, even a large fistula narrows considerably during the immediate postoperative period. The adjacent tissues soften and blood supply improves as swelling resolves and improves the quality of the tissue available for subsequent repair. In an older child, we wait as long as 1 year before reconstruction.

We have noticed that approximately 85% of our complications occur in the 15% of the more complex cases. In the past, these boys would have had a two-stage repair. Although complications are high with the transverse island tube, when we reviewed our complications following the second stage of a two-stage repair, we found them nearly identical to that following the transverse island tube repair. We think that starting with a single-stage repair reduces the number of trips to the operating room without compromising the result.

Chapter 147

Onlay Urethroplasty with Parameatal Foreskin Flap

KOYANAGI REPAIR

The Koyanagi repair uses a meatal-based foreskin flap. This technique is used for patients with severe hypospadias associated with severe penile curvature.

FIGURE 147-1. Place a traction suture in the glans and release any residual preputial adhesions. Insert a 5-F feeding tube into the bladder. Inject lidocaine and epinephrine for hemostasis or be prepared to use a tourniquet.

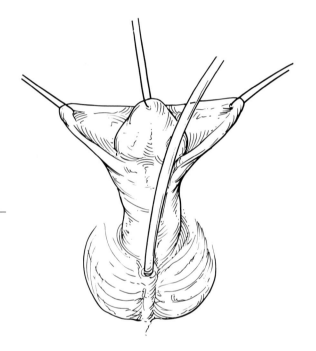

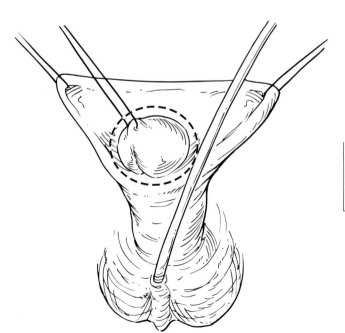

FIGURE 147-2. Mark a skin incision on the inner surface of the prepuce at least 1 cm away from the coronal sulcus, to cross proximally to the meatus and extend laterally on each side to meet in the midline on the dorsum.

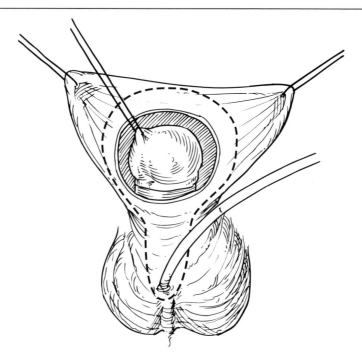

FIGURE 147-3. Mark the incision on the remnant of the distal prepuce by starting from the dorsum on one side and then continuing around the corona down to the urethral plate beneath the glans. Extend the mark all the way along its edge to the most distal end of the glans, at the site of the stay suture. Be sure to make the flap wide enough to cover the plate without tension. On the other side of the prepuce, extend the line from the meatus to the glanular tip, coursing longitudinally along the side of the urethral plate. In the meatal groove, make the lines parallel to each other to keep the meatal plate together with the urethral plate.

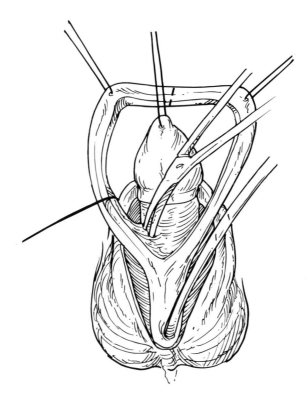

FIGURE 147-4. Deglove the penile shaft proximal to the marked line with curved iris scissors, cutting between Buck's fascia and the dartos fascia. Check by artificial erection for release of the chordee and resect any atretic remnants of the urethra.

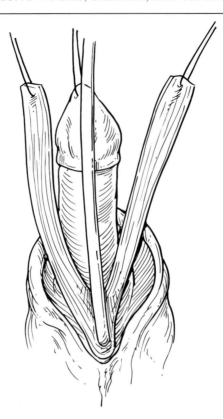

FIGURE 147-5. Cut the marked lines to elevate the parameatal-based "manta-wing" preputial flap, leaving the more central portion in place as the new urethral plate.

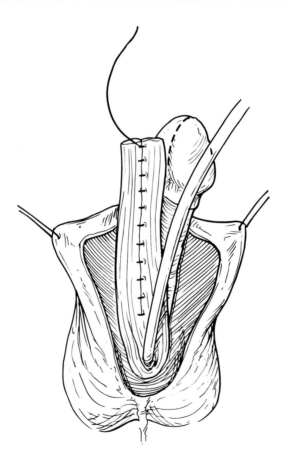

FIGURE 147-6. Make a vertical midline incision into the ventral glans. Deepen the incision to the level of the corpora to free up glans wings. Lay the parameatal foreskin flap on top of the urethral plate. Approximate the loose subcutaneous tissue for a two-layer watertight closure. Anchor the neourethra to the distal edge of the cleft glans. Approximate the glans wings.

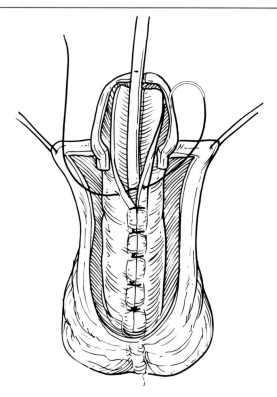

FIGURE 147-7. Divide the prepuce dorsally to form two Byars' flaps.

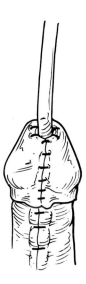

FIGURE 147-8. Swing the flaps ventrally to cover the remaining ventral skin defect.

SABURO TANIKAZE

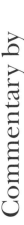

Many novel surgical procedures for hypospadias repair have been described over the last several decades. Now tubularized incised plate (TIP) repair is becoming more popular in many countries. However, there has been debate over whether to preserve the urethral plate in proximal hypospadias with ventral bending. From our experience, untethering of the urethral plate in severe proximal hypospadias brings about improvement of ventral curvature in over 80% of the cases in our series. Koyanagi repair uses meatal-based paracoronal skin flaps, as depicted in the figures, with untethering of the urethral plate down to the base of the penis. After publication of the original paper, many surgeons were concerned by the low success rate and discussed how to preserve the blood supply to the tip of the flaps.

We prefer to do the Koyanagi procedure for penoscrotal or more proximal hypospadias as a one-stage repair. We are not concerned about preserving the subcutaneous tissue of the flap for vascularity. We create a wide flap tip to avoid distal

Continued

shrinkage, while bearing in mind that the neourethra should be covered with enough dartos tissue. Although there is criticism in the use of two suture lines to create the skin tube, thus increasing the potential for fistula formation, meticulous suturing technique overcomes this issue. We use continuous, inverted subcuticular suturing with fine absorbable suture.

In the Koyanagi procedure there is no end-to-end anastomosis; consequently, stenosis around the original meatus is rare. To create the skin tube the dorsal side is closed first, followed by the ventral side; care must be taken that the lowest part of the parameatal flap is closed with tucks such as a purse-string suture to prevent pocket formation. To make a new urethral meatus, we split the glans sharply in the midline. The mucosa of the groove is excised and the neourethra is tucked into the excised edge; then the glans is reapproximated. If the glans is too small to put the neourethra in, a small amount of glanular spongy tissue is excised.

In the case of a small penis, there is often a paucity of lateral skin after harvesting the one-piece skin flap; consequently, a Byars' flap is not enough to cover the ventral surface of the penis, so the flaps are closed in a Z fashion. In general, it is better to close the flaps in the midline to create a central raphe.

We prefer to put an 8-F straight urethral catheter with three holes at the tip for 7 days postoperatively, and to fix the penis with Tegaderm or a DuoActive dressing for several days. We provide a caudal block during the anesthetic process; in general, postoperative pain is not a problem. If necessary, we use a suppository of diclofenac sodium (Voltaren) periodically. For urinary leakage around the catheter, oxybutynin may be effective. Urinary diversion, such as a cystostomy, is not necessary from our experience.

KENNETH GLASSBERG

Commentary by

The Koyanagi repair is very useful for severe hypospadias but should not be done unless there is some urethral plate just distal to the meatus. Since the blood supply is parameatally based, you can safely correct any coexisting penoscrotal transposition under the same anesthetic.

Keep in mind that the Koyanagi repair is an alternative to a staged repair and when done for severe hypospadias, there is at least a 25% incidence of need to repair a fistula or some cosmetic tune-up. I have never seen it associated with postoperative stricture or meatal stenosis.

STEVE KOFF

Commentary by

Proximal hypospadias repair is a challenging undertaking that can be facilitated by ancillary procedures. The first is pretreatment with androgens. I prefer a 5-week (orchiopexy) course of human chorionic gonadotropin (250 to 500 international units twice weekly) and have observed the following advantageous effects that facilitate proximal repairs and improve outcomes: penile lengthening and size increase, movement distally of the meatus away from the scrotum, increased amounts of shaft and preputial skin, increased tissue vascularity, reduction of chordee, and enhanced visualization of hair follicles.

The second is proximal penile shaft vascular control. This is accomplished by making a midline scrotal incision about 2 cm or more proximal to the hypospadiac urethral meatus, dissecting circumferentially around the penile shaft, and passing a rubber band around the shaft for use as a tourniquet.

The most important part of the Koyanagi operative procedure involves maintaining lateral vascular supply to the entire length of the preputial flaps as they are dissected away from the lateral shaft and preputial skin (see Figs. 147-4 to 147-6). This vascularized technique, which is a modification of Koyanagi's original technique, has been shown to significantly reduce the incidence of fistula formation. To reduce the likelihood of fistularization, it is also essential to cover the neourethra with a second layer of tissue that can come either from the tissues supporting the lateral blood supply brought to the midline or from de-epithelialized dartos tissue that is part of the Byars' flaps.

Chapter 148

Free Tube Graft

The free tube graft is appropriate for repair of moderate to severe hypospadias with chordee. Alternatives are onlay grafts, tube repairs, or two-stage procedures.

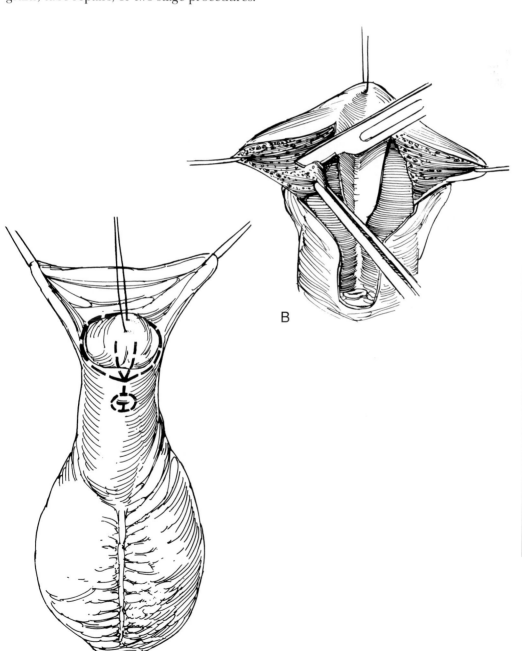

B

A

FIGURE 148-1. A, Place a traction suture in the glans. Mark a V-shaped incision on the glans, and run it around the meatus. Infiltrate the area with 1 mL of 1:100,000 epinephrine solution in 1% lidocaine. Incise the coronal sulcus. B, Elevate the wings of the glans with skin hooks and begin dissection of the ventral tissues that produce chordee. Continue freeing behind the meatus and urethra until the penis can be shown to be straight by artificial erection. Trim and discard the thinned tissue from the terminal urethra and notch it on the ventral edge. Separate the glans from the corpora raising glans wings to a 90-degree angle with the glanular urethral plate.

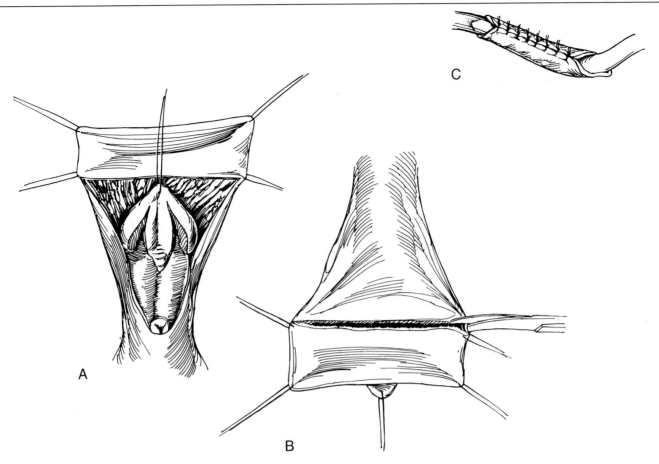

FIGURE 148-2. A, Unfold the dorsal prepuce and place four stay sutures in it at least 1.4 cm apart and at a distance that is 10% longer than the length needed to replace the urethra, since 75% circumferential shrinkage of the graft is expected. **B,** Cut the graft and defat it over the finger or on a board coated with double-surfaced dermatome tape. **C,** Attach the full-thickness, fat-free graft, skin surface inside, to a suitable-size catheter at a site that will allow the end of the catheter to lie in the bladder. Use interrupted 6-0 synthetic absorbable sutures. Cut both ends of the graft obliquely and insert the catheter into the bladder.

FIGURE 148-3. Suture the dorsal side of the proximal end of the graft first, using 6-0 synthetic absorbable sutures, and continue around to the ventrum. Place a suture from the tip of the glans flap through the apex of the oblique cut in the graft.

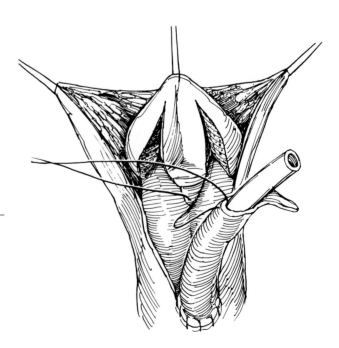

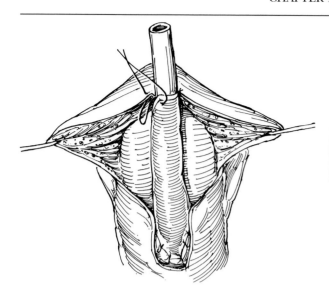

FIGURE 148-4. Complete the approximation of the flap and graft. Place interrupted 6-0 synthetic absorbable sutures along the graft, securing the graft to the corporeal bed.

FIGURE 148-5. Cover the free preputial tube graft by rotation of the remainder of the subcutaneous pedicle flap.

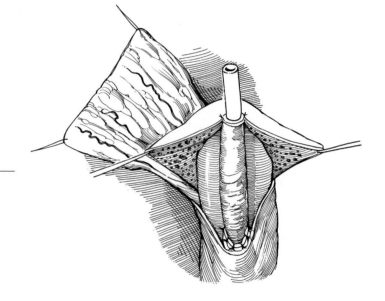

FIGURE 148-6. Close the glans over the graft in two layers with 6-0 synthetic absorbable sutures, and suture the graft to the edges of the glans with 6-0 or 7-0 synthetic absorbable sutures.

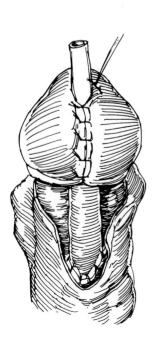

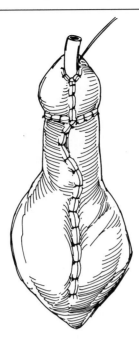

FIGURE 148-7. Split the remaining prepuce and approximate it ventrally, trying to keep from superimposing suture lines. Suture the cutoff catheter to the meatus and leave it in place for 10 to 14 days.

CHARLES J. DEVINE, JR.

Commentary by

When Charlie Horton and I began our experience with genitourinary reconstructive surgery, hypospadias was accomplished in multiple stages, first straightening the penis and moving the extra skin in the prepuce to the ventrum of the penis so that it could be formed into a tube at the next operation. Confidence in our ability to get the penis straight at the first operation encouraged us to develop a one-stage repair of hypospadias using skin grafts. Earlier, surgeons had a great deal of difficulty using split skin grafts for urethroplasty, but Young and Benjamin (1948 and 1949) had demonstrated that full-thickness skin grafts used as skin repairs did not contract. McCormack (1954), applying this knowledge, made a urethra at the time of straightening the penis, but he left a fistula at the junction of the natural urethra and a neourethra to be closed at a later stage. We began to make the anastomosis watertight at the first stage and were very pleased with the results at our first report in 1963. Of our patients, 69% required no further operations. Through the years, this success has improved and, at present, fully 85% to 90% of our patients need no further surgery. We have watched our first patients go through puberty. The grafts, especially those from the penis, have continued to grow with the patients so that later chordee has not been a problem. We feel that placement of the graft onto the straightened penis has helped to ensure this.

Others have had problems with the grafts, which have led to development of techniques of hypospadias repair using flaps of preputial skin. We have used these flaps and find that they work well, but, in our hands, they are no better than grafts. In some special circumstances, however, the graft will still be better, especially when we have had to incise the ventral tunica to release chordee.

The surgeon doing hypospadias repair should have a full armamentarium and should make the procedure fit the patient.

GEORGE W. KAPLAN

Commentary by

I remain a devotee of free preputial skin grafts for repair of moderate to severe hypospadias. Although in the past tube grafts were used, I now try to retain the urethral plate in situ. If the plate can be maintained, I then apply the graft as an onlay rather than using it as a tube. If the plate is intact, I often will elevate the distal aspect of the plate and bury it more deeply in the glans as described by Barcat, which gives a very nice and reliable glanuloplasty producing a slitlike distal meatus. If a tube graft has been used, I will usually merely bivalve the glans so that the graft can be placed deep into the glans, once again producing a slitlike distal meatus. If a free graft is used, it is very important that well-vascularized tissue be brought over it so that it will insulate well. Employing these approaches, the success rate of severe hypospadias repair in a single stage occurs in 85% to 90% of cases.

The success rate of grafts and flaps was the same in our institution. Conceptually, both onlay and tube grafts are much easier to visualize and plan than are some of the flap procedures that have been described. Additionally, free grafts use less of the foreskin than do many of the pedicle flaps. Hence, a one-stage repair of even very severe hypospadias is frequently possible with a graft unless there is severe chordee that necessitates using a dermal or tunica vaginalis graft for the chordee repair. As I am reticent to place a tubed urethral graft on a graft in the corpora cavernosa in the same procedure, I would most likely stage the repair in that scenario.

I stent the repair with a silicone catheter that I leave in place for 7 to 8 days, as experimental studies have shown that re-epithelialization is complete by then.

Chapter 149

Two-Stage Primary Skin Repair

This repair is easy to learn, with few pitfalls for the surgeon, but it does require two stages. It may be a good choice for perineal or scrotal repairs, for previous failures and cases with marginal amounts of prepuce. It may be especially applicable in a boy with a small penis. If a repair had been difficult to complete in one stage, switching to this operation after the chordee had been corrected may be a safe alternative.

FIRST STAGE

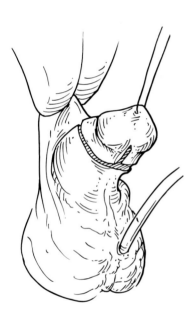

FIGURE 149-1. Make a circumferential incision just proximal to the coronal sulcus and extend it up the midline to the meatus.

FIGURE 149-2. A, Deglove the shaft and excise the chordee. **B,** Apply a tourniquet to the base and create an artificial erection. If the penis is still not straight, consider a midline dorsal plication (see Chapter 133) or, in severe cases, a dermal graft (see Chapter 135).

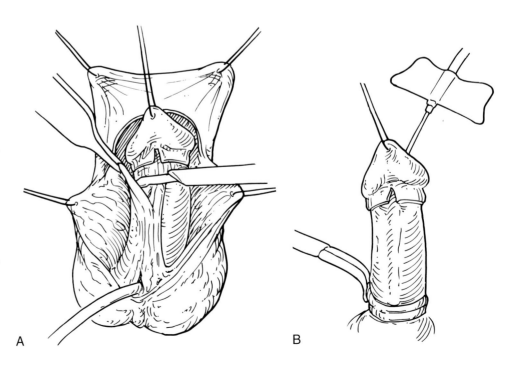

A   B

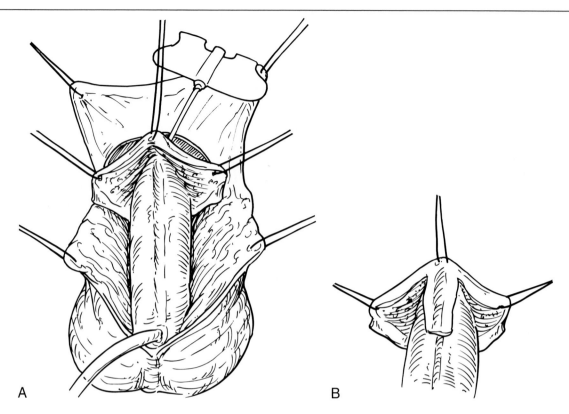

FIGURE 149-3. **A,** Divide the glans deeply in the midline and mobilize glans wings off the corporeal body. **B,** Alternatively, with a deep mucosal groove, make parallel incisions lateral to the groove and preserve the median epithelial portion.

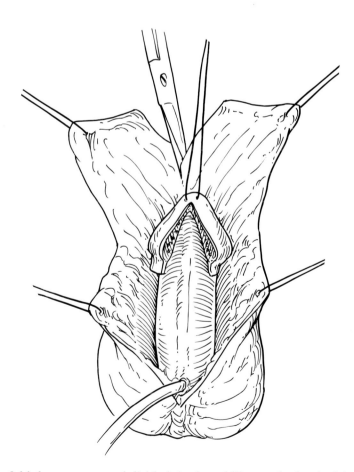

FIGURE 149-4. Carefully unfold the prepuce and divide it in the midline to the level of the coronal sulcus.

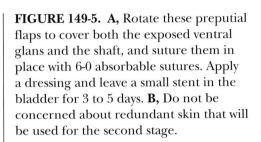

FIGURE 149-5. A, Rotate these preputial flaps to cover both the exposed ventral glans and the shaft, and suture them in place with 6-0 absorbable sutures. Apply a dressing and leave a small stent in the bladder for 3 to 5 days. **B,** Do not be concerned about redundant skin that will be used for the second stage.

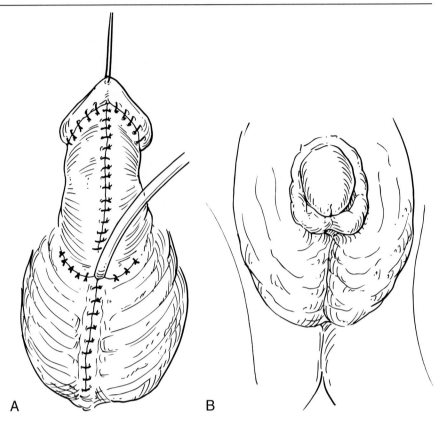

A   B

SECOND STAGE

Allow healing for 6 to 12 months.

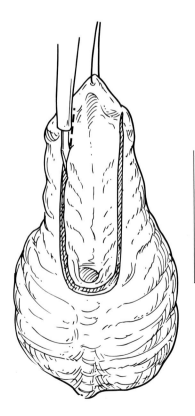

FIGURE 149-6. Mark two parallel lines on the ventrum spaced according to the size of the patient (i.e., 1.5 cm apart in infants, 2.5 cm in children, and 3 cm in adolescents). Try not to include any scrotal skin in the repair; hair, stones, and infection will follow at puberty. Place these incisions eccentrically so that at closure the suture line of the neourethra will not coincide with that of the skin (fistula is the most common complication). Incise along the marks, beginning at one end with a knife, and then proceed with blunt-tipped scissors to cut an edge in the skin at right angles to the surface. Do not mobilize the edges of the strip.

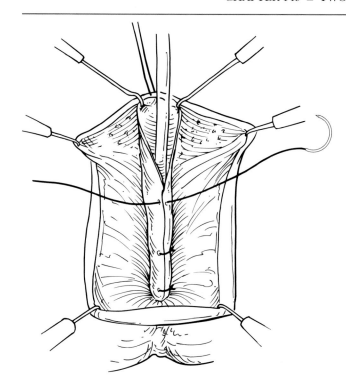

FIGURE 149-7. Mobilize the glans flap and wings as previously described (see Chapter 136). Elevate the edges of the strip with skin hooks, raising the wider side of the strip more than the other side so that the urethral suture line will lie to one side. Tack the edges together in three or four places to maintain orientation. Now run a subcuticular suture of 6-0 polydioxanone to close the strip as a tube over an 8-F feeding tube in babies.

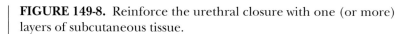

FIGURE 149-8. Reinforce the urethral closure with one (or more) layers of subcutaneous tissue.

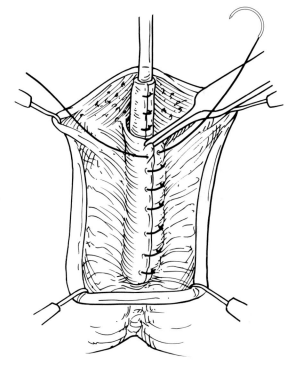

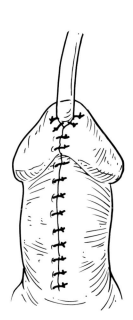

FIGURE 149-9. Approximate the glans with at least one layer of deep sutures. Use fine interrupted 7-0 catgut sutures to encircle the new meatus at the surface. Close the skin with either a running subcuticular suture or with interrupted sutures, trying not to have the suture line in the skin over that of the urethra. Dress the penis appropriately. Remove the catheter in 10 days.

SAUL GREENFIELD

While there are many variations of two-stage hypospadias repair, certain basic principles are shared by all of them. First, the staged approach may have its greatest utility in situations in which it is judged that chordee correction requires transection of the urethral plate and removal of the chordee tissue in the region between the urethra and the glans. Complete elimination of chordee also often requires that the urethra itself be dissected off the underlying corporeal bodies and moved more proximally. Second, small penises can be treated with testosterone injections before both the first and second stages, thereby maximizing whatever response that patient may have to androgen stimulation.

In the first stage, I prefer not to bisect the dorsal foreskin and rotate the flaps ventrally, but rather to place a buttonhole in the penile shaft skin, through which the glans is placed. This transfers the prepuce ventrally without having a midline suture line on the ventral penile shaft. The tissue that is then tubularized into a urethra in the second stage is for the most part virgin and unscarred. In addition, the first stage is an ideal opportunity to recreate a normal-appearing glans. This can be done by resecting the entire glanular urethral groove and re-anastomosing the glans in the midline. The abnormal-appearing ventral mucosal folds, which are lateral to this groove, can then be unfolded and also anastomosed in the midline. These maneuvers eliminate the flattened appearance of the hypospadiac glans, making it conical in shape, and also result in a coronal sulcus that is circumferential and complete ventrally. This glans is then tunneled through at the second stage, and fresh, overlapping suture lines are avoided distally in the glans.

During the second stage the urethra is tubularized and tunneled through the now normal-appearing glans. I use an interrupted 7-0 Vicryl stitch for tubularization. A second interrupted layer in Lembert fashion is placed along the entire neourethra, again using 7-0 Vicryl. To minimize distal stenosis, the glanular tunnel is dilated up to 18 or 20 F, divots of spongy tissue are sharply removed from the interior of the glans, and ellipses of glanular skin are removed from the meatal location, prior to placing the neourethra in position. This also helps to achieve a slitlike urethral meatus. At this point the importance of second layers of tissue and the avoidance of overlapping suture lines cannot be overemphasized. Once the urethra is placed in position, subcutaneous tissue can be harvested from the adjacent penile and scrotal skin and tacked over the urethra to avoid overlapping suture lines. Alternatively, tunica vaginalis can be used. Therefore, even if a portion of the skin closure lines is directly over the urethra, there is healthy, uninterrupted tissue between the urethral and cutaneous suture lines. Urethrocutaneous fistula formation can also be minimized by using mattress sutures to evert the skin edges during skin closure.

Suture choice is important. I have not used long-lasting absorbable sutures for the skin and subcutaneous layers, since they may increase the likelihood of fistulas and cause "suture tracks." My preference is to use 7-0 Vicryl for the urethra and all remaining suturing is done with 6-0 chromic catgut. There are many methods of urinary diversion and stenting. The urine should be diverted for between 10 and 14 days. Since catheters can become dislodged prematurely, I have always used a backup system, whereby a short Silastic stent is placed across the repair and sutured to the glans. A feeding tube is placed through this stent into the bladder and also sutured to the glans. If the feeding tube comes out too soon, it can easily be replaced without causing any trauma to the repair.

Some, but not all, children require anticholinergic medication to prevent bladder spasms and voiding across the repair while at home. We routinely employ caudal anesthesia during surgery and children are sent home with adequate pain medication. Acetaminophen (Tylenol) and codeine combinations work well. Older children and postpubescent boys are in more discomfort after this surgery and they occasionally benefit from epidural or spinal anesthesia for a few days, requiring longer hospital stays. Finally, all children receive intravenous cephalosporin after the induction of anesthesia, followed by 2 weeks of oral cephalosporin.

ALAN B. RETIK

Two-stage repairs in babies with scrotal or perineal hypospadias who have small organs not responding to testosterone should be strongly considered. Although a one-stage repair is possible, the cosmetics are unappealing.

At the first stage, if there is still residual chordee after the usual maneuvers, I will often insert a dermal graft ventrally at the site of the maximum bend. The graft is obtained from the groin. It is important at the first stage to incise the glans deeply and slightly dorsally to be absolutely certain that enough foreskin is placed in the glans to be tubularize at a second stage. I often tack the midline skin closure to the corpora ventrally to eliminate dead space.

Surgery for the second stage is usually done approximately 9 months after the first stage. I tubularize the urethra with a running subcuticular fine absorbable suture. The glans is wrapped loosely around the urethra in layers. The skin is trimmed appropriately and closed with pullout sutures of 4-0 nylon as subcutaneous and subcuticular running sutures. This enables the tissues to adjust for any tension created on the suture lines. The pullout sutures are removed approximately 10 days later.

Chapter 150

Two-Stage Revision Buccal Mucosa Hypospadias Repair

This repair is most appropriate for salvage hypospadias surgery but can be used for severe proximal hypospadias. Provide general anesthesia supplemented with a caudal or penile block.

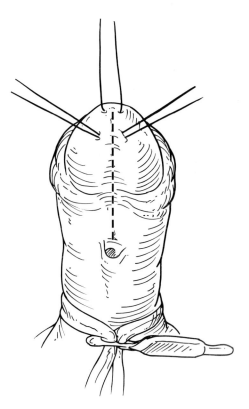

FIGURE 150-1. Place a traction suture in the glans. This illustration depicts a midshaft hypospadias with a paucity of available skin after multiple previous hypospadias repairs. With an iris scissors or #15 blade remove the previous scar tissue exposing the glans and corporeal bodies.

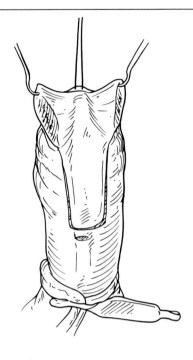

FIGURE 150-2. Check for chordee with an artificial erection. Mobilize glans wings and prepare the meatus, checking for stenosis. Place stay sutures along the glans to facilitate exposure.

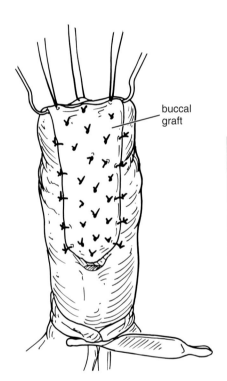

buccal graft

FIGURE 150-3. Harvest a buccal mucosa graft (see Chapter 131) when local tissue is not available. In primary severe cases a preputial graft from the inner layer of the preputial hood can be used and if that is not available, consider a postauricular (Wolfe) graft.

Hold the glans apart with the stay sutures, trim the graft exactly to fit the defect, and suture it in place with 6-0 absorbable sutures. Add quilting sutures within the bed to facilitate graft take.

FIGURE 150-4. Place rolled gauze over the graft and hold it in place by first tying the stay sutures over it, and then adding more fine sutures. Place the knots centrally for easy removal. Place a catheter in the bladder. The catheter can be removed in 3 to 5 days and the dressing in 7 to 10 days.

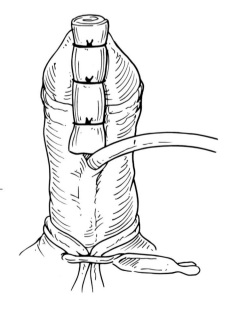

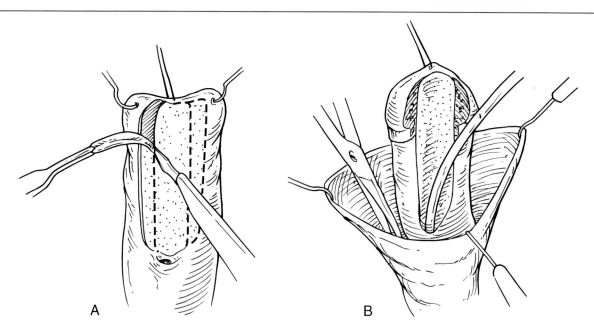

FIGURE 150-5. **A** and **B,** Plan the second-stage surgery for 6 months to 1 year later. Expect 10% to 15% shrinkage of both buccal and skin grafts. Outline a urethroplasty of appropriate size by trimming buccal tissue within the glans and along the corporeal bodies.

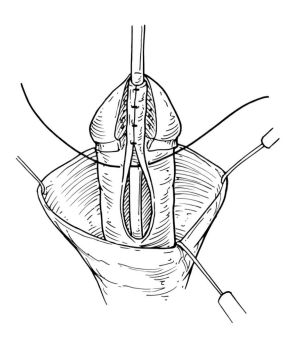

FIGURE 150-6. Perform the urethroplasty with 5-0 or 6-0 absorbable suture. Extra coverage with surrounding dartos tissue will prevent fistula. If the dartos tissue is not available use the tunica vaginalis (see Chapter 129).

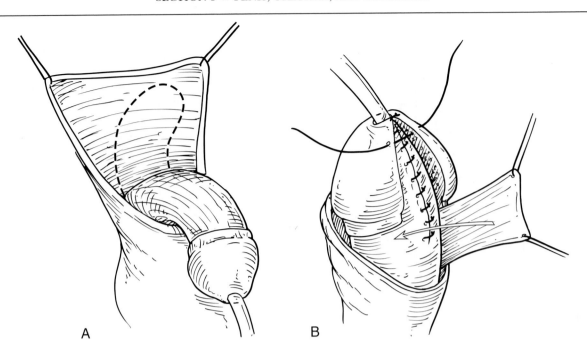

A   B

FIGURE 150-7. A, Create a dartos layer from the dorsal or lateral aspect of the penis. **B,** Cover the urethroplasty preventing opposing suture lines.

FIGURE 150-8. Close the glans in two layers over the urethroplasty.

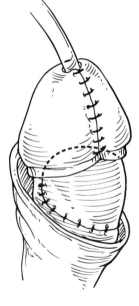

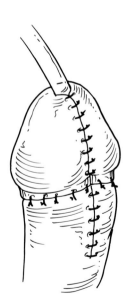

FIGURE 150-9. Organize the skin coverage. A catheter should be left indwelling for 7 to 10 days.

AIVAR BRACKA

Commentary by

For many hypospadias deformities where I would have previously used a two-stage repair, I can now achieve comparable results in a single stage, but the evolution of one-stage surgery still has some way to go before the Philadelphia "one-stage for everything" philosophy becomes a realistic prospect.

I remain puzzled, for instance, as to why urologists are prepared to struggle with one-stage tubed buccal mucosa reconstructions and accept up to 50% complication rates, when doing it in two stages is far easier, safer, free of maintenance postoperatively, and with superior aesthetic results. It is unfortunate that inflexible ideology should prevent the patient from getting the best outcome.

Fortunately, the emerging new generation of pediatric urologists are taking a more enlightened view of two-stage repair and are recognizing that in some situations it still remains the safest and most refined surgical option currently available, and therefore should be part of their armamentarium.

Chapter 151

Penoscrotal Transposition Repair

PENOSCROTAL TRANSPOSITION REPAIR (GLENN-ANDERSON)

The two halves of the scrotum are mobilized to form rotational advancement flaps to fill the space beneath the released penile shaft. If not associated with a hypospadiac meatus, incisions that circle over the top of each scrotal half and meet beneath the base of the penis may be sufficient if the scrotum is widely mobilized and the two wings are rotated beneath the penis, either in the midline or as a Z-plasty.

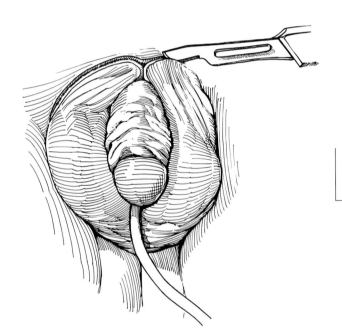

FIGURE 151-1. Insert a silicone balloon catheter in the urethra. Make a curved transverse incision just above the upper scrotal folds.

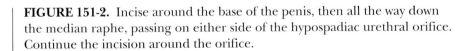

FIGURE 151-2. Incise around the base of the penis, then all the way down the median raphe, passing on either side of the hypospadiac urethral orifice. Continue the incision around the orifice.

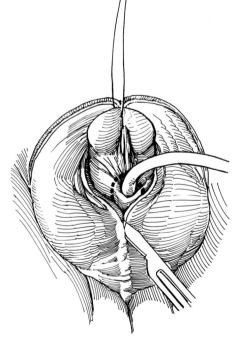

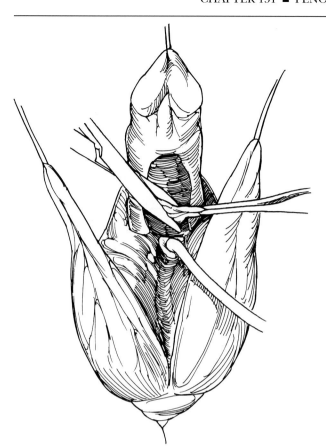

FIGURE 151-3. Free the underlying urethra and excise all the fibrous tissue of the chordee from the ventral surface.

FIGURE 151-4. Draw the lateral scrotal flaps distally into the defect under the penis, bring them underneath the penis, and join them in the midline. Situate the meatus at its distal, most-comfortable spot.

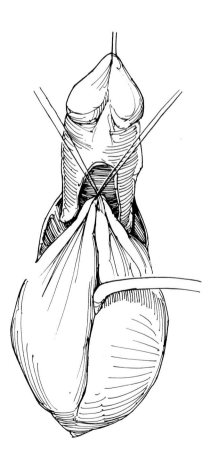

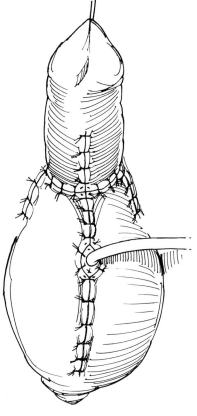

FIGURE 151-5. Close the repair around the new meatus in two layers with 5-0 plain catgut sutures subcutaneously and with interrupted 6-0 chromic catgut sutures for the skin. Remove the catheter in 2 or 3 days. Construct the urethra after complete revascularization of the flaps has occurred.

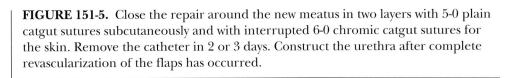

PENOSCROTAL TRANSPOSITION ONE-STAGE REPAIR (PEROVIC)

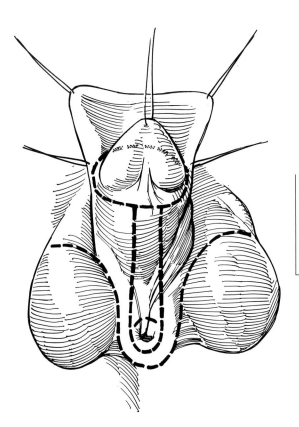

FIGURE 151-6. Mark an incision around the coronal sulcus, continue it along the ventral surface to encircle the hypospadiac meatus and leave a midline strip that will be excised with the chordee. Mark a second incision, beginning below the meatus and continuing up the medial side of the split scrotum and over the anterior aspect at the scrotal base. Incise along the lines.

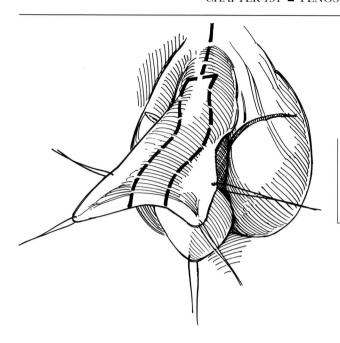

FIGURE 151-7. Deglove the penis. Incise an island flap on the dorsum that will form the new urethra; this leaves a flap of skin on either side of the shaft. Continue the dorsal incision proximally at the base of the penis. Excise the chordee. Correct residual chordee with dorsal midline plication.

FIGURE 151-8. Bluntly make a longitudinal opening in an avascular area, as revealed by transillumination of the vascular pedicle. Free the proximal urethra, and discard the friable tip. Pass the penis through the opening in the dorsal flap.

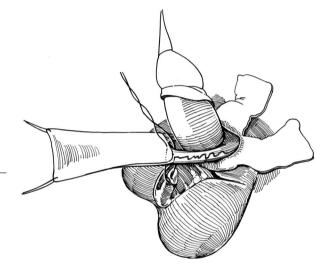

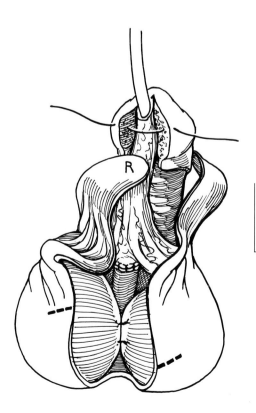

FIGURE 151-9. Tubularize the island flap, and anastomose the stump of the urethra to it. Excise a groove in the ventrum of the glans, and bring the new urethra to the tip. Suture the testes to each other and place traction sutures in each lower pole. Make staggered cuts on either side of the scrotum.

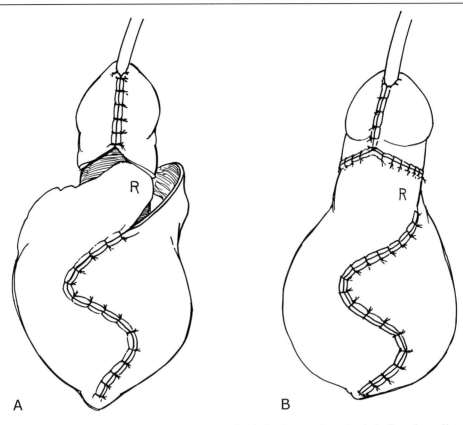

FIGURE 151-10. **A** and **B,** Rotate the right skin flap (R) to the left, then swing the left flap dorsally to cover that aspect of the shaft. Close the scrotum in Z-fashion. Provide drainage. To prevent elevation of the testes, maintain traction on them for a week or two by tying the traction sutures over a bolster.

SAVA PEROVIC

Commentary by

Penoscrotal transposition is characterized by malposition of the penis in relation to the scrotum. In complete transposition the scrotum covers the penis, which emerges from the perineum. In incomplete transposition, which is more common, the penis lies in the middle of the scrotum. Both forms are most often associated with severe forms of hypospadias. Surgical treatment is based on severity of transposition and associated hypospadias. The anomaly is often associated with cryptorchidism as well as disorders of sexual differentiation, which should be identified before surgery.

The goal of surgical treatment is to achieve normal anatomic position of the penis and scrotum with concurrent correction of the severe hypospadias. Since there is no unique operative approach for different forms of penoscrotal transposition with hypospadias, an individual surgical concept is of primary significance.

How do we approach treatment? The first step toward satisfactory outcome is adequate assessment of all characteristics of the anomaly: penile size, size and adequacy of the glans cleft, quality of urethral plate, degree of chordee, available penile skin that is usually present only dorsally as a triangle, and severity of penoscrotal transposition and associated anomalies, especially disorders of sexual differentiation.

Long-term results of one-stage repair of severe hypospadias associated with penoscrotal transposition, using tubularized, dorsal longitudinal penile skin-flaps urethroplasty, showed a complication rate of over 25%. They are related to urethroplasty and penile entrapment as a consequence of insufficient dorsal penile shaft skin. Thus, we abandoned tubularization of dorsal, longitudinal skin flaps, and now we use it only as a ventral onlay. The principle of penoscrotal repair is the same: after creation of a dorsal longitudinal island skin flap for ventral onlay urethroplasty and additional sagittal incision of pubic skin, the hole in the flap pedicle is created as far dorsally as possible and is then transposed ventrally using a buttonhole maneuver. This way, the penis is moved dorsally over the scrotum. Next, two lateral, longitudinal penile skin flaps are fully mobilized together with lateral scrotal flaps as one unit to preserve vascularization. They are moved ventrally and rotated in different ways to cover the penile shaft. This way the penis is moved dorsally in relation to the scrotum, correcting penoscrotal transposition. Lateral scrotal flaps can also be mobilized separately and rotated ventrally to correct the bifid scrotum.

Also, we consider whether a one-stage repair or staged procedure should be done. If the penis has good size and the urethral plate moderate chordee, we prefer one-stage urethroplasty simultaneous with repair of penoscrotal transposition. Concerning urethroplasty, there are several options depending on quality of the urethral plate: simple tubularization, tubularized incised plate (TIP) urethroplasty, TIP urethroplasty augmented with buccal mucosa graft, and onlay flap urethroplasty with or without dissection of urethral plate. In cases with a short urethral plate, inlay-onlay urethroplasty is performed: the gap created after division of the urethral plate is inlayed with buccal mucosa graft quilted to the underlying corpora. Ventral onlay urethroplasty follows. We perform correction of curvature in two ways: simple dorsal plication of the wounded tunica albuginea or dorsal corporoplasty by longitudinal corporotomy with transverse closure (Heineke-Mikulicz principle). In cases with cryptorchidism, simultaneous orchiopexy is performed through the scrotal or additional inguinal incision.

In severe, particularly complete penoscrotal transposition with a small, severely curved penis with an absent or poorly developed urethral plate and penile skin, staged repair is preferred. Two-stage buccal mucosa urethroplasty is performed, while straightening and lengthening of the penis is made by ventral corporotomy and grafting, thus avoiding penile shortening by dorsal corporoplasty. Penoscrotal transposition requires the same principle of correction as incomplete forms but often requires staged repair.

Using current technique the rate of complications is decreased, but it is interestingly similar between one-stage and staged procedures—approximately 12%.

BUTTONHOLE TECHNIQUE FOR CORRECTION OF PENOSCROTAL TRANSPOSITION (REDA)

Patients amenable to correction of penoscrotal transposition by the buttonhole technique have severe chordee typically requiring dermal grafting to correct the curvature.

The chordee is corrected during the first-stage hypospadias repair along with the penoscrotal transposition. Prior to the first-stage repair the size of the phallus is accessed to see if the patient will benefit from possible testosterone therapy. At a second-stage operation 4 to 6 months later the urethroplasty and hypospadias repair are completed.

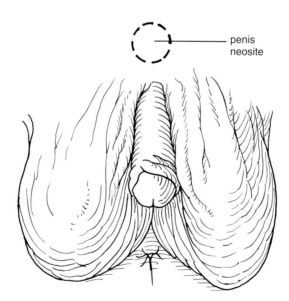

FIGURE 151-11. After placement of a glans-holding suture, perform urethral catheterization to rule out a utricle. Mark the site of the transposed penis in the suprapubic area. The circumference of the proposed site should approximate the circumference of the penis.

FIGURE 151-12. Deglove the penis in routine fashion and perform artificial erection to determine the extent of the chordee. Repair significant chordee by interposition of a dermal graft. Excise a plug of epidermis and underlying subcutaneous fat from the site to create a suprapubic buttonhole or well that will ultimately accommodate the new penis. A bar of skin in subcutaneous tissue separates the buttonhole from the superior margin of the scrotum to lend support and provide dependency to the transposed penis. Use a mosquito clamp to create a passage from the new site of the penis. The size of the buttonhole should not be any larger than the diameter of the penis.

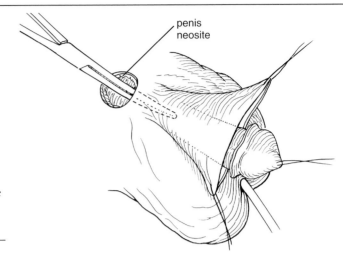

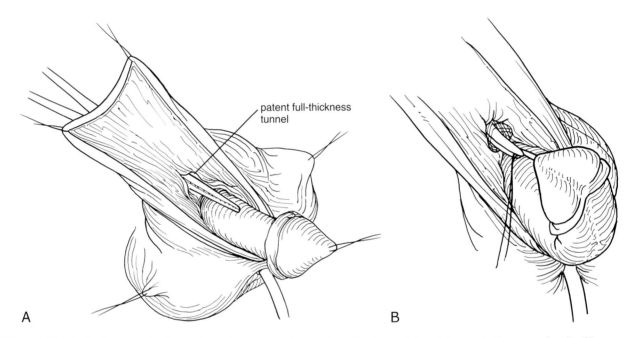

FIGURE 151-13. A, Retract the foreskin and prepare the penis to be brought out through the new site. **B,** Use a mosquito clamp to grab the holding stitch and pull the penis through the new window.

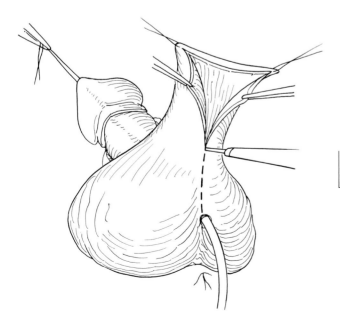

FIGURE 151-14. Split the shaft skin down the ventrum to the proximal urethral meatus.

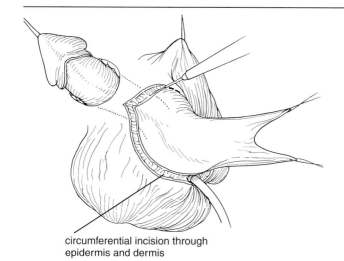

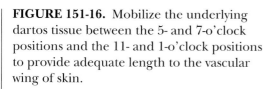

circumferential incision through
epidermis and dermis

FIGURE 151-15. Make a circumferential incision through the epidermis and dermis at the base of the shaft skin.

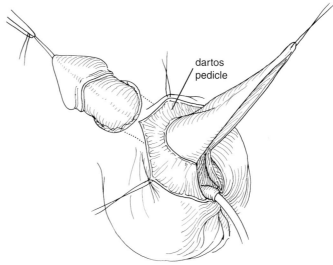

dartos
pedicle

FIGURE 151-16. Mobilize the underlying dartos tissue between the 5- and 7-o'clock positions and the 11- and 1-o'clock positions to provide adequate length to the vascular wing of skin.

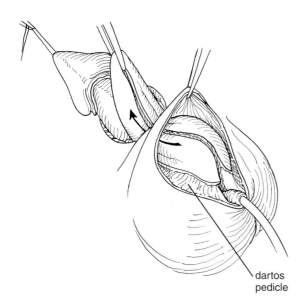

dartos
pedicle

FIGURE 151-17. Deliver the unfurled shaft skin underneath the skin bridge *(arrow)* through the previously created dartos window and out through the buttonhole.

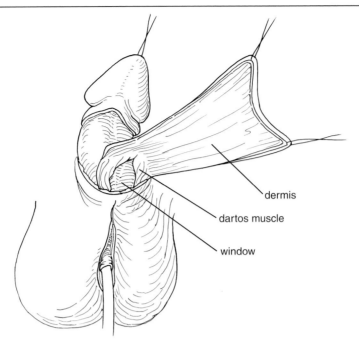

FIGURE 151-18. The penis and shaft skin have been transposed but they are not properly oriented because the epithelial surface of the shaft skin is inferior and flush with a degloved phallus. The penis, therefore, must be delivered through a newly created window in the dartos tissue to achieve proper orientation with the shaft skin.

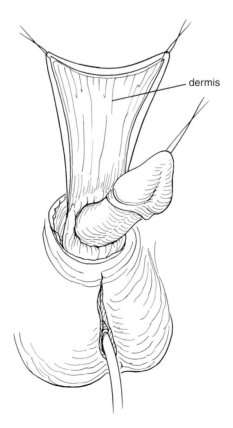

FIGURE 151-19. The penis foreskin and scrotum are now properly oriented spatially and anatomically.

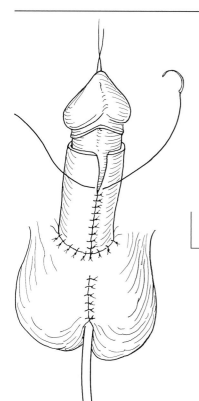

FIGURE 151-20. Resurface the skin to the penis along with a midline scrotoplasty to complete the first-stage hypospadias repair with correction of the penoscrotal transposition.

ISRAEL FRANCO

Commentary by

Correction of penoscrotal transposition can be difficult at times. An excellent review by Husmann and Kramer on their experience with this problem using the Glenn-Anderson technique illustrated the problems that are encountered in complex hypospadias surgery. The complication rate was high in a series of patients who needed penoscrotal transposition repair along with hypospadias repair. We understand that maintenance of a good blood supply to the tissue is critical to the prevention of fistulas and breakdown of skin flaps. The Glenn-Anderson technique requires the creation of multiple flaps that may have compromised the blood supply at their distal edges. In many instances this same tissue that has diminished blood flow may be used to create the urethra later on if the penoscrotal transposition repair is done at the time of the original chordee correction. In other cases this tissue with its decreased blood supply is used to cover the neourethra. In all cases, the multiple flaps with their impaired blood flow are a lightning rod for fistulas and tissue breakdown.

The buttonhole technique created by Ed Reda calls for the maintenance of the blood supply to the flap with little disturbance to the overall blood flow to the penile skin. The dartos tissue is preserved throughout the whole shaft skin, thereby keeping blood flow to the tissue at its maximum. Maintenance of this blood supply allows for an improved success rate in penile reconstruction and prevention of fistulas. Preservation of the penile skin with its normal anatomy can allow for the creation of de-epithelialized flaps in subsequent repairs if there is a need.

The buttonhole technique is a great alternative to the Glenn-Anderson technique, especially when the surgeon has the foresight to anticipate its use in the original surgery. The technique cannot be applied after the chordee correction is done. In many cases when the Glenn-Anderson technique is used it may be necessary to perform three operations in some boys to correct the chordee, hypospadias, and transposition. When you anticipate and use the buttonhole technique only two procedures may be necessary.

We have used the buttonhole technique exclusively for the last 10 years with an excellent cosmetic and functional result. The technique can be used for patients who have penoscrotal transposition without hypospadias, as well as for patients that undergo a one-stage repair of their hypospadias and transposition. The only issue we have seen in some of these patients is shrouding at the base, which was due to wide initial opening when the plug of skin was removed. We have corrected this by making the initial plug of skin no greater than the diameter of the penile shaft. The bar of tissue that is left between penis and scrotum can be removed at the subsequent stage when the penile urethra is reconstructed. Scarring is barely noticeable at the base of the penis, and when the patient goes through puberty and hair covers the mons the scar will be even less noticeable.

Chapter 152

Foreskin Preservation

Foreskin preservation can be successfully performed in patients with hypospadias that do not have significant ventral skin deficiency and chordee. A distal penile shaft coronal or glanular meatus without chordee is best suited for this type of procedure.

Preoperative counseling should include a discussion of postoperative preputial adhesions.

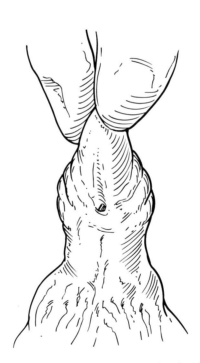

FIGURE 152-1. Place a 5-0 monofilament holding suture for traction in the distal aspect of the glans.

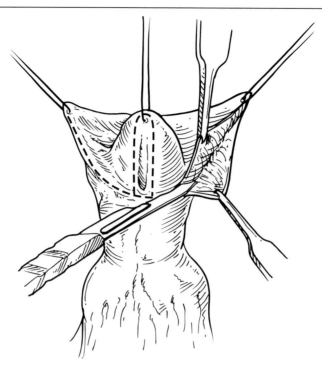

FIGURE 152-2. Make an exaggerated, wide V-shape incision from the corners of the dorsal preputial hood to just underneath the hypospadiac meatus. Place holding sutures to define the abortive prepuce and to aid in placement of the lateral borders of the incision. Make two parallel incisions at the borders of the urethral plate within the glans to define the new urethra.

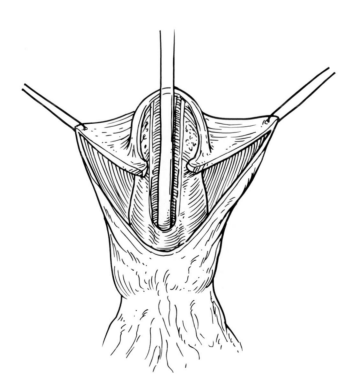

FIGURE 152-3. Proceed with dissection to expose the corporeal bodies as well as glans tissue. Use an iris scissors to facilitate mobilization of the glans wings. Dissect ventrally and laterally along the corporeal body to facilitate a second layer to protect the urethroplasty.

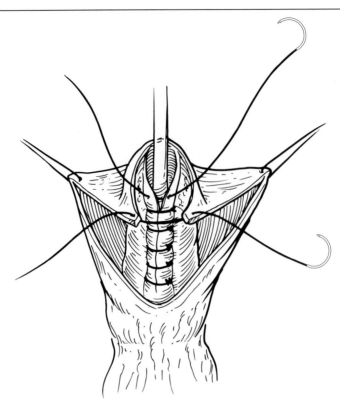

FIGURE 152-4. Tubularize the urethral plate over an 8-F feeding tube. If necessary, perform the Snodgrass modification of the plate in the midline (see Chapter 145). Close the glans wings with 6-0 synthetic absorbable sutures over the urethroplasty in two layers.

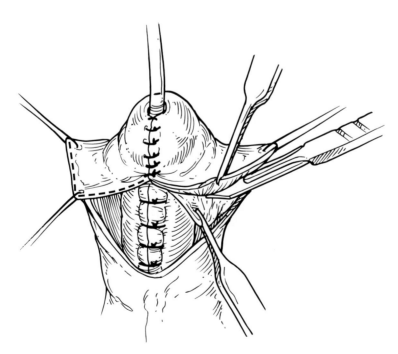

FIGURE 152-5. Carefully dissect from the inner prepuce the subcutaneous tissue that obtains its blood supply from the arteries of the foreskin. Close the outer skin of the glansplasty with interrupted 6-0 or 7-0 sutures.

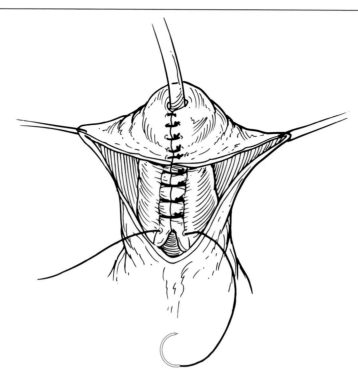

FIGURE 152-6. Bring a second layer of subcutaneous tissue over the urethroplasty. Approximate the foreskin with absorbable 6-0 sutures by closing the inner prepuce, a subcutaneous layer to prevent foreskin fistula and then the outer prepuce.

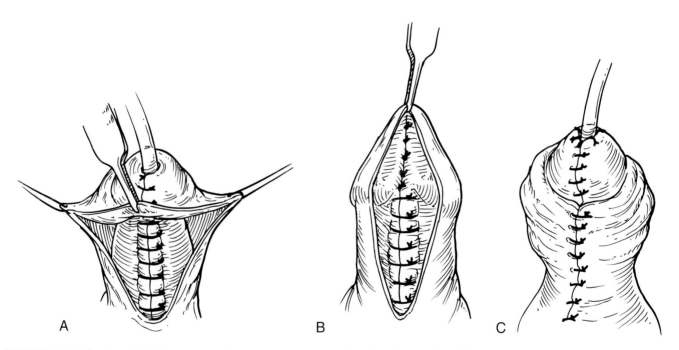

A   B   C

FIGURES 152-7. A to C, Take care to design the reconstructive foreskin so that phimosis will not occur at the completion of the procedure. The foreskin should retract easily over the glans. Dress the completed repair by reducing the reconstructed foreskin over the glans after covering the suture line with antibiotic ointment. Leave a urethral catheter in place for 3 to 5 days, depending on the severity of the urethroplasty.

POSTOPERATIVE PROBLEMS

Foreskin fistula can be prevented by meticulous use of a subcutaneous layer between the reconstructed inner and outer prepuce. Postoperative adhesions and phimosis are avoided by careful attention to the diameter of the new prepuce. After surgery the new prepuce should easily reduce.

ANTHONY A. CALDAMONE

Commentary by

In years past, the excess foreskin at the time of penile reconstructive surgery in children has been routinely excised in the United States, reflecting a cultural bias toward circumcision. However, because the goals of penile reconstructive surgery are to create a functional and normal-appearing penis, expectations of the parents or the patient regarding handling of the foreskin should be considered. Therefore, it is important that pediatric urologists be familiar with this technique, as when planning a hypospadias repair or corrective surgery for prepuce without hypospadias. Ask the parents if they were planning to have their son circumcised at birth. Those who indicate that they would have not requested circumcision should be offered a procedure that preserves the foreskin and reconstructs it to a normal appearance.

Patient selection is critical in the success of this procedure, in terms of both the reconstruction of the foreskin as well as the maintenance of an excellent urethroplasty. The high success rates from this procedure are in those cases of distal hypospadias without significant ventral curvature. Those cases with more proximal hypospadias, or those associated with significant chordee that require complete degloving of the penile shaft, are more likely to result in complications of the preputioplasty or the urethroplasty, or both.

Postoperative management of these children is somewhat controversial. Some reports in the literature suggest that the parents start retracting the foreskin on a regular basis soon after surgery. Others have taken a hands-off approach and do not recommend foreskin retraction until well after the healing process, and induration of the tissues has significantly passed. For those patients in whom the foreskin is difficult to retract postoperatively, steroid cream has been used to facilitate retractability of the foreskin.

In properly selected patients, the incident of complications such as phimosis, foreskin dehiscence, or urethral fistula is very low.

Chapter 153

Closure of Urethrocutaneous Fistula

Fistulas after hypospadias are not uncommon, occurring anywhere along the repair from the perineum, penoscrotal junction, penile shaft, and corona and within the glans in 5% to as many as 55% of patients. One of several factors may be responsible. First, look for distal obstruction, and then consider impaired vascular supply to the neourethra, nonabsorbable suture material in the neourethra, crossed suture lines, poorly vascularized skin flaps covering the neourethra, postoperative wound infection, and urinary extravasation. The success of closure does not appear to be related to stenting, use of loupes, age at time of closure, type of repair, or revision surgery. Three quarters of fistulas can be repaired in one operation, another

two thirds in a second, and all the remainder in a third. Fistula closure should not be performed until 6 months after the previous procedure to allow maximum wound healing and softening of the surrounding tissue.

Small fistulas will rarely close spontaneously. Repair is initiated by dissecting out the fistula, closing the defect by inverting sutures, covering the area with a small skin flap and applying collodion, all as a come-and-go procedure. Always look for obstructive narrowing distal to the leak. Intraurethral injection of dilute methylene blue helps identify the site (there may be more than one) and by staining, identifies the urothelium during the repair.

SIMPLE ADVANCEMENT FLAP CLOSURE

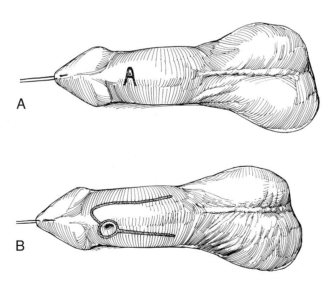

FIGURE 153-1. Small fistula (**A**) and larger fistula (**B**). Place an appropriate-size feeding tube in the urethra to check for stenosis and additional fistulas. Insert a lacrimal probe through the fistula to determine its track, which may be devious. Mark the proposed incision to encircle the fistula on one side and to extend laterally well beyond on the other side to ensure that the suture lines will not be overlapping. Do not be afraid to make a generous incision and wide dissection, but hemostasis must be perfect. For the fistula on the shaft, make the incision longitudinally, and mark a small flap on the adjacent skin in such a direction and shape that the loosest and most normal skin is drawn in for the closure.

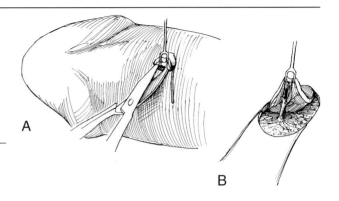

FIGURE 153-2. A, Using a loupe or microscope, elevate one skin edge with fine double-pronged skin hooks. With tenotomy scissors, free the skin generously around the tract. **B,** Continue dissection around the fistula to its base. Use a needle electrode delicately on the bleeders for complete hemostasis.

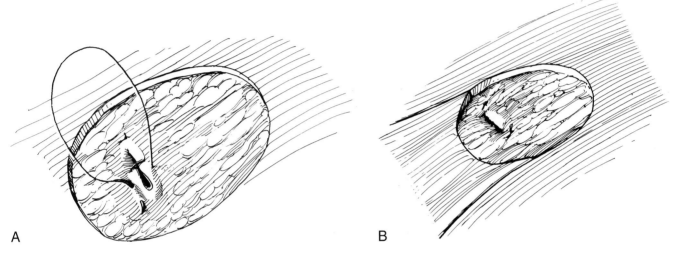

FIGURE 153-3. A and **B,** Divide the fistula very close to the urethral lumen, which can be identified by the catheter and the blue stain of the epithelium (if methylene blue is used). Run a 6-0 or 7-0 synthetic absorbable suture across the fistula subcuticularly, starting and ending the suture well away from the fistula. If the fistula is very small, two or three interrupted sutures may invert it into the urethra. Raise and suture one or two layers of subcutaneous tissue as flaps to interpose between the fistula and the skin flap.

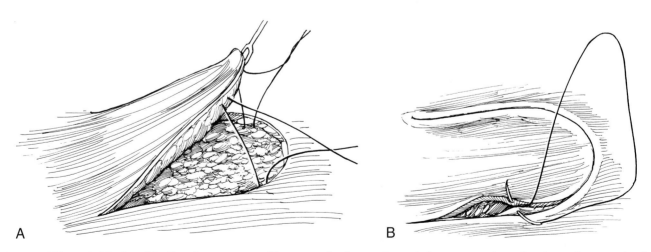

FIGURE 153-4. A, Mark a skin flap for coverage. Elevate and advance it, and then suture it to the deep tissue at the far side of the defect with two subcutaneous 4-0 or 5-0 synthetic absorbable sutures. In large fistulas, use de-epithelialized skin as an intermediate layer (see Fig. 153-6). **B,** Close the skin edges with a 5-0 synthetic absorbable suture running subcuticularly around the perimeter. Remove the catheter. Apply a collodion dressing (this will contract and draw in the skin edges to help the seal).

DE-EPITHELIALIZED FLAP CLOSURE (SMITH)

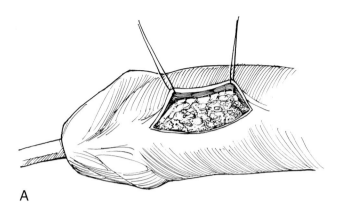

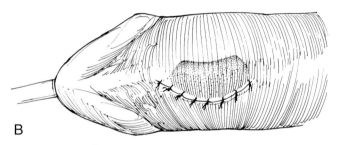

B

FIGURE 153-5. Interpose a de-epithelialized flap for added security. Make the skin incision longer and undermine the flaps laterally, keeping close to the corpora to preserve the blood supply.

   A, After closing the fistula transversely, dissect the epithelium from the dermis of one skin flap to leave a subcutaneous (dermal) flap. Draw the edge of this flap across the fistula, passing it under the opposite free skin flap, and suture the edge to its base with fine interrupted sutures. **B,** Suture the free skin edge to the de-epithelialized margin.

REPAIR OF SMALL CORONAL FISTULA WITH GLANS SUPPORT

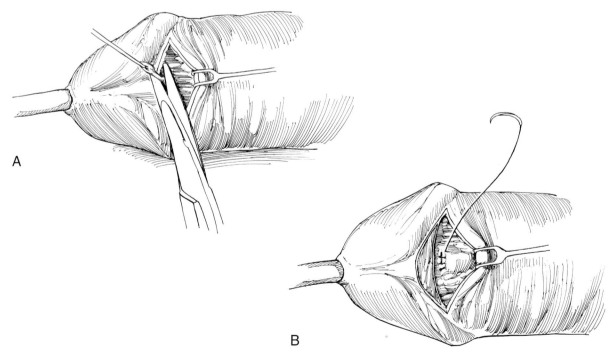

FIGURE 153-6. A, To repair a fistula in the corona, excise the tract through a transverse incision. Free the lateral and proximal skin widely. **B,** Remove the epithelium from the margin of the glans distal to the fistula. Invert the fistula with fine interrupted sutures.

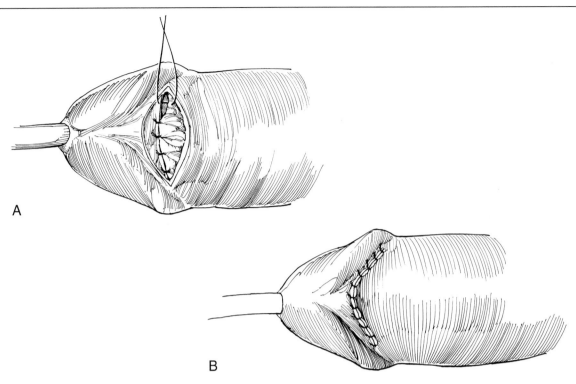

FIGURE 153-7. A, Place a row of 6-0 synthetic absorbable sutures to bring the subcutaneous tissue over the fistula and onto the glans. **B,** Suture the proximal skin edge to the edge of the denuded glans with similar interrupted sutures. Remove the catheter and apply a light dressing.

REPAIR OF CORONAL FISTULA WITH POOR GLANS SUPPORT

Coronal fistulas with poor glans support or large size are best converted to coronal hypospadias. Divide the poorly vascularized glans bridge and proceed with a formal glansplasty.

Options include a Mathieu-style flap or primary tubularization (Thiersch tube) (see Chapter 144), using a midline relaxing incision if needed (see Chapter 145).

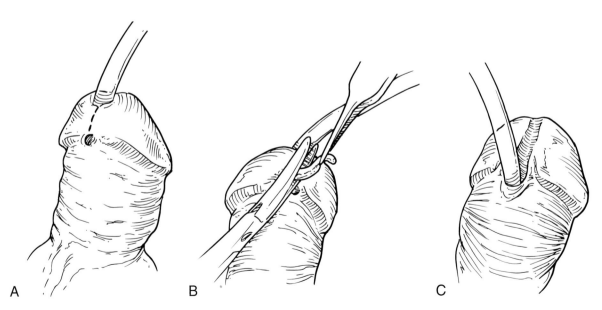

FIGURE 153-8. A, Large coronal fistula at the glans junction. **B,** Excise the glans bridge. **C,** The result is a coronal hypospadias.

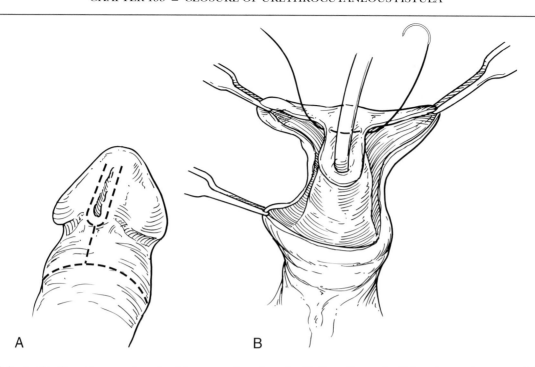

FIGURE 153-9. A, Outline the previous incision now forming the Firlit collar to half the circumference of the penis. In the ventral midline, extend the incision to the base of the fistula and then bring it up along the urethral plate on either side to the tip of the glans. **B,** Preserve the urethral plate for subsequent tubularization. Mobilize the glans wings on each side to an angle of 90 degrees with the urethral plate.

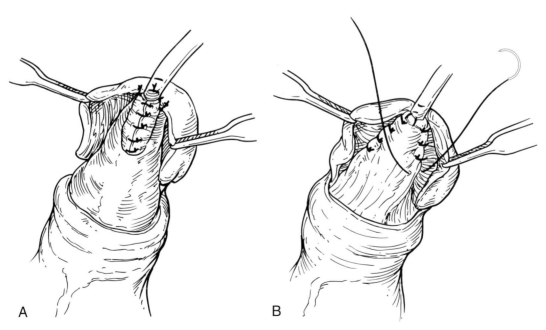

FIGURE 153-10. A, Form the new urethra with 6-0 or 7-0 absorbable sutures. **B,** Place a second layer of subcutaneous tissue over the urethroplasty. Mature the meatus and close the glans and skin. An alternative approach is a vascularized pedicle onlay flap along with a formal glansplasty (see Chapter 136).

REPAIR OF SCROTAL AND PERINEAL FISTULAS

Place the child in a frog-legged position with the soles of the feet held in apposition with tape over the arches. Inject dilute methylene blue through the meatus. Press on the bulb to force the dye through the fistulas to identify all of them. Place a catheter in the urethra.

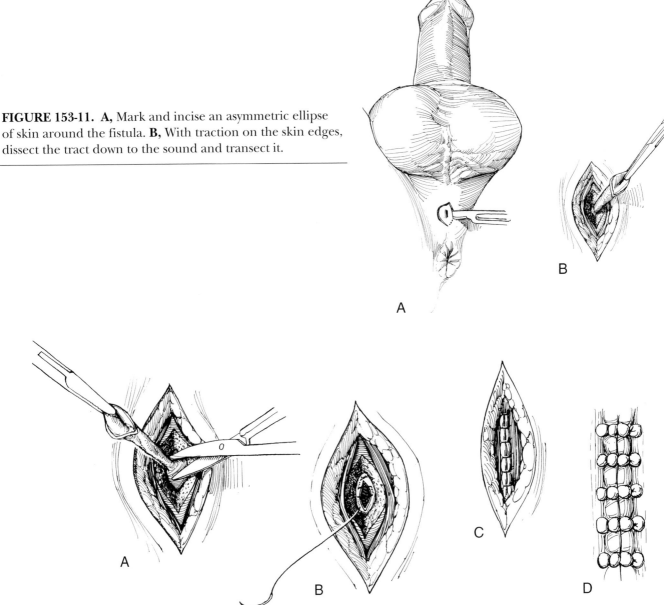

FIGURE 153-11. **A,** Mark and incise an asymmetric ellipse of skin around the fistula. **B,** With traction on the skin edges, dissect the tract down to the sound and transect it.

FIGURE 153-12. **A,** Trim the fistula almost flush with the urethral wall. **B,** Invert the "mucosal" edge with a running 6-0 synthetic absorbable suture as a subcuticular inverting stitch so that it will be flush with the urethral lining. **C,** Free enough subcutaneous tissue on one side to cover the defect without tension, and suture it to the opposite side with 6-0 synthetic absorbable sutures. **D,** Close the skin with interrupted sutures. If under tension, relieve it with mattress sutures bolstered with beads. If the urethral defect was large, drain the urine with a 5-mL silicone balloon catheter inserted into the bladder.

Repair of the large or recurrent fistula: Be sure to calibrate the distal urethra with bougie à boule to check for a stricture distal to the fistula, often an important contributing factor. Compress the urethra proximal to the defect digitally, and then inject dilute methylene blue into the meatus through a blunt adapter on a 10-mL syringe to inflate the urethra. In this way, more than one fistula may be detected, saving later embarrassment. Use optical magnification. In some cases, an operating microscope (×4 to ×16) may be useful.

Resort to flaps for coverage because side-to-side closure, even with undermining, usually fails. Some large fistulas are better managed by a takedown and then complete reconstruction at a second stage (see Chapter 150).

SAUL GREENFIELD

Commentary by

Not all fistulas are created equal. Fistulas at the coronal margin or on the glans present the greatest challenge, while more proximal shaft locations are easier to close. As mentioned, at least 6 months should pass between the hypospadias surgery and attempt at fistula closure. Distal obstruction must be ruled out, either by simple catheterization or cystoscopy. The urine must also be documented to be sterile and there should be no inflammation of the adjacent skin. Antibiotics before surgery may be necessary if there is infection. Prior to beginning the dissection, either methylene blue or betadine solution should be used to inject the urethra to both locate the fistula and make sure that others are not missed.

Distal fistulas are more difficult to correct because there is less subcutaneous tissue to harvest for a second layer and the skin is less maneuverable. Overlapping suture lines are therefore harder to avoid. It is sometimes possible to harvest subcutaneous tissue from the direction of the penile shaft, proximally, and this may be the only source of adjacent tissue for intermediate coverage. Pointed #11 or #12 scalpel blades are often useful in these areas. As mentioned by the author, there should be no hesitancy to make the skin incision longer to accomplish adequate coverage without overlapping suture lines. Hemostasis is important, but cautery can also be damaging to the site of repair if the space is very small. Needle-tip cautery on a lower setting should be used judiciously.

I prefer to use 7-0 Vicryl in an interrupted fashion for the urethra. We use 6-0 chromic catgut for the intermediate and skin layers. Mattress sutures, everting the skin edges, should be used for the final layer. Collodion most often suffices for a dressing. Many authorities will not routinely divert the urine. However, if there is any question about the viability of the repair, the adequacy of the intermediate layer, or the presence of overlapping suture lines, or if the "fistula" is very large, then 1 week to 10 days of catheter drainage may be helpful. I tend to use intraoperative cephalosporins, followed by 1 week of oral cephalosporin. Antibiotic choice may differ if there was a urinary or cutaneous infection documented before the repair.

A. BARRY BELMAN

Commentary by

Urethrocutaneous fistula is the most common complication of hypospadias repair; the incidence of it ranges from 4% to 56%. Meticulous surgical technique and application of the fundamental roles of plastic surgery are mandatory in hypospadias operation, as well as in management of its most common complication. However, closure of a urethrocutaneous fistula is no longer a major undertaking and usually can be accomplished rather easily and highly successfully as an outpatient procedure, without diversion or catheterization.

The principles are quite simple: (1) do not be afraid to free up enough normal tissue to get a good multiple-layered closure; (2) the fistula itself should be closed flush with the urethra, using a fine subcuticular inverting stitch with 6-0 or 7-0 suture; (3) the suture line can be completely covered by application of the de-epithelialized flap technique adapted from Dr. E. Durham Smith's (Smith, 1973) two-stage hypospadias repair; thus three full layers can be closed, including the final skin closure over the actual fistula in most instances; (4) hemostasis must be excellent and can be best achieved using needle-tip electrocautery; and (5) most important, distal obstruction must not exist.

I use collodion as a skin dressing, which tends to seal the wound. As it dries, collodion contracts, compressing the skin edges. With the spectacular success being achieved these days with fistula closure, you really should have no concern about attempting a single-stage hypospadias repair in all but the most severe cases of perineal hypospadias with penoscrotal transposition.

In reviewing our experience, we conclude that repair of urethrocutaneous fistulas can be accomplished with a high degree of success. Although some small fistulas will close spontaneously in the early postoperative period, in our experience, the use of silver nitrate to cauterize the tract locally is of little help. Additionally, to achieve maximum success, we believe that 6 months should elapse between the previous procedure and any attempts at closure to allow resolution of induration and to reduce bleeding when performing the skin-flap mobilization. The techniques are versatile and satisfactory in the more complex as well as in the simple cases. Our more recent experience substantiates that almost all but the most severe fistulas can be closed successfully as an outpatient procedure without the need for urinary diversion or urethral stenting, thus minimizing morbidity, hospitalization, and cost.

Chapter 154

Excision of Male Urethral Diverticulum

Diverticula occur in boys as a complication of hypospadias repair, usually secondary to meatal stenosis or a more distal stricture. They may be secondary to redundant foreskin used as part of an onlay island (see Chapter 143) or transverse tubularized island flap (see Chapter 146). They also occur at the penoscrotal junction in association with anterior urethral valves. Depicted here are two diverticula, one along the penile shaft and the other in the bulbar urethra. An abscessed diverticulum can be endoscopically drained into the urethra.

Clear urinary tract infection if possible and provide intraoperative antibacterial coverage.

PENILE SHAFT DIVERTICULUM

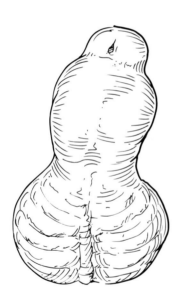

FIGURE 154-1. Diagnosis is suspected when ballooning on urination of the penile shaft, decreased urinary stream, and dribbling are present.

FIGURE 154-2. Check for meatal stenosis with a sound. If the meatus is stenotic, formal repair is necessary (see Chapter 150). If stenosis is not present, deglove the penis through the Firlit collar to the penoscrotal junction.

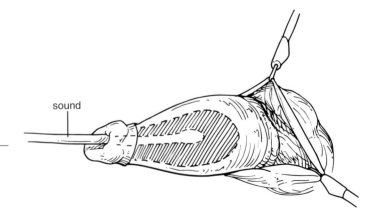

sound

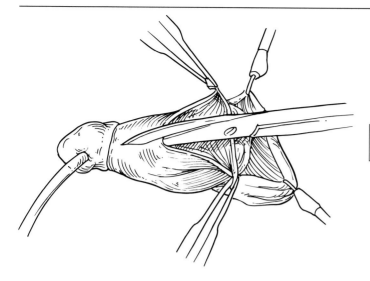

FIGURE 154-3. Open the diverticulum at its maximum diameter. Use a skin hook for exposure.

FIGURE 154-4. Insert a catheter. Define the normal-caliber urethra at the proximal and distal aspects of the diverticulum.

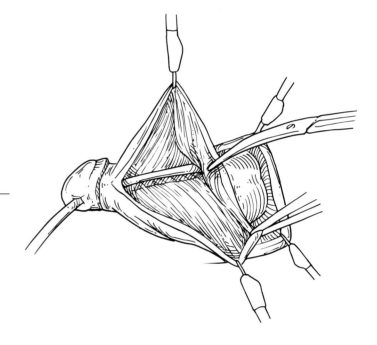

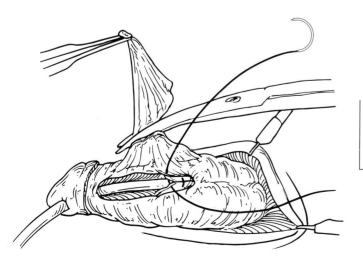

FIGURE 154-5. Aggressively trim the diverticulum and redundant subcutaneous tissue. Close the urethra with interrupted or subcuticular sutures. Use a second layer of subcutaneous tissue to cover the suture line.

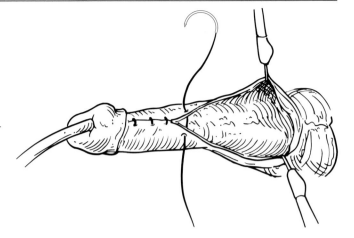

FIGURE 154-6. Trim and close the skin.

BULBAR DIVERTICULUM

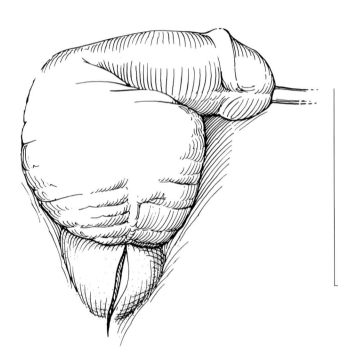

FIGURE 154-7. First, cystoscopically examine the urethra to be sure its caliber is normal. If a septum is found (possibly responsible for development of the diverticulum), consider simple incision with a urethrotome, although that may be only a preliminary step to definitive repair. Inject dilute methylene blue into the meatus to fill and stain the lining of the diverticulum. Try inserting a sound, a bougie à boule, or a Fogarty catheter into the diverticulum; otherwise, place a suitable-size 5-mL silicone balloon catheter into the bladder.

Incision: Incise the skin vertically, on one side of the midline. Dissect the skin and subcutaneous layer laterally as much as possible from the diverticular walls.

FIGURE 154-8. Open into the diverticulum with a longitudinal incision placed to one side. Insert stay sutures on the edges or the ring retractor. If a stricture is still present or if its site is indicated by staining with methylene blue, excise it and cover the defect by swinging a pedicle flap of the diverticular wall.

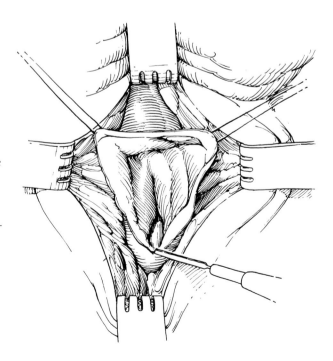

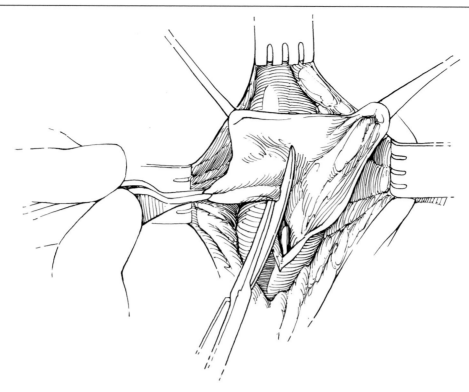

FIGURE 154-9. Trim the walls, but leave a bed for urethral closure, depending on the size of the boy.

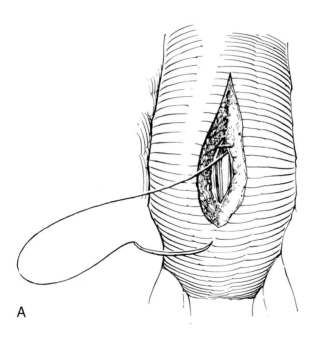

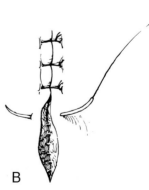

FIGURE 154-10. A, Invert the epithelial edge over an appropriate-size silcone catheter as a mold with a running subepithelial 4-0 chromic catgut suture. Synthetic absorbable sutures are satisfactory but sutures that are absorbed slowly should be avoided for risk of stone formation. Close the remainder of the defect with interrupted 4-0 chromic catgut sutures. **B,** Approximate the fascia and subcutaneous tissue in as many layers as possible with 4-0 chromic catgut sutures, avoiding overlapping suture lines. Close the skin with a fine running subcuticular synthetic absorbable suture. Wound drainage rarely is needed. Leave the catheter in place for 10 days. If there is concern about the suture line, check for extravasation by retrograde instillation of dilute methylene blue or by a urethrogram.

JACK ELDER

Diverticula of the male urethra generally occur following a tubularized transverse preputial hypospadias repair, and result from creating a urethra that is too large or too long, or a urethra associated with delayed urethral obstruction, either meatal stenosis or urethral stricture. A diverticulum is unusual following a tubularized incised plate (Snodgrass) repair or an onlay island flap. Typically there is a slow stream with a bulging fluid-filled mass in the penile shaft or scrotum that appears during voiding. In addition, there is often postvoiding dribbling of urine. The condition is unlikely to improve, and the decision on whether to repair it is based on whether the young man can live with the condition for the rest of his life.

Preoperative evaluation should include either a retrograde urethrogram or voiding cystourethrogram, as distal urethral pathology should be documented.

Surgical management depends on the etiology of the diverticulum. Generally the patient is placed in the supine position. If the diverticulum is in the pendulous urethra, a vertical scrotal incision is made, but if it is in the penile urethra, a circumferential incision 2 cm proximal to the coronal sulcus is made to allow the penis to be degloved and avoid overlapping suture lines. The Scott retractor provides excellent exposure of the urethra. The diverticulum may be identified intraoperatively by filling it through a pediatric feeding tube. Distal urethral caliber should be assessed with a bougie à boule. If a distal urethral stricture is identified, usually the diverticulum may be used as a rotational flap. Otherwise, the diverticulum should be opened longitudinally. I often open it in the midline. The edges of the diverticulum should be trimmed back on each side to minimize any redundant tissue. If there is hair in the urethra, depilation should be performed, or else the tissue should be excised. The urethra is then closed with a running imbricating suture; I generally use 6-0 or 7-0 polydioxanone suture. The periurethral tissue is then closed over the urethra. Even with ideal operative technique, there is a potential for urethral fistula formation. Consequently, another layer of tissue coverage should be added—either tunica vaginalis or vascular tissue from the penile skin or residual foreskin.

If the patient has an anterior urethral valve, the distal lip of the diverticulum must be resected. In some cases, an endoscopic valve incision or ablation procedure is more appropriate.

Postoperatively, an open indwelling 6-F silicone or polyurethral urethral stent is used to drain the bladder for 7 to 10 days. In older boys, a suprapubic tube and a urethral stent are used. Complications are infrequent and include fistula, stricture, and recurrence of the diverticulum.

BRENT SNOW

Diverticula in boys are of two types, congenital and acquired. Congenital diverticula include megalourethra and anterior urethral valves. In both of these circumstances an area of urethra is poorly supported with spongiosal tissue. Generally, anterior urethral valves are due to a ventral flap of tissue obstructing the urine flow causing the diverticulum and are ablated endoscopically. The diverticulum then collapses and usually does not require open surgical repair. If surgical repair is required, if possible, resect the epithelium back to where the spongiosa is normal for the best results.

Acquired urethral diverticula are most often the results of hypospadias repair and can be due to distal urethra (narrowing of the repaired urethra or redundancy of the neourethra at the time of its creation). Avoidance of a diverticulum in hypospadias repair is the best policy; thus, making the neourethra fit snugly around an appropriate-size catheter will ensure the proper caliber and making sure that the catheter as it passes through the glans is of adequate diameter minimizes the chance for a diverticulum.

During repair of a urethral diverticulum, be sure and evaluate carefully for distal urethral stenosis and correct this so that a second diverticulum does not occur. If there is a distal urethral stenosis, I prefer to rotate a flap of the diverticulum into the glanular urethra to add new tissue to the stenotic area, rather than dilating this area or doing an internal urethrotomy.

My personal preference for open diverticular repair is to open the diverticulum laterally, flush with the body of the corpus cavernosum, and then, over an appropriate-size catheter, I trim the rest of the diverticulum. To trim the diverticulum aggressively I find it helpful to trim a portion, sew a short distance, trim some more, and again sew a short distance. That way I avoid overexcision or having an unequal caliber of the urethra.

Because of the poor supporting tissues of a diverticulum, the sutures can include some of the corporeal cavernosal tissue laterally to give good support. This also makes the suture line somewhat off the midline, which is commonly the spot for closure of the penile shaft skin so that the suture lines do not overlap.

If the urethral diverticulum is not too large I have been pleased with the results of urethral plication, infolding the diverticulum over a catheter the same way that a megaureter is plicated in a folding technique (Chapter 48). Without a suture line the risk of fistula formation is minimized.

Part III

Penile Reconstruction

Chapter 155

Meatotomy

Meatal stenosis, often appearing at the time of toilet training, is usually the result of long-tern mild inflammation of the meatal lips in the circumcised child. The patient often needs to hold his penis between his legs to prevent the urinary stream from directing vertically.

Meatotomy can be done under general anesthesia and is the method of choice for both infants and older children. Occasionally, older children may have the procedure performed in the office with topical local agents, short-acting oral agents, and injectable anesthetics.

VENTRAL MEATOTOMY, CLAMP METHOD FOR INFANTS

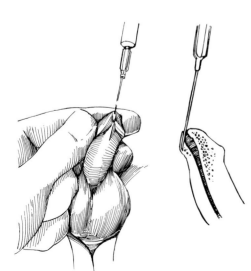

FIGURE 155-1. Instill 1% lidocaine through a 25-gauge needle passed through the meatus and directed at the frenulum.

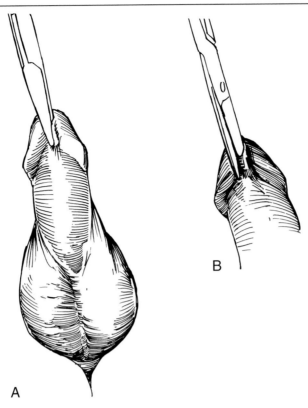

FIGURE 155-2. **A,** Clamp the ventral meatal lip with a fine clamp. Insert it deeply, as healing will reduce the size of the meatus. **B,** Cut the thinned tissue, now avascular, with scissors.

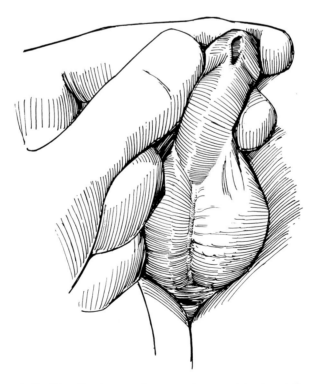

FIGURE 155-3. Apply petroleum jelly (Vaseline) onto the cut edges and instruct the mother or father to do the same at home.

VENTRAL MEATOTOMY, SUTURE METHOD FOR OLDER BOYS

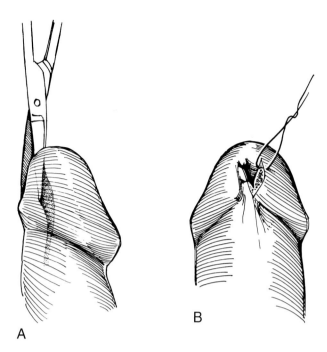

FIGURE 155-4. **A,** Instill 1% lidocaine through a 25-gauge needle passed through the meatus and directed at the frenulum. Divide the ventral rim with scissors, creating a V-shaped defect. Calibrate with an appropriate-size sound. **B,** Place from three to five 6-0 or 7-0 plain catgut or Vicryl sutures to approximate the edges of the V. Apply petroleum jelly twice a day for 3 to 5 days to prevent postoperative adhesions to clothes.

DAVID A. BLOOM

Commentary by

Although meatal stenosis is rather a mundane problem for the surgeon, it can become a matter of great concern to the child and his family. Most cases, I believe, are the long-term consequences of inflammation of the exposed meatal lips. After circumcision, the meatus may become periodically irritated and inflamed from rubbing against urine-soaked diapers. This is why we advise petroleum jelly application to the meatus with every diaper change after circumcision. In the early part of the 20th century this reaction of the meatus was called *ammoniacal meatitis.* This cycle of inflammation and healing with minute cicatrix formation ultimately can lead to meatal stenosis, which typically presents in circumcised boys after toilet training. In most cases meatal stenosis is minimal and is not a clinical problem. I think a legitimate clinical problem exists when two of the three following conditions occur: (1) marked abnormality of the urinary stream (severe angulation, spraying, diminished caliber), (2) stranguria, and (3) inability of the examining physician to evert the meatal lips or pass a 5-F feeding tube. Some boys, however, have a deflecting meatal web that may permit an ample caliber of catheter to pass but still acts as a baffle to the stream. In these instances the problem may be congenital, as I have seen this web in brothers and in fathers and sons. The baffle is often quite elastic and simply needs to be cut rather than dilated.

If meatal stenosis is a significant clinical problem a trial of home dilatation with sequential feeding tubes or meatal dilator to reach an 8-F aperture may solve the problem. In many youngsters, local anesthesia with eutectic mixture of local anesthetics (EMLA) cream may permit an office meatotomy. However, the EMLA cream needs a 1-hour contact time for adequate anesthesia.

Definitive treatment requires two steps: (1) meatotomy or meatoplasty to restore the normal aperture, and (2) a program of intermittent insertion of a catheter every 2 weeks for 1 month, then monthly for 2 months will maintain the opening during the healing period. This second step requires some degree of cooperation from the patient. Our experience has taught us that if the meatotomy was traumatic, the calibration program will be difficult. For that reason, we do not hesitate to use a brief general anesthetic for those few boys with significant meatal stenosis.

Chapter 156

Circumcision

Circumcision is a procedure performed on an organ that becomes of considerable concern to the individual and must be done with precision. The infant should be mature and in good health. Check for hypospadias. With phimosis, consider the simpler (and cheaper) topical steroid therapy of 0.05% betamethasone ointment applied for 4 to 8 weeks, and preserve the prepuce.

Prep the penis with iodophor or betadine solution.

Even in newborns use some form of penile anesthesia to reduce pain and minimize cardiovascular reaction. Give supplemental local anesthesia even if general anesthesia is used.

Four techniques for local anesthesia include:

1. Basal block: Infiltrate the base with 1 mL of 1% or 2% lidocaine (Xylocaine) without epinephrine through a 26-gauge needle.
2. Crural block (best): Palpate the inferior border of the symphysis pubis with the index and middle fingers of one hand. With the other hand, inject 1 to 1.2 mL of 1% lidocaine without epinephrine from a 3-mL syringe, by inserting the needle at this point and directing it 0.25 to 0.5 cm toward the 10-o'clock position just under the symphysis pubis, aiming toward Alcock's canal from which the pudendal nerve exits. Aspirate carefully to avoid accidental intravascular injection. Withdraw the needle and repeat the injection in the 2-o'clock position to the opposite canal. Inject the remaining anesthetic along the ventral surface of the scrotum at the base of the penis.
3. Dorsal penile nerve block: Inject a small volume of bupivacaine into the dorsal nerves through one site in the midline on the dorsum of the shaft.
4. Surface anesthesia: Apply a eutectic mixture of local anesthetics to the outside of the prepuce an hour before operation (safe if the child is older than 1 month).

For hemostasis, apply initially a small tourniquet at the base before draping the area. After excising the prepuce, clamp and then ligate the frenular vessels with fine horizontal mattress sutures. Remove the tourniquet and lightly fulgurate any remaining vessels before approximating the skin edges.

DOUBLE-INCISION TECHNIQUE

A traction suture in the glans aids manipulation. Place it vertically, not coronally, to avoid a snakebite scar.

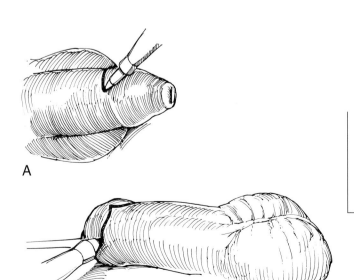

A

B

FIGURE 156-1. A, Mark a slightly oblique incision (one that extends more distally on the ventrum, to provide for advancement of a V-flap) onto the unretracted prepuce over the site of the corona of the glans. **B,** Provide a V-extension on the ventrum to match the groove that will be left by the frenulum. This will prevent it from tethering the penis.

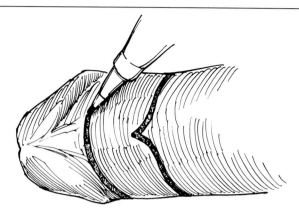

FIGURE 156-2. Retract the prepuce. With a probe and a mosquito clamp, free it completely from the glans. Grasp the glans with moist gauze held over the thumb and fingertips and clear any lumps of smegma. Mark the second incision 0.5 to 1 cm proximal to the coronal sulcus, straight across the base of the frenulum. Be sure to leave a generous cuff at the corona, as this area is highly innervated. The cuff also provides an edge for suturing. Identify the urethral meatus.

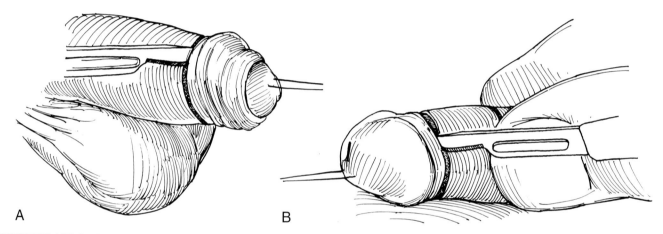

A   B

FIGURE 156-3. A, Incise proximally along the marked lines. **B,** Now incise distally.

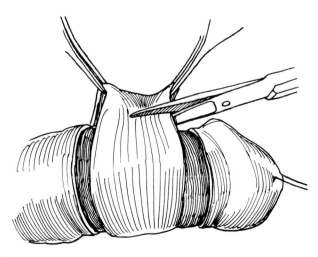

FIGURE 156-4. Divide the two layers of skin on the dorsum with scissors.

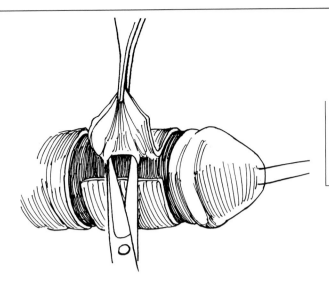

FIGURE 156-5. Elevate the cut edges and free the skin from the dartos fascia. Fulgurate bleeders, or tie them with 6-0 polydioxanone suture. Inspect the frenular area to secure and ligate the artery. Release the tourniquet and complete hemostasis with low-power electrocautery.

FIGURE 156-6. Close the defect with 5-0 Monocryl (older boys) or 6-0 polydioxanone (infants) sutures in interrupted or subcuticular fashion. Dress with Xeroform, gauze, and Tegaderm.

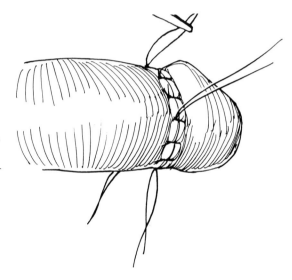

ALTERNATIVE TECHNIQUE FOR SMALL BOYS

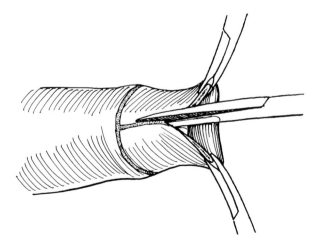

FIGURE 156-7. With the prepuce in place, mark the skin around the level of the corona. Make a dorsal slit to the mark and grasp the skin edges.

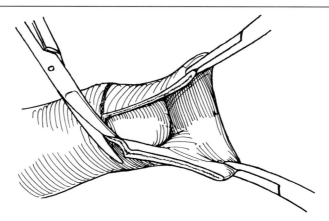

FIGURE 156-8. Divide both layers of the prepuce on the marked line with fine scissors.

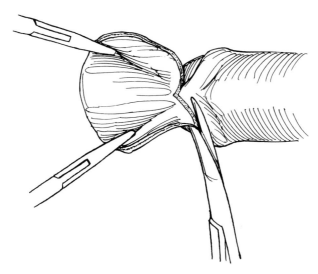

FIGURE 156-9. Provide a V at the frenulum. Reapproximate the edges with sutures as described in Figure 156-6. An alternative is skin adhesive (Dermabond).

POSTOPERATIVE PROBLEMS

Skin necrosis may occur when epinephrine is used in the local anesthetic. Major necrosis may result from electrocoagulation. (If used, apply a saline-soaked sponge around the penis and keep the organ in contact with the body to maximize the path for escape of the current.)

In infants, bleeding and infection occasionally occur. Severe infections with systemic spread are rare but the possibility is a warning that any infection should be treated adequately.

If too much skin is removed, or if too much inner preputial membrane is left while excess outer skin is removed, the penis becomes "buried." Release it by circumcising the junction and covering the defect with the preputial tissue. If insufficient skin has been removed, phimosis may result as the suture line contracts. Recircumcision may be required for a redundant residual prepuce. Skin bridges can usually be divided with small scissors without anesthesia.

If too much preputial skin is excised, that area may reepithelialize, but usually it is the shaft that is denuded. In

a newborn, grafting is seldom if ever needed. Glanular necrosis (or even loss of the corpora) may result from inadvertent contact of the cautery with a clamp. Sagittal division of the glans can occur while making a dorsal slit. Chordee can result from delayed healing on the ventrum. Urethral injury results from sutures hurriedly placed to stop bleeding (see Chapter 157). Urinary retention may occur immediately from a dressing that is too tight, or later from secondary phimosis.

PLASTIBELL TECHNIQUE SUITABLE FOR INFANTS

Wait for 24 hours after birth. Obtain consent. Before starting the procedure, read the printed instructions accompanying the Plastibell device and check the integrity of the instrument. Also have available appropriate-size devices for the penis. Prep and drape the penis and apply local anesthesia, as previously described.

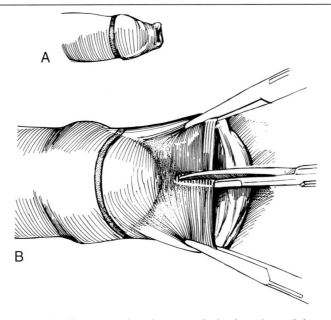

FIGURE 156-10. A, With the prepuce in place over the glans, mark the location of the coronal sulcus on the skin of the shaft with a marking pen. Dilate the preputial ring with a hemostat, and identify the urethral meatus. **B,** Place straight hemostats onto the edge of the prepuce at the 10- and 2-o'clock positions, taking shallow bites. Tease the preputial surface off the dorsum of the glans, freeing adhesions. With a straight hemostat, clamp the prepuce in the midline dorsally for a depth of one third of the distance to the corona for 10 seconds. Divide the crushed line with straight blunt-tipped scissors. Bluntly free the prepuce from the glans with a flexible probe until it can be completely retracted to expose the coronal sulcus.

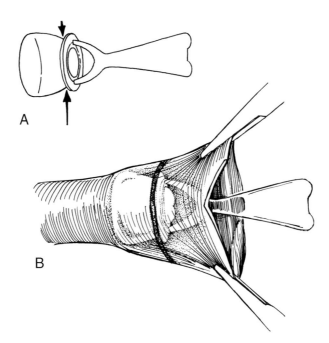

FIGURE 156-11. A, Select the correct size of Plastibell from the six sizes available. The bottom edge of the bell should cover the corona completely. If it is too small, it will exert pressure on the glans and too much prepuce will be left; if it is too large, the glans can slip through the ring and too much prepuce will be removed. Try several sizes for the best fit. The bell should slightly distend the prepuce when it is drawn down over the bell and glans. **B,** Pull the prepuce over the bell until the skin mark made at the coronal sulcus lies over the inner groove in the bell.

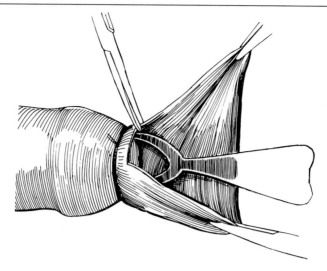

FIGURE 156-12. Pass a suture around the device at the inner groove and tie it tightly. Cut the prepuce with scissors just past the outer groove. Do not use electrocautery. Break off the handle of the bell. Tell the parents that the bell should fall off in 2 to 4 days; if not, they should bring the boy back for its removal.

GOMCO CLAMP TECHNIQUE

Select the correct size of Gomco bell. Fit the parts together to be sure they match (they should be obtained from the same manufacturer) and the instrument has not been damaged. If you find stripped threads, a warped or bent base plate, a bent arm, twisted forks, or a scored or nicked bell, discard the clamp.

Place the clamp as described for the Plastibell in Figure 156-11. Pull the prepuce over the bell and through the plate and yoke portions of the clamp until the skin mark at the coronal sulcus lies at the level of the top of the clamp. Screw the clamp down onto the bell tightly. Cut the prepuce off, close to the top of the plate with a scalpel. Remove the entire clamp and bell with the excised prepuce. Do not use electrocautery around this metal clamp.

In children with hemophilia, applying fibrin glue for hemostasis after Gomco clamp circumcision reduces the need for systemic clotting factor replacement.

POSTOPERATIVE PROBLEMS

Inadequate removal of the foreskin is not uncommon, but excessive removal is unusual. Skin bridges may develop that tether the glans, requiring division later under local anesthesia. Similarly, inclusion cysts at the suture line containing smegma may need unroofing, although they usually clear spontaneously as the prepuce separates from the glans. Circumferential contracture can create phimosis if too much prepuce is left behind, especially in older children with poor attachment of the penile skin to the shaft. This phimosis/ trapped penis phenomenon requires dilatation of the phimotic ring with a fine hemostat, and then regular manual reduction by the parents (see Chapter 158). Significant

infection or bleeding after these techniques is uncommon. However, watch for the development of meatitis involving the newly exposed glans. A urethrocutaneous fistula at the coronal sulcus may result from pulling the urethra into the clamp or from direct injury. (The presence of a megaloure-thra is a hazard here.) Amputation of the glans penis has been reported; treat it by immediate reattachment. Rare but possible complications are penile necrosis, retention of parts of the Plastibell, and denudation of the shaft of the penis.

DORSAL SLIT AND PREPUTIOPLASTY FOR PHIMOSIS AND PARAPHIMOSIS

Try steroids by applying 0.05% betamethasone cream twice daily for 8 weeks. If that fails, make a dorsal slit as a substitute for circumcision (although the cosmetic result may not be acceptable).

For a preputioplasty, mobilize the prepuce by carefully stretching the constriction and separating underlying adhesions. Retract the prepuce and make one or two longitudinal incisions across the constricting band. Close the resulting defect(s) transversely with interrupted, fine plain catgut sutures.

DORSAL SLIT FOR PARAPHIMOSIS

First, try to milk the edema up into the shaft by squeezing the end of the penis, which usually must be done under general anesthesia. Use the fork of the index and middle fingers of both hands, one placed on each side. While pressing with the thumbs on both sides to compress the glans, simultaneously pull the strictured portion of the prepuce over the glans.

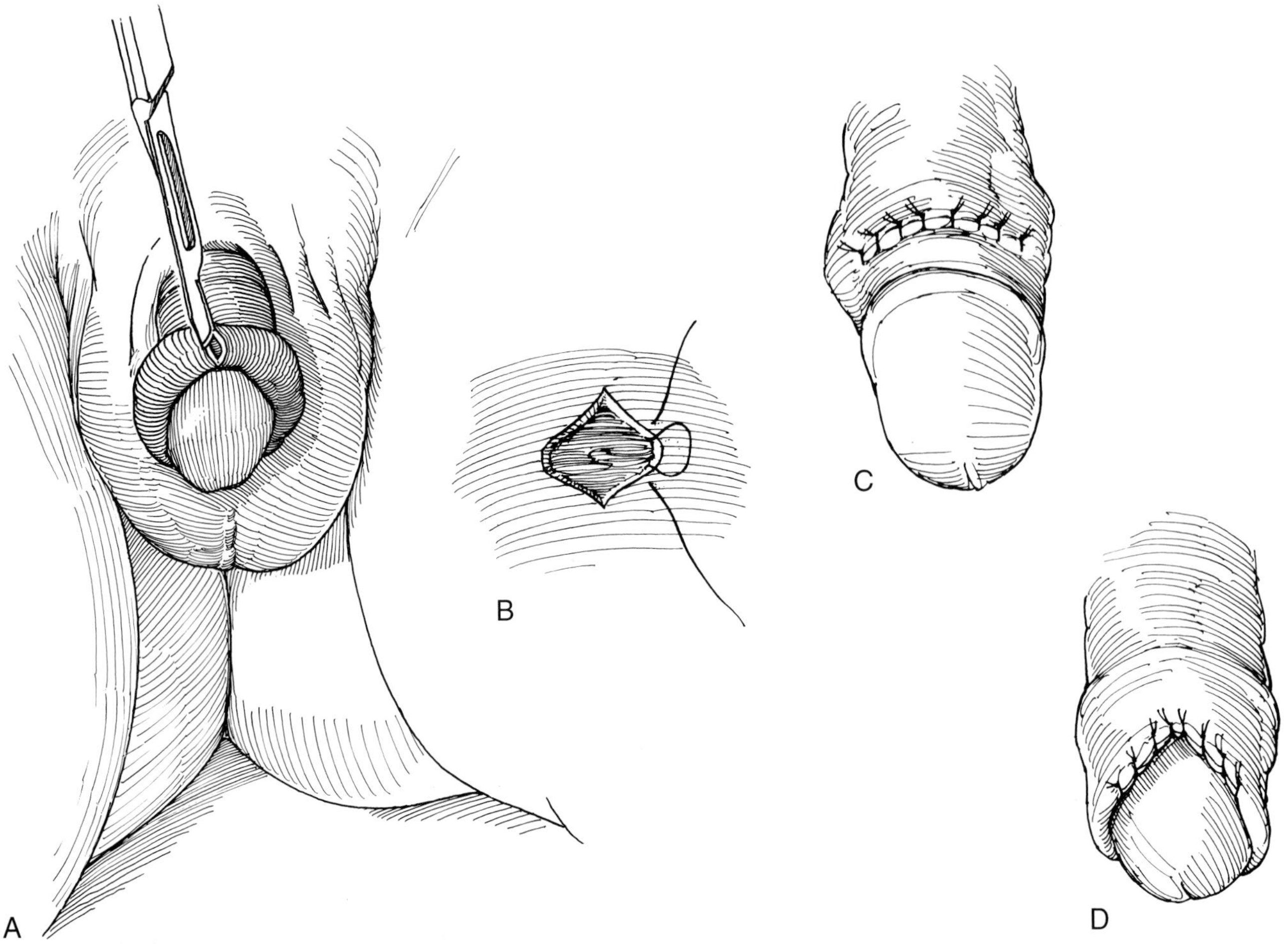

FIGURE 156-13. A, If manual correction fails because the prepuce has become fixed, make a dorsal longitudinal incision sharply through the band, centered at the junction of the shiny inner (preputial) and the duller outer shaft skin. Spread the skin with a small, curved clamp to expose Buck's fascia. Manipulate the prepuce back over the glans to be sure that the incision is adequate for easy passage. **B** and **C,** Approximate the incision transversely with interrupted sutures of 5-0 or 6-0 monofilament suture (a Heineke-Mikulicz-plasty). **D,** Replace the prepuce around the glans and cover it with a medicated gauze dressing. Instruct the parents to mobilize the foreskin regularly after the acute phase has passed. Reserve circumcision for recurrent episodes.

FRENULOPLASTY FOR A SHORT TETHERING FRENULUM

Make a transverse incision at the base of the frenulum. Draw the prepuce out and close the incision longitudinally (Heineke-Mikulicz). Trim the resultant dog-ear. Close the incision with 6-0 fine plain catgut sutures.

ANETTE JACOBSEN

Commentary by

Circumcision is the most common surgical procedure performed on boys. The search for the ancient origin of the procedure takes us back beyond early Egypt where hieroglyphic descriptions of the procedure are found. Current indications for circumcision include religious requirement, recurrent balanitis, severe phimosis, and balanitis xerotica obliterans. Circumcision is also commonly performed for social request. Recent years have seen a surge of anticircumcision activity, the argument being that it is an unnecessary operation with recognized morbidities and it leaves a less sensate glans penis.

In infants and neonates the Plastibell technique is by far the most common. In older boys freehand technique, straight clamp (guillotine method), or other clamp techniques all serve to excise the foreskin to leave an exposed glans, an inner preputial cuff, and a nontented frenulum. In infants and neonates it may be done under regional or local anaesthesia, but to do a circumcision without any anesthetic is not a recommended practice. In older children a general anesthetic is recommended, augmented by a penile block. The most common morbidities include glans scabbing, infection, and bleeding. Glans scabbing is an expected sequela and is proportional to the degree of preputial adhesions separated from the glans. Scabbing should not be mistaken for infection, which is uncommon but easily treated with the use of topical antibiotic cream. It is rare that oral antibiotics are required.

In circumcision a carbon dioxide laser beam can be used as a cutting device. This significantly decreases the incidence of postoperative bleeding and also postoperative edema. The vast majority of boys will experience pain. Sometimes postoperative pain will result in urinary retention. A regional block, topical anesthetic gel, and liberal oral analgesia are required, with pain usually subsiding in 2 to 3 days. On average, a boy will wear pants without any penile dressing after 1 week. Various dressings can be used, with a medicated petroleum jelly gauze and a clear plastic dressing being the most common alternatives. An absorbable suture of a fine caliber, such as 5-0 or 6-0 catgut or undyed 5-0 or 6-0 Vicryl or Dexon provides a nice cosmetic result. Alternatively, a tissue glue supplied with a fine nozzle applicator gives a cosmetically pleasing result.

ADAM HITTELMAN

Commentary by

Although considered a relatively uncomplicated urologic procedure, few surgeries have generated as much controversy and debate. Ranging from advocates arguing medical benefit, to patients following cultural and religious norms, to detractors citing disadvantages and a questionable risk-to-benefit ratio, circumcision clearly evokes strong reaction and contention in both the medical community and the public. The American Academy of Pediatrics acknowledges potential medical benefits of newborn male circumcision; however, they do not feel there is sufficient data to recommend routine neonatal circumcision. Since it is not essential to a child's current well-being, they recommend a thorough discussion of the risks, benefits, and alternatives of the procedure with the pediatrician. Similarly, the American Urological Association recognizes the potential medical benefits and advantages, balanced with disadvantages and risks. While they point out that risks and disadvantages are identified early, the medical benefits and advantages are prospective and may not be appreciated. These statements have clearly influenced recognition and level of compensation by insurance companies.

A variety of benefits have historically been cited in the medical literature. Prevention and reduction in the incidence of penile cancer, phimosis, balanitis, sexually transmitted diseases including HIV, and urinary tract infections are common arguments for circumcision. This is balanced by the low incidence of penile cancer in industrialized countries where genital hygiene is maintained. Phimosis can often be treated with steroid creams and it has been calculated that it takes more than 100 circumcisions to prevent one urinary tract infection. Meatal stenosis is almost solely found in patients who underwent neonatal circumcision.

Circumcision is a surgical intervention and complications can be devastating. Conversely, complication rates are very low and often minor. Advocates point out that the ratio of circumcision complications to urinary tract prevention or to penile cancer prevention is a better indicator and that the prophylactic benefit outweighs the inconvenience of minor complications. Clearly, circumcision in an older patient requires longer recovery. While studies have argued that both sexual advantages as well as sexual dysfunction result from circumcision, it is unlikely that either view will be validated. Needless to say, these arguments are endless and will not be resolved in the scope of this commentary.

There are many approaches to the procedure itself. The best procedure depends on the comfort and experience of the surgeon. We do recommend general anesthesia and in our practice (except for newborns) all children are supplemented with a caudal or penile block; older children receive local anesthesia with penile block. Many providers who perform neonatal circumcision are concerned about removing too much skin. This can lead to excess foreskin and a less than optimal cosmetic result. Circumcision revision is not uncommon and we typically approach this with a dorsal skin incision and wrapping of the edges around ventrally as Byars' flaps. The redundant skin is trimmed ventrally and approximated in the midline. Although we often dress the incisions with sterile gauze sandwiched between an occlusive dressing, the circumcision can also be dressed with bacitracin ointment alone. The dressings commonly fall off and parental anxiety and postoperative calls can be significantly reduced with extra attention placed on meticulous hemostasis.

Chapter 157

Repair of Circumcision Injuries

Circumcision remains the most common operation performed. The most common complication is bleeding. Although rare, injuries to the urethra and glans may occur.

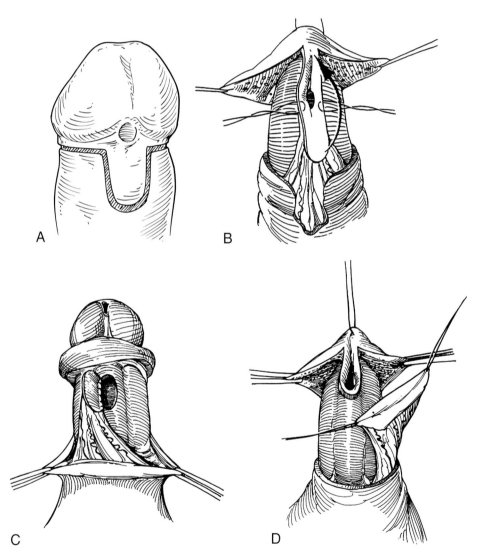

FIGURE 157-1. **A,** Subcoronal urethrocutaneous fistula results when too much traction is placed on the prepuce during incision, or when a portion of the shaft skin is included with the prepuce. **B,** For repair, form a flap by the Mathieu technique (see Chapter 141). **C,** Raise a ventral vascularized pedicle flap. **D,** Place a dorsal vascularized penile pedicle flap. *(From Baskin LS, Canning DA, Snyder HM, Duckett JW: Surgical repair of urethral circumcision injuries. J Urol 158:2269–2271, 1997, Figure 2.)*

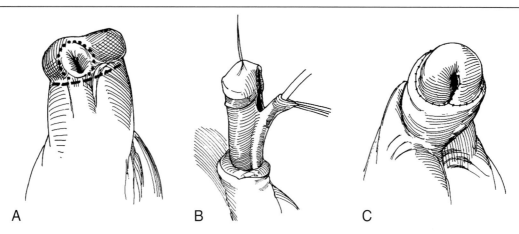

FIGURE 157-2. Partial amputation of the glans may distort the urethra. It is usually caused by its incorporation in a clamp or by division during moments of excessive bleeding before the prepuce and glans have been adequately separated.
   A, The result is urethral deviation. If the amputated segment is present, immediate reattachment is usually successful. If that is not possible, return for repair after 4 to 6 months. **B,** Mobilize the urethra. **C,** Replace it into a normal position on the glans.
   Amputation of the glans at the coronal sulcus can occur during circumcision. Induce general anesthesia. Insert an 8-F balloon catheter though the amputated portion and then into the bladder, to stabilize the glans. Place a small red rubber catheter around the base of the shaft as a tourniquet. Using the operating microscope, anastomose the urethral mucosa end to end with interrupted 6-0 polyglactin sutures. Repair the corpus spongiosum with similar sutures. Close the tunica albuginea with interrupted sutures and then suture the fascial and skin edges. Place a mildly compressive dressing, and give broad-spectrum antibiotics. Remove the catheter in 2 to 3 weeks. The worst complications result from not recognizing hypospadias before circumcision because the resultant loss of preputial skin makes proper repair difficult. *(From Baskin LS, Canning DA, Snyder HM, Duckett JW: Surgical repair of urethral circumcision injuries. J Urol 158:2269–2271, 1997, Figure 3.)*

GEORGE STEINHARDT

Commentary by

Given the current sophistry touting circumcision as an effective mechanism to halt the spread of AIDS, I suspect we are going to continue to experience complications for this, the most common procedure in our country. HIV aside, I spend far more time in the operating room and office taking care of complications of foreskin removal than problems deriving from an intact prepuce. Penile adhesions and meatal stenosis are usually easily managed in the office with eutectic mixture of local analgesia and fine instruments. I have only seen a few fistulas but the techniques illustrated seem reasonable for successful correction. It is a shame that the tip of an inadvertently amputated glans is often discarded, as reattachment as described is straightforward and quite successful. I have never had to reattach a complete amputation of the glans, but believe it possible by following this description. Of course, no surgeon would intentionally circumcise a patient with a penile deformity, but I am often struck with how difficult it is to recognize a normal penis. Perhaps the most common significant problem that I see with increasing frequency (perhaps due to the increased occurrence of the deformity) is a patient with an unrecognized scrotalized penis who is subjected to circumcision. This leads to a paucity of penile skin, which, in my practice, has required full-thickness skin grafting to repair. I harvest two triangles of skin from the groin and suture them together to form a rectangle that is then used to resurface the penis. I deglove the phallus by incising the line of demarcation between the remnant preputial skin and the deficient penile skin and use the graft to bridge the gap. I like Coban and Adaptic as dressings as they firmly support the grafts for the 4 to 5 days necessary for them to heal.

DOUG CANNING

Commentary by

Because the foreskin is gone, there is less tissue available to use in correction of a fistula or severe meatal stenosis. In my experience, it is hard to get a flap based on the tissues surrounding the urethral meatus to work properly under these conditions. I prefer to use a dorsal transverse preputial flap, which we take circumferentially. Before mobilizing the flap, we make a vertical incision on the ventral midline of the penis from the midpoint of the old circumcision scar to the penoscrotal junction. This allows lateral traction to flatten the penile shaft skin to help visualize the pedicle. This augmented view of the dorsal blood supply of the flap provides access to a more consistent plane while separating the vascular pedicle from the dorsal penile shaft skin. The transverse flap provides excellent tissue to correct a urethral meatal injury or a fistula. If the fistula is located at the corona, as is usually the case, the urethral meatus should be opened to the level of the fistula or even proximal to it to allow for complete reconstruction of the urethra or wide mobilization of the fistula before closure. The secret to fistula closure is wide exposure and mobilization of well-vascularized flaps. If the urethral meatus requires mobilization to allow placement deeper within the glans following a glans injury, aggressive dissection proximal to the corona onto the shaft of the penis, or as far as the penoscrotal junction, may be required to provide an effective repair.

Chapter 158

Concealed (Buried) and Webbed Penis

The concealed or buried penis is a relatively rare phenomenon defined as a paucity of ventral foreskin. Patients who have this anatomic abnormality can be repaired by surgically transposing excess dorsal skin ventrally. Symptoms include local infection and foreskin ballooning on urination, secondary to tight phimosis. The phimosis can act as a severe obstruction, causing tissue expansion within the prepuce.

REPAIR OF SEVERE BURIED PENIS

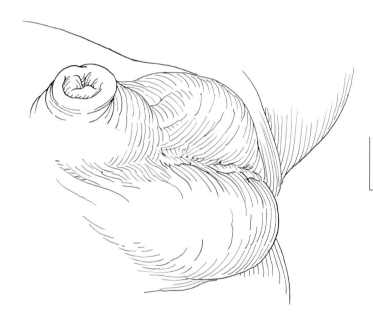

FIGURE 158-1. A ventral skin deficiency and phimosis lead to severe ballooning on urination, with local skin irritation and infection.

FIGURE 158-2. Urine constantly drips from the tight prepuce and the expanded space within the inner prepuce and glans.

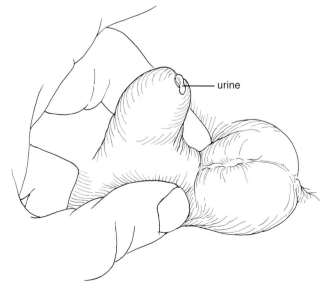

urine

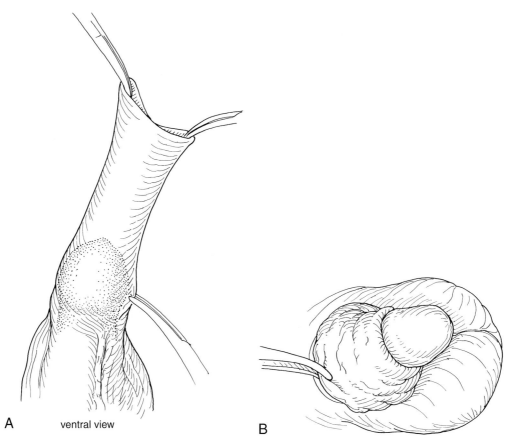

A   ventral view

B

FIGURE 158-3. **A,** Reduce the phimosis by stretching or performing a dorsal slit on the excess foreskin. **B,** This exposes the glans and redundant inner prepuce. Resterilize the now exposed inner prepuce with antiseptic.

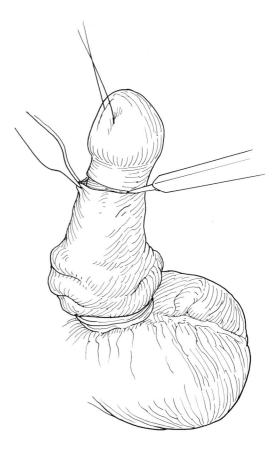

FIGURE 158-4. Make an incision 5 mm below the coronal margin. Deglove the penis to the penoscrotal junction.

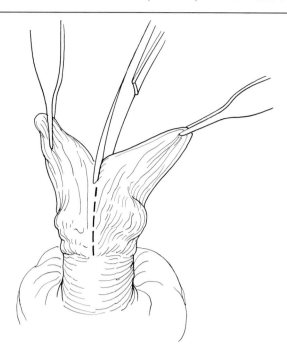

FIGURE 158-5. Perform a dorsal incision through the excess skin, cutting through the phimotic band.

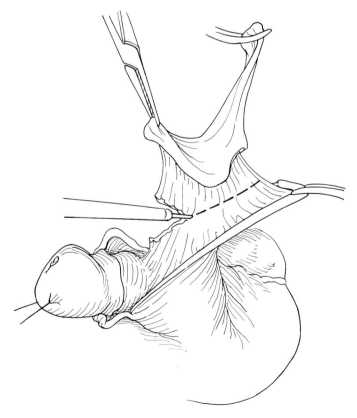

FIGURE 158-6. Trim excess skin and subcutaneous tissue. Use the cautery to prevent bleeding.

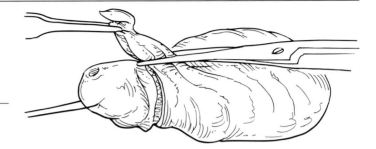

FIGURE 158-7. Transfer excess skin from the dorsal to ventral aspect of the exposed penis, designing a midline seam.

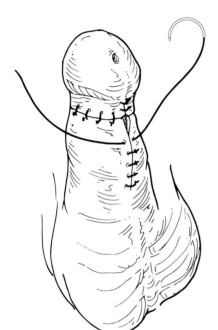

FIGURE 158-8. Close the defect with 6-0 absorbable suture.

INNER PREPUTIAL TECHNIQUE (REDMOND)

For a ventral skin deficiency without severe tissue expansion, the inner preputial technique can be used. The strategy behind the Redmond repair of the buried penis is to remove the phimosis and cover the penile shaft skin with inner prepuce. This will resolve the ventral skin deficiency and clinical symptoms.

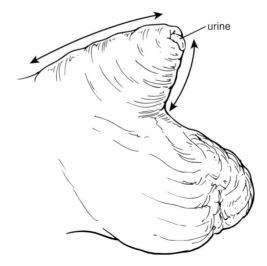

FIGURE 158-9. Note the length difference between the shorter ventral aspect and longer dorsal aspect of the buried or concealed penis *(arrows).*

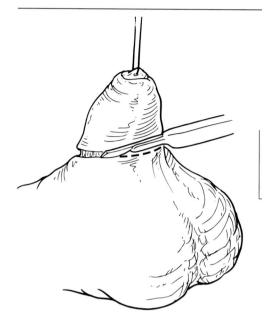

FIGURE 158-10. First, outline an incision on the ventral aspect of the penis at the penoscrotal junction and carry it around to the dorsal aspect of the penis at the base of the shaft skin. Proceed with dissection to relieve tethering tissue along Buck's fascia, exposing the penile shaft.

FIGURE 158-11. In severe cases, open the outer foreskin to relieve the phimosis with the use of a mosquito or dorsal-slit technique. After pulling down the outer and inner prepuce, make a circumcising incision in an appropriate position along the inner prepuce to cover the defect. Design the incision on the inner prepuce to accommodate the ventral skin deficiency.

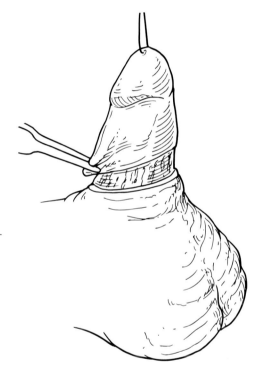

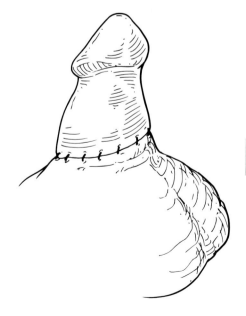

FIGURE 158-12. Then approximate the inner prepuce using absorbable 6-0 sutures to the penoscrotal junction, completing the repair.

POSTOPERATIVE PROBLEMS

In obese children the penis can reconceal. It is important to have the parents push down on tissue surrounding the penis in the immediate postoperative period. Liberal application of antibiotic ointment can facilitate the process.

WEBBED PENIS

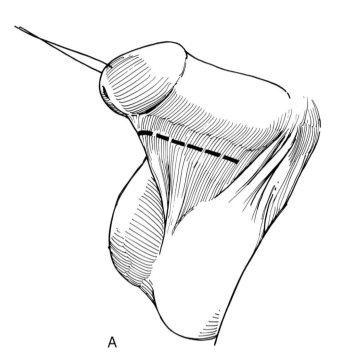
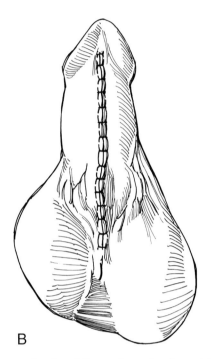

FIGURE 158-13. The webbed penis, from midline bands at the penoscrotal angle, can be freed from the web of scrotal skin. **A,** Place a traction suture in the glans and a second one in the distal edge of the skin fold. Sharply divide the edge, keeping far enough from the shaft to have enough skin for ventral closure. **B,** Approximate the ventral skin edges with 6-0 absorbable suture.

MARK ZAONTZ

Commentary by

Penile concealment has garnered much attention in the last two decades. Prior to this, little attention was paid, if any, to the concealed penis. Unfortunately, many of these children grew up with significant psychosocial issues, especially when no corrective surgery had been undertaken. As seen in this chapter, there are a number of operative techniques to correct the concealed penis, depending on the anatomic causation. In addition to unearthing the phallus to allow full exposure, it is also important for cosmetic improvement to allow the children to mainstream with their peers. While in Chicago we wrote a paper that proposed a classification system consisting of four categories of penile concealment. These included the buried penis, webbed penis, entrapped penis, and micropenis. The etiology of the concealment would often dictate the preferred surgical technique. One caveat that is important to recognize is that not all webbed penises are equal. Also, not all webbed penises require scrotoplasty.

When examining a child with penile concealment and a noted web, I first fully expose the phallus by placing one finger on either side of the penis, pressing downward to see if I can obviate the webbed appearance. If the penis stands up straight and I can visualize a good ventral shaft with this maneuver, then the technique that incorporates three-point fixation at the base of the penis is employed. This was originally described by Cromie and colleagues (1998) and then popularized by Caldamone and colleagues (2004). Essentially that repair includes degloving of the shaft skin with fixation of the penile skin at the penopubic and penoscrotal junctions. Various locations of fixation have been described but I prefer the 12-, 3-, and 9-o'clock positions. The Buck's fascia is very superficially scored and the suture is affixed to the corresponding dermis at the shaft–abdominal wall junction. I generally prefer an absorbable suture and like to use a 4-0 polydioxanone stitch that is long-lasting.

Should there be significant webbing that cannot be obviated by the maneuver described then a scrotoplasty is performed. The technique for this is somewhat different than that described in this chapter. After making an inner preputial incision 1 cm below the corona glandis, the foreskin is reduced over the glans and an Allis clamp grasps the foreskin at its tip while another Allis clamp grasps the midline of the inferior aspect of the scrotum, pulling at a right angle from one another. This delineates the penoscrotal web nicely. A marking pen is used to create an inverted V appearance. The line follows the juncture of the shaft skin with the web. Once the incision is made the scrotum is dropped back proximally and dissection is continued deep to the scrotal tissue, lysing all the bands that are encountered. The dissection is taken directly on top of the urethra for the best results. The remaining ventral prepuce is incised up the midline, and then the dorsal shaft is degloved out to the penopubic junction, lysing all bands and dartos tissue. It is important to stay just above Buck's fascia. This allows maximal unearthing of the phallus. In cases where the penopubic angle is poorly defined, due to either a fat pad or partial penoscrotal transposition, a suture of 4-0 polydioxanone is placed superficially at the 12-o'clock position and Buck's fascia and affixed to the corresponding dermis of the penopubic angle. The dorsal skin is incised and the midline is secured to the mucosal collar with absorbable suture. Byars' flaps are swung ventrally on stay sutures. The ventral shaft is then recreated by transposing the skin medially into the midline. A suture of 4-0 Monocryl is placed deep to the scrotum just outside the urethra and secured to the dartos fascia on each side of the newly created penoscrotal junction. This suture is then run up the dartos layer, creating a median raphe all the way up to the mucosal collar. The midline skin is closed with a running horizontal mattress closure of 5-0 Monocryl, and then the scrotum is generally repaired as a semilunar transverse closure to give a very natural appearance to the scrotum. The remaining excess foreskin is excised over a marking line and closed with absorbable suture. I find this gives an outstanding cosmetic and reproducible result and would recommend this in these situations.

ISRAEL FRANCO

Commentary by

The hidden or buried penis is a very common problem, with the webbed penis being a variant of the aforementioned. In each case the defect is marked by a degree of variability in mobility of the skin. The defect is due to abnormal fixation of the dartos fascia to the shaft of the penis. This allows for the skin to move freely on the shaft, thereby allowing the skin to telescope onto the glans of the penis. Fat tends to accumulate in this loose areolar tissue at the base of the penis, compounding the problem. Normal day-to-day erections are a means for stretching the preputial ring and thus correcting naturally neonatal phimosis. This penile skin is very mobile and not well anchored, allowing the erections to lift the skin; thereby, no pressure is exerted on the phimotic ring. Without this natural stretching the prepuce becomes tighter; the tighter the prepuce gets the more likely that it will entrap urine. This leads to the ballooning of the prepuce that is encountered in some of these cases.

After neonatal circumcision two scenarios can occur. In some cases the penis becomes entrapped by the postoperative cicatrix requiring prompt intervention. In other instances the penile skin telescopes up onto the glans and adheres to the glans. The preputial skin that is naturally elastic and stretches freely. Many parents or pediatricians will say that there was a perfect circumcision with no excess skin for the first month or so. As time goes on, however, the skin appears to have increased in size as the penis becomes more hidden. The excess skin probably is a consequence of penile-to-glanular adhesions that exist in just about all hidden penis cases. The dense adhesions anchor the skin to the glans and the ever-present erections of young boys act as a tissue expander, stretching the penile skin and leading to the occurrence of excess skin. In other cases inaccurate removal of the skin due to hypermobility of the penile skin leads to this excess skin problem. The opposite can occur as well; in boys who were circumcised there will be a paucity of skin on the ventrum of the penis due to excess skin having been removed at the original circumcision.

Pediatricians and obstetricians have learned to identify the child who is likely to have a hidden, buried, or webbed penis, possibly leading to the greater awareness of this problem.

Another means of correcting of this defect can be facilitated by the following technique. After the penis is degloved and the ventral skin is incised down to the penoscrotal junction, the dartos tissue at the base of the penis and the scrotum are released from the corpora. The dartos tissue is then fixed to the base of the penis to recreate the penoscrotal junction with a nonabsorbable suture. The dorsal skin is cut to size, and the flaps are rotated to the ventrum. If the flaps are angled appropriately, they will give additional length and also will correct for the extra skin that is generally present. The midline can be closed with a two-layer continuous closure. The subcoronal skin is trimmed and reapproximated to the mucosal collar. By using this technique, all versions of this deformity can be corrected with excellent cosmetic results; the penis looks like a regular circumcised penis with a recreated midline raphe and normal shaft skin where it belongs. The penoscrotal angle is maintained as well. The technique described in the illustrations leaves a large amount of preputial skin where the shaft skin should be, and this result is less than perfect cosmetically but is a good alternative.

Chapter 159

Penile Torsion

Penile torsion is a well-defined congenital anomaly with a typical 90-degree counterclockwise twist. Torsion is treated by aggressive dissection of the skin and dartos fascia from Buck's fascia to the penoscrotal junction. The skin is then overapproximated in the opposite direction to the torsion.

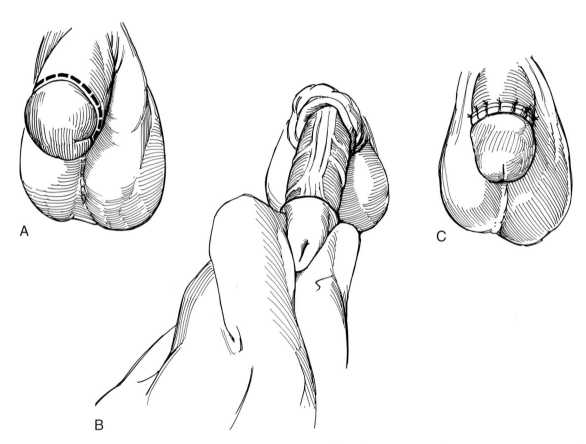

FIGURE 159-1. A, Incise the skin and dartos layer circumferentially at the corona, as for circumcision. **B,** Deglove the shaft and rotate the penis (usually clockwise) to orient the meatus vertically. Slightly overcorrect, because with healing the torsion will tend to reoccur. **C,** Reapproximate the skin with fine interrupted absorbable sutures. The median raphe ideally should be in the midline ventrally, but as noted occasionally may require over-rotation when correcting severe torsion.

MICHAEL DISANDRO

Commentary by

When correcting penile torsion, it must be taken into consideration that the procedure is mainly cosmetic, and as such, at the end of the procedure, not only should the rotation of the penis be correct but the median raphe should be in the midline. With minor torsion, this ideal result can be obtained by rotating the skin as shown above. With more severe torsion, however, simply rotating the skin will "pull" the median raphe off the midline laterally, which cosmetically looks rather bad. To prevent this from happening, in severe cases it is best to free the entire penile skin down to the base of the penis, detorse the penis, and then suture the dorsal Buck's fascia at the base of the corpora cavernosa (avoiding the underlying nerves) to the penile ligaments underneath the pubic skin to keep the penis from twisting back. By using this maneuver, you are not relying on the penile skin alone to detorse the penis, and the median raphe can remain in the midline.

Chapter 160

Epispadias Repair: Penile Disassembly

The epispadiac penis is dissected into three unique and separate parts: (1) urethral plate, (2) right corpus cavernosum with hemiglans, and (3) left corpus cavernosum with hemiglans. After disassembly the urethral plate is tubularized into a new urethra. The corporeal bodies are rotated dorsally, forming a new glans and ventral urethra. In epispadias the family should be aware of abnormal development of the urinary sphincter, which may require future treatment for urinary incontinence.

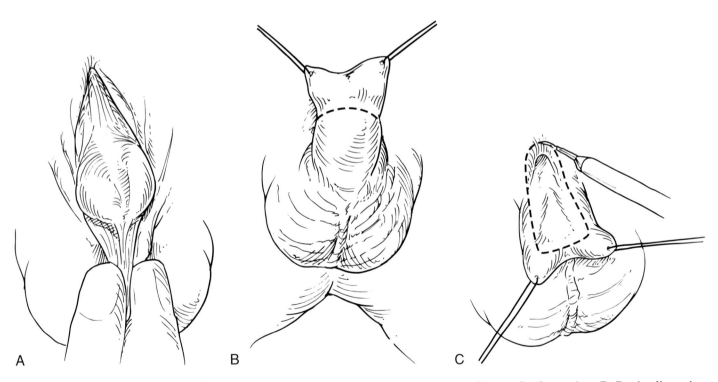

A   B   C

FIGURE 160-1. A, The epispadias defect with the ventral prepuce and a penopubic urethral opening. **B,** Begin dissection by placing two traction sutures into each hemiglans oriented horizontally, not vertically. These stay sutures will become vertical in orientation after later corporeal rotation. **C,** Make a circumcising incision ventrally and outline the urethral plate dorsally (usually about 1.5 cm wide) to allow later tubularization. Extend the urethral plate incisions proximally around the proximal urethral meatus. A fine-tip electrocautery device is useful in making this incision. Taking great care to preserve its blood supply, dissect the shaft skin off the lateral and ventral aspects of the paired corporeal bodies.

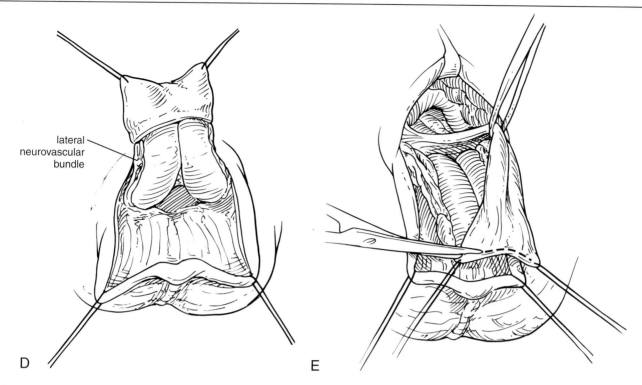

FIGURE 160-1, cont'd. D, The neurovascular bundles are located lateral on the corpora, and should be avoided while degloving the shaft skin. Dissect the urethral plate off of the corporeal bodies. It is useful to dissect the corporeal bodies ventrally and medially to define the appropriate plane between the corpora and urethral plate. The plate should be as thick as possible with dissection directly on Buck's fascia. **E,** Extend the plate incision around the distal tip of the urethral mucosa on the glans. Lift the whole plate based on its proximal blood supply from the glans and corporeal bodies, ready to be tubularized and transferred ventrally. Previous paravesical flap urethroplasty, as performed in primary exstrophy closure, does not preclude dissection of the urethral plate as described.

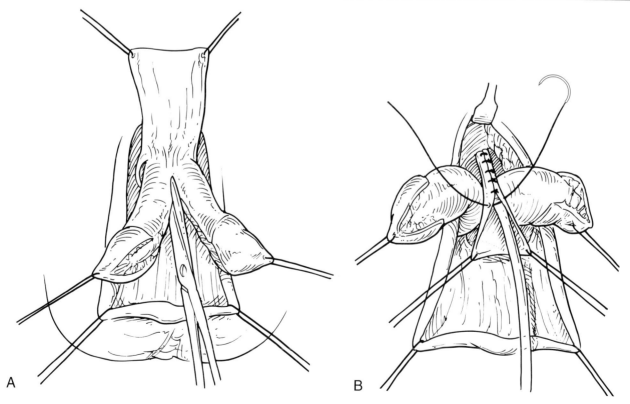

FIGURE 160-2. A, Completely separate the two hemicorporeal glanular bodies in the midline by a vertical incision, beginning distally and extending through the glans, which is divided into two halves that are each supplied by the vessels of the paired dorsal (lateral) neurovascular bundles. Tubularize the urethral plate and position ventrally to the entire length of the corporeal bodies.

Continued

FIGURE 160-2, cont'd. B, Freely rotate the corpus, which is now entirely separated and independent, to correct dorsal chordee. (It is sometimes necessary to correct dorsoventral length discrepancies by dermal graft insertion or suturing together adjacent corporotomies.) Suture together the corpora cavernosa with fine nonabsorbable sutures on the dorsum. Position the urethra in the ventral groove between the corpora cavernosa and suture to each glans half distally to produce an orthotopic urethral meatus. (Glanuloplasty usually includes reduction of glans tissue medially as needed to produce a conical appearance.) Bring together the glans halves with deep 5-0 or 6-0 polydioxanone sutures.

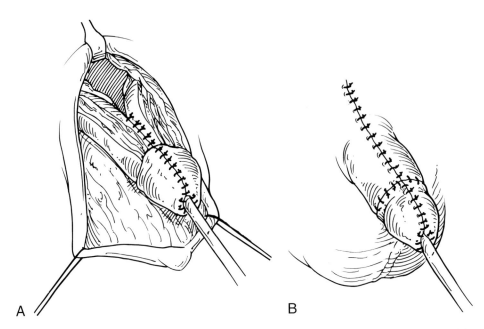

A   B

FIGURE 160-3. A, Advance the urethral neomeatus onto the glans tip and mature, as in standard hypospadias repair. If the tubularized urethra is too short, it can be matured onto the ventral aspect of the penis to form a hypospadias, which is completed later with a second-stage procedure. Alternatively, use a preputial flap for distal urethroplasty (one-stage epispadias repair). **B,** Reconfigure the shaft skin using reverse Byars' flaps for closure as needed. Drain the repair with a feeding tube or stent for 7 to 10 days. Alternatively, if the repair is performed as part of a complete primary closure, the ureteral stents are brought out at the new urethra in lieu of a separate stent.

COMPLICATIONS

A hypospadiac meatus is more the rule than the exception in complete primary closure requiring a second-stage urethroplasty. Fistula and stricture, as in any urethroplasty, are possible although with good technique avoidable if care is taken to preserve the corpora spongiosa ventral to the urethral plate. Residual chordee may not be apparent for many years or until puberty. Expectations must be reasonable in that patients with exstrophy/epispadias have congenitally short penises.

MICHAEL MITCHELL

Commentary by

The technique for disassembly and reconstruction of the epispadias by complete disassembly continues to be very useful, primarily to provide access to the pelvic diaphragm (closure of exstrophy). However, the technique is also very useful in reconstruction of the phallus. What dictates whether complete disassembly or partial disassembly (leaving the glans on the phallus connected to the urethral plate) should be done usually depends on the degree of symphyseal diastasis; the wider the diastasis, the more the requirement for complete disassembly. Therefore, patients with cloacal exstrophy often inherently require complete disassembly as it is not infrequent that the penis is not already separate anyway. The disassembly technique is very useful in those patients in whom the urethral plate is either inherently short or short after some redo cases (in our experience roughly 50% of males with exstrophy have a short urethra) and who ultimately have a urethral meatus somewhere on the ventrum of the reconstructed penis after complete primary repair exstrophy.

A subsequent distal urethroplasty can be performed when the child is approximately 2 years of age. The distal urethroplasty, as an isolated procedure, can usually be done as an outpatient procedure. The Cantwell-Ransley treatment (see Chapter 161) of the distal urethral plate is useful in patients with less separation of the symphyses and adequate length of the urethral plate. In my experience, if there is any question as to the adequacy of the length of the urethral plate then very strong consideration should be given to complete disassembly and placement of the urethral meatus on the ventrum of the phallus.

The neurovascular bundle supplying enervation and the blood supply to the glans or hemiglans is always found lateral to the edge of the urethral plate, is protected by Buck's fascia, and should not be at risk for dissection in complete disassembly. However, extensive lateral dissection to the proximal corpora cavernosa does potentially put this blood supply and enervation at risk. Furthermore, if tension is placed on the closure of the symphyses, the dorsal blood supply may be compromised with subsequent loss of the glans. This usually reflects either a too-aggressive suturing in the symphyseal closure or sometimes failure to recognize the need for osteotomy. If, at the time of closure of the symphyses, a question of blood supply to the glans penis is raised, the closure should be stopped and fascial sutures removed. If osteotomy had not previously been performed it should be done at this point. The sutures should be replaced and closure should be reattempted by closure of the anterior rectus fascia from the cephalad to the caudal end of the incision, followed by gentle closure of the symphyses. If, after these maneuvers, blood supply is still in question then redissection of the pelvic diaphragm should be performed, because it has probably been inadequate. At the completion of closure there should be no question as to blood supply to the glans or to the corpora cavernosa. The blood supply to these structures is obviously completely different and unique and paired side to side.

Chapter 161

Epispadias Repair

Repair the epispadias when the child is 6 months to 1 year of age. Early repair will allow for increased resistance to urinary flow, potentially increasing bladder volume.

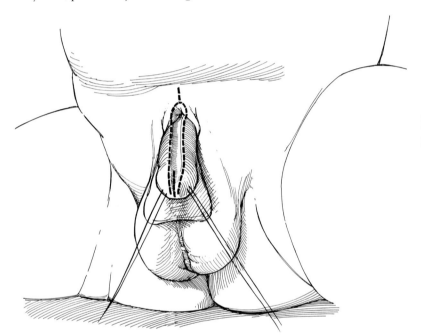

FIGURE 161-1. Place two traction sutures in the glans. Mark two parallel incisions on the dorsum on either side of the urethral plate 1.8 cm apart for the length of the penis *(long dashed line)* with pubic extension. Make a deep incision longitudinally in the urethral plate just proximal to the glans tip *(short dashed line)*.

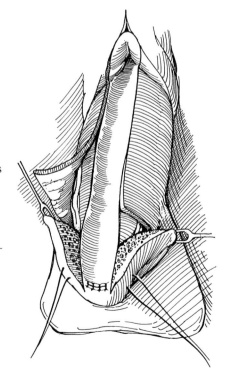

FIGURE 161-2. Close the incision in the urethral plate transversely to bring the plate to the penile tip by the IPGAM (reverse MAGPI) maneuver (see Chapter 138). Excise wedges of glans tissue on either side of the urethral plate to form glans flaps. Dissect the skin of the shaft free throughout its length. Make a Z-incision at the base to release the split suspensory ligaments. Dissect the skin from the entire ventrum, being careful to preserve the proximal mesentery connected to the urethral plate at the base of the penis between the corpora.

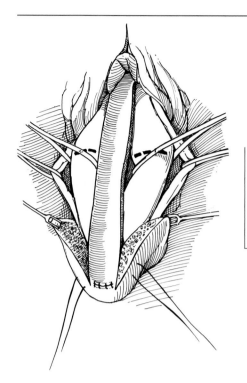

FIGURE 161-3. Expose Buck's fascia ventrally and separate the corporeal bodies in the midline. Retract each corpus with a vessel loop, and develop a plane between the corpora and the urethral plate, extending both proximally and distally to the glans. Dissect the neurovascular bundles from beneath Buck's fascia over the corpora. Retract them in vessel loops. Incise the tunica albuginea of each corpus transversely at the point of greatest angulation *(dashed lines)*.

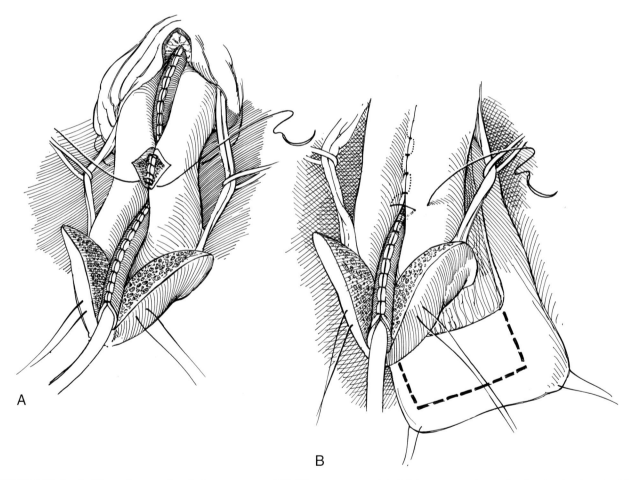

A

B

FIGURE 161-4. A, Close the urethral plate over an 8-F silicone stent with 6-0 interupped, synthetic slowly absorbable sutures. The transverse incisions in the corpora are opened into diamond-shaped defects by traction on the penis. Suture these defects to each other, converting the original transverse incisions into a longitudinal closure. **B,** Suture the corpora to each other using a running Connell stitch of 5-0 Prolene suture, burying the knots. Add additional 5-0 synthetic absorbable sutures between the corpora dorsally to further rotate them and displace the urethra ventrally. This is especially important adjacent to the glans. Outline and incise a rectangular flap on the inner surface of the prepuce.

FIGURE 161-5. **A**, Approximate the glans flaps in two layers and close the epithelium with running subcuticular fine absorbable sutures. It may be necessary to excise redundant glans tissue. Bring the preputial flap to the dorsum, and attach it to the skin as an island. Form flaps from the remainder of the prepuce and ventral skin to cover the rest of the penis. **B**, Alternatively, if there is sufficient ventral skin, bring it around and suture it dorsally. Close the basal Z-incision with interrupted sutures. Suture the stent securely in place and apply a Tegaderm dressing.

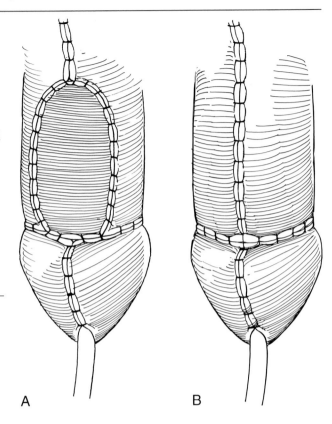

A   B

POSTOPERATIVE PROBLEMS

Fistulas are not uncommon. Avoid tension on the suture lines and prevent infection.

DAVID DIAMOND

Commentary by

The modified Cantwell approach to epispadias repair incorporates certain elements that Cantwell first described in 1895. These include complete mobilization of the urethral plate from the corporeal bodies and ventral transposition of the reconstructed urethral tube with dorsal rotation of the corpora.

Male epispadias most commonly presents in conjunction with classic bladder exstrophy. In the full-term male with adequate phallic size the Cantwell-Ransley technique may be incorporated into the complete primary repair of bladder exstrophy. If the baby is premature and the phallus tiny, defer epispadias repair for 12 to 18 months, which is a traditional, staged approach to bladder exstrophy. Repair of the epispadias has been shown to improve bladder capacity. The male with complete epispadias may undergo repair at 10 to 14 months of age. Preoperative treatment with one or two doses of testosterone enanthate, 25 mg intramuscularly, enlarges the phallus somewhat and improves the quality and suppleness of penile tissue. As penile skin may be in short supply, this can simplify the repair.

Although most male epispadias is complete or penopubic, it may present in milder forms. This has considerable impact on future continence as the bladder neck may be variably involved. Therefore, cystoscopy prior to epispadias repair is important as a diagnostic and prognostic maneuver.

One of the great advantages of the Cantwell-Ransley technique is its maintenance of an intact urethral tube. Over time, these tubes have been found easy to catheterize, making clean intermittent catheterization for those requiring it more straightforward.

Urethrocutaneous fistula has been the most common complication of this repair, occurring in approximately 8% of cases. The areas most vulnerable to fistula formation have been the most proximal portion of the urethral reconstruction as well as the junction of pendulous urethra with glanular urethra at the level of the corona. Urethral stenosis has been an uncommon complication.

RICARDO GONZALEZ

Commentary by

In all cases, with the exception of the more distal glanular epispadias, I now use the Cantwell-Ransley technique. This operation is applicable to all cases of either isolated epispadias or those associated with bladder exstrophy. The important general points of the technique are: (1) use of optical magnification, (2) use of bipolar cautery, (3) use of fine monofilament absorbable suture material, and (4) atraumatic surgery with careful handling of tissues. Specific points include the identification and preservation of the dorsal neurovascular bundles, preservation of the urethral plate whenever possible, and excision of small strips of glans lateral to the urethral plate to avoid leaving a cleft glans.

I begin by placing two traction sutures in the glans; then I perform the IPGAM, which is the reverse meatal advancement and glanuloplasty (MAGPI) procedure. In dissecting the circumference of the corpora, it is important not to injure the neurovascular bundles, but I do not necessarily dissect them and lift them off the corpora as originally described. Medially, during the dissection of the corpora, it is important to preserve the tissue that joins the ventral aspect of the urethral plate to the ventral penile skin to maximize the vascularization of the urethra. In infancy, the age in which I prefer to correct this malformation, excellent straightening of the penis can be obtained by suturing the corpora as shown, without necessarily making corporeal incisions and anastomosing the corpora together. This maneuver may be necessary in older children and adults and in redo cases. However, the proximal dissection of the corpora from the pubic rami is important in all cases. To tubularize the urethra, I prefer a 7-0 running, extraepithelial polydioxanone suture, reinforced by a second layer of the same suture material. I also use 7-0 running polydioxanone suture in the skin, with excellent cosmetic results. At the proximal end of the urethroplasty, avoid leaving a diverticulum that may make catheterization difficult. Remember that in cases of exstrophy, some of these children will need either temporary or permanent intermittent catheterization after the bladder neck reconstruction. In infants, I do all repairs with a 7-F Silastic stent with multiple perforations, with the proximal end just inside the bladder neck. The coverage of the dorsal skin defect is best obtained with an island flap of the ventral prepuce. Rotation of the penis by traction of the subcutaneous vascular pedicle must be avoided. The penis can be left without a dressing, but generally I prefer a double layer of Tegaderm.

Part IV

Genital Repair

Chapter 162

Introduction to Genital Repair in Patients with Disorders of Sex Development

Establish a clinical diagnosis. The most common form of disorders of sex development (DSD) is congenital adrenal hyperplasia or 46,XX DSD secondary to 21-hydroxylase deficiency. Other, less common forms of DSD include mixed gonadal dysgenesis and ovotesticular DSD. Inquire about exposure to maternal androgens; a family history of perinatal deaths (which suggests the salt-losing form of the adrenogenital syndrome), infertility, and operations on the genitalia of family members.

The infant with impalpable gonads requires prompt diagnosis. In addition to looking at the clinical features—family history, chromosomal analysis, biochemical studies, and anatomic appearance—sonogram and MRI will help define the internal anatomy.

The surgeon has a responsibility to outline the surgical sequence and subsequent consequences from infancy to adulthood. Only surgeons with expertise in the care of children and specific training in the surgery of DSD should undertake these

procedures. Parents now appear to be less inclined to choose surgery for less severe clitoromegaly. Surgery should only be considered in cases of severe virilization (Prader 3–5) and should be carried out in conjunction, when appropriate, with repair of the common urogenital sinus. As orgasmic function and erectile sensation may be disturbed by clitoral surgery, the surgical procedure should be anatomically based to preserve erectile function and the innervation of the clitoris. Emphasis is on functional outcome rather than a strictly cosmetic appearance. It is generally felt that surgery that is carried out for cosmetic reasons in the first year of life relieves parental distress and improves attachment between the child and the parents.

TIMING OF SURGERY

Currently there is inadequate evidence in relation to establishment of functional anatomy, to abandon the practice of early separation of the vagina and urethra. The rationale for early reconstruction is based on guidelines on the timing of genital surgery from the American Academy of Pediatrics, the beneficial effects of estrogen on tissue in early infancy, and the avoidance of potential complications from the connection between the urinary tract and peritoneum through the fallopian tubes. It is anticipated that surgical reconstruction in infancy will need to be refined at the time of puberty. Vaginal dilatation should not be undertaken before puberty.

The surgeon must be familiar with several operative techniques in order to reconstruct the spectrum of urogenital sinus disorders. An absent or inadequate vagina (with rare exceptions) requires a vaginoplasty performed in adolescence when the patient is psychologically motivated and a full partner in the procedure. No one technique has been universally successful; self-dilatation, skin substitution, and bowel vaginoplasty each have specific advantages and disadvantages. In the case of a DSD associated with hypospadias, standard techniques for surgical repair such as chordee correction, urethral reconstruction, and the judicious use of testosterone supplementation apply. The magnitude and complexity of phalloplasty in adulthood should be taken into account during the initial counseling period if successful gender assignment is dependent on this procedure. At times this may affect the balance of gender assignment. Patients must not be given unrealistic expectations about penile reconstruction, including the use of tissue engineering.

There is no evidence that prophylactic removal of asymptomatic discordant structures, such as a utriculus or mullerian remnants, is required although symptoms in future may indicate surgical removal. For the male who has a successful neophalloplasty in adulthood, an erectile prosthesis may be inserted but has a high morbidity.

The testes in patients with complete and partial androgen insensitivity syndrome (CAIS) should be removed to prevent malignancy in adulthood. The availability of estrogen replacement therapy allows for the option of early removal at the time of diagnosis, which also takes care of the associated hernia, psychological problems with the presence of testes, and the malignancy risk. Parental choice allows deferment until adolescence, recognizing that the earliest reported malignancy in CAIS is at 14 years of age. The streak gonad in a patient with mixed gonadal dysgenesis who has been raised male should be removed laparoscopically (or by laparotomy) in early childhood. Bilateral gonadectomy is performed in early childhood in females (bilateral streak gonads) with gonadal dysgenesis and Y chromosome material.

In patients with androgen biosynthetic defects raised female, gonadectomy should be undertaken before puberty. A scrotal testis in patients with gonadal dysgenesis is at risk for malignancy. Current recommendations are testicular biopsy at puberty seeking signs of the premalignant lesion termed *carcinoma in situ* or *undifferentiated intratubular germ cell neoplasia*. If positive, the option is sperm banking before treatment with local, low-dose radiotherapy that is curative.

Surgical management in DSD should also consider options that will facilitate the chances of fertility. In patients with a symptomatic utriculus, removal is best undertaken laparoscopically to increase the chance of preserving continuity of the vasa deferentia. Patients with bilateral ovotestes are potentially fertile from functional ovarian tissue. Separation of ovarian and testicular tissue can be technically difficult and should be undertaken, if possible, in early life.

Chapter 163

Vaginoplasty

Review the genitogram to confirm the site of the confluence between the vagina and urethra. Prepare the patient for surgery in consultation with endocrinology. Administer stress steroids.

Position the patient in full-body preparation from the thorax to toe, using stockings for the feet. This will allow turning the patient supine to prone during the procedure for optimal exposure.

LOW–CONFLUENCE FLAP VAGINOPLASTY

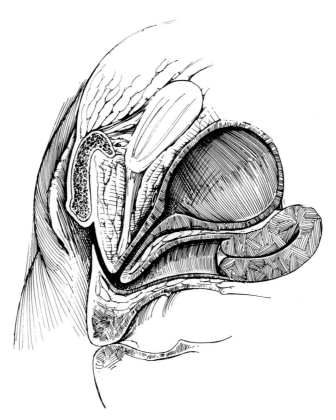

FIGURE 163-1. Perform panendoscopy for orientation. Transilluminate the urogenital sinus with the panendoscope to make sure that the vagina is low enough to be reached by a perineal flap. Insert a small balloon catheter in the urethra. In the rectum, place a 4 × 4 gauze soaked in neomycin solution.

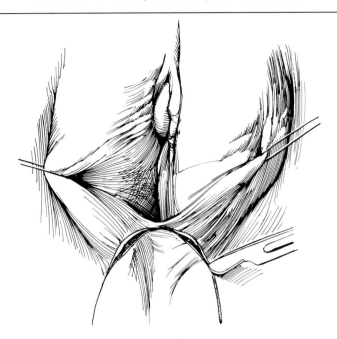

FIGURE 163-2. Incision for the flap: Mark and incise a broad-based, inverted U-shaped flap. Anteriorly it should reach almost to the edge of the sinus, and posteriorly it should end at the posterior margin of the new labia minora. Dissect a thick perineal flap. Be aware that the sinus is surrounded by corpus spongiosum and that the bleeding from the dissection will require fulguration and application of fine figure-eight catgut sutures. A finger in the rectum is not needed for the distal sinus dissection.

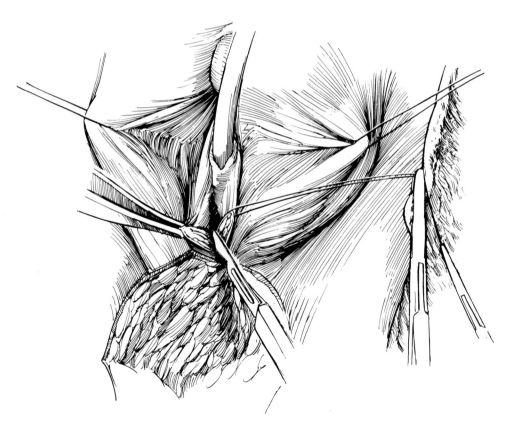

FIGURE 163-3. Incision in the vaginal back wall: Place two traction sutures in the edge of the thin posterior wall of the urogenital sinus and incise it until the vagina is reached. If the vagina is high, pull it down with a small balloon catheter until its thicker wall is exposed. The posterior incision must be deep (at least 1 to 2 cm) to provide adequate caliber for the new introitus. With a high vagina, the incision may be carried as far as the cervix. Be aware that although the rectum lies beneath this incision, the intervening areolar tissue must be incised to accommodate the flap. Place traction sutures in the edges of the vagina and loop them over the tips of clamps on the drapes.

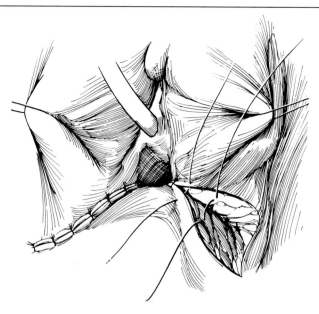

FIGURE 163-4. Insert the apex of the flap into the incision in the vaginal wall, first placing subcutaneous sutures for support. Suture the edges of the flap with 4-0 chromic catgut sutures, beginning at the apex. Postoperatively, start dilatation of the new introitus in 2 weeks with a metal dilator. The parents can continue regular dilatations at home, until they need to be done only monthly.

MID-CONFLUENCE VAGINOPLASTY: VAGINAL DISSECTION

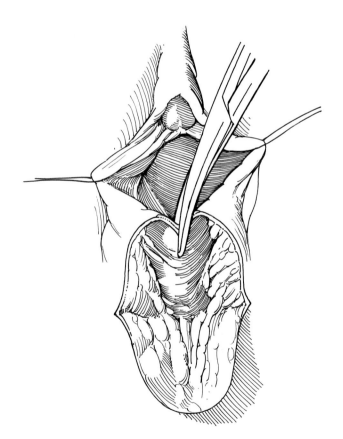

FIGURE 163-5. Form a posterior flap. Incise the posterior wall of the urogenital sinus far enough to expose the urethral meatus. Suture the edges with 5-0 chromic catgut. Place a finger in the rectum and dissect the posterior and lateral walls of the vagina. Incise the back wall deeply and insert the posterior flap. The vagina must be cut back sufficiently to avoid later stenosis, and the flap must neither be too large, producing a shelf, nor too small, resulting in a flat perineum.

HIGH-CONFLUENCE VAGINOPLASTY: PULL-THROUGH PROCEDURE (HENDREN)

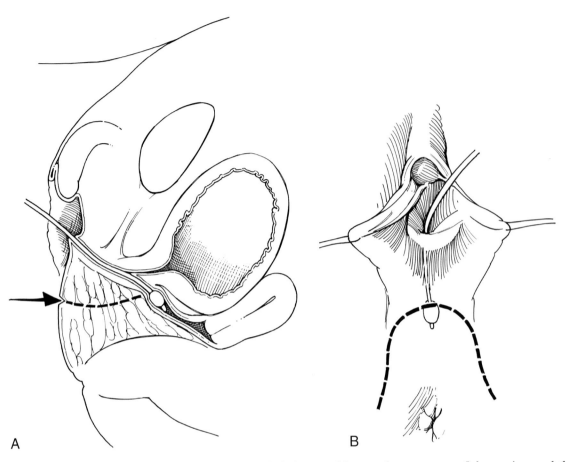

A   B

FIGURE 163-6. A, Perform panendoscopy of the urogenital sinus and locate the entrance of the vagina and the continuation of the urethra. Place a Fogarty catheter into the vagina. The dashed line shows the limit of the cutback incision, stopping at that point to prevent injury to the urethral sphincter. **B,** Incision: Make an inverted U-incision in the perineum with the apex opposite the balloon.

FIGURE 163-7. Place a finger in the rectum and dissect against the rectal wall beneath the external urethral sphincter. Have your assistant gently pull on the balloon so that you can identify the junction of the vagina with the sinus. Incise the vagina almost completely circumferentially about the base of the balloon (*dashed line*). Withdraw the Fogarty catheter. Insert a straight metal sound into the bladder through the urethra and complete the division of the vaginal rim, leaving a little vaginal tissue on the urethra to allow it to be closed without stricture.

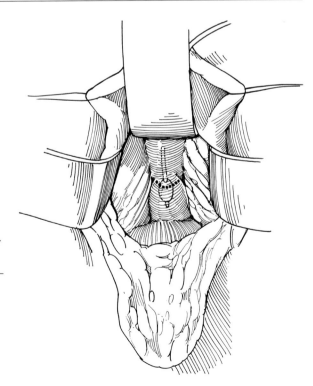

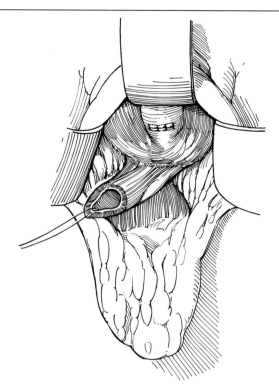

FIGURE 163-8. Close the urethra with interrupted 6-0 chromic catgut sutures. Replace the sound with a balloon catheter. Dissect the vagina from the proximal urethra as high as the back of the trigone.

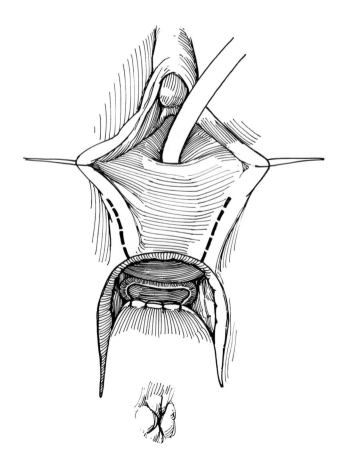

FIGURE 163-9. Suture the posterior flap into the back wall of the vagina with 5-0 chromic catgut sutures. Incise the perineum anterior to the vagina as an inverted U to form a second flap.

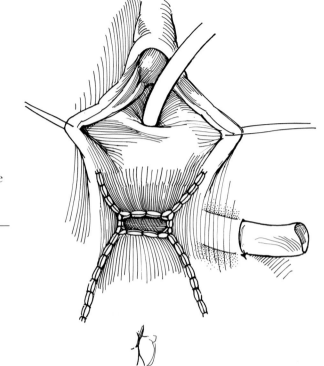

FIGURE 163-10. Mobilize this skin flap anteriorly, and suture it to the vaginal rim. Insert a small suction drain or Penrose drain to exit through a stab wound. Complete the closure by joining the lateral margins of the anterior and the posterior skin flaps to the perineal skin. Place a loose vaginal pack.

REDUNDANT LABIOSCROTAL SKIN

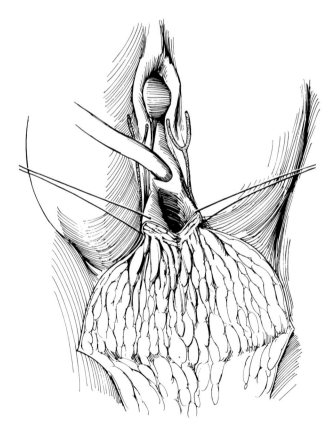

FIGURE 163-11. Mark a Y-shaped incision with the stem extending to the base of the clitoris to form V-shaped flaps on either side of the introitus.

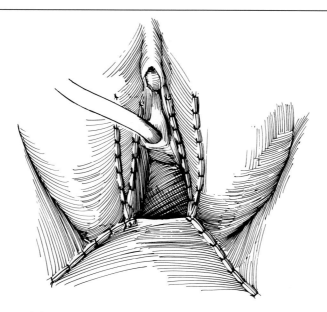

FIGURE 163-12. Raise the flaps and draw them down to meet the upper end of the vaginal incision. Suture them with 4-0 chromic catgut sutures while placing traction on the lateral vaginal tissue. Approximate the posterior flap.

POSTOPERATIVE PROBLEMS

Watch for adrenal insufficiency in the period immediately after operation. Bleeding can be controlled with pressure.

Painful erections may later be a problem if the clitoris is secured to the pubic bone. Vaginal stenosis is common and warrants examination under anesthesia at puberty.

Commentary by ARNOLD H. COLODNY

This section illustrates very nicely several fundamental principles of the surgery on intersex patients who are going to be raised as females.

The preoperative diagnostic modality of choice may eventually be MRI. It does not require injections or radiation and may be more sensitive than either ultrasonography or CT.

It is very important for intersex patients who will be raised as females, which applies to the majority of patients with ambiguity of the genitalia, to carry out surgery early to reduce the visibility of the phallic structure. If the infant is doing well, growing and developing normally, and there are no other medical problems, the operative procedure probably should be done around 2 or 3 months of age.

The surgeon should perform an operative procedure that removes the erectile tissue; preserves the neurovascular bundles and the glans; creates labia minora from the phallic skin, prepuce, or both; has a Y-V plasty to produce labia majora; and has a perineal flap to exteriorize the low vagina.

If the vagina enters the urethra above the external sphincter, the vaginoplasty can be delayed until the child is 2 or 3 years of age.

By freeing up the phallus you can then make an incision on each lateral side through the sheath of the corporeal bodies and remove the erectile tissue without hazard to the neurovascular bundles. When incising the posterior wall of the vagina to allow insertion of a perineal skin flap as illustrated in Figure 163-7, take extreme care to prevent injury to the rectum that lies immediately under the posterior wall of the vagina. The perineal U-shaped flaps should have a wide base.

It may be advantageous to preserve the skin of the shaft of the phallus rather than excising it. The skin can be split in the midline and then draped around the base of the phallus and moved downward to form the labia minora.

RICARDO GONZÁLEZ

To plan an operation to correct the urogenital sinus in a patient with congenital adrenal hyperplasia, it is necessary to understand the anatomy and embryology of the condition. The anatomy of the urogenital sinus in congenital adrenal hyperplasia is more constant and predictable than in cases of primary urogenital sinus or cloaca. The urethra and the vagina always have a confluence below the sphincter mechanism, and the urethra proximal to the confluence is always of adequate length. I agree that endoscopy is useful to define the anatomy except for the vagina, which is invariably present but may be short and thus difficult to visualize if the opening leading to it from the sinus is very small.

The two operations illustrated here have stood the test of time. Patient selection for the Fortunoff-Lattimer flap vaginoplasty is important. If applied to patients other than those with a very low confluence, the patient will be left with an intravaginal urethral meatus.

For cases of high confluence, the vaginal pull-through procedure described by Hendren can be used. However, I have had problems obtaining good tissue for the anterior flap as illustrated. The Passerini technique (1999) uses the urogenital sinus for this purpose. The clitoral prepuce can also be used to create an anterior flap. Another challenging step of the Hendren vaginal pull-through procedure is the dissection of the urethra from the anterior vaginal wall. In 1999 we described the application of total urogenital mobilization to the repair of urogenital sinus not associated with anorectal malformation. This technique had been described by Peña (1997) to repair cloacas with common channels under 3 cm. This technique avoids the separation of the urethra from the vagina and avoids the risk of fistulas. I always combine it with a posterior flap to prevent introital stenosis. With regard to the flap, the cosmetic appearance of the posterior fourchette can be improved by outlining an ω-shaped flap, leaving the subcutaneous pedicle wide. Since the total mobilization follows sound anatomic principles and does not interfere with sphincter innervation, fears of incontinence have been unfounded. When a clitoroplasty is also needed, it should be performed at the same time as the vaginoplasty.

Despite current controversies regarding the timing of female genital surgery, we prefer to correct the problem early in infancy. In patients with congenital adrenal hyperplasia, the gender identity is almost always female; it is easier to perform surgery on infants than on older girls; and no one has proved that operating after puberty decreases the incidence of introital stenosis. All reconstructed girls should be examined under anesthesia at the onset of puberty to detect possible introital stenosis.

Chapter 164

Vaginoplasty Using Urogenital Sinus

TOTAL UROGENITAL SINUS MOBILIZATION

This surgical approach may vary depending on the level of the confluence of the urogenital sinus with the urethra and vagina. Supplement the patient with a stress dose of hydrocortisone.

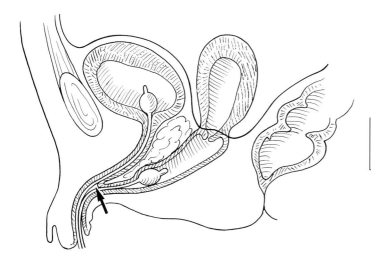

FIGURE 164-1. Cross-sectional schematic drawing of a low to mid confluence *(arrow)* of the urogenital sinus with the urethra and vagina.

FIGURE 164-2. Cross-sectional schematic drawing of a high confluence *(arrow)* of the urogenital sinus with the urethra and vagina. Carry out cystoscopy before the reconstruction. Place a Fogarty catheter in the vagina and a Foley catheter in the bladder.

Prep the patient with a full-bodied surgical preparation from the feet to the thorax, allowing access to the abdomen and perineum. The patient may be rotated to the prone position and back to the supine position during the surgery to optimize exposure.

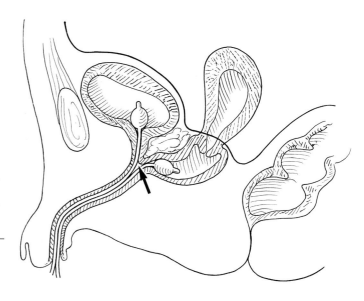

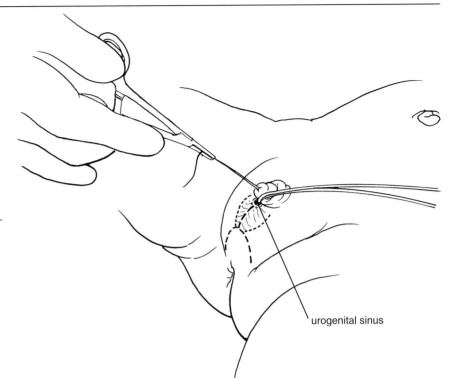

FIGURE 164-3. Place a temporary 5-0 Prolene holding stitch through the clitoris.

urogenital sinus

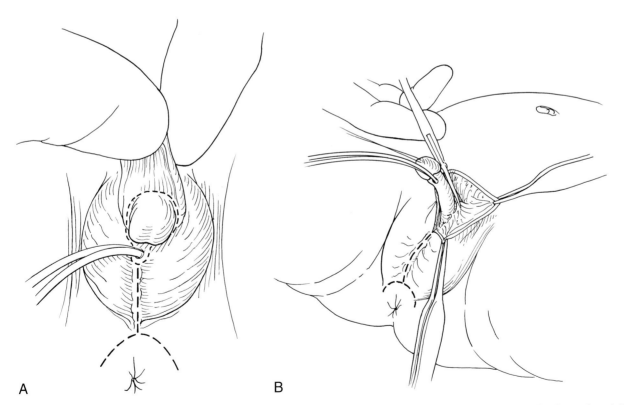

A

B

FIGURE 164-4. A and **B,** Develop an ω-shaped perineal flap extending from the proposed perineal body to the virilized labia. Perform clitoroplasty (see Chapter 165) if indicated for Prader 3–5 virilization at this time. Start the dissection in the midline posteriorly by dividing the attachments between the urogenital sinus and the rectum. With the rectum retracted inferiorly from the urogenital sinus, the entire posterior aspect of the common urogenital sinus and vagina is exposed.

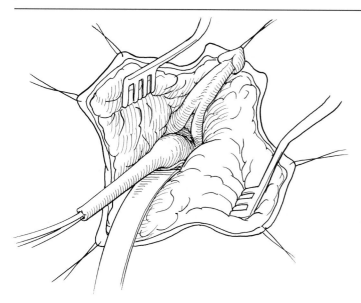

FIGURE 164-5. Separate the urogenital sinus from the virilized clitoris to the level of the pubis. Divide the ligaments, attaching the urogenital sinus to the pubis and thus freeing the urogenital sinus. Identify the vaginal confluence by palpation of the Fogarty catheter.

FIGURE 164-6. Open the vagina posteriorly over the Fogarty catheter. Continue until a normal caliber is encountered, as the distal third of the vagina is typically narrow and prone to stenosis. Complete the anterior dissection of the urogenital sinus from the corpora of the clitoris underneath the pubic bone. This frees the anterior urogenital sinus. Complete the posterior dissection of the vagina, allowing the entire urogenital sinus to become mobile and, in most cases, easily able to reach the perineum.

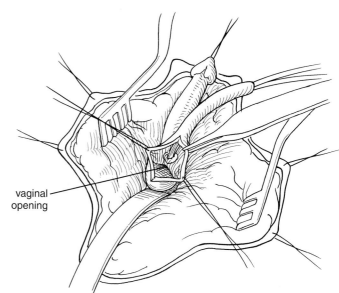

vaginal opening

SPLITTING THE UROGENITAL SINUS VENTRALLY

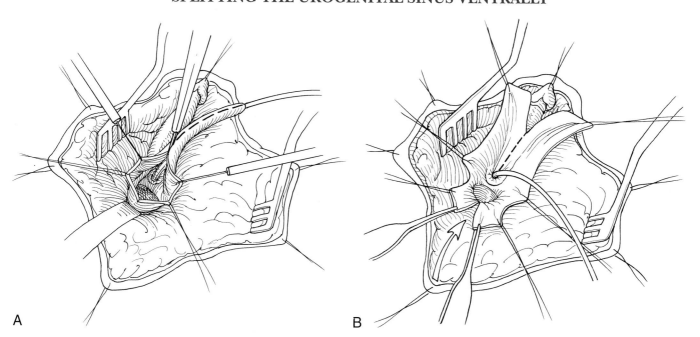

A

B

FIGURE 164-7. A and **B**, With an adequate vaginal opening *(arrow)*, split the common urogenital sinus ventrally and rotate the flap anteriorly to line the vaginal introitus.

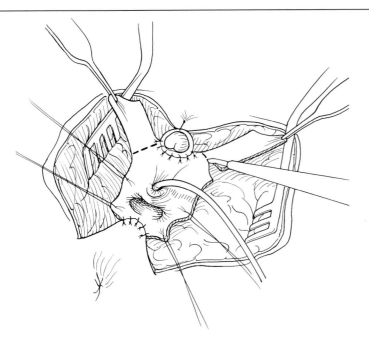

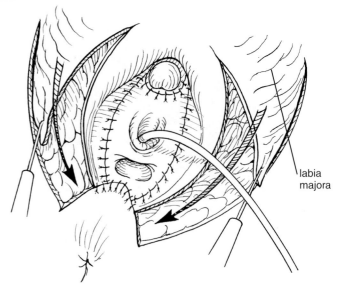

FIGURE 164-9.   Fashion the labia minora from excess clitoral hood preputial skin flaps. Trim the virilized labia majora and anastomose them *(arrows)* to below the vaginal opening.

FIGURE 164-8.   Position the urethral meatus to an orthotopic position beneath the clitoris. Trim excess urogenital sinus tissue and suture to the clitoral collar. Suture the ω-shaped flap to the posterior vaginal wall.

SPLITTING THE UROGENITAL SINUS LATERALLY

FIGURE 164-10.   To avoid excess use of skin in the posterior vagina split the urogenital sinus on its lateral aspect.

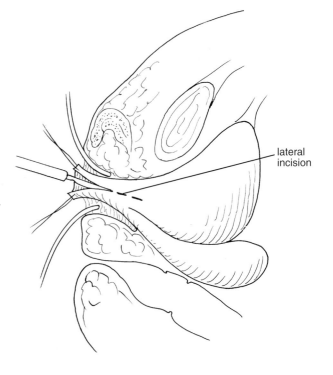

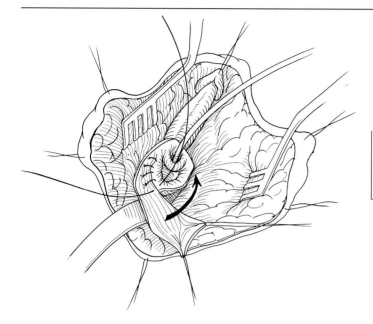

FIGURE 164-11. Rotate the flap *(arrow)* to form the distal vagina with placement of interrupted absorbable sutures. The lateral spiral flap brings excess urogenital sinus tissue to the posterior wall of the vagina.

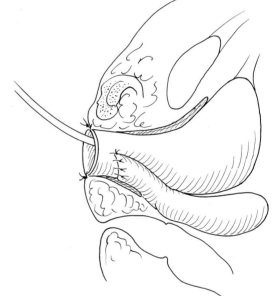

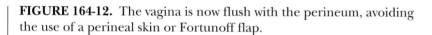

FIGURE 164-12. The vagina is now flush with the perineum, avoiding the use of a perineal skin or Fortunoff flap.

SPLITTING THE UROGENITAL SINUS DORSALLY

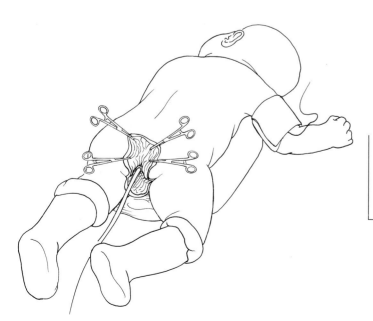

FIGURE 164-13. The urogenital sinus can also be used to create the anterior vaginal wall with the posterior wall composed of a perineal skin flap. With the patient in the prone position, the mobilized urogenital sinus has been separated from the vagina and the fistula closed.

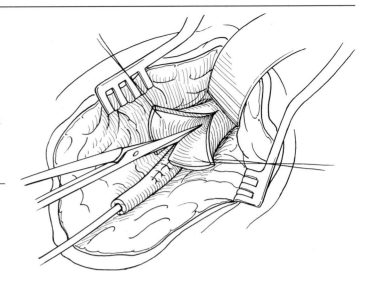

FIGURE 164-14. Split the anterior and posterior vagina in the midline so a normal-caliber vagina is now accessible. Close the defect in the urogenital sinus in several layers, forming the new urethra.

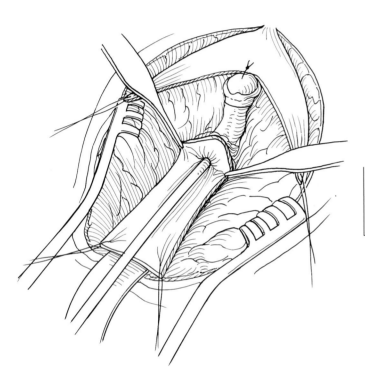

FIGURE 164-15. Flip the patient back to the supine position. Split the urethra at the 12-o'clock position or dorsal aspect, creating a flap of urogenital sinus that is rotated posteriorly to form the anterior vaginal wall.

FIGURE 164-16. Place the urethra in an orthotopic position and form the labia minora from the excess clitoral preputial tissue after fashioning and trimming the virilized labia majora.

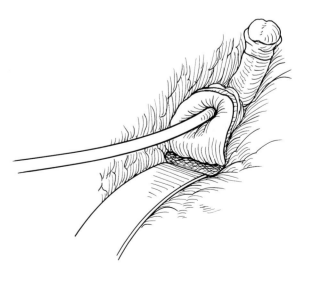

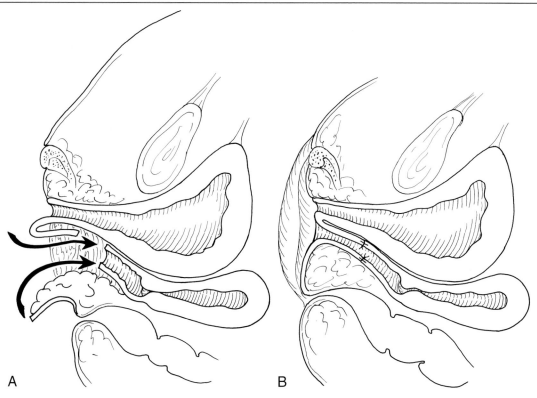

FIGURE 164-17. A and **B**, The anterior vaginal wall is added coverage for separation of the confluence between the vagina and the urethra *(arrow)*, covering the previously closed urethral defect.

RICHARD C. RINK

Commentary by

There are two schools of thought on the timing of repair in congenital adrenal hyperplasia. The most common sequence in the United States has been to do the reconstruction early in a single stage, which would include clitoroplasty, labiaplasty, and vaginoplasty. The advantages of this are that the maternal and placental estrogens will stimulate the growth and vascularity of the genital tissues, and that the vagina is often large at this stage, making the reconstruction easier before any scarring of the tissues.

The other classic sequence has been to do the clitoroplasty early and then do the vaginal reconstruction after puberty. Those who follow this route believe that visibility is better. I do not believe this; in addition, not only is there scarring of tissues but also you are doing a major construction when the child will remember it all.

There is now a third opinion, primarily promoted by the Intersex Society of North America, which is to do nothing and allow the child to determine sex and genital reconstruction when old enough to make the decision. Obviously, this creates a great problem on what to do for sex assignment.

AMICUR FARKAS

Commentary by

The main consideration in planning the right surgical approach is to determine whether the communication of the vagina to the urogenital sinus is above or below the pelvic floor (verumontanum). This can be done by a simple transabdominal ultrasound. The voiding cystourethrogram can be sometimes misleading; when the communication is very small, contrast media will not fill up the vagina. Positioning the baby in the so-called exaggerated lithotomy position with the thighs widely separated will allow a maximal exposure of the perineum and therefore the posterior vaginal wall can be reached without any difficulties in almost all the cases. I prefer to complete the total urogenital sinus mobilization by dissecting it from the corporeal bodies, the pubic arch and rami, and the rectum. Once it is completely free and pulled toward the perineum than to open the posterior vaginal wall over the balloon.

The issue of timing and staging of the genital reconstruction is subject to debate. My preference is to do it as a one-stage operation in early infancy, with the major advantage of using the redundant sinus, phallic, and preputial skin. This excellent

Continued

material is discarded and wasted when clitoral surgery is performed as a separate procedure in infancy and the vaginal reconstruction is postponed until adolescence.

Some have raised the question concerning future urinary continence after the complete urogenital sinus mobilization. In my experience, all the girls who reached toilet training are completely continent.

Intrauterine dexamethasone treatment is now popular in treating congenital adrenal hyperplasia patients. This treatment should be started very early in pregnancy because if it is started later the child can end up with a very small phallus and yet still have a high vaginal insertion. Then functional reconstruction can be difficult, as we do not have the redundant material of phallic and preputial skin.

MODIFICATION AVOIDING THE FORTUNOFF FLAP

The perineal ω- or U-shaped flap, known as the Fortunoff flap, does not reproduce normal female anatomy but shortens the perineum. It also allows hair-bearing skin into the vagina. To obtain mucosal lining of the posterior vaginal fourchette, use excess urogenital sinus for the posterior vagina.

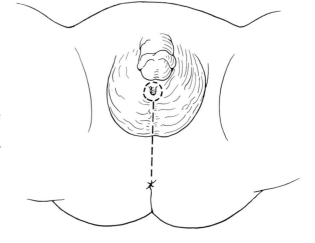

FIGURE 164-18. Make a circumscribing incision around the common urogenital sinus opening, extending the incision posteriorly along the midline toward the anterior margin of the anus.

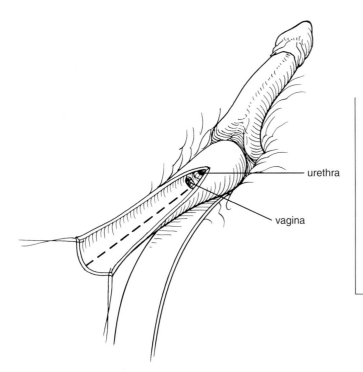

urethra

vagina

FIGURE 164-19. Mobilize the common urogenital sinus, urethra, and vagina extensively until the urethral meatus can be placed in an orthotopic position. Dissect in the plane just outside the urogenital sinus so as not to disrupt the clitoral blood supply. Divide the pubourethral ligaments anteriorly and disrupt the endopelvic fascia to allow caudal displacement of the urethra and bladder neck. Dissect the posterior wall of the vagina above the anterior rectal wall, allowing caudal displacement of the urethral vaginal unit, thereby mobilizing the high urogenital confluence. It is necessary to have 1.2 to 2 cm of urethral length to be able to position the urethral meatus in an orthotopic position.

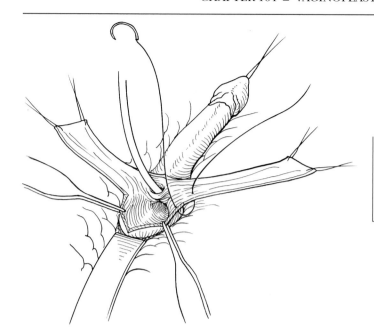

FIGURE 164-20. Incise the urogenital sinus at the 12-o'clock position until the confluence of the urethra and vagina is reached. Next, at the 6-o'clock position incise the common urogenital sinus until the vagina is located. The incision continues until the vaginal opening is of normal caliber.

FIGURE 164-21. Rotate the urogenital sinus flaps downward and medially to form the posterior vaginal wall. Bring the distal end of the flap to the perineum to form the posterior vaginal fourchette, using long-acting absorbable sutures. Reconstruct the perineum in the midline avoiding the use of a Fortunoff skin flap. The labia minora are created from the excess clitoral preputial tissue and the virilized labial majora reconstructed.

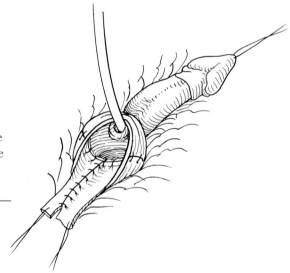

MICHAEL DISANDRO

Commentary by

Although moving the skin to the vagina by means of skin flaps can result in an introitus with a satisfying cosmetic appearance, it does not create an ideal situation. The reason is that normally the vaginal mucosa extends all the way to the end of the introitus, but with skin flaps, the introitus is made up of epithelium. This epithelium does not have the same characteristics of mucosa, and thus, in the long run, could lead to problems with vaginal stenosis and lack of natural lubrication. With any type of vaginoplasty, these risks are a concern, but they can be reduced by creating a large vaginal introitus that is composed of mucosal tissue only. To do this, it is important to first mobilize the vagina and urethra (total urogenital mobilization) enough so that the level at which the vagina inserts into the common urogenital sinus (the confluence) can reach the skin incision without excessive tension. If this can be done, then there is no need for skin flaps. This can be predicted preoperatively with a common urogenital sinogram and cystoscopy. If the distance between the vaginal/urethral confluence and the perineum (measured to the perineum only, not to the end of the common urogenital sinus) is less than 2.5 cm, then this technique should work. It is important to try to determine this preoperatively because the initial skin incision for a technique using skin flaps is different from the skin incision if no skin flap is used.

To create a large vaginal opening, the incision in the posterior urogenital sinus is made in the midline until the vagina is reached, but then it is important to continue to incise a bit into the vagina itself, until the vaginal opening is soft and open. The urogenital flaps, as shown in the illustrations, can then be used to fill the gap.

Chapter 165

Clitoroplasty

To reduce erectile tissue, incise the corpora cavernosa on the ventral surface at the 6-o'clock position to preserve the dorsal nerves. Try to keep much of the tunica of the corporeal bodies to avoid damage to the nerves and to help preserve sensation, which will usually be lost if the nerves are lifted off the bodies at 11- and 1-o'clock. Reduce the tissue of the glans ventrally where the nerves are less dense.

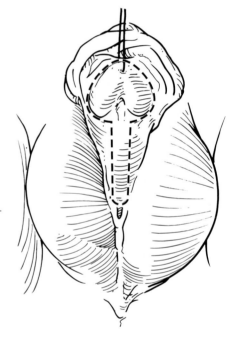

FIGURE 165-1. After anesthesia, prep and position the child as for hypospadias surgery. Place a 5-0 Prolene holding suture in the glans. Inject 1% lidocaine with 1:100,000 epinephrine at the base of the phallus. Make a circumcising incision. Start it 5 mm proximal to the coronal collar dorsally, and extend it ventrally to the opening of the urogenital sinus, thus preserving the urethral plate.

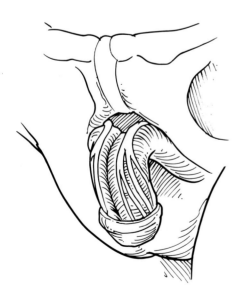

FIGURE 165-2. Elevate the skin and subcutaneous tissue to the junction where the urogenital sinus meets the hilar area of the crural bodies of the clitoris. Take care not to disturb the dorsal neurovascular bundle.

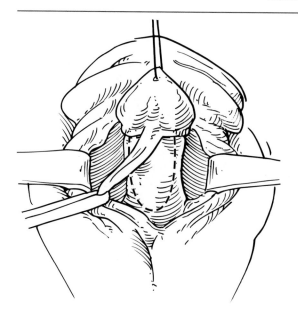

FIGURE 165-3. First mobilize the urethral plate from the corporeal bodies. Make an oval ventral incision *(dashed line)* in the exposed tunica albuginea of the clitoris.

FIGURE 165-4. Dissect the erectile tissue from within the bodies. Close the tunica with a running 5-0 absorbable suture. For reduction clitoroplasty, mark the glans on the ventral aspect where nerves are scarce *(dashed line)*.

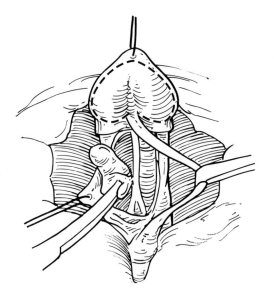

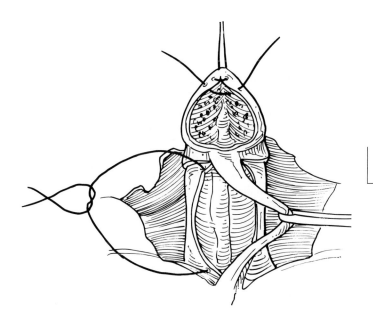

FIGURE 165-5. Excise symmetric wedges of tissue of appropriate size from the glans.

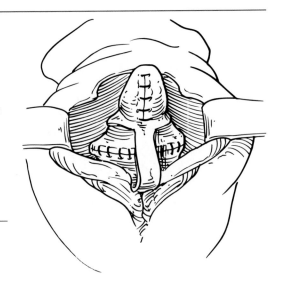

FIGURE 165-6. Approximate the wings of the glans with 5-0 interrupted absorbable sutures. Close the tunica albuginea of the erectile body transversely with 5-0 interrupted absorbable sutures, thereby reducing the length of the clitoris. (Suturing the corporeal body to the symphysis may result in discomfort or pain, especially when the remains of the clitoris grow as the girl matures at puberty.) In some cases the urethral plate is redundant and will need to be excised. During simultaneous vaginoplasty the urethral plate can be used to form the introitus between the reduced clitoris and urethra (separated urogenital sinus).

DIX POPPAS

Commentary by

The techniques used in performing the clitoroplasty, whether as a clitoroplasty alone or in combination with total feminizing genitoplasty, have evolved significantly over the past 2 decades. Initial attempts at performing clitorectomy, clitoral recession, and minor skin arrangements to conceal the clitoris have evolved into more precise approaches that now provide superior function and cosmetic outcomes. Based on our current knowledge of clitoral neural anatomy and the shortcomings of the prior techniques, the approaches used today offer the best opportunity for maximizing functional and cosmetic results. Despite our improved understanding of clitoral anatomy and its inherent impact on current techniques, the most important aspect of successful outcome remains with the surgeon's experience with performing these techniques. Several aspects to providing the patient with the best outcome include maximizing preservation of neurovascular anatomy, leaving enough erectile tissue to provide for appropriate erection during sexual arousal, limited glans clitoris reduction, avoiding attaching the glans clitoris or erectile bodies to the symphysis pubis, and providing skin flaps and rotation flaps to develop labia minora and a clitoral hood for cosmetic and functional optimization.

I presently perform the following operation for clitoroplasty:

Over 90% of patients I have treated underwent single-stage genital reconstruction that included a vaginoplasty and nerve-sparing reduction clitoroplasty. After induction of general anesthesia, the patient is placed in a modified dorsal lithotomy position. Urinary diversion is accomplished using a Foley catheter placed into the bladder through the urethra or urogenital sinus. In patients undergoing combined single-stage restoration, the vaginoplasty is performed first followed by the clitoroplasty.

To begin the nerve-sparing clitoroplasty, a subcoronal circumferential incision is made down to the level of Buck's fascia 0.5 to 1 cm proximal to the glans clitoris. The shaft skin is degloved back to the pubis and sharply bisected in the dorsal midline to create skin flaps for development of labia minora and formation of the clitoral hood. During the degloving, it will be necessary to transect the ventral urethral plate. This will significantly lengthen and straighten the erectile bodies. The erectile body dissection is then carried out to the crural bifurcation between the dartos layer and Buck's fascia.

Buck's fascia is incised using two parallel incisions lateral to the ventral midline in a longitudinal fashion. The lateral edges of Buck's fascia are elevated and sharply dissected off the tunica albuginea circumferentially. Once a plane of dissection has been obtained around the entire corporeal bodies, the neurovascular bundles and Buck's fascia can be easily mobilized for the entire length to approximately 1 to 2 cm distal to the crural bifurcation. Next, the glans clitoris is sharply dissected off of the distal corporeal bodies, leaving the glans attached to Buck's fascia and exposing the entire corporeal bodies. At this point, the neurovascular bundle is irrigated with 1:100,000 papavarine solution to prevent arterial spasm.

The corporeal bodies are then transected approximately 1.5 to 2 cm distal to their bifurcation. By leaving some erectile tissue distal to the bifurcation, clitoral erection during sexual arousal will be maintained, as well as allowing support and elevation of the clitoris beneath the pubis. The transected ends of the corporeal bodies are then oversewn using a 3-0 Maxon suture and the glans clitoris is secured to the end of the corporeal bodies with two 4-0 Byosin sutures. The dorsal aspect of the glans is carefully excluded in these sutures to avoid injuring the nerves and blood supply as they enter the glans. The glans clitoris is rarely ever reduced in size. Once the glans clitoris is secured, the previously bisected preputial skin flaps are rotated posteriorly on each side of the clitoris to create a glans hood and labia minora. The remainder of the genital reconstruction is completed, including any additional procedures necessary for that particular patient (vaginoplasty, labioplasty, etc.).

STANLEY J. KOGAN

Commentary by

The techniques involved with feminizing genital reconstruction have undergone considerable change and refinement. Older techniques of clitoral "amputation" and minor external skin rearrangement fortunately have given way to much more functionally and cosmetically satisfactory techniques of clitoral reduction, vaginoplasty, and labioplasty, sometimes all performed simultaneously. Current techniques now allow for creating completely normal-appearing female external genitalia in most instances in a single-stage operation.

The goals of feminizing genital reconstruction are to (1) create a normal-appearing, sensate clitoris; (2) have an adequately sized and appropriately situated vagina for later female function; and (3) create a normal-appearing female introitus. Subsequent to abandonment of clitoridectomy, clitoral recession under the pubis has been practiced; however, in some girls, painful erections of the restricted shaft occur after puberty, making this a potentially risky choice. Reduction clitoroplasty, in which some of the hypertrophied shaft erectile tissue is excised, while the dorsal neurovascular bundle and glans are preserved, in most circumstances gives a more favorable result. Labioplasty, as described in this chapter, is done simultaneously, making good use of the excess shaft skin left after clitoral reduction to form labia minora. Distal vaginal reconstruction also may be done at the same time, delaying this portion of the repair until 1 or 2 years of age, in those girls with very high junctions of the vagina and urethra.

A radiologic and endoscopic examination of the urogenital sinus is critical in the initial evaluation, defining the location where the takeoff of the vaginal segment occurs from the urogenital sinus. Documentation of a distal urogenital sinus confluence guarantees that a flap vaginoplasty will be satisfactory and that the posterior perineal flap will be long enough to reach the vaginal segment. If a high confluence is present in which the posterior flap will lie, this may damage the bladder neck sphincter, again indicating the need for precise anatomic delineation.

My current preference in performing this repair is to do the entire clitoroplasty, vaginoplasty, and labioplasty simultaneously, unless there is a high confluence. The incisions for each portion of this procedure detail nicely and prevent the subsequent need to operate in scar tissue from the previous procedure. I begin by mobilizing the clitoris circumferentially, much like what is done in degloving the penile shaft in a chordee correction. The ventral mucosa is not preserved, so the erectile bodies can be widely exposed, extending down the descending pubic rami. I then incise the tunica laterally or inferiorly on each erectile body and sharply dissect out the hypertrophied erectile tissue from within, ligating the stumps. Adequate resection of the erectile tissue is important, because engorgement, swelling, and pain in the residual stumps do occur during puberty. This approach leaves the dorsal neurovascular bundle untouched and preserves completely the glans blood supply and sensation. The transverse closure of the ventral tunical tissues is a nice modification, further recessing the glans and aiding in repositioning it properly. The glans is then wedged to reduce its size, as indicated in the figures, and is attached subsequently to the inferior end of the clitoral hood, newly formed from the superior end of the shaft skin brought together in the midline.

Flap vaginoplasty is then performed, cutting back into the urogenital sinus sufficiently to fully exteriorize the vagina. Failure to cut back far enough will lead to vaginal stenosis and the urethral opening will lie on the dorsal wall within the vagina ("female hypospadias"). The flap must be tailored perfectly: a perineal flap that is too short will lead to a flat perineum, and one that is too long may result in a posterior "shelf," sometimes causing trapping of urine within the vagina. The previously mobilized phallic skin is then partially split down the midline to form labia minora and sutured on either side of the urethral meatus. The glans clitoris is sutured to the split phallic skin, which now simulates a clitoral hood, extending over the glans dorsally. Many textbooks show the glans being fixed to the underside of the pubis at this point in the reconstruction; however, positioning the glans here will bring it far from the vagina, an anatomically incorrect location. Rather, it should lie at the inferior portion of the constructed clitoral hood, closer to the urethra and vagina as is encountered naturally. A V-Y posterior advancement of the labioscrotal folds on either side of the vagina is then done, completing the repair. These advancement flaps must be undermined significantly; otherwise, retraction may occur, causing separation and scarring at their apices.

When the vagina enters high, I do the clitoroplasty and labia minora–plasty initially to restore normal external cosmesis, and the vaginoplasty is deferred until the vagina is larger and the vaginal wall is better formed. With this staged approach the labioscrotal tissue is preserved initially for formation of quadrant flaps to be laid in at the time of subsequent high vaginoplasty, because the high detached vagina will not reach down to the perineal surface. When the vagina is detached from the urethra, transverse closure should be done to minimize risk of urethral stricture formation from a longitudinal closure.

A suction drain is helpful, especially if a high dissection is done. The drain should exit away from the labia majora advancement flaps and should not be brought out at their posterior apices. A vaginal packing impregnated with petroleum jelly is left for a few days. A urethral catheter is left for 3 to 5 days, and a compression dressing is used over the repair.

Long-term follow-up in patients undergoing this procedure demonstrates excellent cosmesis and preservation of satisfactory glans sensation. As with many other prepubertal vaginoplasty techniques, a minor introitoplasty is sometimes needed after puberty as the introitus may not enlarge commensurate with the size of the rest of the vagina.

Chapter 166

Vaginal Reconstruction: Skin Inlay

SKIN INLAY VAGINOPLASTY (ABBE-MCINDOE)

For instruments provide a dermatome with cement, a vaginal conformer (Heyer-Schulte prosthesis), condoms, three narrow Deaver retractors, mineral oil, and liquid thrombin.

Place the patient in a low lithotomy position. Thoroughly prep the lower abdomen, upper legs, and perineum, and drape the perineum and one thigh. Insert a 24-F, 5-mL balloon catheter and fill the bladder to allow insertion of a 24-F Malecot cystostomy tube (see Chapter 84). Place sutures in the labia for traction.

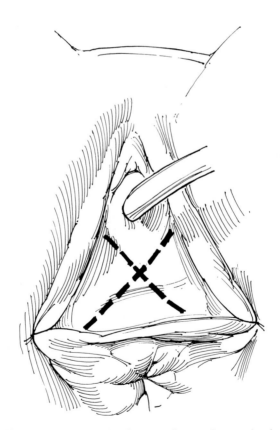

FIGURE 166-1. Incision: Make an X-shaped incision in the anterior perineum in the mucosal plaque, with the crossing of the X below the urethra to create four symmetric mucosal flaps. When infolded into the vaginal canal, they will reduce circumferential scar contraction.

FIGURE 166-2. With a second glove on the left hand, place the index finger in the rectum. Inject a solution of 0.5% lidocaine (Xylocaine) with 1:2000 dilution of epinephrine under the proposed flaps and into the urethrorectal septum, to aid in the dissection and improve hemostasis.

With the right index finger alternating with a knife handle, bluntly tunnel cephaloposteriorly between the rectum and the urethra on alternating sides of the median raphe. Divide the now-conspicuous raphe with Metzenbaum scissors. Identify the anterior rectal wall to avoid accidental perforation but keep closer to the rectum than to the bladder. Take care that the blunt dissection does not force the raphe to tear the rectum. (Should rectal perforation occur, repair the defect, and return for reoperation in several months.) Make the pocket much deeper and wider than you think necessary because it will contract. (In a large patient it should be 21 cm deep and 17 cm wide.) Pack the pocket with roller gauze.

Turn the patient on her side. From the upper thigh, obtain split-thickness skin grafts with the dermatome (see Chapter 169). More than one sweep is usually needed. Alternatively, obtain full-thickness grafts bilaterally from the groin, lateral to the hairline. These will not only leave less scarring in the donor site than split-thickness grafts but will contract less during healing.

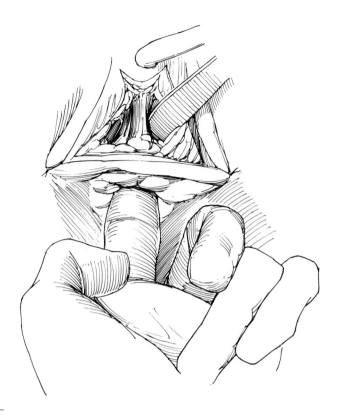

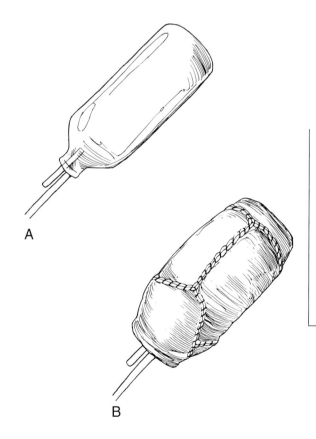

FIGURE 166-3. A and **B**, Trim a piece of rubber foam larger in width than the proposed stent but of appropriate length. Compress the foam into a cylinder of appropriate diameter (usually 3 to 4 cm), and tie it with circular 3-0 synthetic absorbable sutures. Apply two or three condoms over the cylinder, and then suture the graft over the condoms. Alternatively, inflate a commercial vaginal conformer with air and coat it with mineral oil. Its advantage is that it may be deflated and removed painlessly, but it may be too short. Fit the sheets of skin on the stent with the raw side out. Suture the edges to each other with running 5-0 synthetic absorbable sutures, siting the knots against the mold.

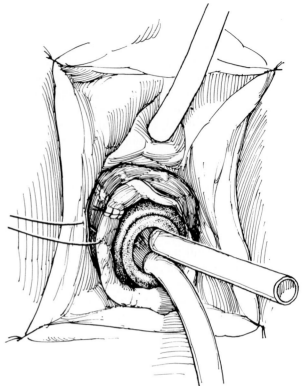

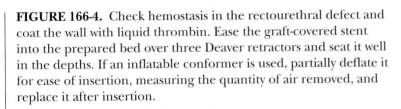

FIGURE 166-4. Check hemostasis in the rectourethral defect and coat the wall with liquid thrombin. Ease the graft-covered stent into the prepared bed over three Deaver retractors and seat it well in the depths. If an inflatable conformer is used, partially deflate it for ease of insertion, measuring the quantity of air removed, and replace it after insertion.

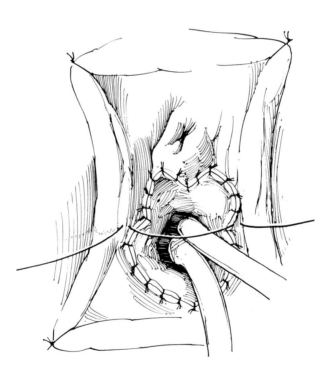

FIGURE 166-5. Make four shallow notches in the exposed end of the graft and insert the four flaps from the X-shaped skin incision into them. Fasten the flaps with 4-0 synthetic absorbable sutures, interrupted to provide a noncircumferential suture line. Place two or three retaining sutures across the vestibule (not across the vulva) to hold the stent in place. Remove the urethral catheter. Apply coated gauze and fluffs held with elastic tape to compress the perineum.

Postoperatively, order bed rest. On the first postoperative day give stool softeners or up to 30 mL of mineral oil orally three times a day, followed by a low-residue diet for several days. Thereafter, have the patient keep the bowel movements loose by taking petroleum agar and stool softeners for 1 to 2 weeks. On the 7th or 8th day postoperatively, sedate the patient to remove the introital sutures and deflate and withdraw the stent. Should the stent hang up, inject mineral oil around it through a small, soft catheter. Cleanse the perineum. Wash, lubricate, replace, and reinflate the stent. Apply a perineal binder to hold it in place. Teach the girl how to remove and reinsert it regularly. It must be retained day and night for 3 months because split-thickness grafts readily contract.

POSTOPERATIVE PROBLEMS

Contraction of the graft is a common and most serious problem, usually caused by poor compliance of the patient in keeping the new vagina dilated. For this reason the candidate must be carefully selected because long-term follow-up is crucial.

In some girls, the use of bowel might be a better choice. The new vagina may be too short, resulting in dyspareunia. Necrosis and sloughing of some of the edge of the graft are usual but major loss should not be expected. Infection is unusual with healthy perineal tissue and good-quality skin. Supply estrogen suppositories to keep the neovagina supple.

JOHN P. GEARHART

Commentary by

It is important initially to make a cruciate incision on the perineum so that the plane between the urethra and the anterior rectal wall can be entered and dissected without injury to either of these structures. I have had only limited experience with the procedure but have been involved in revision of a number of them. Reoperation was needed for correction of three problems: (1) the four perineal flaps were not made large enough to avoid contracture of the introitus; (2) the graft was brought too far distally in the perineum, so that it did not appear as a mucosal opening; and (3) the entire graft contracted. As mentioned in the text, contracture of the graft usually is caused by poor compliance by the patient in keeping the vagina dilated by not using dilators regularly or by infrequent intercourse. Male pseudohermaphrodites, I have found, do better long term using estrogen suppositories on a regular basis, because this seems to keep the graft and introitus supple and aids in preventing contracture.

Chapter 167

Sigmoid Vaginal Reconstruction

Vaginal reconstruction in teenagers is appropriate after the patient and family understand all aspects of the proposed surgery and postoperative care. Pre- and postoperative counseling for the patient and family is a critical adjunct.

Use a sleeve of distal sigmoid colon for vaginal replacement. When this segment is contraindicated, such as when there has been previous pull-through surgery or pelvic irradiation, cecum or ileum is an acceptable alternative. In most patients an 8- to 10-cm sleeve of distal sigmoid colon based on the left colic or superior hemorrhoidal vessels is sufficient for adequate vaginal length. Using segments of greater length can be associated with excessive mucus production and diversion colitis.

Prepare the bowel and administer broad-spectrum antibiotics before the operation.

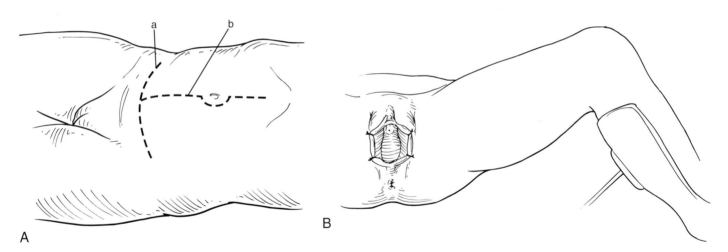

FIGURE 167-1. A, A transverse incision is preferable in most patients who have not had extensive intra-abdominal surgery. Alternatively, a midline lower transperitoneal incision provides access to the bowel. **B**, Perform the operation with the patient supine with legs spread and knees slightly bent, using Allen stirrups. This position affords excellent intra-abdominal exposure as well as wide access to the perineum and introitus.

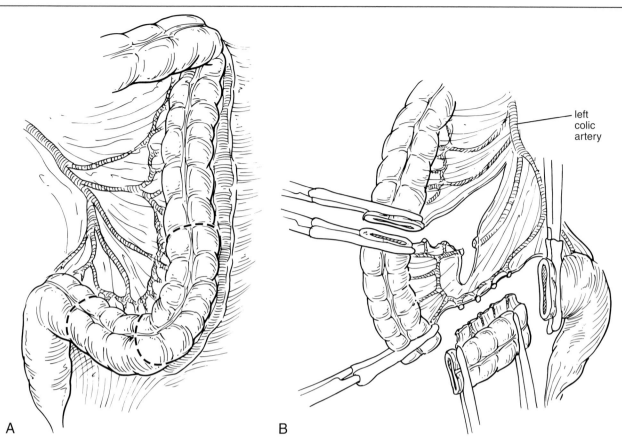

A

B

left
colic
artery

FIGURE 167-2. A, Position the sigmoid segment between noncrushing clamps. Either hand-sew or staple the colon to reestablish bowel continuity. **B**, Discard a short distal sigmoid segment to provide greater length on the mesenteric vasculature for the neovagina.

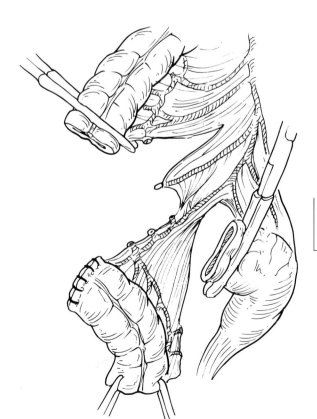

FIGURE 167-3. Rotate the sigmoid segment 180 degrees on its mesentery to allow placement in the perineum. Close the proximal end of the neovagina with two layers of absorbable suture material.

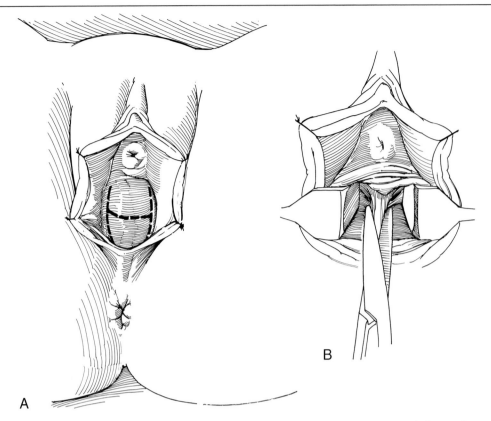

FIGURE 167-4. A and **B**, Make an H-shaped incision in the perineum and, with blunt and sharp dissection through the location of the urogenital diaphragm as for an anorectal pull-through, create a canal to the level of the vesicorectal pouch. The new canal should accommodate at least 3 fingers. Pull the bowel through the perineal tunnel. In patients with an inadequate distal vagina, the bowel segment may be anastomosed directly to the perineum. When a direct perineal anastomosis is required it is important to create a large enough space for the bowel to fit comfortably and enable a capacious, well-vascularized, and tension-free anastomosis.

With both sigmoid and cecal segments provide adequate posterior fixation of the bowel segment to the retroperitoneum. This fixation with nonabsorbable suture prevents wandering of the neovagina as well as prolapse of the segment.

FIGURE 167-5. A and **B**, Suture the colonic margin to the introtius with synthetic absorbable sutures. Stent the neovagina with the barrel of a 5- or 10-mL syringe wrapped in antibiotic-soaked gauze left in place for 5 days. The size of the stent varies with patient age. Examine the patient under anesthesia at 3 to 4 weeks and without anesthesia at 3 months postoperatively. If there is any suggestion of introital stenosis institute manual dilatation at home as necessary.

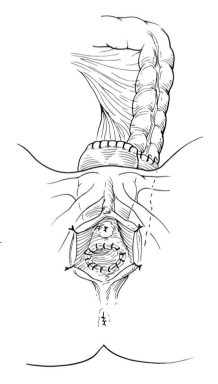

POSTOPERATIVE PROBLEMS

Ileus is avoided by continuing nasogastric suction for 2 or 3 days. Intercourse should not be tried for 6 weeks. Mucus accumulation is managed by douching or by simply having the patient hold the introitus open while in the bath.

Manage redundancy of the neovagina (minor prolapse) by circumferential trimming; major prolapse may require exploration and fixation. Mild stenosis may be treated with manual dilatation, but complete stenosis requires excision and replacement. Sanitary pads or daily douching may be needed for management of mucus secretion.

TERRY HENSLE

Commentary by

The colovaginoplasty is a very acceptable method for vaginal replacement in cases of loss or congenital absence. The advantages of colovaginoplasty include the use of supple, well-vascularized, and resilient tissue as a form of vaginal replacement. In addition, the colon provides natural lubrication and tends to be durable.

The technique that has been described can usually be done with a low transverse incision, which is cosmetically pleasing. Be sure that the blood supply to the sigmoid portion that is used is low enough, concentrating on the left colic or superior hemorrhoidal vessels, and, if the right colon is used, using the ileocolic vessels. Rotating the isolated segment 180 degrees to gain length is also important. Even though elevating the proximal existing vagina into the cul-de-sac to do the anastomosis looks good in pictures, it usually does not work very well. Therefore, bringing the replacement colon segment through the perineum and suturing it in place works much better. Perhaps the most important part of the surgery is to make the perineal opening for the neovagina large enough so that distal stenosis does not take place.

There have been concerns raised about colovaginoplasty because of excess mucus production. Most of the young women in our series do wear a protective pad; however, keeping the segment relatively short, meaning no more than 10 cm in length, decreases the amount of mucus that is produced. Thus, it seems to be manageable. The other concerns, of course, are those of diversion colitis and neoplasia.

Diversion colitis has been reported on numerous occasions and certainly can occur, although, in a review of 25 years of experience, we have had only one documented case of diversion colitis. Neoplasia also has been reported; it is a long-term concern and thus requires gynecologic evaluation on a routine basis, as any female might do who has normal anatomy.

Chapter 168

Thigh Flap Vagina and Tissue Expansion

THIGH FLAP VAGINA AND TISSUE EXPANSION (WEE AND JOSEPH)

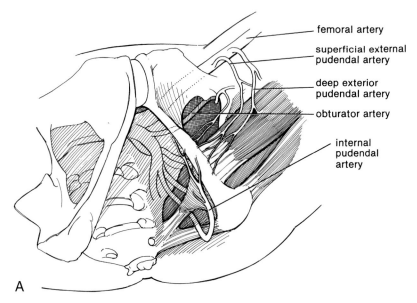

femoral artery

superficial external pudendal artery

deep exterior pudendal artery

obturator artery

internal pudendal artery

A

FIGURE 168-1. A, This technique depends on the blood supply from the posterior labial arteries arising from the perineal artery that also have collateral circulation with the deep external pudendal artery, medial femoral circumflex artery, and anterior branch of the obturator artery. **B**, Position: Lithotomy with the legs in stirrups. Insert a balloon catheter in the bladder. Insert a Hegar dilator in the rectum to develop a plane between it and the base of the bladder large enough to accommodate the new vagina. Incisions: Mark two slightly curved and tapered flaps on either side of the vulva, centered on the crease of the groin. The base in an adult is 6 cm wide, and the length may be up to 15 cm, placing the tip over the femoral triangle.

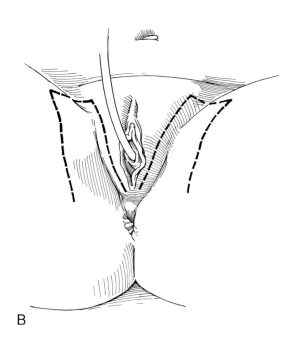

B

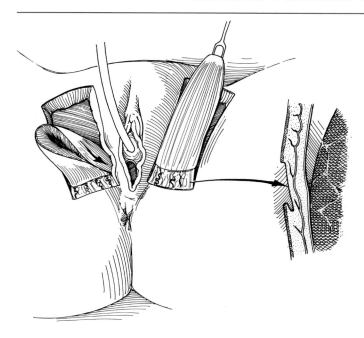

FIGURE 168-2. Incise down to the deep fascia, beginning at the end of the flap, and raise it, taking care to include the perimysium of the adductor muscles to avoid damage to the nerves in the flap. At the base of the flap, divide the skin through the dermis to a depth of 1 to 1.5 cm *(inset)* to allow freedom for the flap to be depressed for passage under the labium.

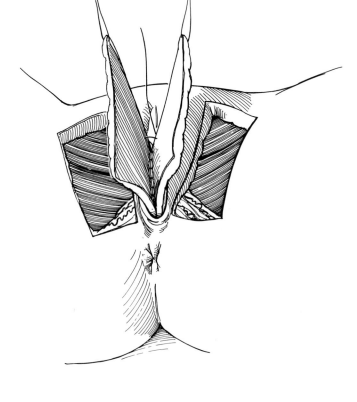

FIGURE 168-3. Form tunnels under the labia by dissecting them from the pubic ramus. Pass the flaps under the labia. With the flaps everted from the introitus, suture the paired flaps together in the midline to close the posterior wall of the new vagina.

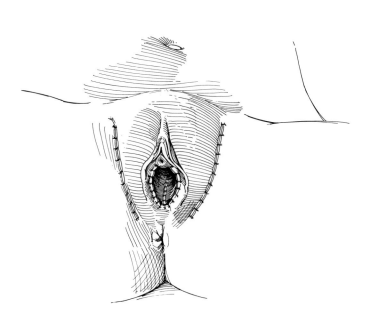

FIGURE 168-4. At the apex, continue suturing to approximate the anterior wall by bringing the lateral borders together to form the vaginal tube. Invert the tube, and fasten the apex to the posterior bladder wall. Close the lateral defects from the graft site. Place it loose pack over gauze impregnated with petroleum jelly.

TISSUE-EXPANSION TECHNIQUE
(PATIL AND HIXSON)

Make a right inguinal incision, and digitally dissect a pocket in the right labium majus. Select a tissue expander of suitable size; 250 mL is suitable for an adolescent. Insert the tissue expander in the labial pocket, and place the filling port subcutaneously in a (future) hair-bearing area, where it can be felt through the skin. Every 2 weeks add up to 20 mL of normal saline through a 25-gauge needle, the volume being dependent on the tolerance of the girl.

When an adequate size is reached (in approximately 6 weeks), give general anesthesia and proceed to bring the vagina toward the perineum.

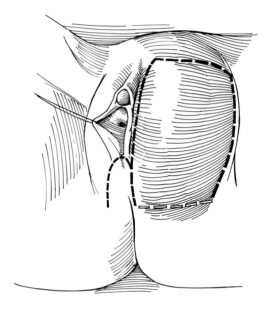

FIGURE 168-5. Mark and raise a 7.5-cm by 10-cm flap on the expanded labium with an incision that circumscribes the area of expansion and also crosses the perineum posterior to the introitus. Remove the expander, but preserve the new vascularized sheath that has formed beneath it.

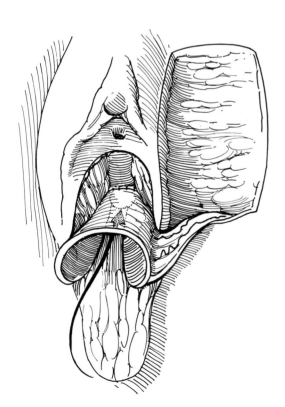

FIGURE 168-6. Rotate the flap and suture the proximal end to the stump of the vagina with 2-0 synthetic absorbable sutures. Because it will not reach completely around the vaginal opening, leave a 1-cm gap at the junction with the vagina to epithelialize.

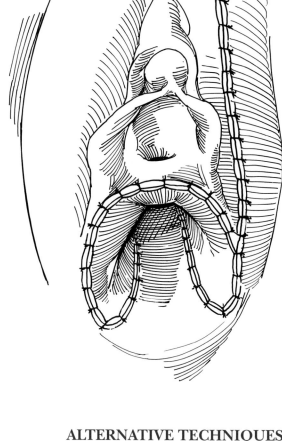

FIGURE 168-7. Suture the distal end to the skin. Insert the initial posterior perineal flap to fill the outer portion of the posterior gap in the tubed flap. Close the labial defect.

ALTERNATIVE TECHNIQUES

Gracilis myocutaneous flaps may be needed if the vaginal defect is large. Raise a flap on both sides, and tunnel them under the intact perineal skin to invaginate them into the new vaginal canal. Suture the two flaps as a tube without a conformer, and close the donor sites.

An ileal segment can be used in cases of congenital vaginal absence. A total of 15 to 20 cm of ileum is opened, folded once, and sutured into a tube, leaving a V-shaped slot to accommodate the inverted V-shaped perineal flap after the segment is tunneled into the perineum. This alternative may be less acceptable to the fastidious patient because of soiling from mucus. A pressure (Ingram) technique is used by some experts with well-motivated patients. Pressure is applied to the perineum 2 hours a day by a bicycle seat stool that holds a plastic dilator. This technique can indent enough skin to form a functional vagina.

Commentary by JOHN P. GEARHART

The subjects treated in this chapter usually are male pseudohermaphrodites who are being raised as females or females with mullerian duct anomalies requiring vaginal construction. Should there be any associated anomalies, they will have been corrected before vaginal construction is done. Certainly, none of the procedures described in this chapter should be undertaken until the patient is fully grown. For practical purposes, this typically means in the later teen years.

SKIN INLAY (ABBE-MCINDOE PROCEDURE)

It is important initially to make a cruciate incision on the perineum, so that the plane between the urethra and the anterior rectal wall can be entered and dissected without injury to either of these structures. I have had only limited experience with the procedure but have been involved in revision of a number of them. Reoperation was needed for correction of three problems: (1) the four perineal flaps were not made large enough to avoid contracture of the introitus; (2) the graft was

Continued

brought too far distally in the perineum, so that it did not appear as a mucosal opening; and (3) the entire graft contracted. As mentioned in the text, contracture of the graft usually is caused by poor compliance by the patient in keeping the vagina dilated by not using dilators regularly, or by infrequent intercourse. Male pseudohermaphrodites, I have found, do better long term using estrogen suppositories on a regular basis, because this seems to keep the graft and introitus supple and aids in preventing contracture.

CECAL VAGINA

Although Turner-Warwick and others have recommended the use of cecum to create a neovagina, I have found that it may be difficult to rotate the cecum downward enough to reach the perineal flaps. I prefer the modified Wagner-Baldwin technique using the sigmoid colon, because it usually is redundant and close to the operative field. When the sigmoid colon is used, I typically bring the omentum down to cover the colonic anastomosis and to separate the anastomosis from the superior suture line of the sigmoid vagina. Whether cecum or sigmoid is used, the difficulties typically lie at the introitus. Although Figure 167-4 (in Chapter 167) shows an H-type incision, with the labia majora and minora present, many male pseudohermaphrodites raised as females have a very flat perineum without an introitus. In this instance, both a large perineally based flap and a flap-based cephalad will be necessary to suitably exteriorize the neovagina. A vaginal pack of iodoform gauze impregnated with petroleum jelly for 2 days postoperatively has proved worthwhile. Although the anastomosis between the perineum and the bowel-vagina usually is quite capacious, care must be taken in the postoperative months to make sure that stenosis does not occur.

PUDENDAL THIGH FLAP VAGINA

Although I have not had personal experience with this procedure, I am a bit concerned about the postoperative appearance of the junction between the upper thigh and the perineal area. This is a large mass of tissue that is being removed. I would have to see the postoperative pictures before I would be convinced that it is superior to bowel interposition.

TISSUE-EXPANDER TECHNIQUE

Although I have not had personal experience with this use of tissue expanders, I find it most intriguing. Certainly tissue expanders have made an impact in reconstructive urology in boys with failed hypospadias repairs and in those with epispadias-exstrophy. It is truly amazing what a few weeks of tissue expansion will do to increase the availability of local skin. I think the wide-based perineal flap shown in Figure 168-5 certainly will aid in preventing stenosis of the neovaginal orifice, and I believe the amount of redundant tissue that is present will allow tension-free closure of the ipsilateral labia majora area.

SUMMARY

Although all of the techniques described certainly are helpful in creating a neovagina, application will be dictated by the surgeon's ability and experience. Hensle has reported excellent results using colonic segments in male pseudohermaphrodites raised as females and those with vaginal agenesis. My results mirror those of Hensle, and I feel that a bowel segment is the best substitute for a vagina and that the sigmoid colon segment is superior to the cecal segment, because the larger diameter of the colon permits anastomosis of the distal end of the straight segment to the perineum, thus requiring less mobilization of the mesentery than with the cecal procedure. Lastly, the colon segment offers the following advantages over the other techniques described, all of which require mobilization of large amounts of skin in the perineal area: (1) the procedure is technically simpler; (2) there is no uncertainty about "take" of the graft; (3) molds are not required to maintain patency; (4) colonic mucosa is more resistant to trauma; (5) adequate spontaneous lubrication is present for sexual intercourse without excessive mucus discharge created by small bowel; and finally, (6) most pediatric urologists are quite familiar with using bowel segments for reconstructive procedures and thus have basic familiarity with the technique.

Chapter 169

Repair of Penile Injuries

AVULSION OR BURN INJURY OF PENIS AND SCROTUM

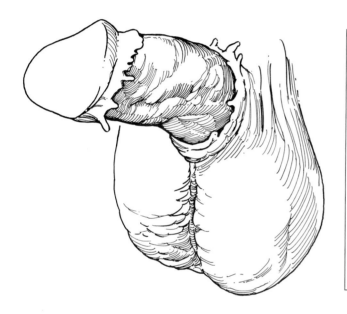

FIGURE 169-1. Avulsion injuries: Repair the defect at once, at least within 8 to 12 hours. Make a circumcising incision around the penis. Remove distal skin remnants from the shaft because they will have lost venous drainage and so be subject to prolonged edema. Cleanse the denuded area thoroughly with saline. Remove foreign bodies and open hematomas. Achieve hemostasis, although bleeding is usually minimal after this type of injury.

Burn injuries: Remove all the skin from the shaft distal to the injury to avoid subsequent lymphedema. Do it at once before infection can set in. It is not necessary to wait for separation of the eschar to see how much skin remains, because the small amount of skin saved in that way is easily made up by a graft.

Immediate care: Place the anesthetized child in the lithotomy position (use the frog-legged position in infants) and insert a balloon catheter. Prep the lower abdomen and genitalia.

FIGURE 169-2. Tack both the coronal and the proximal skin to the shaft with 4-0 synthetic absorbable sutures placed subcutaneously. Wait for formation of a well-vascularized bed.

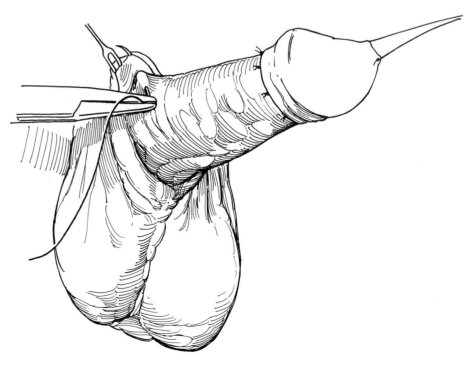

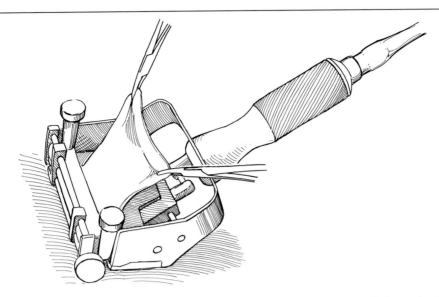

FIGURE 169-3. With an electric dermatome, obtain a medium-thickness split-skin graft from the lower abdomen or from the inner or outer aspect of the thigh in an area least likely to have hair. For primary grafting, make the graft 0.020 to 0.024 inches thick; for grafting after the bed has been infected, obtain a thinner graft, 0.012 to 0.016 inches. For a large graft, especially for the scrotum, mesh the skin on the operating table with a meshing device. Such a graft will contract more but will permit easy escape of exudate. For the penis, do not mesh the graft because that will restrict erection.

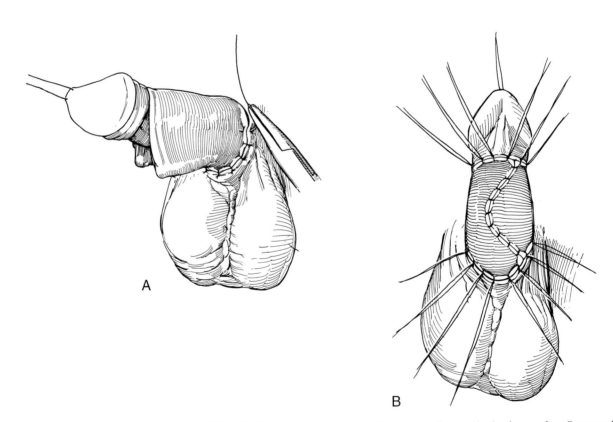

FIGURE 169-4. A, Wrap the graft around the shaft, placing the suture line ventrally to mimic the raphe. Suture the distal and proximal ends of the graft in place with interrupted sutures. Trim the edges of the graft to form a long Z, and close the residual defect with a running 5-0 synthetic absorbable suture. Insert a balloon catheter of suitable size. Bank the excess skin. **B,** Incise the graft in two or three places to lengthen the suture line and reduce the risk of chordee (Z-plasty). Suture the graft to the corona and to the edge of the scrotal skin with interrupted 5-0 synthetic absorbable sutures. Leave these sutures long.

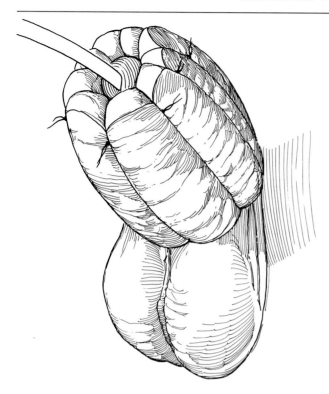

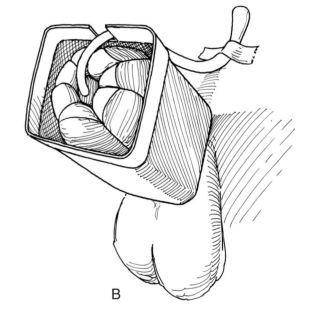

FIGURE 169-5. Apply cotton wool impregnated with glycerin around the penis, and anchor it by tying the sets of long sutures together. Cover with gauze and elastic adhesive tape, and apply tincture of benzoin to fix the tape to the pubic skin.

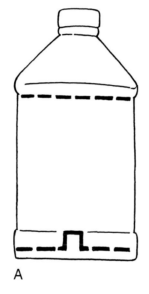

FIGURE 169-6. A and **B,** Suspend the penis inside a section of a plastic bottle that has been cut appropriately and padded with adhesive foam padding.

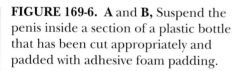

A

B

JAMES M. BETTS

Commentary by

With burns, whether due to flame, hot liquid, or chemical origin, the choice of delayed versus immediate debridement depends on many factors. The depth of the injury, extent of the compromised penile shaft skin, and the condition of the surrounding area will dictate whether immediate excision is possible or a more conservative approach is required, with secondary separation of the injured skin and the demarcation of possibly viable surrounding or juxtaposed skin. In the case of the avulsion of shaft skin, even that which might have been inadvertently excised during a newborn circumcision, if the tissue is intact, it could be reattached to the shaft, with grossly nonviable areas excised. If anything, even if it eventually sloughs, it will have served as a biologic dressing, which can be grafted at a later time.

Chapter 170

Construction of the Penis

Phalloplasty after Puberty

Organize two surgical teams, one to prepare the forearm skin flap, and the other to cover the donor site with a skin graft from the thigh, prepare the recipient site, mobilize the inguinal recipient vessels, and insert a suprapubic cystostomy.

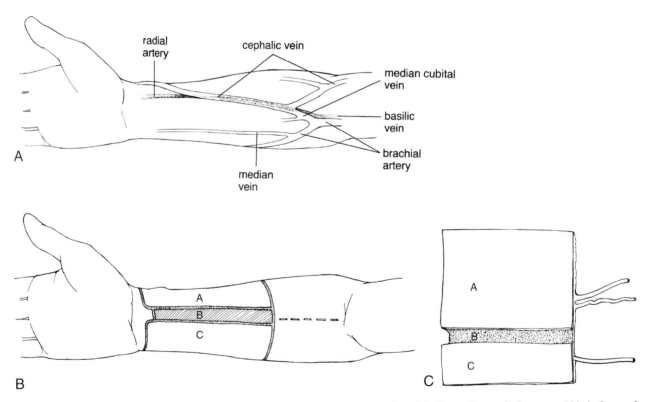

FIGURE 170-1. A, Make certain that the dominant blood supply to the hand is from the radial artery. If it is from the ulnar artery, adapt the procedure by forming the large flap (section A in parts **B** and **C**) medially. Place the boy in the frog-legged position. Prep one arm, the lower abdomen, and the genital area. Study the position of the pertinent vessels on the forearm. **B,** First team: Outline a skin flap on the radial side of the forearm 11 to 12 cm long and 14 to 15 cm wide, the size dependent on the size of the boy. Mark it as a larger section on the radial side (section A) from which to construct the penis; a 1-cm strip, de-epithelialized to increase the area of tissue contact for the prosthesis (section B); and a smaller section on the ulnar side 3.5 to 4 cm in width (section C), which will become the new urethra. A tongue of skin 1 cm in length is provided on sections A and B to shape the glans. **C,** The flap as it appears after removal.

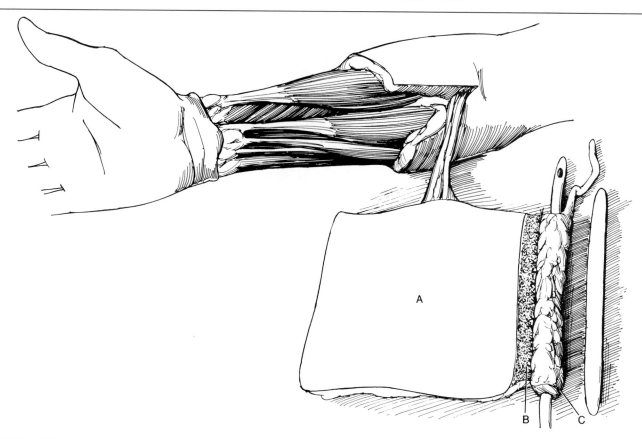

FIGURE 170-2. Press the blood from the forearm with an Esmarch bandage and apply and inflate a sterile tourniquet. Raise a full-thickness flap beginning distally, taking with it the subcutaneous tissue down to, but not including, the epitenon over the distal forearm tendons and the six or seven arteriolar branches of the distal third of the radial artery, as well as the venae comitantes. The vascular pedicle will contain the radial artery and its venae comitantes, cephalic vein, and another forearm vein and should be at least 10 cm in length proximal to the flap. It also will contain the medial and lateral antebrachial cutaneous nerves. Release the tourniquet and secure hemostasis. De-epithelialize the center section B. Roll the narrow section C into a tube around a 16-F silicone balloon catheter, and suture it in place with two layers of interrupted 3-0 synthetic absorbable sutures.

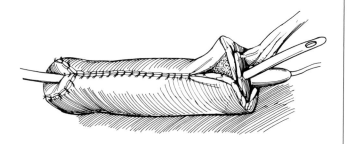

FIGURE 170-3. Cover both the neourethra and raw area with the larger section (section A in Figs. 170-1 and 170-2). Model the extensions to fit the meatus, and model the distal portion into a glans. It is possible at this point to insert a trimmed segment of rib cartilage from the costal cartilage union of the eighth and ninth ribs or a silicone prosthesis inside the skin tube along the raw surface of the tract, although the success of such implants has yet to be shown.

Second team: Cover the donor site with a split-thickness skin graft harvested from the thigh.

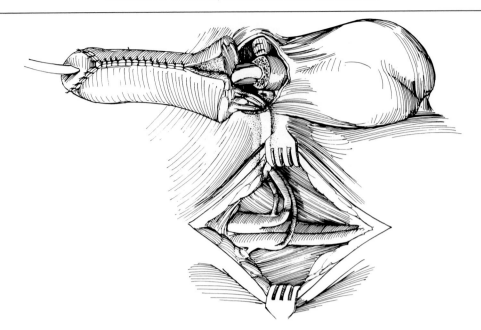

FIGURE 170-4. First team: Divide the vascular pedicle along with the antebrachial nerve(s) and tunnel it subcutaneously under the inguinal region. Using the operating room microscope, anastomose the cephalic vein to the greater saphenous vein or, by a saphenous vein interposition graft, to the femoral vein. Anastomose the superficial flap veins to the saphenous veins on both sides. It is possible to create a third anastomosis between a vena comitans and a saphenous branch. Join the radial artery to the inferior epigastric, lateral circumflex femoral, or deep femoral artery. Anastomose the lateral antebrachial nerve to the erogenous pudendal nerve or the dorsal nerve of the penis or clitoris.

Second team: Anastomose the urethra with interrupted 4-0 chromic catgut sutures. Fasten the prosthesis to the corpus spongiosum, and approximate the skin circumferentially around the base of the new penis. Cover the donor site with a medium split-thickness skin graft from the thigh.

Immobilize the arm at the elbow. Leave the stent in place for 10 days. Clamp the cystostomy tube in 14 days and observe voiding. If satisfactory, remove the tube. An inflatable prosthesis in a GORE-TEX sleeve may be inserted at a second stage, although erosion and extrusion may be a problem.

An alternative to tube flap reconstruction involves the use of a pedicle of scrotal skin wrapped around polyglycolic acid or Marlex mesh, inside of which is placed a small semirigid prosthesis, all anchored into the penile stump (Bissada). Urine will exit from a perineal urethrostomy. If a urethra-sparing penectomy has been performed, place the urethra under the folded scrotal flap.

MONEER HANNA

Commentary by

The ideal timing for pediatric phalloplasty is unknown. Although microsurgical forearm phalloplasty is technically feasible, it is inconceivable that a satisfactory outcome can be achieved during infancy or early childhood.

The width of the radial forearm neurovascular-fascio-cutaneous free flap was originally reported as 13 cm, which in our experience proved to be inadequate for tubularizing the flap and allowing for a tension-free closure. We have found that a flap dimension of 15 cm wide by 13 to 14 cm long to be more appropriate. However, the size of the wrist may limit the width of the flap.

It is possible to divide the forearm fascia into two layers. The superficial layer stays with the flap. The deep layer stays on the forearm donor site and keeps the closely grouped forearm muscles, thus improving the appearance and "take" of the skin graft.

A two-team approach expedites the surgery, which is quite lengthy. The groin team should look for the inferior epigastric artery and vein. However, if they are absent or rudimentary, the saphenous vein is exposed and then serves as a conduit from the common femoral artery to the donor artery of the flap.

At a later date coronal and glanular sculpting can be achieved by harvesting a dermal graft from the area over the iliac crest, and then it can be rolled into a tube and placed under the skin, thus enhancing the coronal and glans penis.

There is a high complication rate of approximately 50%, which includes urethral fistulas and stricture formation; therefore, patients should be advised accordingly. The neophallus can seldom be constructed in one stage. The urethroplasty may require several revisions. A penile prosthetic implant may result in erosion of the prosthesis into the urethra or skin. Furthermore, hyperpigmentation of the graft of the forearm is a common sequel of split-thickness skin grafts and is esthetically unappealing.

Phalloplasty in Infants

Congenital absence of the penis, or penile agenesis or aphallia, is a rare anomaly estimated to occur in one in 30 million males. Early treatment in infancy has the benefits of allowing a young child to feel that he has a male phenotype. In classic penile agenesis, the urethra enters the anterior rectum. An anterior saginal transrectal approach is used to divide the urethra from the rectum. A new urethra is created from a combined bladder–buccal mucosa graft and a new phallus from a quadrangle abdominal skin flap.

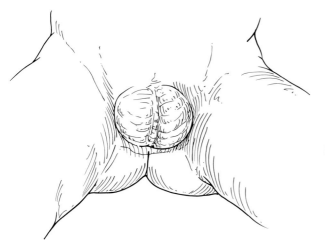

FIGURE 170-5. Classic appearance of penile agenesis.

FIGURE 170-6. Appearance of the perineal location of the urethra with a skin tag. The most common location of the urethral opening is the anterior rectum.

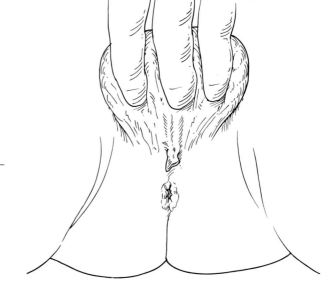

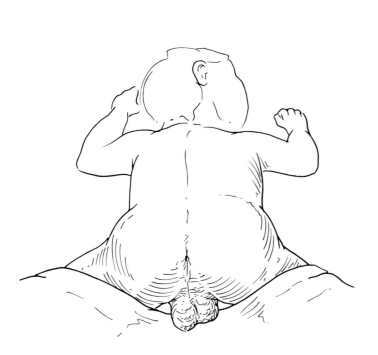

FIGURE 170-7. Place the patient in a prone knee-chest position. Use the anterior saginal transrectal approach to separate the urethra from the rectum.

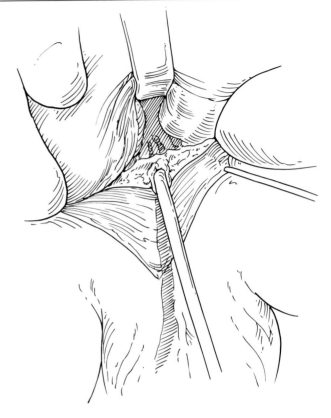

FIGURE 170-8. Proceed to dissect the urethra by splitting the anterior fibers of the rectal wall and separating the urethra from the rectum.

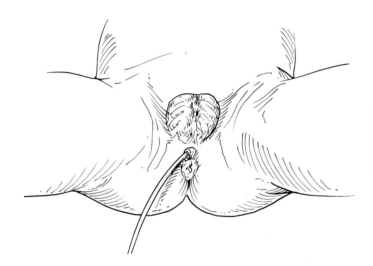

FIGURE 170-9. After the urethra is separated, turn the patient to a supine position. Make an incision in the superior aspect of the scrotum for subsequent neourethra positioning.

FIGURE 170-10. Create a quadrangle of lower abdominal flap 4 × 5 cm in a baby and slightly larger in an older child. Perform a urethroplasty to lengthen the urethra, typically with bladder and buccal mucosa. The length of the reconstructed urethra will be 8 cm.

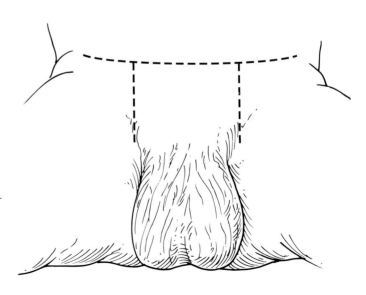

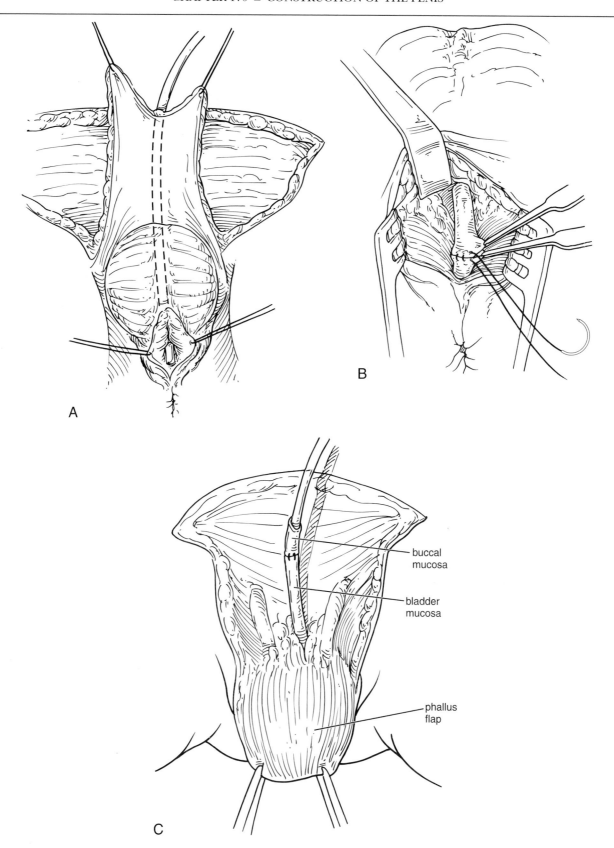

FIGURE 170-11. A, Mobilize the flap off the lower anterior wall to below the level of the symphysis pubis. **B,** Perform the urethroplasty by an interrupted anastomosis of bladder and buccal mucosa to the urethra within the perineum. **C,** Incorporate the urethroplasty into the new phallus.

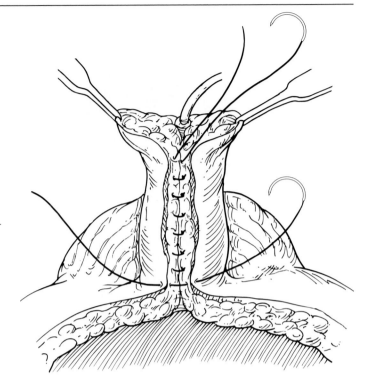

FIGURE 170-12. Wrap the abdominal flap around the urethra, creating a cylinder. Use two layers of interrupted absorbable sutures of 4-0 long-acting material.

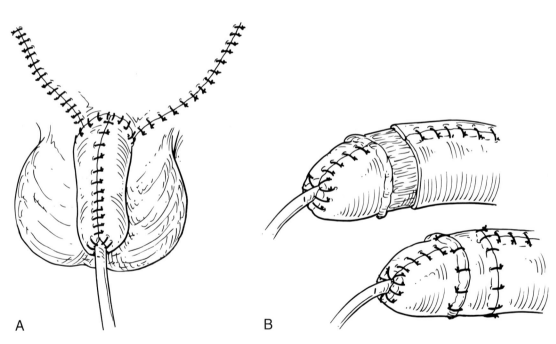

A   B

FIGURE 170-13. A, To form the meatus, mature the urethra circumferentially with 5-0 absorbable sutures. Close the abdominal wall donor site primarily by mobilizing the subcutaneous skin as necessary. Place deep sutures to take the tension off the closure. **B,** Create the glans by denuding 0.5 cm of tissue at the coronal margin and incorporating a strip of folded skin with 6-0 monofilament sutures.

Postoperatively, divert the urine with a urethral stent and suprapubic tube. Alternatively, leave the urethra at the penoscrotal junction for subsequent reconstruction at a later date.

ROBERTO DE CASTRO

Commentary by

There are almost no data on total phallic construction/substitution in infants and children, especially for congenital malformation. The most commonly used procedure for phalloplasty in adolescents and young adults is the microvascular transfer of a radial forearm flap that is generally not recommended before puberty. The limited international experience in phalloplasty in very young patients is the main reason that Western countries tend to assign female gender to infants born with congenital or acquired absence of the penis (aphallia, penile agenesis) or with very poor male external genitalia (cloacal exstrophy). Our early phalloplasty was specially designed to overcome this limitation, allowing preservation of male gender in 46,XY individuals with normal male gonads, despite absence or extreme underdevelopment of the penis and achieving an acceptable male genitalia appearance. Male gender assignment and early phalloplasty might avoid the frequent sexual orientation problems that progress with age and may end with patient-initiated gender reassignment to male, which is likely to occur when these unfortunate individuals have undergone female gender reassignment—including castration—even very early in life.

Experimental data and clinical observations have established the role of androgens in male gender identity formation. Prenatal and early postnatal androgen exposure deeply contributes to male psychosexual development and identity that cannot be changed by neonatal castration, hormonal treatment, phenotypic adjustments, and psychosexual manipulations.

In conclusion, we do believe that patients with congenital or acquired aphallia must be raised as males and any female gender reassignment must be avoided in this particular group of patients.

We start phalloplasty in infants in the prone knee-chest position and use the anterior saginal transrectal approach to detach the urethra from the rectum. We then move the patient to a lithotomy position and develop a quadrangular lower abdominal skin flap for penile construction, adding a bladder-buccal mucosa tube for urethral reconstruction.

The entire abdominal skin flap is reserved for penis and glans replacement, avoiding the complications related to the long-skin-tube new urethra configured from the same abdominal flap (as described by Pryor [2005]), but exposing to the free-graft tube new-urethra complications, experienced in our cases. In general, the procedure has shown reasonable outcomes, especially good for the phalloplasty itself, and it could be the correct treatment for these rare and extreme conditions. The most challenging part of the procedure is the distal urethral and external meatal reconstruction; better results might be achieved with multiple-stage repair.

We first designed our method for infants and as a temporary procedure, anticipating definitive forearm flap phalloplasty after puberty as the final procedure. Obvious social and psychological reasons and possible complications related to the rectal-ending urethra (when present) justify, in our opinion, our early palliative phalloplasty and urethroplasty in infancy. However, we still have to investigate the potential of our procedure in the long term: We will evaluate the growth of the new phallus, with the expectation that it might reach an acceptable size at puberty and be able to accept the insertion of a penile prosthesis, which would allow erection and sexual intercourse.

The same technique was applied for infants affected by cloacal exstrophy with extremely poor external genitalia and bladder exstrophy with severe penile loss after neonatal epispadias repair, and for older children affected by traumatic or iatrogenic-acquired aphallia or in cases of early gender reassignment in disorders of sex development. Any penile or glans remnants are incorporated in the new phallus. In our experience, the maximum size of the lower abdominal skin flap was 11 × 11 cm. Skin expanders might be used in preparation for phalloplasty in cases of previous abdominal surgery and subsequent lower abdominal wall scars.

Finally, we would like to stress that our surgical technique of phalloplasty may improve or be modified or replaced in the future; however, we wish to emphasize again the importance of retaining the male gender in 46,XY individuals affected by congenital or acquired, total or subtotal aphallia, which we strongly believe is the right approach to this complex problem.

ANTONIO MACEDO, JR.

The De Castro neophalloplasty is a strategy to treat infants with congenital aphallia, which is a rare disease, in the most appropriate way in regard to physical and psychological aspects. Female gender reassignment in this situation is a decision that, besides involving gonadectomy and external hormonal administration, will exclude any chance of paternity. As all of us are aware of continuous advancement of assisted reproductive techniques and new prostheses, patients with aphallia will certainly benefit from these technologies in the future.

The technique itself is a combination of the previously discussed anterior saginal transrectal approach to release the posterior urethra from the rectum in a safe and simple way without the need for protective colostomy. Concerning the phallus construction, the mobilization and tubularization of the inferior abdominal flap produce a nice penile aspect without the technical difficulty of microsurgical vascular anastomosis to promote the integration of free forearm grafts, as is frequently done in adults.

One step of the technique that is still to be debated is the neourethroplasty. The recently published series made up of Roberto De Castro's patients and ours in Brazil showed what we could have expected from hypospadias experience: tube grafts of various donor sites such as the bladder and buccal mucosa are particularly prone to complications, mainly strictures. We think that by applying the Bracka two-step strategy in regard to urethral construction we will probably overcome this problem. On the other hand, one question is still left concerning penile growth in proportion to the patient. Our initial psychological results recorded as we have followed patients and families have been extremely encouraging.

Chapter 171

Female Urethrovaginal Fistula

URETHROVAGINAL FISTULA

Culture the urine and give appropriate antibiotics.

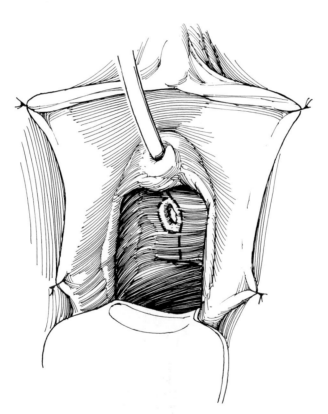

FIGURE 171-1. Position: Lithotomy. Alternatively, place the patient prone in the skydiver position so that the urethra lies directly in view. Examine the area cystoscopically: inspect the defect and attempt passage of a catheter through the fistula. Prep the lower abdomen, vagina, and perineum. Suture the labia laterally. Insert a silicone balloon catheter into the bladder and place a posterior retractor in the vagina (not shown). Infiltrate the vaginal mucosa with dilute epinephrine to reduce bleeding during the dissection.

Incision: Place multiple fine sutures around the fistula for traction (not shown). Incise the vaginal mucosa on one side of the midline.

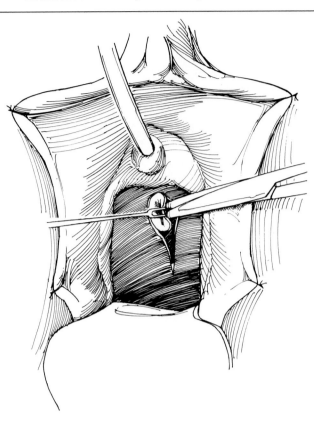

FIGURE 171-2. Dissect the vaginal mucosa laterally, using the sutures for traction. Mobilize a margin of pubocervical fascia asymmetrically. Trim the margins of the fistula back into normal urethral tissue.

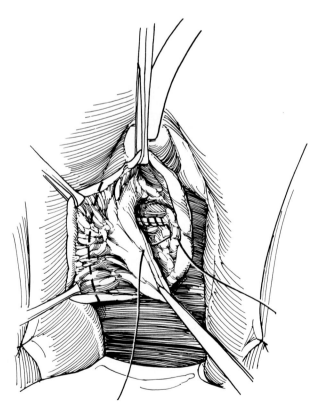

FIGURE 171-3. Close the defect in the urethra transversely with interrupted subepithelial 5-0 synthetic absorbable sutures. Bring the pubocervical fascia over the defect asymmetrically with 4-0 synthetic absorbable sutures. Trim the vaginal mucosa on the opposite side to achieve fit.

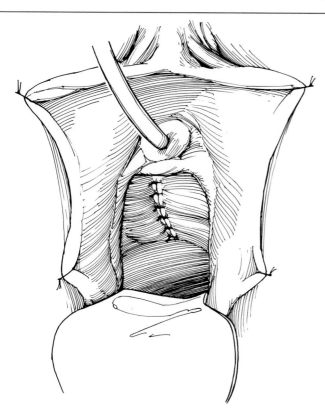

FIGURE 171-4. Bring the vaginal edges together with 4-0 synthetic absorbable sutures. Place a vaginal pack to be left for 24 hours. Insert a catheter and over tincture of benzoin, tape it firmly to the abdomen to prevent traction on the repair, and connect it to sterile drainage to remain for 3 to 5 days.

BULBOCAVERNOSUS MUSCLE SUPPLEMENT (MARTIUS)

Locate the bulbocavernosus muscle by palpating it between the index finger placed just inside the hymeneal ring and the thumb on the labium majus.

FIGURE 171-5. After the fistula has been repaired but before the vaginal mucosa is closed, make a vertical incision in the groove between the labium majus and labium minus.

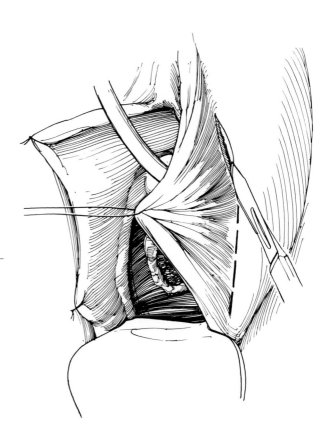

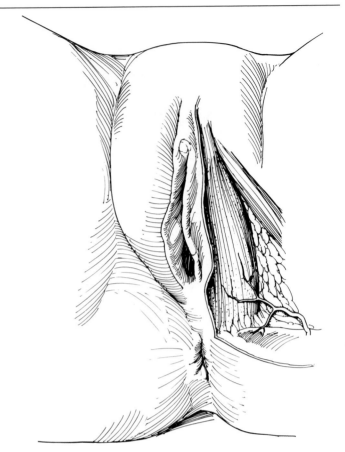

FIGURE 171-6. Expose the bulbocavernosus muscle.

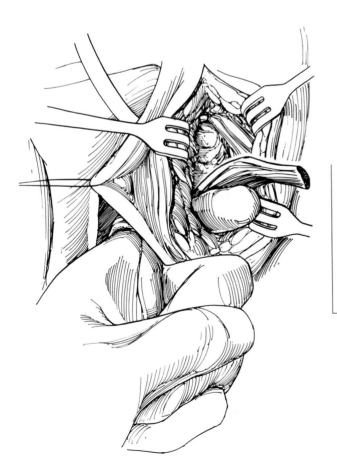

FIGURE 171-7. Dissect the bulbocavernosus muscle free. Take care not to disturb the blood supply that comes from the deep perineal branch of the external pudendal artery and enters the muscle posteriorly close to its origin. Include the fat pad surrounding the muscle. Ligate the tip of the muscle and divide it anteriorly. With a right-angle clamp, develop a tunnel: start lateral to the repair, continue laterally under the labium minus, and end near the dissected muscle. Enlarge the tunnel with the left index finger held against the tip of the clamp.

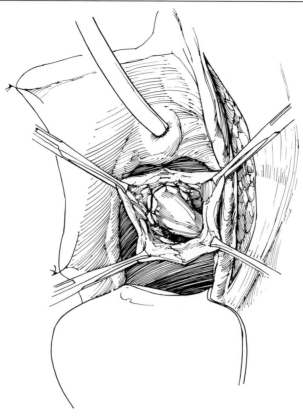

FIGURE 171-8. Grasp the edge of the muscle and draw it through the tunnel. Fix it in place with interrupted 3-0 synthetic absorbable sutures to cover the defect.

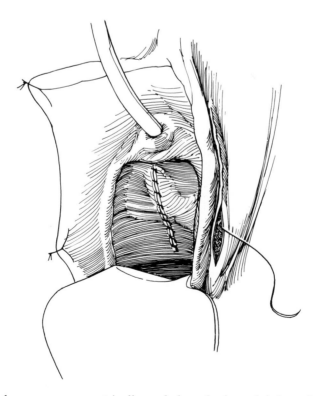

FIGURE 171-9. Trim the vaginal mucosa asymmetrically, and close the lateral defect with a subcuticular 4-0 synthetic absorbable suture.

POSTOPERATIVE PROBLEMS

A hematoma may form following premature removal of the vaginal pack. A fistula may develop if tension persists after repair, if the balloon catheter is forcibly displaced, or if infection supervenes.

JACK ELDER

Commentary by

Urethrovaginal fistulas are rare in girls. They may occur following repair of a cloacal anomaly or urogenital sinus closure. One of the ideal positions for closure is in the prone knee-chest position, allowing direct visualization of the anterior vaginal wall. If there is insufficient healthy tissue for urethroplasty, a buccal mucosa graft often is useful. The bulbocavernosus flap is a nice way to provide vascularized coverage of the urethral repair. Alternatively, we have found that a gracilis flap also may provide excellent coverage.

DAVID DIAMOND

Commentary by

Vesicovaginal fistula is an uncommon problem in the pediatric age group. The differential diagnosis of vesicovaginal fistula includes ureterovaginal fistula and, therefore, evaluation should include an intravenous pyelogram as well as cystoscopy and vaginoscopy. Cystoscopy can enable you to identify the source of the fistula and confirm that it is not near the ureteric orifice. If necessary, at the time of surgery, a ureteral stent may be placed to identify the ureter intraoperatively. If the source of urinary leakage is unclear a dye test may be performed at cystoscopy, in which the vagina is packed with gauze and methylene blue is instilled into the bladder. After a reasonable period of time the pack is removed and blue dye confirms a vesicovaginal fistula. Should the pack be wet with urine but not blue this would support a ureterovaginal fistula.

The principles of fistula repair include a tension-free, watertight, multi-layer closure. Overlapping suture lines should be avoided. A critical component to successful repair of a vesicovaginal fistula is the interposition of healthy vascularized tissue between bladder and vaginal suture lines.

Chapter 172

Female Urethral Construction

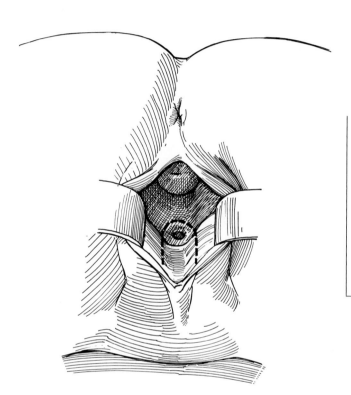

FIGURE 172-1. First stage: Place the girl prone in the skydiver position with the legs spread apart, the knees flexed, and the feet suspended from stirrup holders fixed to the table. Pad the pelvis and shoulders. This unusual position gives ideal exposure of the anterior vaginal wall, from which a urethra or urethral extension will be constructed.

Incise the introitus in a U shape, extending the parallel incisions as far as the clitoris. Its width depends on the size and age of the girl (make them from 2.5 or 3 cm apart to form a 25- or 30-F urethra). Raise the mucosa and paraurethral tissue on either side of the strip.

FIGURE 172-2. Roll the strip into a tube with a running 3-0 synthetic absorbable suture over a straight catheter of appropriate size. There will be ample tissue at the level of the introitus; bring this over to close the distal end of the tube in two or three layers, leaving the opening close to the base of the clitoris.

Technical problem: Because there is usually not enough tissue to cover the proximal tube, use a buttock flap by raising a flap of skin and subcutaneous fat. Make it long enough to reach high in the vagina and wide enough to ensure good blood supply to the end of the flap.

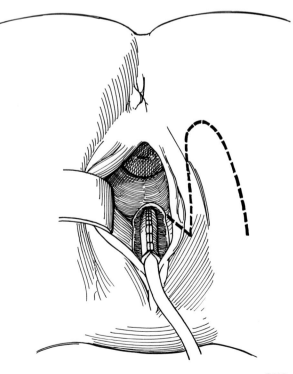

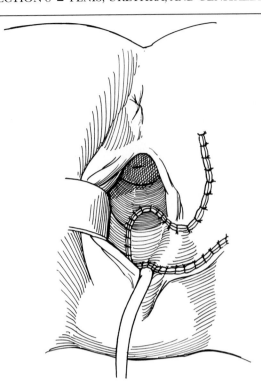

FIGURE 172-3. Open the introitus and lay the flap in place. To avoid overlying suture lines, be sure the end of the flap lies at least 2 cm higher in the vagina than the beginning of the urethral tube. Suture the flap in place with interrupted sutures. Apply a loose dressing (one too tight can compress the blood supply in the base of the flap).

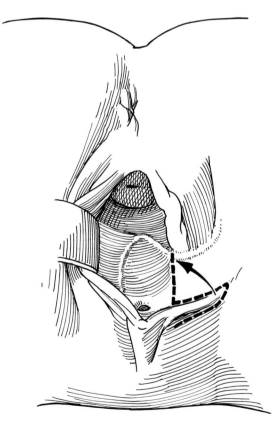

FIGURE 172-4. Second stage (performed several months later): Place the girl supine and divide the base of the flap. Return the flap to its site of origin on the buttock, leaving only that portion covering the vagina in place.

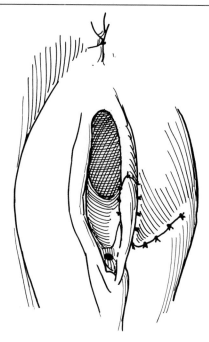

FIGURE 172-5. Close the introitus appropriately, giving it a normal appearance once again, with the isolated end of the flap becoming the anterior vaginal wall.

W. HARDY HENDREN

Commentary by

I first used this operation in 1975 to close a urethral fistula, which resulted from paucity of local tissue when a urethra was made by tubularizing the vaginal wall in this fashion. The fistula was closed and covered with a buttocks flap to prevent its reopening. The buttocks flap was substituted for the vaginal wall to create a urethra. This worked well. Since then, the operation has been used in more than 35 patients, whose urethras were too short from a variety of causes, including congenitally deficient urethras; bilateral, single ectopic ureters with a short urethra; severe pelvic trauma with urethral destruction; cloacal cases; myelodysplasia with short urethras; and vaginectomy (in one adult patient) following radical hysterectomy. The average age of the patients was 13 years, with the youngest being 3 and the oldest 30 years of age. There were two fistulas requiring closure. One was caused by a dressing that was too tight on the base of the flap, resulting in necrosis. The operation was repeated 6 months later. The second fistula was caused by having the tip of the flap too close to the urethral closure. This serves to emphasize that overlying suture lines should be avoided. All of the patients originally had been incontinent. The majority were dry after having one or more operations to narrow the bladder neck and lengthen the urethra upward, with urethral lengthening from below. In some patients, urodynamic study demonstrated additional outlet resistance created by the distal urethra, which is surrounded by introital musculature.

Chapter 173

Urethral Prolapse

Urethral prolapse is typically self-limiting and rarely requires surgical intervention. Presenting symptoms are bleeding or dysuria. In the severe case, in which conservative management with sitz baths and barrier creams is not effective, excision is indicated.

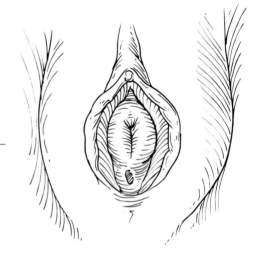

FIGURE 173-1. Place the patient in the lithotomy position and examine the genitalia with attention to the urethra and vagina.

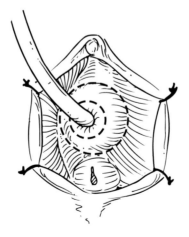

FIGURE 173-2. Insert a urethral catheter into the bladder and outline an incision, leaving a cuff of urethra and a concentric incision at the outlying border of the prolapse. Use 1% lidocaine in 1:100,00 epinephrine for hemostasis.

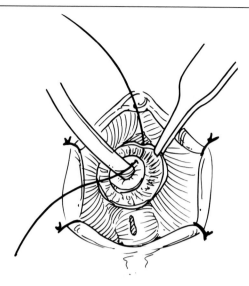

FIGURE 173-3. Incise a doughnut of tissue and approximate the defect using absorbable 5-0 or 6-0 sutures.

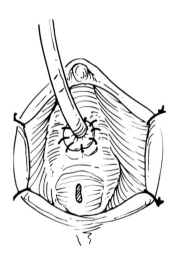

FIGURE 173-4. Leave a urethral catheter in place for 24 to 48 hours. Use antibiotic ointment for comfort and to prevent infection.

COMPLICATIONS

Care should be taken to leave a cuff of urethra, thereby preventing the possibility of urethral stenosis.

JULIAN WAN

Commentary by

Urethral prolapse typically affects two groups of patients: premenarchal girls or postmenopausal elderly women. Children most often have African heritage. Estrogen deficiency has been proposed as a possible common etiology between these groups. Other proposed causes include laxity of the periurethral fascia and redundancy of the urothelium lining the urethra. One significant iatrogenic cause that has been reported in elderly women is the occurrence of prolapse after injection of a periurethral substance for the treatment of stress incontinence. This treatment is also now being used in children so the possibility of postinjection urethral prolapse in children should be kept in mind.

Urethral prolapse in young girls can sometimes be managed with conservative means: warm water sitz baths, topical estrogen cream, and antibiotic ointment. I usually offer this option so long as the child can void and is not in great discomfort. If there is no improvement over the following 3 to 5 days or if there is worsening of the symptoms, surgery is recommended. The typical presentation is dysuria and bleeding. Usually the initial examination is pathognomonic; however, it may be mistaken for a simple urinary tract infection when a physical examination is cursory or skipped over. Duplex prolapsed ureterocele, sarcoma botryoides, and caruncle are the major differential diagnoses. The appearance of urethral prolapse is quite distinctive, having a complete, round buttonlike appearance. The prolapsed ureterocele and sarcoma botryoides do not have a single complete circumferential mass and caruncles are usually laterally placed.

It is often hard to make two concentric incisions in the swollen round surface of the prolapsed urethra. I usually place a suture of 5-0 or 6-0 chromic catgut at the 12- or 6-o'clock position to help stabilize the doughnut of urethra to be resected. You could also place additional sutures at the 3- and 9-o'clock positions but I have found two sutures to be usually adequate. The excess tissue can be cut with a standard scalpel (#15 Bard-Parker) or with a pair of sharp-tipped scissors. The edges of the freshly cut urethra can be sewn together with 5-0 or 6-0 chromic catgut sutures prior to proceeding to the other side. I usually leave the catheter in for 2 to 4 days and ask the family to apply antibiotic ointment to the meatus. When the protruding edges of the prolapsed urethra are very edematous it can be hard to make a clean cut with a scalpel and difficult to engage the blades of the scissors. One method of dealing with this situation is to remove the Foley catheter and place a metal urethral sound. This gives a solid surface on which you can press firmly to make a clean cut with a knife.

Part V

Urethra

Chapter 174

Posterior Urethral Valves

Confirm the diagnosis with a voiding cystourethrogram. A newborn urethra in a full-term infant will be 10 to 12 F and should accept a 7.5 to 8 cystoscope. Premature infants may require placement of a 5-F feeding tube to allow the urethra to dilate. Severely premature infants may require a vesicostomy (see Chapter 85).

The ideal treatment for posterior urethral valves is retrograde endoscopic ablation, avoiding the need for urinary diversion and subsequent reconstruction or blind urethral-valve–disrupting procedures such as hook devices.

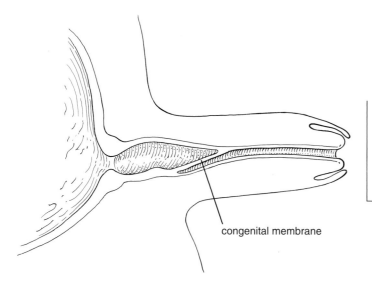

congenital membrane

FIGURE 174-1. The anatomy of the posterior urethral valve has been refined to the present description as a congenital, obstructive posterior urethral membrane. The membrane must have at least a small hole to allow the passage of urine; otherwise, the lack of amniotic fluid would be incompatible with life.

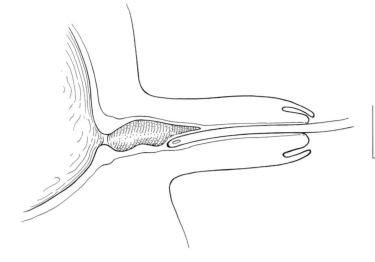

FIGURE 174-2. Passage of a catheter, typically a 5- or 8-F feeding tube after birth, disrupts the membrane, connecting the two lumens into a single channel.

FIGURE 174-3. The edges of the torn membrane heal into the classic type 1 posterior urethral membrane that is visualized at the time of valve ablation. Emanating distally and laterally from the lower portion of the verumontanum are the sail-like folds of the valve, joining anteriorly at the 12-o'clock position. The valve leaflets are most clearly seen at the 5- and 7-o'clock positions. Distal to the valve leaflets is the external sphincter. Proximal to the valve is the bladder neck, which may be exceedingly high, requiring the passage of the endoscope almost directly upward to enter into the bladder.

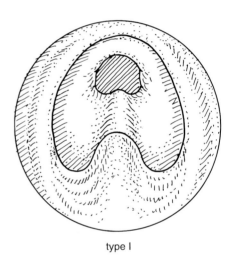

type I

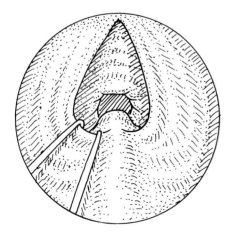

FIGURE 174-4. With the advent of pediatric equipment, valve ablation is now performed with the infant resectoscope loop or endoscopic electrode. Position the resectoscope loop on the leaflets at the 5- and 7-o'clock positions. Set the pure cutting current at 20 to 30 W and then use to destroy the valve tissue. Also check the 12-o'clock position for obstructing valve tissue. Often this tissue has been destroyed by the catheter placement.

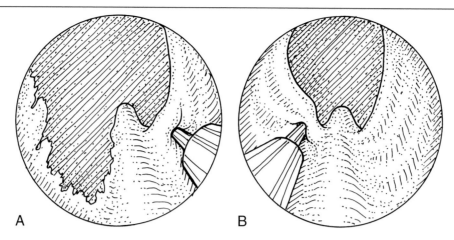

FIGURE 174-5. An alternative approach is to use the endoscopic electrode, which can fit through a 3-F port on the smallest cystoscopes. Set the pure cutting current at 25 W. Apply the electrode to the valve leaflets at the (**A**) 5- and (**B**) 7-o'clock positions. Place a 5- or 8-F feeding tube for 24 to 48 hours.

POSTOPERATIVE CARE

The patient is maintained on prophylactic antibiotics. The upper tracts are monitored with renal bladder sonography. Serum creatinine is periodically checked. A postoperative voiding cystourethrogram is performed at 6 weeks to ensure that the valve has been ablated.

NICHOLAS M. HOLMES

Commentary by

Fetal intervention for posterior urethral valves has greatly evolved since its initial introduction in 1981 at the University of California San Francisco. The most significant improvement has been in the reduction of fetal/maternal morbidity and the use of amnioinfusion at the time of the shunt placement. It is critical to have a well-experienced fetal surgery team (i.e., a fetal ultrasonographer, maternal-fetal medicine specialist, neonatologist, obstetric anesthesiologist, and perioperative obstetric/pediatric nursing staff) in place to facilitate a successful outcome.

Several key studies need to be obtained before considering intervention procedures:

1. Serial fetal urinary electrolytes consistent with hypotonic urine (sodium < 100 mEq/L, chloride < 90 mEq/L, osmolarity < 210 mOsm)
2. Normal-appearing kidneys on ultrasound (normal echotexture, no cortical cysts)
3. Normal fetal karyotype (46,XY)

The use of the shunt is not without complications, such as shunt migration, malposition or malplacement, and shunt blockage. If placed early in the pregnancy, the rate of shunt occlusion is quite high and therefore serial ultrasound monitoring is a must. Repeat shunt placement may be required. At some centers, primary in utero valve ablation is performed via a fetal cystoscope/endoscope, either using laser energy or hydrostatic pressure. No one technique has proven to be superior in securing the survival of the unborn patient or in preventing the associated findings that contribute to early demise after delivery (e.g., renal failure, pulmonary hypoplasia with respiratory failure).

When counseling the families about fetal intervention, focus the discussion on how the process may facilitate carrying the fetus to term, and that the sequelae of posterior urethral valves may not be preventable.

GRAHAME H. H. SMITH

Commentary by

I agree that the ideal treatment for a type 1 posterior urethral valve (COPUM) is endoscopic ablation. I also agree that the diagnosis is best made by a voiding cystourethrogram. Most patients present after an antenatal diagnosis, within the first week of life. Their urine is sterile and their electrolytes are normal. They can usually be readily catheterized using a 5- or 8-F feeding tube and then operated upon on the next available elective list.

I secure the feeding tube using 0.5-inch Steri-Strips, placed longitudinally along the penis and then wrapped around the feeding tube. Liberal amounts of tincture of benzoin aid in the adhesion of the Steri-Strips. Occasionally, a feeding tube will not go up over the bladder neck and into the bladder. This problem can be corrected by using a Coude-tipped catheter, freezing a feeding tube, and bending the tip up slightly, or by placing a gloved little finger in the rectum and pushing the prostate and bladder neck upward during catheterization. Alternatively, an intravenous cannula can be inserted suprapubically and taped in place to drain the bladder.

In the unlikely event that the patient presents with abnormal electrolytes or with sepsis, then these problems need to be corrected before taking the child to the operating room. Usually bladder drainage and intravenous antibiotics are sufficient for this task.

I perform the valve ablation under general anesthesia, using a 9-F resectoscope. The working element is a diathermy knife, rather than a loop. No attempt is made to resect the valve leaflet. The valve leaflets are cut, using a cutting diathermy current set on 25 W at 5-, 7-, and 12-o'clock. Bleeding is usually very minimal. If there is significant bleeding, then it suggests that the cuts have been too deep. Bleeding can be controlled with sparsely applied coagulating current or by inserting a feeding tube catheter and applying perineal pressure. In premature babies, when a 9-F scope will not fit, I use a 7-F cystoscope and an insulated, angled cutting wire placed through the 3-F instrument channel. Technically, it is more difficult to cut the valve leaflet with an angled wire, compared to using a resectoscope. If the procedure goes well, then it is not necessary to replace the feeding tube after surgery. The baby can be left to void spontaneously.

In rare situations in which cystoscopic ablation is not possible, I perform vesicostomy. The valve can be ablated and the vesicostomy closed about 6 months later, once the urethra is large enough to accept a 9-F resectoscope.

The serum creatinine should stabilize and begin to fall within 48 hours of valve ablation. I generally organize a renal and bladder ultrasound 2 weeks after surgery. This should show an improvement in hydronephrosis. A follow-up voiding cystourethrogram 6 weeks after surgery should show a marked reduction in the dilation of the posterior urethra and good filling of the anterior urethra. In my experience, 30% of patients who have had a primary valve ablation need to have a secondary ablation.

A persistently elevated serum creatinine and/or the failure of the hydronephrosis to improve shown on a follow-up ultrasound is an indication to consider further measures to decompress the bladder, such as an indwelling catheter for 1 to 2 weeks or a vesicostomy. If there is no improvement with one or the other of these measures, then an upper-tract diversion is unlikely to help either. A temporary percutaneous nephrostomy will prove this is so.

PADDY DEWAN

Commentary by

Posterior urethral obstruction, like many conditions in pediatric urology, is simplified in most descriptions that discuss its treatment. In reality, the changes in the urethra, bladder, ureters, and kidneys are many, and there is a broad spectrum of both the anatomic lesion and the clinical presentation.

The important facts that affect interpretation and management of these boys' cases are:

1. The posterior urethral anomaly is a membrane with a posterior defect, with paramedian folds back to the crista, best known as COPUM.
2. Passage of a catheter will reduce the degree of obstruction in many cases.
3. The top end of the external sphincter is above the level of the obstruction; the external sphincter is a tube of muscle.
4. Bladder and upper-tract changes do not always directly correlate with the degree of narrowing in the posterior urethra. A significant luminal narrowing may not be associated with adverse renal and bladder changes.
5. The degree of abnormality in the posterior urethra ranges from a minor indentation to severe obstruction, which is a variable expression of the same embryopathy.
6. Bulbar urethral lesions are not in the posterior urethra, and are either a prolapsed COPUM (identified by the attachments to the verumontanum), the distal end of the external sphincter, or a fibrous narrowing (without verumontanum connections), known as Cobb's collar.
7. Ablating the obstruction may be only a minor contribution to the management of a complex patient.

These conclusions are based on extensive review of videotape-recorded endoscopies and an extensive and detailed review of the many hundreds of papers written on the subject of posterior urethral obstruction.

Obstruction of the posterior urethra was first described in 1717 by Morgagni and subsequently by Langenbeck in 1802 in his monograph on stone disease.

The seminal paper of Hugh Hampton Young (1919) was a review of 12 cases, all of which are described in great detail in the text and in Table 4. The cases ranged in age from 11 days to 42 years, with only five being 12 months old or less. Importantly, only three of the 12 cases had been cystoscoped, and these three patients were 17, 26, and 42 years, one of whom had previous venereal infection. In the classification table (Table 1), five were described as type 1 valves, one as type 2 valves, and three were thought to be type 3 valves. The three types were further subdivided, with three subtypes of type 1, one form of type 2, and two variants of the type 3 lesions. Within the type 3 group, one variant was thought to consist of a perforated membrane below the verumontanum, without attachment to it, and the other was thought to be above it. Three of the 12 cases were not specifically classified; thus, a six-part classification was based on nine cases, three of which had only had finger palpation of the lesion. It is also interesting to note that the subtypes presented by Young and colleagues in the 1919 paper differ from those published in the 1929 paper, and that the perforation of the type 3 lesions below the verumontanum was considered either posterior (1919) or central (1929).

Detailed analysis of the cases using the description in the text and Table 4, and in light of recent observations, suggests that type 1A and type 1B are iatrogenic modifications of a congenital posterior urethral obstruction for which there are attachments to the verumontanum. It should be noted that most of Young's type 1 cases were thought to have two valves meeting in the midline, but not fused. Type 2 and type 3 above the verumontanum do not exist, and type 3 obstruction below the verumontanum, without the attachment to the verumontanum, and with a central defect, is probably a remnant of the urogenital diaphragm, if fibrous. This lesion is probably the same as those called Cobb's collar, Moormann's ring, or congenital stricture.

Young made two comments worth highlighting, particularly because they had not been substantiated by detailed study of endoscopic recording. The first was that "cystoscopy furnishes little information regarding the type of urethral anomaly," which most would now find rather contentious, and "little or no difficulty is encountered in passing a catheter, but the ease of the instrumentation is by no means an index of the degree of obstruction."

An additional insight that refutes the original classification is the previous technique of dissection of the specimens. Specimens of the lower urinary tract were opened by a midline anterior approach, leaving the posterior wall intact, splitting the membrane obstruction, giving an impression of a valvular obstruction between two paramedian reinforcements. Jarjavay, in 1856, was the first to give an illustration of a diaphragm that was again highlighted by Lederer in 1911, both papers being quoted by Young and colleagues in 1919.

Young also provided insight into urologic disease in boys when he raised the question of variability of obstruction of the posterior urethra. He and his coauthors wrote, "It should be borne in mind that varying degrees of congenital obstruction may exist, which may result in symptoms so slight that the condition is unrecognised" (p. 297). In contrast, there was little clue to the modern concept of the interrelationship of the external sphincter and the obstructing tissue in the presentation in 1919.

To better understand the conclusions reached on interpretation of the anatomy of posterior urethral obstruction it is necessary to discuss bulbar urethral narrowing.

By consensus, type 3 valves are rare inframontane, bulbar urethral lesions with a central rather than a posterior defect. Cobb and colleagues were the first to describe a significant number of cases of narrowing in the bulbar urethra that appeared to be congenital; hence the term Cobb's collar. They suggested that minor changes could often be seen if the urethra was entered under direct vision. However, the understanding of Cobb's collar appears to have been confused by studies grouping boys with older men; studies of urethrograms without cystoscopy; studies in which prolapsed lesions of the posterior urethra were confused with lesions of the bulbar urethra primarily; and studies regarding all bulbar constrictions as pathologic rather than some as merely anatomic variations. Moormann's ring is another term used for a congenital narrowing in the bulbar urethra. The presence of two separate terms may have added to the confusion.

Cobb thought the lesion could not be muscle, as the 26 children he recorded had a narrowing that was not affected by succinylcholine. Moormann's patients ranged from 21 to 54 years in age. These constricting bulbar urethral lesions in older men may be spasm of intrinsic urethral muscle or spasm of the bulbospongiosus muscle, highlighting that the bulbar urethral findings may be either muscular or membranous, and the delayed presentation of adults suggests that the narrowing is most likely to be muscular in the older patients. Currarino (1986) showed a Cobb's collar impression on radiographs, with variable appearance between patients, and concluded that the radiologic findings were due to contraction of periurethral muscle, which we also identified in 21 boys.

The embryonic origin of Cobb's collar seems to be the result of the persistence of the urogenital membrane, which can be minor or significant, muscular or fibrous. Congenital obstruction of the bulbar urethra has not often been discussed in the literature, possibly because many would agree with Cobb's observation in 1968 that insertion of the cystoscope, while visualizing the urethra, will often show the presence of a ring narrowing of the bulbar urethra, and therefore it is not worthy of recording; a conclusion also reached by Cranston and colleagues. Significant pathology does occur, however, which has been classified according to the degree of encroachment on the lumen (mild, moderate, and severe) and the presence of muscle or a fibrous membrane within the narrowed segment.

Bladder and renal function management are the most important considerations in an infant who has significant upper-tract changes. There are numerous publications debating the pros and cons of various interventions; probably each case is very individual and should be managed with all the armamentarium available, depending on the specific initial findings and the responses to treatment. A fatalistic approach to the outcome for renal function should not be adopted.

Chapter 175

Excision of Utricular (Mullerian Duct) Cyst

Palpate rectally for a midline mass. Use ultrasonography or MRI to detect the cyst and help determine its size. Because cysts open into the posterior urethra, secure a voiding cystourethrogram to evaluate size. In older children assess the caliber of the ostium by endoscopy. Try to obliterate the lumen by thorough endoscopic fulguration of the walls of the cyst. To detect a connection with the vasa deferentia, insert a ureteral catheter into the cyst and inject contrast medium. Resort to vasography if necessary.

TRANSVESICAL APPROACH

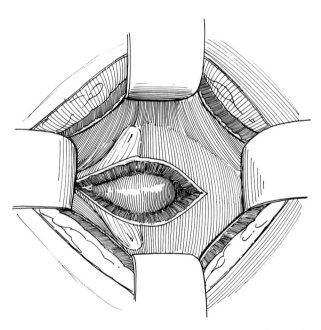

FIGURE 175-1. Make a transverse or vertical lower abdominal incision. (Avoid a perineal approach because of the risk of compromising potency.) Open the bladder and expose the trigone. Place a ring retractor with four blades. Insert an infant feeding tube into each ureter (not shown). Make a vertical incision in the midline through the trigone and posterior bladder wall that extends almost to the vesical neck. Insert stay sutures to hold the incision open. With blunt dissection, expose the anterior wall of the cyst. Use tenotomy scissors to dissect the cyst to its entrance into the posterior urethra. Avoid the orifices of the vasa. Remove the retractor blade at the caudal end of the bladder incision to expose the bladder neck and allow dissection of the cyst to its entrance into the posterior urethra, with or without enlarging it if necessary.

Close the urethra with a running inner layer and an interrupted outer layer of 4-0 polyglycolic suture. Approximate the trigone in two layers. Insert a urethral catheter and a suprapubic tube to remain, with the ureteral catheters, for a week. Close the bladder and the incision.

If the vasa are transected, implant them into the bladder with a nonrefluxing technique, realizing that the prospect of fertility is reduced.

The same approach can be used for a refluxing residual stump of an ectopic ureter after heminephrectomy (see Chapter 28). Use this same approach to avoid the more extensive and possibly damaging dissection required from the previously discussed procedure. An alternative is the transrectal posterior sagittal approach (see Chapter 78). Note: A similar technique is useful for urethrorectal fistula tracts remaining after repair of high imperforate anus.

JACK S. ELDER

Commentary by

Utricular, or mullerian duct, cysts are most common in boys with penoscrotal or perineal hypospadias and in intersex conditions. These cysts vary in size and usually are asymptomatic. However, selected individuals may experience dysuria, perineal discomfort, urinary tract infection, epididymitis, lower abdominal mass, obstructive symptoms, hematuria, incontinence, reduced semen volume, or oligospermia. By definition, these cysts should communicate only with the prostatic urethra. In the literature, however, are reports of mullerian duct cysts that communicate with the vasa deferentia. These latter cysts more appropriately are termed genital duct, or ejaculatory duct, cysts.

Utricular cysts often are palpable on rectal examination. They should be apparent on imaging studies, such as transrectal retrograde urethrogram, or voiding cystourethrogram, which should be done to evaluate the cyst size. Endoscopy is indicated to determine whether the ostium of the cyst is narrow. In addition, a small ureteral catheter should be inserted into the cyst and contrast injected to determine whether the vasa deferentia enter it. In selected cases, it is necessary to perform vasography to learn whether there is communication with the cyst.

Although the ostium of the cyst may be incised endoscopically, signs and symptoms often are not relieved. Consequently, an open surgical approach usually is necessary. The perineal approach should be avoided because of the risk of iatrogenic impotence.

The transtrigonal approach provides the best exposure. After opening the bladder, a Denis Browne retractor is placed. Ureteral catheters or pediatric feeding tubes should be inserted into the ureteral orifices. Next, the trigone is incised in the midline with the cautery. Stay sutures should be placed in the edges of the trigone. The utricle should be immediately apparent and can be dissected out with tenotomy scissors. Extreme care should be taken to avoid the vasa. The cyst may be dissected to its communication with the urethra. At times, opening the cyst is helpful in its mobilization. The urethra should be closed over a urethral catheter with a fine, running, imbricating polyglycolic acid stitch for the inner layer and interrupted sutures in the outer layer. Generally, no drainage of the retrovesical space is necessary. The trigone should be closed in two layers with nonabsorbable suture. I think it is preferable to leave a urethral catheter, a suprapubic tube, and ureteral catheters for 7 to 10 days postoperatively. If the vasa enter the cyst, they will need to be transected. Ideally, they should be implanted into the bladder; usually this can be accomplished in a nonrefluxing manner. However, subsequent fertility would seem unlikely, even with current methods of retrieving sperm from the bladder.

Although this approach has been used mainly for genital duct cysts, it also may be used in excising remnants of fistulous tracts in children born with high imperforate anus.

LAPAROSCOPIC EXCISION

Induce general anesthesia, and place the boy in the lithotomy position with leg support. Cannulate the utricle panendoscopically, and leave the instrument in place for identification and for facilitating mobilization. Insert a 5-mm port into the bladder from above the umbilicus, and two 3- to 5-mm working ports in the right and left mid-abdomen. Hitch the bladder dome to the anterior abdominal wall with a 4-0 polydioxanone suture inserted percutaneously under vision.

With the electrocautery, incise the peritoneal reflection starting immediately behind the bladder. Identify the utricle by the transmitted light from the panendoscope in the bladder. Have your assistant manipulate the panendoscope for countertraction. Visualize and protect the ureters.

Mobilize the utricle completely with the 5-mm electronic scalpel and divide it at its junction with the urethra. Close the defect with fine absorbable sutures or use ultrasonic coagulation. Remove the specimen through the camera port. Leave a urethral catheter in place for 3 days.

CRAIG PETERS

Commentary by

Laparoscopic exposure of the retrovesical space is excellent and offers a much less morbid approach to utricular cysts or mullerian remnants than the traditional transvesical approach. Robotic assistance is now being used to enhance visualization, manipulation, and suturing. We have not found that a cystoscope is needed, as the cysts are readily visible with extraperitoneal dissection. A rectal decompression tube can facilitate exposure. In the cases where the contralateral vas is adherent to the wall of the cyst, leaving a strip of the cyst wall with the vas protects against injury. The mucosa of the cyst wall can be fulgurated to prevent reformation of the cyst. We close with suture any communication with the urethra and do not always leave a bladder catheter.

Bibliography

Section 1
Preparation for Pediatric Operations

Adamson RJ, Musco F, Enquist IF: The clinical dimensions of a healing incision. *Surg Gynecol Obstet* 123:515, 1966.

Adzick NS, Harrison MR, Glick PL, et al: Comparison of fetal, newborn and adult wound healing by histologic, enzyme-histochemical, and hydroxyproline determinations. *J Pediatr Surg* 20:315, 1985.

Adzick NS, Lonaker MT: The biology of fetal wound healing: a review. *Plast Reconstr Surg* 87:788, 1991.

Adzick NS, Lonaker MT (Eds): *Fetal Wound Healing.* New York, Elsevier Scientific Publishing, 1992.

Allen L: Lymphatics and lymphoid tissues. *Ann Rev Physiol* 29:197, 1967.

American Academy of Pediatrics, Section on Anesthesiology: Evaluation and preparation of pediatric patients undergoing anesthesia. *Pediatrics* 98:502, 1996.

Anson BJ, McVay CB: *Surgical Anatomy*, 6th ed. Philadelphia, W. B. Saunders Company, 1984.

Balinsky BI, Fabian BC: *An Introduction to Embryology*, 5th ed. Philadelphia, W. B. Saunders Company, 1981.

Barie PS: Modern surgical antibiotic prophylaxis and therapy: less is more. *Surg Infect* 1: 23, 2000.

Berman SS (Ed): *Vascular Access in Clinical Practice.* New York, Dekker, 2001.

Bhananker SM, Ramamoorthy C, Geiduschek JM, et al: Anesthesia-related cardiac arrest in children: update from the Pediatric Perioperative Cardiac Arrest Registry. *Anesth Analg* 105:344–50, 2007.

Bloch EC: Anesthetic considerations in the neonate. In: King LR (Ed): *Urologic Surgery in Neonates and Young Infants.* Philadelphia, W. B. Saunders Company, 1988, p 119.

Bo WJ, Meschan I, Krueger WA: *Basic Atlas of Cross-Sectional Anatomy.* Philadelphia, W. B. Saunders Company, 1980.

Bohnen JM, Solomkin JS, Dellinger EP, et al: Guidelines for clinical care anti-infective agents for intra-abdominal infection. *Arch Surg* 127:83, 1992.

Borges AF: *Electrical Incisions and Scar Revision.* Boston, Little, Brown & Company, 1973.

Bray L, Sanders C: Preparing children and young people for stoma surgery. *Paediatr Nurs* 18:33–7, 2006. Review.

Breckler FD, Fuchs JR, Rescorla FJ: Survey of pediatric surgeons on current practices of bowel preparation for elective colorectal surgery in children. *Am J Surg* 193:315–8, 2007; discussion 318.

Britt BA: Malignant hyperthermia. *Can Anaesth Soc J* 32:666, 1985.

Broman I: *Normale und Abnormale Entwicklung des Menschen*, Wiesbaden, J. F. Bergman, 1911.

Burns RK: Urogenital system. In: Willier BH, et al (Eds): *Analysis of Development.* Philadelphia, W. B. Saunders Company, 1955, p 462.

Carlson BM: *Patten's Foundations of Embryology*, 5th ed. New York, McGraw-Hill Book Company, 1988.

Cassady JF Jr: Regional anesthesia for urologic procedures. *Urol Clin North Am* 14:43, 1987.

Cook-Sather SD, Litman RS: Modern fasting guidelines in children. *Best Pract Res Clin Anaesthesiol* 20:471–81, 2006.

Crafts RC: Abdominopelvic cavity and perineum. In: Crafts RC (Ed): *A Textbook of Human Anatomy*, 2nd ed. New York, John Wiley & Sons, 1979, pp 269–327.

Crawford MW, Galton S, Abdelhaleem M: Preoperative screening for sickle cell disease in children: clinical implications. *Can J Anaesth* 52:1058–63, 2005.

Crouch JE: The reproductive system. In: Crouch JE (Ed): *Functional Human Anatomy*, 2nd ed. Philadelphia, Lea & Febiger, 1972, pp 430–5.

Crouch JE: The urinary system. In: Crouch JE (Ed): *Functional Human Anatomy*, 2nd ed. Philadelphia, Lea & Febiger, 1972, pp 424–9.

Davis AT: Postoperative infection in surgical patients. In: Raffensperger JG (Ed): *Swenson's Pediatric Surgery*, 5th ed. Norwalk, CT, Appleton and Lange, 1990, p 29.

Deutinger J, Bartl W, Pfersmann C, et al: Fetal kidney volume and urine production in cases of fetal growth retardation. *J Perinat Med* 15:307, 1987.

Elder JS, Longenecker R: Premedication with oral midazolam for voiding cystourethrography in children: safety and efficacy. *AJR Am J Roentgenol* 164:1229, 1995.

Elias H, Pauly JE, Bruns ER: Reproductive system. In: Elias H, et al (Eds): *Histology and Human Microanatomy*, 4th ed. New York, John Wiley & Sons, 1978, p 475.

Emhardt JD, Saysana C, Sirichotvithyakorn P: Anesthetic considerations for pediatric outpatient surgery. *Semin Pediatr Surg* 13:210–21, 2004.

England MA: *Color Atlas of Life Before Birth.* Chicago, Year Book Medical Publishers, 1983.

Engle WD: Development of fetal and neonatal renal function. *Semin Perinatol* 10:113, 1986.

Francis A, Eltaki K, Bash T, et al: The safety of preoperative sedation in children with sleep-disordered breathing. *Int J Pediatr Otorhinolaryngol* 70:1517–21, 2006. Epub 2006 Jul 7.

Franck LS, Allen A, Oulton K: Making pain assessment more accessible to children and parents: can greater involvement improve the quality of care? *Clin J Pain* 23:331–8, 2007.

Fu T, Corrigan NJ, Quinn CT, et al: Minor elective surgical procedures using general anesthesia in children with sickle cell anemia without pre-operative blood transfusion. *Pediatr Blood Cancer* 45:43–7, 2005.

Gerstner T, Teich M, Bell N, et al: Valproate-associated coagulopathies are frequent and variable in children. *Epilepsia* 47:1136–43, 2006.

Gosling JA, Dixon JS, Humpherson JR: *Functional Anatomy of the Urinary Tract.* Baltimore, University Park Press, 1982.

Gray SW, Skandalakis JE: *Embryology for Surgeons: The Embryological Basis for the Treatment of Congenital Defects.* Philadelphia, W. B. Saunders Company, 1972.

Gregory GA: *Pediatric Anesthesia.* New York, Churchill Livingstone, 1983.

Gundeti MS, Godbole PP, Wilcox DT: Is bowel preparation required before cystoplasty in children? *J Urol* 176:1574–6, 2006; discussion 1576–7.

Harting MT, Lally KP: Surgical management of neonates with congenital diaphragmatic hernia. *Semin Pediatr Surg* 16: 109–14, 2007.

Hatch DJ: *Neonatal Anesthesia.* Chicago, Year Book Medical Publishers, 1981.

Hillier SC, Krishna G, Brasoveanu E: Neonatal anesthesia. *Semin Pediatr Surg* 13:142–51, 2004.

Horne B, Reynolds M: Respiratory support. In Raffensperger JG (Ed): *Swenson's Pediatric Surgery,* 5th ed. Norwalk, CT, Appleton and Lange, 1990, p 91.

Ichikawa S, Ishihara M, Okazaki T, et al: Prospective study of antibiotic protocols for managing surgical site infections in children. *J Pediatr Surg* 42:1002–7, 2007.

Jirásek JE: *Atlas of Human Prenatal Morphogenesis.* Boston, Martinus Nijhoff Publishers, 1983.

Jirásek JE: Morphogenesis of the genital system in the human. In: Blandau RJ, Bergsma D (Eds): *Birth Defects: Original Article Series.* New York, Alan R. Liss, 13:13, 1977.

Kain ZN, Caldwell-Andrews AA, Mayes LC, et al: Family-centered preparation for surgery improves perioperative outcomes in children: a randomized controlled trial. *Anesthesiology* 106:65–74, 2007.

Karp G, Berrill NJ: *Development,* 2nd ed. New York, McGraw-Hill Book Company, 1981.

Keibel F: Zur die Entwicklungsgeschichte des menschlichen Urogenitalapparates. *Arch Anat* 55:157, 1896.

Keibel F, Mall FP: *Manual of Human Embryology.* Philadelphia, J. B. Lippincott Company, 1910–1912.

Keith A: *Human Embryology and Morphology,* 4th ed. London, E. Arnold, 1921.

Keith L, Moore P: *L'etre humain en développement.* Quebec, Vigot, 1974.

Khalil SN, Hanna E, Farag A, et al: Presurgical caudal block attenuates stress response in children. *Middle East J Anesthesiol* 18:391–400, 2005.

Koritké JG, Sick H: *Atlas of Sectional Human Anatomy.* Baltimore, Urban and Schwarzenberg, 1988.

Kovac AL: Management of postoperative nausea and vomiting in children. *Paediatr Drugs* 9:47–69, 2007. Review.

Krane RJ, Siroky MD, Fitzpatrick JM: *Operative Urology; Surgical Skills.* New York, Churchill Livingstone, 2000.

Langer CP: Zur Anatomie und Physiologie der Haut. *Sitzungsb Acad Wissensch* 45:223, 1861.

Larsen EH, Gasser TC, Madsen PO: Antimicrobial prophylaxis in urological surgery. *Urol Clin North Am* 13:591, 1986.

Lauder GR: Pre-operative predeposit autologous donation in children presenting for elective surgery: a review. *Transfus Med* 17:75–82, 2007.

Leys CM, Austin MT, Pietsch JB, et al: Elective intestinal operations in infants and children without mechanical bowel preparation: a pilot study. *J Pediatr Surg* 40:978–81, 2005; discussion 982.

Li HC, Lopez V, Lee TL: Psychoeducational preparation of children for surgery: the importance of parental involvement. *Patient Educ Couns* 65:34–41, 2007. Epub 2006 Jul 26.

Little DC, Shah SR, St Peter SD, et al: Urachal anomalies in children: the vanishing relevance of the preoperative voiding cystourethrogram. *Pediatr Surg* 40:1874–6, 2005.

Londergan TA, Hochman HI, Gildberger N: Postoperative pain following outpatient pediatric urologic surgery: a comparison of anesthetic techniques. *Urology* 44: 572, 1994.

Luck SR: Nutrition and metabolism. In: Raffensperger JG (Ed): *Swenson's Pediatric Surgery,* 5th ed. Norwalk, CT, Appleton and Lange, 1990, p 81.

Luck SR: Preoperative evaluation and preparation. In: Raffensperger JG (Ed): *Swenson's Pediatric Surgery,* 5th ed. Norwalk, CT, Appleton and Lange, 1990, p 7.

Lund CH, Nonato LB, Kuller JM, et al: Disruption of barrier function in neonatal skin associated with adhesive removal. *J Pediatr* 131:367, 1997.

Lyon VB: Approach to procedures in neonates. *Dermatol Ther* 18:117–23, 2005.

Mallick MS: Is routine pre-operative blood testing in children necessary? *Saudi Med J* 27:1831–4, 2006.

Moore KL: *The Developing Human: Clinically Oriented Embryology,* 2nd ed. Philadelphia, W. B. Saunders Company, 1977.

Muecke EC: The embryology of the urinary system. In: Harrison JH, Gittes RF, Perlmutter AD, et al. (Eds): *Campbell's Urology.* Philadelphia, W. B. Saunders Company, 1979, p 1286.

Nafiu OO, Reynolds PI, Bamgbade OA, et al: Childhood body mass index and perioperative complications. *Paediatr Anaesth* 17:426–30, 2007.

Page CP, Bohnen JMA, Fletcher JR, et al: Antimicrobial prophylaxis for surgical wounds: guidelines for clinical care. *Arch Surg* 128:79, 1993.

Parrott TS, Woodard JR: Urologic surgery in the neonate. *J Urol* 116:506, 1976.

Perrotti M, Mandel J, Mandell VS: Ethical issues in diagnosis *in utero. Br J Urol* 76 (suppl 2):79, 1995.

Peters JWB, Koot HM, De Boer JB, et al: Major surgery within the first months of life and subsequent biobehavioral pain responses to immunization at a later age: a case comparison study. *Pediatrics* 111:129, 2003.

Pollack SV: Wound healing: a review. *J Dermatol Surg Oncol* 8:667, 1982.

Prentiss CW: *A Laboratory Manual and Textbook of Embryology.* Philadelphia and London, W. B. Saunders Company, 1915.

Raffensperger JG: Fluid and electrolytes. In: Raffensperger JG (Ed): *Swenson's Pediatric Surgery,* 5th ed. Norwalk, CT, Appleton and Lange, 1990, p 73.

Rice HE, Caty MG, Glick PL: Fluid therapy for the pediatric surgical patient. *Pediatr Clin North Am* 45: 719, 1998.

Risau W, Ekblom P: Growth factors and the embryonic kidney. *Prog Clin Biol Res* 226:147, 1986.

Root B, Loveland JP: Pediatric premedication with diazepam or hydroxyzine: oral versus intramuscular route. *Anesth Analg* 52:717, 1973.

Roth DM, Macksood MJ, Perlmutter AD: Outpatient surgery in pediatric urology. *J Urol* 135:104, 1986.

Ryan JF: *A Practice of Anesthesia for Infants and Children.* Orlando, FL, Grune & Stratton, 1986.

Sagi J, Vagman I, David MP, et al: Fetal kidney size related to gestational age. *Gynecol Obstet Invest* 23:1, 1987.

Santamaria LB, Di Paola C, Mafrica F, Fodale V: Preanesthetic evaluation and assessment of children with Down's syndrome. *Scientific World Journal* 19:242–51, 2007.

Sariola H, Holm K, Henke-Fahle S: Early innervation of the metanephric kidney. *Development* 104:589, 1988.

Scanton JW (Ed): *Perinatal Anesthesia.* Boston, Blackwell Scientific Publications, 1985.

Seleny FL, Luck SR: Care of the child in the operating room. In: Raffensperger JG (Ed): *Swenson's Pediatric Surgery,* 5th ed. Norwalk, CT, Appleton and Lange, 1990, p 17.

Shepard B, Hensle TW, Burbige KA, et al: Outpatient surgery in pediatric urology patient. *Urology* 24:581, 1984.

Shields L: Family-centered care in the perioperative area: an international perspective. *AORN J* 85:893–4, 896–902, 2007.

Shikinami J: *Contributions to Embryology,* No. 93, Carnegie Inst. Publicat. 363, 1926.

Silver A, Eichorn A, Kral J, et al: Timeliness and use of antibiotic prophylaxis in selected inpatient surgical procedures. *Am J Surg* 176:548, 1996.

Smith DW: *Recognizable Patterns of Human Malformation.* Philadelphia, W. B. Saunders Company, 1970.

Stephens FD: *Congenital Malformations of the Urinary Tract.* New York, Praeger Publishers, 1983.

Stockman JA III: Hematologic evaluations. In: Raffensperger JG (Ed): *Swenson's Pediatric Surgery,* 5th ed. Norwalk, CT, Appleton and Lange, 1990, p 37.

Theroux MC, Akins RE: Surgery and anesthesia for children who have cerebral palsy. *Anesthesiol Clin North Am* 23:733–43, 2005.

Tuggle DW, Hoelzer DJ, Tunell WP, Smith EI: The safety and cost-effectiveness of polyethylene glycol electrolyte solution bowel preparation in infants and children. *J Pediatr Surg* 22:513, 1987.

Vaughan ED Jr, Middleton GW: Pertinent genitourinary embryology: review for the practising urologist. *Urology* 6:139, 1975.

von Bardenleben K: *Handbuch der Anatomie des Menschen.* Jena, Fischer, 1911.

von Ungern-Sternberg BS, Habre W: Pediatric anesthesia: potential risks and their assessment: Part I. *Paediatr Anaesth* 17:206–15, 2007.

von Ungern-Sternberg BS, Habre W: Pediatric anesthesia: potential risks and their assessment: Part II. *Paediatr Anaesth* 17:311–20, 2007.

Waterman RE: Human embryo and fetus. In: Hafez ESE, Kenemans P (Eds): *Atlas of Human Reproduction by Scanning Electron Microscopy.* Hingham, MA, MTP Press, 1982, p 261.

Wille-Jorgensen P, Guenaga KF, Matos D, Castro AA: Preoperative mechanical bowel cleansing or not? An updated meta-analysis. *Colorectal Dis* 7:304–10, 2005.

Wishnow KI, Johnson DE, Babaian RJ, et al: Effective outpatient use of polyethylene glycol-electrolyte bowel preparation for radical cystectomy and ileal conduit urinary diversion. *Urology* 31:7, 1988.

Wright KD, Stewart SH, Finley GA, Buffett-Jerrott SE: Prevention and intervention strategies to alleviate preoperative anxiety in children: a critical review. *Behav Modif* 31:52–79, 2007.

Section 2
Operating on Neonates, Infants, and Children

American Academy of Pediatrics: Evaluation and preparation of pediatric patients undergoing anesthseia. *Pediatrics* 98:502, 1996.

American Academy of Pediatrics: Prevention and management of pain and stress in the neonate. *Pediatrics* 105(2):454–61, 2000.

Anand KJ, Aranda JV, Berde CB, et al: Summary proceedings from the neonatal pain-control group. *Pediatrics* 117(3 Pt 2): S9–S22, 2006.

Andriole GL, Bettmann MA, Garnick MB, Richie JP: Indwelling double-J ureteral stents for temporary and permanent urinary drainage: experience with 87 patients. *J Urol* 131:239, 1984.

Banowsky LH: Basic microvascular techniques and principles. *Urology* 23:495, 1984.

Barham RE, Butz GW, Ansell JS: Comparison of wound strength in normal, radiated and infected tissue closed with polyglycolic and chromic catgut sutures. *Surg Gynecol Obstet* 146:901, 1978.

Barnes RW: Surgical handicraft: teaching and learning surgical skills. *Am J Surg* 153:422, 1987.

Bartone FF, Shires TK: The reaction of kidney and bladder tissue to catgut and reconstituted collagen sutures. *Surg Gynecol Obstet* 128:1221, 1969.

Bartone FF, Stinson W: Reaction of the urinary tract to polypropylene sutures. *Invest Urol* 14:44, 1976.

Baum NH, Brin E: Use of double-J catheter in pyeloplasty. *Urology* 20:634, 1982.

Berde CB, Sethna NF: Analgesics for the treatment of pain in children. *N Engl J Med* 347(14):1094–1103, 2002.

Bevan PG: The craft of surgery: the anastomosis workshop. *Ann R Coll Surg Engl* 63:405, 1981.

Bhananker SM, Ramamoorthy C, Geiduschek JM, et al: Anesthesia-related cardiac arrest in children: update from the Pediatric Perioperative Cardiac Arrest Registry. *Anesth Analg* 105(2):344–50, 2007.

Blandy J: *Operative Urology,* 2nd ed. Oxford, Blackwell Scientific Publications, 1986.

Borges AF: *Electrical Incisions and Scar Revision.* Boston, Little, Brown & Company, 1973.

Borges AF, Alexander SE: Relaxed skin tension lines, Z-plasties on scars and fusiform excision of lesions. *Br J Plast Surg* 15:242, 1962.

Brigden RJ: *Operating Theatre Technique.* Edinburgh, London, and New York, Churchill Livingstone, 1980.

Burd RS, Mellender SJ, Tobias JD: Neonatal and childhood perioperative considerations. *Surg Clin North Am* 86(2): 227–47, 2006.

Burow CA: *Beschreibung einer neuen Transplantations-methode (Methode der Seitlichen Dreiecke)-zum Wiedersatz Verlorengegangener. Theile des Gesichts.* Berlin, Nauck, 1855.

Case GD, Glenn JE, Postlethwait RW: Comparison of absorbable sutures in urinary bladder. *Urology* 7:165, 1976.

Cassady JF Jr: Regional anesthesia for urologic procedures. *Urol Clin North Am* 14:43, 1987.

Chaffin RC: Drainage. *Am J Surg* 24:100, 1934.

Cheney FW, Domino KB, Caplan RA, Posner KL: Nerve injury associated with anesthesia: a closed claims analysis. *Anesthesiology* 90(4):1062–9, 1999.

Chu CC, Williams DF: Effects of physical configuration and chemical structure of suture material on bacterial absorption. *Am J Surg* 147:197, 1984.

Clark P: *Operations in Urology.* Edinburgh, Churchill Livingstone, 1985.

Clark WR, Furlow W: Use of a balanced bowel preparation solution in urological surgery. *J Urol* 137:455, 1987.

Cockett ATK, Koshiba K: *Manual of Urologic Surgery.* Berlin, Springer-Verlag, 1979.

Cohn I Jr, Dennis C: Segmental resection of the small intestine and "aseptic" end-to-end anastomosis. In: Madden JL (Ed): *Atlas of Technics in Surgery,* 2nd ed. New York, Appleton-Century-Crofts, 1964.

Cook-Sather SD, Harris KA, Chiavacci R, et al: A liberalized fasting guideline for formula-fed infants does not increase average gastric fluid volume before elective surgery. *Anesth Analg* 96(4):965–9, 2003.

Cravero JP, Blike GT, Beach M, et al: Pediatric Sedation Research Consortium: Incidence and nature of adverse events during pediatric sedation/anesthesia for procedures outside the operating room: report from the Pediatric Sedation Research Consortium. *Pediatrics* 118(3):1087–96, 2006.

Daniel RK, Taylor GI: Distant transfer of an island flap by microvascular anastomoses: a clinical technique. *Plast Reconstr Surg* 52:111, 1973.

Daniel RK, Williams HB: The free transfer of skin flaps by microvascular anastomosis: an experimental study and reappraisal. *Plast Reconstr Surg* 52:16, 1973.

Davis DM: The process of ureteral repair: a recapitulation of the splinting question. *Trans Am Assoc Genitourin Surg* 49:71, 1959.

DeHoll D, Rodeheaver G, Edgerton MT, Edlich RF: Potentiation of infection by suture closure of dead space. *Am J Surg* 127:716, 1974.

Douglas DW: Tensile strength of sutures. *Lancet* 2:497, 1949.

Eberhart LH, Geldner G, Kranke P, et al: The development and validation of a risk score to predict the probability of postoperative vomiting in pediatric patients. *Anesth Analg* 99(6):1630–7, 2004.

Eckstein H, Hohenfellner R, Williams DI (Eds): *Surgical Pediatric Urology*. Stuttgart, Thieme, 1977.

Edlich RF, Panek PH, Rodeheaver GT, et al: Physical and chemical configuration of sutures in the development of surgical infection. *Ann Surg* 177:679, 1973.

El-Ghoneimi A, Valla JS, Steyaert H, Aigrain Y: Laparoscopic renal surgery via a retroperitoneal approach in children. *J Urol* 160:1138, 1998.

El-Mahrouky A, McElhaney J, Bartone FF, King L: In vitro comparison of the properties of polydioxanone, polyglycolic acid and catgut sutures in sterile and infected urine. *J Urol* 138:913, 1987.

Feldman D, Reich N, Foster JM: Pediatric anesthesia and postoperative analgesia. *Pediatr Clin North Am* 45(6):1525–37, 1998. Review.

Ferrari LR, Rooney FM, Rockoff MA: Preoperative fasting practices in pediatrics. *Anesthesiology* 90(4):978–80, 1999.

Finney RP: Double-J and diversion stents. *Urol Clin North Am* 9:89, 1982.

Finney RP: Experience with new double-J ureteral catheter stent. *J Urol* 120:678, 1978.

Flick RP, Sprung J, Harrison TE, et al: Perioperative cardiac arrests in children between 1988 and 2005 at a tertiary referral center: a study of 92,881 patients. *Anesthesiology* 106(2):226–37, 2007.

Fowler JE: *Methods of Urologic Surgery*. Chicago, Van Tec, 1987.

Frank JD, Johnston JH: *Operative Pediatric Urology*, Edinburgh, Churchill Livingstone, 1990.

Gambee LP: A single-layer intestinal anastomosis applicable to the small as well as the large intestine. *West J Surg Obstet Gynecol* 59:1, 1951.

Gearhart J, Rink R, Mouriquand P: *Paediatric Urology*. Philadelphia, W. B. Saunders Company, 2001.

Ger R, Duboys E: The prevention and repair of large abdominal-wall defects by muscle transposition: a preliminary communication. *Plast Reconstr Surg* 72:170, 1983.

Gillenwater JY, Grayhack JT, Howards SS, Duckett JW (Eds): *Adult and Pediatric Urology*. Chicago, Year Book Medical Publishers, 1987.

Glenn JF (Ed): *Urologic Surgery*, 3rd ed. Philadelphia and Toronto, J. B. Lippincott Company, 1983.

Golianu B, Krane EJ, Galloway KS, Yaster M: Pediatric acute pain management. *Pediatr Clin North Am* 47(3):559–87, 2000. Review.

Gozal D, Drenger B, Levin PD, et al: A pediatric sedation/anesthesia program with dedicated care by anesthesiologists and nurses for procedures outside the operating room. *J Pediatr* 145(1):47–52, 2004.

Grossfeld JL (Ed): *Common Problems in Pediatric Surgery*. St. Louis, Mosby Year Book, 1991.

Hansen TG, Ilett KF, Reid C, et al: Caudal ropivacaine in infants: population pharmacokinetics and plasma concentrations. *Anesthesiology* 94(4):579–84, 2001.

Hastings JC, Van Winkle H Jr, Barker E, et al: Effect of suture materials on healing wounds of the stomach and colon. *Surg Gynecol Obstet* 140:701, 1975.

Hastings JL: The effect of suture materials on healing wounds of the bladder. *Surg Gynecol Obstet* 140:933, 1975.

Hensle TW, Askanazi J: Metabolism and nutrition in the perioperative period. *J Urol* 139:229, 1998.

Herrmann JB: Tensile strength and knot security of surgical suture materials. *Am J Surg* 37:209, 1971.

Hinman F Jr: Accurate placement of the Penrose drain. *Surg Gynecol Obstet* 102:497, 1956.

Hinman F Jr: Bowel closure techniques: small bowel. Part I. *AUA Update Series*, vol IX, Lesson 35, 1990, p 274.

Hinman F Jr: Bowel closure techniques: large bowel. Part II. *AUA Update Series*, vol IX, Lesson 36, 1990, p 282.

Hinman F Jr: Differential diagnosis of flank pain. In: Tanagho EA (Guest Ed): *Pain of Genitourinary Origin: Problems in Urology*, Vol 3, No 2. Philadelphia: J. B. Lippincott Company, 1989, p 182.

Hinman F Jr: Sources of pain. In: Tanagho EA (Guest Ed): *Pain of Genitourinary Origin: Problems in Urology*, Vol 3, No 2. Philadelphia: J. B. Lippincott Company, 1989, p 179.

Hinman F Jr: Subspecialization and general urology. *J Urol* 141:482, 1989.

Hinman F Jr: Ureteral repair and the splint. *J Urol* 78:376, 1957.

Hoffman GM, Nowakowski R, Troshynski TJ, et al: Risk reduction in pediatric procedural sedation by application of an American Academy of Pediatrics/American Society of Anesthesiologists process model. *Pediatrics* 109(2):236–43, 2002.

Holliday MA, Segar WE: Parenteral fluid therapy. *Pediatrics* 19:823, 1957.

Howard CR, Howard FM, Fortune K, et al: A randomized, controlled trial of a eutectic mixture of local anesthetic cream (lidocaine and prilocaine) versus penile nerve block for pain relief during circumcision. *Am J Obstet Gynecol* 181(6):1506–11, 1999.

Howes EL: Immediate strength of sutured wound. *Surgery* 7:24, 1940.

Howes EL: Strength studies of polyglycolic acid versus catgut sutures of the same size. *Surg Gynecol Obstet* 137:15, 1973.

Hunt TK: *Wound Healing and Wound Infection: Theory and Surgical Practice*. New York, Appleton-Century-Crofts, 1980.

Ireland D: Unique concerns of the pediatric surgical patient: pre-, intra-, and postoperatively. *Nurs Clin North Am* 41(2):265–98, vii, 2006. Review.

Jackson FE, Fleming PM: Jackson Pratt brain drain. *Int Surg* 57:658, 1972.

Jacobson JH II, Suarez EL: Microsurgery in anastomosis of small vessels. *Surg Forum* 2:243, 1960.

Jarowenko MV, Bennett AH: Use of single-J urinary diversion stents in intestinal urinary diversion. *Urology* 22:369, 1983.

Jones PA, Moxon RA, Pittman MR, Edwards L: Double-ended pigtail polyethylene stents in the management of benign and malignant ureteral obstruction. *J R Soc Med* 76:458, 1983.

Joshi GP: Postoperative pain management. *Int Anesthesiol Clin* 32:113, 1994.

Kachko L, Simhi E, Tzeitlin E, et al: Spinal anesthesia in neonates and infants: a single-center experience of 505 cases. *Paediatr Anaesth* 17(7):647–53, 2007.

Krane RJ, Siroky MB, Fitzpatrick JM: *Operative Urology: Surgical Skills*. New York, Churchill Livingstone, 2000.

Kronborg O, Tostergaard A, Steven KG, Toctrik JK: Polyglycolic acid versus chromic catgut in bladder surgery. *Br J Urol* 50:324, 1978.

Kumar M, Kumar R, Hemal AK, Gupta NP: Complications of retroperitoneoscopic surgery at one centre. *BJU Int* 87:607, 2001.

Lang EK: Antegrade ureteral stenting for dehiscence, strictures and fistulae. *AJR Am J Roentgenol* 143:795, 1984.

Larson DL: Musculocutaneous flaps. In: Johnson DE, Boileau MA (Eds): *Genitourinary Tumors: Fundamental Principles and Surgical Techniques*. New York, Grune & Stratton, 1982.

Laufman H, Rickel T: Synthetic absorbable sutures. *Surg Gynecol Obstet* 145:597, 1977.

Leben J, Tryba M, Kura-Muller K, et al: Prevention of intraoperative hypothermia in children. *Anesthetist* 47: 475, 1998.

Lerwick E: Studies on the efficacy and safety of polydioxanone monofilament absorbable sutures. *Surg Gynecol Obstet* 135:497, 1981.

Libertino JA (Ed): *Pediatric and Adult Reconstructive Surgery*, 2nd ed. Baltimore, Williams & Wilkins Company, 1987.

Liebert PS: *Color Atlas of Pediatric Surgery*. New York, Elsevier Scientific Publishing, 1989.

Limberg AA: *The Planning of Local Plastic Operations on the Body Surface*. Lexington, MA, Collamore Press, 1984.

Marshall FF (Ed): *Urologic Complications: Medical and Surgical, Adult and Pediatric*. Chicago, Year Book Medical Publishers, 1986.

Mayor G, Zingg E: *Urologic Surgery*. Stuttgart, Thieme, 1976.

McAninch JW (Guest Ed): Urogenital trauma. In: Blaisdell FW, Trunkey DD (Eds): *Trauma Management*, Vol II, New York, Thieme-Stratton, Inc., 1985.

McCraw JB, Dibbell DG, Carraway JN: Clinical definition of independent myocutaneous vascular territories. *Plast Reconst Surg* 60:341, 1977.

McGregor IA: The theoretical basis of the Z-plasty. *Br J Plast Surg* 9:256, 1957.

McIntyre PB, Ritchie JK, Hawley PR, et al: Management of enterocutaneous fistulas: a review of 132 cases. *Br J Surg* 71:293, 1984.

McMinn RMH, Hutchings RT: *Color Atlas of Human Anatomy*. Chicago, Year Book Medical Publishers, 1977.

Modern technics in surgery. In: Ehrlich RM (Ed): *Urologic Surgery*. Mount Kisco, NY, Future Publishing Company, 1980.

Morris AM: A controlled trial of closed wound suction. *Br J Surg* 60:357, 1973.

Morris KP, Naqvi N, Davies P, et al: A new formula for blood transfusion volume in the critically ill. *Arch Dis Child* 90(7):724–8, 2005.

Morris MC, Baquero A, Redovan E, et al: Urolithiasis on absorbable and non-absorbable suture materials in the rabbit bladder. *J Urol* 135:602, 1986.

Morrow FA, Kogan SJ, Freed SZ, Laufman H: In vivo comparison of polyglycolic acid, chromic catgut and silk in tissue of the genitourinary tract: an experimental study of tissue retrieval and calculogenesis. *J Urol* 112:655, 1974.

Moss JP: Historical and current perspectives on surgical drainage. *Surg Gynecol Obstet* 152:517, 1981.

Murphy GF, Wood DP Jr: The use of mineral oil to manage nondeflating Foley catheter. *J Urol* 149:89, 1993.

Nora PF, Vanecko RM, Brensfield JJ: Prophylactic abdominal drains. *Arch Surg* 105:173, 1972.

Novick AC, Streem SB, Pontes EJ (Eds): *Stewart's Operative Urology*. Baltimore, Williams & Wilkins Company, 1989.

Nyhus LM, Baker RJ (Eds): *Masters of Surgery*, 2nd ed. Boston and Toronto, Little, Brown & Company, 1992.

Olivet RT, Nauss LA, Payne WS: A technique for continuous intercostal nerve block analgesia following thoracotomy. *J Cardiovasc Surg (Torino)* 80:308, 1980.

Oneal RM, Dingman RO, Grabb WC: The teaching of plastic surgical techniques to medical students. *Plast Reconstr Surg* 40:494, 1967.

Parrott TS, Woodard JR: Urologic surgery in the neonate. *J Urol* 116:506, 1976.

Paulson DF (Ed): *Genitourinary Surgery*. New York, Churchill Livingstone, 1984.

Penrose CB: Drainage in abdominal surgery. *JAMA* 14:264, 1890.

Peters CA, Kavoussi LR: Laparoscopy in childen and adults. In: Walsh PC, Retik AB, Vaughan ED Jr, Wein AJ (Eds): *Campbell's Urology*, 7th ed. Philadelphia, W. B. Saunders Company, 1998, pp 2875–911.

Peters JWB, Koot HM, De Boer JB, et al: Major surgery within the first 3 months of life and subsequent behavioral pain responses to immunizations at later age: a case comparison study. *Pediatrics* 111:129, 2003.

Pillo-Blocka F, Adatia I, Sharieff W, et al: Rapid advancement to more concentrated formula in infants after surgery for congenital heart disease reduces duration of hospital stay: a randomized clinical trial. *J Pediatr* 145(6):761–6, 2004.

Pocock RD, Stower MJ, Ferro MA, et al: Double-J stents: a review of 100 patients. *Br J Urol* 58:629, 1986.

Raffensperger JG (Ed): *Swenson's Pediatric Surgery*, 5th ed. Norwalk, CT, Appleton and Lange, 1990.

Ramsay JWA, Payne SR, Gosling PT, et al: The effects of double-J stenting on unobstructed ureters: an experimental and clinical study. *Br J Urol* 57:630, 1985.

Redman JF: An anatomic approach to the pelvis. In: Crawford ED, Borden TA (Eds): *Genitourinary Cancer Surgery*. Philadelphia, Lea & Febiger, 1982, p 126.

Resnick MI, Kursch E (Eds): *Current Therapy in Genitourinary Surgery*. Toronto and Philadelphia, B. C. Decker, 1987.

Rice HE, Caty MG, Glick PL: Fluid therapy for the pediatric surgical patient. *Pediatr Clin North Am* 45(4):719–27, 1998.

Rodeheaver GF, Thacker JG, Edlich RF: Mechanical performance of polyglycolic acid and polyglactin 910 synthetic absorbable sutures. *Surg Gynecol Obstet* 153:835, 1981.

Rowe MI, Rowe SA: The last fifty years of neonatal surgical management. *Am J Surg* 180(5):345–52, 2000. Review.

Singh B, Kim H, Wax SH: Stent versus nephrostomy: is there a choice? *J Urol* 121:268, 1979.

Skandalakis JE, Gray W, Rowe JS Jr: *Anatomical Complications in General Surgery*. New York, McGraw-Hill Book Company, 1983.

Smith AD: Retrieval of ureteral stents. *Urol Clin North Am* 9:109, 1982.

Stephens FD, Smith ED, Hutson J: *Congenital Anomalies of the Kidney, Urinary and Genital Tracts*, 2nd ed. London, Martin Dunitz Publishers, 2002.

Stringer MD, Mouriquand KT, Goward ER (Eds): *Pediatric Surgery and Urology: Long Term Outcomes*. Philadelphia, Harcourt Brace, 1988.

Taddio A, Pollock N, Gilbert-MacLeod C, et al: Combined analgesia and local anesthesia to minimize pain during circumcision. *Arch Pediatr Adolesc Med* 154(6):620–3, 2000.

Taylor BJ, Robbins JM, Gold JI, et al: Assessing postoperative pain in neonates: a multicenter observational study. *Pediatrics* 118(4):e992–1000, 2006.

Ternberg JL, Bell MJ, Bower RJ: *A Handbook for Pediatric Surgery*. Baltimore, Williams & Wilkins, 1980.

Thomas D, Rickwood AMK, Duffy PG: *Essentials of Paediatric Urology*. London, Martin Dunitz Publishers, 2002.

Thomas R, Sharmen G: Urology cart. *Urology* 21:526, 1983.

Trier WC: Considerations in the choice of surgical needles. *Surg Gynecol Obstet* 149:84, 1979.

Trivedi M, Brennan L: Transfusion in pediatric intensive care units. *N Engl J Med* 357(3):301–2, 2007.

Uejima T, Suresh S: Is 0.375% bupivacaine safe in caudal anesthesia in neonates and young infants? *Anesth Analg* 94(4):1041, 2002.

Urology. In: McDougal WS (Ed): *Rob & Smith's Operative Surgery*, 4th ed. St. Louis and Toronto, C. V. Mosby Company, 1983.

Uzzo RG, Bilsky M, Mininberg DT, Poppas DP: Laparoscopic surgery in children with vetriculoperitoneal shunts: effect of pneumoperitoneum on intracranial pressure: preliminary experience. *Urology* 49:753, 1997.

Van Arsdalen KN, Pollack HH, Wein AJ: Ureteral stenting. *Semin Urol* 2:180, 1984.

Van Winkle W Jr, Hastings JC: Considerations in the choice of suture materials for various tissues. *Surg Gynecol Obstet* 135:113, 1972.

Van Winkle W Jr, Hastings J, Barker E, et al: Effect of suture materials on healing skin wounds. *Surg Gynecol Obstet* 140:7, 1975.

Van Winkle W Jr, Salthouse TN: *Biological Response to Sutures and Principles of Suture Selection.* Somerville, MA, Ethicon, Inc., 1976.

Walsh PC, Gittes RF, Perlmutter AD, Stamey TA (Eds): *Campbell's Urology.* Philadelphia, W. B. Saunders Company, 1986.

Walsh-Sukys M, Krug SE: *Procedures in Infants and Children.* Philadelphia, W. B. Saunders Company, 1997.

Wheeless CR: *Atlas of Pelvic Surgery.* Philadelphia, Lea & Febiger, 1981.

Whitehead ED, Leiter E (Eds): *Current Operative Urology*, 2nd ed. Philadelphia, Harper and Row, 1984.

Wieland DE, Bay C, Del Sordi S: Choosing the best abdominal closure by meta-analysis. *Am J Surg* 176:666, 1998.

Williams DI: *Urology in Childhood.* New York, Springer-Verlag, 1974.

Williams RK, Adams DC, Aladjem EV, et al: The safety and efficacy of spinal anesthesia for surgery in infants: the Vermont Infant Spinal Registry. *Anesth Analg* 102(1):67–71, 2006.

Wind GG, Rich NM: *Principles of Surgical Technique: The Art of Surgery.* Baltimore, Urban and Schwarzenberg, 1983.

Woltering EA, Flye MW, Huntley S, et al: Evaluation of bupivacaine nerve blocks in modification of pain and pulmonary function changes after thoracotomy. *Ann Thorac Surg* 30:122, 1980.

Woodman PJ: Topical lidocaine-prilocaine versus lidocaine for neonatal circumcision: a randomized controlled trial. *Obstet Gynecol* 93(5 Pt 1):775–9, 1999.

Wulf H, Peters C, Behnke H: The pharmacokinetics of caudal ropivacaine 0.2% in children: A study of infants aged less than 1 year and toddlers aged 1–5 years undergoing inguinal hernia repair. *Anaesthesia* 55(8):757–60, 2000.

Section 3
Kidney

Abala DM, Grasso M: *Color Atlas of Endourology.* New York, Lippincott-Raven Publishers, 1999.

Abel C, Lendon M, Gough DCS: Histology of the upper pole in complete urinary duplication: does it affect surgical management? *BJU Int* 80:663, 1997.

Abrahams HM, Meng MV, Freise CE, Stoller ML: Laparoscopic donor nephrectomy for pediatric recipients: outcomes analysis. *Urology* 63(1):163–6, 2004.

Adkins KL, Adams MC, Brock JW, Pope JC: Cost and outcome trends in open renal surgery: section on Urology. *Am Acad Pediat*, 2002 (abstract).

Anderson JC, Hynes W: Retrocaval ureter: a case diagnosed pre-operatively and treated successfully by a plastic operation. *Br J Urol* 21:209, 1949.

Anderson RD, Van Savage JG: Laparoscopic nephrectomy of the lower kidney for crossed fused ectopia. *J Urol* 163:1902, 2000.

Anson BJ, Cauldwell EW, Pick JW, Beaton LE: The anatomy of the pararenal system of veins, with comments on the renal arteries. *J Urol* 60:714, 1948.

Anson BJ, Cauldwell EW, Pick JW, Beaton LE: The blood supply of the kidney, suprarenal gland, and associated structures. *Surg Gynecol Obstet* 84:313, 1947.

Anson BJ, Daseler EH: Common variations in renal anatomy, affecting blood supply, form, and topography. *Surg Gynecol Obstet* 112:439, 1961.

Baez-Trinidad LG, Lendvay TS, Broecker BH, et al: Efficacy of nephrectomy for the treatment of nephrogenic hypertension in a pediatric population. *J Urol* 170(4 Pt 2):1655–7, 2003; discussion 1658.

Banerjee GK, Ahlawat R, Dalela D, Kumar RV: Endopyelotomy and pyeloplasty: face to face. *Eur Urol* 26:281, 1994.

Baqi N, Stock J, Lombardo SA, et al: Impact of laparoscopic donor nephrectomy on allograft function in pediatric renal transplant recipients: a single-center report. *Pediatr Transplant* 10(3):354–7, 2006.

Barker AP, Cave MM, Thomas DFM, et al: Fetal pelvi-ureteric junction obstruction: predictor of outcome. *Br J Urol* 76:649, 1995.

Barnett MG, Bruskewitz RC, Belzer FO, et al: Ileocecocystoplasty bladder augmentation and renal transplantation. *J Urol* 138:855, 1987.

Barry JM: Spermatic cord preservation in kidney transplantation. *J Urol* 127:1076, 1982.

Barry JM, Fuchs EF: Right renal vein extension in cadaver kidney transplantation. *Arch Surg* 113:300, 1978.

Barry JM, Hodges CV: The supracostal approach to the kidney and adrenal. *J Urol* 114:666, 1975.

Barry JM, Lawson RK, Strong B, Hodges CV: Urologic complications in 173 kidney transplants. *J Urol* 112:567, 1974.

Bauer JJ, Bishoff JT, Moore RG, et al: Laparoscopic versus open pyeloplasty: assessment of objective and subjective outcome. *J Urol* 162:692, 1999.

Beaton LE: The anatomy of the pararenal system of veins, with comments on the renal arteries. *J Urol* 60:714, 1948.

Belzer FO, Kountz SL, Najarian JS, et al: Prevention of urological complications after renal allotransplantation. *Arch Surg* 101:449, 1970.

Bensimon H: Muscle protective incisions in renal surgery. *Urology* 4:476, 1974.

Berger RE, Ansell JS, Tremann JA, et al: The use of self-retained ureteral stents in the management of urologic complications in renal transplant recipients. *J Urol* 124:781, 1980.

Bergman S, Feifer A, Feldman LS, et al: Laparoscopic live donor nephrectomy: the pediatric recipient in a dual-site program. *Pediatr Transplant* 11(4):429–32, 2007.

Binder C, Bonick P, Ciavarra V: Experience with Silastic U-tube nephrostomy. *J Urol* 106:499, 1977.

Black P, Filipas D, Fichtner J, et al: Nephron sparing surgery for central renal tumors: experience with 33 cases. *J Urol* 163:737, 2000.

Blaivas JG, Pais VM, Spellman RM: Chemolysis of residual stone fragments after extensive surgery for staghorn calculi. *Urology* 6:680, 1975.

Blakely MI, Ritchey MI: Controversies in the management of Wilms' tumor. *Semin Pediatr Surg* 10:127, 2001.

Blandy J: Surgery of renal cast calculi. In: Libertino JA, Zinman L (Eds): *Reconstructive Urologic Surgery.* Baltimore, Williams & Wilkins, 1977, p 17.

Blandy JP, Tresidder GC: Extended pyelolithotomy for renal calculi. *Br J Urol* 39:121, 1967.

Boatman DL, Cornell SH, Kolin CP: The arterial supply of horseshoe kidneys. *Am J Roentgenol Radium Ther Nucl Med* 113:447, 1971.

Borer JG, Cisek LJ, Atala A, et al: Pediatric retroperitoneoscopic nephrectomy using 2 mm instrumentation. *J Urol* 162:1725, 1999.

Borzi PA: A comparison of the lateral and posterior retroperitoneoscopic approach for complete and partial nephroureterectomy in children. *BJU Int* 87:517, 2001.

Borzi PA, Yeung CK: Selective approach for transperitoneal and extraperitoneal endoscopic nephrectomy in children. *J Urol* 171(2 Pt 1):814–6, 2004; discussion 816.

Bowbrick VA, Gold DM: Midline laparotomy incision: a technique with a different slant. *Ann R Coll Surg Engl* 81:113, 1999.

Boyce WH, Elkins IB: Reconstructive renal surgery following anatrophic nephrolithotomy. *J Urol* 111:307, 1974.

Boyce WH, Harrison LH: Complications of renal stone surgery. In: Smith RM, Skinner DG (Eds): *Complications of Urologic Surgery: Prevention and Management.* Philadelphia, W. B. Saunders Company, 1976, p 87.

Brooks J, Kavoussi L, Preminger G, et al: Comparison of open and endourologic approaches to the obstructed ureteropelvic junction. *Urology* 46:791, 1995.

Browse NL, Hurst P: Repair of long, large midline incisional hernias using reflected flaps of anterior rectus sheath reinforced with Marlex mesh. *Am J Surg* 138:738, 1979.

Brynger H, Claes G, Gelin LE, et al: Extracorporeal resection for parenchymatous renal tumours. *Scand J Urol Nephrol Suppl* 60:27, 1981.

Buntain WL, Lynn HB: Splenorrhaphy! Changing concepts for traumatized spleen. *Surgery* 86:748, 1979.

Butarazzi PJ, Devine PC, Devine CJ, et al: The indications, complications, and results of partial nephrectomy. *J Urol* 99:376, 1968.

Cadeddu JA, Kavoussi LR: Laparoscopic pyeloplasty using an automated suturing device. *Curr Techn Urol* 10(3), 1997.

Cadeddu JA, Moore RG: Laparoscopic pyeloplasty. In: *Glenn's Urology,* 5th ed. Philadelphia, W. B. Saunders Company, 1998.

Cain MP, Rink RC, Thomas AC, et al: Symptomatic ureteropelvic junction obstruction in the era of prenatal ultrasonography: is there a higher incidence of crossing vessels? *Urology* 57: 338, 2001.

Capolicchio G, Homsey YL, Houle A-M, et al: Long-term results of percutaneous endopyelotomy in the treatment of children with failed open pyeloplasty. *J Urol* 158:1534, 1997.

Carini M, Selli C, Grechi G, Masini G: Pyelovesicostomy: an alternative to ureteropelvic junction-plasty in pelvic ectopic kidneys. *Urology* 26:125, 1983.

Carlton CE Jr, Scott R Jr, Goldman M: The management of penetrating injuries of the kidney. *J Trauma* 8:1071, 1968.

Carpiniello VL, Malloy TR, Wein AJ: Toward bloodless nephrectomy during Gil-Vernet pyelolithotomy. *Urology* 26:187, 1985.

Cass AS, Luxenberg M: Conservative or immediate surgical management of blunt renal injuries. *J Urol* 130:11, 1983.

Chan DY, Cadeddu JA, Jarrett J, et al: Laparoscopic radical nephrectomy: cancer control for renal carcinoma. *J Urol* 166:2095, 2002.

Chandhoke PS, Clayman RV, Stone AM, et al: Endopyelotomy and endoureterotomy with the Acucise ureteral cutting balloon device: preliminary experience. *J Endourol* 7:45, 1993.

Chang R, Marshall FF, Mitchell S: Percutaneous management of benign ureteral strictures and fistulas. *J Urol* 137:1126, 1987.

Chen RN, Moore RG, Kavoussi LR: Laparoscopic pyeloplasty. Indications, technique and long-term outcome. *Urol Clin North Am* 25: 323, 1998.

Chertin B, Rolle U, Farkas A, Puri P: Does delaying pyeloplasty affect renal function in children with a prenatal diagnosis of pelvi-ureteric junction obstruction? *BJU Int* 90:72, 2002.

Chute R: The thoracoabdominal incision in urological surgery. *J Urol* 65:784, 1951.

Chute R, Baron JA, Olsson CA: The transverse upper abdominal "chevron" incision in urological surgery. *Trans Am Assoc Genitourin Surg* 29:14, 1967.

Cieslik R, Cerkownik L: Management of the posterior peritoneum after transperitoneal renal surgery. *Br J Urol* 57:279, 1985.

Clayman RV, Basler JW, Kavoussi L, Picus DD: Ureteronephroscopic endopyelotomy. *J Urol* 144: 246, 1990.

Clayman RV, Garske GL, Lange PH: Total nephroureterectomy with ureteral intussusception and transurethral ureteral detachment and pull-through. *Urology* 21:482, 1983.

Clayman RV, Kavoussi LR, Soper NJ, et al: Laparoscopic nephrectomy: initial case report. *J Urol* 146: 278, 1991.

Clayman RV, Sheldon CA, Gonzales R: Wilms' tumor: an approach to vena caval intrusion. *Prog Pediatr Surg* 15:285, 1982.

Cloix P, Martin X, Pangaud C, et al: Surgical management of complex renal cysts: a series of 32 cases. *J Urol* 156:28, 1996.

Cockrell SN, Hendren WH: The importance of visualizing the ureter before performing a pyeloplasty. *J Urol* 144:588, 1990; discussion 593.

Cole AT, Fried FA: Experience with the thoraco-abdominal incision for nephroblastoma in children less than 3 years old. *J Urol* 114:114, 1975.

Collins GM, Green RD, Boyer D, et al: Protection of kidneys from warm ischemic injury: dosage and timing of mannitol administration. *Transplantation* 29:83, 1980.

Congdon ED, Edson JN: The cone of renal fascia in the adult white male. *Anat Rec* 80:289, 1941.

Constant DL, Florman SS, Mendez F, et al: Use of the LigaSure vessel sealing device in laparoscopic living-donor nephrectomy. *Transplantation* 78(11):1661–4, 2004.

Cook A, Lorenzo AJ, Salle JL, et al: Pediatric renal cell carcinoma: single institution 25-year case series and initial experience with partial nephrectomy. *J Urol* 175(4):1456–60, 2006; discussion 1460.

Cook JH III, Lytton B: Intraoperative localization of renal calculi during nephrolithotomy by ultrasound scanning. *J Urol* 117:546, 1979.

Cooper MJ, Williams RC: Splenectomy: indications, hazards and alternatives. *Br J Surg* 71:173, 1984.

Copolicchio G, Homsey YL, Houle A-M, et al: Long-term results of percutaneous endopyelotomy in the treatment of children with failed open pyelotomy. *J Urol* 158:1534, 1997.

Cornford PA, Rickwood AMK: Functional results of pyeloplasty in patients with antenatally diagnosed pelvi-ureteric junction obstruction. *Br J Urol* 81:152, 1998.

Corriere JN, Perloff LJ, Barker CF, et al: The ureteropyelostomy in human renal transplantation. *J Urol* 110:24, 1973.

Cox PJ, Ausobsky JR, Ellis H, Pollack AV: Towards no incisional hernias: lateral paramedian versus midline incisions. *J R Soc Med* 79:711, 1986.

Cozzi F, Schiavetti A, Morini F, et al: Renal function adaptation in children with unilateral renal tumors treated with nephron sparing surgery or nephrectomy. *J Urol* 174(4 Pt 1): 1404–8, 2005.

Crawford ED, Skinner DG, Capparell DB: Intercostal nerve block with thoracoabdominal incision. *J Urol* 121:290, 1978.

Crissey MM, Gittes RF: Dissolution of cystine ureteral calculus by irrigation with tromethamine. *J Urol* 121:811, 1979.

Cromie WJ: Complications of pyeloplasty. *Urol Clin North Am* 10:385, 1983.

Culp OS: Anterior nephroureterectomy: advantages and limitations of a single incision. *J Urol* 85:193, 1961.

Culp OS, DeWeerd JH: A pelvic flap operation for certain types of ureteropelvic obstruction: preliminary report. *Proc Staff Meet Mayo Clin* 26:483, 1951.

Culp OS, Winterringer JR: Surgical treatment of horseshoe kidney: a comparison of results after various types of operations. *J Urol* 73:747, 1955.

Cummings KB, Li W-I, Ryan JA, et al: Intra-operative management of renal cell carcinoma with supradiaphragmatic caval extension. *J Urol* 122:829, 1979.

Damone AA: Abdominal masses in children. In: Resnick MI, Caldamone AA, Spinak JP (Eds): *Decision Making in Urology*. St. Louis, C. V. Mosby Company, 1985.

D'Angio GJ, Breslow N, Beckwith JB, et al: Treatment of Wilms' tumor: results of the Third National Wilms' Tumor Study. *Cancer* 64:349, 1989.

D'Angio GJ, Evans A, Breslow N, et al: The treatment of Wilms' tumor: results of the Second National Wilms' Tumor Study. *Cancer* 47:2302, 1981.

Danuser H, Ackermann DK, Böhlen D, Studer UE: Endopyelotomy for primary ureteropelvic junction obstruction: risk factors determine the success rate. *J Urol* 159: 56, 1998.

Das S: Radical nephrectomy: thoracoabdominal intrapleural approach. In: Crawford ED, Borden TA (Eds): *Genitourinary Cancer Surgery*. Philadelphia, Lea & Febiger, 1982, p 30.

Davis DM: Intubated ureterotomy: a new operation for ureteral and ureteropelvic stricture. *Surg Gynecol Obstet* 76:513, 1943.

Davis RA, Milloy FJ Jr, Anson BJ: Lumbar, renal and associated parietal and visceral veins based upon a study of 100 specimens. *Surg Gynecol Obstet* 107:122, 1958.

DeKernion JB: Lymphadenectomy for renal cell carcinoma: therapeutic implications. *Urol Clin North Am* 7:697, 1980.

DeKernion JB: Radical nephrectomy. In: Ehrlich RM (Ed): *Modern Technics in Surgery (Urologic Surgery)*. New York, Futura, 1980.

Delany HM, Porreca F, Mitsudo S, et al: Splenic capping: an experimental study of a new technique for splenorrhaphy using woven polyglycolic acid mesh. *Ann Surg* 196:187, 1982.

Delmas P, Ravasse P, Mallet JF, Pheline Y: Anatomical basis of the surgical approach to the kidney in children. *Anat Clin* 7:267, 1985.

Dénes FT, Danilovic A, Srougi M: Outcome of laparoscopic upper-pole nephrectomy in children with duplex systems. *J Endourol* 21(2):162–8, 2007.

Desai MM, Gill IS, Carvalhal EF, et al: Percutaneous endopyeloplasty: a novel technique. *J Endourol* 16:431, 2002.

DeWeerd JH, Paulk SC, Tomera FM, et al: Renal autotransplantation for upper ureteral stenosis. *J Urol* 116:23, 1976.

Diamond DA, Price HM, McDougall EM, Bloom DA: Retroperitoneal laparoscopic nephrectomy in children. *J Urol* 153: 1966, 1995.

Dixon JS, Gosling JA: The musculature of the human renal calices, pelvis and upper ureter. *J Anat* 135:129, 1982.

Djurhuus JC, Nerström B, Rask-Andersen H: Dynamics of upper urinary tract in man. *Acta Chir Scand* 472:49, 1976.

Dodds WJ: Retroperitoneal compartmental anatomy. *AJR Am J Roentgenol* 148:829, 1987.

Dodds WJ, Darweesh RMA, Lawson TL, et al: The retroperitoneal spaces revisited. *AJR Am J Roentgenol* 147:1155, 1986.

Doménec-hMateu JM, Gonzalez-Compta X: Horseshoe kidney: a new theory on its embryogenesis based on the study of a 16-mm human embryo. *Anat Rec* 222:408, 1988.

Donahoe PK, Hendren WH: Pelvic kidney in infants and children: experience with 16 cases. *J Pediatr Surg* 15:486, 1980.

Donohue JP, Hostetter M, Glover J, Madura J: Ureteroneocystostomy versus ureteropyelostomy: a comparison in the same renal allograft series. *J Urol* 114:202, 1975.

Douville E, Hollingshead WH: The blood supply of the normal renal pelvis. *J Urol* 73:906, 1955.

Dretler SP, Pfister RC, Newhouse JH: Renal stone dissolution via percutaneous nephrostomy. *N Engl J Med* 300:341, 1979.

Duckett JW, Lifland JJ, Peters PC: Resection of the vena cava for adjacent malignant disease. *Surg Gynecol Obstet* 136:711, 1973.

Duckett JW, Pfister RR: Ureterocalicostomy for renal salvage. *J Urol* 128:98, 1982.

Duel B, Vates T, Heiser D, et al: The utility of antegrade pyelography prior to pyeloplasty via dorsal lumbotomy. *J Urol* 162:174–6, 1999.

Eckstein HB, Kamal I: Hydronephrosis due to pelvi-ureteric obstruction in children: an assessment of the anterior transperitoneal approach. *Br J Surg* 58:663, 1971.

Eden CG: Treatment options for pelvi-ureteric junction obstruction: implications for practice and training. *Br J Urol* 80:365, 1997.

Eden CG, Sultana SR, Murray KHA, Carruthers RK: Extraperitoneal laparoscopic dismembered fibrin-glued pyeloplasty: medium term results. *Br J Urol* 80:382, 1997.

Edwards EA: The anatomy of collateral circulation. *Surg Gynecol Obstet* 107:183, 1958.

Edwards EA: Clinical anatomy of lesser variations of the inferior vena cava; and a proposal for classifying the anomalies of this vessel. *Angiology* 2:85, 1951.

Ehrlich RM, Gerschman A, Fuchs G: Laparoscopic renal surgery in children. *J Urol* 151:735, 1994.

Ehrlich RM, Goodwin WE: The surgical treatment of nephroblastoma (Wilms' tumor). *Cancer* 32:1145, 1973.

Elashry OM, Makada SY, McDougall M, Clayman RV: Laparoscopic nephropexy: Washington University experience. *J Urol* 154:1655, 1995.

El-Ghoneimi A, Farhat W, Bolduc S, et al: Retroperitoneal laparoscopic vs. open partial nephroureterectomy in children. *BJU Int* 91(6):532–5, 2003.

El-Ghoneimi A, Valla JS, Steyaert H, Algrain Y: Laparoscopic renal surgery via a retroperitoneal approach in children. *J Urol* 160:1138, 1998.

Erbagci A, Yaĝi F, Sarica K, Bakir K: Predictve value of renal histological changes for postoperative renal function improvement in children with congenital ureteropelvic junction stenosis. *Int J Urol* 9:279, 2992.

Escala JM, Keating MA, Boyd G, et al: Development of elastic fibers in the upper urinary tract. *J Urol* 141:969, 1989.

Facer MJ, Lynch RD, Evans HO, Chin FK: Inferior vena cava duplication: demonstration by computed tomography. *Radiology* 130:707, 1979.

Faerber GJ, Ritchey ML, Bloom DA: Percutaneous endopyelotomy in infants and young children after failed open pyeloplasty. *J Urol* 154:1495, 1995.

Fahlenkamp D, Winfield HN, Schonberger B, et al: *Eur Urol* 32:75, 1997.

Farhat W, Khoury A, Bagli D, et al: Mentored retroperitoneal laparoscopic renal surgery in children: a safe approach to learning. *BJU Int* 92(6):617–20, 2003; discussion 620.

Feldman RA, Shearer JK, Shield DE, et al: Sensitive method for intraoperative roentgenograms. *Urology* 9:695, 1977.

Feller I, Woodburne RT: Surgical anatomy of the abdominal aorta. *Ann Surg* 154 (suppl):239, 1961.

Figenshau RS, Clayman RV: Endourology options for management of ureteropelvic junction obstruction in children. *Urol Clin North Am* 25:199, 1998.

Figenshau RS, Yu MK: Laparoscopic nephrectomy and nephroureterectomy in the pediatric patient. *Urol Clin North Am* 28:53, 2001.

Fine H, Keen EN: The arteries of the human kidney. *J Anat* 100:881, 1966.

Flatmark A, Albrechtsen D, Södal G, et al: Renal autotransplantation. *World J Surg* 13:206, 1989.

Foley FEB: New plastic operation for stricture at ureteropelvic junction: report of 20 operations. *J Urol* 38:643, 1937.

Foote JW, Blennerhasset JB, Eiglesworth FW, MacKinnon KJ: Observations on the ureteropelvic junction. *J Urol* 104:252, 1970.

Fourman J, Moffat DB: *The Blood Vessels of the Kidney.* Oxford, Blackwell Scientific Publications, 1971.

Freed SZ, Veith FJ, Soberman R, Gliedman ML: Simultaneous bilateral posterior nephrectomy in transplant recipients. *Surgery* 68:468, 1970.

Friedland GW, DeVries P: Renal ectopia and fusion: embryologic basis. *Urology* 5:698, 1975.

Gaur DD: Laparoscopic operative retroperitoneoscopy: use of a new device. *J Urol* 148:1137, 1992.

Gaur DD: Retroperitoneal laparoscopy: a simple technique of balloon insertion and establishment of the primary port. *Br J Urol* 77:458, 1996.

Gaur DD: Retroperitoneal laparoscopy: some technical modifications. *Br J Urol* 77:304, 1996.

Gaur DD, Agarwal DK, Purohit KC: Retroperitoneal laparoscopic nephrectomy: initial case report. *J Urol* 149:103, 1993.

Gelin LE, Claes G, Gustafsson A, Storm B: Total bloodlessness for extracorporeal organ repair. *Rev Surg* 28:305, 1971.

Gibbons RP, Correa RJ Jr, Cummings KB, Mason JT: Surgical management of renal lesions using in situ hypothermia and ischemia. *J Urol* 115:12, 1976.

Gil Vernet JM: New surgical concepts in removing renal calculi. *Urol Int* 20:255, 1965.

Gill IS: Hand-assisted laparoscopy: con. *Urology* 58:313, 2001.

Gill IS: Retroperitoneal laparoscopic nephrectomy. *Urol Clin North Am* 25:43, 1998.

Gill IS, Delworth MG, Munch LC: Laparoscopic retroperitoneal partial nephrectomy. *J Urol* 152:1539, 1994.

Gill IS, Desai MM, Kouk JH, et al: Laparoscopic partial nephrectomy for renal tumor: duplicating open surgical techniques. *J Urol* 167:469, 2002.

Gill IS, Kavoussi LR, Clayman RV, et al: Complications of laparoscopic nephrectomy in 185 patients: a multi-institutional review. *J Urol* 154:479, 1995.

Gill IS, Liao JC: Pelvi-reteric junction obstruction treated with Acucise retrograde endopyelotomy. *Br J Urol* 82:8, 1998.

Gill IS, Rassweiler JJ: Retroperitoneoscopic renal surgery: our approach. *Urology* 54:734, 1999.

Gill IS, Schweizer D, Hobart MG, et al: Laparoscopic radical nephrectomy: the Cleveland experience. *J Urol* 163:1665, 2000.

Gill IS, Sung GT, Hsu TH: Robotic remote laparoscopic nephrectomy and adrenalectomy: the initial experience. *J Urol* 164:2082, 2000.

Gillou CR, Hall TJ, Donaldson DR, et al: Vertical abdominal incisions: a choice? *Br J Surg* 67:395, 1980.

Giordano JM, Trout HH III: Anomalies of the inferior vena cava. *J Vasc Surg* 3:924, 1986.

Gittes RF: Partial nephrectomy and bench surgery: techniques and applications. In: Libertino R, Zinman L (Eds): *Reconstructive Urologic Surgery: Pediatric and Adult.* Baltimore, Williams & Wilkins, 1977, p 45.

Golbus MS, Harrison MR, Filly RA, et al: In utero treatment of urinary tract obstruction. *Am J Obstet Gynecol* 142:383, 1982.

Goldfischer ER, Jabbour ME, Stravodimos KG, et al: Review: techniques in endopyelotomy. *Br J Urol* 82:1, 1998.

González R: Extraperitoneal midline approach to the retroperitoneum in children. *Urology* 20:13, 1982.

González R, Aliabadi H: Posterior lumbotomy for pediatric pyeloplasty. *J Urol* 137:468, 1987.

Gordon MR, Carrion HM, Politano VA: Dissolution of uric acid calculi with THAM irrigation. *Urology* 12:393, 1978.

Gorey TF, Bonadio D: Laparoscopic-assisted surgery. *Semin Laparosc Surg* 4:102–9, 1997.

Gosling JA: The musculature of the upper urinary tract. *Acta Anat (Basel)* 75:408, 1970.

Gosling JA, Dixon JS: The structure of the normal and hydronephrotic upper urinary tract. In: O'Reilly PH, Gosling JA (Eds): *Idiopathic Hydronephrosis.* London, Springer-Verlag, 1982.

Graham SD Jr, Glenn JF: Enucleative surgery for renal malignancy. *J Urol* 122:546, 1979.

Graves FT: The aberrant renal artery. *J Anat* 90:553, 1956.

Graves FT: The anatomy of the intrarenal arteries and its application to segmental resection of the kidney. *Br J Surg* 43:132, 1954.

Graves FT: The anatomy of the intra-renal arteries in health and disease. *Br J Surg* 43:605, 1956.

Graves FT: The arterial anatomy of the congenitally abnormal kidney. *Br J Surg* 56:533, 1969.

Graves FT: Renal hypothermia: an aid to partial nephrectomy. *Br J Surg* 50:362, 1963.

Greenall MJ, Evans M, Pollock AV: Midline or transverse laparotomy? A random controlled clinical trial: I. Influence on healing. *Br J Surg* 67:188, 1980.

Greenberg SH, Wein AJ, Perloff LF, Barker CF: Ureteropyelostomy and ureteroneocystostomy in renal transplantation: postoperative urological complications. *J Urol* 118:17, 1977.

Griffiths DA: A reappraisal of the Pfannenstiel incision. *Br J Urol* 48:469, 1976.

Guerriero WG, Carlton CE Jr, Scott R Jr, Beall AC Jr: Renal pedicle injuries. *J Trauma* 11:53, 1971.

Gundeti MS, Taghizaedh A, Mushtaq I: Bilateral synchronous posterior prone retroperitoneoscopic nephrectomy with simultaneous peritoneal dialysis: a new management for end-stage renal disease in children. *BJU Int* 99(4):904–6, 2007. Epub 2007 Jan 16.

Gupta M, Tuncay O, Smith A: Open surgical exploration after failed endopyelotomy: a 12-year perspective. *J Urol* 157:1613, 1997.

Hadar H, Gadoth N: Positional relationships of the colon and kidney determined by perirenal fat. *Am J Roentgenol Radium Ther Nucl Med* 143:773, 1984.

Hamilton BD, Gatti JM, Cartwright PC, Snow BW: Comparison of laparoscopic versus open nephrectomy in the pediatric population. *J Urol* 163:937, 2000.

Hamm FC, Weinberg SR: Renal and ureteral surgery without intubation. *J Urol* 73:475, 1955.

Hanna MK, Jeffs RD, Sturgess JM, Barkin M: Ureteral structure and ultrastructure: Part 1. The normal human ureter. *J Urol* 116:718, 1976.

Hanna MK, Jeffs RD, Sturgess JM, Barkin M: Ureteral structure and ultrastructure: Part 2. Congenital ureteropelvic junction obstruction and primary obstructive megaureter. *J Urol* 116:725, 1976.

Harper JD, Shah SK, Baldwin DD, Moorhead JD: Laparoscopic nephrectomy for pediatric giant hydronephrosis. *Urology* 70(1):153–6, 2007.

Harrell WB, Snow BW: Minimally invasive pediatric nephrectomy. *Curr Opin Urol* 15(4):277–81, 2005.

Harrison MR, Golbus MS, Filly RA, et al: Management of the fetus with congenital hydronephrosis. *J Pediatr Surg* 17:728, 1982.

Hassein S, Frank JD: Complications and length of hospital stay following stented and non-stented paediatric pyeloplasties. *Br J Urol* 73:87, 1994.

Hatch DA, Koyle MA, Baskin LS, et al: Kidney transplantation in children with urinary diversion or bladder augmentation. *J Urol* 165:2265, 2001.

Hedican SP, Adams JB II: Laparoscopic surgery of the ureter. In: Marshall FF: *Textbook of Urologic Surgery*. Philadelphia, W. B. Saunders Company, 1996, p 144.

Hegedüs V: Arterial anatomy of the kidney: a three-dimensional angiographic investigation. *Acta Radiol* 12:604, 1972.

Hemal AK, Aron M, Gupta NP, et al: The role of retroperitoneoscopy in the management of renal and adrenal pathology. *BJU Int* 83:929, 1999.

Hemal AK, Kumar M: Extracorporeal renal retraction as an adjunct during retroperitoneoscopic renal surgery. *BJU Int* 83:136, 1999.

Hendren WH, Radharkrishnan J, Middleton AW Jr: Pediatric pyeloplasty. *J Pediatr Surg* 15:133, 1980.

Henriksson C, Brynger H, Nilsson AE, et al: Reconstruction of urinary outflow obstructions by renal autotransplantation. *Scand J Urol Nephrol* suppl 59:1980.

Hewitt CB: Nephroureterectomy with bladder cuff in the treatment of transitional cell carcinoma of the upper urinary tract. In: Scott R (Ed): *Current Controversies in Urologic Management*. Philadelphia, W. B. Saunders Company, 1972.

Heynes CF, van Gelderen WFC: Three-dimensional imaging of the pelviocaliceal system by computerized tomographic reconstruction. *J Urol* 144:1335, 1990.

Hinman F Jr: Ballottement of peripelvic cyst for operative diagnosis and localization. *J Urol* 97:7, 1967.

Hinman F Jr: Dismembered pyeloplasty without urinary diversion. In: Scott R (Ed): *Current Controversies in Urologic Management*. Philadelphia, W. B. Saunders Company, 1972, p 253.

Hinman F Jr: Peripelvic extravasation during intravenous urography: evidence for an additional route for backflow after ureteral obstruction. *J Urol* 85:385, 1961.

Hinman F Jr: Techniques for ureteropyeloplasty. *Arch Surg* 71:790, 1955.

Hinman F Jr, Belzer FO: Urinary tract infection and renal homotransplantation: I. Effect of antibacterial irrigations on defenses of the defunctionalized bladder. *J Urol* 101:477, 1969.

Hinman F Jr, Cattolica EV: Branched calculi: shapes and operative approaches. *J Urol* 126:291, 1981.

Hinman F Jr, Oppenheimer R: Ureteral regeneration: VI. Delayed urinary flow in the healing of unsplinted ureteral defects. *J Urol* 78:138, 1957.

Hinman F Jr, Schmaelzle JF, Belzer FO: Urinary tract infection and renal homotransplantation: II. Post-transplantation bacterial invasion. *J Urol* 101:673, 1969.

Hodges CV, Lawson RK, Pearse HD, Stranburg CO: Autotransplantation of the kidney. *J Urol* 110:20, 1973.

Hoeltl W, Hruby W, Aharinejad S: Renal vein anatomy and its implications for retroperitoneal surgery. *J Urol* 143:1108, 1990.

Hohenfellner R, Wulf AD: Urologie. In: Kunz H (Ed): *Operationen des Kindesalters*, Vol II. Stuttgart, Thieme, 1975.

Hollenbeck BK, Wolf JS: Laparoscopic partial nephrectomy. *Semin Urol Oncol* 19:114, 2001.

Homsy Y, Simard J, Debs C, et al: Pyeloplasty: to divert or not to divert? *Urology* 16:577, 1980.

Horowitz M, Shah SM, Ferzli G, et al: Laparoscopic partial upper pole nephrectomy in infants and children. *BJU Int* 87:514, 2001.

Horwitz JR, Ritchey JM, Moksness J, et al: Renal salvage procedures in patients with synchronous bilateral Wilms' tumors: a report from the National Wilms' Tumor Study Group. *J Pediatr Surg* 31:1020, 1996.

Howard FS, Hinman, F Jr: The ureteral splint in the repair of ureteropelvic avulsion. *J Urol* 68:148, 1952.

Hsu TH, Su LM, Trock BJ, et al: Laparoscopic adult donor nephrectomy for pediatric renal transplantation. *Urology* 61(2):320–2, 2003.

Huesman JK, Kaplan GQ, Brock WA, Packer MG: Ipsilateral ureteroureterostomy and pyeloureterostomy: a review of 15 years of experience with 52 patients. *J Urol* 138:1207, 1987.

Hureau J, Hidden G, Thanh Minh TA: The vascularisation of the suprarenal glands. *Anat Clin* 2:127, 1980.

Immergut MA, Jacobson JJ, Culp DA: Cutaneous pyelostomy. *J Urol* 101:276, 1969.

Jackman SV, Caddeddu JA, Chen RN, et al: Utility of harmonic scalpel for laparoscopic partial nephrectomy. *J Endourol* 12:441, 1998.

Jackman SV, Hedican SF, Peters CA, Docimo SG: Percutaneous nephrolithotomy in infants and preschool age children: experience with a new technique. *Urology* 52:697, 1998.

Janetschek G, Peschel R, Altarac D, Bartsch G: Laparoscopic and retroperitoneoscopic repair of ureteropelvic junction obstruction. *Urology* 47:311, 1996.

Janetschek G, Seibold J, Radmayer C, Bartsch G: Laparoscopic heminephroureterectomy in pediatric patients. *J Urol* 158:1928, 1997.

Jarrett TW, Chan DY, Charambura TC, et al: Laparoscopic pyeloplasty: the first 100 cases. *J Urol* 167:1253, 2002.

Jeong BC, Lim DJ, Lee SC, et al: Laparoscopic nephrectomy for a single-system ectopic ureter draining a small, dysplastic and poorly functioning kidney in children. *Int J Urol* 14(2):104–7, 2007.

Jesch NK, Metzelder ML, Kuebler JF, Ure BM: Laparoscopic transperitoneal nephrectomy is feasible in the first year of life and is not affected by kidney size. *J Urol* 176(3):1177–9, 2006.

Jordan GH, Winslow DH: Laparo-endoscopic upper pole partial nephrectomy with ureterectomy. *J Urol* 150:940, 1993.

Kadir S, White RI Jr, Engel R: Balloon dilatation of a ureteropelvic junction obstruction. *Radiology* 143:263, 1982.

Kaneto H, Orikasa S, Chiba T, Takahashi T: Three-D muscular arrangement at the ureteropelvic junction and its changes in congenital hydronephrosis: a stereo-morphometric study. *J Urol* 146:909, 1991.

Kark RM: Renal biopsy. *JAMA* 105:220, 1968.

Karlin GS, Badlani GH, Smith AD: Endopyelotomy versus open pyeloplasty: comparison in 88 patients. *J Urol* 140:476, 1988.

Karlin GS, Smith AD: Endopyelotomy. *Urol Clin North Am* 15:439, 1988.

Karsburg W, Leary FJ: Nephrostomy tube replacement. *Urology* 13:301, 1979.

Kaufman BH, Telander RL, van Heerden JA, et al: Pheochromocytoma in the pediatric age group: current status. *J Pediatr Surg* 18:879, 1983.

Kavoussi LR, Abala DM, Clayman RV: Outcome of secondary open surgical procedures in patients who failed primary endopyelotomy. *Br J Urol* 72:157, 1993.

Kavoussi LR, Meretyk SM, Dierks SM, et al: Endopyelotomy for secondary ureteropelvic junction obstruction in children. *J Urol* 145:345, 1991.

Kavoussi LR, Peters CA: Laparoscopic pyeloplasty. *J Urol* 150:1891, 1993.

Keeley FX Jr, Bagley DH, Kulp-Hughes D, Gomella LG: Laparoscopic division of crossing vessels at the ureteropelvic junction. *Endourol* 10:163, 1996.

Keeley FX, Moussa SA, Miller J, Tolley DA: A prospective study of endoluminal ultrasound versus computerized tomography angiography for detecting crossing vessels at the ureteropelvic junction. *J Urol* 162:1938, 1999.

Keeley FX, Tolley DA: Retroperitoneal laparoscopy. *BJU Int* 84:212, 1999.

Kessler O, Franco I, Jayabose S, et al: Is contralateral exploration of the kidney necessary in patients with Wilms' tumor? *J Urol* 156:693, 1996.

Kim DY, Stegall MD, Prieto M, et al: Hand-assisted laparoscopic donor nephrectomy for pediatric kidney allograft recipients. *Pediatr Transplant* 8(5):460–3, 2004.

Kim YS, Do SH, Hong CH, et al: Does every patient with ureteropelvic junction obstruction need voiding cystourethrography? *J Urol* 165:2305, 2001.

King LR: Management of multicystic kidney and ureteropelvic junction obstruction. In: King LR (Ed): *Urologic Surgery in Neonates and Young Infants.* Philadelphia, W. B. Saunders Company, 1988, p 140.

Koff SA, Campbell KD: The nonoperative management of unilateral neonatal hydronephrosis: natural history of poorly functioning kidneys. *J Urol* 152:593, 1994.

Koff SA, Hayden LJ, Cirulli C, Shore R: Pathophysiology of ureteropelvic obstruction: experimental and clinical observations. *J Urol* 136:336, 1986.

Koff SA, Thrall JH, Keyes JW Jr: Diuretic radionuclide urography: a non-invasive method for evaluating nephroureteral dilatation. *J Urol* 121:153, 1979.

Konda R, Sakai K, Shozo O, et al: Ultrasound grade of hydronephrosis and severity of renal cortical damage on 99m technetium dimercaptosuccinic acid renal scan in infants with unilateral hydronephrosis during follow-up and after pyeloplasty. *J Urol* 167:2159, 2002.

Koop CE, Schnaufer L: The management of abdominal neuroblastoma. *Cancer* 35:905, 1975.

Koyle MA, Ehrlich RM: Wilms' tumor in neonates and young infants: current considerations and controversies. In: King LR (Ed): *Urologic Surgery in Neonates and Young Infants.* Philadelphia, W. B. Saunders Company, 1988, p 429.

Ku JH, Byun SS, Choi H, Kim HH: Laparoscopic nephrectomy for congenital benign renal diseases in children: comparison with adults. *Acta Paediatr* 94(12):1752–5, 2005.

Ku JH, Yeo WG, Choi H, Kim HH: Comparison of retroperitoneal laparoscopic and open nephrectomy for benign renal diseases in children. *Urology* 63(3):566–70, 2004; discussion 570.

Ku JH, Yeo WG, Kim HH, Choi H: Laparoscopic nephrectomy for renal diseases in children: is there a learning curve? *Pediatr Surg* 40(7):1173–6, 2005.

Kumar R, Fitzgerald R, Breatnach F: Conservative surgical management of bilateral Wilms' tumor: results of the United Kingdom Children's Cancer Study Group. *J Urol* 160:1450, 1998.

Kusunoki T: Partial nephrectomy. *Urol Int* 1:243, 1955.

Lam JP, MacKinlay GA, Munro FD, Aldridge LM: Endoscopic nephrectomy in children: is retro the way forward? *J Laparoendosc Adv Surg Tech A* 16(1):59–62, 2006.

Leape LL, Breslow NE, Bishop HC: The surgical management of Wilms' tumor. *Ann Surg* 187:351, 1978.

Lee CT, Katz J, Shi W, et al: Surgical management of renal tumors 4 cm. or less in a contemporary cohort. *J Urol* 163:730, 2000.

Lee RS, Retik AB, Borer JG, et al: Pediatric retroperitoneal laparoscopic partial nephrectomy: comparison with an age matched cohort of open surgery. *J Urol* 174(2):708–11, 2005; discussion 712.

Lee WJ, Badlani GH, Karlin GS, et al: Treatment of ureteropelvic strictures with percutaneous pyelotomy: experience in 62 patients. *AJR Am J Roentgenol* 151:515, 1988.

Longo JA, Netto NR Jr: Extracorporeal shock-wave lithotripsy in children. *Urology* 46:550, 1995.

Lottman HB, Traxer O, Archambaud F, Mercier-Pageyral B: Monotherapy extracorporeal shock wave lithotripsy for the treatment of staghorn calculi in children. *J Urol* 165:2324, 2001.

Love L, Meyers MA, Churchill RJ, et al: Computed tomography of the extraperitoneal spaces. *AJR Am J Roentgenol* 136:781, 1981.

Lowe RK, Kogan BA, Stoller ML: Intraluminal wire retrieval of proximally migrated pediatric double-J stent. *J Urol* 154:223, 1995.

Lyon R: An anterior extraperitoneal incision for kidney surgery. *J Urol* 79:383, 1958.

Mahoney EM, Crocker DW, Friend DG, et al: Adrenal and extra-adrenal pheochromocytomas: localization by vena cava. *J Urol* 108(1):4–8, 1972.

Marshall FF: Intraoperative localization of renal calculi. *Urol Clin North Am* 10:629, 1983.

Marshall M Jr, Johnson SH III: A simple direct approach to the renal pedicle. *J Urol* 84:24, 1960.

Marshall VR, Singh M, Tresidder GC, Blandy JP: The place of partial nephrectomy in the management of renal calyceal calculi. *Br J Urol* 47:759, 1976.

Martin LW, Schaffner DP, Cox JA, et al: Retroperitoneal lymph node dissection for Wilms' tumor. *J Pediatr Surg* 14:704, 1979.

Marx WJ, Patel SK: Renal fascia: its radiographic importance. *Urology* 13:1, 1979.

Masaki Z, Iguchi A, Kinoshita N, et al: Intrasinusal pyelolithotomy with lower pole nephrotomy for removal of renal stones. *Urology* 26:461, 1985.

Mayo WJ: The incision for lumbar exposure of the kidney. *Ann Surg* 55:63, 1912.

McAninch JW, Carroll PR: Renal trauma: kidney preservation through improved vascular control: a refined approach. *J Trauma* 22:285, 1982.

McClure CFW, Butler EG: The development of the vena cava inferior in man. *Am J Anat* 35:331, 1925.

McDougall EM, Clayman RV: Laparoscopic nephrectomy for benign disease: comparison of the transperitoneal and retroperitoneal approach. *J Endourol* 10:45,1996.

McDougall EM, Clayman RV, Elashry OM: Laparoscopic radical nephrectomy for renal tumor: the Washington University experience. *J Urol* 155:1180, 1996.

McLaren CJ, Simpson ET: Vesico-ureteric reflux in the young infant with follow-up direct radionuclide cystograms: the medical and surgical outcome at 5 years old. *BJU Int* 90:721, 2002.

McLean PA, Gawley WF, Gorey TP: Technical modifications of Anderson-Hynes pyeloplasty for congenital pelviureteric junction obstruction. *Br J Urol* 57:114, 1985.

McVay CB, Anson BJ: Aponeurotic and fascial continuities in the abdomen, pelvis and thigh. *Anat Rec* 76:213, 1940.

McVay CB, Anson BJ: Composition of the rectus sheath. *Anat Rec* 77:213, 1940.

Meretyk I, Meretyk S, Clayman RV: Endopyelotomy: comparison of ureteroscopic retrograde and antegrade percutaneous techniques. *J Urol* 148:775, 1992.

Merklin RJ, Michels NA: The variant renal and suprarenal blood supply with data on the inferior phrenic, ureteral and gonadal arteries. *J Int Coll Surg* 29:41, 1958.

Merrill DC: Modified thoracoabdominal approach to the kidney and retroperitoneal tissue. *J Urol* 117:15, 1977.

Mesrobian H-G J: Wilms' tumor: past, present and future. *J Urol* 140:231, 1988.

Metzelder ML, Kübler J, Petersen C, et al: Laparoscopic nephroureterectomy in children: a prospective study on LigaSure versus clip/ligation. *Eur J Pediatr Surg* 16(4):241–4, 2006.

Milloy FJ, Anson BJ, Cauldwell EW: Variations in the inferior caval veins and in their renal and lumbar communications. *Surg Gynecol Obstet* 115:131, 1962.

Mitchell GAG: The renal fascia. *Br J Surg* 37(3):257, 1950.

Moore R, Averch T, Schulum P, et al: Laparoscopic pyeloplasty: experience with the initial 30 cases. *J Urol* 157:459, 1997.

Moore RG, Brooks JD: Ureteropelvic junction obstruction: assessment of minimally invasive therapies. *Contemp Urol* 7:47, 1995.

Mor Y, Mouriquand PD, Quimby GF, et al: Lower pole heminephrectomy: its role in treating nonfunctioning lower pole segments. *J Urol* 156:683, 1996.

More RH, Duff GL: The renal arterial vasculature in man. *Am J Pathol* 27:95, 1950.

Morey AF, Bruce JE, McAninch J: Efficacy of radiographic imaging in pediatric blunt renal trauma. *J Urol* 156:2014, 1996.

Motola JA, Badlani GH, Smith AD: Results in 212 consecutive pyelotomies: an 8-year follow-up. *J Urol* 149:453, 1993.

Motola JA, Freid R, Badlani GH, Smith AD: Failed endopyelotomy: implications for future surgery on the ureteropelvic junction. *J Urol* 150:821, 1993.

Mulholland TL, Kropp BP, Wong C: Laparoscopic renal surgery in infants 10 kg or less. *J Endourol* 19(3):397–400, 2005.

Murnaghan GF: The dynamics of the renal pelvis and ureter with reference to congenital hydronephrosis. *Br J Urol* 30:321, 1958.

Murnaghan GF: Mechanisms of congenital hydronephrosis with reference to factors influencing surgical treatment. *Ann R Coll Surg Engl* 23:25, 1958.

Murphy DP, Gill IS: Energy-based renal tumor ablation: a review. *Semin Urol Oncol* 19:133, 2001.

Murphy JJ, Glantz W, Schoenberg HW: The healing of renal wounds: III. A comparison of electrocoagulation and suture ligation for hemostasis in partial nephrectomy. *J Urol* 85:882, 1961.

Nagai A, Nasu Y, Hashimoto H, et al: Retroperitoneoscopic pyelotomy combined with transposition of crossing vessels for ureteropelvic junction obstruction. *J Urol* 165:23, 2001.

Nakada S, McDougall E, Clayman RV: Laparoscopic pyeloplasty for secondary ureteropelvic junction obstruction: preliminary experience. *Urology* 46:257, 1995.

Nakada S, Moon TD, Gist M, Mahvi D: Use of the Pneumo Sleeve as an adjunct to laparoscopic nephrectomy. *Urology* 49:612, 1997.

Nesbit RM: Elliptical anastomosis in urologic surgery. *Ann Surg* 130:796, 1949.

Nicholls G, Hrouda D, Kellett MJ, Duffy PJ: Endopyelotomy in the symptomatic older child. *BJU Int* 87:525, 2001.

Notley RG, Beaugle JM: The long-term follow-up of Anderson-Hynes pyeloplasty for hydronephrosis. *Br J Urol* 45:464, 1973.

Novick A: Posterior surgical approach to the kidney and ureter. *J Urol* 124:192, 1980.

O'Brien WM, Maxted WC, Pahora LL: Ureteral stricture: experience with 32 cases. *J Urol* 140:737, 1988.

O'Conor VJ, Logan DJ: Nephroureterectomy. *Surg Gynecol Obstet* 122:601, 1966.

Odiase V, Whitaker RH: Dynamic evaluation of the results of pyeloplasty using pressure-flow studies. *Eur Urol* 7:324, 1981.

O'Flynn K, Hehir M, McKelvie G, et al: Endoballoon rupture and stenting for pelviureteric junction obstruction. *Br J Urol* 64:574, 1989.

Onen A, Kaya M, Cigdem MK, et al: Blunt renal trauma in children with previously undiagnosed pre-existing renal lesions and guideline for effective initial management of kidney injury. *BJU Int* 89:936, 2002.

Oppenheimer R, Hinman F Jr: Ureteral regeneration: contracture vs. hyperplasia of smooth muscle. *J Urol* 74:476, 1955.

Oravisto KJ: Transverse partial nephrectomy. *Acta Chir Scand* 130:331, 1965.

O'Reilly PH, Brooman PJC, Mak S, et al: The long-term results of Anderson-Hynes pyeloplasty. *BJU Int* 87:287, 2001.

Orland SM, Snyder HM, Duckett JW: The dorsal lumbotomy incision in pediatric urological surgery. *J Urol* 138:963, 1987.

Ossandon F, Androulakakis P, Ransley PG: Surgical problems in pelviureteral junction obstruction of the lower moiety in incomplete duplex systems. *J Urol* 125:871, 1981.

Ostling K: The genesis of hydronephrosis particularly with regard to the changes at the ureteropelvic junction. *Acta Chir Scand* 86 (suppl):72, 1942.

Parker RM, Rudd RG, Wonderly RK, et al: Ureteropelvic junction obstruction in infants and children: functional evaluation of the obstructed kidney preoperatively and postoperatively. *J Urol* 126:509, 1981.

Parry WL, Finelli JF: Some consideration in the technique of partial nephrectomy. *J Urol* 82:562, 1959.

Passerotti C, Peters CA: Pediatric robotic-assisted laparoscopy: a description of the principal procedures. *Scientific World Journal* 6:2581–8, 2006.

Patas K, Moor RG: Laparoscopic pyeloplasty. *J Endourol* 14:895, 2000.

Patil U, Mathews R: Minimal surgery with renal preservation in anomalous complete duplicated systems: is it feasible? *J Urol* 154:727, 1995.

Perez CA, Kaiman HA, Keith J, et al: Treatment of Wilms' tumor and factors affecting prognosis. *Cancer* 32:609, 1973.

Perlmutter AD, Kroovand RL, Lai Y-W: Management of ureteropelvic obstruction in the first year of life. *J Urol* 123:535, 1980.

Persky L, McDougal WS, Kedia O: Management of initial pyeloplasty failure. *J Urol* 125:695, 1981.

Peters CA, Schlussel RN, Retik AB: Pediatric laparoscopic dismembered pyeloplasty. *J Urol* 153:1962, 1995.

Peters PC, Bright TC III: Blunt renal injuries. *Urol Clin North Am* 4:17, 1977.

Petit T, Ravsse P, Delmas P: Does the endoscopic incision of ureteroceles reduce the indications for partial nephrectomy? *BJU Int* 83:675, 1999.

Piaggio L, Franc-Guimond J, Figueroa TE, et al: Comparison of laparoscopic and open partial nephrectomy for duplication anomalies in children. *J Urol* 175(6):2269–73, 2006.

Pietrow PK, Pope JC, Adams MC, et al: Clinical outcome of pediatric stone disease. *J Urol* 167:670, 2002.

Pitts WR Jr, Muecke EC: Horseshoe kidneys: a 40-year experience. *J Urol* 113:743, 1975.

Pohl HG, Rushton HG, Park J-S, et al: Early diuresis renogram findings predict success following pyeloplasty. *J Urol* 165:2311, 2001.

Potter EL: *Normal and Abnormal Development of the Kidney.* Chicago, Year Book Medical Publishers, 1972.

Poutasse EF: Anterior approach to the upper urinary tract. *J Urol* 85:199, 1961.

Poutasse EF: Partial nephrectomy: new techniques, approach, operative indications, and review of 51 cases. *J Urol* 88:153, 1962.

Pressman D: Eleventh intercostal space incision for renal surgery. *J Urol* 74:578, 1955.

Provet JA, Hanna MK: Simultaneous repair of bilateral ureteropelvic junction obstruction. *Urology* 33:390, 1989.

Ramsay JWA, Miller RA, Kellett MJ, et al: Percutaneous pyelolysis: indications, complications and results. *Br J Urol* 56:586, 1984.

Rassweller J, Henkel T, Petempa D, et al: The technique of transperitoneal laparoscopic nephrectomy, adrenalectomy and nephroureterectomy. *Eur Urol* 23:425, 1993.

Richter S, Ringet A, Shalev M, Nissenkorn I: The indwelling ureteric stent: a "friendly" procedure with unfriendly high morbidity. *BJU Int* 85:408, 2000.

Rickwood AM, Phadke D: Pyeloplasty in infants and children with particular reference to the method of drainage postoperatively. *BJU Int* 50:217, 1978.

Riehle RA Jr, Lavengood R: The eleventh rib transcostal incision: technique for an extrapleural approach. *J Urol* 132:1089, 1984.

Ritchey ML: Primary nephroectomy for Wilms' tumor: approach of the National Wilms' Tumor Study Group. *Urology* 47:787,1996.

Ritchey ML, Kelalis PP, Breslow N: Intracaval and atrial involvement with nephroblastoma: review of National Wilms' Tumor Study: III. *J Urol* 140:1113, 1988.

Robinson BC, Snow BW, Cartwright PC, et al: Comparison of laparoscopic versus open partial nephrectomy in a pediatric series. *J Urol* 169(2):638–40, 2003.

Robson WJ, Rudy SM, Johnston JH: Pelviureteric obstruction in infancy. *J Pediatr Surg* 11:57, 1976.

Rodriguez Netto N Jr, Esteves SC, D'Ancona CA: Antegrade endopyelotomy for pelviureteric junction obstruction in children. *Br J Urol* 78:607, 1996.

Rohrman D, Snyder HM, Duckett JW Jr, et al: The operative management of recurrent ureteropelvic junction obstruction. *J Urol* 158:1257, 1997.

Ross JH, Kay R, Knipper NS, Streem SB: The absence of crossing vessels in association with ureteropelvic junction obstruction detected by prenatal ultrasonography. *J Urol* 160:973, 1998.

Rushton HG, Salem Y, Belman AB, Majd M: Pediatric pyeloplasty: is routine retrograde pyelography necessary? *J Urol* 152:604, 1994.

Sampaio FJB, Aragao AHM: Anatomical relationship between the intrarenal arteries and the kidney collecting system. *J Urol* 143:679, 1990.

Sampaio FJB, Mandarim-De-Lacerda CA: Anatomic classification of the kidney collecting system for endourologic procedures. *Endourol* 2:247, 1988.

Sandler CM, Toombs BD: Computed tomographic evaluation of blunt renal injuries. *Radiology* 141:461,1981.

Scardino PL, Prince CL: Vertical flap ureteropelvioplasty: preliminary report. *South Med J* 46:325, 1953.

Schenkman EM, Tarry WF: Comparison of percutaneous endopyelotomy with open pyeloplasty for pediatric ureteropelvic junction obstruction. *J Urol* 159:1013, 1998.

Schuessler WW, Grune MT, Tecuanhuey LV, Preminger GN: Laparoscopic dismembered pyeloplasty. *J Urol* 150:1795, 1993.

Schuster T, Diwtz HG, Schutz S: Anderon-Hynes pyeloplasty in horseshoe kidney in children: is it effective without symphysiotomy? *Pediatr Surg Int* 15:230, 1999.

Segura JW, Kellis Burke EC: Horseshoe kidney in children. *J Urol* 108:333, 1972.

Seibold J, Janetschek G, Bartsch G: Laparoscopic surgery in pediatric urology. *Eur Urol* 30(3):394–9, 1996.

Sekaran P, MacKinlay GA, Lam J: Comparative evaluation of laparoscopic versus open nephrectomy in children. *Scott Med J* 51(4):15–7, 2006.

Selikowitz SM, Curtis MR: Hemostatic control with flexible compression tape used during partial nephrectomy and organ salvage. *J Urol* 162:458, 1999.

Semb C: Conservative renal surgery. *J R Coll Surg Edinb* 10:9, 1964.

Shah J, Mackay S, Rockall T, et al: "Urobotics" in urology. *BJU Int* 88:313, 2001.

Shamberg AM, Sandersdon K, Rajpoot D, Duel B: Laparoscopic retroperitoneal renal and adrenal surgery in children. *BJU Int* 87:321, 521, 2001.

Shukla AR, Hoover DL, Homsy YL, et al: Urolithiasis in the low birth weight infant: the role and efficacy of extracorporeal shock wave lithotripsy. *J Urol* 165:2320, 2001.

Siegfried MS, Rochester D, Bernstein JR, Miller JW: Diagnosis of inferior vena cava anomalies by computerized tomography. *Comput Radiol* 7:119, 1983.

Simforoosh N, Basiri A, Tabibi A, et al: Comparison of laparoscopic and open donor nephrectomy: a randomized controlled trial. *BJU Int* 95(6):851–5, 2005.

Siqueira TM, Nadu A, Kuo RL, et al: Laparoscopic treatment for ureteropelvic junction obstruction. *Urology* 60:973, 2002.

Smith FL, Ritchie EL, Maizels M, et al: Surgery for duplex kidneys with ectopic ureters: ipsilateral ureteroureterostomy versus polar nephrectomy. *J Urol* 142(Pt 2):532, 1989.

Smith JM, Butler MR: Splinting in pyeloplasty. *Urology* 8:218, 1976.

Smith MJV, Boyce WH: Anatrophic nephrotomy and plastic calyrhaphy. *J Urol* 99:521, 1968.

Smith P, Roberts M, Whitaker RH, et al: Primary pelvic hydronephrosis in children: a retrospective study. *Br J Urol* 48:549, 1976.

Snyder HM III, Lebowitz RL, Colodny AH, et al: Ureteropelvic junction obstruction in children. *Urol Clin North Am* 7:273, 1980.

Song SH, Lee SB, Yoo DS, Kim KS: Fluoroscopy-assisted retroperitoneal laparoscopic renal surgery in children. *J Endourol* 2006 20(4):256–9, 2006.

Soulie M, Salomon L, Patard JJ, et al: Extraperitoneal laparoscopic pyeloplasty: a multicenter study of 55 procedures. *J Urol* 166:48, 2001.

Steinbrecher HA, Malone PSJ: Wilms' tumors and hypertension: incidence and outcome. *Br J Urol* 76:241, 1995.

Sugita Y, Clarnette TD, Hutson JM: Retrograde balloon dilatation for primary pelvi-ureteric junction stenosis in children. *Br J Urol* 77:587, 1996.

Sung GT, Gill IS, Hsu TH: Laparoscopic pyeloplasty: a pilot study. *Urology* 53:1099, 1999.

Sydorak RM, Shaul DB: Laparoscopic partial nephrectomy in infants and toddlers. *J Pediatr Surg* 40(12):1945–7, 2005.

Sykes D: The arterial supply of the human kidney with special reference to accessory renal arteries. *Br J Surg* 50:368, 1963.

Sykes D: The morphology of renal lobulations and calices, and their relationship to partial nephrectomy. *Br J Surg* 51:294, 1964.

Tan HL: Laparoscopic Anderson-Hynes dismembered pyeloplasty in children. *J Urol* 162:1045, 1999.

Tan HL, Roberts JO, Grattan-Smith D: Retrograde balloon dilation of ureteropelvic obstructions in infants and children: early results. *Urology* 46:89, 1995.

Tash JA, Stock JA, Hanna MK: The role of partial nephrectomy in the treatment of pediatric renal hypertension. *J Urol* 169(2):625–8, 2003.

Thomas R: Endopyelotomy for ureteropelvic junction obstruction and ureteral stricture disease: a comparison of antegrade and retrograde techniques. *Curr Opin Urol* 4:174, 1994.

Thomas R, Monga M: Endopyelotomy: retrograde ureteroscopic approach. *Urol Clin North Am* 25:305, 1998.

Thomas R, Monga M, Klein EW: Ureteroscopic retrograde endopyelotomy for management of ureteropelvic junction obstruction. *J Endourol* 2:141, 1996.

Thomas R, Ortenberg J, Lee BR, Harmon EP: Safety and efficacy of pediatric ureteroscopy for management of calculus disease. *J Urol* 149:1082, 1993.

Thompson IM, Latourette H, Montie JE, Ross G Jr: Results of nonoperative management of blunt renal trauma. *J Urol* 118:522, 1977.

Thornbury JR: Perirenal anatomy: normal and abnormal. *Radiol Clin North Am* 17:321, 1979.

Thüroff JW, Frohneberg D, Riedmiller R, et al: Localisation of segmental arteries in renal surgery by Doppler sonography. *J Urol* 127:863, 1982.

Tobin CE: The renal fascia and its relation to the transversalis fascia. *Anat Rec* 89:295, 1944.

Towbin RB, Wacksman J, Ball WS: Percutaneous pyeloplasty in children: experience in three patients. *Radiology* 163:381, 1987.

Turner-Warwick R: The supracostal approach to the renal area. *Br J Urol* 37:671, 1965.

Turner-Warwick R: The use of pedicle grafts in the repair of urinary tract fistulae. *Br J Urol* 44:644, 1972.

Turner-Warwick R, Wynne EJ, Ashken MH: The use of the omental pedicle graft in the repair and reconstruction of the urinary tract. *Br J Surg* 54:849, 1967.

Vancaillie T, Schuessler W, Preminger G: Laparoscopic dismembered pyeloplasty. *J Endourol* 7:117, 1993.

Wagget J, Koop CE: Wilms' tumor: preoperative radiotherapy and chemotherapy in the management of massive tumors. *Cancer* 26:338, 1970.

Wallis MC, Khoury AE, Lorenzo AJ, et al: outcome analysis of retroperitoneal laparoscopic heminephrectomy in children. *J Urol* 175(6):2277–80, 2006; discussion 2280–2.

Ward JP, Smart CJ, O'Donoghue EPN, et al: Synchronous bilateral lumbotomy. *Eur Urol* 2:102, 1976.

Watts HG: Heminephrectomy: a simplified technique. *Aust N Z J Surg* 37:256, 1968.

Wein AJ, Carpiniello VL, Murphy JJ: A simple technique for partial nephrectomy. *Surg Gynecol Obstet* 146:620, 1978.

Wein AJ, Murphy JJ, Mulholland SG, et al: A conservative approach to the management of blunt renal trauma. *J Urol* 117:425, 1977.

Whitfield HN, Mills V, Miller RA, Wickham JEA: Percutaneous pyelolysis: an alternative to pyeloplasty. *Br J Urol* 53(suppl):93, 1983.

Williams DF, Schapiro AE, Arconti JS, et al: A new technique of partial nephrectomy. *J Urol* 97:955, 1967.

Williams DI, Cromie WJ: Ring ureterostomy. *Br J Urol* 47:789, 1975.

Williams DI, Karlaftis CM: Hydronephrosis due to pelviureteric obstruction in the newborn. *Br J Urol* 38:138, 1969.

Winfield HN, Donovan JF, Godet AS, Clayman RV: Laparoscopic partial nephrectomy: initial case report for benign disease. *J Endourol* 7:521, 1993.

Witherington R: Improving the supracostal loin incisions. *J Urol* 124:73, 1980.

Wolf JS Jr: Hand-assisted laparoscopy: pro. *Urology* 58:310, 2001.

Wolf JS Jr, Seifman BD, Montie JE: Nephron sparing surgery for suspected malignancy: open surgery compared with laparoscopy with selected use of hand assiatance. *J Urol* 193:1659, 2000.

Wollin M, Duffy PG, Diamond DA, et al: Priorities in urinary diversion following pyeloplasty. *J Urol* 142:573, 1989.

Wolpert JJ, Woodard JR, Parrott TS: Pyeloplasty in the young infant. *J Urol* 142:576, 1989.

Woo HH, Farnsworth RH: Dismembered pyeloplasty in infants under the age of 12 months. *Br J Urol* 77:449, 1996.

Woodruff MFA, Doig A, Donald KW, Nolan B: Renal autotransplantation. *Lancet* 1:433, 1966.

Woodside JR, Stephens GF, Stark GI, et al: Percutaneous stone removal in children. *J Urol* 134:1166, 1985.

Yao D, Poppas DP: A clinical series of laparoscopic nephrectomy, nephroureterectomy and heminephroureterectomy in the pediatric population. *J Urol* 163:1531, 2000.

Yeung CK, Liu KW, Ng WT, et al: Laparoscopy as the investigation and treatment of choice for urinary incontinence caused by small "invisible" dysplastic kidneys with infrasphincteric ureteric ectopia. *BJU Int* 84:324, 1999.

Yeung CK, Tam YH, Sihoe JDY, et al: Retroperitoneoscopic dismembered pyeloplasty for pelvi-ureteric junction obstruction in infants and children. *BJU Int* 87:509, 2001.

Yohannes P, Smith AD: The endourological management of complications associated with horseshoe kidney. *J Urol* 168:5, 2002.

Young HH: A technique for simultaneous exposure and operation on the adrenals. *Surg Gynecol Obstet* 54:179, 1936.

Zargooshi J: Open stone surgery in children: is it justified in the era of minimally invasive therapies. *BJU Int* 88:928, 2001.

Zincke H, Kelalis PP, Culp OS: Ureteropelvic obstruction in children. *Surg Gynecol Obstet* 139:873, 1974.

Zisman A, Pantuck AJ, Belldegrun AS, et al: Laparoscopic radical nephrectomy. *Semin Urol Oncol* 19:114, 2001.

Section 4
Adrenal Gland

Aird I: Bilateral anterior transabdominal adrenalectomy. *Br Med J* 2:708, 1955.

Castilho LN, Castillo OA, Denes FT, et al: Laparoscopic adrenal surgery in children. *J Urol* 168(1):221–4, 2002.

Castillo OA, Vitagliano G, Villeta M, et al: Laparoscopic resection of adrenal teratoma. *JSLS* 10(4):522–4, 2006.

Caty MG, Coran AG, Geagan M, Thompson NW: Current diagnosis and treatment of pheochromocytoma in children: experience with 22 consecutive tumors in 14 patients. *Arch Surg* 125:978, 1990.

Chino ES, Thomas CG: An extended Kocher incision for bilateral adrenalectomy. *Am J Surg* 149:292, 1985.

Das NK, Lyngdoh BT, Bhakri BK, et al: Surgical management of pediatric Cushing's disease. *Surg Neurol* 67(3):251–7, 2007.

de Lagausie P, Berrebi D, Michon J, et al: Laparoscopic adrenal surgery for neuroblastomas in children. *J Urol* 170(3):932–5, 2003.

Del Pizzo JJ: Laparoscopic adrenalectomy in children. *Curr Urol Rep* 7(1):68, 2006.

Del Pizzo JJ, Shichman SJ, Sosa RE: Laparoscopic adrenalectomy: The New York–Presbyterian Hospital experience. *J Endocrinol* 16:591, 2002.

Doherty GN, Skogseid B: *Surgical Endocrinology.* Philadelphia, Lippincott, Williams and Wilkins, 2001.

Fonkalsrud EW: Adrenal pheochromocytoma in childhood. *Progr Pediatr Surg* 26:103, 1991.

Gagner M, Inabnet W III: *Minimally Invasive Endocrine Surgery.* Philadelphia, Lippincott, Williams and Wilkins, 2002.

Gagner M, Lacroix A, Bolte E: Laparoscopic adrenalectomy in Cushing's syndrome and pheochromocytoma. *N Engl J Med* 327:1033, 1992.

Hernandez FC, Sanchez M, Alvarez A, et al: A five-year report on experience in the detection of pheochromocytoma. *Clin Biochem* 33:649, 2000.

Hume DM: Pheochromocytoma in the adult and in the child. *Am J Surg* 99:458, 1960.

Kadamba P, Habib Z, Rossi L: Experience with laparoscopic adrenalectomy in children. *J Pediatr Surg* 39(5):764–7, 2004.

Lenders JWM, Pacak K, Walther MM, et al: Biochemical diagnosis of pheochromocytoma: which is the best test? *JAMA* 287(11):1427–34, 2002.

Michalkiewicz E, Sandrini R, Figueiredo B, et al: Clinical and outcome characteristics of children with adrenocortical tumors: a report from the International Pediatric Adrenocortical Tumor Registry. *J Clin Oncol* 22(5):838–45, 2004.

Misseri R: Adrenal surgery in the pediatric population. *Curr Urol Rep* 8(1):89–94, 2007. Review.

Pacak K, Linehan WM, Eisenhofer G, et al: Recent advances in genetics, diagnosis, localization, and treatment of pheochromocytoma. *Ann Intern Med* 134:315, 2001.

Salomon L, Soule M, Mouly P, et al: Experience with retroperitoneal laparoscopic adrenalectomy in 115 procedures. *J Urol* 166:38, 2001.

Scott HW Jr, Dean RH, Oates JA, et al: Surgical management of pheochromocytoma. *Am Surg* 47:6, 1981.

Shandling B, Wesson D, Filler RM: Recurrent pheochromocytoma in children. *J Pediatr Surg* 25:1063, 1990.

Shulkin BL, Wieland DM, Schwaiger M, et al: PET scanning with hydroxyephedrine: an approach to the localization of pheochromocytoma. *J Nucl Med* 33:1125, 1992.

Skarsgard ED, Albanese CT. The safety and efficacy of laparoscopic adrenalectomy in children. *Arch Surg* 140(9):905–8, 2005.

Soulie M, Mouly P, Caron P, et al: Retroperitoneal laparoscopic adrenalectomy: clinical experience in 52 procedures. *Urology* 50:921, 2000.

Stanford A, Upperman JS, Nguyen N, et al: Surgical management of open versus laparoscopic adrenalectomy: outcome analysis. *J Pediatr Surg* 37(7):1027–9, 2002.

Vaughan ED, Blumenfeld J, Del Pizzo JJ, et al: Surgical approach to the adrenal gland. In: Walsh PC, Retik AB, Vaughan ED, Wein AP (Eds): *Campbell's Urology,* 8th ed. Philadelphia, W. B. Saunders Company, pp 3507–69, 2002.

Vaughan ED Jr, Phillips H: Modified posterior approach for right adrenalectomy. *Surg Gynecol Obstet* 165:453, 1987.

Walther MC, Herring J, Choyke PL, Linehan WM: Laparoscopic partial adrenalectomy in patients with hereditary forms of pheochromocytoma. *J Urol* 163:14, 2000.

Whalen RK, Althausen AF, Daniels GH: Extra-adrenal pheochromocytoma. *J Urol* 147:1, 1992.

Winfield HN, Hamilton BD, Bravo EL: Technique of laparoscopic adrenalectomy. *Urol Clin North Am* 24:459, 1997.

Witteles RM, Kaplan EL, Roizen MF: Sensitivity of diagnostic and localization tests for pheochromocytoma in clinical practice. *Arch Intern Med* 160:2521, 2000.

Young HH: A technique for simultaneous exposure and operation on the adrenals. *Surg Gynecol Obstet* 54:179, 1936.

Section 5
Ureter

Aboutaleb H, Bolduc S, Upadhyay J, et al: Subureteral polydimethylsiloxane injection versus extravesical reimplantation for primary low grade vesicoureteral reflux in children: a comparative study. *J Urol* 169(1):313–6, 2003.

Abrahamsson K, Hansson E, Sillen U, et al: Bladder dysfunction: an integral part of the ectopic ureterocele complex. *J Urol* 160:1468,1998.

Agran MA, Kratzman EA: Inferior vena cava on the left side: its relationship to the right ureter. *J Urol* 101:149, 1969.

Al-Hunayan AA, Kehinde EO, Elsalam MA, Al-Mukhtar RS: Outcome of endoscopic treatment for vesicoureteral reflux in children using polydimethylsiloxane. *J Urol* 168(5):2181–3, 2002.

Ali-el-Dein B, Ghoneim MA: Bridging long ureteral defects using the Yang-Monti principle. *J Urol* 169:1074, 2003.

Allen TD: Congenital ureteral strictures. *J Urol* 104:196, 1970.

Amar AD: Reimplantation of completely duplicated ureters. *J Urol* 107:230, 1972.

Amar AD, Egan RM, Das S: Ipsilateral ureteroureterostomy combined with ureteral reimplantation for treatment of disease in both ureters in a child with complete ureteral duplication. *J Urol* 125:581, 1981.

Amin H: Experience with the ileal ureter. *Br J Urol* 48:19, 1976.

Anderson JC, Hynes W: Retrocaval ureter: a case diagnosed preoperatively and treated successfully by plastic operation. *Br J Urol* 21:209, 1949.

Atala A, Kavoussi LR, Goldstein DS, et al: Laparoscopic correction of vesicoureteral reflux. *J Urol* 150:748, 1993.

Barrett DM, Malek RS, Kelalis PP: Problems and solutions in surgical treatment of 100 consecutive ureteral duplications in children. *J Urol* 114:126, 1975.

Barrieras D, Lapointe S, Reddy PP, et al: Urinary retention after bilateral extravesical ureteral reimplantation: does dissection distal to the ureteral orifice have a role? *J Urol* 162(3 Pt 2):1197–200, 1999.

Barry JM, Hatch DA: Parallel incision, unstented extravesical ureteroneocystostomy: follow-up of 203 kidney transplants. *J Urol* 134:249, 1985.

Basiri A, Otookesh H, Simforoosh N, et al: Does pre-transplantation antireflux surgery eliminate post-renal transplantation pyelonephritis in children? *J Urol* 175(4):1490–2, 2006.

Baskin LS, Zderic SA, Snyder HM, Duckett JW: Primary dilated megaureter: long-term follow-up. *J Urol* 152:618, 1994.

Baum WC: The clinical use of terminal ileum as a substitute ureter. *J Urol* 72:16, 1954.

Beganovic A, Klijn AJ, Dik P, De Jong TP: Ectopic ureterocele: long-term results of open surgical therapy in 54 patients. *J Urol* 178(1):251–4, 2007. Epub 2007 May 17.

Bellman GC, Smith AD: Special considerations in the technique of laparoscopic ureterolithotomy. *J Urol* 151:146, 1994.

Belman AB, Filmer RB, King LR: Surgical management of duplication of the collecting system. *J Urol* 112:316, 1974.

Benoit RM, Peele PB, Docimo SG: The cost-effectiveness of dextranomer/hyaluronic acid copolymer for the management of vesicoureteral reflux: 1. substitution for surgical management. *J Urol* 176(4 Pt 1):1588–92, 2006.

Bieri M, Smith CK, Smith AY, Borden TA: Ipsilateral ureteroureterostomy for single ureteral reflux or obstruction in a duplicate system. *J Urol* 159(3):1016–8, 1998.

Bischoff P: Operative treatment of megaureter. *J Urol* 85:268, 1961.

Bishop MC, Askew AR, Smith JC: Reimplantation of the wide ureter. *Br J Urol* 50:383, 1978.

Blok C, Van Venroolj EPM, Mokhless I, Coolsaet BLRA: Dynamics of the ureterovesical junction: its fluid transport mechanism in the pig. *J Urol* 134:175, 1985.

Boari A: Chirurgia dell'uretere. In: *Societa Editrice Dante Alighieri.* Rome, 1900, pp 176–7.

Bomalski MD, Hirschl RB, Bloom DS: Vesicoureteral reflux and ureteropelvic junction obstruction: association, treatment of options and outcome. *J Urol* 157:969, 1997.

Boxer RJ, Fritzsche P, Skinner DG, et al: Replacement of the ureter by small intestine: clinical applications and results of ileo-ureter in 89 patients. *J Urol* 121:128, 1979.

Brown S: Open versus endoscopic surgery in the treatment of vesicoureteral reflux. *J Urol* 142:499, 1989.

Burbridge KA, Miller M, Connor JP: Extravesical ureteral reimplantation: results in 128 patients. *J Urol* 155:1721, 1996.

Burno DK, Glazier DB, Zaontz MR: Lessons learned about contralateral reflux after unilateral extravesical ureteral advancement in children. *J Urol* 160:995, 1998.

Cain MP, Pope JC, Casale AJ, et al: Natural history of refluxing distal ureteral stumps after nephrectomy and partial ureterectomy for vesicoureteral reflux. *J Urol* 160(3 Pt 2):1026–7, 1998.

Caldamone AA, Diamond DA: Long-term results of the endoscopic correction of vesicoureteral reflux in children using autologous chondrocytes. *J Urol* 165(6 Pt 2):2224–7, 2001.

Canning DA: Laparoscopic extravesical reimplantation for post-pubertal vesicoureteral reflux. *J Urol* 174(3):1103–4, 2005.

Canon SJ, Jayanthi VR, Patel AS: Vesicoscopic cross-trigonal ureteral reimplantation: a minimally invasive option for repair of vesicoureteral reflux. *J Urol* 178(1):269–73, 2007.

Capozza N, Caione P: Dextranomer/hyaluronic acid copolymer implantation for vesico-ureteral reflux: a randomized comparison with antibiotic prophylaxis. *J Pediatr* 140(2):230–4, 2002.

Capozza N, Caione P, de Gennaro M, et al: Endoscopic treatment of vesico-ureteric reflux and urinary incontinence: technical problems in the paediatric patient. *Br J Urol* 75:538, 1995.

Capozza N, Lais A, Matarazzo E, et al: Influence of voiding dysfunction on the outcome of endoscopic treatment for vesicoureteral reflux. *J Urol* 168(4 Pt 2):1695–8, 2002.

Carini M, Selli C, Lenzi R, et al: Surgical treatment of vesicoureteral reflux with bilateral medialization of the ureteral orifices. *Eur Urol* 11:181, 1985.

Carrion H, Safewood J, Politano V, et al: Retrocaval ureter: report of 8 cases and their surgical management. *J Urol* 121:514, 1979.

Cartwright PC, Snow BW, Mansfield JC, et al: Percutaneous endoscopic trigonoplasty: a minimally invasive approach to correct vesico-ureteral reflux. *J Urol* 156:661, 1996.

Casale P, Grady RW, Lee RS, et al: Symptomatic refluxing distal ureteral stumps after nephroureterectomy and heminephroureterectomy: what should we do? *J Urol* 173(1):204–6, 2005.

Cass AS, Schmaelzle JF, Hinman F Jr: Ureteral anastomosis in the dog: comparing continuous with interrupted sutures. *Invest Urol* 6:94, 1968.

Caulk JR: Megaloureter: the importance of the ureterovesical valve. *J Urol* 9:315, 1923.

Cendron J, Melin Y, Valayer J: Simplified treatment of ureterocele with pyelo-ureteric duplication. *Eur Urol* 7:321, 1981.

Chang SS, Koch MO: The use of an extended spiral bladder flap for treatment of upper ureteral loss. *J Urol* 156:1981, 1996.

Chen HW, Lin GJ, Lai CH, et al: Minimally invasive extravesical ureteral reimplantation for vesicoureteral reflux. *J Urol* 167(4):1821–3, 2002.

Chertin B, Colhoun E, Velayudham M, Puri P: Endoscopic treatment of vesicoureteral reflux: 11 to 17 years of follow-up. *J Urol* 167(3):1443–5, 2002; discussion 1445–6.

Chilton CP, Vordermark JS, Ransley PG: Transuretero-ureterostomy: a review of its use in modern pediatric urology. *Br J Urol* 56:604, 1984.

Choi H, Oh S-J: The management of children with complete ureteric duplication: selective use of uretero-ureterostomy as a primary and a salvage procedure. *BJU Int* 86:508, 2000.

Chow S-H, LaSalle MD, Stock JA, Hanna MK: Ureterocystostomy: to drain or not to drain. *J Urol* 160:1001, 1998.

Cohen SJ: Vesicoureteral reflux: a new surgical approach. *Int Urol Pediatr* 6:20, 1975.

Cooper CS, Passerini-Glazel G, Hutcheson JC, et al: Long-term follow-up of endoscopic incision of ureteroceles: intravesical versus extravesical. *J Urol* 164(3 Pt 2):1097–9, 2002; discussion 1099–100.

Coplen DE, Barthold JS: Controversies in the management of ectopic ureteroceles. *Urology* 56:665, 2000.

Couvelaire R, Auvert J, Moulonguet A, et al: Implantations et anastomoses urétéro-calicielles: techniques et indications. *J Urol Nephrol* 70:437, 1964.

Creevy CD: The atonic distal ureteral segment (ureteral achalasia). *J Urol* 97:457, 1969.

Creevy CD: Misadventures following replacement of ureters with ileum. *Surgery* 58:497, 1965.

Daines SI, Hodgson NB: Management of reflux in total duplication anomalies. *J Urol* 105:720, 1971.

David S, Kelly C, Poppas DP: Nerve sparing extravesical repair of bilateral vesicoureteral reflux: description of technique and evaluation of urinary retention. *J Urol* 172(4 Pt 2): 1617–20, 2004.

Dawrant MJ, Mohanan N, Puri P: Endoscopic treatment for high-grade vesicoureteral reflux in infants. *J Urol* 176(4 Pt 2): 1847–50, 2006.

De Caluwe D, Chertin B, Puri P: Fate of the retained ureteral stump after upper pole heminephrectomy in duplex kidneys. *J Urol* 168(2):679–80, 2002.

De Jong TPVM, Dik P, Klijn AJ, et al: Ectopic ureterocele: results of open surgical therapy in 40 patients. *J Urol* 164:2040, 2000.

de Kort LM, Klijn AJ, Uiterwaal CS, de Jong TP: Ureteral reimplantation in infants and children: effect on bladder function. *J Urol* 167(1):285–7, 2002.

Decter RM, Sprunger JK, Holland RJ: Can a single individualized procedure predictably resolve all the problematic aspects of the pediatric ureterocele? *J Urol* 165:2308, 2001.

Diamond DA, Caldamone AA, Bauer SB, Retik AB: Mechanisms of failure of endoscopic treatment of vesicoureteral reflux based on endoscopic anatomy. *J Urol* 170(4 Pt 2):1556–8, 2003; discussion 1559.

Diamond DA, Parulkar BG: Ureteral tailoring in situ: a practical approach to persistent reflux in the dilated re-implanted ureter. *J Urol* 160:998, 1998.

Diamond DA, Rabinowitz R, Hoenig D, Caldamone AA: The mechanism of new onset contralateral reflux following unilateral ureteroneocystostomy. *J Urol* 156 (2 pt 2):665,1996.

Donohue JP, Hostetter M, Glover J, Madura J: Ureteroneocystostomy versus ureteropyelostomy: a comparison in the same renal allograft series. *J Urol* 114:202, 1975.

Dowd JB, Chen F: Ileal replacement of the ureter in the solitary kidney. *Surg Clin North Am* 51:739, 1971.

Duckett JW, Pfister RR: Ureterocalicostomy for renal salvage. *J Urol* 128:98, 1982.

Duong DT, Parekh DJ, Pope JC 4th, et al: Ureteroneocystostomy without urethral catheterization shortens hospital stay without compromising postoperative success. *J Urol* 170(4 Pt 2): 1570–3, 2003.

Ehrlich RM: Success of transvesical advancement technique for vesicoureteral reflux. *J Urol* 128:554, 1982.

Ehrlich RM: The ureteral folding technique for megaureter surgery. *J Urol* 134:668, 1986.

Ehrlich RM, Skinner DG: Complications of transuretero-ureterostomy. *J Urol* 113:467, 1975.

Elder JS, Diaz M, Caldamone AA, et al: Endoscopic therapy for vesicoureteral reflux: a meta-analysis: I. Reflux resolution and urinary tract infection. *J Urol* 175(2):716–22, 2006.

Ellsworth PI, Lim DJ, Walker RD, et al: Common sheath reimplantation yields excellent results in the treatment of vesicoureteral reflux in duplicated collecting systems. *J Urol* 155:1407, 1996.

Elmore JM, Kirsch AJ, Perez-Brayfield MR, et al: Salvage extravesical ureteral reimplantation after failed endoscopic surgery for vesicoureteral reflux. *J Urol* 176(3):1158–60, 2006.

El-Sherbiny MT, Hafez AT, Ghoneim MA, Greenfield SP: Ureteroneocystostomy in children with posterior urethral valves: indications and outcome. *J Urol* 168(4 Pt 2):1836–9, 2002; discussion 1839–40.

Ericsson NO: Ectopic ureterocele in infants and children: a clinical study. *Acta Chir Scand* 197(suppl):1–93, 1954.

Fort KF, Selman SH, Kropp KA: A retrospective analysis of the use of ureteral stents in children undergoing ureteroneocystostomy. *J Urol* 129:545, 1983.

Frey P, Lutz N, Jenny P, et al: Endoscopic subureteral collagen injection for the treatment of vesicoureteral reflux in infants and children. *J Urol* 154:804, 1995.

Fung LCT, McLorie GS, Jain U, et al: Voiding efficiency after ureteral implantation: a comparison of extravesical and intravesical techniques. *J Urol* 153:1972, 1995.

Gaur DD: Laparoscopic operative retroperitoneoscopy: use of a new device. *J Urol* 148:1137, 1992.

Gaur DD: Retroperitoneal laparoscopic ureterolithotomy. *World J Urol* 11:175, 1993.

Gaur DD, Trevidi MR, Prabhudesai MR, et al: Laparoscopic ureterolithotomy: technical considerations and long-term follow-up. *BJU Int* 89:339, 2002.

Gearhart JP, Woolfenden KA: The vesico-psoas hitch as an adjunct to megaureter repair in childhood. *J Urol* 127:505, 1982.

Gill HS, Liao JC: Pelvi-ureteric junction obstruction treated with Acusize® retrograde endopyelotomy. *Br J Urol* 82:8, 1998.

Gill IS, Ponsky LE, Desai M, Kay R, Ross JH: Laparoscopic cross-trigonal Cohen ureteroneocystostomy: novel technique. *J Urol* 166(5):1811–4, 2001.

Gil-Vernet JM: A new technique for surgical correction of vesicoureteral reflux. *J Urol* 131:456, 1984.

Glassberg KI, Laungani G, Wasnick RJ, Waterhouse K: Transverse ureteral advancement technique of ureteroneocystostomy (Cohen re-implant) and a modification for difficult cases (experience with 121 ureters). *J Urol* 134:306, 1985.

Gonzales ET Jr, Decter RM: Management of ureteroceles in the newborn. In: King LR (Ed): *Urologic Surgery in Neonates and Young Infants.* Philadelphia, W. B. Saunders Company, 1988, p 204.

Gonzalez R, Piaggio L: Initial experience with laparoscopic ipsilateral ureteroureterostomy in infants and children for duplication anomalies of the urinary tract. *J Urol* 177(6):2315–8, 2007.

Goodwin WE, Burke DE, Muller WH: Retrocaval ureter. *Surg Gynecol Obstet* 104:337, 1957.

Goodwin WE, Winter CC, Turner RD: Replacement of the ureter by small intestine: clinical application and results of the ileal ureter. *J Urol* 81:406, 1959.

Gosalbez R Jr, Gousse AE: Reconstruction and undiversion of the short or severely dilated ureter: the antireflux ileal nipple revisited. *J Urol* 159(2):530–4, 1998.

Gow JG: *Color Atlas of Boari Bladder Flap Procedure.* Oradell, NJ, Medical Economics Books, 1983.

Gregoir W: Lich-Gregoir operation. In: Epstein HB, Hohenfellner R, Williams DI (Eds): *Surgical Pediatric Urology.* Stuttgart, Thieme, 1977, p 265.

Gregoir W, Schulman CC: Die extravesikale Antirefluxplastik. *Urologe A* 16:124, 1977.

Gregoir W, Van Regemorter GV: Le reflux vésico-urétéral congenital. *Urol Int* 18:122, 1964.

Gross M, Peng B, Waterhouse L: Use of the mobilized bladder to replace the pelvic ureter. *J Urol* 101:40, 1969.

Grossklaus DJ, Pope JC IV, Adams MC, Brock JW: Is postoperative cystography necessary after ureteral implantation? *Urology* 58:1041, 2001.

Gutierrez J, Chang CY, Nesbit RM: Ipsilateral ureteroureterostomy for vesicoureteral reflux in duplicated ureter. *J Urol* 101:36, 1969.

Gylys-Morin VM, Minevich E, Tackett LD, et al: Magnetic resonance imaging of the dysplastic renal moiety and ectopic ureter. *J Urol* 164:2034, 2000.

Hagg MJ, Mourachov PV, Snyder HM, et al: The modern endoscopic approach to ureterocele. *J Urol* 163:940, 2000.

Halpern GN, King LR, Belman AB: Transureteroureterostomy in children. *J Urol* 109:504, 1973.

Hanna MK: Megaureter. In: King LR (Ed): *Urologic Surgery in Neonates and Young Infants.* Philadelphia, W. B. Saunders Company, 1988, p 160.

Hanna MK: New surgical method for one-stage total remodeling of massively dilated and tortuous ureter: tapering in situ technique. *Urology* 14:453, 1979.

Harrill HC: Retrocaval ureter: report of a case with operative correction of the defect. *J Urol* 44:450, 1940.

Hawthorne NJ, Zincke H, Kelalis PP: Ureterocalycostomy: an alternative to nephrectomy. *J Urol* 115:583, 1976.

Hayashi Y, Yamataka A, Kaneyama K, et al: Review of 86 patients with myelodysplasia and neurogenic bladder who underwent sigmoidocolocystoplasty and were followed more than 10 years. *J Urol* 176(4 Pt 2):1806–9, 2006.

Hendren WH: Complications of megaureter repair in children. *J Urol* 113:238, 1975.

Hendren WH: Complications of ureteral reimplantation and megaureter repair. In: Smith RB, Skinner DC (Eds): *Complications of Urologic Surgery: Prevention and Management.* Philadelphia, W. B. Saunders Company, 1976, pp 151–208.

Hendren WH: Functional restoration of decompensated ureters in children. *Am J Surg* 119:477, 1970.

Hendren WH: A new approach to infants with severe obstructive uropathy: early complete reconstruction. *J Pediatr Surg* 5:184, 1970.

Hendren WH: Operative repair of megaureter in children. *J Urol* 101:49, 1969.

Hendren WH: Technical aspects of megaureter repair. *Birth Defects* 13:21, 1977.

Hendren WH, Hensle TW: Transureteroureterostomy: experience with 75 cases. *J Urol* 123:826, 1980.

Hendren WH, McLorie GA: Late stricture of intestinal ureters. *J Urol* 129:584, 1983.

Hendren WH, Mitchell ME: Surgical correction of ureteroceles. *J Urol* 121:590, 1979.

Hendren WH, Monfort GJ: Surgical correction of ureteroceles in childhood. *J Pediatr Surg* 6:235, 1971.

Hendren WH, Radhakrishnan J, Middleton RW: Pediatric pyeloplasty. *J Pediatr Surg* 15:133, 1980.

Hensle TW, Burbige KA, Levin RK: Management of the short ureter in urinary tract reconstruction. *J Urol* 137:707, 1987.

Herz D, Hafez A, Bagli D, et al: Efficacy of endoscopic subureteral polydimethylsiloxane injection for treatment of vesicoureteral reflux in children: a North American clinical report. *J Urol* 166:1880, 2001.

Higgins CC: Transuretero-ureteral anastomosis. *J Urol* 34:349, 1935.

Higham-Kessler J, Reinert SE, Snodgrass WT, et al: A review of failures of endoscopic treatment of vesicoureteral reflux with dextranomer microspheres. *J Urol* 177(2):710–4. 2007.

Hinman F Jr: Ureteral repair and the splint. *J Urol* 78:376, 1957.

Hinman F Jr, Baumann FW: Complications of vesicoureteral operations from incoordination of micturition. *J Urol* 116:638, 1976.

Hinman F Jr, Miller ER: Mural tension in vesical disorders and ureteral reflex. *J Urol* 91:33, 1964.

Hinman F Jr, Miller ER, Hutch JA, et al: Low pressure reflux: relation of vesicoureteral reflux to intravesical pressure. *J Urol* 88:758–65, 1962; reprinted *J Urol* 167:1063, 2002.

Hirschorn RC: The ileal sleeve: II. Surgical technique in clinical application. *J Urol* 92:120, 1964.

Hodges CV, Barry JM, Fuchs EF, et al: Transureteroureterostomy: 25 years experience with 100 patients. *J Urol* 123:834, 1980.

Hodges CV, Moore RJ, Lehman TH, Benham AM: Clinical experiences with transureteroureterostomy. *J Urol* 90:552, 1963.

Hodgson NB: Urinary tract infections in childhood. In: Kendall AR, Karafin L (Eds): *Urology,* vol 1, p 22. Philadelphia, Harper and Row, 1982.

Hodgson NB, Thompson LW: Technique of reductive ureteroplasty in the management of megaureter. *J Urol* 113:118, 1975.

Houle AM, McLorie GA, Heritz DM, et al: Extravesical non-dismembered ureteropyleoplasty with detrusorrhaphy: a renewed technique to correct vesicoureteral reflux in children. *J Urol* 148:704, 1992.

Huisman TK, Kaplan GW, Brock WA, Packer MG: Ipsilateral ureteroureterostomy and pyeloureterostomy: a review of 15 years of experience with 25 patients. *J Urol* 138:1207, 1987.

Husman DA, Ewalt DH, Glenski WJ, Bernier PA: Ureterocele associated with ureteral duplication and a nonfunctioning upper pole segment: management by partial nephroureterectomy alone. *J Urol* 154:723, 1995.

Hutch JA: *The Uretero-vesical Junction.* Berkeley and Los Angeles, University of California Press, 1958.

Hutch JA, Hinman F, Miller ER: Reflux as a cause of hydronephrosis and chronic pyelonephritis. *J Urol* 88:169, 1962.

Jameson SG, McKinney JS, Rushton JF: Ureterocalycostomy: a new surgical procedure for correction of ureteropelvic stricture associated with an intrarenal pelvis. *J Urol* 77:135, 1957.

Janetschek G, Radmayer C, Bartsch G: Laparoscopic ureteral anti-reflux plasty reimplantation: first clinical experience. *Ann d'Urol* 29:101, 1995.

Jayanthi VR, Churchill BM, Khoury AE, et al: Bilateral single ureteral ectopia: difficulty attaining continence using standard bladder neck repair. *J Urol* 158:1933, 1997.

Jayanthi VR, Churchill BM, Khoury AE, et al: Reconstructive surgery of mega-ureter in childhood. *Br J Urol* 39:17, 1967.

Jayanthi VR, Koff S: Long-term outcome of transurethral puncture of ectopic ureteroceles: initial success and late problems. *J Urol* 162:1077, 1999.

Jayanthi VR, McLorie GA, Khoury AE, Churchill BM: Extravesical detrusorrhaphy for refluxing ureters associated with paraureteral diverticula. *Urology* 45:664, 1995.

Johnston JH, Farkas A: The congenital refluxing megaureter: experiences with surgical reconstruction. *Br J Urol* 47:153, 1975.

Johnston JH, Heal MR: Reflux in complete duplicated ureters in children: management and techniques. *J Urol* 105:881, 1971.

Johnston JH, Johnson LM: Experiences with ectopic ureteroceles. *Br J Urol* 41:61, 1971.

Jung C, DeMarco RT, Lowrance WT, et al: Subureteral injection of dextranomer/hyaluronic acid copolymer for persistent vesicoureteral reflux following ureteroneocystostomy. *J Urol* 177(1):312–5, 2007.

Juskiewenski S, Vaysse P, Moscovici J, et al: The ureterovesical junction. *Anat Clin* 5:251, 1984.

Kalicinski ZH, Kansy J, Kotarbínska B, Joszt W: Surgery of megaureters: modification of Hendren's operation. *J Pediatr Surg* 12:183, 1977.

Kehinde EO, Rotimi VO, Al-Awadi KA, et al: Factors predisposing to urinary tract infection after J ureteral stent insertion. *J Urol* 167:1334, 2002.

Kennelly MJ, Bloom DA, Richey ML, Panzl AC: Outcome analysis of bilateral Cohen cross-trigonal ureteroneocystostomy. *Urology* 46:393, 1995.

King LR: Megaloureter: definition, diagnosis and management. *J Urol* 123:222, 1980.

Kirsch AJ, Perez-Brayfield MR, Scherz HC: Minimally invasive treatment of vesicoureteral reflux with endoscopic injection of dextranomer/hyaluronic acid copolymer: the Children's Hospitals of Atlanta experience. *J Urol* 170(1):211–5, 2003.

Kirsch AJ, Perez-Brayfield M, Smith EA, Scherz HC: The modified sting procedure to correct vesicoureteral reflux: improved results with submucosal implantation within the intramural ureter. *J Urol* 171(6 Pt 1):2413–6, 2004.

Kitchens D, Minevich E, DeFoor W, et al: Endoscopic injection of dextranomer/hyaluronic acid copolymer to correct vesicoureteral reflux following failed ureteroneocystostomy. *J Urol* 176(4 Pt 2):1861–3, 2006.

Kobelt G, Canning DA, Hensle TW, Lackgren G: The cost-effectiveness of endoscopic injection of dextranomer/hyaluronic acid copolymer for vesicoureteral reflux. *J Urol* 169(4):1480–4, 2003; discussion 1484–5.

Koff SA, Wagner TT, Jayanthi VR: The relationship among dysfunctional elimination syndromes, primary vesicourethral reflux, and urinary tract infections in children. *J Urol* 160:1019, 1998.

Kogan BA, Baskin LS, Allison MJ: Length of stay for specialized pediatric urologic care. *Arch Pediatr Adolesc Med* 152(11):1126–31, 1998.

Krishnan A, Swana H, Mathias R, Baskin LS: Redo ureteroneocystostomy using an extravesical approach in pediatric renal transplant patients with reflux: a retrospective analysis and description of technique. *J Urol* 176(4 Pt 1):1582–7, 2006.

Lackgren G, Skoldenberg E, Stenberg A: Endoscopic treatment with stabilized nonanimal hyaluronic acid/dextranomer gel is effective in vesicoureteral reflux associated with bladder dysfunction. *J Urol* 177(3):1124–8, 2007.

Lackgren G, Wahlin N, Skoldenberg E, et al: Endoscopic treatment of vesicoureteral reflux with dextranomer/hyaluronic acid copolymer is effective in either double ureters or a small kidney. *J Urol* 170(4 Pt 2):1551–5, 2003.

Lackgren G, Wahlin N, Skoldenberg E, Stenberg A: Long-term follow-up of children treated with dextranomer/hyaluronic acid copolymer for vesicoureteral reflux. *J Urol* 166:1887, 2001.

Lapides J: The physiology of the intact human ureter. *J Urol* 59:501, 1948.

Lapointe SP, Barrieras D, Leblanc B, Williot P: Modified Lich-Gregoir ureteral reimplantation: experience of a Canadian center. *J Urol* 159(5):1662–4, 1998.

Leissner J, Allhoff EP, Wolff W, et al: The pelvic plexus and antireflux surgery: topographical finding and clinical consequences. *J Urol* 165:1652, 2001.

Lich R Jr, Howerton LW, Davis LA: Recurrent urosepsis in children. *J Urol* 86:554, 1961.

Lipski BA, Mitchell ME, Burns MW: Voiding dysfunction after bilateral extravesical ureteral reimplantation. *J Urol* 159(3):1019–21, 1998.

Lipsky H: Endoscopic treatment of vesicoureteral reflux with bovine collagen. *Eur Urol* 18:52, 1990.

Liu HYA, Dhillon HK, Yeung CK, et al: Clinical outcome and management of prenatally diagnosed primary megaureters. *J Urol* 152:614, 1994.

Liu HYA, Yeung CK, Diamond DA, et al: Clinical outcome and management of prenatally diagnosed primary megaureters. *J Urol* 152:614, 1994.

Lorenzo AJ, Pippi Salle JL, Barroso U, et al: What are the most powerful determinants of endoscopic vesicoureteral reflux correction? Multivariate analysis of a single institution experience during 6 years. *J Urol* 176(4 Pt 2):1851–5, 2006.

Lyon RP, Marshall S, Tanagho EA: The ureteral orifice: its configuration and competency. *J Urol* 102:504, 1969.

Malek RS, Kelalis PP, Burke EC, et al: Simple and ectopic ureterocele in infancy and childhood. *Surg Gynecol Obstet* 134:611, 1972.

Marberger M, Altwein JE, Straub E, et al: The Lich-Gregoire antireflux plasty: experiences with 371 children. *J Urol* 120:216, 1978.

Marotte JB, Smith DP: Extravesical ureteral reimplantations for the correction of primary reflux can be done as outpatient procedures. *J Urol* 165(6 Pt 2):2228–31, 2001.

Marr L, Skoog SJ: Laser incision of ureterocele in the pediatric patient. *J Urol* 167(1):280–2, 2002.

Mathews R, Smith PA, Fishman EK, Marshall FF: Anomalies of the inferior vena cava and renal veins: embryologic and surgical considerations. *Urology* 53:873, 1999.

Mathisen W: Vesicoureteral reflux and its surgical correction. *Surg Gynecol Obstet* 118:965, 1964.

McAchran SE, Palmer JS: Bilateral extravesical ureteral reimplantation in toilet-trained children: is 1-day hospitalization without urinary retention possible? *J Urol* 174(5):1991–3, 2005.

McMann LP, Scherz HC, Kirsch AJ: Long-term preservation of dextranomer/hyaluronic acid copolymer implants after endoscopic treatment of vesicoureteral reflux in children: a sonographic volumetric analysis. *J Urol* 177(1):316–20, 2007.

Merguerian PA, Byun E, Chang B: Lower urinary tract reconstruction for duplicated renal units with ureterocele: is excision of the ureterocele with reconstruction of the bladder base necessary? *J Urol* 170(4 Pt 2):1510–3, 2003; discussion 1513.

Mering JM, Steel JF, Gittes RF: Congenital ureteral valves. *J Urol* 107:737, 1972.

Mevorach RA, Hulbert WC, Rabinowitz R, et al: Results of a 2-year multicenter trial of endoscopic treatment of vesicoureteral reflux with synthetic calcium hydroxyapatite. *J Urol* 175(1):288–91, 2006.

Miller DC, Bloom DA, McGuire EJ, Park JM: Temporary perineal urethrostomy for external sphincter dilation in a male patient with high risk myelomeningocele. *J Urol* 170(4 Pt 2):1606–8, 2003.

Minevich E, Aronoff D, Wacksman J, Sheldon CA: Voiding dysfunction after bilateral extravesical detrusorrhaphy. *J Urol* 160:1004, 1998.

Minevich E, Tackett L, Wacksman J, Sheldon CA: Extravesical common sheath detrusorrhaphy (ureteroneocystotomy) and reflux in duplicated collecting systems. *J Urol* 167(1):288–90, 2002.

Minevich E, Wacksman J, Lewis AG, Sheldon CA: Incidence of contralateral vesicoureteral reflux following unilateral extravesical detrusorrhaphy (ureteroneocystostomy). *J Urol* 159:2126, 1998.

Mollard P, Braun P: Primary ureterocalycostomy for severe hydronephrosis in children. *J Pediatr Surg* 15:87, 1980.

Moore EV, Weber R, Woodward ER, et al: Isolated ileal loops for ureteral repair. *Surg Gynecol Obstet* 102:87, 1956.

Nesbit RM: Elliptical anastomosis and urologic surgery. *Ann Surg* 130:796, 1949.

Neuwirt K: Implantation of the ureter into the lower calyx of the renal pelvis. In: *VII Congrés de la Société Internationale d'Urologie*, Part 2, 1947, p 253.

Noe HN: The risk and risk factors of contralateral reflux following repair of simple unilateral primary reflux. *J Urol* 160:849, 1998.

Noe H: The role of dysfunctional voiding in failure or complication of ureteral reimplantation for primary reflux. *J Urol* 134:1172, 1985.

Ockerblad N: Reimplantation of the ureter into the bladder by a flap method. *J Urol* 57:845, 1947.

O'Donnell B, Puri P: Treatment of vesicoureteral reflux by endoscopic injection of Teflon. *Br Med J* 148:7, 1984.

Okamura K, Yamada Y, Tsuji Y: Endoscopic trigonoplasty in pediatric patients with primary vesicoureteral reflux: preliminary report. *J Urol* 156:198, 1996.

Paquin AJ Jr: Ureterovesical anastomosis: the description and evaluation of a technique. *J Urol* 82:573, 1959.

Perez-Brayfield M, Kirsch AJ, Hensle TW, et al: Endoscopic treatment with dextranomer/hyaluronic acid for complex cases of vesicoureteral reflux. *J Urol* 172(4 Pt 2):1614–6, 2004.

Peters CA: Robotically assisted surgery in pediatric urology. *Urol Clin North Am* 31(4):743–52, 2004.

Petit T, Ravasse P, Delmas P: Does endoscopic incision of ureteroceles reduce the indications for partial nephrectomy? *BJU Int* 83:675, 1999.

Pfister C, Ravasse P, Barret E, et al: The value of endoscopic treatment of ureteroceles during the neonatal period. *J Urol* 159:1006, 1998.

Pohl HG, Joyce GF, Wise M, Cilento BG Jr: Vesicoureteral reflux and ureteroceles. *J Urol* 177(5):1659–66, 2007.

Politano VA, Leadbetter WF: An operative technique for the correction of ureteric reflux. *J Urol* 79:932, 1958.

Prout GR Jr, Stuart WT, Witus WS: Utilization of ileal segments to substitute for extensive ureteral loss. *J Urol* 90:541, 1963.

Puri P: Ten-year experience with subureteric Teflon (polytetrafluoroethylene) injection (STING) in the treatment of vesico-ureteric reflux. *Br J Urol* 75:126, 1995.

Puri P, Chertin B, Velayudham M, et al: Treatment of vesicoureteral reflux by endoscopic injection of dextranomer/hyaluronic acid copolymer: preliminary results. *J Urol* 170 (4 Pt 2):1541–4, 2003.

Puri P, Pirker M, Mohanan N, et al: Subureteral dextranomer/hyaluronic acid injection as first line treatment in the management of high grade vesicoureteral reflux. *J Urol* 176(4 Pt 2):1856–9, 2006.

Putman S, Wicher C, Wayment R, et al: Unilateral extravesical ureteral reimplantation in children performed on an outpatient basis. *J Urol* 174(5):1987–9, 2005.

Quilan D, O'Donnell B: Unilateral ureteric reimplantation for primary vesicoureteric reflux in children. *Br J Urol* 57:406, 1985.

Raboy A, Fergli GS, Iofreda R, Albert PS: Laparoscopic ureterolithotomy. *Urology* 39:223, 1992.

Reha WC, Gibbons MD: Neonatal ascites and ureteral valves. *Urology* 33:468, 1989.

Reid R, Schneider K, Fruchtman B: Closure of the bladder neck in patients undergoing continent vesicostomy for urinary incontinence. *J Urol* 120:40, 1978.

Reinberg Y, Aliabadi H, Johnson P, et al: Congenital ureteral valves in children: case report and review of the literature. *J Pediatr Surg* 22:379, 1987.

Retik AB, McEvoy JP, Bauer SB: Megaureters in children. *Urology* 11:231, 1978.

Riccabona JOM, Lusuardi I, Bartsch G, Radmayr C: Prospective comparison and 1-year follow-up of single endoscopic subureteral polydimethylsiloxane versus dextranomer/hyaluronic acid copolymer injection for treatment of vesicoureteral reflux in children. *Urology* 60:894, 2002.

Rickwood AMK, Reiner I, Jones M, Pournaras C: Current management of duplex-system ureteroceles: experience with 41 patients. *Br J Urol* 70:196, 1992.

Roberts WW, Cadeddu JA, Micali S, et al: Ureteral stricture formation after removal of impacted calculi. *J Urol* 159:723, 1998.

Ruano-Gil D, Coca-Payeras A, Tejedo-Mateu A: Obstruction and normal recanalization of the ureter in the human embryo: its relation to congenital ureteric obstruction. *Eur Urol* 1:287, 1975.

Sant GR, Barbalias GA, Klauber GT: Congenital ureteral valves: an abnormality of ureteral embryogenesis? *J Urol* 133:427, 1985.

Scherz HC, Kaplan GW, Packer MG, Brock WA: Ectopic ureteroceles: surgical management with preservation of continence: review of 60 cases. *J Urol* 142:538, 1989.

Schulman CC, Gregoir W: Ureteric duplication. In: Eckstein HB, Hohenfellner R, Williams DI (Eds): *Surgical Pediatric Urology.* Stuttgart and Philadelphia, Georg Thieme Verlag, 1977, p 244.

Schwarz R, Stephens FD: The persisting mesonephric duct: high junction of vas deferens and ureter. *J Urol* 120:592, 1978.

Shankar KR, Vishwanath N, Rickwood AMK: Outcome of patients with prenatally detected duplex system ureteroceles: natural history of those managed expectantly. *J Urol* 165:1226, 2001.

Shapiro SR, Peckler MS, Johnston JH: Transureteroureterostomy for urinary diversion in children. *Urology* 8:35, 1976.

Shehata R: A comparative study of the urinary bladder and the intramural portion of the ureter. *Acta Anat* 98:380, 1977.

Shekarriz B, Upadhyay J, Fleming P, et al: Long-term outcome based on the initial surgical approach to ureterocele. *J Urol* 162:1072, 1999.

Shokeir AA, El-Hammady S: Extravesical seromuscular tunnel: a new technique of ureteroneocystotomy. *BJU Int* 82:749, 1998.

Shokeir AA, Nijman RJM: Primary megaureter: current trends in diagnosis and treatment. *BJU Int* 86:861, 2000.

Simforoosh N, Tabibi A, Basiri A, et al: Is ureteral reimplantation necessary during augmentation cystoplasty in patients with neurogenic bladder and vesicoureteral reflux? *J Urol* 168(4 Pt 1):1439–41, 2002.

Slaton JW, Kropp KA: Proximal ureteral stent migration: an avoidable complication. *J Urol* 155:58, 1996.

Smith AD: Management of iatrogenic ureteral strictures after urological procedures. *J Urol* 140:1372, 1988.

Smith C, Gosalbez R, Parrott TS, et al: Transurethral puncture of ectopic ureteroceles in neonates and infants. *J Urol* 152:2110, 1994.

Smith JA Jr, Lee RE, Middleton RG: Ventriculoureteral shunt for hydrocephalus without nephrectomy. *J Urol* 123:224, 1980.

Sparr KE, Balcom AH, Mesrobian H-G O: Incidence and natural history of contralateral vesicoureteral reflux in patients presenting with unilateral disease. *J Urol* 160:1023, 1998.

Starr A: Ureteral plication: a new concept in ureteral tailoring for megaureter. *Invest Urol* 17:153, 1979.

Stenberg A, Larsson E, Lackgren G: Endoscopic treatment with dextranomer-hyaluronic acid for vesicoureteral reflux: histological findings. *J Urol* 169(3):1109–13, 2003.

Stephens FD: Treatment of megaureters by multiple micturition. *Aust N Z J Surg* 27:130, 1957.

Stephens FD: The vesicoureteral hiatus and para ureteral diverticula. *J Urol* 121:786, 1979.

Stephens FD, Lenaghan D: The anatomical basis and dynamics of vesicoureteral reflux. *J Urol* 87:669, 1962.

Strup SE, Sindelar WF, Walther MM: The use of transureteroureterostomy in the management of complex ureteral problems. *J Urol* 156:1572, 1996.

Tanagho EA: A case against incorporation of bowel segments into the closed urinary system. *J Urol* 113:796, 1975.

Tanagho EA: Anatomy and management of ureteroceles. *J Urol* 107:729, 1972.

Tanagho EA: Embryologic basis for lower ureteral anomalies: a hypothesis. *Urology* 7:451, 1976.

Tanagho EA: Ureteral tailoring. *J Urol* 106:194, 1971.

Tanagho EA, Meyers FH, Smith DR: The trigone: anatomical and physiological considerations in relation to the ureterovesical junction. *J Urol* 100:623, 1968.

Tanagho EA, Pugh RCB: The anatomy and function of the ureterovesical junction. *Br J Urol* 35:151, 1963.

Thompson RH, Chen JJ, Pugach J, et al: Cessation of prophylactic antibiotics for managing persistent vesicourethra reflux. *J Urol* 166:1465, 2001.

Turner-Warwick R: Lower pole pyelocalycotomy, retrograde partial nephrectomy and ureterocalycostomy. *Br J Urol* 37:673, 1965.

Udall DA, Hodges CV, Pearse HM, Burns AB: Transuretero-ureterostomy: a neglected procedure. *J Urol* 109:817, 1973.

Upadhyay J, Bolduc S, Braga L, et al: Impact of prenatal diagnosis on the morbidity associated with ureterocele management. *J Urol* 167(6):2560–5, 2002.

Upadhyay J, Shekarriz B, Fleming P, et al: Ureteral reimplantation in infancy: evaluation of long-term voiding function. *J Urol* 162(3 Pt 2):1209–12, 1999.

Van Gool JD, Hjalmas K, Mobius T, et al: Historical clues to the complex of dysfunctional voiding, urinary tract infection and vesicoureteral reflux: The International Reflux Study in Children. *J Urol* 148:1699, 1992.

Vandersteen DR, Routh JC, Kirsch AJ, et al: Postoperative ureteral obstruction after subureteral injection of dextranomer/hyaluronic acid copolymer. *J Urol* 176(4 Pt 1):1593–5, 2996.

Wacksman J, Gilbert A, Sheldon CA: Results of the renewed extravesical reimplant for surgical correction of vesicoureteral reflux. *J Urol* 148:359, 1992.

Waldeyer W: Ureter-scheide. *Verh Anat Ges* 6:259, 1892.

Wallis MC, Khoury AE, Lorenzo AJ, et al: Outcome analysis of retroperitoneal laparoscopic heminephrectomy in children. *J Urol* 175(6):2277–80, 2006.

Weinstein AJ, Bauer SB, Retik AB, et al: The surgical management of megaureters in duplex systems: the efficacy of ureteral tapering and common sheath reimplantation. *J Urol* 139:328, 1988.

Wesolowski S: Corrective operative procedure after unsuccessful pelvi-ureteric plastic surgery. *Br J Urol* 43:679, 1971.

Wesolowski S: Ureterocalycostomy. *Eur Urol* 1:18, 1975.

Wickramasinghe SF, Stephens FD: Paraureteral diverticula: associated renal morphology and embryogenesis. *Invest Urol* 14:381, 1977.

Williams DI, Eckstein HB: Surgical treatment of reflux in children. *Br J Urol* 37:13, 1965.

Williams DI, Woodard JR: Problems in the management of ectopic ureteroceles. *J Urol* 92:635, 1964.

Woodhouse CRJ: Transureterostomy. In: Krane RJ, Siroky MB, Fitzpatrick JM: *Operative Urology: Surgical Skills*. New York, Edinburgh, London, and Philadelphia, Churchill Livingstone, 2000, pp 89–92.

Yeung CK, Liu KW, Ng WT, et al: Laparoscopy as the investigation and treatment for urinary incontinence caused by small "invisible" dysplastic kidneys with infrasphincteric ureteric ectopia. *BJU Int* 84:324, 1999.

Yu TJ: Extravesical diverticuloplasty for repair of a paraureteral diverticulum and the associated refluxing ureter. *J Urol* 168(3):1135–7, 2002.

Yucel S, Tarcan T, Simsek F: Durability of a single successful endoscopic polytetrafluoroethylene injection for primary vesicoureteral reflux: 14-year follow-up results. *J Urol* 178(1):265–8, 2007.

Zaontz MR, Maizels M, Sugar EC, Firlit CF: Detrusorrhaphy: extravesical ureteral advancement to correct vesicoureteral reflux in children. *J Urol* 138:947, 1987.

Section 6
Bladder

Abrahamsson A: Bladder dysfunction: an integral part of the ectopic ureterocele complex. *J Urol* 160:1468, 1998.

Abrams JS: *Abdominal Stomas: Indications, Operative Techniques and Patient Care.* Boston, Wright, 1984.

Adams JT: Z-stitch suture for inversion of appendiceal stump. *Surg Gynecol Obstet* 127:1320, 1968.

Adams MC, Mitchell ME, Rink RC: Gastrocystoplasty: an alternative solution to the problem of urological reconstruction in the severely compromised patient. *J Urol* 140:1152, 1988.

Admire AA, Greenfeld JI, Cosentino CM, et al: Repair of cloacal exstrophy, omphalocele, and gastroschisis using porcine small-intestinal submucosa or cadaveric skin homograft. *Plast Reconstr Surg* 112(4):1059–62, 2003.

Agarwal SK, Fisk NM: In utero therapy for lower urinary tract obstruction. *Prenat Diagn* 21:970, 2001.

Ahlering TE, Weinberg AC, Razor B: A comparative study of the ileal conduit, Kock pouch and modified Indiana pouch. *J Urol* 142:1193, 1989.

Albert DJ, Persky L: Conjoined end-to-end uretero-intestinal anastomosis. *J Urol* 105:201, 1971.

Albouy B, Grise P, Sambuis C, et al: Pediatric urinary incontinence: evaluation of bladder wall wraparound sling procedure. *J Urol* 177(2):716–9, 2007.

Alday ES, Goldsmith HS: Surgical technique for omental lengthening based on arterial anatomy. *Surg Gynecol Obstet* 135:103, 1972.

Allen TD: Vesicostomy for the temporary diversion of the urine in small children. *J Urol* 123:929, 1980.

Allen TD, Husman DS, Bucholz RW: Exstrophy of the bladder: primary closure after iliac osteotomies without external or internal fixation. *J Urol* 147:438, 1992.

Allen TD, Spence HM, Salyer KE: Reconstruction of the external genitalia in exstrophy of the bladder: preliminary communication. *J Urol* 11:830, 1974.

Althausen AF, Hagen-Cook K, Hendren WH III: Non-refluxing colon conduit: experience with 70 cases. *J Urol* 120:35, 1978.

Ambrose SS, O'Brien DP III: Surgical embryology of the exstrophy-epispadias complex. *Surg Clin North Am* 54:1379, 1974.

Anderl H, Jaske G, Marberger H: Reconstruction of abdominal wall and mons pubis in females with bladder exstrophy. *Urology* 22:247, 1983.

Ansell JS: Exstrophy and epispadias. In: Glenn JF (Ed): *Urologic Surgery*, 3rd ed. Philadelphia, J. B. Lippincott Company, 1983.

Ansell JS: Surgical treatment of exstrophy of bladder with emphasis on neonatal primary closure: personal experience with 28 consecutive cases treated at University of Washington Hospitals from 1962 to 1977: technique and results. *J Urol* 121:650, 1979.

Arai Y, Kawakita M, Terachi T, et al: Long-term follow-up of Kock and Indiana pouch procedures. *J Urol* 150:51, 1993.

Arap S, Giron AM: Complete reconstruction of bladder exstrophy: experimental program. *Urology* 7:413, 1976.

Arap S, Giron AM: Initial results of the complete reconstruction of bladder exstrophy. *Urol Clin North Am* 7:477, 1980.

Ariyoshi A, Fujisawa Y, Ohshima K: Catheterless cutaneous ureterostomy. *J Urol* 114:533, 1975.

Arnarson O, Straffon RA: Clinical experience with the ileal conduit in children. *J Urol* 102:768, 1969.

Ashken MH: An appliance-free ileocaecal urinary diversion: preliminary communication. *Br J Urol* 46:631, 1974.

Ashken MH: Stomas continent and incontinent. *Br J Urol* 59:203, 1987.

Ashken MH: *Urinary Diversion.* Berlin, Heidelberg, and New York, Springer-Verlag, 1982.

Atala A, Bauer SB, Hendren WH, Retik AB: The effect of gastric augmentation on bladder function. *J Urol* 149:1099, 1993.

Austin JC, Canning DA, Johnson MP, et al: Vesicoamniotic shunt in a female fetus with the prune belly syndrome. *J Urol* 166(6):2382, 2001.

Austin PF, Westney OL, Leng WW, et al: Advantages of rectus fascial slings for urinary incontinence in children with neuropathic bladders. *J Urol* 165(Pt 2):2369–71, 2001.

Avni EF, Matos C, Diard F, Schulman CC: Midline omphalocele anomalies in children: contribution of ultrasound imaging. *Urol Radiol* 10:189–94, 1988.

Bagley DH, Glazier W, Osias M, et al: Retroperitoneal drainage of uretero-intestinal conduits. *J Urol* 121:271, 1979.

Baird AD, Mathews RI, Gearhart JP: The use of combined bladder and epispadias repair in boys with classic bladder exstrophy: outcomes, complications and consequences. *J Urol* 174(4 Pt 1):1421–4, 2005.

Barrett DM, Furlow WL: The management of severe urinary incontinence in patients with myelodysplasia by implantation of the AS 791/792 urinary sphincter device. *J Urol* 128:484, 1982.

Barrett DM, Malek RS, Kelalis P: Observations on vesical diverticulum in childhood. *J Urol* 116:234, 1976.

Barrington JW, Fulford S, et al: Tumors in bladder remnants after augmentation enterocystoplasty. *J Urol* 157:482, 1997.

Barroso U Jr, Duel B, Barthold JS, González R: Orthotopic urethral substitution in female patients using the Mitrofanoff principle. *J Urol* 161(1):251–3, 1999.

Barry JM, Pitre TM, Hodges CV: Ureteroileourethrostomy: 16-year follow-up. *J Urol* 115:29, 1976.

Basmajian JV: The main arteries of the large intestine. *Surg Gynecol Obstet* 101:585, 1959.

Bau MO, Younes S, Aupy A, et al: The Malone antegrade colonic enema isolated or associated with urologic incontinence procedures: evaluation from patient point of view. *J Urol* 165:2399, 2001.

Bauer SB, Hendren WH, Kozakewich H, et al: Perforation of the augmented bladder. *J Urol* 148:699, 1992.

Bauer SB, Retik AB: Urachal anomalies and related umbilical disorders. *Urol Clin North Am* 5:195, 1978.

Beckley S, Wajsman W, Pontes JE, Murphy G: Transverse colon conduit: a method of urinary diversion after pelvic irradiation. *J Urol* 128:464, 1982.

Begg RC: The urachus and umbilical fistulae. *Surg Gynecol Obstet* 45:165, 1927.

Bejany DE, Politano VA: Stapled and nonstapled tapered distal ileum for construction of a continent colonic urinary reservoir. *J Urol* 140:491, 1988.

Beland G, Laberge I: Cutaneous transureterostomy in children. *J Urol* 114:588, 1975.

Bellinger MF: Ureterocystoplasty: a unique method for vesical augmentation in children. *J Urol* 149:811, 1993.

Bellinger MF: Ureterocystoplasty update. *World J Urol* 16:251, 1998.

Belman AB, King LR: Urinary tract abnormalities associated with imperforate anus. *J Urol* 108:823, 1972.

Benchekroun A: Continent caecal bladder. *Br J Urol* 54:505, 1982.

Benchekroun A: The ileocecal continent bladder. In: King LR, Stone AR, Webster GD (Eds): *Bladder Reconstruction and Continent Urinary Diversion.* Chicago, Mosby Year Book, 1991, p 324.

Benjamin JA, Tobin CE: Abnormalities of the kidneys, ureters, and perinephric fascia: anatomic and clinical study. *J Urol* 65:715, 1951.

Bennett RC, Duthie HL: The functional importance of the internal anal sphincter. *Br J Surg* 51:355, 1964.

Berglund B, Kock NG, Norlen L, Philipson BM: Volume capacity and pressure characteristics of the continent ileal reservoir used for urinary diversion. *J Urol* 137:29, 1987.

Biard JM, Johnson MP, Carr MC, Wilson RD, et al: Long-term outcomes in children treated by prenatal vesicoamniotic shunting for lower urinary tract obstruction. *Obstet Gynecol* 106(3):503–8, 2005.

Bissada NK: Characteristics and use of in situ appendix as continent catheterization stoma for continent urinary diversion in adults. *J Urol* 150:151, 1993.

Blichert-Toft M, Nielson OV: Congenital patent urachus and acquired variants. *Acta Chir Scand* 137:807, 1971.

Blocksom BH Jr: Bladder pouch for prolonged tubeless cystostomy. *J Urol* 78:398, 1957.

Bloom DA, Lieskovsky G, Rainwater G, et al: The Turnbull loop stoma. *J Urol* 129:715, 1983.

Bloom DA, Turner WRJ, Skinner DG: Urological stomas. In: Ehrlich RM (Ed): *Modern Techniques in Surgery: Urologic Surgery.* Mount Kisco, NY, Futura, 1981.

Bolduc S, Capolicchio G, Upadhyay J, et al: The fate of the upper urinary tract in exstrophy. *J Urol* 168(6):2579–82, 2002.

Borer JG, Gargollo PC, Hendren WH, et al: Early outcome following complete primary repair of bladder exstrophy in the newborn. *J Urol* 174(4 Pt 2):1674–8, 2005.

Borer JG, Gargollo PC, Kinnamon DD, et al: Bladder growth and development after complete primary repair of bladder exstrophy in the newborn with comparison to staged approach. *J Urol* 174(4 Pt 2):1553–7, 2005.

Borzyskowski M, Mundy E (Eds): *Neuropathic Bladder in Childhood.* New York, Cambridge University Press, 1991.

Boucher BJ: Sex differences in the fetal pelvis. *Am J Phys Anthropol* 15:581, 1957.

Boyce WH, Kroovand RL: The Boyce-Vest operation for exstrophy of the bladder: 35 years later. *Urol Clin North Am* 13:307, 1986.

Boyce WH, Vest SA: A new concept concerning treatment of exstrophy of the bladder. *J Urol* 67:503, 1952.

Bozkurt P, Kilic N, Kaya G, et al: The effects of intranasal midzolam on urodynamic studies in children. *Br J Urol* 78:282, 1996.

Braren V, Bishop MR: Laparoscopic retropubic autoaugmentation in children. *Urol Clin North Am* 25:533, 1998.

Bricker EM: Bladder substitution after pelvic evisceration. *Surg Clin North Am* 30:1511, 1950.

Bricker EM: The evolution of the ileal segment bladder substitution operation. *Am J Surg* 135:834, 1978.

Bricker EM: The technique of ileal segment bladder substitution. In: Meigs JV, Sturgis SH (Eds): *Progress in Gynecology,* vol 3. New York, Grune & Stratton, 1957.

Brock WA: Anorectal malformations: urologic implications. *Dial Ped Urol* 10:1, 1987.

Browne D: Congenital deformities of the anus and the rectum. *Arch Dis Child* 30:42, 1955.

Browning GG, Parks AG: A method and the results of loop colostomy. *Dis Colon Rectum* 26:223, 1983.

Bruce RB, Gonzales ET: Cutaneous vesicostomy: a useful form of temporary diversion in children. *J Urol* 123:927, 1980.

Bryniak SR, Bruce AW, Awad SA: Skin flap technique in formation of urinary conduit stoma. *Urology* 15:275, 1980.

Bukowski TP, Perlmutter AD: Reduction cystoplasty in the prune belly syndrome: a long-term follow-up. *J Urol* 152:2113, 1994.

Bukowski TP, Smith CA: Monfort abdominoplasty with neoumbilical modification. *J Urol* 164(5):1711–3, 2000.

Burbige KA, Hensle TW: The complications of urinary tract reconstruction. *J Urol* 136(Pt 2):292, 1986.

Burki T, Hamid R, Duffy P, et al: Long-term follow-up of patients after redo bladder neck reconstruction for bladder exstrophy complex. *J Urol* 176(3):1138–41, 2006.

Bystrom J: Early and later complications of ileal conduit urinary diversion. *Scand J Urol Nephrol* 12:233, 1978.

Cain MP, Casale AJ, King SJ, Rink RC: Appendicovesicostomy and newer alternatives for the Mitrofanoff procedure: results in the last 100 patients at Riley Children's Hospital. *J Urol* 162(5):1749–52, 1999.

Cain MP, Casale AJ, Rink RC: Initial experience using a catheterizable ileovesicostomy (Monti procedure) in children. *Urology* 52:870, 1998.

Cain MP, Rink RC, Yerkes EB, et al: Long-term follow-up and outcome of continent catheterizable vesicocostomy using the Rink modification. *J Urol* 168(6):2583–5, 2002.

Caione P, Capozza N, Lais A, Matarazzo E: Periurethral muscle complex reassembly for exstrophy-epispadias repair. *J Urol* 164(6):2062–6, 2000.

Canales BK, Fung LC, Elliott SP: Miniature intravesical urethral lengthening procedure for treatment of pediatric neurogenic urinary incontinence. *J Urol* 176(6 Pt 1):2663–6, 2006.

Capolicchio G, McLorie GA, Farhat W, et al: A population-based analysis of continence outcomes and bladder exstrophy. *J Urol* 165:2418, 2001.

Carney M, Richard F, Botto H: Bladder replacement by ileocystoplasty. In: King LR, Stone AR, Webster GD (Eds): *Bladder Reconstruction and Continent Urinary Diversion*. Chicago, Year Book Medical Publishers, 1987.

Cartwright PC, Snow BW: Autoaugmentation cystoplasty. In: Dewan P, Mitchell ME (Eds): *Bladder Augmentation*. London, Arnold Publishers, 2000, p 83.

Cartwright PC, Snow BW: Bladder augmentation: partial detrusor excision to augment the bladder without the use of bowel. *J Urol* 142:1050, 1989.

Casale AJ: A long continent ileovesicostomy using a single piece of bowel. *J Urol* 162(5):1743–5, 1999.

Casale AJ, Metcalfe PD, Kaefer MA, et al: Total continence reconstruction: a comparison to staged reconstruction of neuropathic bowel and bladder. *J Urol* 176(4 Pt 2):1712–5, 2006.

Castellan M, Gosalbez R, Labbie A, et al: Bladder neck sling for treatment of neurogenic incontinence in children with augmentation cystoplasty: long-term follow-up. *J Urol* 173(6):2128–31, 2005.

Castellan MA, Gosalbez R Jr, Labbie A, Monti PR: Clinical applications of the Monti procedure as a continent catheterizable stoma. *Urology* 54:152, 1999.

Castera R, Podesta MI, Ruarte A, et al: 10-year experience with artificial urinary sphincter in children and adolescents. *J Urol* 165:2373, 2001.

Cauldwell EW, Anson BJ: The visceral branches of the abdominal aorta: topographical relationships. *Am J Anat* 73:27, 1943.

Chadwick Plaire J, Snodgrass WT, Grady RW, Mitchell ME: Long-term follow-up of the hematuria-dysuria syndrome. *J Urol* 164(3 Pt 2):921–3, 2000.

Chan SL, Ankenman GJ, Wright JE, McLoughlin MG: Cecocystoplasty in the surgical management of the small contracted bladder. *J Urol* 124:338, 1980.

Chandna S, Bruce J, Dickson A, Gough D: The Whitaker hook in the treatment of posterior urethral valves. *Br J Urol* 78:783, 1996.

Chevrel JP, Gueraud JP: Arteries of the terminal ileum: diaphanization study and surgical applications. *Anat Clin* 1:95, 1979.

Chin-Peuckert L, Pippi Salle JL: A modified biofeedback program for children with detrusor-sphincter dyssynergia: 5-year experience. *J Urol* 166:1470, 2001.

Churchill BM, Aliabadi H, Landau EH, et al: Ureteral bladder augmentation. *J Urol* 150:716, 1993.

Churchill BM, Jayanthi VR, Landau EH, et al: Ureterocystoplasty: importance of the proximal blood supply. *J Urol* 154:197, 1995.

Clark SS: Electrolyte disturbance associated with jejunal conduit. *J Urol* 112:42, 1974.

Clark T, Pope JC 4th, Adams C, et al: Factors that influence outcomes of the Mitrofanoff and Malone antegrade continence enema reconstructive procedures in children. *J Urol* 168(4 Pt 1):1537–40, 2002.

Coffey RC: Transplantation of the ureters into the large intestine in the absence of the functioning urinary bladder. *Surg Gynecol Obstet* 32:383, 1921.

Cohen JS, Harbach LB, Kaplan GW: Cutaneous vesicostomy for temporary diversion in infants with neurogenic bladder dysfunction. *J Urol* 119:120, 1978.

Cole EE, Adams MC, Brock JW 3rd, Pope JC 4th: Outcome of continence procedures in the pediatric patient: a single institutional experience. *J Urol* 170(2 Pt 1):560–3, 2003.

Colodny AJ: An improved surgical technique for intravesical resection of bladder diverticulum. *Br J Urol* 47:399, 1975.

Colvert JR 3rd, Kropp BP, Cheng EY, et al: The use of small intestinal submucosa as an off-the-shelf urethral sling material for pediatric urinary incontinence. *J Urol* 168(4 Pt 2):1872–5, 2002.

Comer MT, Thomas DF, et al: Construction of the urinary bladder by auto-augmentation, enterocystoplasty, and composite enterocystoplasty. *Adv Exp Med Biol* 462:43, 1999.

Connar RG, Sealy WC: Gastrostomy and its complications. *Am Surg* 138:732, 1979.

Cook AJ, Farhat WA, Cartwright LM, et al: Simplified mons plasty: a new technique to improve cosmesis in females with the exstrophy-epispadias complex. *J Urol* 173(6):2117–20, 2005.

Coppa GF, Eng K, Gouge TH, et al: Parenteral and oral antibiotics in elective colon and rectal surgery: a prospective, randomized trial. *Am J Surg* 145:62–65, 1983.

Cordonnier JJ: Ureterosigmoid anastomosis. *J Urol* 63:275, 1950.

Cordonnier JJ: Urinary diversion. *Arch Surg* 71:818, 1955.

Courtney H: Anatomy of the pelvic diaphragm and anorectal musculature as related to sphincter preservation in anorectal surgery. *Am J Surg* 79:155, 1950.

Couvelaire R: "La petite vessie" des tuberculeaux genitourinaires: essae de classification place et varidentes des cysto-intestino-plasties. *J Urol* 56:381, 1950.

Creevy CD: Facts about ureterosigmoidostomy. *JAMA* 151:120, 1953.

Dager JE, Sanford EJ, Rohner TJ Jr: Complications of the nonrefluxing colon conduit. *J Urol* 123:585, 1980.

Daniel O, Shackman R: The blood supply of the human ureter in relation to ureterocolic anastomosis. *Br J Urol* 24:334, 1952.

David FDR: A new surgical procedure for revision of the ileal conduit stoma in children. *J Urol* 115:188, 1976.

Davidsson T, Barker SB, Mansson W: Tapering of intussuscepted ileal nipple valve or ileocecal valve to correct secondary incontinence in patients with urinary reservoir. *J Urol* 147:144, 1992.

DeCambre M, Casale P, Grady R, et al: Modified bladder neck reconstruction in patients with incontinence after staged exstrophy/epispadias closures. *J Urol* 176(1):288–91, 2006.

DeKernion JB, DenBesten L, Kaufman JJ, Ehrlich R: The Kock pouch as a urinary reservoir: pitfalls and perspectives. *Am J Surg* 150:83, 1985.

Deklerk JN, Lambrechts W, Viljoen I: The bowel as substitute for the bladder. *J Urol* 121:22, 1979.

Demirbilek S, Shekarriz B, Upadhyay J, et al: Complications of bladder augmentation requiring reoperation. *Urology* 55:123–8, 2000.

DeVries PA, Peña A: Posterior sagittal anorectoplasty. *J Pediatr Surg* 17:638, 1982.

Dewan P, Anderson P: Ureterocystoplasty: the latest developments. *BJU Int* 88:744, 2001.

Dewan P, Mitchell ME (Eds): *Bladder Augmentation*. London, Arnold Publishers, 2000.

Diamond DA, Ransley PG: Bladder neck reconstruction with omentum, silicone and augmentation cystoplasty: a preliminary report. *J Urol* 136:252, 1986.

Dodson JL, Surer I, Baker LA, et al: The newborn exstrophy bladder inadequate for primary closure: evaluation, management and outcome. *J Urol* 165:1656, 2001.

Donnahoo KK, Rink RC, Cain MP, Casale AJ: The Young-Dees-Leadbetter bladder neck repair for neurogenic incontinence. *J Urol* 161(6):1946–9, 1999.

Dounis A, Abel BJ, Gow JG: Cecocystoplasty for bladder augmentation. *J Urol* 123:164, 1980.

Dretler SP: The pathogenesis of urinary tract calculi occurring after ileal conduit diversion: I. Clinical study. II. Conduit study. III. Prevention. *J Urol* 109:204, 1973.

Dretler SP, Hendren WH, Leadbetter WF: Urinary tract reconstruction following ileal conduit diversion. *J Urol* 109:217, 1973.

Droes JTPM: Observations on the musculature of the urinary bladder and the urethra in the human foetus. *Br J Urol* 46:179, 1974.

Duckett JW: Editorial comment in Van Savage JG et al: Outcome analysis of Mitrofanoff principle: applications using appendix and ureter to umbilical or lower quadrant stomal sites. *J Urol* 156:1794, 1996.

Duckett JW: Ureterosigmoidostomy: the pros and cons. *Dial Pediatr Urol* 5:4, 1982.

Duckett JW Jr: Cutaneous vesicostomy in childhood: the Blocksom technique. *Urol Clin North Am* 1:485, 1974.

Duckett JW Jr: Epispadias. *Urol Clin North Am* 5:107, 1978.

Duckett JW Jr: Use of paraexstrophy skin pedicle grafts for correction of exstrophy and epispadias repair. *Birth Defects* 13:175, 1977.

Duckett JW, Gazak JM: Complications of ureterosigmoidostomy. *Urol Clin North Am* 10:473, 1983.

Duckett JW, Lofti A-H: Appendicovesicostomy (and variations) in bladder reconstruction. *J Urol* 149:567, 1993.

Duckett JW, Snyder HM III: Use of the Mitrofanoff principle in urinary reconstruction. *World J Urol* 3:191, 1985; *Urol Clin North Am* 13:271, 1986.

Dwoskin JY: Management of the massively dilated urinary tract in infants by temporary diversion and single-stage reconstruction. *Urol Clin North Am* 1:515, 1974.

Dyber R, Jeter K, Lattimer JK: Comparison of intraluminal pressures in ileal and colon conduits in children. *J Urol* 108:477, 1972.

Eagle JR Jr, Barrett GS: Congenital deficiency of abdominal musculature with associated genitourinary abnormalities: a syndrome: report of nine cases. *Pediatrics* 6:721, 1950.

Eckstein HB: Cutaneous ureterostomy. *Proc R Soc Med* 56:749, 1963.

Edgerton MT, Gillenwater JY: A new surgical technique for phalloplasty in patients with exstrophy of the bladder. *Plast Reconstr Surg* 78:399, 1986.

Ehrlich RM, Lesavoy MA: Umbilicus preservation with total abdominal wall reconstruction in the prune belly syndrome. *Urology* 41:231, 1993.

Ehrlich RM, Lesavoy MA, Fine RN: Total abdominal reconstruction in the prune belly syndrome. *J Urol* 136:282, 1986.

Eiseman B, Bricker EM: Electrolyte absorption following bilateral ureteroenterostomy into an isolated intestinal segment. *Ann Surg* 136:761, 1952.

Ekman H, Jacobsson B, Kock N, Sundin T: The functional behavior of different types of intestinal urinary bladder substitutes. *Proc Cong Soc Int Urol* 11:213, 1964.

Elder JS, Longenecker R: Premedication with oral midzolam for voiding cystourethrography in children: safety and efficacy. *AJR Am J Roentgenol* 164:1229, 1995.

Elder JS, Snyder HM, Hulbert WC, Duckett JW: Perforation of the augmented bladder in patients undergoing clean intermittent catheterization. *J Urol* 140:1159, 1988.

El-Sherbiny MT, Hafez AT, Ghoneim MA: Complete repair of exstrophy: further experience with neonates and children after failed initial closure. *J Urol* 168(4 Pt 2):1692–4, 2002.

Emmett D, Noble MJ, Mebust WK: A comparison of end versus loop stomas for ileal conduit urinary diversion. *J Urol* 133:588, 1985.

Englemann UH, Light JK, Scott FB: Use of artificial urinary sphincter with lower urinary tract reconstruction and continent urinary diversion: clinical and experimental studies. In: King LR (Ed): *Bladder Reconstruction and Continent Urinary Diversion*. Chicago, Year Book Medical Publishers, 1986.

English SF, Pisters LL, McGuire EJ: The use of the appendix as a continent catheterizable stoma. *J Urol* 159:747, 1998.

Enhörning G, Miller ER, Hinman, F Jr: Urethral closure studied with cine-roentgenography and simultaneous bladder urethral pressure recording. *Surg Gynecol Obstet* 118:507, 1964.

Erich JB: Plastic repair of the female perineum in a case of exstrophy of the bladder. *Proc Staff Meet Mayo Clin* 34:235, 1959.

Esho J, Cass AS: Management of stomal encrustations in children. *J Urol* 108:797, 1972.

Fallat ME, Skoog SJ, Belman AB, et al: The prune belly syndrome: a comprehensive approach to management. *J Urol* 142:802, 1989.

Fallon B, Latini JM: Urinary diversion. *Urology Board Review Manual, Hospital Physician*. Vol 11, Pt 1, February 2003. (Good references.)

Fasth S, Hulten L: Loop ileostomy: a superior diverting stoma in colorectal surgery. *World J Surg* 8:401, 1984.

Faxén A, Kock NG, Sundin T: Long-term functional results after ileocystoplasty. *Scand J Urol Nephrol* 7:127, 1973.

Feneley RCL: The management of female incontinence by suprapubic catheterisation, with or without urethral closure. *Br J Urol* 55:203, 1983.

Feng WC, Casale P, Grady RW, et al: The ureter as a pedicle for construction of a ureteral urethra: the double tunnel. *J Urol* 172(3):1089–91, 2004.

Ferris DO, Odel HM: Electrolyte pattern of the blood after bilateral ureterosigmoidostomy. *JAMA* 142:634, 1950.

Filmer RB: Malignant tumors arising in bladder augmentations, and ileal and colon conduits. *Society for Pediatric Urology Newsletter*, Dec. 9, 1986.

Firlit CF, Sommer JT, Kaplan WE: Pediatric urinary undiversion. *J Urol* 123:748, 1980.

Fisch M, Wammack R, Müller SC, Hohenfellner R: The Mainz pouch II (sigma rectum pouch). *J Urol* 149:258, 1993.

Flinn RA, King LR, McDonald JH, et al: Cutaneous ureterostomy: an alternative urinary diversion. *J Urol* 105:358, 1971.

Flocks RH, Boldus R: The surgical treatment and prevention of urinary incontinence associated with disturbance of the internal sphincter mechanism. *J Urol* 109:279, 1973.

Fox M, Power RF, Bruce AW: Diverticulum of the bladder: presentation and evaluation of treatment of 115 cases. *Br J Urol* 34:286, 1962.

Frimberger D, Gearhart JP, Mathews R: Female exstrophy: failure of initial reconstruction and its implications for continence. *J Urol* 170(6 Pt 1):2428–31, 2003.

Gadacz TR, Kelly KA, Phillips SF: The continent ileal pouch: absorptive and motor features. *Gastroenterology* 72:1287, 1977.

Garcia VF, Bloom DA: Inversion appendectomy. *Urology* 28:142, 1986.

Gearhart JP: Complete repair of bladder exstrophy in the newborn: complications and management. *J Urol* 165: 2431, 2001.

Gearhart JP, Baird AD: The failed complete repair of bladder exstrophy: insights and outcomes. *J Urol* 174(4 Pt 2):1669–72, 2005.

Gearhart JP, Canning DA, Jeffs RD: Failed bladder neck reconstruction: options for management. *J Urol* 146:1082, 1991.

Gearhart JP, Mathews R, Taylor S, Jeffs RD: Combined bladder closure and epispadias repair in the reconstruction of bladder exstrophy. *J Urol* 160(3 Pt 2):1182–5, 1998.

Gearhart JP, Peppas DS, Jeffs RD: The failed exstrophy closure: strategy for management. *Br J Urol* 71:217, 1993.

Gecelter L: Transanorectal approach to the posterior urethra and bladder neck. *J Urol* 109:1011, 1973.

Gerharz EW, Kohl UN, Weingartner K, et al: Experience with the Mainz modification of ureterosigmoidostomy. *Br J Surg* 85(11):1512–6, 1998.

Gerharz EW, Riedmiller H, Woodhouse CR: Re: Strategies for reconstruction after unsuccessful or unsatisfactory primary treatment of patients with bladder exstrophy or incontinent epispadias. *J Urol* 162(5):1706–7, 1999.

Gerharz EW, Tassaque T, Pickard RS, et al: Transverse retubularized ileum: early clinical experience with a new second line Mitrofanoff tube. *J Urol* 159:525, 1998.

Gershbaum MD, Stock JA, Hanna MK: Gracilis muscle sling for select incontinent "bladder exstrophy cripples." *J Urol* 165(6 Pt 2):2422–4, 2001.

Gersuny R: Officielles protokoll der k.k. gesellshaft der Aerzte in Wien. *Wien Klin Wochenschr* 11:990, 1898. Cited in Foges.

Ghoneim MA, Kock NG, Lycke G, Shehab El-Din AB: An appliance-free sphincter-controlled bladder substitute: the urethral Kock pouch. *J Urol* 138:1150, 1987.

Ghoneim MA, Shehab-El-Din AB, Ashamallah AK, Gaballah MA: Evolution of the rectal bladder as a method for urinary diversion. *J Urol* 126:737, 1981.

Giertz G, Franksson C: Construction of a substitute bladder with preservation of urethral voiding after subtotal or total cystectomy. *Acta Clin Scand* 113:218, 1957.

Gil-Vernet JM: A new technique for surgical correction of vesicoureteral reflux. *J Urol* 131:456, 1984.

Gil-Vernet JM Jr: The ileocolic segment in urologic surgery. *J Urol* 94:418, 1965.

Gil-Vernet JW, Escarpenter JM, Perez-Trujillo G, Bonet Vic J: A functioning artificial bladder: results of 41 consecutive cases. *J Urol* 87:825, 1962.

Gilchrist RK, Merricks JW, Hamlin HH, et al: Construction of a substitute bladder and urethra. *Surg Gynecol Obstet* 90:752, 1950.

Gittes RF: Augmentation cystoplasty. In: Libertino J (Ed): *Reconstructive Surgery in Urology*. Philadelphia, W. B. Saunders Company, 1976.

Gittes RF: Carcinogenesis in ureterosigmoidostomy. *Urol Clin North Am* 13:201, 1986.

Goepel M, Sperling H, Stohrer M, et al: Management of neurogenic fecal incontinence in melodysplastic children by a modified continent appendiceal stoma and antegrade colonic enema. *Urology* 49:758, 1997.

Goldman HJ: A rapid, safe technique for removal of a large vesical diverticulum. *J Urol* 106:380, 1971.

Goligher JC, Leacock AG, Brossy JJ: The surgical anatomy of the anal canal. *Br J Surg* 43:51, 1955.

Goligher JC, Morris C, McAdam WAF, et al: A controlled trial of inverting versus everting suture in clinical large bowel surgery. *Br J Surg* 57:817, 1970.

Golomb J, Klutke CG, Raz S: Complications of bladder substitution and continent urinary diversion. *Urology* 34:329, 1989.

Gonsalbez R, Gousse A, Labbie A: Refashioned short bowel segments for construction of efferent catheterizable channels (Monti procedure): early clinical experience. *Pediatrics* 100:563, 1997; abstract 77.

Gonsalbez R Jr, Kim CO Jr: Ureterocystoplasty with preservation of ispsilateral renal function. *J Pediatr Surg* 31:970, 1996.

González R: Bladder augmentation with sigmoid or descending colon. In: Webster GD, Kirby R, King LR, Goldwasser B (Eds): *Reconstructive Urology*. Boston, Blackwell Scientific, 1992, p 443.

González R: Reconstruction of the female urethra to allow intermittent catheterization for neurogenic bladders and urogenital sinus anomalies. *J Urol* 133:478, 1985.

González R: Sigmoid cystoplasty. In: King LR, Stone AR, Webster GD (Eds): *Bladder Reconstruction and Continent Urinary Diversion*. Chicago, Mosby Year Book, 1991, p 88.

González R, Jednak R, Franc-Guimond J, Schimke C: Treating neuropathic incontinence in children with seromuscular colocystoplasty and an artificial urinary sphincter. *BJU Int* 90(9):909–11, 2002.

González R, Koleilat N, Austin C, et al: The artificial sphincter AS 800 in congenital urinary incontinence. *J Urol* 142:512, 1989.

González R, LaPointe S, Sheldon CA, Mauer SM: Undiversion in children with renal failure. *J Pediatr Surg* 19:632, 1984.

González R, Myers S, Franc-Guimond J, Piaggio L: Surgical treatment of neuropathic urinary incontinence in 2005. *J Pediatr Urol* 1(6):378–82, 2005.

González R, Sheldon CA: Artificial sphincters in children with neurogenic bladders: long-term results. *J Urol* 128:1270, 1982.

González R, Sidi AA: Preoperative prediction of continence after enterocystoplasty or undiversion in children with neurogenic bladder. *J Urol* 134:705, 1985.

Goodwin WE: Ileocystoplasty. In: Cooper P (Ed): *Craft of Surgery*. Boston, Little, Brown & Company, 1964, p 1139.

Goodwin WE, Harris AP, Kaufman JJ, Beal JM: Open, transcolonic ureterointestinal anastomosis: a new approach. *Surg Gynecol Obstet* 97:295, 1953.

Goodwin WE, Scardino PT: Ureterosigmoidostomy. *J Urol* 118:169, 1977.

Goodwin WE, Smith RB, Skinner DG (Eds): Complications of ureterosigmoidostomy. In: Smith RB, Skinner PD (Eds): *Complications of Urologic Surgery, Prevention and Management*. Philadelphia, W. B. Saunders Company, 1976, p 229.

Goodwin WE, Turner RD, Winter CC: Results of ileocystoplasty. *J Urol* 80:461, 1958.

Goodwin WE, Winter CC: Technique of sigmoidocystoplasty. *Surg Gynecol Obstet* 108:370, 1959.

Gorsch RV: *Perineopelvic Anatomy*. New York, Tilghman, 1941.

Gosling JA: The structure of the bladder and urethra in relation to function. *Urol Clin North Am* 6:31, 1979.

Gosling JA, Dixon JS, Humpherson JR: *Functional Anatomy of the Urinary Tract.* Baltimore, University Park Press, 1982.

Grady R, Carr MC, Mitchell ME: Complete primary closure of bladder exstrophy: epispadias and bladder exstrophy repair. *Urol Clin North Am* 26:95, 1999.

Grady RW, Mitchell ME: Complete primary repair of exstrophy surgical technique. *Urol Clin North Am* 27(3):569–78, xi, 2000.

Green D, Mitcheson HD, McGuire EJ: Management of the bladder by augmentation ileocecocystoplasty. *J Urol* 130:133, 1981.

Griffiths DM, Malone PS: The Malone antegrade continence enema. *J Pediatr Surg* 30:68, 1995.

Gruenwald P: The relation of the growing Müllerian duct to the Wolffian duct and its importance for the genesis of malformations. *Anat Rec* 81:1, 1941.

Grunberger I, Catanese A, Hanna MK: Total replacement of bladder and urethra by cecum and appendix in bladder exstrophy. *Urology* 6:497, 1986.

Gugenheim JJ, Gonzales ET Jr, Roth DR, Montagnino BA: Bilateral posterior pelvic resection osteotomies in patients with exstrophy of the bladder. *Clin Orthop Relat Res* (364): 70–5, 1999.

Gundeti MS, Godbole PP, Wilcox DT: Is bowel preparation required before cystoplasty in children? *J Urol* 176(4 Pt 1): 1574–6, 2006.

Hafez AT, El-Sherbiny MT: Complete repair of bladder exstrophy: management of resultant hypospadias. *J Urol* 173(3):958–61, 2005.

Hafez AT, Elsherbiny MT, Dawaba MS, et al: Long-term outcome analysis of low pressure rectal reservoir in 33 children with bladder exstrophy. *J Urol* 165:2414, 2001.

Hafez AT, Elsherbiny MT: Ghoneim MA: Complete repair of bladder exstrophy: preliminary experience with neonates and children with failed initial closure. *J Urol* 162(5):1749–52, 1999; 165(6 Pt 2):2428–30, 2001.

Hafez AT, McLorie G, Bagli D, Khoury A: A single-centre long-term outcome analysis of artificial urinary sphincter placement in children. *BJU Int* 89:82, 2003.

Hammond G, Iglesias L, Davis JE: The urachus, its anatomy and associated fasciae. *Anat Rec* 80:271, 1941.

Hammouda HM: Results of complete penile disassembly for epispadias repair in 42 patients. *J Urol* 170(5):1963–5, 2003.

Hanna MK: Reconstruction of umbilicus during functional closure of bladder exstrophy. *Urology* 27:340, 1986.

Hanna MK, Richter F, Stock JA: Salvage continent vesicostomy after enterocystoplasty in the absence of the appendix. *J Urol* 162(3 Pt 1):826–8, 1999.

Harris CF, Cooper CS, Hutcheson JC, Snyder HM 3rd: Appendicovesicostomy: the Mitrofanoff procedure: a 15-year perspective. *J Urol* 163(6):1922–6, 2000.

Harrison MR, Glick PL, Nakayama DL, et al: Loop colon rectovaginoplasty for high cloacal anomaly. *J Pediatr Surg* 18:885, 1983.

Hartmann RE, Egghart G, Frohneberg D, Miller K: The ileal neobladder. *J Urol* 139:39, 1988.

Hasan ST, Marshall C, Neal DE: Continent urinary diversion using the Mitrofanoff principle. *Br J Urol* 74:454, 1994.

Hautmann RE, Egghart G, Frohneberg D, Miller K: The ileal neobladder. *J Urol* 139:39, 1988.

Hautmann RE, Miller K, Steiner U, Wenderoth U: The ileal neobladder: 6 years of experience with more than 200 patients. *J Urol* 150:40, 1993.

Hawley PR, Hunt TK, Dunphy JE: Etiology of colonic anastomotic leaks. *Proc R Soc Med* 63:28, 1970.

Hays DM, Powell TO: Various intestinal segments utilized for bladder enlargement in pediatric patients with reference to the management of exstrophy. *Surgery* 47:999, 1960.

Heitz-Boyer M, Hovelacque A: Création a une nouvelle vessie et un nouvel uretre. *J d'Urol* 1:237, 1912.

Hendren WH: Cloacal malformations: experience with 105 cases. *J Pediatr Surg* 27:890, 1992.

Hendren WH: Complications of ureterostomy. *J Urol* 120:269, 1978.

Hendren WH: Exstrophy of the bladder: an alternative method of management. *J Urol* 115:195, 1976.

Hendren WH: Exstrophy of the bladder. *Birth Defects* 13:207, 1977.

Hendren WH: Further experience in reconstructive surgery for cloacal anomalies. *J Pediatr Surg* 17:695, 1982.

Hendren WH: Ileal nipple for continence in cloacal exstrophy. *J Urol* 148:372, 1992.

Hendren WH: Non-refluxing colon conduit for temporary or permanent urinary diversion in children. *J Pediatr Surg* 10:381, 1975.

Hendren WH: Reconstruction of previously diverted urinary tracts in children. *J Pediatr Surg* 8:135, 1973.

Hendren WH: Repair of cloacal anomalies: current techniques. *J Pediatr Surg* 21:1159, 1986.

Hendren WH: Some alternatives to urinary diversion in children. *J Urol* 119:652, 1978.

Hendren WH: Surgical management of urogenital sinus abnormalities. *J Pediatr Surg* 12:339, 1977.

Hendren WH: Ureterocolic diversion of urine: management of some difficult problems. *J Urol* 129:719, 1983.

Hendren WH: Urinary diversion and undiversion in children. *Surg Clin North Am* 56:425, 1976.

Hendren WH: Urinary tract re-functionalization after long-term diversion: a 20-year experience with 177 patients. *Ann Surg* 212:478, 1990; discussion 494.

Hendren WH: Urinary tract refunctionalization after prior diversion in children. *Ann Surg* 180:494, 1974.

Hendren WH: Urinary undiversion and augmentation cystoplasty. In: Kelalis PP, King LR, Belman AB (Eds): *Clinical Pediatric Urology*, 2nd ed, vol 1. Philadelphia, W. B. Saunders Company, 1985, p 620.

Hendren WH, Hendren RB: Bladder augmentation: experience with 129 children and young adults. *J Urol* 144:445, 1990; discussion 460.

Hendren WH, Radopoulous D: Complications of ileal loop and colon conduit urinary diversion. *Urol Clin North Am* 10:451, 1983.

Hensle TW, Burbige KA: Bladder replacement in children and young adults. *J Urol* 133:1004, 1985.

Hensle TW, Connor JP, Burbige KA: Continent urinary diversion in childhood. *J Urol* 143:981, 1990.

Hensle TW, Dean GE: Complications of urinary tract reconstruction. *Urol Clin North Am* 18:755, 1991.

Hensle TW, Kirsch AJ, Kennedy WA, Reiley EA: Bladder neck closure in association with continent urinary diversion. *J Urol* 154:883, 1995.

Hensle TW, Reiley EA, Chang DT: The Malone antegrade continence enema procedure in the management of patients with spina bifida. *J Am Coll Surg* 186:669, 1998.

Herndon CD, Rink RC, Shaw MB, et al: The Indiana experience with artificial urinary sphincters in children and young adults. *J Urol* 169(2):650–4, 2003.

Herschorn S, Hewitt RJ: Patient perspective of long-term outcome of augmentation cystoplasty for neurogenic bladder. *Urology* 52:672, 1998.

Hinman F Jr: Functional classification of conduits for continent diversion. *J Urol* 144:27, 1990.

Hinman F Jr: The Garage Door Syndrome. *Neurourol Urodynamics* 5:515, 1986.

Hinman F Jr: Leakage and reflux in uretero-intestinal anastomosis: I. The free peritoneal graft. *J Urol* 70:419, 1953.

Hinman F Jr: The non-neurogenic neurogenic bladder (the Hinman syndrome): fifteen years later. *J Urol* 136:769, 1986.

Hinman F Jr: Obstruction to voiding. In: Resnick MI (Ed): *Current Therapy in Genitourinary Surgery.* Hamilton, Ontario: B. C. Decker, 1987.

Hinman F Jr: Overview: the choice between ureterosigmoidostomy with perineal (Gersuny, Heitz-Boyer) or abdominal (Mauclaire) colostomy. In: Whitehead ED, Leiter E (Eds): *Current Operative Urology,* 2nd ed. Philadelphia, Harper and Row, 1984, p 783.

Hinman F Jr: Pascal, Laplace and a length of bowel. *J d'Urol* 95:11, 1989.

Hinman F Jr: Patent urachus and urachal cysts. In: Gellis SS, Kogan BM (Eds): *Current Pediatric Therapy,* 12th ed. Philadelphia, W. B. Saunders Company, 1986, p 391.

Hinman F Jr: Reservoirs and continent conduits. *Int Urogynecol* 3:208, 1992.

Hinman F Jr: Selection of intestinal segments for bladder substitution: physical and physiological characteristics. *J Urol* 139:519, 1988.

Hinman F Jr: Surgical disorders of the bladder and umbilicus of urachal origin. *Surg Gynecol Obstet* 113:605, 1961.

Hinman F Jr: The technique of the Gersuny operation (ureterosigmoidostomy with perineal colostomy) in vesical exstrophy. *J Urol* 80:126, 1959.

Hinman F Jr: Ureteral implantation: II. Clinical results from a method of open submucosal anastomosis. *J Urol* 64:567, 1950.

Hinman F Jr: Urinary conduction versus storage by isolated ileal segment. In: *Proceedings of the 11th Congress of the International Society of Urology,* Stockholm, June 25–30, 1958, p 37.

Hinman F Jr: Urologic aspects of alternating urachal sinus. *Am J Surg* 102:339, 1961.

Hinman F, Weyrauch HM: A critical study of the different principles of surgery which have been used in uretero-intestinal implantation. *Int Abstracts Med* 64:313, 1937.

Hinman F Jr, Baumann FW: Complications of vesicoureteral operations from incoordination of micturition. *J Urol* 116:638, 1976.

Hinman F Jr, Baumann FW: Vesical and ureteral damage from voiding dysfunction in boys without neurogenic or obstructive disease. *J Urol* 109:727, 1973.

Hinman F Jr, Hinman F Sr: Ureteral implantation: I. Experiments on the surgical principles involved in an open submucosal method of ureterointestinal anastomosis. *J Urol* 64:457, 1950.

Hinman F Jr, Oppenheimer R: Functional characteristics of the ileal segment as a valve. *J Urol* 80:448, 1958.

Hodges CV: Surgical anatomy of the urinary bladder and pelvic ureter. *Surg Clin North Am* 44:1327, 1964.

Hoebeke P, Van Laecke E, Van Camp C, et al: One thousand video-urodynamic studies in children with non-neurogenic bladder sphincter dysfunction. *Br J Urol Int* 87: 575, 2001.

Hohenfellner R: Ureterosigmoidostomy. In: Eckstein HB, Hohenfellner R, Williams DL (Eds): *Surgical Pediatric Urology.* Stuttgart, Thieme, 1977.

Hollowell JG, Ransley PG: Surgical management of incontinence in bladder exstrophy. *Br J Urol* 68:543, 1991.

Holmes N, Harrison MR, Baskin LS: Fetal surgery for posterior urethral valves: long-term postnatal outcomes. *Pediatrics* 108(1):E7, 2001.

Holmes NM, Kogan BA, Baskin LS: Placement of artificial urinary sphincter in children and simultaneous gastrocystoplasty. *J Urol* 165(6 Pt 2):2366–8, 2001.

Howell C, Caldamone A, Snyder H, et al: Optimal management of cloacal exstrophy. *J Pediatr Surg* 18:365, 1983.

Hurwitz RS, Manzoni GAM, Ransley PG, Stephens FD: Cloacal exstrophy: a report of 34 cases. *J Urol* 138:1060, 1987.

Hurwitz RS, Woodhouse CRJ, Ransley P: The anatomical course of the neurovascular bundles in epispadias. *J Urol* 136:68, 1986.

Husmann DA, Gearhart JP: Loss of the penile glans and/or corpora following primary repair of bladder exstrophy using the complete penile disassembly technique. *J Urol* 172(4 Pt 2):1696–700, 2004.

Husmann DA, McLorie GA, Churchill BM: Closure of the exstrophic bladder: an evaluation of the factors leading to its success and its importance in urinary continence. *J Urol* 142:522, 1989.

Husmann DA, Snodgrass WT, Koyle MA, et al: Ureterocystoplasty: indications for a successful augmentation. *J Urol* 171(1): 376–80, 2004. Erratum in: *J Urol* 171(3):1247, 2004.

Husmann OA, Cain MP: Fecal and urinary continence after ileal cecal cystoplasty for the neurogenic bladder. *J Urol* 165(3):922–5, 2001.

Hutcheson JC, Cooper CS, Canning DA, et al: The use of vesicostomy as permanent urinary diversion in the child with myelomeningocele. *J Urol* 166(6):2351–3, 2001.

Ikeguchi EF, Stifelman MD, Hensle TW: Ureteral tissue expansion for bladder augmentation. *J Urol* 159:1665, 1998.

Issa MM, Oesterling JE, Canning DA, Jeffs RD: A new technique of using the in situ appendix as a catheterizable stoma for continent urinary reservoirs. *J Urol* 141:1385, 1989.

Jacobs A, Stirling WB: The late results of ureterocolic anastomoses. *Br J Urol* 24:259, 1952.

Jaffe BM, Bricker EM, Butcher HR Jr: Surgical complications of ileal segment urinary diversion. *Ann Surg* 167:367, 1968.

Jaramillo D, Lebowitz RL, Hendren WH: The cloacal malformation: radiologic findings and imaging recommendations. *Radiology* 177:441, 1990.

Jayanthi VR, Churchill BM, McLorie GA, Khoury, AF: Concomitant bladder neck closure and Mitrofanoff diversion for the management of intractable urinary incontinence. *J Urol* 154:886, 1985.

Jayanthi VR, Koff SA: Long-term outcome of transurethral puncture of ectopic ureteroceles: initial success and late problems. *J Urol* 162:1077, 1999.

Jednak R, Schimke CM, Barroso U Jr, et al: Further experience with seromuscular colocystoplasty lined with urothelium. *J Urol* 164(6):2045–9, 2000.

Jeffs RD: Exstrophy. In: Harrison JH, Gittes RI, Perlmutter AD, et al. (Eds): *Campbell's Urology,* vol 2. Philadelphia, W. B. Saunders Company, 1979, p 1672.

Jeffs RD: Exstrophy and cloacal exstrophy: congenital anomalies of the lower genitourinary tract. *Urol Clin North Am* 5:127, 1978.

Jeffs RD: Exstrophy, epispadias and cloacal and urogenital sinus abnormalities. *Pediatr Clin North Am* 34:1233, 1987.

Jeffs RD, Charrois R, Many M, et al: Primary closure of the exstrophied bladder. In: Scott R Jr, Gordon HL, Scott FB, et al (Eds): *Current Controversies in Urologic Management.* Philadelphia, W. B. Saunders Company, 1972, p 235.

Jeffs RD, Guice SL, Oesch I: The factors in successful exstrophy closure. *J Urol* 127:974, 1982.

Jeter K, Lattimer JK: Common stomal problems following ileal conduit urinary diversion. *Urology* 3:399, 1974.

Jeter KF: Care of the ostomy patient. In: Kaufman JJ (Ed): *Current Urologic Therapy.* Philadelphia, W. B. Saunders Company, 1980.

Jeter KF: The flush versus the protruding urinary stoma. *J Urol* 116:424, 1976.

Johnston JH: The genital aspects of exstrophy. *J Urol* 113:701, 1975.

Johnston JH: Temporary cutaneous ureterostomy in the management of advanced congenital urinary obstruction. *Arch Dis Child* 38:161, 1963.

Kajbafzedeh AM, Duffy PJ, Carr B, et al: A review of 100 Mitrofanoff stomas and report on the VQZ technique for prevention of complications at stoma level. Paper presented at the 6th annual meeting of the European Society of Pediatric Urology, Toledo, Spain, April 27–29, 1995.

Kajbafzedeh AM, Hubak N: Simultaneous Malone antegrade continent enema and Mitrofanoff principle using divided appendix: report of a new technique for prevention of stoma complications. *J Urol* 185:2404, 2001.

Kajbafzedeh AM, Tajik P: A novel technique for approximation of the symphysis pubis in bladder exstrophy without pelvic osteotomy. *J Urol* 175(2):692–7, 2006.

Kalloo NB, Jeffs RD, Gearhart JP: Long-term nutritional consequences of bowel segment use for lower urinary tract reconstruction in pediatric patients. *Urology* 50:967, 1997.

Kandemir U, Yazici M, Tokgozoglu AM, Alanay A: Distraction osteogenesis (callotasis) for pelvic closure in bladder exstrophy. *Clin Orthop Relat Res* 418:231–6, 2004.

Kass EJ, Koff SA: Bladder augmentation in the pediatric neuropathic bladder. *J Urol* 129:552, 1983.

Kaufman JJ: Repair of parastomal hernia by translocation of the stoma without laparotomy. *J Urol* 129:278, 1983.

Kay R, Tank ES: Principle of management of the persistent cloaca in the female newborn. *J Urol* 117:102, 1977.

Keisling VJ, Tank ES: Postoperative intussusception in children. *Urology* 33:387, 1989.

Kelalis PP: Urinary diversion in children by the sigmoid conduit: its advantages and limitations. *J Urol* 112:666, 1974.

Kelly JH: Soft tissue repair of vesical exstrophy. *Pediatr Surg Int* 10:298, 1995.

Kelly JH, Eraklis AJ: The procedure for lengthening the phallus in boys with exstrophy of the bladder. *J Pediatr Surg* 6:645, 1971.

Kennedy HA, Adams MC, Mitchell ME, et al: Chronic renal failure and bladder augmentation: stomach versus sigmoid colon in the canine model. *J Urol* 140:1138, 1988.

Khoury AE, Agarwal SK, Bagli D, et al: Concomitant modified bladder neck closure and Mitrofanoff urinary diversion. *J Urol* 162:1746, 1999.

Khoury AE, Papanikolaou F, Afshar K, Zuker R: A novel approach to skin coverage for epispadias repair. *J Urol* 173(4):1332–3, 2005.

Khurana S, Borzi PA: Laparoscopic management of complicated urachal disease in children. *J Urol* 168(4 Pt 1):1526–8, 2002.

Kiddoo DA, Carr MC, Dulczak S, Canning DA: Initial management of complex urological disorders: bladder exstrophy. *Urol Clin North Am* 31(3):417–26, vii–viii, 2004. Review.

Kim KS, Susskind MR, King LR: Ileocecal ureterosigmoidostomy: an alternative to conventional ureterosigmoidostomy. *J Urol* 140:1494, 1988.

King LR: Technique of ileal conduit: evolution of the Brady method. Papers presented in honor of W. W. Scott. New York, Plenum Publications, 1972.

King LR, Scott WW: Pyeloileocutaneous anastomosis. *Surg Gynecol Obstet* 119:281, 1964.

King LR, Stone AR, Webster GD (Eds): *Bladder Reconstruction and Continent Urinary Diversion.* Chicago, Year Book Medical Publishers, 1987.

King LR, Wendel EF: Primary cystectomy and permanent urinary diversion in the treatment of exstrophy of the urinary bladder. In: Scott R (Ed): *Current Controversies in Urologic Management.* Philadelphia, W. B. Saunders Company, 1972, p 244.

Kiricuta I: *Use of the Omentum in Plastic Surgery.* Romania, Editura Medicala, 1980.

Kitchens DM, Minevich E, DeFoor WR, Reddy P, Wacksman J, Koyle M, Sheldon CA: Incontinence following bladder neck reconstruction: is there a role for endoscopic management? *J Urol* 177:302–6, 2007.

Klauber GT: Posterior bladder tube for CIC. *Society for Pediatric Urology Newsletter,* May 20, 1992, p 9.

Koch MO, McDougal WS: Nicotinic acid: treatment for the hyperchloremic acidosis following urinary diversion through intestinal segments. *J Urol* 134:162, 1985.

Kock NG: Ileostomy without external appliance: a survey of 25 patients provided with intestinal reservoir. *Ann Surg* 173:545, 1971.

Kock NG, Hultén L, Leandoer L: A study of the motility in different parts of the human colon: resting activity, response to feeding and to prostigmine. *Scand J Gastroenterol* 3:163, 1968.

Kock NG, Nilson AE, Nilsson LO et al: Urinary diversion via a continent ileal reservoir: clinical results in 12 patients. *J Urol* 128:469, 1982.

Koff SA: Abdominal neourethra in children: technique and long-term results. *J Urol* 133:244, 1985.

Koff SA, Wagner TT, Jayanthi VR: The relationship among dysfunctional elimination syndromes, primary vesicourethral reflux, and urinary tract infections in children. *J Urol* 160:1019, 1998.

Koraitim MM, Khalil MR, Ali GA, Foda MK: Micturition after gastrocystoplasty and gastric bladder replacement. *J Urol* 161(5):1480–4, 1999.

Kosko JW, Kursh ED, Resnick MI: Metabolic complications of urologic intestinal substitutes. *Urol Clin North Am* 13:193, 1986.

Koyle MA, Kaji DW, Duque M, et al: The Malone antegrade continence enema for neurogenic and structure fecal incontinence and constipation. *J Urol* 154:759,1995.

Kretschner KP: The intestinal stoma. *Major Probl Clin Surg* 24:98, 1978.

Kronner KM, Casale AJ, Cain MP, et al: Bladder calculi in the pediatric augmented bladder. *J Urol* 160(3 Pt 2):1096–8, 1998.

Kroovand RL, Al-Ansari RM, Perlmutter AD: Urinary and genital malformations in prune belly syndrome. *J Urol* 127:94, 1982.

Kropp BP, Cheng EY: Total urogenital complex mobilization in female patients with exstrophy. *J Urol* 164(3 Pt 2):1035–9, 2000.

Kropp KA, Angwafo FF: Urethral lengthening and reimplantation for neurogenic incontinence in children. *J Urol* 135:534, 1986.

Kryger JV, Barthold JS, Fleming P, González R: The outcome of artificial sphincter placement after a mean 15-year follow-up in a paediatric population. *BJU Int* 83:1026, 1999.

Kryger JV, González R: Urinary continence is well preserved after total urogenital mobilization. *J Urol* 172(6 Pt 1):2384–6, 2004.

Kryger JV, Leverson G, González R: Long-term results of artificial urinary sphincters in children are independent of age of implantation. *J Urol* 165:2377, 2001.

Kurzrock EA, Baskin LS, Kogan BA: Gastrocystoplasty: long-term follow-up. *J Urol* 160(6 Pt 1):2182–6, 1998.

Kurzrock EA, Skinner DG, Stein JP: Hemi-T pouch modification for pediatric urinary diversion. *J Urol* 170(3):949–51, 2003.

Ladd WE, Gross RE: Congenital malformations of the anus and rectum: report of 162 cases. *Am J Surg* 23:167, 1934.

Lailas NG, Cilento B, Atala A: Progressive ureteral dilation for subsequent ureterocystoplasty. *J Urol* 156:1151, 1996.

Landau EH, Jayanthi VR, Khoury AE, et al: Bladder augmentation: ureterocystoplasty versus ileocystoplasty. *J Urol* 152:716, 1984.

Lapides J: The abdominal neourethra. *J Urol* 95:350, 1966.

Lapides J: Butterfly cutaneous ureterostomy. *J Urol* 88:735, 1962.

Lapides J, Ajemian EP, Lichtwardt JR: Cutaneous vesicostomy. *J Urol* 84:609, 1960.

Lapides J, Diokno AC, Gould FR, et al: Clean intermittent self-catheterization in the treatment of urinary tract disease. *J Urol* 107:458, 1972.

Lattimer JK: Congenital deficiency of the abdominal musculature and associated genitourinary anomalies: a report of 22 cases. *J Urol* 79:343, 1958.

Le Duc A, Camey M, Teillac P: An original antireflux ureteroileal implantation technique: long-term follow-up. *J Urol* 137:1156, 1987.

Leadbetter GW Jr, Leadbetter WF: Ureteral reimplantation and bladder neck reconstruction. *JAMA* 175:676, 1976.

Leadbetter GW Jr, Zickermin P, Pierce E: Ureterosigmoidostomy and carcinoma of the colon. *J Urol* 121:732, 1979.

Leadbetter WF: Considerations of problems incident to performance of uretero-enterostomy: report of a technique. *J Urol* 68:818, 1951.

Leadbetter WF, Clarke BG: Five years experience with uretero-enterostomy by the "combined" technique. *J Urol* 73:67, 1954.

Leclair MD, Gundetti M, Kiely EM, Wilcox DT: The surgical outcome of total urogenital mobilization for cloacal repair. *J Urol* 177(4):1492–5, 2007.

Lee RS, Grady R, Joyner B, et al: Can a complete primary repair approach be applied to cloacal exstrophy? *J Urol* 176(6 Pt 1): 2643–8, 2006.

Leisinger HJ: Continent urinary diversion: review of the intussuscepted ileal valve. *World J Urol* 4:231, 1986.

Leissner EP, Allhoff W, Wolff C, et al: The pelvic plexus and antireflux surgery: topographical findings and clinical consequences. *J Urol* 165:1652, 2001.

Lemelle JL, Simo AK, Schmitt M: Comparative study of the Yang-Monti channel and appendix for continent diversion in the Mitrofanoff and Malone principles. *J Urol* 172(5 Pt 1): 1907–10, 2004.

Leng WW, Blalock HJ, Fredriksson WH, et al: Enterocystoplasty or detrusor myectomy? Comparison of indications and outcomes for bladder augmentation. *J Urol* 161(3):758–63, 1999.

Leng WW, Faerber G, Del Terzo M, McGuire EJ: Long-term outcome of incontinent ileovesicostomy management of severe lower urinary tract dysfunction. *J Urol* 161:1803, 1999.

Leonard MP, Dharamsi N, Williot PE: Outcome of gastrocystoplasty in tertiary pediatric urology practice. *J Urol* 164(3 Pt 2): 947–50, 2000.

Leonard MP, Gearhart JP, Jeffs RD: 50 continent urinary reservoirs in pediatric urological practice. *J Urol* 144(Pt 2):330, 1990.

Leonard MP, Quinlan DM: The Benchekroun ileal valve. *Urol Clin North Am* 18:717, 1991.

Leong CH: Use of the stomach for bladder replacement and urinary diversion. *Ann R Coll Surg Engl* 60:283, 1978.

Lepor H, Jeffs RD: Primary bladder closure and bladder with reconstruction in classical bladder exstrophy. *J Urol* 130:1142, 1983.

Lepor H, Shapiro E, Jeffs RD: Urethral reconstruction in boys with classical bladder exstrophy. *J Urol* 131:512, 1984.

Liard A, Seguier-Lipszyc E, Mathiot A, Mitrofanoff P: The Mitrofanoff procedure: 20 years later. *J Urol* 165(6 Pt 2): 2394–8, 2001.

Libertino JA, Zinman L: Ileocecal antirefluxing conduit. *Surg Clin North Am* 62:999, 1982.

Lierse W: *Applied Anatomy of the Pelvis*. Berlin, Springer-Verlag, 1987.

Lieskovsky G, Bloom DA: Creation of a Turnbull loop stoma. In: Skinner DG (Ed): *Genitourinary Cancer*. Philadelphia, W. B. Saunders Company, 1987.

Lieskovsky G, Boyd SD, Skinner DG: Cutaneous Kock pouch urinary diversion. *Probl Urol* 5:256, 1991.

Light JK: Enteroplasty to ablate bowel contractions in the reconstructed bladder: a case report. *J Urol* 134:958, 1985.

Light JK, Flores FN, Scott FB: Use of the AS792 artificial sphincter following urinary undiversion. *J Urol* 129:548, 1983.

Lilien OM, Camey M: 25-year experience with replacement of the human bladder (Camey procedure). *J Urol* 132:886, 1984.

Linder A, Leach GE, Raz S: Augmentation cystoplasty in the treatment of neurogenic bladder dysfunction. *J Urol* 129:491, 1983.

Lockhart JL, Davies R, Cox C, et al: Gastroileoileal pouch: alternative continent urinary reservoir for patients with short bowel, acidosis and/or extensive pelvic radiation. *J Urol* 150:46, 1993.

Lockhart JL, Pow-Sang JM, Persky L, et al: A continent colonic urinary reservoir: the Florida pouch. *J Urol* 144:864, 1990.

Loughlin KR, Retik AB, Weinstein HJ, et al: Genitourinary rhabdomyosarcoma in children. *Cancer* 63:1600, 1989.

Limpi HD, Khubchandovic IT, Sheets JA, Stasik JJ: Advances in intestinal anastomoses. *Dis Colon Rectum* 20:107, 1977.

Lynch AC, Beasley SW, Robertson RW, Morreua PN: Comparison of results of laparoscopic and open antegrade continence enema procedures. *Pediatr Surg Int* 15:343, 1999.

Lytton B, Weiss RM: Cutaneous vesicostomy for temporary urinary diversion in infants. *J Urol* 105:888, 1971.

Magnus R, Stephens FD: Imperforate anal membrane. *Austral Pediat* 2:431, 1966.

Malone PS, Ransley PG, Kiely EM: Preliminary report: the antegrade continence enema. *Lancet* 336:1217, 1990.

Malone PS, Curry JI, Osborne A: The antegrade continence enema procedure: why, when and how? *World J Urol* 16:274, 1998.

Mansi MK: Re: Simplified technique with short and long-term follow-up of conversion of an ileal conduit to an Indiana pouch. *J Urol* 165(1):192, 2001.

Mansson W: The continent cecal reservoir for urine. *Scand J Urol* 85(suppl):1, 1984.

Mansson W, Mattiasson A, White T: Acute effects of full urinary bladder and full caecal urinary reservoir on regional renal function: a study with scintillation camera renography. *Scand J Urol Nephrol* 18:299, 1984.

Manzoni GA, Ransley PG, Hurwitz RS: Cloacal exstrophy and cloacal exstrophy variants: a proposed system of classification. *J Urol* 138:1065, 1987.

Marconi F, Messina P, Pavanello P, Castro RD: Cosmetic reconstruction of the mons veneris and lower abdominal wall by skin expansion as the last stage of the surgical treatment of bladder exstrophy: a report of three cases. *Plast Reconstr Surg* 91:551, 1993.

Markland C, Fraley EE: Management of infants with cloacal exstrophy. *J Urol* 109:740, 1973.

Marshall FF, Leadbetter WF, Dretler SP: Ileal conduit parastomal hernias. *J Urol* 144:40, 1975.

Marshall VF, Muecke EC: Functional closure of typical exstrophy of the bladder. *J Urol* 104:205, 1970.

Marshall VF, Muecke EC: Variations in exstrophy of the bladder. *J Urol* 88:766, 1962.

Martin EC, Fankuchen EI, Casarella WJ: Percutaneous dilation of ureteroenteric strictures or occlusions in ileal conduit. *Urol Radiol* 4:19, 1982.

Mathews R, Gearhart JP, Bhatnagar R, Sponseller P: Staged pelvic closure of extreme pubic diastasis in the exstrophy-epispadias complex. *J Urol* 176(5):2196–8, 2006.

Mathisen W: A new method of ureterointestinal anastomosis: preliminary report. *Surg Gynecol Obstet* 96:255, 1953.

Mathisen W: Open-loop sigmoido-cystoplasty. *Acta Chir Scand* 110:227, 1955.

Mayo ME, Chapman WH: Management of ileal conduit obstruction: a urodynamic study. *J Urol* 125:828, 1981.

Mayo ME, Chapman WH: Stomal obstruction of ileal conduits in children: a urodynamic study. *J Urol* 121:68, 1979.

McDougal WS: Editorial: the continent urinary diversion. *J Urol* 137:1214, 1987.

McDougal WS: Use of intestinal segments in urinary diversion. In: Walsh P (Ed): *Campbell's Urology*, 8th ed. Philadelphia, W. B. Saunders Company, 2002, pp 3745–88.

McGuire EJ, Cespedes RD, O'Connell HE: Leak-point pressures. *Urol Clin North Am* 23:253–62, 1996.

McLeod RS, Fazio VW: Quality of life with the continent ileostomy. *World J Surg* 8:90, 1984.

Menville JG, Nix JT, Pratt AM II: Cecocystoplasty. *J Urol* 79:78, 1958.

Mesrobian H-G J: Exstrophy of the bladder. In: King LR (Ed): *Urologic Surgery in Neonates and Young Infants.* Philadelphia, W. B. Saunders Company, 1988, p 265.

Metcalfe PD, Casale AJ, Kaefer MA, et al: Spontaneous bladder perforations: a report of 500 augmentations in children and analysis of risk. *J Urol* 175(4):1466–70, 2006; discussion 1470–1.

Michie AJ, Borns P, Ames MD: Improvement following tubeless suprapubic cystostomy of myelomeningocele patients with hydronephrosis and recurrent acute pyelonephritis. *J Pediatr Surg* 1:347, 1966.

Middleton RG: Further experience with the Young-Dees procedure for urinary incontinence in selected cases. *J Urol* 115:159, 1976.

Mildenberger H, Kluth D, Dziuba M: Embryology of bladder exstrophy. *J Pediatr Surg* 23:166, 1988.

Miller A: The aetiology and treatment of diverticulum of the bladder. *Br J Urol* 30:43, 1958.

Miller EA, Mayo M, Kwan D, Mitchell M: Simultaneous augmentation cystoplasty and artificial urinary sphincter placement: infection rates and voiding mechanisms. *J Urol* 160 (3 Pt 1):750–2, 1998.

Mingin GC, Nguyen HT, Mathias RS, et al: Growth and metabolic consequences of bladder augmentation in children with myelomeningocele and bladder exstrophy. *Pediatrics* 110(6):1193–8, 2002.

Mingin GC, Stock JA, Hanna MK: Gastrocystoplasty: long-term complications in 22 patients. *J Urol* 162(3 Pt 2):1122–5, 1999.

Mingin GC, Stock JA, Hanna MK: The Mainz II pouch: experience in 5 patients with bladder exstrophy. *J Urol* 162(3 Pt 1): 846–8, 1999.

Mingin GC, Youngren K, Stock JA, Hanna MK: The rectus myofascial wrap in the management of urethral sphincter incompetence. *BJU Int* 90:550, 2002.

Mininberg DT, Genvert HP: Posterior urethral valves: role of temporary and permanent urinary diversion. *Urology* 33:205, 1989.

Misseri R, Cain MP, Casale AJ, et al: Small intestinal submucosa bladder neck slings for incontinence associated with neuropathic bladder. *J Urol* 174(4 Pt 2):1680–2, 2005.

Mitchell ME: The role of bladder augmentation in undiversion. *J Pediatr Surg* 16:790, 1981.

Mitchell ME: Urinary tract diversion and undiversion in the pediatric age group. *Surg Clin North Am* 61:1147, 1981.

Mitchell ME: Use of bowel in undiversion. *Urol Clin North Am* 13:349, 1986.

Mitchell ME, Adams MC, Rink RC: Urethral replacement with ureter. *J Urol* 139:1282, 1988.

Mitchell ME, Brito CG, Rink RC: Cloacal exstrophy reconstruction for urinary continence. *J Urol* 144:554, 1990; discussion 562.

Mitchell ME, Hensle TW, Crooks KK: Urethral reconstruction in the young female using a perineal pedicle flap. *J Pediatr Surg* 17:687, 1982.

Mitchell ME, Rink RC: Urinary diversion and undiversion. *Urol Clin North Am* 12:111, 1985.

Mitchell ME, Yoder IC, Pfister RC, et al: Ileal loop stenosis: a late complication of urinary diversion. *J Urol* 118:957, 1977.

Mitrofanoff P: Cystostomie continente trans-appendiculaire dans le traitement des vessies neurologiques. *Chir Ped* 21:297, 1980.

Mogg RA: The result of urinary diversion using the colonic conduit. *Br J Urol* 97:684, 1967.

Mollard P, Mouriquand P, Joubert P: Urethral lengthening for neurogenic urinary incontinence (Kropp's procedure): results of 16 cases. *J Urol* 143:95, 1990.

Monfort G, Guys JM, Bocciardi A, et al: A novel technique for reconstruction of the abdominal wall in the prune-belly syndrome. *J Urol* 146:361, 1991.

Monfort G, Guys JM, Morrisson-Lacombe G: Appendicovesicostomy: an alternative urinary diversion in the child. *Eur Urol* 10:361, 1984.

Monie IW, Monie BJ: Prune belly syndrome and fetal ascites. *Teratology* 19:111, 1979.

Monti PR, de Carvalho JR, Arap S: The Monti procedure: applications and complications. *Urology* 55:616, 2000.

Monti PR, Lara RC, Dutra MA, Carvalho JR: New techniques for construction of efferent conduits based on the Mitrofanoff principle. *Urology* 49:112, 1997.

Moorcraft J, DuBoulay CEH, Isaacson P, Atwell JD: Changes in the mucosa of colon conduits with particular reference to the risk of malignant change. *Br J Urol* 55:185, 1983.

Mor Y, Kajbafzedeh AM, German K, et al: The role of the ureter in the creation of Mitrofanoff channels in children. *J Urol* 152:635, 1997.

Mor Y, Quinn FM, Carr B, et al: Combined Mitrofanoff and antegrade continence enema for urinary and fecal incontinence. *J Urol* 158:192, 1997.

Mor Y, Ramon J, Raviv G, et al: Low loop cutaneous ureterostomy and subsequent reconstruction: 20 years of experience. *J Urol* 147:1595, 1992.

Mostwin JL: Current concepts of female pelvic anatomy and physiology. *Urol Clin North Am* 18:175, 1991.

Muecke EC: Exstrophy, epispadias and other anomalies of the bladder. In: Walsh PC, Gittes RF, Perlmutter AD, Stamey TA (Eds): *Campbell's Urology*, 5th ed. Philadelphia, W. B. Saunders Company, 1986.

Muecke EC: The role of the cloacal membrane in exstrophy: the first successful experimental study. *J Urol* 92:659, 1964.

Nande JH: The hidden vesicostomy. *Br J Urol* 541:686, 1982.

Naryanaswami B, Wilcox DT, Cuckow PM, et al: The Yang-Monti ileovesicostomy: a problematic channel? *BJU Int* 87:861, 2001.

Nesbit RM: Ureterosigmoid anastomosis by direct elliptical connection: a preliminary report. *J Urol* 61:728, 1949.

Netto NR Jr, Lemos GC, de Almeida Claro JF, Hering FLO: Congenital diverticulum of male urethra. *Urology* 24:239, 1984.

Nguyen HT, Baskin LS: The outcome of bladder neck closure in children with severe urinary incontinence. *J Urol* 169(3):1114–6, 2003.

Nichols G, Duffy PG: Anatomical correction of the exstrophy-epispadias complex: analysis of 34 patients. *Br J Urol* 82:865, 1998.

Nix JT, Menville JG, Albert M, Wendt DL: Congenital patent urachus. *J Urol* 79:264, 1958.

Noh PH, Cooper CS, Winkler AC, et al: Prognostic factors for long-term renal function in boys with the prune-belly syndrome. *J Urol* 162(4):1399–401, 1999.

Norlén L, Trasti H: Functional behavior of the continent ileum reservoir for urinary diversion: experimental and clinical study. *Scand J Urol Nephrol* 49(suppl):33, 1978.

Nurse DE, Mundy AR: Metabolic complications of cystoplasty. *Br J Urol* 63:165, 1988.

Oesterling JE, Gearhart JP: Utilization of an ileal conduit in construction of a continent urinary reservoir. *Urology* 36:15, 1990.

Overstreet EW, Hinman F Jr: Some gynecologic aspects of bladder exstrophy: with report of an illustrative case. *West J Surg Obstet Gynecol* 64:131, 1956.

Owsley JQ Jr, Hinman F Jr: One-stage reconstruction of the external genitalia in the female with exstrophy of the bladder. *Plast Reconstr Surg* 50:227, 1972.

Pahernik S, Beetz R, Schede J, et al: Rectosigmoid pouch (Mainz Pouch II) in children. *J Urol* 175(1):284–7, 2006.

Parekh DJ, Pope JC, Adams MC, Brock JW III: The use of radiography, urodynamic studies and cystoscopy in the evaluation of voiding dysfunction. *J Urol* 165:215, 2001.

Parkash S, Bhandari M: Rectus abdominis myocutaneous island flap for bridging defect after cystectomy for bladder exstrophy. *Urology* 20:536, 1982.

Parra RO: A simplified technique for continent urinary diversion: an all-stapled colonic reservoir. *J Urol* 146:1496, 1991.

Parrott TS, Woodard JR: The Monfort operation for abdominal wall reconstruction in the prune belly. *J Urol* 148:688, 1992.

Patil KK, Duffy PG, Woodhouse CR, Ransley PG: Long-term outcome of Fowler-Stephens orchiopexy in boys with prune-belly syndrome. *J Urol* 171(4):1666–9, 2004.

Patten BM, Barry A: The genesis of exstrophy of the bladder and epispadias. *Am J Anat* 90:35, 1952.

Paul M, Kanagasuntheram R: The congenital anomalies of the lower urinary tract. *Br J Urol* 28(Pt 1):64, 1956; 28(Pt 2):118, 1956.

Pegum JM, Loly PCM, Falkiner NM: Development and classification of anorectal anomalies. *Arch Surg* 89:481, 1964.

Peña A: Anatomical considerations relevant to fecal incontinence. *Semin Surg Oncol* 3:1141, 1987.

Peña A: Posterior sagittal anorectoplasty as a secondary operation for the treatment of fecal incontinence. *J Pediatr Surg* 18:762, 1983.

Peña A: Posterior sagittal approach for the correction of anorectal malformations. *Adv Surg* 19:69, 1986.

Peña A: Surgical treatment of high imperforate anus. *World J Surg* 9:236, 1985.

Perlmutter AD: Reduction cystoplasty in prune belly syndrome. *J Urol* 116:356, 1976.

Perlmutter AD: Spiral advancement skin flap for stomal revision. *J Urol* 114:131, 1975.

Perlmutter AD, Tank ES: Loop cutaneous ureterostomy. *J Urol* 99:559, 1968.

Perlmutter AD, Weinstein MD, Reitelman C: Vesical neck reconstruction in patients with epispadias-exstrophy complex. *J Urol* 146:613, 1991.

Perovic SV, Vukadinovic VM, Djordjevic MIJ: Augmentation ureterocystoplasty could be performed more frequently. *J Urol* 164:924, 2000.

Persky L: Relocation of ileal stomas. *J Urol* 96:702, 1966.

Peters CA, Mandell J, Lebowitz RL, et al: Congenital obstructed megaureters in early infancy: diagnosis and treatment. *J Urol* 142(Pt 2):641, 1989; discussion 667.

Piaggio L, Myers S, Figueroa T, et al: Influence of type of conduit and site of implantation on the outcome of continent catheterizable channels. *J Pediatr Urol* 3(3):230–4, 2007.

Pinto PA, Stock JA, Hanna MK: Results of umbilicoplasty for bladder exstrophy. *J Urol* 164(6):2055–7, 2000.

Pitts WR, Muecke EC: A 20-year experience with ileal conduit: the fate of the kidneys. *J Urol* 122:154, 1979.

Pohlmann AG: The development of the cloaca in human embryos. *Am J Anat* 12:1, 1911.

Pokorny M, Pontes JE, Pierce JM Jr: Ureterostomy in-situ. *Urology* 8:447, 1976.

Pope JC 4th, Keating MA, Casale AJ, Rink RC: Augmenting the augmented bladder: treatment of the contractile bowel segment. *J Urol* 160(3 Pt 1):854–7, 1998.

Poppas DP, Uzzo RG, Britanisky RG, Mininberg DT: Laparoscopic laser assisted auto-augmentation of the pediatric neurogenic bladder: early experience with urodynamic follow-up. *J Urol* 155:1057, 1996.

Potter JM, Duffy PG, Gordon EM, Malone PR: Detrusor myotomy: a 5-year review in unstable and non-compliant bladders. *BJU Int* 89:932, 2002.

Powers JC, Fitzgerald JF, McAhranah MJ: The anatomic basis for the surgical detachment of the greater omentum from the transverse colon. *Surg Gynecol Obstet* 143:105, 1976.

Quek ML, Ginsberg DA: Long-term urodynamics follow-up of bladder augmentation for neurogenic bladder. *J Urol* 169(1):195–8, 2003.

Quinlan DM, Leonard MP, Brendler CB, et al: Use of the Benchekroun hydraulic valve as a catheterizable continence mechanism. *J Urol* 145:1151, 1991.

Rabinowitz R, Barkin M, Schillinger JF, et al: Surgical treatment of the massively dilated ureter in children: Part I. Management by cutaneous ureterostomy. *J Urol* 117:658, 1977.

Rabinowitz R, Barkin M, Schillinger JF, et al: Upper tract management when posterior urethral valve ablation is insufficient. *J Urol* 122:370, 1979.

Randolph J, Cavett C, Eng G: Abdominal wall reconstruction in the prune belly syndrome. *J Pediatr Surg* 16:960, 1981.

Rané A, Jones DA: Seromuscular myotomy to help eversion of an urostomy. *Br J Urol* 80:668, 1997.

Ransley PG, Duffy PG, Wollin M: Bladder exstrophy closure and epispadias repair. In: Spitz L, Nixon HH (Eds): *Operative Surgery (Paediatric Surgery)*. London, Butterworth-Heinemann, 1988, p 620.

Ravitch MM: Observations on the healing of wounds of the intestines. *Surgery* 77:665, 1975.

Raz S: *Atlas of Transvaginal Surgery*, 2nd ed. Philadelphia, W. B. Saunders Company, 2002.

Redman JF: An anatomic approach to the pelvis. In: Crawford ED, Borden TA (Eds): *Genitourinary Cancer Surgery*. Philadelphia, Lea & Febiger, 1982, p 126.

Redman JF: Extensive shortening of ileal conduit through peristomal incision. *Urology* 9:45, 1977.

Reid R, Schneider K, Fruchtman B: Closure of the bladder neck in patients undergoing continent vesicostomy for urinary incontinence. *J Urol* 120:40, 1978.

Reidmiller H, Bürger R, Müller S, et al: Continent appendix stoma: a modification of the Mainz pouch technique. *J Urol* 143:1115, 1990.

Reidmiller H, Thüroff J, Stöckle M, et al: Continent urinary diversion and bladder augmentation in children: the Mainz pouch procedure. *Pediatr Nephrol* 3:68, 1989.

Reiner WG, Gearhart JP: Discordant sexual identity in some genetic males with cloacal exstrophy assigned to female sex at birth. *N Engl J Med* 350(4):333–41, 2004.

Resnick MJ, Caldamone AA (Eds): Use of large and small bowel in urologic surgery. *Urol Clin North Am* 13:177, 1986.

Retik AB, Bauer SB: Bladder and urachus. In: Kelalis PP, et al (Eds): *Clinical Pediatric Urology*. Philadelphia, W. B. Saunders Company, 1976.

Reynolds EL: The bony pelvis in prepubertal childhood. *Am J Phys Anthropol NS* 5:165, 1947.

Rich RH, Hardy BE, Filler RM: Surgery for anomalies of the urachus. *J Pediatr Surg* 18:4, 1983.

Richardson JR Jr, Linton PC, Leadbetter GW Jr: A new concept in the treatment of stomal stenosis. *J Urol* 108:159, 1972.

Richie JP: Colonic and jejunal conduits. In: Johnson DE, Boileau MA (Eds): *Genitourinary Tumo rs*. New York, Grune & Stratton, Inc, 1982.

Richie JP: Nonrefluxing sigmoid conduit for urinary diversion. *Urol Clin North Am* 6:469, 1979.

Rickham PP: Vesicointestinal fissure. *Arch Dis Child* 35:97, 1960.

Rickwood AMK: Urinary diversion in children. In: Ashken MH (Ed): *Urinary Diversion*. Berlin, Springer-Verlag, 1982, p 22.

Rink RC: Bladder augmentation: options, outcomes, future. *Urol Clin North Am* 26(1):111–23, viii–ix, 1999.

Rink RC, McLaughlin RP, Adams MC, Keating MA: Modification of the Casale vesicostomy: continent diversion without the use of bowel. *J Urol* 153(Pt 2):339A, 1995. Abstract 442.

Rink RC, Retik AB: Ureteroileocecal sigmoidostomy and avoidance of carcinoma of the colon. In: King LR, Stone AR, Webster GD (Eds): *Bladder Reconstruction and Continent Urinary Diversion*. Chicago, Mosby Year Book, 1991, p 221.

Roberts JP, Moon S, Malone PS: Treatment of neuropathic urinary and faecal incontinence with synchronous bladder reconstruction and antegrade continence enema procedure. *Br J Urol* 75:386, 1994.

Robertson CN, King LR: Bladder substitution in children. *Urol Clin North Am* 13:333, 1986.

Rosenberg ML: The physiology of hyperchloremic acidosis following ureterosigmoidostomy: a study of urinary reabsorption with radioactive isotopes. *J Urol* 70:569, 1953.

Rowland RG: Continent urinary diversion. *J Urol* 136:76, 1986.

Rowland RG, Mitchell ME, Bihrle R, et al: Indiana continent urinary reservoir. *J Urol* 137:1136, 1987.

Ruiz E, Puigdevall J, Moldes J, et al: 14 years of experience with the artificial urinary sphincter in children and adolescents without spina bifida. *J Urol* 176(4 Pt 2):1821–5, 2006.

Rukhoff NJ, Wijkstra H, Van Kerrebroeck PE, Debruyne FM: Urinary bladder control by electrical stimulation techniques in spinal cord injury. *Neurourol Urodyn* 16:39, 1997.

Sagalowsky A: Mechanisms of continence in urinary reconstructions. *AUA Update Series*, vol XI, lesson 4, 1991.

Salley R, Bucher RM, Rodring CB: Colostomy closure: morbidity reduction employing a semi-standardized protocol. *Dis Colon Rectum* 26:319, 1983.

Saltzman B, Mininberg DT, Muecke EC: Exstrophy of bladder: evolution of management. *Urology* 26:383, 1985.

Scardino PT, Bagley DH, Javadpour N, Ketchom AS: Sigmoid conduit urinary diversion. *Urology* 6:167, 1975.

Scheidler DM, Klee LW, Rowland RG, et al: Update on the Indiana continent urinary reservoir. *J Urol* 141(Pt 2):302A, 1989.

Scherster T: Studies of the motorial function in the ileal segment in cutaneous uretero-ileostomy. *Acta Clin Scand* 124:149, 1962.

Schlegel PN, Gearhart JP: Neuroanatomy of the pelvis in an infant with cloacal exstrophy: a detailed microdissection with histology. *J Urol* 141:583, 1989.

Schlesinger RE, Berman ML, Ballon SC, et al: The choice of an intestinal segment for a urinary conduit. *Surg Gynecol Obstet* 148:45, 1979.

Schmidbauer CP, Chiang H, Raz S: Compliance of tubular and detubularized ileal reservoirs. *J Urol* 137:171A, 1987.

Schmidt JD, Buchsbaum HJ, Jacobo EC: Transverse colon conduit for supravesical urinary tract diversion. *Urology* 8:542, 1976.

Schmidt JD, Buchsbaum HJ, Nachtsheim DA: Long-term follow-up, further experience with and modifications of the transverse colon conduit in urinary tract diversion. *Br J Urol* 57:284, 1985.

Schneider KM, Reid RE, Fruchtman B: Closure of the bladder neck in patients undergoing continent vesicostomy. *J Urol* 120:40, 1978.

Schreck WR, Campbell WA: The relationship of bladder outlet obstruction to urinary umbilical fistula. *J Urol* 108:641, 1972.

Schrock TR, Deveney CW, Dunphy JE: Factors contributing to leakage of colonic anastomoses. *Ann Surg* 177:513, 1973.

Schunke GB: The anatomy and development of the sacro-iliac joint in man. *Anat Rec* 72:313, 1938.

Scott FB, Light JK, Fishman I, et al: Implantation of an artificial sphincter for urinary incontinence. *Contemp Surg* 18:11, 1981.

Senn E, Thüroff JW, Barandhauer K: Urodynamics of ileal conduits in adults. *Eur Urol* 10:401, 1984.

Shafik A: Stomal stenosis after cutaneous ureterostomy: etiology and management. *J Urol* 105:65, 1971.

Shaw MB, Rink RC, Kaefer M, et al: Continence and classic bladder exstrophy treated with staged repair. *J Urol* 172 (4 Pt 1):1450–3, 2004.

Shaw PJR: Supravesical bladder neck closure. In: Whitfield HH (Ed): *Genitourinary Surgery*. Oxford, Butterworth-Heinemann, 1993.

Sheldon CA, Minevich E, Wacksman J: Modified technique of antegrade continence enema using a stapling device. *J Urol* 163(2):589–91, 2000.

Shimada K, Matsumoto F, Tohda A, et al: Surgical management of urinary incontinence in children with anatomical bladder-outlet anomalies. *Int J Urol* 9:561, 2002.

Shire R, Kiely EM, Varr B, et al: The clinical application of the Malone antegrade colonic enema. *J Pediatr Surg* 28:1012, 1993.

Sidi AA, Reinberg Y, González R: Influence of intestinal segment and configuration on the outcome of augmentation enterocystoplasty. *J Urol* 136:1201, 1986.

Silver PHS: The role of the peritoneum in the formation of the septum recto-vesicale. *J Anat* 90:538, 1956.

Silver RI, Sponseller PD, Gearhart JP: Staged closure of the pelvis in cloacal exstrophy: first description of a new approach. *J Urol* 161(1):263–6, 1999.

Simon J: Ectopia vesicae (absence of the anterior walls of the bladder and pubic abdominal parietes): operation for directing the orifices of the ureters into the rectum. Temporary success: subsequent death. Autopsy. *Lancet* 2:568, 1852.

Singh G, Thomas DG: Artificial urinary sphincter in patients with neurogenic bladder dysfunction. *Br J Urol* 77:252, 1996.

Skinner DG: Further experience with the ileocecal segment in urinary reconstruction. *J Urol* 128:252, 1982.

Skinner DG: Secondary urinary reconstruction: use of the ileocecal segment. *J Urol* 112:48, 1974.

Skinner DG, Boyd SD, Lieskovsky G, et al: Lower urinary tract reconstruction following cystectomy: experience and results in 126 patients using the Kock ileal reservoir with bilateral uretero-ileo-urethrostomy. *J Urol* 146:756, 1991.

Skinner DG, Gottesman JE, Richie JP: The isolated sigmoid segment: its value in temporary urinary diversion and reconstruction. *J Urol* 113:614, 1975.

Skinner DG, Lieskowsky G, Boyd S: Continent urinary diversion. *J Urol* 141:1323, 1989.

Skobeiko-Wlodarska L, Strulak K: Bladder autoaugmentation in myelodysplastic children. *Br J Urol* 81:(suppl 3):114, 1998.

Smith ED: Follow-up study on 150 ileal conduits in children. *J Pediatr Surg* 7:1, 1972.

Smith GI, Hinman F Jr: The intussuscepted ileal cystostomy. *J Urol* 73:261, 1955.

Smith GI, Hinman F Jr: The rectal bladder (colostomy with ureterosigmoidostomy): experimental and clinical aspects. *J Urol* 74:354, 1955.

Smith RB, Van Cangh P, Skinner DG, et al: Augmentation enterocystoplasty: a critical review. *J Urol* 118:35, 1977.

Snodgrass WT, Elmore J, Adams R: Bladder neck sling and appendicovesicostomy without augmentation for neurogenic incontinence in children. *J Urol* 177(4):1510–4, 2007.

Snow BW, Cartwright PC: Bladder autoaugmentation. *Urol Clin North Am* 23:323, 1996.

Snyder HM III: Continent reconstruction of the lower urinary tract: variations of the Mitrofanoff principle. In: *Advances in Urology*, 2nd ed. Chicago, Year Book Medical Publishers, 1989.

Snyder HM III: Foreword. In: King LR, Stone AR, Webster GD (Eds): *Bladder Reconstruction and Continent Urinary Diversion*. Chicago, Year Book Medical Publishers, 1986, p xi.

Soper RT, Kilger K: Vesico-intestinal fissure. *J Urol* 92:490, 1964.

Soygur T, Arikan N, Zumrutbas AE, Gulpinar O: Serosal lined extramural tunnel (Ghoneim) principle in the creation of a catheterizable channel in bladder augmentation. *J Urol* 174(2):696–9, 2005.

Spence HM: Ureterosigmoidostomy for exstrophy of the bladder: results in a personal series of 31 cases. *Br J Urol* 38:36, 1966.

Spence HM, Allen TD: Vaginal vesicostomy for empyema of the defunctionalized bladder. *J Urol* 106:862, 1971.

Spence HM, Hoffman WW, Fosmire GP: Tumour of the colon as a late complication of ureterosigmoidostomy for exstrophy of the bladder. *Br J Urol* 51:466, 1978.

Spence HM, Hoffman WW, Pate VA: Exstrophy of the bladder: I. Long-term results in a series of 37 cases treated by ureterosigmoidostomy. *J Urol* 114:133, 1974.

Spindel MR, Winslow BH, Jordan GH: The use of paraexstrophy flaps for urethral construction in neonatal girls with classical exstrophy. *J Urol* 140:574, 1988.

Sponseller PD, Jani MM, Jeffs RD, Gearhart JP: Anterior innominate osteotomy in repair of bladder exstrophy. *J Bone Joint Surg Am* 83(2):184–93, 2001.

Steiner MS, Morton RA, Marshall FF: Vitamin B12 deficiency in patients with ileocolic neobladders. *J Urol* 149:255, 1993.

Stephens FD: Congenital imperforate rectum, rectourethral and rectovaginal fistulae. *Aust N Z J Surg* 22:161, 1953.

Stephens FD: *Congenital Malformations of the Rectum, Anus and Genitourinary Tracts*. London, E & S Livingstone, 1963.

Stephens FD: Form of stress incontinence in children: another method for bladder neck repair. *Aust N Z J Surg* 40:124, 1970.

Stephens FD: Imperforate anus. *Med J Aust* 2:803, 1959.

Stephens FD, Smith ED: *Anorectal Malformations in Children*. Chicago, Year Book Medical Publishers, 1971.

Stevens PS, Eckstein HB: Ileal conduit diversion in children. *Br J Urol* 49:379, 1977.

Stohrer M, Goepel M, et al: Detrusor myomectomy (autoaugmentation) in the treatment of hyperreflexive low compliance bladder. *Urologe Q* 38:30, 1999.

Stone AR: Ileocystoplasty. In: King LR, Stone AR, Webster GD (Eds): *Bladder Reconstruction and Continent Urinary Diversion*. Chicago and London, Year Book Medical Publishers, 1991, p 58.

Stower MJ, Massey JA, Feneley RCL: Urethral closure in management of urinary incontinence. *Urology* 34:246, 1989.

Straffon RA, Kyle K, Corvalan J: Techniques of cutaneous ureterostomy and results in 51 patients. *J Urol* 103:138, 1970.

Strand WR: Initial management of complex pediatric disorders: prune belly syndrome, posterior urethral valves. *Urol Clin North Am* 31(3):399–415, vii, 2004. Review.

Strothers L, Johnson J, Arnold W, et al: Bladder augmentation by vesicomyotomy in the pediatric neurogenic bladder. *Urology* 44:110, 1994.

Suber I, Baker LA, Jeffs RD, Gearhart JP: Combined bladder neck reconstruction and epispadias repair for exstrophy-epispadias complex. *J Urol* 165:2425, 2001.

Sugarman ID, Malone PS, Terry TR, Koyle MA: Transversely tubularized ileal segments for the Mitrofanoff or Malone antegrade colonic enema procedures: the Monti principle. *Br J Urol* 81:253, 1998.

Sujijantararat PA, Chotivichit A: Surgical construction of exstrophy-epispadias complex: analysis of 13 patients. *Int J Urol* 9:377, 2002.

Sumfest JM, Burns MW, Mitchell ME: The Mitrofanoff principle in urinary reconstruction. *J Urol* 150:1875, 1993.

Surer I, Baker LA, Jeffs RD, Gearhart JP: The modified Cantwell-Ransley repair for exstrophy and epispadias: 10-year experience. *J Urol* 164(3 Pt 2):1040–2, 2000; discussion 1042–3.

Surer I, Baker LA, Jeffs RD, Gearhart JP: Modified Young-Dees-Leadbetter bladder neck reconstruction in patients with successful primary bladder closure elsewhere: a single institution experience. *J Urol* 165(6 Pt 2):2438–40, 2001.

Surer I, Ferrer FA, Baker LA, Gearhart JP: Continent urinary diversion and the exstrophy-epispadias complex. *J Urol* 169(3):1102–5, 2003.

Swami KS, Feneley RCL, Hammonds JC, Abrams P: Detrusor myomectomy for detrusor overactivity: a minimum 1-year follow-up. *Br J Urol* 81:68, 1998.

Sweat SD, Itano NB, Clemens JQ, Bushman W, et al: Polypropylene mesh tape for stress urinary incontinence: complications of urethral erosion and outlet obstruction. *J Urol* 168:144–6, 2002.

Syme RRA: Bladder neck closure for neurogenic incontinence. *Aust N Z J Surg* 51:197, 1981.

Tackett LD, Minevich W, Benedict JF, et al: Appendiceal versus ileal segment for antegrade continence enema. *J Urol* 167:683, 2002.

Tanagho EA: Bladder neck reconstruction for total urinary incontinence: 10 years of experience. *J Urol* 125:321, 1981.

Tanagho EA: Urethrosphincteric reconstruction for congenitally absent urethra. *J Urol* 116:237, 1976.

Tanagho EA, Smith DR, Meyers FH, Fisher R: Mechanism of urinary continence: II. Technique for surgical correction of incontinence. *J Urol* 101:305, 1969.

Tank ES, Lindenauer SM: Principles of management of exstrophy of the cloaca. *Am J Surg* 119:95, 1970.

Tasker JH: Ileo-cystoplasty: a new technique (an experimental study with report of a case). *Br J Urol* 25:349, 1953.

Tekgul S, Oge O, Bal K, et al: Ureterocystoplasty: an alternative reconstructive procedure to enterocystoplasty in suitable cases. *J Pediatr Surg* 35:577, 2000.

Thüroff JW, Alken P, Riedmiller H, et al: The Mainz-pouch (mixed augmentation ileum'n zecum) for bladder augmentation and continent diversion. *World J Urol* 11:152, 1985.

Thüroff JW, Alken P, Riedmiller H, et al: 100 cases of Mainz pouch: continuing experience and evolution. *J Urol* 140:283, 1988.

Turial S, Hueckstaedt T, Schier F, Fahlenkamp D: Laparoscopic treatment of urachal remnants in children. *J Urol* 177(5):1864–6, 2007.

Turner WR Jr, Ransley PG, Bloom DA, et al: Variants of the exstrophic complex. *Urol Clin North Am* 7:493, 1980.

Turner-Warwick R: Cystoplasty. In: Blandy JP (Ed): *Urology.* Oxford, Blackwell Scientific Publications, 1976, p 840.

Turner-Warwick R: The use of the omental pedicle graft in urinary tract reconstruction. *J Urol* 16:341, 1976.

Turner-Warwick R, Ashken MH: The functional results of partial, subtotal and total cystoplasty with special reference to ureterocaecocystoplasty, selective sphincterotomy and cystocystoplasty. *Br J Urol* 39:3, 1967.

Turner-Warwick R, Wynne EJ, Ashken MH: The use of the omental pedicle graft in the repair and reconstruction of the urinary tract. *Br J Surg* 54:849, 1967.

Uhlenhuth E, Wolfe WM, Smith EM: The rectogenital septum. *Surg Gynecol Obstet* 86:148, 1948.

Van den Beviere H, Vossaert R, DeRoose J, Derom F: Our experience in the treatment of imperforate anus: anterior Mollard's technique versus posterior approach (Stephen's technique). *Acta Chir Belg* 82:205, 1983.

Van Savage JG, Yepuri JN: Transverse retubularized sigmoid-ovesicostomy continent urinary diversion to the umbilicus. *J Urol* 166(2):644–7, 2001.

VanderBrink BA, Stock JA, Hanna MK: Aesthetic aspects of bladder exstrophy: results of puboplasty. *J Urol* 176(4 Pt 2):1810–5, 2006.

Vose SN, Dixey GM: Ureterostomy in-situ. *J Urol* 69:503, 1953.

Wallace DM: Ureteric diversion using a conduit: simplified technique. *Br J Urol* 38:522, 1966.

Walsh A: Ureterostomy in-situ. *Br J Urol* 39:744, 1967.

Warne SA, Godley ML, Wilcox DT: Surgical reconstruction of cloacal malformation can alter bladder function: a comparative study with anorectal anomalies. *J Urol* 172(6 Pt 1):2377–81, 2004.

Warne SA, Wilcox DT, Creighton S, Ransley PG: Long-term gynecological outcome of patients with persistent cloaca. *J Urol* 170(4 Pt 2):1493–6, 2003.

Weakley FL, Turnbull RB Jr: Special intestinal procedures. In: Stewart BH (Ed): *Operative Urology.* Baltimore, Williams & Wilkins Company, 1975.

Wear JB Jr, Barquin OP: Ureterosigmoidostomy: long-term results. *Urology* 1:192, 1973.

Webster GD (Guest Ed): Problems in reconstructive urology. In: Paulson DF (Series Ed): *Problems in Urology, vol 1.* Philadelphia, J. B. Lippincott Company, 1987.

Webster GD, Goldwasser B: Management of incontinence after cystoplasty. In: King LR, Stone AR, Webster GD (Eds): *Bladder Reconstruction and Continent Urinary Diversion.* Chicago and London, Year Book Medical Publishers, 1986, p 75.

Webster GD, Goldwasser B (Eds): *Urinary Diversion.* Oxford, Isis Medical Media 22, 1995.

Wedderburn A, Lee RS, Denny A, Steinbrecher HA, et al: Synchronous bladder reconstruction and antegrade continence enema. *J Urol* 165(6 Pt 2):2392–3, 2001.

Wein AJ, Malloy TR, Greenberg SH, et al: Omental transposition as an aid in genitourinary reconstructive procedures. *J Trauma* 10:473, 1980.

Weingarten JL, Cromie WJ: The Mitrofanoff principle: an alternative form of continent urinary diversion. *J Urol* 140:1529, 1998.

Weiss JP: Sigmoidocystoplasty to augment bladder capacity. *Surg Gynecol Obstet* 159:377, 1984.

Wells CA: The use of the intestine in urology. *Br J Urol* 28:335, 1956.

Wespes E, Stone AR, King LR: Ileocaecocystoplasty in urinary tract reconstruction in children. *J Urol* 58:266, 1986.

Wesselhoeft CWJ, Perlmutter AD, Berg S, et al: Pathogenesis and surgical treatment of diverticulum of the bladder. *Surg Gynecol Obstet* 116:719, 1963.

Weyrauch HM, Young BW: Evaluation of common methods of uretero-intestinal anastomosis: an experimental study. *J Urol* 67:880, 1952.

Whitmore WF III, Gittes RF: Reconstruction of the urinary tract by cecal and ileocecal cystoplasty: review of a 15-year experience. *J Urol* 130:494, 1983.

Wilbert DM, Hohenfellner R: Colonic conduit: preoperative requirements, operative techniques, postoperative management. *World J Urol* 2:159, 1984.

Williams DI, Cromie WJ: Ring ureterostomy. *Br J Urol* 47:789, 1976.

Williams DI, Keeton JE: Further progress with reconstruction of the exstrophied bladder. *Br J Surg* 60:203, 1973.

Williams DI, Rabinovitch HH: Cutaneous ureterostomy for the grossly dilated ureter of childhood. *Br J Urol* 39:696, 1967.

Williams DI, Snyder H: Anterior detrusor tube repair for urinary incontinence in children. *Br J Urol* 48:671, 1976.

Woodard JR: Editorial: Lessons learned in 3 decades of managing the prune-belly syndrome. *J Urol* 159:1680, 1998.

Woodard JR, Marshall VF: Reconstruction of the female urethra to reduce post-traumatic incontinence. *Surg Gynecol Obstet* 113:687, 1961.

Woodard JR, Parrott TS: Reconstruction of the urinary tract in prune belly uropathy. *J Urol* 119:824, 1978.

Woodhouse CRJ, Kellett MJ, Williams DI: Minimal surgical interference in the prune belly syndrome. *Br J Urol* 51:475, 1979.

Woodhouse CRJ, MacNeily, AE: The Mitrofanoff principle: expanding upon a versatile technique. *Br J Urol* 74:447, 1994.

Woodhouse CRJ, Malone PR, Cumming J, Reilly TM: The Mitrofanoff principle for continent urinary diversion. *Br J Urol* 63:53, 1989.

Yang WH: Yang needle tunneling technique in creating antireflux and continent mechanisms. *J Urol* 150:830, 1993.

Yerkes EB, Rink RC, Cain MP, Luerssen TG, et al: Shunt infection and malfunction after augmentation cystoplasty. *J Urol* 165(6 Pt 2):2262–4, 2001.

Yerkes EB, Rink RC, King S, et al: Tap water and the Malone antegrade continence enema: a safe combination. *J Urol* 166:1476, 2001.

Yohannes P, Hanna M: Current trends in the management of posterior urethral valves in the pediatric population. *Urology* 60:953, 2002.

Young HH: Exstrophy of the bladder: the first case in which a normal bladder and urinary control have been obtained by plastic operations. *Surg Gynecol Obstet* 74:729, 1942.

Zimmern PE, Hadley HR, Leach GE, Raz S: Transvaginal closure of the bladder neck and placement of a suprapubic catheter for destroyed urethra after long-term indwelling catheterization. *J Urol* 134:554, 1985.

Zingg E, Tscholl R: Continent cecoileal conduit: preliminary report. *J Urol* 118:724, 1977.

Zinman L, Libertino JA: The ileo-cecal conduit for temporary and permanent urinary diversion. *J Urol* 113:317, 1975.

Zinman L, Libertino JA: The ileocecal segment: an antirefluxing colonic conduit form of urinary diversion. *Surg Clin North Am* 56:733, 1976.

Section 7
Testes and Groin

Abbassian A: A new surgical technique for testicular implantation. *J Urol* 107:618, 1972.

Aceland RD: Instrumentation for microsurgery. *Orthop Clin North Am* 8:281, 1977.

Action Committee on Surgery on the Genitalia of Male Children: The timing of elective surgery on the genitalia of male children with particular reference to undescended testes and hypospadias. *Pediatrics* 56:479, 1975.

Alfert HJ, Gillenwater JY: Ectopic vas deferens communicating with lower ureter: embryological considerations. *J Urol* 108:172, 1972.

Alukal JP, Zurakowski D, Atala A, et al: Testicular hypotrophy does not correlate with grade of adolescent varicocele. *J Urol* 174(6):2367–70, 2005; discussion 2370.

Al-Zahem A, Shun A: Routine contralateral orchiopexy for children with a vanished testis. *Eur J Pediatr Surg* 16(5):334–6, 2006.

Arda IS, Ozyaylali I: Testis tissue bleeding as an indicator of gonadal salvageability in testicular torsion surgery. *BJU Int* 87:89, 2001.

Backhouse KM: Embryology of the normal and cryptorchid testis. In: Fonkelsrud EW, Mengel W (Eds): *The Undescended Testis.* Chicago, Year Book Medical Publishers, 1981.

Backhouse KM: The gubernaculum testis Hunteri: testicular descent and maldescent. *Ann R Coll Surg* 35:15, 1964.

Baker LA, Docimo SG, Surer I, et al: A multi-institutional analysis of laparoscopic orchiopexy. *BJU Int* 87:484, 2001.

Bassel YS, Scherz HC, Kirsch AJ: Scrotal incision orchiopexy for undescended testes with or without a patent processus vaginalis. *J Urol* 177(4):1516–8, 2007.

Beck EM, Schlegel PN, Goldstein M: Intraoperative varicocele anatomy: a macroscopic and microscopic study. *J Urol* 148:1190, 1992.

Belman AB: The adolescent varicocele. *Pediatrics* 114(6):1669–70, 2004. No abstract available.

Belman AB, Rushton HG: Is an empty left hemiscrotum and hypertrophied right descended testis predictive of perinatal torsion? *J Urol* 170(4 Pt 2):1674–5, 2003; discussion 1675–6.

Belman AB, Rushton HG: Is the vanished testis always a scrotal event? *BJU Int* 87:480, 2001.

Ben-Meir D, Hutson JM: Re: Successful outpatient management of the nonpalpable intra-abdominal testis with staged Fowler-Stephens orchiopexy. *J Urol* 173(6):2206–7, 2005.

Bloom DA: Two-step orchiopexy with pelviscopic clip ligation of the spermatic vessels. *J Urol* 145:1030, 1991.

Bloom DA, Ayers JW, McGuire EJ: The role of laparoscopy in management of undescended testes. *J d'Urol* 94:465, 1988.

Bloom DA, Guiney EJ, Richey ML: Normal and abnormal pelviscopic anatomy at the internal inguinal ring and the vasal triangle in boys. *Urology* 44:905, 1994.

Bogaert GA, Kogan BA, Mevorach RA: Therapeutic laparoscopy for the intra-abdominal testis. *Urology* 42:182,1993.

Bong GW, Koo HP: The adolescent varicocele: to treat or not to treat. *Urol Clin North Am* 31(3):509–15, 2004.

Borten M: *Laparoscopic Complications: Prevention and Management.* Boston, B C Decker, 1986.

Browne D: Diagnosis of undescended testicle. *Br Med J* 2:168, 1938.

Browne D: Some anatomical points in the operation for undescended testicle. *Lancet* 1:460, 1933.

Burton CC: A description of the boundaries of the inguinal rings and scrotal pouches. *Surg Gynecol Obstet* 104:142, 1957.

Burton CC: The embryologic development and descent of the testis in relation to congenital hernia. *Surg Gynecol Obstet* 107:294, 1958.

Cabot H, Nesbit RM: Undescended testis. *Arch Surg* 22:850, 1931.

Caldamone AA, Amaral J: Laparoscopic 2-stage Fowler-Stephens orchiopexy. *J Urol* 152:1253, 1994.

Cartwright PC, Snyder HM III: Obstacles in reoperative orchiopexy—and a method to master them. *Contemp Urol* 15:56, 1993.

Cartwright PC, Velagapudi S, Snyder HM III, Keating MA: A surgical approach to reoperative orchiopexy. *J Urol* 149:817, 1993.

Casale AJ, Austin PF, Cain MP, et al: Nonpalpable undescended testis: does the order of procedure affect outcome and cost? A prospective randomized analysis of laparoscopy and groin exploration. *Pediatrics* 104:819, 1999.

Cattolica EV, Karol JB, Rankin KN, Klein RS: High testicular salvage rate in torsion of the spermatic cord. *J Urol* 128:66, 1982.

Cayan S, Acar D, Ulger S, Akbay E: Adolescent varicocele repair: long-term results and comparison of surgical techniques according to optical magnification use in 100 cases at a single university hospital. *J Urol* 174(5):2003–6, 2005; discussion 2006–7.

Cayan S, Akbay E, Bozlu M, Doruk E, et al: The effect of varicocele repair on testicular volume in children and adolescents with varicocele. *J Urol* 168(2):731–4, 2002.

Cendron M, Huff DS, Keating MA, et al: Anatomical, morphological and volumetric analysis: review of 759 cases of testicular maldescent. *J Urol* 149:570, 1983.

Chang B, Palmer LS, Franko I: Laparoscopic orchiopexy: a review of a large clinical series. *BJU Int* 87:490, 2001.

Chrouser K, Vandersteen D, Crocker J, Reinberg Y: Nerve injury after laparoscopic varicocelectomy. *J Urol* 172(2):691–3, 2004; discussion 693.

Cisek LJ, Peters CA, Atala A, et al: Current findings in diagnostic laparoscopic evaluation of the nonpalpable testis. *J Urol* 160:1145, 1998.

Clatworthy HW Jr, Hollabaugh RS, Grosfeld JL: The "long loop vas" orchiopexy for high undescended testis. *Am Surg* 38:69, 1972.

Cohen TD, Kay R, Knipper N: Reoperation for cryptorchid testis in the prepubertal child. *Urology* 42:437, 1993.

Coolsaet BLRA: The varicocele syndrome: venography determining the optimal level for surgical management. *J Urol* 124:833, 1980.

Cooper BJ, Little TM: Orchidopexy: theory and practice. *Br Med J* 291:706, 1985.

Cooper JF, Leadbetter WF, Chute R: The thoracoabdominal approach for retroperitoneal gland dissection: its application to testis tumors. *Surg Gynecol Obstet* 90:496, 1950.

Coplen DE, Manley CG: Timing of genital surgery. In: Ehrlich RM, Alter GJ: *Reconstructive and Plastic Surgery of the External Genitalia: Adult and Pediatric.* Philadelphia, W.B. Saunders Company, 1999, p 19.

Corkery JJ: Staged orchiopexy: a new technique. *J Pediatr Surg* 10:515, 1975.

Cortesi N, Ferrari P, Zambarda E, et al: Diagnosis of bilateral abdominal cryptochidism by laparoscopy. *Endoscopy* 8:33, 1976.

Dahl DS, Singh M, O'Conor VJ Jr, et al: Lord's operation for hydrocele compared with conventional techniques. *Arch Surg* 104:40, 1972.

Dajani AM: Transverse ectopia of the testis. *Br J Urol* 41:80, 1969.

Davits RJAM, Van Den Aker ESS, Scholtmeijer RJ, et al: Effect of parenteral testosterone therapy on penile development in boys with hypospadias. *Br J Urol* 71:593, 1993.

De Luna AM, Ortenberg J, Craver RD: Exploration for testicular remnants: implications of residual seminiferous tubules and crossed testicular ectopia. *J Urol* 169(4):1486–9, 2003.

DeBoer A: Inguinal hernia in infants and children. *Arch Surg* 75:920, 1957.

Dewbury KC: Scrotal ultrasonography: an update. *BJU Int* 86(suppl 1):143, 2000.

Diamond DA, Caldamone AA: The value of laparoscopy for 106 impalpable testes relative to clinical presentation. *J Urol* 148:632, 1992.

Diamond DA, Zurakowski D, Atala A, et al: Is adolescent varicocele a progressive disease process? *J Urol* 172(4 Pt 2):1746–8, 2004; discussion 1748.

Docimo SG : Improved technique for open laparoscopic access. *J Endocrinol* 121(suppl):S185, 1998.

Docimo SG: The results of surgical therapy for cryptorchidism: a literature review and analysis. *J Urol* 154:1148, 1995.

Docimo SG, Moore RG, Adams J, Kavoussi LR: Laparoscopic orchiopexy for high palpable undescended testis: preliminary experience. *J Urol* 154:1513, 1995.

Docimo SG, Moore RG, Kavoussi LR: Laparoscopic orchiopexy. *Urology* 46:715, 1995.

Driver CP, Losty PD: Neonatal testicular torsion. *Br J Urol* 82:855, 1998.

Dwoskin JY, Kuhn JP: Herniograms in undescended testes and hydroceles. *J Urol* 109:520, 1973.

Eaton SH, Cendron MA, Estrada CR, et al: Intermittent testicular torsion: diagnostic features and management outcomes. *J Urol* 174(4 Pt 2):1532–5, 2005; discussion 1535.

Elder JS: The failed orchiopexy. In: Cohen MS, Resnick MI (Eds): *Reoperative Urology.* Philadelphia, Lippincott-Raven Publications,1994, p 251.

Elder JS: Laparoscopy and Fowler-Stephens orchiopexy in the management of the impalpable testis. *Urol Clin North Am* 16:399, 1989.

Elder JS: Laparoscopy for impalpable testes: significance of the patent processus vaginalis. *J Urol* 152:776, 1994.

Elder JS: Ultrasonography is unnecessary in evaluating boys with a nonpalpable testis. *Pediatrics* 110:748, 2002.

Elder JS, Keating MA, Duckett JW: Infant testicular prostheses. *J Urol* 141:1413, 1989.

Elkabir JJ, Smith GL, Dinneen MD: Testicular prosthesis placement: a new technique. *BJU Int* 84:867–8, 1999.

Esposito C, Garipoli V: The value of 2-step laparoscopic Fowler-Stephens orchiopexy for intra-abdominal testes. *J Urol* 158:1952, 1997.

Esposito C, Valla JS, Najmaldin A, et al: Incidence and management of hydrocele following varicocele surgery in children. *J Urol* 171(3):1271–3, 2004.

Ewert EE, Hoffman HA: Torsion of the spermatic cord. *J Urol* 51:551, 1944.

Ferrer FA, Cadeddu JA, Schulam P, et al: Orchiopexy using 2-mm laparoscopic instruments: two techniques for delivering the testis into the scrotum. *J Urol* 164:160, 2000.

Firor HV: Two-stage orchiopexy. *Arch Surg* 102:598, 1971.

Flinn RA, King LR: Experiences with the midline transabdominal approach in orchiopexy. *Surg Gynecol Obstet* 133:285, 1971.

Fowler R, Stephens FD: The role of testicular vascular anatomy in the salvage of the high undescended testis. *Aust N Z J Surg* 29:92, 1959.

Fowler R, Stephens FD: The role of testicular vascular anatomy in the salvage of the high undescended testis. In: Stephens FD (Ed): *Congenital Malformations of Rectum, Anus and Genitourinary Tract.* Edinburgh, E & S, 1963, pp 306–20.

Franc-Guimond J, Kryger J, González R: Experience with the Bailez technique for laparoscopic access in children. *J Urol* 170(3):936–8, 2003.

Frank JD, O'Brien M: Fixation of the testis: review. *BJU Int* 89:331, 2002.

Garibyan H, Hazebroek FWJ, Schulkes JAR, et al: Microvascular surgical orchiopexy in the treatment of high-lying undescended testes. *Br J Urol* 56:326, 1984.

Gatti JM, Cooper CS, Kirsch AJ: Bimanual digital rectal exam in the evaluation of the non-palpable testis. AUA, South Central Section, 2002. Abstract.

Gauer DD, Agarwal DK, Purohit K, et al: Laparoscopic orchidopexy for the intra-abdominal testis. *J Urol* 153:481, 1995.

Gearhart JB, Jeffs RD: The use of parenteral testosterone therapy in genital reconstructive surgery. *J Urol* 138:1077, 1987.

Gill IS, Ross JH, Sung GT, Kay R: Needlescopic surgery for cryptorchidism: the initial series. *J Pediatr Surg* 35:1426, 2000.

Goldberg LM, Skaist LB, Morrow JW: Congenital absence of testes: anorchism and monorchism. *J Urol* 111:840, 1974.

Goldstein M, Gilbert BR, Dicker AP, et al: Microsurgical inguinal varicocelectomy with delivery of the testis: an artery and lymphatic sparing technique. *J Urol* 148:1608, 1992.

Greenfield SP, Seville P, Wan J: Experience with varicoceles in children and young adults. *J Urol* 168(4 Pt 2):1684–8, 2002; discussion 1688.

Gross RE: *The Surgery of Infancy and Childhood: Its Principles and Techniques.* Philadelphia, W. B. Saunders Company, 1953.

Gross RE, Jewett TC Jr: Surgical experiences from 1,222 operations for undescended testes. *JAMA* 160:634, 1956.

Gulanikar AC, Anderson PAM, Schwarz R, Giacomantonio M: Impact of diagnostic laparoscopy in the management of the unilateral impalpable testis. *Br J Urol* 77:455, 1996.

Hack WW, Sijstermans K, van der Voort-Doedens LM: Correction of cryptorchidism and testicular cancer. *N Engl J Med* 357(8):825–7, 2007.

Hadziselimovic F, Kogan SJ: Testicular development. In: Gillenwater JY, Grayhack JT, Howards SS, Duckett JW (Eds): *Adult and Pediatric Urology.* Chicago, Year Book Medical Publishers, 1987.

Halachmi S, El-Ghoneimi A, Bissonnette B, et al: Hemodynamic and respiratory effect of pediatric urological laparoscopic surgery: a retrospective study. *J Urol* 170(4 Pt 2):1651–4, 2003; discussion 1654.

Han WK, Kim JH, Hong CH, Han SW: Structural evidence against hormonal therapy for cryptorchid testis: abnormal gubernacular attachment. *J Urol* 171(6 Pt 1):2427–9, 2004.

Harkins HN: *Hernia.* Philadelphia, J. B. Lippincott Company, 1964.

Harrison RG: The distribution of the vasal and cremasteric arteries to the testis and their functional importance. *J Anat* 83:267, 1949.

Harrison RG, McGregor GA: Anomalous origin and branching of the testicular arteries. *Anat Rec* 129:401, 1957.

Hart RR, Rushton HG, Belman AB: Intraoperative spermatic venography during varicocele surgery in adolescents. *J Urol* 148:1514, 1992.

Hass JA, Carrion HM, Sharkey J, Politano VA: Operative treatment of hydrocele: another look at Lord's procedure. *Urology* 12:578, 1978.

Hassan JM, Adams MC, Pope JC 4th, Demarco RT, et al: Hydrocele formation following laparoscopic varicocelectomy. *J Urol* 175(3 Pt 1):1076–9, 2006.

Hazebroeck FWJ, Molenaar JC: The management of the impalpable testis by surgery alone. *J Urol* 148:629, 1993.

Hill EC: The vascularisation of the human testis. *Am J Anat* 9:463, 1909.

Hinman F Jr: The case for primary orchiectomy for the unilateral abdominal testis. In: Carlton CE Jr (Ed): *Controversies in Urology.* Chicago: Year Book Medical Publishers, 1989, p 42.

Hinman F Jr: Indications and contraindications for orchiopexy and orchiectomy. In: Fonkalsrud EW, Mengel W (Eds): *The Undescended Testis.* Chicago and London, Year Book Medical Publishers, 1981.

Hinman F Jr: Indications and contraindications for orchiopexy. In: Hadziselimovic F (Ed): *Cryptorchidism: Management and Implications.* Berlin and Heidelberg, Springer-Verlag, 1983, p 99.

Hinman F Jr: Management of the intra-abdominal testis. *Eur J Pediatr* 146:549, 1987.

Hinman F Jr: Optimum time for orchiopexy in cryptorchidism. *Fertil Steril* 6:206, 1955.

Hinman F Jr: Survey: localization and operation for nonpalpable testes. *Urology* 30:193, 1987.

Hinman F Jr: Unilateral abdominal cryptorchidism. *J Urol* 122:71, 1979.

Holcomb GR, Brock JR, Neblett WR, et al: Laparoscopy for the nonpalpable testis. *Am Surg* 60:143, 1994.

Hopps CV, Lemer ML, Schlegel PN, Goldstein M: Intraoperative varicocele anatomy: a microscopic study of the inguinal versus subinguinal approach. *J Urol* 170(6 Pt 1):2366–70, 2003.

Humke U, Siemer S, Bonnet L, et al: Pediatric laparoscopy for nonpalpable undescended testes. *J Endourol* 12:445, 1998.

Hunt JB, Witherington R, Smith AM: The midline preperitoneal approach to orchiopexy. *Am Surg* 47:184, 1981.

Ivanissevich O: Left varicocele due to reflux: experience with 4,470 operative cases in 42 years. *J Int Coll Surg* 34:742, 1918.

Ivanissevitch O, Gregorini H: A new operation for the cure of varicocele. *Semana Med* 25:575, 1918.

Janecka IP, Romas NA: Microvascular free transfer of human testes. *J Plast Reconstr Surg* 63:42, 1979.

Jirásek JE: The relationship between differentiation of the testicle, genital ducts and external genitalia in fetal and postnatal life. In: Rosenberg E, Paulsen AC (Eds): *The Human Testis.* New York, Plenum Press, 1970.

Jordan GH, Robey EL, Winslow BH: Laparo-endoscopic surgical management of the abdominal/transinguinal undescended testicle. *J Endocrinol* 6:159, 1992.

Jordan GH, Winslow BH: Laparoscopic single stage and staged orchiopexy. *J Urol* 152:1249, 1994.

Juskiewenski S, Vaysse P: Arterial vascularisation of the testes and surgery for undescended testicles (testicular ectopia). *Anat Clin* 1:127, 1979.

Kalfa N, Veyrac C, Baud C, et al: Ultrasonography of the spermatic cord in children with testicular torsion: impact on the surgical strategy. *J Urol* 172(4 Pt 2):1692–5, 2004; discussion 1695.

Kanemoto K, Hayashi Y, Kojima Y, et al: The management of nonpalpable testis with combined groin exploration and subsequent transinguinal laparoscopy. *J Urol* 167(2 Pt 1):674–6, 2002.

Kass EJ, Belman AB: Reversal of testicular growth failure by varicocele ligation. *J Urol* 137:475, 1987.

Kass EJ, Chandra RS, Belman AB: Testicular histology in the adolescent with a varicocele. *Pediatrics* 79:996, 1987.

Kass EJ, Freitas JE, Bour JB: Pituitary-gonadal function in adolescents with a varicocele. *J Urol* 139:207, 1988.

Kavoussi LR: Pediatric applications of laparoscopy. In: Clayman RV, McDougall EM (Eds): *Laparoscopic Urology.* St. Louis, Quality Medical Publishing, 1993, p 209.

Kavoussi LR, Sosa RE, Capelouto C: Complications of laparoscopic surgery. *J Endocrinol* 6:95, 1992.

Kaye KW, Lange PH, Fraley EE: Spermatic cord block in urologic surgery. *J Urol* 128:720, 1982.

Kelalis PP, King LR, Belman AB (Eds): *Clinical Pediatric Urology,* 2nd ed. Philadelphia, W. B. Saunders Company, 1985.

Khamesra HL, Gupta AS, Malpani NK: Transverse testicular ectopia. *Br J Urol* 50:283, 1978.

Kiddoo DA, Wollin TA, Mador DR: A population-based assessment of complications following outpatient hydrocelectomy and spermatocelectomy. *J Urol* 171(2 Pt 1):746–8, 2004.

King LM, Sekaran SK, Sauer D, et al: Untwisting in delayed treatment of torsion of the spermatic cord. *J Urol* 112:217, 1974.

Kocvara R, Dvoracek J, Sedlacek J, et al: Lymphatic sparing laparoscopic varicocelectomy: a microsurgical repair. *J Urol* 173(5):1751–4, 2005.

Koff SA: Does compensatory testicular enlargement predict monorchism? *J Urol* 146:632, 1991.

Koff SA, Sethi PS: Treatment of high undescended testes by low spermatic cord ligation: an alternative to the Fowler-Stephens technique. *J Urol* 156(Pt 2):799,1996.

Kogan SJ, Houman BZ, Reda EF, Levitt SB: Orchiopexy of the high undescended testis by division of the spermatic vessels: a critical review of 38 selected transections. *J Urol* 141:1416, 1989.

Kolon TF, Miller OF: Comparison of single versus multiple dose regimens for human chorionic gonadotropin stimulatory test. *J Urol* 166:1451, 2001.

Koyle MA, Oottamasathien S, Barqawi A, et al: Laparoscopic Palomo varicocele ligation in children and adolescents: results of 103 cases. *J Urol* 172(4 Pt 2):1749–52, 2004; discussion 1752.

Lakhoo K, Thomas FM, Najmeldin AS: Is inguinal exploration for impalpable testis an outdated operation? *Br J Urol* 77:452, 1996.

LaPointe SP, Wei DC, Hricak H, et al: Magnetic resonance imaging in the evaluation of congenital anomalies of the external genitalia. *Urology* 58:452, 2001.

Lattimer JK, Vakili BF, Smith AM, et al: A natural-feeling testicular prosthesis. *J Urol* 110:81, 1973.

Lee LY, Tzeng J, Grosman M, Unger PD: Prostate gland-like epithelium in the epididymis: a case report and review of the literature. *Arch Pathol Lab Med* 128(4):e60–2, 2004. Review.

Lemoh CN: A study of the development and structural relationships of the testis and gubernaculum. *Surg Gynecol Obstet* 110:164, 1960.

Levitt SB, Kogan SJ, Engel RM, et al: The impalpable testis: a rational approach to management. *J Urol* 120:515, 1978.

Lewis EL: The Ivanissevich operation. *J Urol* 63:165, 1950.

Lindgren BW, Darby EC, Faiella L, et al: Laparoscopic orchiopexy: procedure of choice for the nonpalpable testis? *J Urol* 159:2132, 1998.

Lindgren BW, Franco I, Blick S, et al: Laparoscopic Fowler-Stephens orchiopexy for the high abdominal testis. *J Urol* 162:990, 1999.

Livne PM, Savir A, Servadio C: Re-orchiopexy: advantages and disadvantages. *Eur Urol* 18:137, 1990.

Lord PH: A bloodless operation for the radical cure of idiopathic hydrocele. *Br J Surg* 51:914, 1964.

Lord PH: A bloodless operation for spermatocoele or cyst of the epididymis. *Br J Surg* 57:641, 1970.

Loughlin KR, Brooks DC: The use of a Doppler probe to facilitate laparoscopic varicocele ligation. *Surg Gynecol Obstet* 174:326, 1992.

Loughlin KR, Brooks DC: The use of a Doppler probe in laparoscopic surgery. *J Laparoendosc Surg* 2:191, 1992.

Luker CD, Siegel MJ: Pediatric testicular tumors: evaluation with gray-scale and color Doppler US. *Radiology* 191:561, 1994.

Lyon RP: Torsion of the testicle in childhood: a painless emergency requiring contralateral orchiopexy. *JAMA* 178:702, 1961.

MacMahon RA, OBrien BM, Cussen LJ: The use of microsurgery in the treatment of the undescended testis. *J Pediatr Surg* 11:52, 1976.

MacMillan EW: The blood supply of the epididymis in man. *Br J Urol* 26:60, 1954.

Maizels M, Gomez F, Firlit CF: Surgical correction of failed orchiopexy. *J Urol* 130:955, 1983.

Mansbach JM, Forbes P, Peters C: Testicular torsion and risk factors for orchiectomy. *Arch Pediatr Adolesc Med* 159(12):1167–71, 2005.

Margews R, Docimo SG: Laparoscopy for the management of the undescended testis. *Urol Clin North Am* 8:91, 2000.

Marshall FF, Elder JS: *Cryptorchidism and Related Anomalies.* New York, Praeger, 1982.

Marshall FF, Shermeta DW: Epididymal abnormalities associated with undescended testis. *J Urol* 121:341, 1979.

Martin DC, Menck HR: The undescended testis: management after puberty. *J Urol* 114:77, 1975.

McVay CB: The anatomic basis for inguinal and femoral hernioplasty. *Surg Gynecol Obstet* 139:931, 1974.

Mesrobian HG: Evaluation and management of the undescended testis and failed orchiopexy. *Prob Urol* 2:87, 1988.

Metcalfe PD, Farivar-Mohseni H, Farhat W, et al: Pediatric testicular tumors: contemporary incidence and efficacy of testicular preserving surgery. *J Urol* 170(6 Pt 1):2412–5, 2003; discussion 2415–6.

Metwalli AR, Cheng EY: Inguinal hernia after laparoscopic orchiopexy. *J Urol* 168(5):2163, 2002.

Mitchell ME: Urinary tract diversion and undiversion in the pediatric age group. *Surg Clin North Am* 61:1147, 1981.

Moorcraft J, DuBoulay CEH, Isaacson P, Atwell JD: Changes in the mucosa of colon conduits with particular reference to the risk of malignant change. *Br J Urol* 55:185, 1983.

Moore RG, Peters CA, Bauer SB, et al: Laparoscopic evaluation of the nonpalpable testis: a prospective assessment of accuracy. *J Urol* 151:728, 1994.

Mor Y, Pinthus JH, Nadu A, et al: Testicular fixation following torsion of the spermatic cord: does it guarantee prevention of recurrent torsion events? *J Urol* 175(1):171–3, 2006; discussion 173–4.

Morse TS, Hollebaugh RS: The window orchiopexy for prevention of testicular torsion. *J Pediatr Surg* 12:237, 1977.

Moul JW, Belman AB: A review of surgical treatment of undescended testes with emphasis on anatomical position. *J Urol* 140:125, 1988.

Murnaghan GF: The appendages of the testis and epididymis: a short review with case reports. *Br J Urol* 31:190, 1959.

Nadelson EJ, Cohen M, Warner R, Leiter E: Update: varicocelectomy: a safe outpatient procedure. *Urology* 14:259, 1984.

Nunn LN, Stephens FD: The triad syndrome: a composite anomaly of the abdominal wall, urinary system, and testis. *J Urol* 86:782, 1961.

Nyhus LM: The preperitoneal approach and iliopubic tract repair on inguinal hernia. In: Nyhus LM, Condon RE (Eds): *Hernia,* 2nd ed. Philadelphia, J. B. Lippincott Company, 1978, pp 212–35.

O'Brien BM, Rao VK, MacLeod AM, et al: Microvascular testicular transfer. *Plast Reconstr Surg* 71:87, 1983.

Odiase V, Whitaker RH: Analysis of cord length obtained during steps of orchiopexy. *Br J Urol* 54:308, 1982.

Oh J, Landman J, Evers A, et al: Management of the postpubertal patient with cryptorchidism: an updated analysis. *J Urol* 1767:1329, 2002.

Ombredanne L: Sur l'orchiopexie. *Bull Soc Pediatr (Paris)* 25:473, 1927.

Ottenheimer EJ: Testicular fixation in torsion of the spermatic cord. *JAMA* 101:116, 1933.

Pakzad K, MacLennan GT, Elder JS, et al: Follicular large cell lymphoma localized to the testis in children. *J Urol* 168(1):225–8, 2002.

Paloma A: Radical cure of varicocele by a new technique: preliminary report. *J Urol* 61:604, 1949.

Parkash S, Ramakrishnan K, Bagdi RK: Orchiopexy: trans-septal ipsilateral positioning. *Br J Urol* 55:79, 1982.

Parker RM, Robison JR: Anatomy and diagnosis of torsion of the testicle. *J Urol* 106:243, 1971.

Parkinson MC, Swerdlow AJ, Pike MC: Carcinoma in situ in boys with cryptorchidism: when can it be detected? *Br J Urol* 63:431, 1994.

Parsons JK, Ferrer F, Docimo SG: The low scrotal approach to the ectopic or ascended testicle: prevalence of a patent processus vaginalis. *J Urol* 169(5):1832–3, 2003; discussion 1833.

Pascual JA, Villanueva-Meyer J, Salido E, et al: Recovery of testicular blood flow following ligation of the testicular vessels. *J Urol* 142:549, 1989.

Patil KK, Duffy PG, Woodhouse CR, Ransley PG: Long-term outcome of Fowler-Stephens orchiopexy in boys with prune-belly syndrome. *J Urol* 171(4):1666–9, 2004.

Pearse I, Grick RD, Abramson AB, et al: Testicular sparing surgery for benign testicular tumors. *J Pediatr Surg* 34:100, 1999.

Persky L, Albert DJ: Staged orchiopexy. *Surg Gynecol Obstet* 132:43, 1971.

Peters CA: Laparoscopic and robotic approach to genitourinary anomalies in children. *Urol Clin North Am* 31(3):595–605, xi. Review.

Pettersson A, Richiardi L, Nordenskjold A, et al: Age at surgery for undescended testis and risk of testicular cancer. *N Engl J Med* 356(18):1835–41, 2007.

Pinsolle J, Drouillard J, Bruneton JN, Grenier FN: Anatomical bases of testicular vein catheterization and phlebography. *Anat Clin* 2:191, 1980.

Plottzker ED, Rushton HG, Belman AN, Skoog SJ: Laparoscopy for nonpalpable testes in childhood: is inguinal exploration also necessary when the vas and vessels exit the external ring? *J Urol* 148:635, 1992.

Poppas DP, Lemack GE, Mininberg DT: Laparoscopic orchiopexy: clinical experience and description of technique. *J Urol* 155:708, 1996.

Poppas DP, Wei JT, Mingin GC: The concealed laparoscopic orchidopexy. *Br J Urol* 86:138, 2000.

Prentiss RJ, Boatwright DC, Pennington RD, et al: Testicular prosthesis: materials, methods and results. *J Urol* 90:208, 1963.

Prentiss RJ, Weickgenant CJ, Moses JJ, Frazier DB: Undescended testis: surgical anatomy of spermatic vessels, spermatic surgical triangles and lateral spermatic ligament. *J Urol* 83:686, 1960.

Radmayr C, Oswald J, Schwentner C, et al: Long-term outcome of laparoscopically managed nonpalpable testes. *J Urol* 170 (6 Pt 1):2409–11, 2003.

Raijfer J, Pickett S, Klein SR: Laparoscopic occlusion of testicular veins for clinical varicocele. *Urology* 40:113, 1992.

Ransley PG, Vordermark JS, Caldamone AA, et al: Preliminary ligation of the gonadal vessels prior to orchiopexy for the intra-abdominal testicle: a staged Fowler-Stephens procedure. *World J Urol* 2:266, 1984.

Redman JF: Reoperative orchiopexy: approach through the cremasteric fascia. *Dial Ped Urol* 16(5):5, 1983.

Redman JF: Simplified technique for scrotal pouch orchiopexy. *Urol Clin North Am* 17:9, 1990.

Redman JF, Barthold SJ: A technique for atraumatic scrotal pouch orchiopexy in the management of testicular torsion. *J Urol* 154:1511, 1995.

Riccabona M, Oswald J, Koen M, et al: Optimizing the operative treatment of boys with varicocele: sequential comparison of 4 techniques. *J Urol* 169(2):666–8, 2003.

Riquelme M, Aranda A, Rodriguez C, et al: Incidence and management of the inguinal hernia during laparoscopic orchiopexy in palpable cryptoorchidism: preliminary report. *Pediatr Surg Int* 23(4):301–4, 2007. Epub 2007 Feb 8.

Robertson SA, Munro FD, Mackinlay GA: Two-stage Fowler-Stephens orchiopexy preserving the gubernacular vessels

and a purely laparoscopic second stage. *J Laparoendosc Adv Surg Tech A* 17(1):101–7, 2007.

Rolnick D, Kawanoue S, Szanto P, et al: Anatomical incidence of testicular appendages. *J Urol* 100:755, 1968.

Rosito NC, Koff WJ, da Silva Oliveira TL, et al: Volumetric and histological findings in intra-abdominal testes before and after division of spermatic vessels. *J Urol* 171(6 Pt 1):2430–3, 2004.

Rushton HG, Belman AB: Testis sparing surgery for benign lesions of the prepubertal testis. *Urol Clin North Am* 20:27, 1933.

Russinko PJ, Siddiq FM, Tackett LD, Caldamone AA: Prescrotal orchiopexy: an alternative surgical approach for the palpable undescended testis. *J Urol* 170(6 Pt 1):2436–8, 2003.

Scardino PT: Thoracoabdominal retroperitoneal lymphadenectomy for testicular carcinoma. In: Crawford ED, Borden TA (Eds): *Genitourinary Cancer Surgery.* Philadelphia, Lea & Febiger, 1982, p 27.

Schwentner C, Oswald J, Kreczy A, et al: Neoadjuvant gonadotropin-releasing hormone therapy before surgery may improve the fertility index in undescended testes: a prospective randomized trial. *J Urol* 173(3):974–7, 2005.

Schwentner C, Oswald J, Lunacek A, et al: Optimizing the outcome of microsurgical subinguinal varicocelectomy using isosulfan blue: a prospective randomized trial. *J Urol* 175(3 Pt 1):1049–52, 2006.

Scorer CG: The descent of the testis. *Arch Dis Child* 39:605, 1964.

Scorer CG, Farrington GH: *Congenital Deformities of the Testis and Epididymis.* London, Butterworth and Company, 1971.

Semm BK: *Operative Manual for Endoscopic Abdominal Surgery.* Friedrich ER (Trans). Chicago, Year Book Medical Publishers, 1987.

Sessions AE, Rabinowitz R, Hulbert WC, et al: Testicular torsion: direction, degree, duration and disinformation. *J Urol* 169:663, 2003.

Shafik A: Obturator foramen approach: II. A new surgical approach for management of the short-pedicled undescended testis. *Am J Surg* 144:381, 1982.

Shafik A, Moftah A, Olfat S, et al: Testicular veins: anatomy and role in varicocelogenesis and other pathologic conditions. *Urology* 35:175, 1990.

Shan CJ, Lucon AM, Arap S: Comparative study of sclerotherapy with phenol and surgical treatment for hydrocele. *J Urol* 169(3):1056–9, 2003.

Sharlip ID: Surgery of scrotal contents. *Urol Clin North Am* 14:145, 1987.

Silber S, Kelly J: Successful autotransplantation in an intra-abdominal testis to the scrotum by microvascular technique. *J Urol* 115:452, 1976.

Skandalakis JE: *Hernia: Surgical Anatomy and Technique.* New York, McGraw-Hill Book Company, 1989.

Skinner DG: Considerations for management of large retroperitoneal tumors: use of the modified thoracoabdominal approach. *Urology* 117:605, 1977.

Smith SP, King LR: Torsion of the testis: techniques of assessment. *Urol Clin North Am* 6:429, 1979.

Snodgrass W, Chen K, Harrison C: Initial scrotal incision for unilateral nonpalpable testis. *J Urol* 172(4 Pt 2):1742–5, 2004; discussion 1745.

Snyder WH Jr: Inguinal hernia complicated by descended testis. *Am J Surg* 94:325, 1955.

Soble JJ, Gill IS: Needlescopic urology: incorporating 2-mm instruments in laparoscopic surgery. *Urology* 52:187, 1998.

Solomon AA: The extrusion operation for hydrocele. *N Y State J Med* 55:1885, 1955.

Solomon AA: Testicular prosthesis: a new insertion operation. *J Urol* 108:436, 1972.

Steiner H, Hoeltl L, Maneschg C, et al: Frozen section analysis-guided organ-sparing approach in testicular tumors: technique, feasibility and long-term results. *Urology* 62:508, 2003.

Steinhardt GF, Kroovand RL, Perlmutter AD: Orchiopexy: planned 2-stage technique. *J Urol* 133:434, 1985.

Stephens FD: Embryopathy of malformations. *J Urol* 127:13, 1982.

Swerdlow AJ, Higgins CD, Pike MC: Risk of testicular cancer in cohort of boys with cryptorchidism. *Br Med J* 314:1507, 1997.

Taskinen D, Taavitsainen M, Wikström S: Measurement of testicular volume: comparison of 3 different methods. *J Urol* 155:930, 1996.

Tennenbaum SY, Lerner SE, McAleer IM, et al: Preoperative laparoscopic localization of the nonpalpable testis: a critical analysis of a 10-year experience. *J Urol* 151:732, 1994.

Thayyil S, Shenoy M, Agrawal K: Delayed orchidopexy: failure of screening or ascending testis. *Arch Dis Child* 89(9):890, 2004.

Thomas JC, Elder JS: Testicular growth arrest and adolescent varicocele: does varicocele size make a difference? *J Urol* 168(4 Pt 2):1689–91, 2002; discussion 1691.

Thorup J, Haugen S, Kollin C, et al: Surgical treatment of undescended testes. *Acta Paediatr* 96(5):631–7, 2007. Epub 2007 Mar 23. Review.

Thorup JM, Cortes D, Visfeldt J: Germ cells may survive clipping and division of the spermatic vessels in surgery for intra-abdominal testes. *J Urol* 162:872, 1999.

Tsujihata M, Miyake O, Yoshimura K, et al: Laparoscopic diagnosis and treatment of nonpalpable testis. *Int J Urol* 8:693, 2001.

Turek PJ, Ewalt DG, Snyder HM III, et al: The absent cryptorchid testis: surgical findings and their implications for diagnosis and etiology. *J Urol* 151:718, 1994.

Turek PJ, Master VA: Testicular Prosthesis Study Group. Safety and effectiveness of a new saline filled testicular prosthesis. *J Urol* 172(4 Pt 1):1427–30, 2004.

Valla JS for the Group d'Etude en Urologie Pédiatrique: Testis-sparing surgery for benign testicular tumors in children. *J Urol* 165:2280, 2001.

Vergnes P, Midy D, Bondonny JM, Cabanie H: Anatomical basis of inguinal surgery in children. *Anat Clin* 7:257, 1985.

Viidik T, Marshall DG: Direct inguinal hernias in infancy and early childhood. *J Pediatr Surg* 15:646, 1980.

Wacksman J, Dinner M, Handler M: Results of testicular auto-transplantation using microvascular technique: experience with 8 intra-abdominal testes. *J Urol* 128:1319, 1982.

Wacksman J, Dinner M, Straffon R: Technique of testicular autotransplantation using microvascular anastomosis. *Surg Gynecol Obstet* 150:399, 1980.

Waldron R, James M, Clain A: Technique and results of trans-scrotal operations for hydrocele and scrotal cysts. *Br J Urol* 58:303, 1986.

Weiss RM, Seashore JH: Laparoscopy in the management of the nonpalpable testis. *J Urol* 138:385, 1997.

Weissbach L: Alloplastic testicular prostheses. In: Wagenknecht LV, Furlow WL, Auvert J (Eds): *Genitourinary Reconstruction with Prostheses*. Stuttgart, Georg Thieme Verlag, 1981, p 173.

Weissbach L: Organ preserving surgery of malignant germ cell tumors. *J Urol* 153:90, 1995.

Winfield HN, Donovan JF, See WA, et al: Urological laparoscopic surgery. *J Urol* 146:941, 1991.

Woodard JR, Parrot TS: Orchiopexy in the prune-belly syndrome. *Br J Surg* 50:348, 1978.

Yasbeck S, Patiquin HB: Accuracy of Doppler sonography in the evaluation of acute conditions of the scrotum in children. *J Pediatr Surg* 29:1270, 1994.

Youngson GG, Jones PF: Management of the impalpable testis: long-term results of the preperitoneal approach. *J Pediatr Surg* 26:618, 1991.

Yuzpe AA: Pneumoperitoneum needle and trocar injuries in laparoscopy: a survey on possible contributing factors and prevention. *J Reprod Med* 25:485, 1990.

Zer M, Wolloch Y, Dintsman M: Staged orchiorrhaphy: therapeutic procedure in cryptorchid testicle with a short spermatic cord. *Arch Surg* 110:387, 1975.

Zilberman D, Inbar Y, Heyman Z, et al: Torsion of the cryptorchid testis: can it be salvaged? *J Urol* 175(6):2287–9, 2006; discussion 2289.

Section 8
Penis, Urethra, and Genitalia

Aaronson IA: Micropenis: medical and surgical implications. *J Urol* 152:4, 1994.

Abbé R: New method of creating a vagina in a case of congenital absence. *Med Rec*, Dec 10, 1898.

Allen LE, Hardy BE, Churchill BM: The surgical management of the enlarged clitoris. *J Urol* 128:351, 1982.

Allen TD: Microphallus: clinical and endocrinological characteristics. *J Urol* 119:750, 1978.

Allen TD, Spence HM: The surgical treatment of coronal hypospadias and related problems. *J Urol* 100:504, 1968.

Alter GJ, Ehrlich RM: A new technique for the correction of the hidden penis in children and adults. *J Urol* 161:455, 1999.

American Academy of Pediatrics, Section on Urology: Timing of elective surgery on the genitalia of male children with particular reference to the risks, benefits, and psychological effects of surgery and anesthesia. *Pediatrics* 97:590, 1996.

Amukele SA, Lee GW, Stock JA, Hanna MK: 20-year experience with iatrogenic penile injury. *J Urol* 170(4 Pt 2):1691–4, 2003.

Amukele SA, Stock JA, Hanna MK: Management and outcome of complex hypospadias repairs. *J Urol* 174(4 Pt 2):1540–2, 2005.

Amukele SA, Weiser AC, Stock JA, Hanna MK: Results of 265 consecutive proximal hypospadias repairs using the Thiersch-Duplay principle. *J Urol* 172:2382–3, 2004.

Ansell JS, Rajfer J: A new and simplified method for concealing the hypertrophied clitoris. *J Pediatr Surg* 16:681, 1984.

Arap S, Giron AM: Urinary tract reconstruction in exstrophy and epispadias. In: Thuroff JW, Hohenfellner M (Eds): *Reconstructive Surgery of the Lower Urinary Tract in Children*. Oxford, ISIS Medical Media, 1995, p 88.

Arap S, Mitre A, de Góes GM: Modified meatal advancement and glanuloplasty for distal hypospadias. *J Urol* 131:1140, 1984.

Arneri V: Reconstruction of the male genitalia. In: Converse JM (Ed): *Reconstructive and Plastic Surgery*, 2nd ed, vol 7. Philadelphia, W. B. Saunders Company, 1977, p 3902.

Asopa HS, Elhence IP, Atri SP, Bansal NK: One-stage correction of penile hypospadias using a foreskin tube: a preliminary report. *Int Surg* 55:435, 1971.

Asopa R, Asopa HS: One-stage repair of hypospadias using double island preputial skin tube. *Indian J Urol* 1:41, 1984.

Atala A, Retik AB: Hypospadias. In: Libertino JA, Zinman L (Eds): *Reconstructive Urologic Surgery*. St. Louis, C. V. Mosby, 1988.

Atala A, Retik AB: Late complications of hypospadias repair. In: Horton CA, Elder JC (Eds): *Reconstructive Surgery of External Genitalia*. Boston, Little, Brown. In press.

Atala A, Retik AB: Two-stage hypospadias repair. In Ehrlich RM, Alter GJ (Eds): *Reconstructive and Plastic Surgery of the External*

Genitalia: Adult and Pediatric. Philadelphia, W. B. Saunders Company, 1999, p 113.

Atikeler MK, Onur R, Gecit I, et al: Increased morbidity after circumcision from a hidden complication. *BJU Int* 88:938, 2001.

Austin JC, Clement MR, Canning DA: Modified tubular transverse preputial island flap for repair of severe hypospadias. Paper presented at the annual meeting of the AUA, 2002. Program Abstracts, p 91.

Avanoglu A, Celik A, Ulman I, et al: Safer circumcision in patients with haemophilia: the use of fibrin glue for local hemostasis. *BJU Int* 83:91, 1999.

Azmy A, Eckstein HB: Surgical correction of torsion of the penis. *Br J Urol* 53:378, 1981.

Bagshaw HA, Flynn JT, James AN, et al: The use of thioglycolic acid in hair-bearing skin inlay urethroplasty. *Br J Urol* 52:346, 1980.

Bailez MM, Gearhart JP, Migeon C, Rock J: Vaginal reconstruction after initial construction of the external genitalia in girls with salt-wasting adrenal hyperplasia. *J Urol* 148:680, 1992.

Baldwin JF: The formation of an artificial vagina by intestinal transplantation. *Ann Surg* 40:398, 1904.

Bale PM, Lochhead A, Martin HC, et al: Balanitis xerotica obliterans in children. *Pediatr Pathol* 7:617, 1987.

Ballesteros JJ: Personal technique for surgical repair of balanic hypospadias. *J Urol* 118:983, 1977.

Bar Yosef Y, Binyamini J, Matzkin H, Ben-Chaim J: Midline dorsal plication technique for penile curvature repair. *J Urol* 172(4 Pt 1):1368–9, 2004.

Barcat J: Current concepts of treatment. In: Horton CE (Ed): *Plastic and Reconstructive Surgery of the Genital Area.* Boston, Little, Brown & Company, 1973, p 249.

Barcat J: L'hypospadias: III. Les urethroplasties, le resultats – le complications. *Ann Chir Infant* 10:310, 1969.

Barrett TM, Gonzales ET Jr: Reconstruction of the female external genitalia. *Urol Clin North Am* 7:455, 1980.

Barthold JS, Teer TL, Redman JF: Modified Barcat balanitic groove technique for hypospadias repair: experience with 296 cases. *J Urol* 155:1735, 1996.

Bartone F, Shore N, Newland J, et al: The best suture for hypospadias? *Urology* 29:517, 1987.

Baskin LS: Fetal genital anatomy reconstructive implications. *J Urol* 162:527, 1999.

Baskin LS: Hypospadias: anatomy, embryology, and reconstructive techniques. *J Urol* 26:621, 2000.

Baskin LS: Hypospadias: a critical analysis of cosmetic outcomes using photography. *BJU Int* 87:534, 2001.

Baskin LS: Penile curvature (chordee). In: Ehrlich RM, Alter GJ (Eds): *Reconstructive and Plastic Surgery of the External Genitalia: Adult and Pediatric.* Philadelphia, W. B. Saunders Company, 1999, p 22.

Baskin LS, Duckett JW: Buccal mucosal grafts in hypospadias surgery: review article. *Br J Urol* 76(suppl 3):23, 1995.

Baskin LS, Duckett JW: Dorsal tunica albuginea plication for hypospadias curvature. *J Urol* 151:1668, 1994.

Baskin LS, Duckett JW: Mucosal grafts in hypospadias and stricture management. *AUA Update Series* 13:270, 1994.

Baskin LS, Duckett JW, Ueoka K, et al: Changing concepts of hypospadias curvature lead to more island flap onlay procedures. *J Urol* 151:191, 1994.

Baskin LS, Erol A, et al: Anatomical studies of hypospadias. *J Urol* 160(3):1108, 1998; discussion 1137.

Baskin LS, Erol A, Li YW, et al: Anatomic studies of the human clitoris. *J Urol* 162:1015, 1999.

Baskin LS, Erol A, Li YW, Cunha G: Neuro and vascular anatomy of hypospadias. *J Urol* 160:1108, 1998.

Baskin LS, Lue TF: The correction of congenital penile curvature in young men. *Br J Urol* 81:895, 1998.

Beck C: Hypospadias and its treatment. *Surg Gynecol Obstet* 24:511, 1917.

Beemer W, Hopkins MP, Morley GW: Vaginal reconstruction in gynecologic oncology. *Obstet Gynecol* 72:911, 1988.

Bellinger MF: Embryology of the male external genitalia. *Urol Clin North Am* 8:375, 1981.

Belman AB: De-epithelialized skin flap coverage in hypospadias repair. *J Urol* 140:1273, 1988.

Belman AB: The de-epithelialized skin flap and its influence on hypospadias repair. *J Urol* 152:2332, 1994.

Belman AB: The modified Mustardé hypospadias repair. *J Urol* 127:88, 1982.

Belman AB, King LR: Urinary tract abnormalities associated with imperforate anus. *J Urol* 108:823, 1972.

Bennett AH, Gittes RF: Congenital penile curvature without hypospadias. *Urology* 16:364, 1980.

Berdeu D, Sauze L, Ha-Vinh P, Blum-Boisgard C: Cost-effectiveness analysis of treatments for phimosis: a comparison of surgical and medicinal approaches and their economic effect. *BJU Int* 87:239, 2001.

Berg R, Berg G: Penile malformation, gender identity and sexual orientation. *Acta Psychiatr Scand* 68:154, 1983.

Bergman R, Howard AH, Barnes RW: Plastic reconstruction of the penis. *J Urol* 59:1174, 1948.

Bevan AD: A new operation for hypospadias. *JAMA* 68:1032, 1917.

Bhandari M, Kumar S: Modified single-stage hypospadias repair using double island preputial skin tube. *Br J Urol* 62:189, 1988.

Blalock HJ, Vemulakonda V, Ritchey Ml, Ribbeck MR: Outpatient management of phimosis following newborn circumcision. *J Urol* 169:2332, 2003.

Blandy JP: Circumcision. In: Chamberlain GVP (Ed): *Contemporary Obstetrics and Gynaecology.* London, Northwood, 1977, p 240.

Blandy JP: Urethral stricture. *Postgrad Med J* 56:383, 1980.

Blandy JP, Singh M: The technique and results of one-stage island patch urethroplasty. *Br J Urol* 47:83, 1975.

Blandy JP, Tresidder GC: Meatoplasty. *Br J Urol* 39:633, 1967.

Boemers TML, De Jong TPVM: The surgical correction of buried penis: a new technique. *J Urol* 154:550, 1995.

Boxer JB: Reconstruction of the male genitalia. *Surg Gynecol Obstet* 141:939, 1975.

Bracka A: Hypospadias repair: the two-stage alternative. *Br J Urol* 76(suppl):31, 1995.

Bracka A: Sexuality after hypospadias repair. *Br J Urol* 83(suppl):29–33, 1999.

Brannan W, Ochsner M, Fuselier HA, Goodlet JS: Free full-thickness skin graft urethroplasty for urethral stricture: experience with 66 patients. *J Urol* 115:677, 1976.

Broadbent TR, Woolf RM, Toksu E: Hypospadias: one-stage repair. *Plast Reconstr Surg* 27:154, 1961.

Brock JW III: Autologous buccal mucosal graft for urethral reconstruction. *Urology* 44:753, 1994.

Brough RJ, Betts CD, Payne SR: EMLA cream anaesthesia for frenuloplasty. *Br J Urol* 76:653, 1995.

Browne D: A comparison of the Duplay and Denis Browne techniques for hypospadias operation. *Surgery* 34:787, 1953.

Browne D: An operation for hypospadias. *Lancet* 1:141, 1936.

Bulmer D: The development of the human vagina. *J Anat* 91:490, 1957.

Burbige KA: Simplified post-operative management of hypospadias repairs. *Urology* 43:719, 1994.

Burbige KA: Transpubic-perineal urethral reconstruction in boys using a substitution graft. *J Urol* 148:1235, 1992.

Bürger RA, Müller SC, El-Damanhoury H, et al: The buccal mucosal graft for urethral reconstruction: a preliminary report. *J Urol* 147:662, 1992.

Bürger RA, Riedmiller H, Knapstein PG, et al: Ileocecal vaginal construction. *Am J Obstet Gynecol* 161:162, 1989.

Burkholder GV, Newell ME: New surgical treatment for micropenis. *J Urol* 129:832, 1983.

Byars LT: Technique for consistently satisfactory repair of hypospadias. *Surg Gynecol Obstet* 100:184, 1955.

Cabral BHP, González R: Use of urethral drainage tube and dressing in hypospadias repair. *Urology* 33:327, 1989.

Caesar RE, Caldamone AA: The use of free grafts for correcting penile chordee. *J Urol* 164:1691, 2000.

Caione P, Capozza N: Evolution of male epispadias repair: 16 year experience. *J Urol* 165:2410, 2001.

Caione P, Capozza N, Lais A, et al: Periurethral muscle complex reassembly in exstrophy-epispadias repair. *J Urol* 151:457, 2000.

Cantwell FV: Operative treatment of epispadias by transplantation of the urethra. *Ann Surg* 22:689, 1895.

Casale AJ: Genitourinary trauma in children. In: King LR (Ed): *Urologic Surgery in Neonates and Young Infants*. Philadelphia, W. B. Saunders Company, 1988, p 284.

Cecil AB: Repair of hypospadias and urethral fistula. *J Urol* 56:237, 1946.

Cecil AB: Surgery of hypospadias and epispadias in the male. *J Urol* 67:1006, 1932.

Cendron J, Melin Y: Congenital curvature of the penis without hypospadias. *Urol Clin North Am* 8:398, 1981.

Chandna S, Bruce J, Dickson A, Gough D: The Whitaker Hook in the treatment of posterior urethral valves. *Br J Urol* 78:783, 1996.

Chang T-S, Hwang W-Y: Forearm flap in one-stage reconstruction of the penis. *Plast Reconstr Surg* 74:251, 1984.

Cheng EY, Kropp BP, Pope JC 4th, Brock JW 3rd: Proximal division of the urethral plate in staged hypospadias repair. *J Urol* 170(4 Pt 2):1580–3, 2003; discussion 1584.

Chibber AK, Perkins FM, Rabinowitz R, et al: Penile block for postoperative analgesia of hypospadias repair in children. *J Urol* 158:1156, 1997.

Chuang JH: Penoplasty for the buried penis. *J Pediatr Surg* 30:1256, 1995.

Churchill BM, Van Savage JG, Khoury AE, McLorie GA: The dartos flap as an adjunct in preventing urethrocutaneous fistulas in repeat hypospadias surgery. *J Urol* 156:2047, 1996.

Coleman JW: The bladder mucosal graft technique for hypospadias repair. *J Urol* 125:708, 1981.

Coleman JW, McGovern JH, Marshall VF: The bladder mucosal graft technique for hypospadias repair. *Urol Clin North Am* 8:457, 1981.

Conway H, Stark RB: Construction and reconstruction of the vagina. *Surg Gynecol Obstet* 97:573, 1953.

Cook AJ, Farhat WA, Cartwright LM, et al: Simplified mons plasty: a new technique to improve cosmesis in females with the exstrophy-epispadias complex. *J Urol* 173(6):2117–20, 2005.

Coran AG, Polley TZ Jr: Surgical management of ambiguous genitalia in the infant and child. *J Pediatr Surg* 26:812, 1991.

Crawford BS: Buried penis. *Br J Plast Surg* 30:96, 1977.

Crawford ED: Technique of ilioinguinal lymph node dissection. In: Skinner DG, Lieskovsky G (Eds): *Diagnosis and Management of Genitourinary Cancer*. Philadelphia, W. B. Saunders Company, 1988.

Cromie WJ, Bellinger MF: Hypospadias dressing and diversions. *Urol Clin North Am* 8:545, 1981.

Cromie WJ, Ritchey ML, Smith RC, Zagaja GP: Anatomical alignment for correction of buried penis. *J Urol* 160:1482, 1998.

Cuckow PM, Rix G, Mouriquand PD: Preputial plasty: a good alternative to circumcision. *J Pediatr Surg* 29:561, 1994.

Culp DA: Genital injuries: etiology and initial management in genitourinary trauma. *Urol Clin North Am* 4:143, 1977.

Das S, Brosman SA: Duplication of male urethra. *J Urol* 117:452, 1977.

Davis RS, Linke CA, Kraemer GK: Use of labial tissue in repair of urethrovaginal fistula and injury. *Arch Surg* 115:628, 1980.

De Castella H: Prepuce plasty: an alternative to circumcision. *Ann R Coll Surg Engl* 76:257, 1994.

De Castro R, Merlini E, Rigamonti W, Macedo A Jr: Phalloplasty and urethroplasty in children with penile agenesis: preliminary report. *J Urol* 177(3):1112–6, 2007; discussion 1117.

De la Rosette JJMCH, de Vries JDM, Lock MTWT, Debruyne FMJ: Urethroplasty using the pedicled island flap technique in complicated urethral strictures. *J Urol* 146:40, 1991.

Decter RM: M inverted V glansplasty: a procedure for distal hypospadias. *J Urol* 146:641, 1991.

Decter RM: The M inverted V glansplasty: a variation of the MAGPI procedure. In: Ehrlich RM, Alter GJ (Eds): *Reconstructive and Plastic Surgery of the External Genitalia: Adult and Pediatric*. Philadelphia, W. B. Saunders Company, 1999, p 35.

Decter RM, Franzoni DF: Distal hypospadias repair by the modified Thiersch-Duplay technique with or without hinging the urethral plate: a near ideal way to correct distal hypospadias. *J Urol* 162:1156, 1999.

DeFoor W, Wacksman J: Results of single staged hypospadias surgery to repair penoscrotal hypospadias with bifid scrotum or penoscrotal transposition. *J Urol* 170(4 Pt 2):1585–8, 2003; discussion 1588.

DeJong TP, Boemers TN: Improved Mathieu repair for coronal and distal shaft hypospadias with moderate chordee. *Br J Urol* 72:927, 1993.

Desautel MG, Stock J, Hanna MK: Müllerian duct remnants: surgical management and fertility issues. *J Urol* 162:1008, 1999.

Dessanti A, Iannuccelli M, Ginesu G, Feo C: Reconstruction of hypospadias and epispadias with buccal mucosa free graft as primary surgery: more than 10 years of experience. *J Urol* 170(4 Pt 2):1600–2, 2003.

Dessanti A, Rigamonti W, Merulla V, et al: Autologous buccal mucosa graft for hypospadias repair: an initial report. *J Urol* 147:1081, 1992.

DeSy WA: Aesthetic repair of meatal strictures. *J Urol* 132:678, 1984.

DeSy WA, Oosterlinck W: Partial pubectomy: technique and indications. *Br J Urol* 58:464, 1986.

DeSy WA, Verbaeys A, Roelandt R, Osterlinck W: A simple approach to the entire urethra. *Br J Urol* 58:344, 1986.

Devine CJ Jr: Editorial comment. *J Urol* 144:283, 1990.

Devine CJ Jr: Embryology of the male external genitalia. *Clin Plast Surg* 7:141, 1980.

Devine CJ Jr, Blackley SK, Horton CE, Gilbert DA: The surgical treatment of chordee without hypospadias and associated anomalies: review of 400 cases. *J Urol* 96:339, 1991.

Devine CJ Jr, Franz JP, Horton CE: Evaluation and treatment of patients with failed hypospadias repairs. *J Urol* 119:223, 1978.

Devine CJ Jr, Gonzalez-Serva L, Stecker JF Jr, et al: Utricular configuration in hypospadias and intersex. *Trans Am Assoc Genitourin Surg* 71:154, 1979.

Devine CJ Jr, Horton CE: Chordee without hypospadias. *J Urol* 110:264, 1973.

Devine CJ Jr, Horton CE: A one-stage hypospadias repair. *J Urol* 85:166, 1961.

Devine CJ Jr, Horton CE, Snyder HM III, et al: Chordee without hypospadias. In: Hurwitz RS, Ehrlich RM (eds): *Dial Ped Urol* 9:2, 1986.

Devine PC, Devine CJ, Horton CE: Anterior urethral injuries: secondary reconstruction. *Urol Clin North Am* 4:157, 1977.

Devine PC, Horton CE: Hypospadias repair. *J Urol* 118:188, 1977.

Devine PC, Horton CE, Devine CJ Jr, et al: Use of full-thickness skin grafts in repair of urethral strictures. *J Urol* 90:67, 1963.

Devine PC, Wendelken JR, Devine CJ Jr: Free full-thickness skin graft urethroplasty: current technique. *J Urol* 121:282, 1979.

Dewan PA: Distal hypospadias repair with preputial reconstruction. *J Paediatr Child Health* 29:183, 1993.

Dewan PA, Dinneen MD, Duffy PG, et al: Pedicle patch urethroplasty. *Br J Urol* 67:420, 1991.

Diagnosis and therapy of micropenis. *Dialogues in Pediatric Urology* 7(1), 1984.

Diamond DA, Ransley PG: Male epispadias. *J Urol* 154:2150, 1995.

Disandro M, Palmer JM: Stricture incidence related to suture material in hypospadias surgery. *J Pediatr Surg* 131:881, 1996.

Dodson JL, Baird AD, Baker LA, et al: Outcomes of delayed hypospadias repair: implications for decision making. *J Urol* 178(1):278–81, 2007. Epub 2007 May 17.

Donahoe PK, Keating MA: Preputial unfurling to correct the buried penis. *J Pediatr Surg* 21:1055, 1986.

Donnahoo KK, Cain MP, Pope JC, et al: Etiology, management and surgical complications of congenital chordee without hypospadias. *J Urol* 160:1120, 1998.

Dreger AD (Ed): *Intersex in the Age of Ethics.* Ethics in Clinical Medicine Series. University Publishing Group, 1999.

Duckett JW: Hypospadias. In: Walsh PC, Retik AB, Vaughan ED, Wein AJ (Eds): *Campbell's Urology,* 7th ed. Philadelphia, W. B. Saunders Company, 1998, p 2093.

Duckett JW: The island flap technique for hypospadias repair. *Urol Clin North Am* 8:503, 1981.

Duckett JW Jr: MAGPI (meatoplasty and glanuloplasty): a procedure for subcoronal hypospadias. *Urol Clin North Am* 8:513, 1981.

Duckett JW Jr: Transverse preputial island flap technique for repair of severe hypospadias. *Urol Clin North Am* 7:423, 1980.

Duckett JW, Baskin LS: Hypospadias. In: Gillenwater JY, Grayhack JT, Howards SS, Duckett JW (Eds): *Adult and Pediatric Urology,* 3rd ed. St. Louis, Mosby Year Book, 1996.

Duckett JW, Coplen D, Ewalt D, et al: Buccal mucosa in urethral reconstruction. *J Urol* 153:1660, 1995.

Duckett JW, Keating MA: Technical challenge of the megameatus intact prepuce hypospadias variant: the pyramid procedure. *J Urol* 141:1407, 1989.

Duckett JW, Smith GHH: Urethral lesions in infants and children. In: Gillenwater JY, Grayhack JT, Howards SS, Duckett JW (Eds): *Adult and Pediatric Urology,* 3rd ed. St. Louis, Mosby Year Book, 1996, p 2411.

Duckett JW, Snyder HM III: The MAGPI hypospadias repair in 1111 patients. *Ann Surg* 213:620, 1991.

Duckett JW, Snyder HM III: Meatal advancement and glanuloplasty hypospadias repair after 1,000 cases: avoidance of meatal stenosis and regression. *J Urol* 147:665, 1992.

Duel BP, Barthold JS, González R: Management of urethral strictures after hypospadias repair. *J Urol* 160:170, 1998.

Duffy PG, Ransley PG, Malone PS, et al: Combined free autologous bladder mucosa/skin tube for urethral reconstruction: an update. *Br J Urol* 61:505, 1988.

Duplay S: Sur le traitement chirurgical del hypospadias, et la: epispadias. *Arch Gen Med* 5:257, 1880.

Eardley I, Whitaker RH: Surgery for hypospadias fistula. *Br J Urol* 69:306, 1992.

Ebbehoj J, Metz P: New operation for "Krummerik" (penile curvature). *Urology* 26:76–8, 1985.

Ehrlich RM, Alter GJ: *Reconstructive and Plastic Surgery of the External Genitalia: Adult and Pediatric.* Philadelphia, W. B. Saunders Company, 1999.

Ehrlich RM, Alter GJ: Split-thickness skin graft urethroplasty and tunica vaginalis flaps for failed hypospadias repairs. *J Urol* 155:131, 1996.

Ehrlich RM, Gershman A, Fuchs G: Selected topics in pediatric urology. *Pediatr Urol Corresp Club Letter,* Feb 28, 1993.

Ehrlich RM, Reda EF, Koyle MA, et al: Complications of bladder mucosal graft. *J Urol* 142:626, 1989.

Ehrlich RM, Scardino PT: Surgical correction of scrotal transposition and perineal hypospadias. *J Pediatr Surg* 17:175, 1982.

Elder JS: Influence of glans morphology on choice of island flap technique in children with proximal hypospadias. *J Urol* 147:317A, 1992.

Elder JS, Duckett JW, Snyder HM, et al: Onlay island flap in the repair of mid- and distal penile hypospadias without chordee. *J Urol* 138:376, 1987.

Elder JS, Mostwin JL: Cyst of the ejaculatory duct/urogenital sinus. *J Urol* 132:768, 1984.

El-Kasaby AW, Fath-Alla M, Noweir AM, et al: The use of buccal mucosa patch graft in the management of anterior urethral strictures. *J Urol* 149:276, 1993.

Epstein A, Strauss B: Prolapse of the female urethra with gangrene. *Am J Surg* 35:563–5, 1937.

Erol A, Baskin LS, Li YW, Liu WH: Anatomical studies of the urethral plate: why preservation of the urethral plate is important in hypospadias repair. *BJU Int* 85:728, 2000.

Farkas A, Chertin SB, Hadas-Halpren I: One-stage feminizing genitoplasty: 8 years experience with 49 cases. *J Urol* 165:2341, 2001.

Feldman KW, Smith DW: Fetal phallic growth and penile standards for newborn male infants. *J Pediatr* 86:395, 1975.

Ferlise VJ, Ankem MK, Batone JG: Use of cyanoacrylate tissue adhesive under a diaper. *Br J Urol* 87:672, 2001.

Fichtner J, Filipas D, Fisch M, et al: Long-term follow-up of buccal mucosa onlay graft for hypospadias repair: analysis of complications. *J Urol* 172(5 Pt 1):1970–2, 2004.

Fichtner J, Filipas D, Mottrie AM, et al: Analysis of meatal location in 500 men: wide variation questions need for meatal advancement in all pediatric anterior hypospadias cases. *J Urol* 154:833, 1995.

Filipas D, Fisch M, Fichtner J, et al: The histology and immunohistochemistry of free buccal mucosa and full-skin grafts after exposure to urine. *BJU Int* 84:108, 1999.

Firlit CF: The mucosal collar in hypospadias surgery. *J Urol* 137:80, 1987.

Flack CE, Walker RD: Onlay-tube-onlay urethroplasty technique in primary perineal hypospadias surgery. *J Urol* 154:837, 1995.

Fraser ID, Goede AC: Sutureless circumcision. *BJU Int* 90:467, 2002.

Freitas Filho LG, Carnevale J, Melo ML, Silva MC: A posterior-based omega-shaped flap vaginoplasty in girls with congenital adrenal hyperplasia caused by 21-hydroxylase deficiency. *BJU Int* 91:263, 2003.

Frey P, Cohen SJ: Reconstruction of the foreskin in distal hypospadias repair. *Prog Pediatr Surg* 23:192,1989.

Garibay JT, Reid C, González R: Functional evaluation of the results of hypospadias surgery with uroflowmetry. *J Urol* 154:835, 1995.

Gaylis FD, Zaontz MR, Dalton D, et al: Silicone foam dressing for penis after reconstructive pediatric surgery. *Urology* 33:296, 1989.

Gearhart JP, Borland RN: Onlay island flap urethroplasty: variation on a theme. *J Urol* 148:1507, 1992.

Ghonium GM, Khater U: Urethral prolapse after durasphere injection. *Int Urogynecol J* 17:297–8, 2006.

Gibbons MD, Gonzalez ET Jr: The subcoronal meatus. *J Urol* 130:739, 1983.

Gilbert DA, Jordan GH, Devine CJ Jr, et al: Phallic construction in prepubertal and adolescent boys. *J Urol* 149:1521, 1993.

Gilbert DA, Jordan GH, Devine CJ Jr, Winslow BH: Microsurgical forearm "cricket bat-transformer" phalloplasty. *Plast Reconstr Surg* 90:711, 1992.

Gillett MD, Rathbun SR, Husmann DA, et al: Split-thickness skin graft for the management of concealed penis. *J Urol* 173(2):579–82, 2005.

Gilpin D, Clements WDB, Boston VE: GRAP repair: single-stage reconstruction of hypospadias as an outpatient procedure. *Br J Urol* 71:226, 1993.

Glassberg KI: Augmented Duckett repair for severe hypospadias. *J Urol* 138:380, 1988.

Glassberg KI, Hansbrough F, Horwitz M: The Koyanagi-Nonomura 1-stage bucket repair of severe hypospadias with and without penoscrotal transposition. *J Urol* 160 (Pt 2):1104,1998.

Glenister TW: The origin and fate of the urethral plate in man. *J Anat* 288:413, 1954.

Gonzales ET Jr, Veeraraghavan KA, Delaune J: The management of distal hypospadias with meatal-based vascularized flaps. *J Urol* 129:119, 1983.

González R, Fernandes E: Feminization genitoplasty. *J Urol* 143:776, 1989.

González R, Fernandes ET: Single-stage feminization genitoplasty. *J Urol* 143:776, 1990.

Goodwin WE: Partial (segmental) amputation of the clitoris for female pseudohermaphroditism. *Society for Pediatric Urology Newsletter*, 1981.

Gonsalbez R, Castellan M, Ibrahim E, et al: New concepts in feminizing genitoplasty: is the Fortunoff flap obsolete? *J Urol* 174(6):2350–3, 2005; discussion 2353.

Grady RW, Mitchell ME: Complete primary repair of exstrophy. *J Urol* 162:1415, 1999.

Hafez AT, El-Assmy A, Dawaba MS, et al: Long-term outcome of visual internal urethrotomy for the management of pediatric urethral strictures. *J Urol* 173(2):595–7, 2005.

Hagerty RC, Vaughn TR, Lutz MH: The perineal artery axial flap in reconstruction of the vagina. *Plast Reconstr Surg* 82:344, 1988.

Hammouda HM: Results of complete penile disassembly for epispadias repair in 42 patients. *J Urol* 170(5):1963–5, 2003; discussion 1965.

Hanna MK: Vaginal construction. *Urology* 29:272,1987.

Harris RL, Cundiff GW, Coates KW, et al: Urethral prolapse after collagen injection. *Am J Obstet Gynecol* 178:614–5, 1998.

Heaton BW, Snow BW, Cartwright PC: Repair of urethral diverticulum by plication. *Urology* 44:749, 1994.

Hendren WH: Construction of a female urethra from vaginal wall and perineal flap. *J Urol* 123:657, 1980.

Hendren WH: Penile lengthening after previous repair of epispadias. *J Urol* 121:527, 1979.

Hendren WH: Reconstructive problems of the vagina and female urethra. *Clin Plast Surg* 7:207, 1980.

Hendren WH: Surgical management of urogenital sinus abnormalities. *J Pediatr Surg* 12:339, 1977.

Hendren WH, Atala A: Repair of the high vagina in girls with severely masculinized anatomy from the adrenogenital syndrome. *J Pediatr Surg* 30:91, 1995.

Hendren WH, Caesar RE: Chordee without hypospadias: experience with 33 cases. *J Urol* 147:107, 1992.

Hendren WH, Crawford JD: Adrenogenital syndrome: the anatomy of the anomaly and its repair: some new concepts. *J Pediatr Surg* 4:49, 1969.

Hendren WH, Crawford JD: The child with ambiguous genitalia. *Curr Probl Surg* 1:64, 1972.

Hendren WH, Donahoe PK: Correction of congenital abnormalities of the vagina and perineum. *J Pediatr Surg* 15:751, 1980.

Hendren WH, Keating MA: Use of dermal grafts and free urethral grafts in penile reconstruction. *J Urol* 140(Pt 2):1265, 1988.

Hendren WH, Reda EF: Bladder mucosa graft in construction of male urethra. *J Pediatr Surg* 21:189, 1986.

Hensle TW, Chang DT: Vaginal reconstruction. *Urol Clin North Am* 26:39, 1999.

Hensle TW, Dean GE: Vaginal replacement in children. *J Urol* 148:677, 1992.

Hensle TW, Kearney MC, Bingham JB: Buccal mucosa grafts for hypospadias surgery: long-term results. *J Urol* 168(4 Pt 2):1734–6, 2002; discussion 1736–7.

Hensle TW, Reiley EA: Vaginal reconstruction in children and adults. *J Urol* 159:1035, 1998.

Hensle TW, Seaman EK: Vaginal reconstruction in children and adults. In: Libertino JA (Ed): *Reconstructive Urologic Surgery*, 3rd ed. St. Louis, Mosby Year Book, 1998, p 661.

Herndon CD, Casale AJ, Cain MP, Rink RC: Long-term outcome of the surgical treatment of concealed penis. *J Urol* 170(4 Pt 2):1695–7, 2003; discussion 1697.

Hester TR, Hill HL, Jurkewicz MJ: One-stage reconstruction of the penis. *Br J Plast Surg* 31:279, 1978.

Hill GA, Wacksman J, Alfor GL, Curtis AS: The modified pyramid hypospadias procedure: repair of megameatus and deep glanular groove variants. *J Urol* 150:1208, 1993.

Hinderer JT: Secondary repair of hypospadias failures. *Plast Reconstr Surg* 50:13, 1972.

Hinderer U: New one-stage hypospadias repair (technique of penile tunnelization). In: Hueston JT (Ed): *Transactions of the 5th International Congress of Plastic and Reconstructive Surgery*, Melbourne, Australia, 1971. Stoneham, MA, Butterworths, 1971, pp 283–305.

Hinman F Jr: The blood supply to preputial island flaps. *J Urol* 145:1232, 1991.

Hinman F Jr: A method of lengthening and repairing the penis in exstrophy of the bladder. *J Urol* 79:237, 1958.

Hinman F Jr: Microphallus: characteristics and choice of treatment from a study of 20 cases. *J Urol* 107:499, 1972.

Hinman F Jr: Microphallus: distinction between anomalous and endocrine types. *J Urol* 123:412, 1980.

Hinman F Jr: Penis and male urethra. In: Hinman F Jr (Ed): *Atlas of Urosurgical Anatomy*. Philadelphia, W. B. Saunders Company, 1993, p 418.

Hinman F Jr: Surgical reversal of the female adrenal intersex. *Urol Int* 19:211, 1965.

Hinman F Jr, Spence HF, Culp OS, et al: Panel discussion: anomalies of external genitalia in infancy and childhood. *J Urol* 93:1, 1965.

Hodgson NB: Editorial comment. *J Urol* 149:816, 1993.

Hodgson NB: Hypospadias and urethral duplications. In: Harrison JH, et al (Eds): *Campbell's Urology*, 4th ed. Philadelphia, W. B. Saunders Company, 1979, p 1566.

Hodgson NB: One-stage hypospadias repair. *J Urol* 118:188, 1977.

Hodgson NB: Use of vascularized flaps in hypospadias repair. *Urol Clin North Am* 8:471, 1981.

Hoepffner W, Rothe K, Bennek J: Feminizing reconstructive surgery for ambiguous genitalia: the Leipzig experience. *J Urol* 175(3 Pt 1):981–4, 2006.

Hollowell JG, Keating MA, Snyder HM III, Duckett JW: Preservation of the urethral plate in hypospadias repair: extended applications and further experience with the onlay island flap urethroplasty. *J Urol* 143:98, 1990.

Horton CE, Devine CJ Jr: A one-stage repair for hypospadias cripples. *Plast Reconstr Surg* 66:407, 1970.

Horton CE, Devine CJ Jr: Plication of the tunica albuginea to straighten the curved penis. *Plast Reconstr Surg* 52:32, 1973.

Horton CE, McCraw JB, Devine CJ Jr, Devine PC: Secondary reconstruction of the genital area. *Urol Clin North Am* 4:133, 1977.

Horton CE, Vorstman B, Teasley D, Winslow B: Hidden penis release: adjunctive suprapubic lipectomy. *Ann Plast Surg* 19:131, 1987.

Howard CR, Howard FM, Garfunkel LC, et al: Neonatal circumcision and pain relief: current training practices. *Pediatrics* 101:423, 1998.

Howard FS: Hypospadias with enlargement of the prostatic utricle. *Surg Gynecol Obstet* 86:307, 1948.

Howard FS: The surgery of intersexuals. *J Urol* 65:636, 1951.

Hsiao KC, Baez-Trinidad L, Lendvay T, et al: Direct vision internal urethrotomy for the treatment of pediatric urethral strictures: analysis of 50 patients. *J Urol* 170(3):952–5, 2003.

Huffman WC, Culp DA, Flocks RH: Injuries of the external male genitalia. In: Converse JM (Ed): *Reconstructive Plastic Surgery*. Philadelphia, W. B. Saunders Company, 1964.

Huffman WC, Culp DA, Greenleaf JS, et al: Injuries to the male genitalia. *Plast Reconstr Surg* 18:344, 1956.

Husmann DA, Allen TG: Endoscopic management of infected enlarged prostatic utricles and remnants of rectourethral fistula tracts of high imperforate anus. *J Urol* 157:1902, 1997.

Issa MM, Gearhart JP: The failed MAGPI: management and prevention. *Br J Urol* 64:169, 1989.

Jackson ND, Rosenblatt PL: Use of Intercede® absorbable adhesion barrier for vaginoplasty. *Obstet Gynecol* 84:1048, 1994.

Jayanthi VR: The modified Snodgrass hypospadias repair: reducing the risk of fistula and meatal stenosis. *J Urol* 170(4 Pt 2):1603–5, 2003; discussion 1605.

Jayanthi VR, Koff S: Urethral plate mobilization: the modified Barcat hypospadias repair. In: Ehrlich RM, Alter GJ (Eds): *Reconstructive and Plastic Surgery of the External Genitalia: Adult and Pediatric*. Philadelphia, W.B. Saunders Company, 1999, p 54.

Jednak R, Hernandez N, Barthold JS, González R: Correcting chordee without hypospadias and with deficient ventral skin: a new technique. *Br J Urol Int* 87:528, 2001.

Jednak R, Ludwikowski B, González R: Total urogenital mobilization: a modified perineal approach for feminizing genitoplasty and urogenital sinus repair. *J Urol* 165(Pt 2):2347–9, 2001.

Jerkins G, Verheeck K, Noe HN: Treatment of girls with urethral prolapse. *J Urol* 132:733–4, 1994.

Johanson B: Reconstruction of the male urethra in strictures: application of the buried intact epithelium technic. *Acta Chir Scand* 176(suppl):3, 1953.

Johnson N, Lilford RJ, Batchelor A: The free flap vaginoplasty: a new surgical procedure for the treatment of vaginal agenesis. *Br J Obstet Gynaecol* 98:184, 1991.

Jones FW: The development and malformations of the glans and prepuce. *Br Med J* 1:137, 1910.

Jones HW Jr, Garcia SC, Klingensmith GJ: Secondary surgical treatment of the masculinized external genitalia of patients with virilizing adrenal hyperplasia. *Obstet Gynecol* 48:73, 1976.

Jordan GH: Reconstruction of the fossa navicularis. *J Urol* 138:102, 1987.

Jordan GH, Devine PC: Application of tissue transfer techniques to the management of urethral strictures. *Semin Urol* 5:228, 1987.

Jordan GH, Schlossberg SM: Surgery of the penis and urethra. In: Walsh PC, et al (Eds): *Campbell's Urology*, 8th ed., 2002, p 3886.

Joseph VT: A new approach to the surgical correction of buried penis. *J Pediatr Surg* 30:727, 1995.

Juskiewenski S, Vaysse P, Moscovici J: A study of the blood supply to the penis. *Anat Clin* 4:101, 1982.

Kajbafzedeh AM, Sina A, Payabvash S: Management of multiple failed repairs of the phallus using tissue expanders: long-term postpubertal results. *J Urol* 177(5):1872–7, 2007.

Kaplan GW: Repair of proximal hypospadias using a preputial free graft for neourethral covering and a preputial pedicle flap for ventral skin coverage. *J Urol* 140:1270, 1988.

Kaplan GW, Brock WA: Urethral strictures in children. *J Urol* 129:1200, 1983.

Kaplan GW, Lamm DL: Embryogenesis of chordee. *J Urol* 114:768, 1975.

Kaplan I, Wesser D: A rapid method for constructing a functional sensitive penis. *Br J Plast Surg* 24:342, 1971.

Kass EJ: Dorsal corporeal rotation: an alternative technique for the management of severe chordee. *J Urol* 150:635, 1993.

Keating MA, Cartwright PC, Duckett JW: Bladder mucosa in urethral reconstructions. *J Urol* 144:827, 1990.

Keating MA, Duckett JW Jr: Failed hypospadias repair. In: Cohen MS, Resnick MI (Eds): *Reoperative Urology*. Boston, Little, Brown, 1995, p 187.

Keating MA, Rich MA: Onlay and tubularized preputial island flaps. In: Ehrlich RM, Alter GJ (Eds): *Reconstructive and Plastic Surgery of the External Genitalia: Adult and Pediatric*. Philadelphia, W. B. Saunders Company, 1999, p 70.

Kelami A: Congenital penile deviation and its treatment with the Nesbit-Kelami technique. *Br J Urol* 60:261, 1987.

Kessler SJ: *Lessons from the Intersex*. Piscataway, NY, Rutgers University Press, 1998.

Khen-Dunlop N, Lortat-Jacob S, Thibaud E, et al: Rokitansky syndrome: clinical experience and results of sigmoid vaginoplasty in 23 young girls. *J Urol* 177(3):1107–11, 2007.

Khoury AE, Papanikolaou F, Afshar K, Zuker R: A novel approach to skin coverage for epispadias repair. *J Urol* 173(4):1332–3, 2005.

Kim KS, King LR: Method for correcting meatal stenosis after hypospadias repair. *Urology* 39:545, 1992.

King LR: Hypospadias: a one-stage repair without skin graft based on a new principle: chordee is sometimes produced by skin alone. *J Urol* 103:660, 1970.

Kirsch AJ, Duckett JW: Appropriate stenting in hypospadias repair. In: Yacchia D (Ed): *Stenting the Urinary System*. Oxford, Isis Medical Media, 1998, pp 1–6.

Klauber GT, Williams DI: Epispadias with incontinence. *J Urol* 111:110, 1974.

Klijn AJ, Dik P, De Jong TPVM: Results of preputial reconstruction in 77 boys with distal hypospadias. *J Urol* 165:1255, 2001.

Klimberg I, Walker RD: Comparison of Mustardé and Horton-Devine flip-flap techniques of hypospadias repair. *J Urol* 134:103, 1985.

Koff SA: Mobilization of the urethra in the surgical treatment of hypospadias. *J Urol* 125:394, 1981.

Koff SA, Eakins M: The treatment of penile chordee using corporal rotation. *J Urol* 131:931, 1984.

Koff SA, Jayanth VR: Preoperative treatment with human chorionic gonadotropin in infancy decreases the severity of proximal hypospadias and chordee. *J Urol* 162:1435, 1999.

Kogan BA: Intraoperative pharmacological erection as an aid to pediatric hypospadias repair. *J Urol* 164:2058, 2000.

Kogan BA: Treatment options for posterior urethral valves in neonates. In: King LR (Ed): *Urologic Surgery in Neonates and Young Children*. Philadelphia, W. B. Saunders Company, 1988, p 238.

Kogan BA: Urethral diverticula in males. In: Resnick MI, Kursh ED (Eds): *Current Therapy in Genitourinary Surgery*. St. Louis, C. V. Mosby, 1992, p 313.

Kogan SJ: Technical nuances in intersex surgery: clitoroplasty. In: Ehrlich RM, Alter GJ (Ed): *Reconstructive and Plastic Surgery of the External Genitalia: Adult and Pediatric*. Philadelphia, W. B. Saunders Company, 1999, p 269.

Kogan SJ, Smey P, Leavitt S: Subtunical total reduction clitoroplasty: a safe modification of existing techniques. *J Urol* 130:746, 1983.

Kojima Y, Hyashi Y, Maruyama T, et al: Comparison between ultrasonography and retrograde urethrography for detection of prostatic utricle associated with hypospadias. *Urology* 57:1151, 2001.

Koyanagi T, Nonomura K, Asano Y, et al: Onlay urethroplasty with parameatal foreskin flaps for distal hypospadias. *Eur Urol* 19:221, 1991.

Koyanagi T, Nonomura K, Gotoh T, et al: One-stage repair of perineal hypospadias and scrotal transposition. *Eur Urol* 19:364, 1984.

Koyanagi T, Nonomura K, Kakizaki H, et al: Experience with a one-stage repair of severe proximal hypospadias: operative technique and results. *Eur Urol* 24:106, 1993.

Koyanagi T, Nonomura K, Kakizaki H, et al: One-stage total repair of severe hypospadias with scrotal transposition: experience in 18 cases. *J Pediatr Surg* 23:177, 1988.

Koyanagi T, Nonomura K, Kanagawa K, Yamashita T: Hypospadias repair. In: Thuroff JW, Hohenfellner M (Eds): *Reconstructive Surgery of the Lower Urinary Tract in Children*. Oxford, ISIS Medical Media, 1995, p 1.

Koyle MA, Ehrlich RM: The bladder mucosal graft for urethral reconstruction. *J Urol* 138:1093, 1987.

Kramer SA, Aydin G, Kelalis PP: Chordee without hypospadias in children. *J Urol* 128:559, 1982.

Kramer SA, Mesrobian HG, Kelalis PP: Long-term follow-up of cosmetic appearance and genital function in male epispadias: review of 70 cases. *J Urol* 135:543, 1986.

Kryger J, González R: Urinary continence is well preserved after total urogenital mobilization. *J Urol* 172:2384–6, 2004.

Kubota Y, Ishii N, Watanabe H, et al: Buried penis: a surgical repair. *Urol Int* 46:61, 1991.

Kukreja RA, Desai RM, Sabnis RB, et al: The urethral instillation of depilatory cream for hair removal after scrotal urethroplasty. *BJU Int* 87:708, 2001.

Lam PN, Greenfield SP, Williot P: 2-stage repair in infancy for severe hypospadias with chordee: long-term results after puberty. *J Urol* 174(4 Pt 2):1567–72, 2005.

Landau EH, Gofrit ON, Meretyk S, et al: Outcome analysis of tunica vaginalis flap for the correction of recurrent urethrocutaneous fistula in children. *J Urol* 170(4 Pt 2):1596–9, 2003; discussion 1599.

Lander J, Brady-Freyer B, Metcalfe JB, et al: Comparison of ring block, dorsal penile nerve block, and topical anesthesia for neonatal circumcision: a randomized controlled trial. *JAMA* 278:2157, 1997.

Larson DL: Musculocutaneous flaps. In: Johnson DE, Boileau MA (Eds): *Genitourinary Tumors: Fundamental Principles and Surgical Techniques*. New York, Grune & Stratton, 1982.

Lattimer JK: Relocation and recession of the enlarged clitoris with preservation of the glans: an alternative to amputation. *J Urol* 86:113, 1961.

Lattimer JK, MacFarlane MT: A urethral lengthening procedure for epispadias and exstrophy. *J Urol* 123:544, 1980.

Lau JTK, Ong GB: Subglandular urethral fistula following circumcision: repair by the advancement method. *J Urol* 126:702, 1981.

Leadbetter GW, Leadbetter WF: Urethral strictures in male children. *J Urol* 87:409, 1962.

Lesavoy MA: Vaginal reconstruction. *Urol Clin North Am* 12:369, 1985.

Li Q, Li S, Chen W, et al: Combined buccal mucosa graft and local flap for urethral reconstruction in various forms of hypospadias. *J Urol* 174(2):690–2, 2005.

Li ZC, Zheng ZH, Sheh YX, et al: One-stage urethroplasty for hypospadias using a tube constructed with bladder mucosa: a new procedure. *Urol Clin North Am* 8:463, 1981.

Livne PM, Gibbons MD, Gonzales ET Jr: Correction of disproportion of corpora cavernosa as cause of chordee in hypospadias. *Urology* 22:608, 1983.

Ludwikowski B, Hayward IO, González R: Total urogenital sinus mobilization: an easier way to repair cloacas. *BJU Int* 83:820, 1999.

Ludwikowski B, Oesch-Hayward I, González R: Total urogenital mobilization: expanded applications. *BJU Int* 83:820–22, 1999.

Maizels M, Zaontz M, Donovan J, et al: Surgical correction of the buried penis: description of a classification system and a technique to correct the disorder. *J Urol* 136:268, 1986.

Malament M: Repair of the recurrent fistula of the penile urethra. *J Urol* 106:704, 1971.

Marberger H, Pauer W: Experience in hypospadias repair. *Urol Clin North Am* 8:403, 1981.

Marshall M Jr, Beh WP, Johnson SH III, et al: Etiologic considerations in penoscrotal hypospadias repair. *J Urol* 120:229, 1978.

Marshall VF, Spellman RM: Construction of urethra in hypospadias using vesical mucosal grafts. *J Urol* 73:335, 1955.

Mathews R, Gearhart JP, Bhatnagar R, Sponseller P: Staged pelvic closure of extreme pubic diastasis in the exstrophy-epispadias complex. *J Urol* 176(5):2196–8, 2006.

Mathieu P: Traitement en un temps de l'hypospadias balanique et juxtabalanique. *J Chir (Paris)* 39:481, 1932.

Mays HB: Epispadias: a plan of treatment. *J Urol* 107:251, 1972.

McAninch JW (Guest Ed): Trauma management. In: Blaisdell FW, Trunkey DD (Eds): *Urogenital Trauma*, vol 2. New York, Thieme-Stratton, 1985.

McAninch JW, Kahn RI, Jeffrey RB, et al: Major traumatic and septic genital injuries. *J Trauma* 24:291, 1984.

McCormack RM: Simultaneous chordee repair and urethral reconstruction for hypospadias. *Plast Reconstr Surg* 13:257, 1954.

McCraw J, Massey F, Shankin K, Horton C: Vaginal reconstruction using gracilis myocutaneous flaps. *Plast Reconstr Surg* 58:176, 1970.

McDougal WS: Vaginal construction using sigmoid colon in children and young adults. *J Urol* 173(6):2145–6, 2005.

McFarlane RM: The use of continuous suction under skin flaps. *Br J Plast Surg* 17:77, 1959.

McGowan AJ, Waterhouse K: Mobilization of the anterior urethra. *Bull N Y Acad Med* 40:776, 1964.

McGraw JB, Myers B, Shanklin KD: The value of fluorescein in predicting the viability of arterialized flaps. *Plast Reconstr Surg* 60:710, 1977.

McGuire EJ, Weiss RM: Scrotal flap urethroplasty for strictures of the deep urethra in infants and children. *J Urol* 110:599, 1973.

McIndoe A: The treatment of congenital absence and obliterative conditions of the vagina. *Br J Plast Surg* 2:254, 1950.

McKinley GA: Save the prepuce: painless separation of preputial adhesions in the out-patient department. *Br Med J* 297:590, 1988.

McLorie GA, Joyner BD, Herz D, et al: A prospective randomized clinical trial to evaluate methods of postoperative care of hypospadias. *J Urol* 165:1669, 2001.

McMillan RDH, Churchill BM, Gilmore RF: Assessment of urinary stream after repair of anterior hypospadias by meatoplasty and glanuloplasty. *J Urol* 134:100, 1985.

Mettauer JP: Practical observations on those malformations of the male urethra and penis, termed hypospadias and epispadias, with an anomalous case. *Am J Med Sci* 4:43, 1842.

Michalowski E, Modelski W: The surgical treatment of epispadias. *Surg Gynecol Obstet* 117:465, 1963.

Micheli E, Ranieri A, Peracchia G, Lembro A: End-to-end urethroplasty: long-term results. *BJU Int* 90:68, 2002.

Mininberg DT: Phalloplasty in congenital adrenal hyperplasia. *J Urol* 128:355, 1982.

Mitchell ME, Bagli DJ: Complete penile disassembly for epispadias repair: the Mitchell technique. *J Urol* 155:300, 1996.

Mitchell ME, Hensle TW, Crooks KK: Urethral reconstruction in the young female using a perineal pedicle flap. *J Pediatr Surg* 17:687, 1982.

Mollard P, Castagnola C: Hypospadias: the release of chordee without dividing the urethral plate and onlay island flap (92 cases). *J Urol* 152:1238, 1994.

Mollard P, Juskiewenski S, Sarkissian J: Clitoroplasty in intersex: a new technique. *Br J Urol* 53:371, 1981.

Mollard P, Mouriquand P, Bringeon G, et al: Repair of hypospadias using bladder mucosal graft in 76 cases. *J Urol* 142:1548, 1989.

Mollard P, Mouriquand P, Felfela T: Application of the onlay island-flap urethroplasty to penile hypospadias with severe chordee. *Br J Urol* 68:317, 1991.

Money J, Mazur T: Microphallus: the successful use of a prosthetic phallus in a 9-year-old boy. *J Sex Marital Ther* 3:187, 1977.

Monfort G: Transvesical approach to utricular cyst. *J Pediatr Surg* 17:406, 1982.

Monfort G, Bretheau D, diBenedetto V, Bankole R: Posterior hypospadias repair: a new technical approach: mobilization of the urethral plate and Duplay urethroplasty. *Eur Urol* 22:137, 1992.

Monfort G, Bretheau D, diBenedetto V, et al: Urethral stricture in children: treatment by urethroplasty with bladder mucosa graft. *J Urol* 145:1504, 1992.

Monfort G, Morisson-Lacombe G, Guys JM, Coquet M: Transverse island flap amd double flap procedure in the treatment of congenital epispadias in 32 patients. *J Urol* 138:1069, 1987.

Morey AF, Lin HC, DeRosa CA, Griffith BC: Fossa navicularis reconstruction: impact of stricture length on outcomes and assessment of extended meatotomy (first stage Johanson) maneuver. *J Urol* 177(1):184–7, 2007; discussion 187.

Morey AF, McAninch JW: Technique of harvesting buccal mucosa for urethral reconstruction. *J Urol* 155:1696, 1996.

Moscona AR, Govrin-Yehudain J, Hirshowitz B: Closure of urethral fistulae by transverse Y-V advancement flap. *Br J Urol* 56:313, 1984.

Mufti GR, Aitchison M, Bramwell SP, et al: Corporeal plication for surgical correction of Peyronie's disease. *J Urol* 144:281, 1990.

Mundy AR, Stephenson TP: Pedicled preputial patch urethroplasty. *Br J Urol* 61:48, 1988.

Mureau MA, Slijper FH, Nijman RJ, et al: Psychosexual adjustment of children and adolescents after different types of hypospadias surgery. *J Urol* 154:1902, 1995.

Mustardé JC: One-stage correction of distal hypospadias and other people's fistulae. *Br J Plast Surg* 18:413, 1965.

Nelson CP, Bloom DA, Kinast R, et al: Long-term patient reported outcome and satisfaction after oral mucosa graft urethroplasty for hypospadias. *J Urol* 174(3):1075–8, 2005.

Nesbit RM: Congenital curvature of the phallus: report of 3 cases with description of corrective operation. *J Urol* 93:230, 1965.

Nesbit RM: Operation for correction of distal penile ventral curvature with or without hypospadias. *J Urol* 97:470, 1967.

Nesbit RM: Plastic procedure for correction of hypospadias. *J Urol* 45:699, 1941.

Nesbit RM, MacKinney CC, Dingman R: Z-plasty for correction of meatal ureteral stricture after hypospadias repair. *J Urol* 72:681, 1954.

Netto NR Jr: Surgical repair of posterior urethral strictures by transpubic urethroplasty or pull-through technique. *J Urol* 133:411, 1985.

Nguyen MT, Snodgrass WT: Tubularized incised plate hypospadias reoperation. *J Urol* 171(6 Pt 1):2404–6, 2004.

Nonomura K, Kakizaki H, Yamashita T, et al: Vaginoplasty with bilateral labioscrotal flap: a new flap vaginoplasty. In: Thuroff JW, Hohenfellner M (Eds): *Reconstructive Surgery of the Lower Urinary Tract in Children.* Oxford, ISIS Medical Media, 1995, p 236.

Nonomura K, Koganagi T, Imanaka K, et al: One stage total repair of severe hypospadias with scrotal transposition: experience in 18 cases. *J Pediatr Surg* 23:177, 1988.

Nuininga JE, De Gier RP, Verschuren R, Feitz WF: Long-term outcome of different types of 1-stage hypospadias repair. *J Urol* 174(4 Pt 2):1544–8, 2005.

O'Brien A, Shapiro AMJ, Frank JD: Phimosis or congenital megaprepuce. *Br J Urol* 73:719, 1994.

O'Connell HE, Hutson JM, Anderson CR, Plenter RJ: Anatomical relationship between urethra and clitoris. *J Urol* 159:1892, 1998.

Oesch IL, Pinter A, Ransley PG: Penile agenesis: report of six cases. *J Pediatr Surg* 22:172, 1987.

Oesterling JE, Gearhart JP, Jeffs RD: A unified approach to early reconstructive surgery of the child with ambiguous genitalia. *J Urol* 138:1079, 1987.

Oesterling JE, Gearhart JP, Jeffs RD: Urinary diversion after hypospadias surgery. *Urology* 29:513, 1987.

Orandi A: One-stage urethroplasty. *Br J Urol* 40:717, 1968.

Orticochea M: A new method of total reconstruction of the penis. *Br J Plast Surg* 25:347, 1972.

Osegbe DN, Ntia I: One-stage urethroplasty for complicated urethral strictures using axial penile skin island flap. *Eur Urol* 17:79, 1990.

Pansadoro V, Emiliozzi P: Internal urethrotomy in the management of anterior urethral strictures: long-term follow-up. *J Urol* 156:73, 1996.

Park JK, Min JK, Kim HJ: Reimplantation of an amputated penis in prepubertal boys. *J Urol* 165:585, 2001.

Parrott TS, Scheflan M, Hester TR: Reduction clitoroplasty and vaginal construction in a single operation. *Urology* 14:367, 1980.

Pascual LA, Benegas JC, Cuevas CR, Vega Perugorria JM: Tissue expander enhanced onlay island flap in the repair of severe hypospadias. *J Urol* 169(2):606, 2003.

Passerini-Glazel G: A new 1-stage procedure for clitorovaginoplasty in severely masculinized female pseudohermaphrodites. *J Urol* 142:565, 1989.

Passerini-Glazel G, Maio G, Cisternino A, et al: One-stage repair of severe hypospadias. Paper presented at the International Congress of Pediatric Urology, Florence, Italy, 1986. Quoted in: Gillenwater JY, Grayhack JT, Howards SS, Duckett JW (Eds): *Adult and Pediatric Urology*. Chicago, Year Book Medical Publishers, 1986, p 1902.

Patel RP, Shukla AR, Leone NT, et al: Split onlay skin flap for the salvage hypospadias repair. *J Urol* 173(5):1718–20, 2005.

Patel RP, Shukla AR, Snyder HM 3rd: The island tube and island onlay hypospadias repairs offer excellent long-term outcomes: a 14-year follow-up. *J Urol* 172(4 Pt 2):1717–9, 2004.

Peña A: *Atlas of Surgical Management of Anorectal Malformations.* New York, Springer-Verlag, 1990.

Perovic S: Phalloplasty in children and adolescents using the extended pedicle island groin flap. *J Urol* 154:848, 1995.

Perovic SV, Djordjevic ML: A new approach to hypospadias repair. *World J Urol* 16:195, 1988.

Perovic S, Djordjevic M, Djakovic N: Natural erection induced by prostaglandin-E1 in the diagnosis and treatment of congenital penile anomalies. *Br J Urol* 79:43, 1997.

Perovic SV, Perovic S: Hypospadias sine hypospadias. *World J Urol* 10:85, 1992.

Perovic SV, Radojicic ZI: Vascularization of the hypospadiac prepuce and its impact on hypospadias repair. *J Urol* 169:1098, 2002.

Perovic S, Radojicic ZI, Djordjevic ML, Vukadinovic VV: Enlargement and sculpturing of a small and deformed glans. *J Urol* 170(4 Pt 2):1686–90, 2003; discussion 1690.

Perovic S, Vukadinovic F: Onlay island-flap urethroplasty for severe hypospadias. *J Urol* 151:711, 1994.

Perovic S, Vukadinovic F: Penoscrotal transposition with hypospadias: 1-stage repair. *J Urol* 148:1510, 1992.

Persky L, Resnick M, Desprez J: Penile reconstruction with gracilis pedicle grafts. *J Urol* 129:603, 1983.

Peters CA, Hendren WH: Splitting the pubis for exposure in difficult reconstructions for incontinence. *J Urol* 142(Pt 2):527, 1989; discussion 542.

Peters KM, Kass EJ: Electrosurgery for routine pediatric penile procedures. *J Urol* 157:1453, 1997.

Peters PC: Complications of penile surgery. In: Smith RB, Skinner DG (Eds): *Complications of Urologic Surgery: Prevention and Management*. Philadelphia, W. B. Saunders Company, 1976, p 420.

Peterson AC, Joyner BD, Allen RC Jr: Plastibell template circumcision: a new technique. *Urology* 58:603, 2001.

Pippi Salle JL, Jednak R, Capolicchio JP, et al: A ventral rotational skin flap to improve cosmesis and avoid chordee recurrence in epispadias repair. *BJU Int* 90:918, 2002.

Pond HS, Brannan W: Correction of congenital curvature of the penis: experiences with the Nesbit operation at Ochsner Clinic. *J Urol* 112:491, 1974.

Prado NG, Ide E, Batista AK: Micropenis: evaluation and approach. In: Thuroff JW, Hohenfellner M (Eds): *Reconstructive Surgery of the Lower Urinary Tract in Children.* Oxford, ISIS Medical Media, 1995, p 64.

Presman D, Greenfield DL: Reconstruction of the perineal urethra with a free full-thickness skin graft from the prepuce. *J Urol* 69:677, 1953.

Quartey JKM: One-stage penile/preputial cutaneous island flap urethroplasty for urethral stricture: a preliminary report. *J Urol* 129:284, 1983.

Quartey JKM: One-stage penile/preputial island flap urethroplasty for urethral stricture. *J Urol* 134:474, 1985.

Rabinowitz R: Outpatient management of hypospadias and the complications of repair. *Probl Urol* 2:109, 1988.

Radhakkrishnan J: Colon interposition vaginoplasty: a modification of the Wagner-Baldwin technique. *J Pediatr Surg* 22:1175, 1987.

Rahman A, Khan N, Ali M, et al: Hypospadias repairs: surgeons, techniques and results. Paediatric Urology Poster Session. *BJU Int* 85(suppl 5):44, 2000.

Randolph JG, Hung W: Reduction clitoroplasty in females with hypertrophied clitoris. *J Pediatr Surg* 5:224, 1970.

Randolph JG, Hung W, Rathlev MC: Clitoroplasty for females born with ambiguous genitalia: a long-term study of 37 patients. *J Pediatr Surg* 16:882, 1981.

Rangecroft L: Surgical management of ambiguous genitalia. British Association of Paediatric Surgeons Working Party on the Surgical Management of Children Born with Ambiguous Genitalia. *Arch Dis Child* 88(9):799–801, 2003. Review.

Ransley PG: Epispadias repair. In: Spitz L, Homewood NH (Eds): *Operative Surgery: Paediatric Surgery*, 4th ed. London, Butterworths, 1988, p 624.

Ransley PG, Duffy PG, Oesch IL, et al: The use of bladder mucosa and combined bladder mucosa/preputial skin grafts for urethral reconstruction. *J Urol* 138:1096, 1987.

Redman JF: The Barcat balanic groove technique for the repair of distal hypospadias. *J Urol* 137:83, 1987.

Redman JF: Dorsal curvature of the penis. *Urology* 21:479, 1983.

Redman JF: Extended application of Nesbit ellipses in the correction of childhood penile curvature. *J Urol* 119:122, 1978.

Redman JF: A favorable experience with rotational flap techniques for fashioning the Firlit preputial collar. *J Urol* 176(2):715–7, 2006.

Redman JF: A technique for correction of penoscrotal fusion. *J Urol* 133:432, 1985.

Redman JF: Technique for phalloplasty. *Urology* 27:360, 1986.

Redman JF, Bissada NK: One-stage correction of chordee and 180-degree penile rotation. *Urology* 7:632, 1976.

Retik AB, Bauer SB, Mandell J, et al: Management of severe hypospadias with a 2-stage repair. *J Urol* 152:749, 1994.

Retik AB, Keating M, Mandell J: Complications of hypospadias repair. *Urol Clin North Am* 15:223, 1988.

Rich MA, Keating MA, Snyder HM, Duckett JW: "Hinging" the urethral plate in hypospadias meatoplasty. *J Urol* 142:1551, 1989.

Richter F, Pinto PA, Stock JA, Hanna MK: Management of recurrent urethral fistulas after hypospadias repair. *Urology* 61:448, 2003.

Rickwood AMK, Anderson PAM: One-stage hypospadias repair: experience with 367 cases. *Br J Urol* 67:424, 1991.

Rink RC, Pope JC, Kropp BP, et al: Reconstruction of the high urogenital sinus: early perineal prone approach without division of the rectum. *J Urol* 158:1293, 1997.

Ritchie ML: Management of phimosis/trapped penis after newborn circumcision.

Roberts AHN: A new operation for the repair of hypospadias fistulae. *Br J Plast Surg* 35:386, 1982.

Roberts JP, Hutson JM: Reduction of scrotalized skin improves the cosmetic appearance of feminizing genitoplasty. *Pediatr Surg Int* 12:228, 1997.

Rogers BO: History of external genital surgery. In: Horton CE (Ed): *Plastic and Reconstructive Surgery of the Genital Area.* Boston, Little, Brown, 1973, pp 3–47.

Ross JH, Kay R: Use of de-epithelialized local skin flap in hypospadias repairs accomplished by tubularization of the incised urethral plate. *Urology* 50:110, 1997.

Rossi F, De Castro RO, Ceccarelli PL, Domini R: Anterior sagittal transanorectal approach to the posterior urethra in the pediatric age group. *J Urol* 160:1173, 1998.

Routh JC, Wolpert JJ, Reinberg Y: Tunneled tunica vaginalis flap is an effective technique for recurrent urethrocutaneous fistulas following tubularized incised plate urethroplasty. *J Urol* 176(4 Pt 1):1578–80, 2006.

Rushton HG, Belman B: The split prepuce in situ onlay hypospadias repair. *J Urol* 160:1134, 1998.

Saad MN, Khoo CTK, Lochaitis AS: A simple technique for repair of urethral fistula by Y-V advancement. *Br J Plast Surg* 33:410, 1980.

Sadlowski RW, Belman AB, King LR: Further experience with one-stage hypospadias repair. *J Urol* 112: 677, 1974.

Santangelo K, Rushton HG, Belman AB: Outcome analysis of simple and complex urethrocutaneous fistula closure using a de-epithelialized or full thickness skin advancement flap for coverage. *J Urol* 170(4 Pt 2):1589–92, 2003; discussion 1592.

Scherz HC, Kaplan GW, Packer MG, et al: Post-hypospadias repair of urethral strictures: a review of 30 cases. *J Urol* 140:1253, 1988.

Schober JM: Feminizing genitoplasty for intersex. In: Stringer, Oldham, Mariquand, et al (Eds): *Pediatric Surgery: Urology Long-term Outcomes.* London, W. B. Saunders Company, 1998, pp 549–58. (A good review.)

Schober JM: Long-term outcomes and changing attitudes to intersexuality. *BJU Int* 83(suppl 3):39, 1999.

Schreiter F, Noll F: Mesh graft urethroplasty using split thickness skin graft or foreskin. *J Urol* 142:1223–6, 1989.

Schuhrke TD, Kaplan GW: Prostatic utricle cysts (müllerian duct cysts). *J Urol* 119:765, 1978.

Schultz JR, Klykylo WM, Wacksman J: Timing of elective hypospadias repair in children. *Pediatrics* 71:342, 1983.

Schwentner C, Gozzi C, Lunacek A, et al: Interim outcome of the single stage dorsal inlay skin graft for complex hypospadias reoperations. *J Urol* 175(5):1872–6, 2006.

Scuderi N, Chiummariello S, De Gado F: Correction of hypospadias with a vertical preputial island flap: a 23-year experience. *J Urol* 175(3 Pt 1):1083–7, 2006.

Secrest CL, Jordan GH, Winslow BH, et al: Repair of complications of hypospadias surgery. *J Urol* 150:1415, 1993.

Sensoz O, Ortak T, Baran CN, Unlu RE: A new technique for distal hypospadias repair: advancement of a distally deepithelialized urethrocutaneous flap. *Plast Reconstr Surg* 112(3):840–3, 2003.

Shahbandi PM, Cuckow PM, Smeulders N: The buried penis: an anatomic approach: Paediatric Urology Poster Session. *BJU Int* 85(suppl 5):44, 2000.

Shanberg AM, Sanderson K, Duel B: Re-operative hypospadias repair using the Snodgrass incised plate urethroplasty. *BJU Int* 87:344, 2001.

Shankar KR, Losty PD, Hopper M, et al: Outcome of hypospadias fistula repair. *Br J Urol* 89:103, 2002.

Shapiro SR: Surgical treatment of the "buried" penis. *Urology* 30:554, 1987.

Sharp RJ, Holder TM, Howard CD, Grunt JA: Neonatal genital reconstruction. *J Pediatr Surg* 22:168, 1987.

Shaw A: Subcutaneous reduction clitoroplasty. *J Pediatr Surg* 112:331, 1977.

Shepard GH, Wilson CS, Sallade RL: Webbed penis. *Plast Reconstr Surg* 66:46, 1980.

Sherman J, Borer JG, Horowitz M, Glassberg KL: Circumcision: successful glanular reconstruction and survival following traumatic amputation. *J Urol* 156:342, 1996.

Simmons GR, Cain MP, Casale AJ, et al: Repair of hypospadias complications using a previously utilized urethral plate. *Urology* 54:724, 1999.

Sislow JG, Ireton RCM, Onsell JS: Treatment of congenital penile curvature due to disparate corpora cavernosa by the Nesbit technique: a rule of thumb for the number of wedges required to achieve correction. *J Urol* 141:92, 1989.

Slawin KM, Nagler HM: Treatment of congenital penile curvature with penile torsion: a new twist. *J Urol* 147:152, 1992.

Smeulders N, Wilcox DT, Cuckow PM: The buried penis: an anatomical approach. *BJU Int* 86:523, 2000.

Smith ED: Commentary: multiple stage repair of hypospadias. In: Whitehead ED, Leiter E (Eds): *Current Operative Urology,* 2nd ed. Philadelphia, Harper & Row, 1984, p 1251.

Smith ED: A de-epithelialized overlap technique in the repair of hypospadias. *Br J Plast Surg* 26:106, 1973.

Smith ED: Durham-Smith repair of hypospadias. *Urol Clin North Am* 8:451, 1981.

Smith ED: Malformations of the bladder, urethra and hypospadias. In: Holder TM, Ashcraft KW (Eds): *Pediatric Surgery.* Philadelphia, W. B. Saunders Company, 1990, p 752.

Smith ED: Timing of surgery in hypospadias repair. *Aust N Z J Surg* 53:396, 1983.

Smith JA Jr, Middleton RG: Surgical approach to large müllerian duct cysts. *Urology* 14:44, 1979.

Snodgrass W: Does tubularized incised plate hypospadias repair create neourethral strictures? *J Urol* 162:1150, 1999.

Snodgrass W: Suture tracks after hypospadias repair. *BJU Int* 84:843, 1999.

Snodgrass W: Tubularized, incised plate urethroplasty. In: Ehrlich RM, Alter GJ (Eds): *Reconstructive and Plastic Surgery of the External Genitalia: Adult and Pediatric.* Philadelphia, W. B. Saunders Company, 1999, p 66.

Snodgrass W: Tubularized, incised plate urethroplasty for distal hypospadias. *J Urol* 151:464, 1994.

Snodgrass W, Elmore J: Initial experience with staged buccal graft (Bracka) hypospadias reoperations. *J Urol* 172 (4 Pt 2):1720–4, 2004.

Snodgrass W, Koyle M, Manzoni G, et al: Tubularized incised plate hypospadias repair for proximal hypospadias. *J Urol* 159:2129, 1998.

Snodgrass W, Koyle M, Manzoni G, et al: Tubularized incised plate urethroplasty: results of a multicenter experience. *J Urol* 156:839, 1966.

Snodgrass W, Yucel S: Tubularized incised plate for mid shaft and proximal hypospadias repair. *J Urol* 177(2):698–702, 2007.

Snodgrass WT, Khavari R: Prior circumcision does not complicate repair of hypospadias with an intact prepuce. *J Urol* 176(1):296–8, 2006.

Snodgrass WT, Koyle MA, Baskin LS, Caldamone AA: Foreskin preservation in penile surgery. *J Urol* 176: 711, 2006.

Snow BW: Transverse corporeal plication for persistent chordee. *Urology* 34:360, 1989.

Snow BW, Cartwright PC: The Yoke hypospadias repair. *J Pediatr Surg* 29:557, 1994.

Snow BW, Cartwright PC, Unger K: Tunica vaginalis blanket wrap to prevent urethrocutaneous fistula: an eight year experience. *J Urol* 153:472, 1995.

Snow BW, Georges LS, Tarry WF: Techniques for outpatient hypospadias surgery. *Urology* 35:327, 1990.

Snyder HM: Does glans configuration indicate the type of chordee present in hypospadias? *Society for Pediatric Urology Newsletter*, May 24,1991, pp 38–39.

Snyder HM III: Management of ambiguous genitalia in the neonate. In: King LR (Ed): *Urologic Surgery in Neonates and Young Infants*. Philadelphia, W. B. Saunders Company, 1988, p 346.

Snyder HM III, Retik AB, Bauer SB, Colodny AH: Feminizing genitoplasty: a synthesis. *J Urol* 129:1024, 1983.

Soderdahl DW, Brosman SA, Goodwin WE: Penile agenesis. *J Urol* 108:496, 1972.

Sommerton DJ, McNally J, Denny AJ, Malone PSJ: Congenital megaprepuce: an emerging condition: how to recognize and treat it. *BJU Int* 86:519, 2000.

Spaulding MH: The development of external genitalia in the human embryo. *Contr Embryol Carnegie Inst Publ* 276:67, 1921.

Speakman MJ, Azmy AF: Skin chordee without hypospadias: an unrecognized entity. *Br J Urol* 69:428, 1992.

Spence HM, Allen TD: Genital reconstruction in the female with the adrenogenital syndrome. *Br J Urol* 45:126, 1973.

Spence HM, Duckett JW Jr: Diverticulum of the female urethra: clinical aspects and presentation of a simple operative technique for cure. *J Urol* 104:432, 1970.

Standoli L: One-stage repair of hypospadias: preputial island-flap technique. *Ann Plast Surg* 9:81, 1982.

Steckler RE, Zaontz MR: Stent-free Thiersch-Duplay hypospadias repair with the Snodgrass modification. *J Urol* 158:1178, 1997.

Stephens FD: Congenital imperforate rectum, rectourethral and rectovaginal fistulae. *Aust N Z J Surg* 22:161, 1953.

Stock JA, Cortez J, Sherz HC, Kaplan WC: The management of proximal hypospadias repair with a preputial free graft for neourethral reconstruction and a preputial pedicle flap for ventral skin coverage. *J Urol* 152:2335, 1994.

Surer I, Ferrer FA, Baker LA, Gearhart JP: Continent urinary diversion and the exstrophy-epispadias complex. *J Urol* 169:1102, 2002.

Tanagho EA: Male epispadias: surgical repair of urethropenile deformity. *Br J Urol* 48:127, 1976.

Taylor JR, Lockwood AP, Taylor AJ: The prepuce: specialized mucosa of the penis and its loss in circumcision. *Br J Urol* 77:291, 1996.

Terzioglu A, Gokrem S, Aslan G: A modification of the pyramid procedure: the correction of subcoronal hypospadias with complete prepuce. *Plast Reconstr Surg* 112(3):922–3, 2003.

Thomalla JV, Mitchell ME: Ventral preputial island flap technique for the repair of epispadias with or without exstrophy. *J Urol* 132:985, 1984.

Thuroff JW, Hohenfellner M (Eds): *Reconstructive Surgery of the Lower Urinary Tract in Children*. Oxford, ISIS Medical Media, 1995.

Turner-Warwick R: The management of traumatic urethral strictures and injuries. *Br J Surg* 60:775, 1973.

Turner-Warwick R: Observations upon techniques for reconstruction of the urethral meatus, the hypospadiac glans deformity and the penile urethra. *Urol Clin North Am* 6:643, 1979.

Turner-Warwick R: The use of pedicle grafts in repair of urinary fistulae. *Br J Urol* 44:644, 1972.

Turner-Warwick R, Kirby RS: The construction and reconstruction of the vagina with the colocecum. *Surg Gynecol Obstet* 170:132, 1990.

Turner-Warwick R, Parkhouse H, Chapple CR: Bulbar elongation anastomotic meatoplasty (BEAM) for subterminal and hypospadiac urethroplasty. *J Urol* 158:1160, 1997.

Ulman I, Avanoglu A, Herek O, et al: A simple method of treating priapism in children. *Br J Urol* 77:460, 1996.

Van der Meulen JC: Correction of hypospadias. *Br J Plast Surg* 8:403, 1982.

Van Savage JG, Palanca LG, Slaughterhoupt BL: Prospective randomized trial of dressings versus no dressings in hypospadias repair. *J Urol* 164:981, 2000.

Vela D, Mendez R, Tellado MG, et al: Lengthening the urethral plate with a double flap technique: a new procedure for correction of primary hypospadias with chordee. *J Urol* 167(1):306–8, 2002.

Von Horn AC, Kass EL: Glanuloplasty and in situ tubularization of the urethral plate: simple reliable technique for the majority of boys with hypospadias. *J Urol* 154:1505, 1995.

Wacksman J: Modification of the one stage flip-flap procedure to repair distal penile hypospadias. *Urol Clin North Am* 8:527, 1981.

Wacksman J: Use of the Hodgson XX (modified Asopa) procedure to correct hypospadias with chordee: surgical technique and results. *J Urol* 136:1264, 1986.

Walker RD: Outpatient repair of urethral fistulae. *Urol Clin North Am* 8:582, 1981.

Walsh PC, Wilson JD, Allen TD, et al: Clinical and endocrinological evaluation of patients with congenital microphallus. *J Urol* 120:90, 1978.

Wang Y, Hadley HR: The use of rotated vascularized pedicle flaps for complex transvaginal procedures. *J Urol* 149:590, 1993.

Waterhouse K: The surgical repair of membranous urethral strictures in children. *Trans Am Assoc Genitourin Surg* 67:81, 1975.

Waterman BJ, Renschler T, Cartwright PC, et al: Variables in successful repair of urethrocutaneous fistula after hypospadias surgery. *J Urol* 168: 726, 2002.

Webster G, Kirby R, King L, Goldwasser B: *Reconstructive Urology*. Boston, Blackwell Scientific Publications, 1993.

Webster GD, Robertson CN: The vascularized skin island urethroplasty: its role and results in urethral stricture management. *J Urol* 133:31, 1985.

Wehrbein HL: Hypospadias. *J Urol* 50:335, 1943.

Weiser AC, Franco I, Herz DB, et al: Single layered small intestinal submucosa in the repair of severe chordee and complicated hypospadias. *J Urol* 170(4 Pt 2):1593–5, 2003; discussion 1595.

Williams DI: The development and abnormalities of the penile urethra. *Acta Anat* 15:176, 1952.

Wilson MC, Wilson CL, Thickstein JN: Transposition of the external genitalia. *J Urol* 94:600, 1965.

Winter CC: Priapism cured by creation of a fistula between the glans penis and the corpora cavernosa. *J Urol* 119:227, 1978.

Wise HA II, Berggren RB: Another method of repair for urethrocutaneous fistulae. *J Urol* 118:1054, 1977.

Wolin M, Duffy PG, Malone PS, Ransley PG: Buried penis: a novel approach. *Br J Urol* 65:97, 1990.

Woodhouse CRJ: Penile reconstruction in exstrophy and epispadias. In: Thuroff JW, Hohenfellner M (Eds): *Reconstructive Surgery of the Lower Urinary Tract in Children.* Oxford, ISIS Medical Media, 1995, p 71.

Woods JE, Alter G, Meland B, Podratz K: Experience with vaginal reconstruction utilizing the modified Singapore flap. *Plast Reconstr Surg* 90:270, 1992.

Yachia D: Congenital penile curvature in childhood. In: Thuroff JW, Hohenfellner M (Eds): *Reconstructive Surgery of the Lower Urinary Tract in Children.* Oxford, Isis Medical Media, 1995, p 59.

Yachia D: Early assessment of penile curvature in infants. *J Urol* 145:103, 1991.

Yachia D: Modified corporoplasty for the treatment of penile curvature. *J Urol* 143:80, 1990.

Yachia D: Pedicled scrotal skin advancement for one-stage anterior urethral reconstruction in circumcised patients. *J Urol* 139:1007, 1988.

Yang CC, Bradley WE: Peripheral distribution of the human dorsal nerve of the penis. *J Urol* 159:1912, 1998.

Yeoman PM, Cooke R, Hain WR: Penile block for circumcision? A comparison with caudal block. *Anesthesia* 38:862, 1983.

Yeung CK, Sihoe JDY, Tam YH, Lee KH: Laparoscopic excision of prostatic utricles in children. *BJU Int* 87:505, 2001.

Young F, Benjamin JA: Preschool age repair of hypospadias with free inlay skin graft. *Surgery* 26:384, 1949.

Young F, Benjamin JA: Repair of hypospadias with free inlay skin graft. *Surg Gynecol Obstet* 5:86, 1948.

Young HH: *Genital Abnormalities.* Baltimore, Williams & Wilkins Company, 1937.

Young HH, Davis DN: Operations on the penis: circumcision. In: *Young's Practice of Urology*, vol II. Philadelphia, W.B. Saunders Company, 1926, pp 643–5.

Yu TJ, Shu K, Kung FT, et al: Use of laparoscopy in intersex patients. *J Urol* 154:1190, 1995.

Yucel S, Sanli A, Kukul E, et al: Midline dorsal plication to repair recurrent chordee at reoperation for hypospadias surgery complication. *J Urol* 175(2):699–702, 2006.

Zagula EM, Braren V: Management of urethrocutaneous fistulas following hypospadias repair. *J Urol* 130:743, 1983.

Zaontz MR: The GAP (glans approximation procedure) for glanular/coronal hypospadias. *J Urol* 141:359, 1989.

Zaontz MR, Dean GE: Glanular hypospadias repair. *J Urol* 176(4 Pt 1):1578–80, 2006.

Zaontz MR, Kaplan WE, Maizels M: Surgical correction of anterior urethral diverticula after hypospadias repair in children. *Urology* 33:40, 1989.

Zhong-Chu L, Yu-Hen Z, Ya-Xiong S, Yu-Feng C: One-stage urethroplasty for hypospadias using a tube constructed with bladder mucosa: a new procedure. *Urol Clin North Am* 8:463, 1981.

Index

Note: Page numbers followed by *f* indicate figures; those followed by *t* indicate tables.